PEDIATRIC EMERGENCIES

PEDIATRIC EMERGENCIES

A Practical, Clinical Guide

EDITED BY

EMILY ROSE, MD

Director for Pre-Health Undergraduate Studies
Keck School of Medicine of the University of Southern California
Associate Professor of Clinical Emergency Medicine (Educational Scholar)
Department of Emergency Medicine
Los Angeles County + USC Medical Center
Los Angeles, CA

OXFORD
UNIVERSITY PRESS

OXFORD
UNIVERSITY PRESS

Oxford University Press is a department of the University of Oxford. It furthers the University's objective of excellence in research, scholarship, and education by publishing worldwide. Oxford is a registered trade mark of Oxford University Press in the UK and certain other countries.

Published in the United States of America by Oxford University Press
198 Madison Avenue, New York, NY 10016, United States of America.

Library of Congress Cataloging-in-Publication Data
Names: Rose, Emily, MD, editor.
Title: Pediatric emergencies : a practical, clinical guide / [edited by] Emily Rose.
Other titles: Pediatric emergencies (Rose)
Description: New York, NY : Oxford University Press, [2021] |
Includes bibliographical references and index.
Identifiers: LCCN 2020016474 (print) | LCCN 2020016475 (ebook) |
ISBN 9780190073879 (hardback) | ISBN 9780190073893 (epub) | ISBN 9780190073909
Subjects: MESH: Pediatric Emergency Medicine—methods | Emergencies |
Emergency Treatment—methods | Child | Infant | Adolescent
Classification: LCC RJ370 (print) | LCC RJ370 (ebook) | NLM WS 205 |
DDC 618.92/0025—dc23
LC record available at https://lccn.loc.gov/2020016474
LC ebook record available at https://lccn.loc.gov/2020016475

3 5 7 9 8 6 4 2

Printed by Integrated Books International, United States of America

This book is dedicated to all providers entrusted with care of children. May you heal, protect, and advocate for this special population with wisdom.

People were bringing little children to Jesus for him to place his hands on them, but the disciples rebuked them. When Jesus saw this, he was indignant. He said to them, "Let the little children come to me, and do not hinder them, for the kingdom of God belongs to such as these. Truly I tell you, anyone who will not receive this kingdom of God like a little child will never enter it." And he took the children in his arms, placed his hands on them and blessed them.

—Mark 10:13–16

CONTENTS

CONTRIBUTORS

Chisom Agbim, MD
Pediatric Emergency Medicine Fellow
Emergency Medicine and Trauma Center
Children's National Health System
Washington, DC

Shilpa Agraharkar, MD
Clinical Assistant Professor
Child and Adolescent Psychiatry
Hassenfeld Children's Hospital at NYU Langone Medical Center
New York, NY

Christopher S. Amato, MD
Director, Pediatric Emergency Medicine Fellowship
Pediatric Medical Director, Atlantic Ambulance
Goryeb Children's hospital/Morristown Medical Center
Princeton, NJ

Katie Bakes, MD
Medical Director of PreHealth
Denver Health Medical Center
Denver, CO
Professor of Emergency Medicine
University of Colorado School of Medicine
Morrison, CO

Jacquelyn Baskin, MD
Associate Professor of Pediatrics
Department of Pediatrics
Division of Hematology–Oncology
University of North Carolina at Chapel Hill
Chapel Hill, NC

Samuel R. Beckerman, MD, PhD
Resident Physician
Emergency Medicine
Los Angeles County + USC Medical Center
Los Angeles, CA

Solomon Behar, MD
Director, Pediatric Medical Education
Long Beach Memorial & Miller Children's Hospital
Los Angeles, CA
Volunteer Faculty/Pediatrics
University of California at Irvine School of Medicine
Irvine, CA

Ryan H. Belcher, MD
Assistant Professor
Pediatric Otolaryngology Division
Vanderbilt Department of Otolaryngology–Head and Neck Surgery
Vanderbilt University
Nashville, TN

Meghan R. Cain, MD
Instructor of Pediatrics and Emergency Medicine
Mayo Clinic College of Medicine and Science
Department of Emergency Medicine
Division of Pediatric Emergency Medicine
Rochester, MN

Vincent Calleo, MD
Assistant Professor of Emergency Medicine
Emergency Medicine
State University of New York Upstate Medical University
Syracuse, NY

Richard Cantor, MD, FAAP, FACEP
Professor of Emergency Medicine and Pediatrics
Emeritus Director, Upstate Poison Center
Syracuse, NY

Nam S. Cho, MD, DDS, FACS
Assistant Professor
Program Director, Oral & Maxillofacial Surgery Residency
University of Southern California
Los Angeles, CA

Ilene Claudius, MD
Associate Professor
Emergency Medicine
David Geffen School of Medicine at UCLA
Los Angeles, CA

Angelica W. DesPain, MD
Pediatric Emergency Medicine Fellow
Emergency Medicine
Children's National Hospital
Washington, DC

Ann M. Dietrich, MD, FAAP, FACEP
Associate Professor of Pediatrics
Ohio University Heritage College of Medicine
Columbus, OH

Ellen Duncan, MD, PhD
Pediatric Emergency Medicine Fellow
Emergency Medicine
NYU Medical Center/Bellevue Hospital Center
New York, NY

Joshua Easter, MD, MSc
Associate Professor
Emergency Medicine
University of Virginia
Charlottesville, VA

Ara Festekjian, MD, MS
Associate Professor of Pediatrics
Children's Hospital Los Angeles Division of Emergency Medicine and Transport
Keck School of Medicine of the University of Southern California
Los Angeles, CA

Eron Friedlaender, MD, MPH
Attending Physician
Pediatrics
The Children's Hospital of Philadelphia
Philadelphia, PA

Julie Furmick, DO
Pediatric Emergency Medicine Fellow
Emergency Medicine
Carolinas Medical Center, Atrium Health
Charlotte, NC

Henrik Galust, MD
Resident Physician
Department of Emergency Medicine
Denver Health
Denver, CO

Molly Hartrich, MD, MPH
Emergency Ultrasound Fellow
Department of Emergency Medicine
University of Illinois at Chicago Hospital and Health Sciences Center
Chicago, IL

Davida Hemmy, MD, MS
Resident Physician
Department of Emergency Medicine
Denver Health
Denver, CO

Annique Hogan, MD
Assistant Professor of Clinical Pediatrics, Medical Director, Care Management and CHOP Compass Care
Medical Director, Complex Care Service Blue Team
Attending Physician, Care Network–CHOP Campus
Division of General Pediatrics
University of Pennsylvania Perelman School of Medicine
Philadelphia, PA

Rosalia Holzman, MD
Department of Emergency Medicine
University of Wisconsin
Pleasant Prairie, WI

James L. Homme, MD
Assistant Professor of Pediatrics and Emergency Medicine
Mayo Clinic College of Medicine and Science
Department of Emergency Medicine
Division of Pediatric Emergency Medicine
Rochester, MN

Anneka Hooft, MD, MPH, FAAP
Clinical Fellow
Pediatric Emergency Medicine
University of California, San Diego
San Diego, CA

Paul Ishimine, MD
Program Director, Pediatric Emergency Medicine Fellowship Training Program
Rady Children's Hospital–San Diego
Director, Pediatric Emergency Medicine
UC San Diego Heath
Clinical Professor of Emergency Medicine and Pediatrics
University of California, San Diego School of Medicine
La Jolla, CA

Shweta R. Iyer, MD
Assistant Professor of Pediatrics and Emergency Medicine
Division of Pediatric Emergency Medicine
NewYork–Presbyterian/Weill Cornell Medical Center
New York, NY

Laura Jacobson, MD
Child Abuse Pediatrics Fellow
Loma Linda University Medical Center and Children's Hospital
Loma Linda, CA

Madeline Joseph, MD, FAAP, FACEP
Associate Dean for Inclusion and Equity-College of Medicine Jacksonville
Professor of Emergency Medicine and Pediatrics
Assistant Chair of Pediatric Emergency Medicine Quality Improvement
Department of Emergency Medicine
University of Florida College of Medicine
Jacksonville, FL

Kate Kaufman, MD
Attending Physician
Department of Emergency Medicine
LAC + USC Medical Center
Los Angeles, CA

Liza Kearl, MD
Associate Professor of Emergency Medicine
Keck School of Medicine of the University of Southern California
Director, Pediatric Emergency Medicine
Department of Emergency Medicine
LAC + USC Medical Center
Los Angeles, CA

Thomas M. Kennedy, MD
Pediatric Emergency Medicine Ultrasound Fellow
Department of Emergency Medicine
NewYork–Presbyterian Morgan Stanley Children's Hospital/Columbia University Irving Medical Center
New York, NY

Erica Kiemele, MD, MSc
Resident Physician
Emergency Medicine
University of Southern California, LAC + USC Medical Center
Los Angeles, CA

Scott Kobner, MD
Resident Physician
Department of Emergency Medicine
LAC + USC Medical Center
Los Angeles, CA

Ioannis Koutroulis, MD, PhD, MBA
Attending Physician
Assistant Professor of Pediatrics, Emergency Medicine, Genomics and Precision Medicine
Emergency Medicine
Children's National Hospital
Washington, DC

C. Anthoney Lim, MD
Director, Pediatric Emergency Medicine
Associate Professor, Emergency Medicine, Pediatrics and Medical Education
Mount Sinai Health System
New York, NY

Deborah R. Liu, MD
Associate Division Head
Division of Emergency and Transport Medicine
Children's Hospital Los Angeles
Associate Professor of Pediatrics
USC Keck School of Medicine
Los Angeles, CA

Mimi Lu, MD
Associate Clinical Professor
Emergency Medicine
University of California, San Francisco
San Francisco, CA

Sharon E. Mace, MD
Professor of Medicine
Cleveland Clinic Lerner College of Medicine at Case Western Reserve University
Cleveland Clinic
Cleveland, OH

Emily MacNeill, MD
Associate Professor
Emergency Medicine
Carolinas Medical Center, Atrium Health
Charlotte, NC

Rhiannon Main, DO
Pediatric Emergency Medicine Fellow
Loma Linda University Medical Center and Children's Hospital
Loma Linda, CA

Meghan Maloney, MD
Clinical Instructor
Pediatric Emergency Medicine
Mount Sinai Beth Israel
New York, NY

Mark S. Mannenbach, MD
Assistant Professor of Pediatrics and Adolescent Medicine
Mayo Clinic College of Medicine and Science
Department of Emergency Medicine
Division of Pediatric Emergency Medicine
Rochester, MN

Maureen McCollough, MD
Associate Professor of Emergency Medicine
David Geffen School of Medicine at UCLA
Department of Emergency Medicine
Olive View–UCLA Medical Center
Pasadena, CA

Taylor McCormick, MD, MSc
Staff Physician and Assistant Professor
Department of Emergency Medicine
Denver Health and the University of Colorado School of Medicine
Denver, CO

Anna McFarlin, MD, FAAP, FACEP
Assistant Professor of Pediatrics and Emergency Medicine
Program Director, Combined Pediatrics/Emergency Medicine Residency
Pediatrics and Internal Medicine
Louisiana State University, New Orleans
New Orleans, LA

Matthew Mendes, MD
Chief Resident
Denver Health Residency in Emergency Medicine
Denver Health and Hospital Authority
Denver, CO

Kelsey A. Miller, MD
Chief Fellow
Division of Emergency Medicine
Boston Children's Hospital
Boston, MA

Jennifer Mitzman, MD
Assistant Professor
Emergency Medicine and Pediatrics
The Ohio State University
Columbus, OH

Ameer P. Mody, MD, MPH
Associate Division Director
Division of Emergency and Transport Medicine
Children's Hospital Los Angeles
Los Angeles, CA

Neal Moehrle, MD
Resident Physician
Department of Emergency Medicine
LAC + USC Medical Center
Los Angeles, CA

Patrick Munson, MD
Assistant Professor of Pediatric Otolaryngology
Sanford Children's Hospital
University of South Dakota School of Medicine
Sioux Falls, SD

Joshua Nagler, MD, MHPEd
Associate Division Chief and Fellowship Director
Division of Emergency Medicine
Boston Children's Hospital
Associate Professor of Pediatrics and Emergency Medicine
Harvard Medical School
Boston, MA

Kim Newton, MD
Associate Clinical Professor of Emergency Medicine
Keck School of Medicine of the University of Southern California
LAC + USC Medical Center
Los Angeles, CA

Jeranil Nunez, MD
Assistant Medical Director
Pediatric Emergency Department
Mount Sinai Beth Israel
Site-Director, Pediatric Emergency Medicine Education
Associate Professor of Emergency Medicine and Pediatrics
Icahn School of Medicine at Mount Sinai
New York, NY

Nicholas M. Orozco, MD, MS
Physician
Emergency Medicine
Los Angeles County + USC Medical Center
Los Angeles, CA

Jessica Lange Osterman, MS, MD
Associate Professor of Clinical Emergency Medicine
Assistant Program Director
Department of Emergency Medicine
LAC + USC Medical Center
Los Angeles, CA

Garrett S. Pacheco, MD
Assistant Professor
Departments of Emergency Medicine and Pediatrics
Residency Associate Program Director
EM and Combined EM & Pediatrics
University of Arizona
Tucson, AZ

Christian D. Pulcini, MD, MEd, MPH
Attending Physician, Pediatric Emergency Medicine
Assistant Professor of Surgery & Pediatrics
University of Vermont Medical Center and Children's Hospital
Burlington, VT

Jeremy M. Rose, MD, MPH
Assistant Professor of Emergency Medicine
Icahn School of Medicine at Mount Sinai
New York, NY

Emily Rose, MD
Director for Pre-Health Undergraduate Studies
Associate Professor of Clinical Emergency Medicine (Educational Scholar)
Department of Emergency Medicine
Keck School of Medicine of the University of Southern California
LAC + USC Medical Center
Los Angeles, CA

Jerri A. Rose, MD
Associate Professor
Division of Pediatric Emergency Medicine
Pediatrics
University Hospitals Rainbow Babies and Children's Hospital
Cleveland, OH

Genevieve Santillanes, MD
Department of Emergency Medicine
Keck School of Medicine of the University of Southern California
Los Angeles, CA

Janet Semple-Hess, MD
Attending Physician
Division of Emergency Medicine
Children's Hospital Los Angeles
Associate Professor of Pediatrics (Retired)
Keck School of Medicine of the University of Southern California
Chatsworth, CA

Seema Shah, MD
Medical Director
Division of Emergency Medicine
Rady Children's Hospital–San Diego
Clinical Professor of Pediatrics
University of California, San Diego
San Diego, CA

Ghazala Q. Sharieff, MD, MBA
Chief Medical Officer, Clinical Excellence and Experience
Scripps Health
San Diego, CA
Clinical Professor
University of California, Carlsbad
Carlsbad, CA

Ee Tein Tay, MD
Site Chief, Pediatric Emergency Medicine
Assistant Professor of Emergency Medicine and Pediatrics
Department of Emergency Medicine
NYU Langone Health/Bellevue Medical Center
New York, NY

Rachel Whitney, MD
Assistant Professor
Pediatric Emergency Medicine
Mount Sinai Beth Israel
New York, NY

Emily L. Willner, MD
Attending Physician
Emergency Medicine and Trauma Center
Children's National Medical Center
Washington, DC

Dale Woolridge, MD, PhD
Professor Emergency Medicine/Pediatrics/Chemistry-Biochemistry
Department of Emergency Medicine
University of Arizona
Tucson, AZ

Loren G. Yamamoto, MD, MPH, MBA, FAAP, FACEP
Professor of Pediatrics
University of Hawaii John A. Burns School of Medicine
Chief of Staff and Pediatric Emergency Physician
Kapiolani Medical Center for Women & Children
Honolulu, HI

Thomas A. Yamamoto, DDS
Chief Resident, Oral and Maxillofacial Surgery
University of Southern California
Los Angeles, CA

Sheryl Yanger, MD
Assistant Professor of Pediatrics
Emergency Medicine
Lurie Children's Hospital of Chicago, Northwestern University
Chicago, IL

F. Kyle Yip, MS, DDS, MD
Assistant Professor
Associate Program Director, Oral & Maxillofacial Surgery Residency
University of Southern California
Los Angeles, CA

Amy Young, MD
Program Director
Child Abuse Pediatrics Fellowship
Loma Linda University Medical Center and Children's Hospital
Loma Linda, CA

Kelly D. Young, MD, MS, FAAP
Program Director
Pediatric Emergency Medicine Fellowship
Harbor–UCLA Medical Center
Torrance, CA

Tim Young, MD
Program Director
Pediatric Emergency Medicine Fellowship
Loma Linda University Medical Center and Children's Hospital
Loma Linda, CA

Mark Zhang, MD
Resident Physician
Emergency Medicine
LAC + USC Medical Center
Los Angeles, CA

ACKNOWLEDGMENTS

A heartfelt thank you to the many outstanding educators who contributed to this text. It is an honor and privilege to collaborate with you on this book. Thank you for your time and dedication to improving the care of children.

To my husband and our precious daughters: You are my home, my delight, and my joy in life. And to my extended family—my parents, parents-in-law, sisters, friends, and colleagues (who, gratefully, are too numerous to name): Thank you for your love and inspiration.

—Emily Rose

INTRODUCTION

The majority of children seen in the emergency department (ED) are cared for by providers without pediatric subspecialty training. Due to significant exposure and experience, most emergency physicians are relatively comfortable with both medical and traumatic resuscitation in adults. However, caring for the sick (or possibly sick) child is a high-stakes event and often is more stressful than caring for the critically ill adult patient. Dosing and equipment sizes differ, differential diagnoses vary based on age, physician knowledge base may have less breadth and depth of less common conditions, and there is often a lack of experience resuscitating children. Training and experience provide a specialized relative comfort in critically ill adults. But emergency trainees, physicians, and other providers without additional specialty pediatric training commonly express a distinct discomfort in the care of common pediatric conditions as well as in the evaluation and management of critically ill children.

As an emergency medicine trained physician, I was distinctly aware of the gaps in my pediatric knowledge and experience. I had incredible training and experience at the Los Angeles County + University of Southern California (LAC + USC) Medical Center Emergency Medicine residency program, but I graduated from an outstanding 4-year residency acutely aware of a deficiency in my ability to care for children with the same excellence as my training in adults. This led me to complete a fellowship in pediatric emergency medicine at Loma Linda University prior to returning to LAC + USC as faculty. Throughout my training, I had searched for a textbook to fill in my knowledge gaps in caring for children as an emergency physician. I never found one that completely satisfied what I needed. The best books covered emergencies well but left me wanting for more basic pediatrics (since I did not complete a pediatric residency). After fielding similar requests from my EM residents and colleagues for years, I decided to finally organize that book—the one I always wished that I had during my training. I knew what I did not know after emergency medicine residency and what is not commonly taught/understood about children in general emergency medicine education. I also have the distinct privilege of working with some of the smartest, hardest working emergency medicine residents in both our adult ED pods and Peds ED and am familiar with their comfort and knowledge base gaps when caring for children. I get to see these amazing physicians orchestrate difficult resuscitations in adults practically without batting an eye but then see the same physicians be quite nervous or insecure about managing the fairly stable infant with bronchiolitis. I wanted this book for them as well—to help give them greater clarity, confidence, and empowerment in caring for children.

This book was created by a group of experts as a relatively comprehensive but succinct review of important pediatric emergencies. We have meticulously tailored this book to those of you, like me, with general emergency training [prior to a fellowship and many more years of painstaking literature review; residency Pediatric Emergency Medicine (PEM) curriculum creation; development of hundreds of lectures; and several courses on PEM, including a PEM Bootcamp with HIPPO EM]. In many cases, the authors presume a relative comfort with these topics in adults and spend time highlighting unique features of illness and injury in children. All authors were selected based on their expertise and experience in caring for children. Well-known educators from academic institutions throughout the United States were invited to author chapters. Most authors have reviewed hundreds of peer-reviewed articles throughout years of practices to distill the essentials in a practical clinically applicable manner. References were requested to be minimal, only citing controversial or cutting-edge sources or recommendations for further reading on topics.

Acute resuscitation of a critically ill child is a high-stakes and stressful event for everyone, no matter how much training and experience one may have. It is the hope of this team that this book can ease discomfort, increase the knowledge base, and improve the care of children.

1

Common Neonatal Presentations

KELLY D. YOUNG

INTRODUCTION

Caring for neonates in the emergency department (ED) requires knowledge of newborn-specific conditions as well as the range of normal behaviors. Common chief complaints include jaundice, feeding difficulties, vomiting, irritability and crying, breathing difficulty, and rash. Fewer than one-third are admitted, with the most common diagnoses being jaundice, fever, vomiting, and respiratory infections.

Birth and perinatal history are key data when evaluating neonates. Practitioners should ask about gestational age; vaginal versus cesarean birth; birth weight; prenatal, birth, and postnatal complications; and age at discharge (often 48 hours if no complications). The newborn's clothes must be removed to adequately examine for findings such as increased work of breathing, bruises and sentinel injuries of non-accidental trauma, and umbilical cord abnormalities. In addition, while addressing the parents' specific concern, the ED provider should also assess common areas of concern, such as feeding, stooling, sleeping, breathing patterns, and umbilical cord issues. If possible, neonates should be isolated from other ED patients with potential infections, particularly respiratory infections.

Parents are commonly concerned about a behavior or physical finding in the newborn. New parents may be wondering if the finding is "normal," and even experienced parents may be worried if their newborn differs from older siblings.

FEEDING, GROWTH, AND STOOLING PATTERNS

Diagnosis

Assess growth by comparing current weight to birth weight. Neonates initially lose 5–10% of their birth weight, and they typically regain birth weight by age 10–14 days. Once birth weight is regained, neonates are expected to gain a minimum of 30 g/day.

A feeding history should include breast versus bottle versus mixed, any difficulties encountered, how the parent is mixing powdered or concentrated formula if used, frequency and amount (minutes per side for breastfeeding and ounces for bottle feeding) of feeds, and total feeds in a 24-hour period. Most newborns feed every 2 or 3 hours, or 8–12 times in a 24-hour period—10 minutes per side for breastfed infants and 1 or 2 oz for bottle-fed infants, increasing to 2 or 3 oz by age 2 weeks. Adequacy of feeding can also be assessed by quantifying the number of wet diapers (for urine) in a 24-hour period. A history of delayed time to passage of first meconium stool after birth, particularly >48 hours, raises concerns for Hirschsprung disease.

Breastfeeding infants initially feed colostrum; the milk "comes in" at approximately 3 or 4 days of life. Early on, infants may not completely empty the mother's breast, causing engorgement. The rapid letdown of engorged breasts can cause infants to sputter and choke at the initiation of feeds. If this is occurring, mothers can be instructed to allow the rapid letdown to flow into a container or cloth and then put the infant back on to breastfeed.

Formula-fed infants can be given ready-to-feed formula without any mixing required, but it is expensive. Liquid concentrated formula is mixed with 1 oz of formula concentrate to 1 oz of water. The most commonly used form is powdered formula, which is mixed one scoop formula to 2 oz of water (must use the scoop that comes with the can of formula). Sometimes parents are mixing the formula incorrectly, often overdiluting because of perceived constipation or to save money, which may result in electrolyte abnormalities.

Assess outputs such as spit up, urine, and stools. Overfed neonates (>3 or 4 oz at a time) may spit up. A small amount of spit up, often with burping, is common and normal. Adequately fed neonates should have five or six wet (urine) diapers per day (although they may have only two or three in the first few days of life). Initially, neonates have thick, dark green–black meconium stools. By day of life 2–4, the stools start to transition. Breastfed infants' stools are yellow, seedy, and runny, and breastfed infants often stool six or more times a day, sometimes after every feed. Parents may mistake this normal stool pattern for diarrhea. Formula-fed infants' stools are pastier, yellow to tan, less frequent, and become more malodorous. Stool frequency usually lessens as neonates age, to a mean of four per day by 1 month of age and sometimes as infrequent as one per week in the second month of life.

Treatment and Disposition

Any neonate not back to birth weight by 14 days of age, or not gaining 30 g/day after that, should be followed up closely (1 or 2 days) with the pediatrician. If weight gain is extremely abnormal, such as well below birth weight at 14 days of age, gaining <30 g/day, or losing weight, admit the patient for further evaluation and monitoring. Further workup and possible admission are warranted if there have been no wet diapers for 8 hours. If the neonate is feeding well, not vomiting excessively, has a benign abdominal examination without distension, and has normal vital signs, reassurance and close follow-up with the pediatrician are all that is generally needed for concerns about stool frequency.

SLEEPING

Diagnosis

Neonates sleep the majority of the day but wake frequently to feed, resulting in parental exhaustion despite the total amount of time newborns spend sleeping. Recommended sleep duration for infants aged 0–3 months is 14–17 hours per day (range, 11–19 hours). Initially, neonates often have day–night reversal, where they sleep more in the daytime and are awake at night, which can also be challenging for parents.

Treatment and Disposition

Reassurance and education regarding sleeping norms are generally all that are needed. Assess support for the primary caregiver, such as spouse, grandparent, other relative, or even hired aides, to reduce parental frustration and exhaustion from lack of sleep. Sometimes parents' concerns are the opposite—their infant is sleeping too much. Newborns not waking for feeds can be stimulated through diaper changes, undressing and re-dressing, gentle rubbing, and baby "exercises" such as bicycling the legs or lifting the arms. Parents can slowly change day–night reversal by working to keep the infant awake during the day. Parents should be told to place the infant to sleep on their back and to avoid co-sleeping or placement of fluffy items such as blankets, thick bumpers, or stuffed animals in the sleeping area because these are important measures to reduce sudden infant death syndrome (see Chapter 4).

CRYING AND COLIC

Diagnosis

Crying is normal in newborns; it is a primary method of communication. The median number of hours per day spent crying at age 2 weeks is 1.75 hours, and this usually increases to a peak of 2.75 hours at age 6–8 weeks and then slowly declines by age 3 or 4 months. Crying tends to be most frequent in the late afternoon and evening hours. There is considerable variation in frequency, duration, and character of crying bouts from infant to infant, and parents may be concerned because a newborn's crying bouts are different from those of an older sibling when the sibling was a newborn.

Colic is excessive crying beyond the standard and is classically described by Wessel's rule of threes: crying for more than 3 hours per day, more than 3 days per week, with these episodes occurring for more than 3 weeks. Approximately 10–20% of infants are "colicky" by this definition. Similar to normal crying, colic tends to begin at 3 or 4 weeks of age, peak at 6–8 weeks of age, and improve by 3 or 4 months of age. Parents often think their child has gas pains or another cause of pain. Some breastfeeding mothers alter their own diet and parents who formula feed their infants change formula types and brands in an effort to reduce colic. These treatments, however, have not been shown to be uniformly helpful.

Pathologic crying must be excluded before diagnosing colic. A thorough history and physical examination should be performed to rule out treatable causes of crying, such as otitis media; ocular foreign body; glaucoma; frenulum tear (which is a sentinel injury for child abuse in a nonmobile child); oral thrush; acute abdomen; hair tourniquet on a digit or penis or, very rarely, clitoris; testicular torsion; incarcerated inguinal hernia; anal fissure; trauma and fracture; neonatal drug withdrawal; hydrocephalus; meningitis; and rash. Corneal abrasions have classically been taught as a potential cause of excessive crying, although Shope et al. found that 49% of asymptomatic infants seen at well-child visits had corneal abrasions. Fluorescein examination should be reserved for infants with corroborating signs, such as conjunctival injection or apparent eye pain, or as part of the workup of the inconsolable infant.

Treatment and Disposition

If the infant is still feeding and growing well, has a normal physical examination and no concerning historical factors, and is either consoled by the motion of the ride to the ED, as commonly happens, or is consolable in the ED, reassurance and education are all that is needed. Assess for support and availability of other caretakers to help the parent(s). Parents can be taught Dr. Harvey Karp's "5 S's" for soothing colicky infants: swaddling, side or stomach positioning (with the caveat that infants should sleep or be left alone in the crib only on their backs), shushing noises (or white noise), swinging and other motion (car ride, baby swing, walk in stroller, rocking, or carried by parent), and suck (on a pacifier or parent's clean pinky finger). Parents should be warned to never shake the infant and instructed that if they become very frustrated, they should either place the crying infant in a safe place such as a crib or hand the infant off to another caretaker. They can be reassured that a period of crying will not be harmful to the newborn. Medications such as simethicone or anticholinergics and herbal remedies such as chamomile tea have not shown efficacy and should not be recommended by ED providers. Similarly, changes in maternal diet or formula type or brand should be left to the primary care provider.

If the infant is not consolable in the ED, perform an initial abbreviated workup such as fluorescein examination and urine to rule out infection and for toxicologic screen, and observe the infant while continuing attempts to console through the 5 S's, feeding, burping, and changing the diaper. If the infant remains inconsolable despite a period of observation and attempts to console, consider expanding the workup to include laboratory tests, blood culture, lumbar puncture, electrocardiogram (ECG), abdominal ultrasound, and skeletal survey. In addition, consider head computed tomography and admitting the patient for empiric antibiotics for possible sepsis. It is extremely rare to get to this step, however.

HEAD BUMPS AND BALD SPOTS

Diagnosis

The newborn's soft, flexible skull and lack of fused sutures allow for molding with gravitational pressure. In addition to open sutures, the anterior fontanelle is widely patent and does not close until 18–24 months of age, and the posterior fontanelle is also patent, closing in the first few months of life or as late as 12–24 months.

Deformational plagiocephaly, an abnormally shaped head due to pressure forces on the skull, may be birth related (i.e., from the birth canal or from forceps) or related to sleep positioning, particularly due to the campaign to encourage sleeping supine only. Excessive supine positioning, particularly in combination with torticollis leading to a fixed neck position, can lead to flattening of the occiput and/or a bald spot in that area.

Several birth-related head swellings may not be noticed by parents until after nursery discharge. Caput succedaneum is a soft subdermal or subcutaneous edema that can cross midline and suture lines, occurring due to pressure applied to the head during vaginal birth and/or from vacuum extraction. There may be overlying skin discoloration with erythema or even petechiae. Caput succedaneum usually self-resolves during the first week of life.

Cephalohematoma is a collection of blood from ruptured subperiosteal veins that occurs in 1% or 2% of newborns, particularly those delivered using vacuum or forceps. It is usually unilateral, more discrete than caput succedaneum, and does not cross midline nor suture lines. Due to slow accumulation of blood, size peaks in the middle of the first week of life. The hematoma then organizes and becomes firmer, and it is slowly resorbed during the first 1 or 2 months of life. Rarely, cephalohematomas can become infected, most commonly with *Escherichia coli*. Suspect infected cephalohematoma if a previously stable hematoma is enlarging and/or the infant is ill-appearing or febrile.

Subgaleal hemorrhage, also more common in vacuum-assisted deliveries, collects between the galea aponeurotica and the periosteum of the skull. This is a large potential space, and bleeding significant enough to cause anemia and even shock can occur. Suspect subgaleal hemorrhage when there is a large fluctuance ballooning out the scalp that is easily moved to other parts of the head as in a fluid wave, signs of anemia, or a rapid increase in head circumference in the first 24–48 hours. Hematocrit should be checked and followed.

Treatment and Disposition

If the timeline fits one of the previously discussed diagnoses and the patient is hemodynamically stable, neurologically normal, and does not have a rapidly growing head circumference, reassurance and close follow-up with the primary care provider are all that is needed. Imaging is not indicated unless there is a suspicion for infected cephalohematoma, hydrocephalus, or non-accidental trauma or a new swelling developing several days beyond birth. Differential diagnosis of a new enlarging swelling includes growing skull fracture, or leptomeningeal cyst, a rare complication of a previously unrecognized skull fracture. Infants with infected cephalohematomas require a complete sepsis workup and admission for empiric broad-spectrum antibiotics. Consult a neurosurgeon for neonates with subgaleal hemorrhage who are not hemodynamically stable. Counsel parents of infants with deformational plagiocephaly to place their infant in supervised “tummy time” prone positioning while awake and to alternate which end of the crib the infant’s head is in to encourage variation in head positioning.

EYE DISCHARGE

Diagnosis

Neonatal conjunctivitis can have several causes, which are differentiated by time of onset and physical examination findings.

Chemical conjunctivitis is less common now that silver nitrate is not used in the United States for ocular prophylaxis after birth. However, silver nitrate is more effective for gonorrhea prophylaxis than the erythromycin ointment recommended in the United States, and silver nitrate may be used in areas with high rates of gonorrhea. The trade-off is that silver nitrate is ineffective against chlamydia. Silver nitrate-induced chemical conjunctivitis starts a few hours after application of the drops and lasts for 24–36 hours, presenting as conjunctival injection and watery eye discharge/tearing.

Gonococcal conjunctivitis carries the most morbidity of the various causes of neonatal conjunctivitis. It typically presents in the first week of life, often within 48 hours of birth. In addition to conjunctival injection, there can be erythema and edema of the eyelids and chemosis. There is typically profuse purulent discharge.

Chlamydial conjunctivitis presents in the second week of life (5–14 days) up to 1 month of age as either unilateral or bilateral conjunctival injection, sometimes with eyelid edema, pseudomembrane formation, or papillary conjunctival involvement. Discharge is initially watery, unlike gonococcal conjunctivitis, but becomes more mucopurulent over time. Chlamydia pneumonitis concomitantly occurs in up to half of infected neonates.

Herpes simplex virus (HSV) conjunctivitis presents at age 6–14 days with conjunctival injection and sometimes eyelid redness and swelling. Discharge is watery. Vesicles may be present around the eye. There may be no known history of maternal HSV. Perform a fluorescein examination to look for dendritic lesions.

Bacterial conjunctivitis caused by a multitude of other bacteria, such as *Staphylococcus* species, *Streptococcus pneumonia*, or *Moraxella catarrhalis*, is more frequent than the previously mentioned causes.

Nasolacrimal duct stenosis is a common disorder affecting up to 20% of newborns. Initial presentation is in the first weeks to months of life with excessive tearing, particularly in the medial canthal area. If the child has a viral upper respiratory infection, the discharge can become mucoid and more evident. If the eye becomes superinfected, there may be purulent discharge.

Dacrocystitis (Figure 1.1), an infection of the nasolacrimal system, is a rare serious complication of nasolacrimal duct stenosis. Infants present with acute-onset redness, swelling, tenderness, and fluctuance around the medial canthal area, sometimes with purulent discharge. Infants may be febrile, and the infection can progress to periorbital or orbital cellulitis. Mean age of onset is in the first 1–3 weeks of life. Diagnosis is clinical, and the infecting organism is confirmed through bacterial culture of purulent discharge (expressed if necessary).

Confirmatory testing (culture and polymerase chain reaction) should be performed for all suspected infectious causes of conjunctivitis.

Treatment and Disposition

If gonococcal conjunctivitis is suspected, the infant should be admitted for intravenous (IV) antibiotics and frequent ocular lavage with normal saline. Intramuscular 50 mg/kg of ceftriaxone may be considered if IV access is difficult. Similarly, if HSV is suspected, infants should undergo testing of other sites (oral, nasopharyngeal, rectal swabs, and lumbar puncture) and be admitted for IV acyclovir. For the rare case of dacryocystitis, patients should be admitted for broad-spectrum IV antibiotics. All three of these suspected diagnoses warrant emergent consultation with an ophthalmologist.

Chemical conjunctivitis will resolve spontaneously, but it is often treated with a topical antibiotic ointment for prophylaxis and emollient purposes. Chlamydial conjunctivitis should be treated with *oral* erythromycin for at least 14 days due to the common involvement of other sites such as the lungs; additional topical antibiotics are not needed. Routine bacterial conjunctivitis can be treated with topical erythromycin ointment. Ointment is preferred to drops for young infants because it is easier to apply and is not as easily washed out.

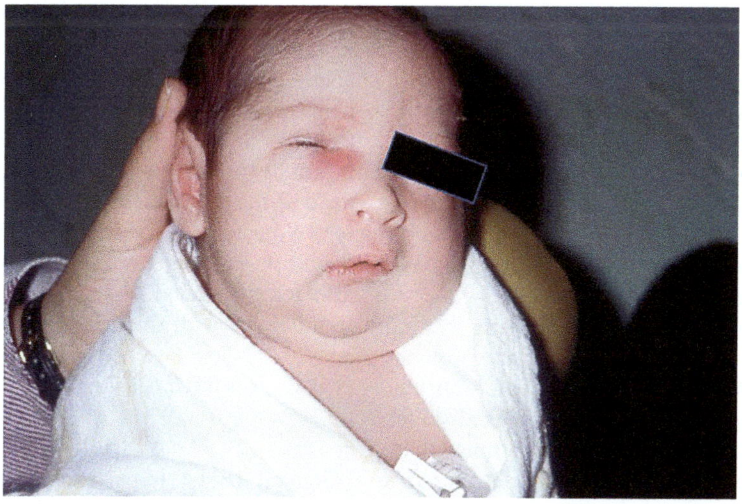

FIGURE 1.1 Dacrocystitis.

Source: Photo courtesy of Dr. Stan Inkelis.

ORAL FINDINGS

Diagnosis

Oral thrush is a very common problem in neonates due to the ubiquity of *Candida* species and the neonate's weaker immune system. It presents as patchy white exudate commonly on the buccal mucosa and tongue. Infants may be noted to have poorer feeding. It is differentiated from residual milk in that it cannot be scraped off with a tongue depressor. There may or may not be an associated candida diaper rash. Breastfeeding mothers may have infection evidenced by red, cracked, sore, or itchy nipples.

Ankyloglossia, commonly called "tongue-tie," is a shortened lingual frenulum that inserts near the tip of the tongue. In neonates, it may impair feeding, particularly breastfeeding.

Several benign oral findings may concern parents. Natal teeth are present at birth, and neonatal teeth emerge during the neonatal period. Both can be an early eruption of normal primary teeth or an extra supernumary tooth. Epstein pearls are tiny firm white bumps on the midline palate or sometimes the gums that stem from entrapment of keratin during development. Bohn nodules are small, <3-mm gray–white cystic nodules on the alveolar gums and occasionally the palate.

Treatment and Disposition

Oral thrush is treated with oral nystatin, 100,000 units/mL, 0.5 mL in each buccal pouch (right and left side), four times a day for 5–10 days (or until a few days after no further white exudate is seen). Any concomitant candidal diaper rash should also be treated. Instruct parents to sterilize bottle nipples and pacifiers by cleaning them in a hot dishwasher or placing them briefly in boiling water. Breastfeeding mothers with evidence of nipple candidiasis can be given topical nystatin or clotrimazole to apply to the nipples *after* each feed (it should be absorbed into the skin by the next feed).

Ankyloglossia that is not inhibiting feeding can be followed by the primary care provider and will often resolve spontaneously. Consider consultation with a lactation specialist for breastfeeding infants or an occupational therapist for other feeding issues. Sometimes frenectomy is performed, but not by emergency physicians.

Reassurance and follow-up with the primary care provider are sufficient for natal and neonatal teeth, Epstein pearls, and Bohn nodules. Only very loose teeth that pose an aspiration risk need to be managed emergently; these can be removed with a simple pull if they are very loose, or a dental or oral and maxillofacial surgery specialist can be consulted. Ensure that the patient has received vitamin K prophylaxis before removing any teeth.

TORTICOLLIS

Diagnosis

Congenital muscular torticollis is a common newborn abnormality, particularly in cases in which the birth was difficult. It is due to shortening and fibrosis of one of the sternocleidomastoid muscles (SCMs), which is sometimes palpable as a firm mass at 3 or 4 weeks of age. The shortened muscle causes the head to be tilted toward the affected SCM and rotated such that the chin points away from the affected SCM. There is decreased passive range of motion when tilting the chin toward the affected SCM or rotating the head away from the affected SCM (any movement that requires stretching of that SCM). Because the infant prefers to hold the head in a position that does not stretch the affected SCM, positional plagiocephaly and facial asymmetry can occur. The diagnosis is clinically made, and the infant should be otherwise well-appearing, afebrile, feeding normally, and neurologically normal.

Treatment and Disposition

Initial management is conservative, including gentle passive stretching exercises—three sets held for 30–60 seconds at a time, performed six to eight times per day—and placement of the infant in the crib so as to encourage turning the head in the direction opposite preferred in order to see out toward the middle of the room/door. Prone positioning tummy time while awake is also recommended. Patients can be discharged to follow up with the primary care provider.

BREAST ISSUES

Diagnosis

Neonatal breast hypertrophy occurs in both female and male infants as a result of exposure to maternal estrogen in utero. There may even be a few drops of milky discharge ("witch's milk"). Hypertrophy is typically noticed in the first 1 or 2 weeks of life, and it resolves within a few weeks in male infants and within a few months in female infants.

Mastitis must be differentiated from benign breast hypertrophy. It presents as erythematous, tender, indurated breast tissue that is usually unilateral. Mastitis also occurs in both females and males, and incidence peaks at age 2 weeks. It may progress to abscess formation, and there may be associated purulent nipple discharge or systemic symptoms such as fever.

Treatment and Disposition

Reassurance and education are all that is needed for benign neonatal breast hypertrophy. Parents should be instructed to avoid stimulating the area, such as palpating it to check for resolution or squeezing the nipple to express discharge, because this may prolong hypertrophy through a hormonal feedback loop, irritate the area, and increase the risk of mastitis.

Neonates with mastitis should be admitted for parenteral broad-spectrum antibiotics, and a pediatric surgeon should be consulted to follow the patient in case of abscess formation.

PERIODIC BREATHING

Diagnosis

Parents sometimes present with concerns that their neonate has stopped breathing. True apnea is defined as cessation of breathing for 20 seconds or longer, often associated with bradycardia, cyanosis and oxygen desaturation, pallor, and/or hypotonia. True apnea is more common in preterm infants and can be associated with respiratory syncytial virus infection.

Periodic breathing is a much more common finding in neonates through age 6 months, consisting of alternating short 5- to 10-second periods of normal respirations or even tachypnea followed by a short period of lack of breathing. There should be no hypoxia, cyanosis, bradycardia, or tone changes. Parents often overestimate the duration of lack of breathing, so timing with a stopwatch can be useful.

Treatment and Disposition

A short period of observation on a cardiorespiratory monitor to rule out true apnea and to reassure the parents is warranted. Once periodic breathing is identified and confirmed, parental education and reassurance are all that is needed.

HEART MURMUR

Diagnosis

During examination for another chief complaint, an incidental heart murmur may be heard. Or, less commonly, the infant may be referred by an outside provider for heart murmur assessment. Innocent heart murmurs are very common in pediatrics, and less than 1% of all pediatric murmurs are due to a congenital heart defect. Characteristics concerning for pathologic murmur include grade 4–6, harsh, diastolic (except venous hum) or holosystolic. Associated findings concerning for congenital heart disease include gallop rhythm, poor feeding or poor weight gain, sweating with feeding, increased work of breathing, liver edge palpable more than 2 or 3 cm below the right subcostal margin, cyanosis or hypoxemia, and pulse or blood pressure or oxygen saturation differential between preductal (right upper extremity) and postductal (either lower extremity).

Treatment and Disposition

If a pathologic heart murmur is suspected, ECG and chest radiograph may be helpful. Infants with normal feeding, growth, oxygen saturation, ECG for age, and chest radiograph can be followed by primary care and cardiologist referral as needed. Consultation with a pediatric cardiologist should occur if a congenital lesion is suspected.

VOMITING

Diagnosis

The differential diagnosis for vomiting in a neonate is broad, ranging from normal spit up or overfeeding to highly morbid conditions such as midgut volvulus. Other serious conditions that can present with vomiting in the neonate include pyloric stenosis, necrotizing enterocolitis, inborn error of metabolism, neonatal withdrawal syndrome, tracheoesophageal fistula, salt-wasting congenital adrenal hyperplasia, hydrocephalus and increased intracranial pressure, non-accidental trauma, Hirschsprung disease, urinary tract infection, sepsis, meningitis, and omphalitis. Any of the following findings warrant further workup and potentially admission to rule out a serious etiology of vomiting: bilious vomiting (concerning for volvulus), projectile vomiting (concerning for pyloric stenosis), hematemesis, inability to tolerate any oral intake, dehydration or reduced number of wet diapers, abnormal abdominal examination including even mild distension, poor growth, abnormal vital signs (especially fever or hypotension), and lethargy or irritability. Demonstrating tolerance of a small oral intake trial (e.g., 0.5–1 oz) is useful. When in doubt, screening urinalysis, electrolytes, and abdominal radiography to assess for signs of obstruction, free air, pneumatosis intestinalis, and evidence of malrotation or toxic megacolon, and also a period of observation while awaiting results of this abbreviated workup, may aid the assessment.

Gastroesophageal reflux is a very common finding in neonates and infants due to developmental laxity in the gastroesophageal sphincter. This natural reflux peaks at approximately age 4 months and often resolves by age 1 year. It is not termed gastroesophageal disease unless there are pathologic consequences such as poor weight gain, recurrent aspiration pneumonia, or esophagitis.

Treatment and Disposition

Neonates with concerning history, physical examination, laboratory, or radiography findings should be admitted for further evaluation and management. If borderline, a period of observation either in the ED or as an inpatient is warranted; vomiting in the neonate is a symptom to take seriously, and high morbidity entities often progress rapidly. Ondansetron is not recommended for this age group.

If the neonate is growing well, has no red flag history or physical examination findings, is not unusually irritable (i.e., is a "happy spitter"), and tolerates an oral intake trial in the ED, the parents can be reassured and sent home to follow up with the primary care provider. Conservative interventions such as smaller, more frequent, and sometimes thickened feeds and also keeping the infant upright for 20–30 minutes after feeds may be trialed. Or, management trials can be left to the primary care provider. If the parents are giving >2 oz per feed, overfeeding is a possibility, and these infants may also benefit from smaller, more frequent feeds.

JAUNDICE

Diagnosis

Jaundice (icterus), manifested by a yellow tinge to the skin and the sclerae of the eyes, is one of the most common complaints for which neonates are brought to medical attention. There are several benign etiologies, but very high levels can cause kernicterus, neurologic sequelae from bilirubin crossing the blood–brain barrier, and direct central nervous system toxicity. Also, conjugated (direct) hyperbilirubinemia carries a wide differential of pathologic causes, most notably biliary atresia.

Physiologic jaundice is due to immature development of liver enzymes that conjugate excess bilirubin, among other developmentally related causes. Bilirubin level peaks in the first 3–5 days of life, usually at <6 mg/dL, but higher at 10 mg/dL in Asian neonates, and the bilirubin is unconjugated (indirect). A bilirubin level >17 mg/dL in an infant 96 hours old or older should not be attributed to benign physiologic jaundice.

Breastfeeding jaundice differs from breast milk jaundice and is due to inadequate oral intake from either breast milk not fully coming in or difficulties with breastfeeding. It typically potentiates the effect of physiologic jaundice in the first week of life, contributing to an elevated unconjugated (indirect) bilirubin level. Dehydration may be present. Assess adequacy of breastfeeding (should be 8–12 times per day), wet diapers, and weight gain. Offer mothers support and/or consultation with a lactation specialist. Formula supplementation may be needed.

Breast milk jaundice is a separate entity of unknown mechanism, but it is thought to be due to some component of human breast milk inhibiting liver enzyme conjugation of bilirubin. This type of jaundice presents as an unconjugated (indirect) hyperbilirubinemia that starts in the second week of life (days 6–14) and may continue for up to 3 months. A brief pause in breastfeeding (with the mother pumping and saving breast milk so her production is not impaired) can be diagnostic and therapeutic—the bilirubin level should decline by 3 mg/dL per day.

Cholestasis is indicated by conjugated (direct) hyperbilirubinemia, and although the differential diagnosis for the underlying etiology is broad, biliary atresia is one of the most important causes to identify. These infants develop jaundice in the first few weeks of life. They remain well-appearing, with normal feeding and growth, but become jaundiced and have acholic or clay-colored stools. Jaundice thought to be physiologic but persisting beyond 2 weeks of life or acholic stools should prompt a laboratory workup including direct bilirubin level, liver enzymes, and γ-glutamyltransferase to identify cholestasis.

Treatment and Disposition

Well-appearing low-risk infants can be screened with a transcutaneous bilirubin measurement ("bilimeter"). Although transcutaneous measurements correlate well with serum bilirubin, they are less accurate at higher serum bilirubin levels. If the value is >13 mg/dL or ≥70% of the serum bilirubin level requiring intervention, then a serum bilirubin level should be obtained to confirm.

Standard laboratory studies when drawing blood include total and indirect bilirubin and hemoglobin. If not previously found to be normal, direct bilirubin should also be measured; an abnormal level should prompt admission and further workup for cholestatic disease. If hemoglobin reveals anemia or if there is potential for isoantibodies (particularly with mother blood type O or Rh negative), perform a complete blood count, type and screen, and direct antibody (Coomb's) test. For significantly jaundiced infants, urinalysis to rule out urinary tract infection, reticulocyte count, and glucose-6-phosphate dehydrogenase level are recommended.

Most physiologic jaundice requires no specific treatment. If breastfeeding jaundice is present, offer mothers support and/or consultation with a lactation specialist. Formula supplementation may be needed. Close follow-up to ensure adequate intake is important. Breast milk jaundice can be treated by a brief pause in breastfeeding (while the mother pumps her milk), but providers should not suggest that the mother stop breastfeeding. Sunlight exposure, thought to work similarly to phototherapy, has previously been recommended but carries the risk of overexposure and sunburn.

If the unconjugated bilirubin level approaches 25 mg/dL in a term infant or 20 mg/dL in an infant with other risk factors, kernicterus may develop. Infants at intermediate or high risk for such complications should be admitted for phototherapy, and if the level is very high, exchange transfusion should be considered. A 2004 American Academy of Pediatrics nomogram for infants born at ≥35 weeks of gestation uses gestational age, hours since birth, total bilirubin level (not just indirect), and the presence of other risk factors such as hemolysis to define the threshold level for intervention. Bilitool, a useful online calculator, returns the results from this nomogram (http://www.bilitool.org). If the level is in the moderate- to high-risk zone, phototherapy should be begun in the ED if inpatient admission cannot occur immediately.

UMBILICUS CONCERNS

Diagnosis

Umbilical granuloma results from inflamed granulation tissue, and it presents as a 3- to 10-mm round, pink, sometimes pedunculated lesion that may be moist. Umbilical granuloma is a clinical diagnosis.

Urachal abnormalities arise in the urachus, an embryologic connection between the umbilicus and the bladder that normally closes and forms a fibrous cord. Urachal abnormalities can often be assessed by ultrasound.

Patent urachus allows free flow of urine to the umbilicus and results in an umbilical cord area that is constantly wet or draining. It occasionally results in urinary tract infection.

Urachal sinus is closed at one end (either bladder or umbilical) and may present with periumbilical redness, pain, and drainage at the umbilicus. In sinuses opening to the bladder, urinary tract infection can occur.

Urachal cyst is a mid-remnant cyst, as the urachus closes on both ends but not completely in the middle. It presents as a palpable periumbilical mass and, if infected, as a red, tender, usually infraumbilical swelling associated with abdominal pain.

Omphalomesenteric (vitelline) duct patent remnant connecting the intestinal tract and the umbilicus may result in fecal drainage at the umbilicus.

Delayed cord separation becomes a concern when a neonate reaches 3 weeks of age without cord separation. Mean cord separation is usually 7–15 days. The significance is that delayed cord separation may be a harbinger of leukocyte adhesion disorder, a rare immunologic disease.

Treatment and Disposition

Umbilical granulomas are treated with silver nitrate applications. Take care to apply only to the granuloma because the silver nitrate can burn and discolor the surrounding skin. Additional applications by the primary care provider will be required.

Suspicion of urachal or omphalomesenteric remnants or delayed cord separation requires subspecialty referral (by the primary care provider). A bacterial superinfection requires admission and parenteral antibiotics.

The cord should be kept clean and dry, and the diaper should be folded down below the level of the cord. The base of the stump can be gently cleaned with rubbing alcohol several times a day to help dry it out. Avoid application of large amounts of liquid alcohol, which can be systemically absorbed.

GENITAL AND INGUINAL COMPLAINTS

Diagnosis

Inguinal hernia occurs when the processus vaginalis does not fully close, allowing bowel to pass through. It typically presents as an inguinal or scrotal swelling that comes out with Valsalva, such as when crying, and returns into the abdomen when the infant is relaxed. Inguinal hernias are more common in male and preterm infants. Vomiting and intolerance of oral intake, redness and tenderness overlying the mass, inability to push the mass back into the abdomen, and ill appearance may indicate incarceration.

Hydrocele occurs when the processus vaginalis closes enough to exclude bowel, but fluid passes through into the scrotum. It presents as a nonreducible fluid-filled scrotal swelling that is palpable separate from the almond-sized testis and that transilluminates with a bright light source. The swelling of hydroceles is typically more discrete than that of hernia.

Vaginal withdrawal bleeding sometimes occurs in the first few weeks of life. The female fetus may develop an endometrial lining due to stimulation from maternal estrogen in utero. Once the infant is born and that hormonal influence wanes, shedding of the lining results in a light bloody discharge that can be distressing to parents.

Treatment and Disposition

Easily reduced inguinal hernias can be non-urgently referred to a surgeon for elective herniorrhaphy. Return instructions include signs and symptoms of incarceration. Trendelenburg positioning, continuous gentle pressure, and sometimes sedation are required to reduce incarcerated hernias. If unsuccessful, consult a surgeon emergently.

Hydroceles usually resolve spontaneously during the first few years of life. Vaginal withdrawal bleeding is a single self-limited event. For both of these diagnoses, reassurance and parental education are sufficient.

DIAPER RASH

Diagnosis

Irritant diaper dermatitis (Figure 1.2) is the most common diaper rash. It is caused either by the soiled diaper chafing the infant's skin or by a contact dermatitis reaction to diaper or wipe material. Erythematous papules, plaques, and erosions are on the parts of the skin that touch the diaper; the skin creases are spared. Parents should be asked about a recent increase in stool volume and about a change in brand of diapers or wipes used.

Candidal diaper dermatitis is another common presentation, with erythematous patches, plaques, and erosions. Differentiating from irritant etiology, candidal rashes tend to be brighter red, more moist appearing, involve the skin creases, and have satellite lesions—small discrete papules around the borders of the main rash. Recent antibiotic therapy disrupts the normal skin flora and is a risk factor for candidiasis.

Seborrheic dermatitis can cause a diaper rash in addition to rash on the scalp, face, ears, and neck. Etiology may be due to *Malassezia* yeast species. The rash consists of scaly red papules and plaques and can be mistaken for psoriasis. Unlike irritant diaper dermatitis, the rash does involve the skin creases. There may be greasy yellow scales similar to scalp seborrheic dermatitis.

Treatment and Disposition

Parents of infants with irritant diaper dermatitis should be instructed to check the diaper

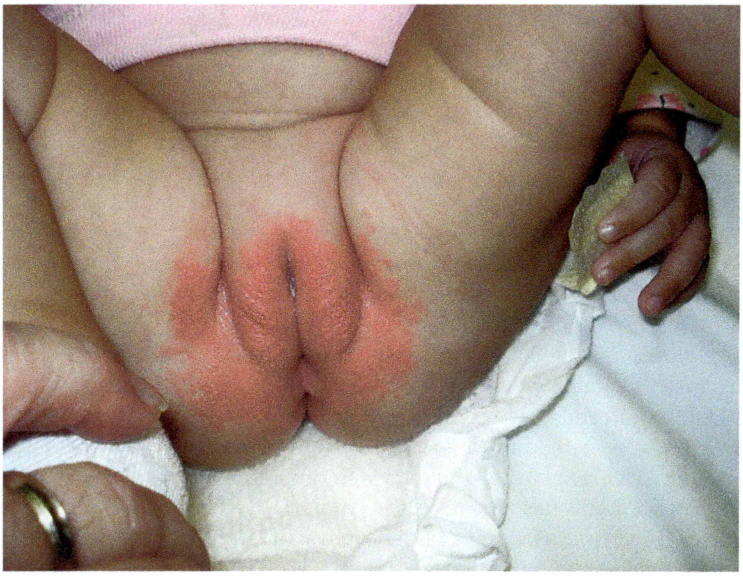

FIGURE 1.2 Irritant diaper dermatitis.
Source: Photo courtesy of Dr. Stan Inkelis.

every few hours for soiling and to change the diaper frequently. Scented wipes, soaps, and other potential irritants should be avoided; severe rash should be cleansed with a clean towel and warm water only. A thick layer of zinc oxide-based diaper rash cream should be applied with each diaper change to act as a barrier between the infant's skin and the diaper. When the infant is sleeping, the diaper can be removed entirely and the infant laid on a cloth diaper. Severe inflammation may benefit from low-potency topical steroid cream (e.g., 1% hydrocortisone) applied in a thin layer twice daily. Combination steroid and antifungal creams should be avoided because the steroid component is too potent for neonatal skin.

Candidal diaper dermatitis is treated with topical antifungal creams, such as nystatin or clotrimazole, applied four times per day. Treat any concomitant oral thrush.

Seborrheic dermatitis is treated with topical steroid cream as for irritant and/or topical ketoconazole cream, applied once a day.

JERKS AND JITTERINESS

Diagnosis

Moro (startle) reflex is a normal newborn reflex in which, when the infant is held in supine position and then the head is suddenly dropped back a few inches, the infant abducts both arms and then brings them back in toward midline. Parents who have elicited a Moro reflex from their infant may be concerned as to whether it is normal. The Moro reflex usually extinguishes by 3 or 4 months of age.

Benign sleep myoclonus presents as symmetric, bilateral extremity jerks occurring during non-rapid eye movement sleep, typically starting in the first 2 weeks of life. They occur in rhythmic clusters and may be multiple or single; they occur only when the infant is falling asleep or sleeping. They may be difficult to differentiate from true epileptic seizures, and a normal electroencephalogram (EEG) is useful in establishing the diagnosis. Benign sleep myoclonus typically self-resolves by age 4 months.

Neonatal jitteriness may be a normal finding in response to overstimulation. The jitteriness presents as typically symmetric bilateral tremors with oscillations of equal amplitude and frequency. Unlike with seizures, tremors can be reduced with consoling the neonate or holding the affected extremity. Although common in normal newborns, the differential diagnosis includes pathologic conditions such as hypoglycemia, hypocalcemia, neonatal drug withdrawal, and hypoxic–ischemic encephalopathy.

Neonatal seizures can be subtle in presentation and can involve eye twitching, nystagmus, lip smacking or rhythmic chewing movements, tongue protrusion, bicycling/swimming movements or thrashing of extremities, and salaam bowing-style infantile spasms.

Treatment and Disposition

Unless history and physical examination clearly support the diagnosis of benign Moro reflex or benign sleep myoclonus, it is wise to check glucose, sodium, and calcium levels to rule out immediately treatable hypoglycemia, hyponatremia, or hypocalcemia. Also consider obtaining an ECG to screen for rare long QT syndrome producing seizures. If the infant is feeding and growing normally, has normal vital signs and an otherwise normal physical examination (especially neurologic examination), has no periods of apnea or cyanosis, and there are no historical factors that place the infant at high risk for a pathologic process (e.g., birth asphyxia), the patient can be discharged home with close primary care follow-up. Outpatient imaging and EEG may be indicated. If these discharge criteria are not met, or if the movements are frequent and distressing, admission for monitoring and inpatient neurology consultation may be warranted.

NEONATAL SKIN FINDINGS

Cutis marmorata is flat symmetric reticular mottling of the trunk and extremities exacerbated by cold. It is usually relieved by warming the skin.

Harlequin color change, reddening of one half of the body with a clear demarcation at midline, occurs when the infant lies on one side. Onset is sudden, and the discoloration lasts seconds to minutes, resolving with increased activity or crying. It is most commonly seen from day of life 2 to 5, and it may continue to occur for the first 3 weeks of life.

Acrocyanosis peripherally of the feet, hands, and lips is common in cold temperatures, and it resolves with warming. Central cyanosis requires investigation, but isolated acrocyanosis is benign.

Erythema toxicum is a common neonatal rash characterized by pink macules, papules, and pustules on a blotchy erythematous base. Lesions typically develop on day of life 2 or 3 and resolve spontaneously over 5–7 days. Lesions are found on the face, trunk, and extremities, but not the palms and soles. Recurrences can occur during the next several weeks.

Transient neonatal pustular melanosis (TNPM) is an uncommon benign vesiculopustular rash seen more often in Black neonates. Lesions include pustules and hyperpigmented macules, often surrounded by a fine collarette of scale, and can be diffuse, including on the palms and soles. Differentiation from more severe causes of vesicles and pustules (e.g., HSV infection) can be difficult, and thus TNPM is generally an ED diagnosis of exclusion.

Neonatal acne (Figure 1.3) is a common finding due to the effects of maternal hormones. Acneiform comedones are found most often on the forehead, nose, and cheeks, although they may also occur on the chest and back. Neonatal acne usually resolves spontaneously during the first year of life, but severe lesions may require treatment.

Seborrheic dermatitis has unknown etiology, although *Malassezia furfur* yeast may play a role. It causes the very common "cradle cap" rash consisting of thick, greasy, yellow adherent scales on the scalp. Rash may also occur on the face, ears, neck, and diaper area, consisting of erythematous papules and plaques, sometimes with scale. The plaques may have a shiny, moist appearance. Seborrheic dermatitis typically resolves spontaneously during the first year of life.

Milia are tiny, pearly white to yellow papules commonly found on the nose, forehead, cheeks, and chin due to retained keratin. They resolve spontaneously during the first month of life.

Miliaria crystallina occur due to retained sweat in eccrine ducts. They present as tiny vesicles with no surrounding erythema on the head, neck, and trunk.

Miliaria rubra (heat rash) occurs due to a similar mechanism but with inflammation. It presents as small erythematous prickly appearing papules and vesicles, typically on areas of the body covered by clothing. A history of bundling or overheating may be obtained.

Dermal melanosis, previously termed "Mongolian spots," presents as flat irregular patches of blue-gray discoloration, commonly on the lower back and buttocks. It is more common in Asian, Native American, Hispanic,

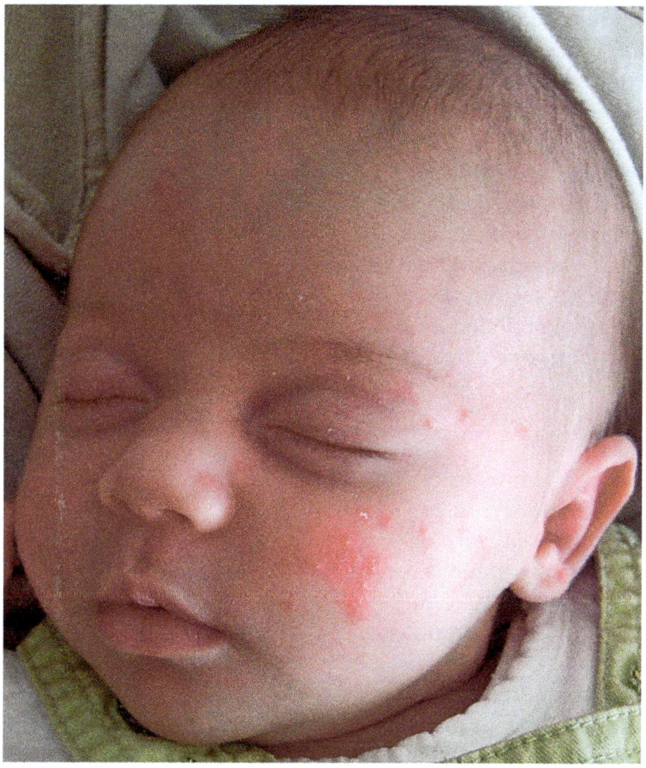

FIGURE 1.3 Neonatal acne.

and Black infants. It should not be mistaken for bruising.

Nevus simplex, or "stork bite" or "salmon patch," presents as a blanchable, flat, salmon-colored pink macule commonly seen on the nape of the neck, eyelid, nose, and scalp. Lesions can be bilateral and symmetric, and they typically fade during the first year of life.

Nevus flammeus, or "port-wine stain," presents as a unilateral, blanchable, flat, dark red to purple, often large, macule. If it involves the part of the face innervated by the trigeminal nerve ophthalmic portion (V1), there may be associated Sturge–Weber syndrome, glaucoma, and seizures. Nevus flammeus, unlike nevus simplex, does not fade over time.

Hemangiomas are usually not present at birth but appear in the first days to months of life. They first appear as a subtle telangiectasia and then proliferate during the next 6–12 months into a larger bright red (strawberry hemangioma) or bluish (deep subcutaneous hemangioma) swelling. They spontaneously involute during the next several years of life. Unless complicated by infection, bleeding, or obstructing vision or airway, no acute treatment is needed.

Treatment and Disposition

Most of the benign skin findings require no more than reassurance, parental education, and follow-up with the primary care provider. Significant seborrheic dermatitis may respond to low-potency topical steroid (e.g., 1% hydrocortisone cream) or topical ketoconazole applied once daily. Parents of infants with miliaria rubra should be instructed to avoid overheating. Parents can be reassured that the amount of clothing a newborn requires is similar to what is comfortable for a parent in the current environmental temperatures. When pustules or vesicles are present, practitioners must consider more serious skin conditions such as HSV.

KEY POINTS

- Neonates have a narrow range of behaviors: sleeping, feeding, urinating and defecating, and some quiet alert time. ED practitioners must be familiar with the typical normal patterns for these behaviors.

- When evaluating the neonate, obtaining a prenatal, perinatal, and birth history is key.
- Weight gain compared to birth weight should be assessed for adequacy.
- ED providers must be familiar with common physical examination findings and benign diagnoses seen in neonates. With this familiarity, providers can avoid unnecessary diagnostic testing and admission.

PITFALLS

- Not fully removing the infant's clothing during examination may result in missing signs of increased work of breathing, problems with umbilical cord healing, sentinel injuries concerning for non-accidental trauma, and other important findings.
- Not checking the umbilical cord may result in missing evidence of infection, congenital abnormality, or delayed cord separation.
- Even if not the chief complaint, jaundiced infants should be assessed to ensure that they do not meet criteria for phototherapy.

Further Reading

Aby, J. Photo Gallery. Stanford Medicine Newborn Nursery at Lucile Packard Children's Hospital. https://med.stanford.edu/newborns/professional-education/photo-gallery.html. Accessed April 24, 2019.

Burgos T, Turner S. BiliTool. http://www.bilitool.org. Accessed April 27, 2019.

Karp, H. The 5 S's for Soothing Babies. Happiest Baby. https://www.happiestbaby.com/blogs/baby/the-5-s-s-for-soothing-babies. Accessed April 24, 2019.

Lowe MC, Woolridge DP. The normal newborn exam, or is it? *Emerg Med Clin North Am.* 2007;25:921–946.

Maisels MJ, Bhutani VK, Bogen D, et al. Hyperbilirubinemia in the newborn infant ≥35 weeks' gestation: An update with clarifications. *Pediatrics* 2009;124(4):1193–1198.

Shope TR, Rieg TS, Kathiria NN. Corneal abrasions in young infants. *Pediatrics* 2010 Mar;125(3):e565–e569. PMID 20142290.

2

The Crashing Neonate

THOMAS M. KENNEDY AND GHAZALA Q. SHARIEFF

INTRODUCTION

Several studies have demonstrated an increasing incidence of newborn emergency department (ED) visits in the United States, which may be due to a higher number of home births and hospital policies directing earlier discharge of newborns from nurseries. Although many of these visits are for benign conditions, it is imperative that the emergency physician know how to manage a critically ill neonate (a newborn in the first 28 days of life). The mnemonic, THE MISFITS, provides a method for remembering many of the serious conditions that present acutely in the neonatal period, including trauma (accidental trauma and child abuse), heart disease (structural and nonstructural) and hypovolemia, endocrinopathies, metabolic abnormalities (electrolyte imbalances), inborn errors of metabolism, sepsis, formula mishaps (under- or overdilution), intestinal catastrophes (e.g., necrotizing enterocolitis and midgut volvulus), toxic exposures, and seizures (Table 2.1). This chapter provides the essential clinical information for several of these conditions; others are discussed in-depth elsewhere in this book.

TABLE 2.1 CAUSES OF THE CRASHING NEONATE: THE MISFITS MNEMONIC

T	Trauma (accidental trauma and child abuse)
H	Heart disease and hypovolemia
E	Endocrinopathies
M	Metabolic disturbances
I	Inborn errors of metabolism
S	Sepsis
F	Formula mishaps (under- or overdilution)
I	Intestinal catastrophes
T	Toxins
S	Seizures

CRITICAL CONGENITAL HEART DISEASE

Background

Critical congenital heart disease (CHD) refers to lesions requiring surgery or catheter-based interventions in the first year of life. Ill neonates presenting to the ED with critical CHD may have left-sided obstructive lesions, right-sided obstructive lesions, dextro-transposition

TABLE 2.2 OBSTRUCTIVE CRITICAL CONGENITAL HEART DISEASE LESIONS

Left-Sided Obstructive Lesions	Right-Sided Obstructive Lesions
Aortic valve stenosis	Pulmonary atresia with intact ventricular septum
Coarctation of the aorta	Pulmonic stenosis
Hypoplastic left heart syndrome	Severe neonatal Ebstein anomaly
Interrupted aortic arch	Tetralogy of Fallot with pulmonary atresia
	Tetralogy of Fallot
	Tricuspid atresia

of the great arteries (d-TGA), truncus arteriosus, or total anomalous pulmonary venous return (TAPVR). Table 2.2 displays the left- and right-sided obstructive lesions of concern. Several of these conditions are ductal dependent and therefore present acutely as the ductus arteriosus closes in the first several days to weeks of life.

Clinical Presentation

A crashing neonate with critical CHD generally presents in one of two ways: gray (circulatory collapse caused by a left-sided obstructive lesion) or blue (central cyanosis caused by a right-sided obstructive lesion, d-TGA, truncus arteriosus, or TAPVR). Central cyanosis is distinguished from peripheral cyanosis by involvement of the lips and oral mucosa. It is most often caused by pulmonary disease or CHD, whereas peripheral cyanosis may be due to sepsis, acrocyanosis, or cold exposure. Vital signs suggestive of CHD include a lack of fever; a pulse oximetry reading <90% in any extremity or a 3% differential between the right upper extremity (preductal) and a lower extremity (postductal); and a higher blood pressure in the right upper extremity than a lower extremity, often by 10 mmHg or more. Physical examination findings concerning for CHD include auscultation of a pathologic heart murmur, absent femoral pulses, and hepatomegaly more than 2.5 cm below the right costal margin. Differential cyanosis, in which the upper half of the body is pink and the lower half is cyanotic, may be encountered in patients with coarctation of the aorta and interrupted aortic arch.

Diagnostic Confirmation

The likelihood of critical CHD in an undifferentiated crashing neonate depends on the findings of a sequence of diagnostic screening tests. The hyperoxia test is used to distinguish CHD with right-to-left shunting from other causes of cyanosis. Classically, this test is performed by obtaining an arterial blood gas (ABG) to measure the partial pressure of oxygen, then administering 100% oxygen for 10 minutes, and lastly obtaining another ABG. If the lungs are already fully oxygenated, then administration of oxygen will have no effect on the partial pressure of arterial oxygen (it will remain <150 mmHg). This suggests that the hypoxia is due to a cardiac lesion. Although potentially less reliable, pulse oximetry can be used in place of ABG measurements for this purpose. If the pulse oximetry reading does not increase by at least 10%, then a cardiac abnormality is favored. Keep in mind that oxygen is a potent vasodilator and may worsen respiratory distress in patients with some ductal-dependent lesions by decreasing pulmonary vascular resistance and thus causing pulmonary overcirculation and resultant pulmonary edema. For this reason, some practitioners argue against performing this test if echocardiography can be done in a reasonable time frame. In addition, hypoxia allows the patent ductus arteriosus to remain open, which can be lifesaving for neonates awaiting definitive care.

Electrocardiography (ECG) may reveal findings that increase the probability of a cardiac abnormality. At birth, the right ventricular muscle is thicker than the left. Left axis deviation is always pathologic in the neonatal period. A normal axis may be within normal limits during the first month of life considering that the normal range is 65–161° in the first 1–3 weeks of life; however, it should still raise concern in a critically ill neonate because the axis is more often deviated rightward. Assess the ECG for signs of ventricular hypertrophy and atrial enlargement, which also raise suspicion for CHD.

There are several findings on chest radiography that are concerning for CHD. First, it may reveal one of the classic patterns: a boot-shaped heart [tetralogy of Fallot (TOF)], the snowman or figure of 8 sign (TAPVR type 1), or the egg on a string appearance (d-TGA). Next, there are four radiographic features to look for that increase the likelihood of CHD: (1) the presence of cardiomegaly, (2) increased pulmonary vascular markings suggestive of pulmonary overcirculation or lack of expected markings (black lungs) suggestive of pulmonary vascular obstruction, (3) the presence of a right-sided aortic arch (associated with TOF, truncus arteriosus, and tricuspid atresia), and (4) the presence of situs inversus (associated with d-TGA).

Consult a pediatric cardiologist and have a formal echocardiogram performed as soon as possible once the diagnosis is suspected. Currently, a limitation of focused cardiac ultrasound (FoCUS) performed by emergency medicine physicians is the diagnosis or exclusion of CHD due to a paucity of evidence in the literature. However, there are case reports of FoCUS resulting in the rapid identification of critical CHD by revealing gross anatomic abnormalities in neonates presenting in extremis and thereby expediting management.

Treatment

Attention to the airway, breathing, and circulation is the first step for all ED patients. Critically ill neonates are at risk for upper airway obstruction, due to altered mental status, and apnea. If intubation is necessary, administer atropine intravenously (IV), fentanyl IV, and rocuronium IV followed by initiation of a fentanyl IV infusion for post-intubation sedation. A minimum atropine dose of 0.1 mg is no longer advised. Table 2.3 displays the recommended medication doses for neonates with critical CHD.

It is important to keep the physiologic consequences of positive pressure ventilation in mind because the resulting decrease in preload has unpredictable effects in a patient with undifferentiated CHD. If time permits, administer a normal saline 10 mL/kg IV bolus prior to intubation and have a vasopressor infusion ready at the bedside to administer if needed to maintain a target mean arterial pressure of 40 mmHg. Begin mechanical ventilation with a low positive end-expiratory pressure, and titrate settings to achieve a pulse oximetry reading of 75–85%. As previously stated, oxygen is a potent vasodilator, and hyperoxygenation can result in pulmonary overcirculation with some types of CHD.

Initiate a prostaglandin E_1 (PGE_1) infusion as soon as critical CHD is suspected.

TABLE 2.3 NEONATAL CRITICAL CONGENITAL HEART DISEASE THERAPIES

Category	Medication	Dose
Endotracheal intubation	Atropine	0.02 mg/kg IV
	Fentanyl	2-4 µg/kg IV 0.5–1 µg/kg/min IV
	Rocuronium	1 mg/kg IV
Circulatory support	Dobutamine	2–20 µg/kg/min
	Dopamine	15–20 µg/kg/min
	Milrinone	0.25–0.75 µg/kg/min
	Prostaglandin E_1	0.05–0.1 µg/kg/min
Tet spell management	Esmolol	500 µg/kg IV 50–300 µg/kg/min IV
	Fentanyl	1–2 µg/kg IN
	Morphine	0.1 mg/kg IV
	Phenylephrine	10–20 mcg/kg IV 2–5 µg/kg/min

IN, intranasally; IV, intravenously.

This infusion helps keep the ductus arteriosus open with life-saving blood flow. It requires a dedicated intravenous site to ensure continuous infusion. The initial dose is 0.05 μg/kg/min and can be increased every 15 minutes to a maximum of 0.1 μg/kg/min. Once a therapeutic response is achieved, indicated by an increase in systemic blood pressure and pH for the gray neonate with restricted systemic blood flow or an increase in oxygenation with improvement in cyanosis for the blue neonate with restricted pulmonary blood flow, reduce the rate to the lowest effective dose.

Adverse reactions are common with administration of PGE_1. Apnea occurs in 10–12% of neonates, and the risk is dose dependent. It can occur at any time during the infusion. Other adverse effects of this medication include fever, flushing, hypotension, bradycardia, tachycardia, and seizures. Consider a diagnosis of d-TGA with an intact ventricular septum or restricted atrial or ventricular communication if cyanosis fails to improve after starting a PGE_1 infusion. This condition may require an emergent atrial septostomy. If there is clinical deterioration after starting a PGE_1 infusion, the newborn may have an obstructed form of TAPVR that requires discontinuation of the infusion because opening the ductus arteriosus results in worsening pulmonary edema.

Several additional medications may be necessary to stabilize an ill neonate with critical CHD. An essential therapeutic goal is to balance systemic and pulmonary blood flow. For the gray neonate, use dobutamine and/or milrinone to decrease systemic vascular resistance and thereby increase systemic circulation. In contrast, for the blue neonate, use high-dose dopamine to increase systemic vascular resistance and thereby promote pulmonary circulation.

The neonate with known TOF presenting with a cyanotic tet spell is managed uniquely. If it is the first episode in a newborn with undiagnosed TOF, it can be treated as previously described for a blue infant with a right-sided obstructive lesion. However, if the diagnosis is known and the tet spell occurs while awaiting surgical correction, a stepwise management approach is recommended. The goal is to decrease pulmonary vascular resistance and increase systemic vascular resistance. Initially, administer oxygen and place the newborn in a knees-to-chest position. If this fails, then administer morphine IV (intranasal fentanyl is an alternative option for a patient without intravenous access) and a normal saline IV bolus. If the tet spell is refractory to these therapies, then administer an esmolol IV bolus followed by a continuous infusion and, if necessary, a phenylephrine IV bolus followed by a continuous infusion. Immediate surgical intervention is needed if these therapies are ineffective.

Disposition

All neonates with critical CHD causing acute illness require admission to an intensive care unit (ICU) and emergent pediatric cardiology consultation.

Key Points

- Critical CHD can be distinguished from other etiologies of acute illness in a newborn, such as sepsis and endocrinopathies, by preductal and postductal pulse oximetry and blood pressure differentials, ECG abnormalities, and findings on chest radiography. Although there is a paucity of evidence, perform FoCUS to look for gross cardiac malformations.
- It is not necessary to diagnose the specific cardiac lesion in the ED. Management of the acutely ill neonate with critical CHD can be simplified by categorizing the newborn as either gray with circulatory collapse caused by a left-sided obstructive lesion or blue with central cyanosis caused by a right-sided obstructive lesion, d-TGA, truncus arteriosus, or TAPVR.
- The indications for prostaglandin infusion are hypoxic neonates (blue) who are not responsive to oxygen and neonates in shock (gray) who are not responsive to fluids.
- Early recognition of clinical deterioration after starting a PGE_1 infusion is crucial because obstructed forms of TAPVR worsen with this treatment. Discontinue the infusion and continue supportive therapy until rapid transfer to a higher level of care can be achieved.

Pitfalls

- Forgetting to palpate femoral pulses and the liver edge during the newborn examination.

- Failing to administer antibiotic and antiviral therapies when CHD is suspected. Sepsis is always the first consideration in the differential diagnosis for a critically ill neonate.
- Delayed initiation of a PGE_1 infusion due to diagnostic uncertainty. Maintain a low threshold to start this treatment empirically, and consider ordering it simultaneously with antibiotics due to the time it may take the pharmacy to prepare.
- Transferring a newborn to another facility on a PGE_1 infusion without a secure airway.

ENDOCRINOPATHIES

Congenital Adrenal Hyperplasia

Background

Congenital adrenal hyperplasia is a group of autosomal recessive disorders in which there is a deficiency of an enzyme necessary for cortisol synthesis. Deficiency of other steroids distal to the disrupted enzymatic step may occur as well, depending on the enzyme involved. The most common type is due to 21-hydroxylase deficiency, accounting for more than 90% of all cases. The three phenotypes of this enzyme deficiency are the classic salt wasting form, the classic non-salt wasting form, and the nonclassic, or late-onset, form. Approximately 75% of patients with the classic form have aldosterone deficiency with salt wasting that may present with adrenal crisis in the neonatal period. The remaining 25% of patients have aldosterone deficiency without salt wasting (the simple virilizing variant) caused by low, but detectable, enzyme activity. Notably, all newborn screens in the United States include congenital adrenal hyperplasia, but the test is not 100% sensitive.

Clinical Presentation

The classic salt wasting form is usually discovered at the time of birth in females because of genital ambiguity. However, in males, it presents with adrenal crisis between 1 and 4 weeks of life if undetected by newborn screening. Adrenal crisis manifests with nonspecific symptoms such as vomiting and poor feeding. The newborn may progress to hypovolemic or cardiogenic shock due to dehydration or dysrhythmias caused by hyperkalemia, respectively. Hypoglycemic or hyponatremic seizures can also occur. Physical examination may demonstrate phallic enlargement and scrotal hyperpigmentation.

Diagnostic Confirmation

The serum chemistry panel may reveal hyponatremia, hypoglycemia, and hyperkalemia. Perform an ECG if hyperkalemia is present. Peaked T waves with shortening of the QT interval are initially seen, and then increased PR and QRS intervals develop as hyperkalemia worsens. Neonates in shock will have a metabolic acidosis. A random cortisol level will be low (usually <10 μg/dL). Diagnosis is based on a high random serum concentration of 17-hydroxyprogesterone, often >3,500 ng/dL. An adrenocorticotropic hormone (ACTH) stimulation test and genetic testing can be used for equivocal cases in the inpatient or outpatient setting.

Treatment

For the newborn presenting in adrenal crisis, the cornerstone of treatment is stress dosing of hydrocortisone. Ideally, obtain blood samples to test the concentrations of 17-hydroxyprogesterone, ACTH, aldosterone, renin, and cortisol prior to hydrocortisone administration. Treat hypovolemia with normal saline 10 mL/kg IV boluses. Due to the mineralocorticoid effect of stress dose hydrocortisone, electrolyte derangements usually improve rapidly after administration. However, additional treatment for these derangements is warranted in the setting of ECG changes caused by hyperkalemia and seizures caused by hypoglycemia or hyponatremia. For hyperkalemia, administer calcium gluconate 10% IV over 5–10 minutes to stabilize the myocardium and a regular insulin IV infusion with a dextrose 10% IV infusion to drive potassium intracellularly and maintain euglycemia. Nebulized albuterol may also be used. Electrolytes must be monitored frequently during treatment. Treat hypoglycemic seizures with a dextrose 10% IV bolus. Seizures caused by hyponatremia often respond to administration of a normal saline IV bolus. Treat refractory hyponatremic seizures with a hypertonic (3%) saline IV bolus. Table 2.4 displays the recommended doses for these medications.

TABLE 2.4 NEONATAL ADRENAL CRISIS THERAPIES

Condition	Medication	Dose
Hyperkalemia	Calcium gluconate 10%	60–100 mg/kg IV
	Insulin	0.1–0.6 U/kg/hr IV
	Dextrose 10% infusion	5–10 mL/kg/hr IV
	Nebulized albuterol	0.4–2.5 mg in 2 mL of saline
Hypocortisolemia	Hydrocortisone	25 mg IV/IM
Hypoglycemia	Dextrose 10%	2 mL/kg IV
Hyponatremia	Hypertonic (3%) saline	3 mL/kg IV

IM, intramuscularly; IV, intravenously.

Disposition

Admit all patients presenting with adrenal crisis to a hospital. Whether they require admission to a general inpatient unit or an ICU depends on the severity of their presentation. In general, patients with electrolyte imbalances not promptly responding to treatment and those with ECG abnormalities should be admitted to an ICU. Consultation with a pediatric endocrinologist is necessary.

Complications

The most dangerous complications of adrenal crisis are hypovolemic shock, cardiogenic shock caused by dysrhythmias, and seizures resulting from hypoglycemia or hyponatremia.

Key Points

- Include adrenal crisis in the differential diagnosis for neonates presenting with vomiting, dehydration, dysrhythmias, and seizures.
- Hydrocortisone 25 mg IV or intramuscularly is the cornerstone of treatment. If possible, obtain blood samples for diagnostic tests prior to administration.
- ECG changes caused by hyperkalemia warrant administration of a calcium gluconate IV bolus and insulin with dextrose IV infusions.

Pitfall

- Forgetting to check a rapid bedside glucose test immediately upon arrival to the ED.

Thyrotoxicosis

Background

Most cases of neonatal thyrotoxicosis are caused by neonatal Graves' disease. This is a transient condition seen in 1–5% of newborns born to women with Graves' disease. It is caused by transplacental passage of immunoglobulins that stimulate the newborn's thyroid gland. Neonatal thyrotoxicosis can also be caused by genetic activating mutations that result in a permanent state of hyperthyroidism. This should be suspected if there is no maternal history of Graves' disease.

Clinical Presentation

Neonates with symptomatic hyperthyroidism may present with poor weight gain or weight loss, irritability, difficulty sleeping, flushing, sweating, and diarrhea. Vital signs may reveal hyperthermia, tachycardia, hypertension, and tachypnea. Important physical examination findings include a small fontanelle, microcephaly caused by craniosynostosis, and exophthalmos. Severe cases can result in heart failure, pulmonary hypertension, hepatomegaly, and jaundice.

In the case of neonatal Graves' disease, the timing of symptoms depends on whether the mother was taking an antithyroid medication. If she was not, then the symptoms are present at the time of birth. However, if she was taking a medication, then the neonate will be euthyroid at birth and begin to develop symptoms between 1 and 3 weeks of life. Newborns with genetic mutations causing hyperthyroidism are symptomatic at birth.

Diagnostic Confirmation

The diagnosis is confirmed by measurements of serum free thyroxine (T_4), total triiodothyronine (T_3), and thyroid-stimulating hormone.

TABLE 2.5 REFERENCE RANGES FOR THYROID FUNCTION TESTS IN TERM INFANTS

Age (Days)	Free T_4 (ng/dL)	Total T_3 (ng/dL)	TSH (mU/L)
7	2.7 ± 0.6	148 ± 50	2.6 ± 1.8
14	2.03 ± 0.3	167 ± 31	2.5 ± 2.0
28	1.65 ± 0.3	176 ± 32	1.8 ± 0.9

T_3, triiodothyronine; T_4, thyroxine; TSH, thyroid-stimulating hormone.
Source: Adapted from Williams FL, Simpson J, Delahunty C, et al. Developmental trends in cord and postpartum serum thyroid hormones in preterm infants. *J Clin Endocrinol Metab.* 2004;89(11): 5314–5320.

Normal reference ranges for these laboratory tests are provided in Table 2.5.

Treatment

Consultation with a pediatric endocrinologist is essential. Treatment in the ED consists of administering methimazole (0.2–0.5 mg/kg/day divided every 12 hours) and propranolol (2 mg/kg/day divided every 12 hours). Symptomatic improvement requires a few weeks of therapy. In severe cases, potassium iodide may be indicated. Hydrocortisone 2.5–10 mg/kg/day divided every 8 hours may also be beneficial because it inhibits thyroid hormone secretion and decreases peripheral conversion of T_4 to T_3. Neonates with heart failure may require dobutamine and/or milrinone IV infusions for cardiovascular support.

Disposition

All neonates with thyrotoxicosis require admission to the hospital. Whether an ICU is required depends on the patient's hemodynamic stability.

Complication

If left untreated, neonatal thyrotoxicosis has a mortality rate of 12%, with most deaths caused by heart failure.

Key Point

- It is essential to obtain a maternal history for a neonate presenting in extremis because it may reveal a history of Graves' disease.

INBORN ERRORS OF METABOLISM

Background

More than 5,000 different types of inborn errors of metabolism (IEM) have been identified. Fortunately, with regard to the acute management of a neonatal metabolic crisis, the emergency physician only needs to know how to identify and manage two categories of IEM: carbohydrate metabolism disorders and protein metabolism disorders. The latter group is subdivided into aminoacidopathies, organic acidemias, and urea cycle defects. Table 2.6 displays examples of each category.

Clinical Presentation

In the neonatal period, these conditions present with poor feeding, vomiting, diarrhea, and lethargy that can progress to coma. Several of the organic acidemias manifest with unusual urine or body odors. Physical

TABLE 2.6 INBORN ERRORS OF METABOLISM THAT CAUSE NEONATAL METABOLIC CRISES

Category	Examples
Carbohydrate metabolism disorders	Galactosemia
Protein metabolism disorders	
Aminoacidopathies	Maple syrup urine disease
	Tyrosinemia type 1
Organic acidemias	Glutaric acidemia type 1
	Methylmalonic acidemia
Urea cycle defects	Ornithine transcarbamylase deficiency

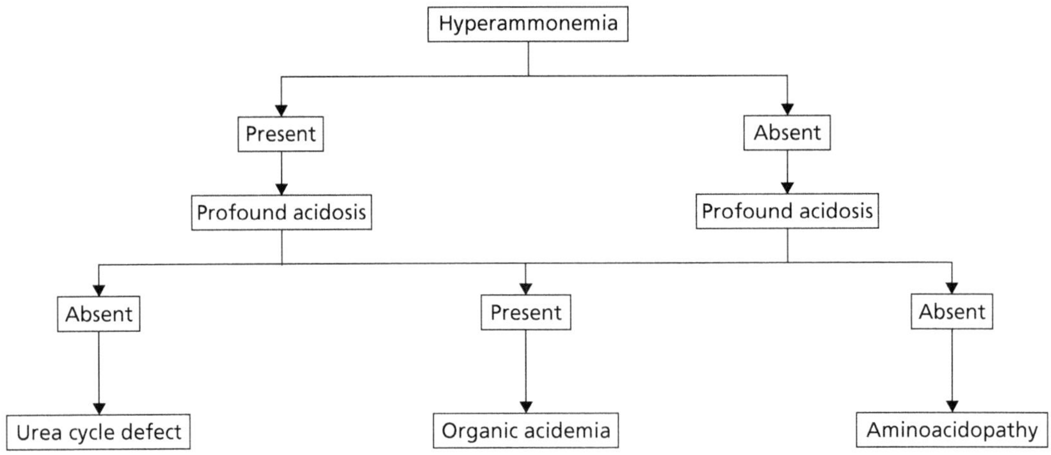

FIGURE 2.1 Algorithm for the diagnosis of neonatal inborn errors of protein metabolism.

examination may reveal hepatomegaly or jaundice. Newborns with classic galactosemia, a carbohydrate metabolism disorder, often have cataracts. Patients with this condition are notorious for developing *Escherichia coli* sepsis. Cerebral edema may develop from toxic concentrations of organic acids or ammonia caused by an organic acidemia or urea cycle defect, respectively.

Diagnostic Confirmation

Hypoglycemia and liver dysfunction are commonly seen with IEM. The hallmark of urea cycle disorders is severe hyperammonemia, often >1,000 μg/dL. Newborns with this condition may present with respiratory alkalosis due to the direct stimulating effect of ammonia on the respiratory center. Organic acidemias can also cause hyperammonemia, but not as severe (usually <500 μg/dL). Metabolic acidosis with a large anion gap, frequently >30–50, is the hallmark of organic acidemias. Aminoacidopathies that present in the neonatal period typically do so with severe, progressive central nervous system dysfunction without hyperammonemia or metabolic acidosis. Figure 2.1 is an easy-to-follow algorithm that can assist with differentiating between the types of protein metabolism defects. Table 2.7 shows the laboratory tests, in addition to a rapid bedside glucose test, to obtain for a critically ill neonate with a suspected IEM. A urinalysis can be helpful in the diagnosis because spindle-shaped crystals may be seen with urea cycle defects. Basic cerebrospinal fluid (CSF) studies are included in the evaluation because infection is always considered in the differential diagnosis for a critically ill neonate.

Treatment

There are five main steps in the management of a metabolic crisis:

1. Remove the inciting metabolic substrate by making the patient NPO.
2. Restore circulatory volume by administering normal saline 10 mL/kg IV boluses.

TABLE 2.7 LABORATORY STUDIES FOR A SUSPECTED INBORN ERROR OF METABOLISM

Ammonia (arterial sample)	Cerebrospinal fluid studies
Blood culture	Urinalysis
Blood gas with lactate	Urine culture
Complete blood count	Urine amino acids
Complete metabolic panel	Urine organic acids
Plasma amino acids	Urine reducing substances

3. Provide an energy substrate to halt catabolism by administering a dextrose 10% in normal saline IV infusion at 1.5 times maintenance rate.
4. Treat severe metabolic acidosis.
5. Eliminate ammonia.

Aggressive guidelines recommend treatment of a pH ≤ 7.2 with 1 or 2 mEq/kg/hr of sodium bicarbonate. In contrast, due to the potential adverse effects of sodium bicarbonate, conservative guidelines recommend initiating treatment for a pH ≤ 7.0 at a rate of 0.25–0.5 mEq/kg/hr. Hemodialysis is indicated for intractable acidosis.

There are three methods of treating hyperammonemia. Ammonia scavengers, sodium phenylacetate and sodium benzoate (Ammonul), are used to directly reduce the ammonia concentration in the blood. A urea cycle intermediate, arginine hydrochloride, reduces the production of ammonia. Administer Ammonul through a central venous line. Arginine hydrochloride may be administered through an IV or a central venous line. These medications are indicated for an ammonia concentration >100 µg/dL. Their recommended doses are shown in Table 2.8. The third method to treat hyperammonemia is dialysis. It should be prepared for use, in case the previously mentioned therapies fail, if the newborn's ammonia concentration is between 200 and 300 µg/dL and immediately performed for concentrations >300 µg/dL.

Disposition

Admit a newborn with a metabolic crisis caused by an IEM to an ICU.

Complication

The severity of neurologic morbidity for patients with urea cycle defects and organic acidemias is strongly associated with the duration of time the ammonia concentration is elevated.

Key Point

- IEM are a complex group of disorders, but their management can be simplified by following the five key steps (listed previously).

Pitfall

- Failing to consider IEM in newborns presenting with lethargy.

SEPSIS

Background

Sepsis is a clinical syndrome of life-threatening organ dysfunction caused by a dysregulated host response to infection. Neonatal sepsis is divided into early onset, occurring before 7 days of life, and late-onset disease. Early onset sepsis is caused by the vertical transmission of a pathogen from the mother to the newborn. In contrast, late-onset sepsis is due to horizontal transmission from the newborn's environment.

Clinical Presentation

A newborn with sepsis may present with subtle signs or in extremis. Common symptoms include irritability, lethargy, poor feeding, vomiting, and diarrhea. Apnea and seizures may also occur. Vital sign abnormalities including fever (≥38.0°C), hypothermia (<36.5°C), tachycardia, bradycardia, and tachypnea are often encountered. Physical examination may reveal a bulging anterior fontanelle in the setting of meningitis, respiratory distress (e.g., nasal flaring and grunting), an erythematous umbilicus with or without discharge consistent with omphalitis, hepatomegaly, mottling of the extremities, decreased

TABLE 2.8 MEDICATIONS FOR HYPERAMMONEMIA

Medication	Dose
Ammonul	250 mg/kg in 10% glucose via CVL over 90–120 minutes followed by a continuous infusion at 250 mg/kg/day
Arginine hydrochloride	600 mg/kg IV in 10% glucose over 90-120 minutes followed by a continuous infusion at 600 mg/kg/day

CVL, central venous line.

capillary refill time, weak pulses, jaundice, or abnormal tone. Cutaneous vesicles may be encountered with herpes simplex virus (HSV) infection but are frequently not present. Neonatal HSV infection may manifest as skin, eyes, and mouth (SEM) disease, disseminated disease, or meningoencephalitis.

Diagnostic Confirmation

Obtain a complete blood count (CBC), complete metabolic panel (CMP), blood gas with lactate, and blood culture in all patients with concern for sepsis. In addition, perform an HSV polymerase chain reaction (PCR) blood test and HSV PCR testing of surface swabs of the conjunctivae, nasopharynx, mouth, cutaneous vesicles (if present), and rectum. A peripheral white blood cell (WBC) count >15,000 or <5,000 × 10^9/L, an abnormal platelet count, and metabolic acidosis are concerning for sepsis. Hypoglycemia commonly occurs as well. Transaminitis can be seen in the setting of disseminated HSV infection or hepatic injury from septic shock. C-reactive protein and procalcitonin are other inflammatory markers that may also be obtained to help determine the likelihood of an infectious process.

A urinalysis and urine culture must be performed. Bagged urine specimens are not acceptable due to a high rate of false-positive results. A urinary tract infection is diagnosed by a urine culture obtained by bladder catheterization growing a pathogenic bacterium with ≥50,000 colony-forming units (CFU)/mL or between 10,000 and 50,000 CFU/mL with pyuria (≥5 WBC/high power field) detected on urinalysis. Suprapubic aspiration is an alternative method of obtaining urine but is rarely necessary.

If the neonate is stable, perform a lumbar puncture. Always have a pulse oximeter in place during lumbar puncture due to the risk of apnea. Order CSF cell count, protein and glucose concentrations, bacterial gram stain and culture, and HSV PCR tests. Notably, the normal ranges for CSF WBC count, protein concentration, and glucose concentration differ for neonates. Table 2.9 displays age-specific CSF parameters that can be used to interpret results for a newborn. Last, obtain a chest radiograph to evaluate for pneumonia.

Treatment

Attention to the airway and breathing may reveal a need for endotracheal intubation. Treat

TABLE 2.9 PERCENTILE DISTRIBUTION OF CEREBROSPINAL FLUID PARAMETERS BASED ON AGE

Age (Days)	Percentile		
	5th	50th	95th
WBC count (cells/mm^3)			
7	0.7	5	19.1
14	0.6	4	16
21	0.4	3.4	13.7
28	0.3	3	11.9
Protein concentration (mg/dL)			
7	47	78.4	130.7
14	39.6	66.9	113.1
21	34.9	60	103.1
28	32.1	56.2	98.4
Glucose concentration (mg/dL)			
7	34.7	44.9	60.6
14	34.7	44.6	59.7
21	34.8	44.5	59.2
28	35.2	44.8	59.5

WBC, white blood cell.
Source: Adapted from Thomson J, Sucharew H, Cruz AT, et al. Cerebrospinal fluid reference values for young infants undergoing lumbar puncture. *Pediatrics.* 2018;141(3).

TABLE 2.10 THERAPIES FOR ILL-APPEARING NEONATES WITH SUSPECTED SEPSIS

Therapy	Medication	Dose
Antibiotics	Cefepime	50 mg/kg IV
	Vancomycin	20 mg/kg IV
Antiviral	Acyclovir	20 mg/kg IV
Vasopressors	Dopamine	5–9 μg/kg/min IV
	Epinephrine	0.05–0.3 μg/kg/min IV

IV, intravenously.

poor perfusion with normal saline 10 mL/kg IV boluses up to 40 mL/kg. Perform lung auscultation and liver edge palpation after each bolus to assess for signs of fluid overload. For fluid-refractory shock, begin a dopamine IV infusion. Initiate an epinephrine IV infusion for fluid-refractory, dopamine-resistant shock. Treat hypoglycemia with a dextrose 10% IV bolus followed by initiation of a dextrose 10% IV infusion at 1.5 times maintenance rate to provide a glucose infusion rate of 6–8 mg/kg/min. Aggressively manage hypothermia with an infant radiant warmer.

Immediately treat an ill-appearing neonate with suspected sepsis with broad-spectrum antibiotic therapy based on local resistance patterns and antiviral therapy. An example regimen is the combination of acyclovir IV, cefepime IV, and vancomycin IV. Table 2.10 shows recommended medication doses for neonatal sepsis.

Disposition

Admit a critically ill neonate with sepsis to an ICU.

Complications

- Mortality rates for late preterm (born between 34 and 36 weeks of gestation) and term neonates with sepsis range from 1% to 10%.
- Neonatal bacterial meningitis has a mortality rate of 10%; 20% of survivors have severe disability, and another 35% have mild to moderate disability.
- Disseminated HSV infection has a mortality rate of 29%, often due to pneumonia or liver failure. HSV meningoencephalitis has a mortality rate of 4%, and HSV SEM disease has a mortality rate of <1%.

Key Point

- Immediate administration of broad-spectrum antibiotic and antiviral therapy is essential for the management of a critically ill neonate with suspected sepsis.

Pitfalls

- Failing to aggressively manage hypothermia.
- Forgetting pulse oximetry monitoring while performing a lumbar puncture.

INTESTINAL CATASTROPHES

Congenital Diaphragmatic Hernia

Background

A congenital diaphragmatic hernia (CDH) is a condition in which intra-abdominal contents herniate into the thoracic cavity due to a defect of the diaphragm. The defects occur on the left side in 85% of cases, the right side in 13% of cases, and bilaterally in 2% of cases. The presence of intra-abdominal contents in the thorax during development leads to pulmonary hypoplasia and pulmonary hypertension. The diagnosis may be missed prenatally. If so, patients usually present in extremis at birth or, less commonly, later in life.

Classic Clinical Presentation

Newborns most often present within the first 24 hours after birth with respiratory distress, unilateral absence of breath sounds, and a scaphoid-shaped abdomen. With left-sided defects, the heart sounds may be displaced to the right side of the chest. Compression of the mediastinum can result in decreased cardiac output with hypotension and poor perfusion.

Atypical Presentation

When the defect is less severe, newborns may be asymptomatic at birth. They can present later in the neonatal period, in infancy, or as a toddler with recurrent respiratory distress, chronic pulmonary infections, or bowel obstruction caused by a volvulus.

Diagnostic Confirmation

Chest radiography will reveal intra-abdominal contents in the thoracic cavity. Late-presenting CDH is frequently misdiagnosed radiographically, often as a pneumothorax or pleural effusion. Case reports suggest that the use of point-of-care ultrasound (PoCUS) can help identify this condition more rapidly and accurately. Echocardiography is indicated to assess the degree of pulmonary hypertension and to evaluate for CHD. Approximately 10% of newborns with CDH have hemodynamically significant CHD.

Treatment

Insert a nasogastric or orogastric tube to decompress the intestines. Depending on the severity of respiratory distress, endotracheal intubation may be necessary. If so, ventilation with a low peak inspiratory pressure of <25 cm H_2O is recommended to minimize lung injury. A dopamine infusion may be indicated if cardiac output is significantly compromised. Interestingly, a large proportion of newborns with CDH also have adrenal insufficiency. Consider administration of hydrocortisone IV for patients with suspicious electrolyte derangements or refractory hypotension. Advanced therapies such as inhaled nitric oxide and extracorporeal membrane oxygenation may be required for management of pulmonary hypertension. Once medically stabilized, definitive treatment is surgery.

Disposition

All newborns diagnosed with CDH require hospital admission.

Complication

The overall mortality rate for neonates born alive with CDH is approximately 10–30%.

Key Points

- Although usually symptomatic at birth, CDH can present later in life.
- PoCUS can assist in the diagnosis of CDH.

Pitfall

- Mistaking radiographic findings of CDH for a pneumothorax and inserting a chest tube resulting in bowel perforation.

NECROTIZING ENTEROCOLITIS

Background

Necrotizing enterocolitis (NEC) is primarily a disease of premature newborns. However, up to 10% of cases occur in late preterm and term neonates. Usually, these more mature newborns present in the first week of life and often have associated risk factors such as CHD or a history of perinatal asphyxia. The pathogenesis of this condition is poorly understood. It is the primary cause of short bowel syndrome in the pediatric population.

Clinical Presentation

Newborns commonly present with vomiting, abdominal distension, abdominal tenderness, and bloody stools. Apnea, bradycardia, and temperature instability may develop. Advanced disease can present with abdominal discoloration, intestinal perforation, peritonitis, circulatory compromise with shock, and respiratory failure. Laboratory evaluation may demonstrate metabolic acidosis, thrombocytopenia, and disseminated intravascular coagulation (DIC).

Diagnostic Confirmation

The diagnosis is made by visualizing pneumatosis intestinalis, portal venous gas, or pneumoperitoneum on a two-view abdominal radiograph. The two former findings can help differentiate this condition from neonatal midgut volvulus, which presents similarly. Laboratory evaluation should include a CBC, CMP, blood gas with lactate, and coagulation studies. Due to the risk of bacterial translocation in the setting of ischemic bowel, obtain a blood culture as well.

Treatment

Endotracheal intubation may be necessary. Provide circulatory support with normal saline IV boluses and, if needed, a vasopressor infusion. Initiate bowel rest and gastric decompression with low-intermittent nasogastric or orogastric suction. Due to the potential for bacterial translocation in the setting of bowel ischemia and necrosis, administer broad-spectrum antibiotic therapy based on local resistance patterns. An example regimen is the combination of cefepime 50 mg/kg IV, metronidazole 15 mg/kg IV, and vancomycin 20 mg/kg IV. Blood product transfusions are indicated for DIC. Surgical intervention is necessary if there is evidence of intestinal perforation. Advanced disease without perforation, such as in patients with severe acidosis and thrombocytopenia, may also warrant surgery. This decision should be made in consultation with a pediatric surgeon.

Disposition

All newborns with NEC require admission to an ICU or, if indicated, an operating room.

Complications

- The mortality rate ranges between 15% and 30%.
- Survivors are at substantially increased risk for neurodevelopmental delay.
- An acquired small bowel stricture can develop several months after recovery.

Key Point

- Findings on abdominal radiography can help differentiate NEC from midgut volvulus.

Pitfall

- Failing to consider NEC in the differential diagnosis for term newborns.

MIDGUT VOLVULUS

Background

Malrotation of the intestines is caused by abnormal rotation and fixation of the bowel during embryonic development. The most devastating complication that can occur with intestinal malrotation is a midgut volvulus.

Clinical Presentation

Midgut volvulus typically presents in the first month of life with bilious vomiting and crying due to abdominal pain. Hematochezia may develop as a result of bowel ischemia and necrosis. Newborns can rapidly decompensate and progress to cardiovascular collapse. Physical examination may reveal a tender abdomen with or without distension. Signs of peritonitis are a late finding. Perform a rectal examination to evaluate for the presence of blood.

Diagnostic Confirmation

In a stable patient with a suspected midgut volvulus, an upper gastrointestinal series is the study of choice. However, this study is incompletely sensitive, and consultation with a pediatric surgeon is recommended in all cases of bilious vomiting, even if the patient is initially well-appearing. In an ill-appearing neonate, immediate exploratory laparotomy is indicated. Obtain a CBC, CMP, blood gas with lactate, type and screen, and blood culture. The latter is recommended due to the risk of bacterial translocation in the setting of ischemic bowel.

Treatment

Insert a nasogastric or orogastric tube to decompress the bowel. Surgical consultation for an emergent exploratory laparotomy is necessary for an ill-appearing neonate with a suspected midgut volvulus. If transfer to a pediatric hospital is desired but cannot be accomplished within 1 hour, a laparotomy must be performed without delay at the hospital of initial presentation. Administer normal saline IV boluses for signs of shock. A vasopressor infusion may be necessary for cardiovascular support. Due to the potential for bacterial translocation in the setting of bowel ischemia and necrosis, administer broad-spectrum antibiotic therapy based on local resistance patterns. An example regimen is the combination of cefepime 50 mg/kg IV, metronidazole 15 mg/kg IV, and vancomycin 20 mg/kg IV.

Disposition

- All cases of bilious vomiting in neonates should ideally be evaluated by a pediatric surgeon due to the significant associated risk of morbidity and potential mortality of a midgut volvulus. An ill-appearing neonate with a suspected midgut volvulus must be taken to an operating room immediately.

Complication

- Within hours, a midgut volvulus can result in the loss of the entire small bowel and ascending colon.

Key Points

- Bilious vomiting in a neonate is a surgical emergency until proven otherwise.

- For a critically ill neonate with a suspected midgut volvulus, bypass diagnostic imaging and consult a surgeon for an emergent exploratory laparotomy.

Pitfalls

- Failure to rapidly and thoroughly evaluate a neonate with bilious vomiting due to initially appearing well.
- Delaying an exploratory laparotomy in an ill-appearing neonate with a suspected midgut volvulus for more than 1 hour while waiting for transfer to a pediatric hospital.

SEIZURES

Background

Seizures in the neonate often present subtly due to incomplete myelination of the motor pathways. They are rarely idiopathic and have an extensive differential diagnosis to consider. Their management significantly differs from that of seizures in other pediatric age groups and adults.

Clinical Presentation

Neonatal seizures are classified as subtle, clonic, tonic, and myoclonic. Subtle seizures are the most common and manifest as oral–buccal–lingual movements, ocular movements, or stereotypic bicycling or stepping movements of the lower extremities. They can also manifest as isolated autonomic dysfunction, such as abnormal heart rate and blood pressure. Neonatal seizures uncommonly present as generalized tonic–clonic movements.

Differential Diagnosis

The differential diagnosis is detailed in Table 2.11.

TABLE 2.11 NEONATAL SEIZURE ETIOLOGIES

Etiology	Examples
Acute electrolyte derangements	Hypernatremia Hypocalcemia Hypoglycemia Hypomagnesemia Hyponatremia
Cerebral dysgenesis	
Hypertensive encephalopathy	
Hypoxic ischemic encephalopathy	
Inborn errors of metabolism	Aminoacidopathies Organic acidemias Urea cycle disorders
Infection	Encephalitis
Intracranial hemorrhage or thrombosis	Intraventricular hemorrhage Traumatic brain injury
Mitochondrial disorders	
Neonatal epileptic syndromes	Benign familial neonatal seizures Benign idiopathic neonatal seizures Early infantile epileptic encephalopathy Early myoclonic encephalopathy
Neurocutaneous disorders	Incontinentia pigmenti Neurofibromatosis Sturge–Weber syndrome Tuberous sclerosis
Peroxisomal disorders	Neonatal adrenoleukodystrophy Zellweger syndrome
Pyridoxine dependency	
Toxins	Kernicterus Maternal (e.g., cocaine and heroin)

Diagnostic Confirmation

Initially, perform a rapid bedside glucose test. Then obtain blood for a CBC, CMP, blood gas with lactate, magnesium, ammonia, and blood culture. Lumbar puncture is necessary if there is concern for an infection. Magnetic resonance imaging (MRI) of the brain is indicated. If there is an expected delay in obtaining an MRI, consider ordering a cranial ultrasound to evaluate for hydrocephalus or an intracranial hemorrhage. A computed tomography scan of the head is warranted if there are signs of a traumatic head injury. Emergent consultation with a pediatric neurologist is essential to perform an electroencephalogram (EEG). Importantly, subclinical seizure activity may persist after resolution of clinical seizures, which is known as electroclinical dissociation.

Treatment

Electrolyte derangements, if identified, must be corrected. Table 2.12 displays the recommended therapies and their doses. Hypoglycemia is treated with a dextrose 10% IV bolus followed by initiation of a dextrose 10% IV infusion at 1.5 times maintenance rate to provide a glucose infusion rate of 6–8 mg/kg/min. Seizures caused by hyponatremia and hypernatremia often respond to administration of a normal saline IV bolus. Treat refractory hyponatremic seizures with a hypertonic (3%) saline IV bolus. Seizures caused by hypocalcemia are treated with a calcium gluconate IV bolus followed by initiation of an IV infusion. Importantly, calcium levels may not normalize if serum magnesium is low. Therefore, treat concurrent hypomagnesemia with magnesium sulfate IV.

Due to the potential for electroclinical dissociation, continuous EEG monitoring is necessary if antiepileptic medications are used to treat seizures in newborns. Clinically apparent seizures in the neonate should be treated with antiepileptic medications if they last more than 3 minutes or are brief serial seizures. Traditionally, phenobarbital has been the first-line antiepileptic medication of choice for neonatal seizures. Despite growing evidence of potential harm from neonatal exposure, it remains the most widely used medication for seizures in this age group. Fosphenytoin and phenytoin are commonly used as second-line agents, but they have also been shown to have undesirable side effect profiles. There is growing evidence that levetiracetam is effective and safe for newborn seizures. Ahmad and colleagues published data in 2017 demonstrating that it has surpassed phenytoin as the most common second-line antiepileptic medication administered in the United States.

Administration of pyridoxine for refractory neonatal seizure activity is recommended due to the possibility of pyridoxine-dependent epilepsy, an autosomal recessive condition. Benzodiazepines, such as midazolam, are often avoided in newborns because of the potential for respiratory suppression, hypotension, and apoptotic neurodegeneration. Figure 2.2 displays a management algorithm for neonatal seizures. Of note, the phenobarbital loading dose can be maximized at 40 mg/kg, but this significantly increases the risk of respiratory depression.

Disposition

All neonates presenting with seizures require hospital admission. The decision to place the patient in the general inpatient unit or an ICU

TABLE 2.12 TREATMENTS FOR NEONATAL ELECTROLYTE DERANGEMENTS

Condition	Medication	Doses
Hypocalcemia	Calcium gluconate 10%	100–200 mg/kg IV over 5–10 minutes 500–800 mg/kg/day IV infusion
Hypoglycemia	Dextrose 10%	2 mL/kg IV 1.5 times maintenance rate IV infusion
Hypomagnesemia	Magnesium sulfate	50–100 mg/kg IV over 1–2 hours
Hyponatremia	Hypertonic (3%) saline	3 mL/kg IV

IV, intravenously.

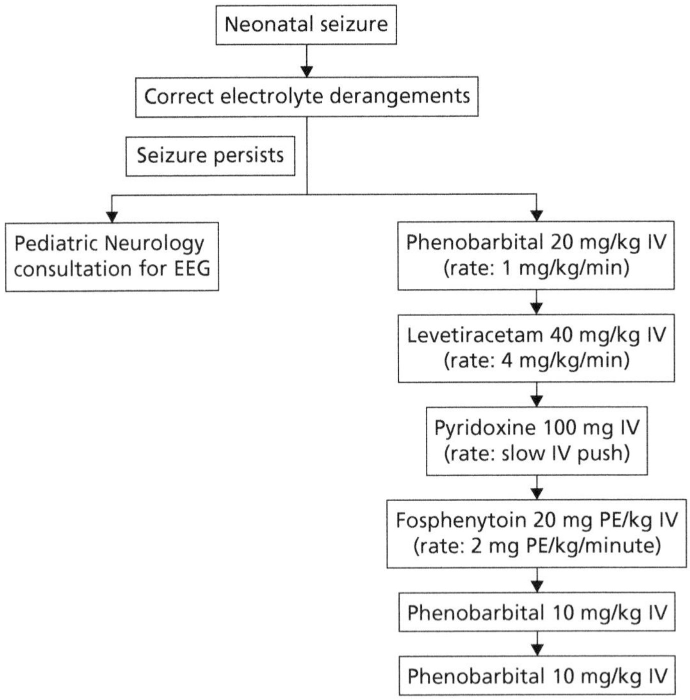

FIGURE 2.2 Management algorithm for neonatal seizures. PE, phenytoin sodium equivalents.

depends on the etiology and initial response to treatment.

Complications

- Phenobarbital may cause apnea (especially with rapid IV administration), hypoventilation, bradycardia, and hypotension.
- Fosphenytoin and phenytoin may induce cardiac dysrhythmias, hypotension, and apnea.

Key Points

- Emergency physicians must be aware of the subtle manifestations of neonatal seizures.
- Clinically apparent seizures in the neonate should be treated with antiepileptic medications if they last more than 3 minutes or are brief serial seizures.

Pitfalls

- Failure to concurrently treat hypomagnesemia, if present, when treating hypocalcemia.
- Omission of EEG monitoring when treating neonatal seizures with antiepileptics.

Further Reading

Ahmad KA, Desai SJ, Bennett MM, et al. Changing antiepileptic drug use for seizures in US neonatal intensive care units from 2005 to 2014. *J Perinatol.* 2017;37(3):296–300.

Ahrens S, Ream MA, Slaughter LA. Status epilepticus in the neonate: Updates in treatment strategies. *Curr Treat Options Neurol.* 2019;21(2):8.

Davis AL, Carcillo JA, Aneja RK, et al. The American College of Critical Care Medicine clinical practice parameters for hemodynamic support of pediatric and neonatal shock: Executive summary. *Pediatr Crit Care Med.* 2017;18(9):884–890.

Nehra D, Goldstein AM. Intestinal malrotation: Varied clinical presentation from infancy through adulthood. *Surgery.* 2011;149(3):386–393.

Strobel AM, Lu LN. The critically ill infant with congenital heart disease. *Emerg Med Clin North Am.* 2015;33(3):501–518.

Weiner DL. Metabolic emergencies. In: Shaw KN, Bachur RG, eds. *Fleisher & Ludwig's Textbook of Pediatric Emergency Medicine.* 7th ed. Philadelphia, PA: Wolters Kluwer; 2016:894–913.

3

Brief Resolved Unexplained Event

ILENE CLAUDIUS

INTRODUCTION

Brief resolved unexplained event (BRUE), or a transient and resolved change in color, breathing, tone, or mental status in an infant, supplanted the term apparent life-threatening event (ALTE) after the publication of a 2016 American Academy of Pediatrics guideline. Due to the novelty of the condition BRUE, minimal literature exists to inform incidence or risk. Although the overlap between ALTE and BRUE is not complete, historic data on ALTE can be used to fill these gaps. The estimated incidence of an ALTE ranges from 0.46 to 10 per 1,000 births, depending on whether coding data or parental report is used. ALTE was thought to account for 0.6–1.7% of emergency visits for children younger than age 1 year and 2% of hospitalizations, with a median age of 1–3 months. A few retrospective studies have examined the application of the BRUE criteria to records of patients previously admitted to the emergency department (ED) or inpatient unit. Between 23% and 58% of patients admitted with an ALTE met criteria for a BRUE. No clear adult equivalent exists, and the diagnosis of BRUE is limited to patients younger than age 1 year.

The obvious concern when an infant presents with a period of breathing irregularity or cyanosis is the potential for a recurrent event. The patient was lucky once and survived; will there be a next episode? Will the next episode be terminal? Is this the manifestation of a life-threating pathology that we, in the ED, cannot afford to miss? Will this infant succumb to sudden infant death syndrome (SIDS)? Conversely, 80–90% of ALTE patients look well at the time of ED presentation, and with studies citing mean admit times of 4.4 days and charges of $15,567 per admission, is this an acceptable use of resources and is the level of family disruption and exposure to hospital pathogens acceptable? From 12% to 14% of historic ALTE patients will have a subsequent event or condition requiring hospitalization. The BRUE risk-stratification criteria (discussed later) were designed with identified recurrence risk factors in mind, and the risk of a recurrent event in a patient deemed to have had a low-risk BRUE approaches the baseline age-matched population risk of such an event. ALTE mortality is low, with a recent meta-analysis identifying 12 post-ALTE deaths reported, 8 of which were within 4 months of the event and 4 of which occurred while in the hospital. This represents a 1 in 800–1,200 patient mortality risk, near baseline for age. Using the BRUE criteria, particularly the low-risk BRUE criteria, likely lowers this number further. Although ALTE was once thought to be a precursor to SIDS, it is now clear from the epidemiologic differences that these two conditions are unrelated.

The change from ALTE to BRUE was predicated on the fact that the classic ALTE definition of an episode that is "frightening to the observer and that is characterized by some combination of apnea (central or occasionally obstructive), color change (usually cyanotic or pallid but occasionally erythematous or plethoric), marked change in muscle tone (usually marked limpness), choking, or gagging" was too vague. It relied too heavily on the observation and diagnostic decision-making capability of the parent. In addition, the broad reach of the definition made it difficult to provide clinicians with guidance to the evaluation and management of these patients, and the default became near ubiquitous admission.

CLASSIC CLINICAL PRESENTATION

The classic patient is a young infant who appears well to the provider, with normal vital signs and examination, and who is reported to have gone flaccid and apneic at home.

A BRUE is defined as a sudden, brief (<1 minute), resolved event in an infant younger than age 1 year, that remains of unclear etiology after evaluation. including one or more of the following:

- Cyanosis or pallor
- Absent, decreased, or irregular breathing
- Marked change in tone (hyper- or hypotonia)
- Altered level of responsiveness

A low-risk BRUE is a BRUE that also meets the following criteria:

- Age >60 days
- Born ≥32 weeks of gestation and corrected age ≥45 weeks
- No cardiopulmonary resuscitation (CPR) by trained medical provider
- Event <1 minute
- First and single event
- No concerns identified from the history and physical

A higher risk BRUE is a BRUE that does not meet one or more of the low-risk criteria.

ATYPICAL CLINICAL PRESENTATION

As mentioned previously, there are a number of patients who would have met the definition for ALTE but do not meet the definition for BRUE. In many cases, this is due to an examination abnormality or a clear explanatory diagnosis. In a recent study, in which the minority of ALTE patients met BRUE criteria, 70% of the patients discharged from the ED were given an explanatory diagnosis. Therefore, although the occasional patient may still represent an idiopathic ALTE, in most non-BRUE cases, a specific pathology is suspected or proven. Alternatively, a patient may not meet the BRUE definition because of a lack of symptom resolution, thus requiring further inpatient evaluation.

DIFFERENTIAL DIAGNOSIS

Common

- Gastroesophageal reflux disease (GERD)
- Seizure
- Respiratory infection (e.g., pertussis, bronchiolitis)
- Benign mimics (e.g., vasomotor instability, dense perioral venous plexus, periodic breathing)
- Child abuse (suffocation, non-accidental trauma, poisoning)
- Breath-holding spell

Uncommon

- Serious bacterial infection
- Inborn error of metabolism
- Swallowing dysfunction
- Non-abusive intracranial pathology (e.g., mass, hydrocephalus)
- Foreign body
- Cardiovascular causes (e.g., channelopathy, accessory pathway)
- Accidental intoxication
- Craniofacial abnormalities

DIAGNOSTIC CONFIRMATION

For a patient with a low-risk BRUE, implying a resolved event and a normal examination, minimal further evaluation is needed. Although the guidelines recommend against most routine testing (complete blood count, cultures, cerebrospinal fluid, electrolytes, metabolic workup, chest X-ray, echocardiogram, electroencephalogram, GERD studies, respiratory viral panel, lactate, urinalysis, and neuroimaging), they do allow for an electrocardiogram (ECG) and pertussis testing to be performed at clinician discretion. Regarding ECG, the incidence of cardiac disease in ALTE patients is 0–4%; however, because channelopathies are associated with 9.5–13% of SIDS cases, if easily available, an ECG is a reasonable intervention. In the clinic setting without a readily available ECG, a patient does not need to be transferred for the purposes of obtaining an ECG unless the history and physical examination are concerning for a cardiac pathology or toxin. Pertussis is a potential cause of BRUE symptoms, and clinicians should consider testing if the patient has an exposure, inadequate vaccine status, or there is a high community prevalence. Certainly, if symptoms exist, the patient would no longer be considered as having a BRUE, but testing would be indicated.

For a patient with a higher risk BRUE without any localizing symptoms (e.g., staccato cough indicating pertussis), the literature is less clear regarding evaluation. Routine screening labs and radiographs are unlikely to yield valuable information. However, often a period of inpatient observation can either ensure the patient is stable or allow providers to witness the concerning events and target the evaluation accordingly.

TREATMENT

If the cause of an event is identified, appropriate disease-specific treatment should be rendered. For a BRUE, implying no etiology is found, no specific treatment is advised. In fact, a number of treatments for conditions that may underlie an event have historically been given to patients, with little basis for use. Therefore, the current guidelines recommend against the use of acid suppression therapy or antiepileptic medications and against home monitoring for a low-risk BRUE. Although there certainly are patients who initially present with a BRUE but are eventually found to have conditions requiring these treatments, for the typical low-risk BRUE, they should not be prescribed.

CLINICAL ALGORITHM

Figure 3.1 presents a clinical algorithm for BRUE.

DISPOSITION

Patients with a low-risk BRUE and reliable caregivers can be discharged home, and these patients should not be admitted merely for cardiopulmonary monitoring. If there is any concern on the part of the clinician or family, a 1- to 4-hour period of monitoring and serial examinations in the ED can be reassuring, as well as quickly identify symptom progression or early recurrence. Caregivers should be instructed to return for any concerning behavior and to follow up in 24 hours, preferably with a primary care provider. Both education regarding BRUE and resources for CPR training should be given to families.

Higher risk BRUE patients are a pleomorphic group that may be more likely to have a serious underlying cause, recurrent event, or an adverse outcome. Until the literature exists to provide further guidance, infants may warrant increased observation to better document the events or contextual factors. In summary, the disposition of these patients remains at the discretion of the clinician.

KEY POINTS

- Most low-risk BRUE patients require no evaluation beyond a careful history and physical examination.
- Parental response to BRUE and to discharge home is mixed; it is imperative to address parental concerns and consider a brief period of observation if needed.
- Higher risk BRUE patients represent a more pleomorphic group for whom guidelines do not yet exist. Often, a brief period of inpatient observation can be helpful.

PITFALLS

The major pitfall in the evaluation of BRUE is failure to consider child abuse. Although routine toxicology screening and cranial imaging are not suggested, appropriate attention to the tenents of history taking and physical examination for a patient at risk for abuse must be followed. In fact, of ALTE patients who expired following the event, half were victims of inflicted head injury, poisoning, or suffocation. Look for signs of familial instability or violence, evidence of trauma on the patient (remembering that even simple bruising is unusual in a child who is too young to cruise or walk), and facial petechiae or nasal bleeding to indicate suffocation. There is also some literature indicating a higher than baseline risk of

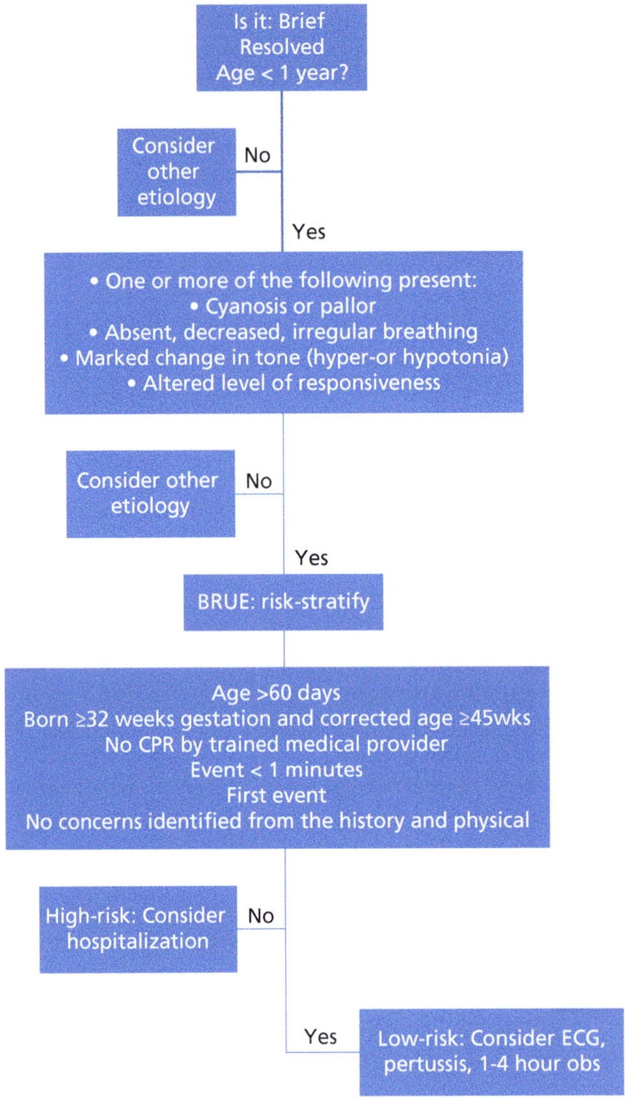

FIGURE 3.1 Clinical algorithm for assessing patients with BRUE.

abuse in the years after discharge, highlighting that this is a vulnerable population who will require ongoing pediatric care and assessment of family social support.

Further Reading

Brand DA, Fazzari MJ. Risk of death in infants who have experienced a brief resolved unexplained event: A meta-analysis. *J Pediatr.* 2018; 197:63–67.

Colombo M, Katz ES, Bosco A, Melzi ML, Nosetti L. Brief resolved unexplained events: Retrospective validation of diagnostic criteria and risk stratification. *Pediatr Pulmonol.* 2019;54(1):61–65.

McFarlin A. What to do when babies turn blue: Beyond the basic brief resolved unexplained event. *Emerg Med Clin North Am.* 2018;36:335–347.

Meyer JS, Stensland EG, Murzycki J, Gulen CR, Evindar A, Cardoso MZ. Retrospective application of BRUE criteria to patients presenting with ALTE. *Hosp Pediatr.* 2018;8(12):740–745.

Tieder JS, Bonkowsky JL, Etzel RA, et al. Clinical practice guideline: Brief resolved unexplained events (formerly apparent life-threatening events) and evaluation of lower-risk infants: Executive summary. *Pediatrics.* 2016:137(5):e20160591. http://pediatrics.aappublications.org/cgi/doi/10.1542/peds.2016-1488.

4

Sudden Infant Death Syndrome

SHERYL YANGER

Sudden infant death syndrome (SIDS) is the third leading cause of infant mortality in the United States. SIDS is defined as the sudden death of an infant younger than age 1 year that cannot be explained after a thorough investigation, including autopsy, scene investigation, and clinical history. Despite research and advances in understanding of SIDS, it remains a diagnosis of exclusion after ruling out accidental causes such as suffocation/strangulation and cardiac, infectious, metabolic, or traumatic etiologies.

SIDS is the leading cause of death in infants aged 1 month to 1 year. The incidence is approximately 0.5 deaths per 1,000 live births, and approximately 3,500 infants die from sleep-related deaths in the United States each year. The Back to Sleep campaign in the early 1990s, which encouraged parents to place infants to sleep on their backs, effectively halved the rate of SIDS, but there has been no further decline since the mid-2000s.

Although the exact pathogenesis is unknown, a working model of SIDS includes a combination of exogenous factors, such as overbundling, prone sleep position, airway obstruction, and intrinsic factors such as immature cardiorespiratory or arousal systems.

SIDS disparately affects different races and ethnicities despite the decline in rates overall. The rates for non-Hispanic Black and American Indian/Alaska Natives are more than double that for non-Hispanic white infants. Ninety percent of deaths occur in the first 6 months of life; SIDS is uncommon after age 8 months. Side and prone sleep positions increase risk of hypercapnia and hypoxia, thought to be one of the mechanisms of SIDS. Parents are often concerned about the risk of aspiration or reflux with infants on their backs, but studies have shown no increased incidence of aspiration with supine sleeping. Similarly, bed sharing and soft bedding increase the risk of SIDS. Other risk factors include preterm and low-birth-weight infants and maternal smoking, either in utero or after birth.

PREVENTION

Infants should be placed on a safe sleep surface on their backs. This includes a flat sleep surface free from any soft bedding such as pillows, loose blankets, crib bumpers, stuffed animals, or toys. Wearable blankets and sleep clothing are acceptable alternatives. Sofas have also been found to be one of the most dangerous sleep surfaces, and parents should take care not to place infants to sleep or to fall asleep with an adult on a sofa, couch, or cushioned surface. Infants also should not be placed to sleep in car seats, infant carriers, swings, or inclined sleepers because infants do not have sufficient head control to maintain their airway in these devices. Other recent studies have found pacifier use and breastfeeding to be protective measures.

KEY POINTS

- SIDS is the leading cause of death in young infants.
- Infants should be placed to sleep on their backs on a firm, flat sleep surface free from loose bedding.
- Risk factors for SIDS include non-supine sleep positions, unsafe sleep surfaces, maternal smoking, prematurity, and low birth weight.
- Additional protective factors for SIDS include breastfeeding and pacifier use.

Further Reading

Carlin RF, Moon RY. Risk factors, protective factors, and current recommendations to reduce sudden infant death syndrome. *JAMA Pediatr.* 2017;171(2):175–180.

De Luca F, Hinde A. Effectiveness of the "Back-to-Sleep" campaigns among healthcare professionals in the past 20 years: A systematic review. *BMJ Open.* 2016;6(9):e011435.

Task Force on Sudden Infant Death Syndrome. SIDS and other sleep-related infant deaths: Updated 2016 recommendations for a safe infant sleeping environment. *Pediatrics.* 2016;138(5):e20162938.

5

Emergent Airway Management in Pediatrics

KELSEY A. MILLER AND JOSHUA NAGLER

INTRODUCTION

Airway management is the cornerstone to resuscitation efforts for many critically ill pediatric patients presenting for emergency care. The etiology of arrest in children is more commonly from a respiratory than a cardiac process, and early and effective airway management can be life-saving. However, only a small proportion of pediatric patients ultimately require advanced airway management: The need for endotracheal intubation in children presenting to the emergency department (ED) ranges from 0.6 to 3.3 cases per 1,000 visits. In addition to its rarity, lack of familiarity with predictable differences in pediatric airway management can further complicate performance of this critical procedure. This chapter reviews current best practices in pediatric airway management. We review relevant anatomic and physiologic differences in children and offer strategies to optimize procedural success, including tips for effective bag mask ventilation (BMV), laryngoscopy (direct and video) and intubation, use of pharmacologic agents, and approaches to predict and manage difficult pediatric airways.

Characteristics of children requiring intubation are variable, with median reported ages ranging from 2 to 7 years, although a disproportionate number are aged 1 year or younger. Broadly, there are approximately equal numbers of intubations for trauma and medical indications in children, although proportions vary by institution given differences in patient populations and trauma center designations.

ANATOMIC AND PHYSIOLOGIC DIFFERENCES IN PEDIATRIC AIRWAY MANAGEMENT

A number of predictable anatomic and physiologic differences in children affect airway management, and various strategies can be employed to address each of these (Table 5.1).

Infants have a large occiput causing natural flexion of the airway in neutral position, and using a shoulder roll helps align their airways. Toddlers and school-age children are often well anatomically aligned when supine without support, whereas older children and adolescents frequently benefit from elevation of the head, similar to adults. To obviate the need to remember position by age group, proceduralists should align the external auditory meatus with the sternal notch (Figure 5.1).

The larynx in children is anatomically high in the neck. Although commonly referred to as anterior, it is this superior position that can

TABLE 5.1 ANATOMIC AND PHYSIOLOGIC DIFFERENCES IN CHILDREN AND STRATEGIES TO ADDRESS THEM

Anatomic and Physiologic Differences	Strategies to Address Differences
Large occiput	Position patient appropriately (align external auditory meatus with sternal notch).
Superior airway	Look "up" during laryngoscopy.
Large epiglottis	Lift with straight blade. Engage the hypoepiglottic ligament.
Airway shape (elliptical, not funneled)	Consider cuffed endotracheal tubes.
Smaller lung volume	Use the "pop-off" valve during mask ventilation to avoid inadvertent barotrauma.
Rapid desaturation	Preoxygenation. Apneic oxygenation. Limit duration of attempts.

create the acute angle needed to see the glottis, often making visualization with direct laryngoscopy challenging. If using a traditional direct laryngoscope, the proceduralist should anticipate the glottic opening will be located at the top of the visual field.

The epiglottis in children is commonly large, floppy, and can obstruct visualization. The common teaching is to utilize a straight Miller blade to lift the epiglottis directly. However, curved Macintosh blades can also be used in pediatric airway management. The curved blade should be placed along the base of the tongue to indirectly lift the epiglottis by engaging the hyoepiglottic ligament within the vallecula to elevate the epiglottis (Figure 5.2).

Historically, the airway in children was described as funnel-shaped, with the narrowest portion at the cricoid cartilage. This understanding contributed to the recommendation for using uncuffed endotracheal tubes in children. More recently, a series of studies using bronchoscopy, magnetic resonance imaging, and airway computed tomography have demonstrated that cross-sectional areas of the subglottis are not smaller than adjacent areas of the airway. The difference, however, is a narrower transverse dimension, resulting in an elliptical shape. This recognition, combined with changes in the size and design of endotracheal tubes, has contributed to increased utilization of cuffed endotracheal tubes in pediatric patients. Cuffed endotracheal tubes reduce the need for tube exchange without increasing the risk of tracheal injury, and they may decrease the risk of aspiration. According to current Pediatric Advanced Life Support (PALS) guidelines, cuffed and uncuffed tubes are safe for use in children, but cuffed tubes may be preferable in cases in which high airway pressure or

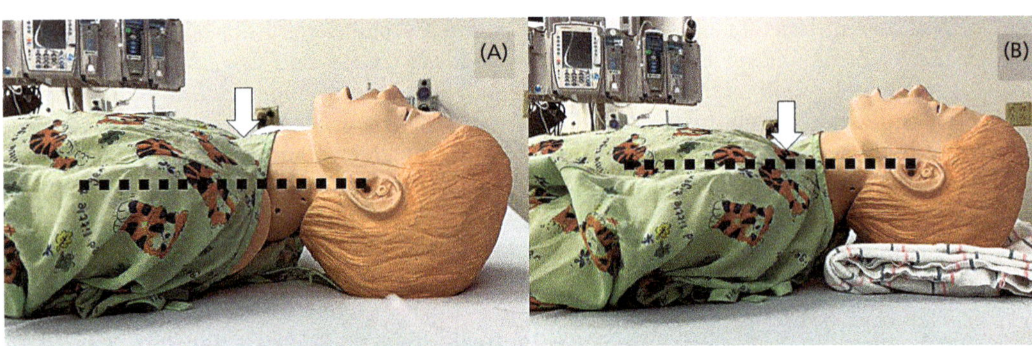

FIGURE 5.1 Patient positioning for airway alignment. Line up the external auditory canal (or tragus) with the sternal notch (arrows). In older children, this often requires a head roll (as shown in A and B); in infants, a shoulder roll is often necessary.

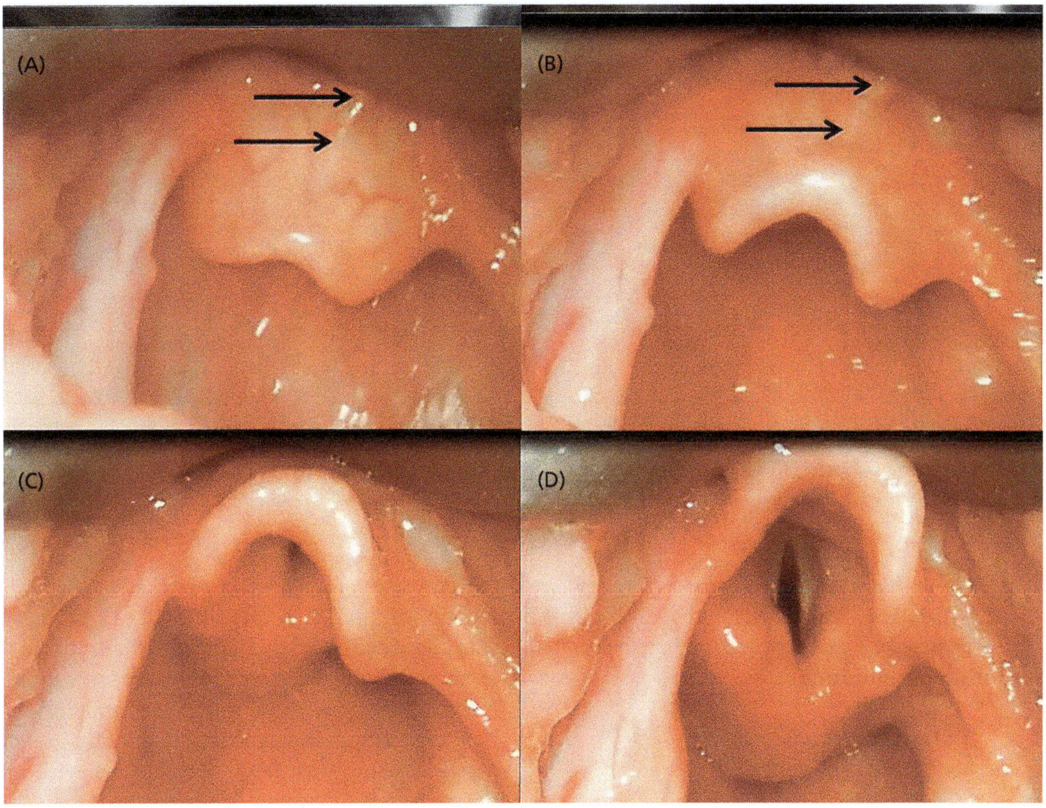

FIGURE 5.2 Engaging the hyoepiglottic ligament. When the laryngoscope blade is placed in the vallecula, pressure on the hyoepiglottic ligament (arrows) can lift the epiglottis up and out of line of sight, helping expose the glottic inlet (A–D).

poor lung compliance are anticipated. The vast majority of intubations in emergency medicine will be for airway obstruction (i.e., high airway pressure), lung disease (i.e., often with poor lung compliance), or altered/depressed mental status (i.e., loss of protective airway reflexes and risk of aspiration), all of which are included in these "cuffed preferred" conditions. Therefore, it is our practice to use cuffed endotracheal tubes in essentially all pediatric intubations in the ED, with careful attention paid to correct positioning of the endotracheal tube and avoidance of overinflation of the cuff.

Children have smaller lungs and tidal volumes than adults. When children need assisted ventilation, the size of breaths should be adjusted to provide the lowest pressure needed to achieve adequate chest rise. Motor memory among providers who care primarily for adult patients might result in excessive volumes when providing assisted ventilation in children. To help minimize the risk of barotrauma, many pediatric self-inflating bags have built-in "pop-off" valves (Figure 5.3) to limit the maximum pressure being inadvertently delivered during stressful clinical scenarios in which providers may themselves be in highly adrenergic states.

The most critical physiologic differences between children and adults relevant to airway management is the more rapid rate of desaturation. Children have a relatively smaller functional residual capacity. Even with appropriate preoxygenation, the stores of oxygenated airspace from which to draw are smaller. In addition, children have a higher metabolic rate and consume oxygen at approximately twice the rate of adults, on a per kilogram basis. These factors combine to create a relatively shorter safe apnea time for infants and young children. Data show that the time to desaturation to 90% in fully preoxygenated healthy children in the operating room setting is approximately 90 seconds for children younger than age 6 months compared to more than 6 minutes for adolescents. It is important to note that the time to hypoxemia will likely be significantly

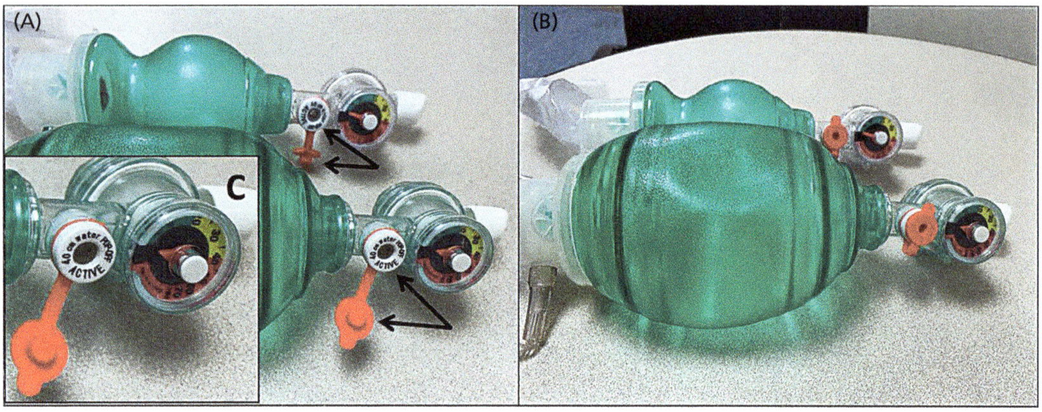

FIGURE 5.3 (A) There are many different versions of pop-off valves (arrows) to help prevent excessive pressure when the valve is open. (B) Generated pressures are not limited when the valve is closed. (C) The equipment shown in this figure has an upper pressure limit of 40 cm H_2O when the valve is open.

faster in pediatric emergency medicine practice in children with underlying lung and cardiac symptomatology and less comprehensive preintubation optimization.

CLINICAL APPLICATION

Indications

Indications for advanced airway management in children are similar to those in adult patients, namely acute respiratory failure (hypoxic, hypercarbic, or both), cardiovascular collapse/arrest, inability to maintain or protect the airway for patients with altered mental status, or expected clinical course.

Alternatives to Endotracheal Intubation

In considering airway management in pediatric patients, providers should evaluate whether there are alternative modalities to support a patient. This is particularly the case for patients in whom the primary indication for increased ventilatory support is hypoxic or hypercarbic respiratory failure or in patients predicted to have difficult airways. Examples include high-flow nasal cannula and noninvasive ventilation. See Chapter 6 on noninvasive ventilation for further details and indications.

CLINICAL ALGORITHM

Equipment

When preparing for emergent pediatric airway management, selection of the appropriately sized equipment is key. Oxygen delivery for preoxygenation can occur through a nonrebreather (pediatric or adult-sized). A nasal cannula (neonatal, pediatric, or adult-sized) is also beneficial as an alternative or supplemental source of oxygen delivery and for the delivery of apneic oxygenation. Finally, either a self-inflating or a flow-inflating bag with an appropriately sized mask is necessary for providing assisted ventilation. In case of difficult ventilation, providers should have oral and nasal airways available. The appropriately sized nasal airway can be selected by choosing the size that extends from the tip of the patient's nose to the tragus of the ear (i.e., rule to T's), whereas an appropriately sized oral airway should extend from the corner of the mouth to the angle of the mandible (rule of M's).

To perform laryngoscopy and intubation, providers must select the appropriately sized blade and endotracheal tube. In general, the Miller 1 straight blade is used for infants and children younger than age 2 years. Starting at age 2 years, children will likely require a size 2 blade ("switch to size 2 at age 2"), regardless of whether the straight Miller or curved Macintosh blade is used. The decision to upsize to a size 3 blade is more subjective: Once a child is approaching the size of a small adult, they will require a size 3 blade, generally around the time of puberty.

In terms of endotracheal tube size, weight-based guidelines such as a length-based system (e.g., Broselow tape) can help providers select the appropriate-sized tube. Age-based formulas are also helpful in estimating the correct size (Table 5.2).

TABLE 5.2 SIZING FOR SELECT PEDIATRIC AIRWAY EQUIPMENT

Equipment	Guidelines for Selecting Appropriate Size
Nasopharyngeal airway	Rule of T's: Measure from tip of nose to tragus of ear
Oropharyngeal airway	Rule of M's: Measure from corner of mouth to angle of mandible
Laryngoscope blade size	Neonate (preterm): Size 0
	Neonate (term)–2 years old: Size 1 (switch to size 2 at age 2 years)
	2 years old–puberty: Size 2
	Puberty–adolescent: Size 3
	Large adolescent: Size 4
Endotracheal tube	3.5 + age in years/4 and 4+age in years/4
Cuffed (preferred)	
Uncuffed	

In general, it is best practice to also have available the endotracheal tubes that are one half-size above and below the estimated size. The provider should obtain the stylet and syringe for cuff inflation and check the cuff to ensure it appropriately inflates and deflates.

Bag Mask Ventilation

Bag mask ventilation can be provided with either a self-inflating bag or a flow-inflating bag. Self-inflating bags have a one-way valve, and providers must remember that spontaneously breathing infants and young children may not have the inspiratory force to open the one-way valve in these devices. If using a self-inflating bag, positive pressure breaths must be applied (synchronized to the patient's breaths when possible) to facilitate oxygen delivery. Alternatively, flow-inflating bags such as Mapleson and Jackson–Rees bags do not have a one-way valve and can be used to provide increased fraction of inspired oxygen (FiO_2) without delivery of assisted breaths or to provide ventilatory support in patients with absent or inadequate respiratory effort.

Effective BMV requires an adequate seal with the mask, a patent airway, and squeezing the bag to deliver breaths. In pediatric patients, choosing the appropriately sized mask in key to effective BMV. The mask should cover the nares and mouth without covering the orbital region or extending beyond the lower border of the mandible to avoid leak or injury to anatomic structures. If a child is between sizes, choosing the smaller size is preferred to minimize air leak. Providers also need to be aware of their hand and finger positioning to avoid inadvertently occluding the airway. The first and second digits can be used to make a "C" to provide gentle downward pressure on the mask over the nose and mouth, with the third through fifth digits placed under the lower border of the mandible, avoiding the soft tissues, to elevate the face into the mask and open the airway (the C–E technique). Alternatively, the thumb(s) can be used to provide the gentle downward pressure to achieve mask seal; this is called the thenar approach (Figure 5.4). If providers have difficulty achieving an effective seal with a one-handed technique, they should immediately switch to a two-handed mask seal and recruit a second person to squeeze the bag. Two-person BMV has been shown to be more effective than single-person efforts.

In squeezing the bag to provide assisted ventilation, it is important to remember that children have smaller tidal volumes than adults. Whether BVM is being performed as the primary procedure for transient respiratory support or in the context of endotracheal intubation, delivering effective but safe breaths is key. Many pediatric bags are equipped with pop-off valves designed to limit maximal pressure to a preset limit (often 35–40 cm H_2O) (see Figure 5.3). This valve can be opened to create a maximal allowable pressure (preferred in most patients to avoid barotrauma or overventilation) or closed so there is no limit to the pressure that can be delivered (may be necessary in patients with poor lung compliance or high airway resistance).

Endotracheal Intubation Technique

Preparing for Intubation

Maximizing preoxygenation and utilizing apneic oxygenation can help avoid or limit desaturation in pediatric patients undergoing intubation. Preoxygenation in children in the

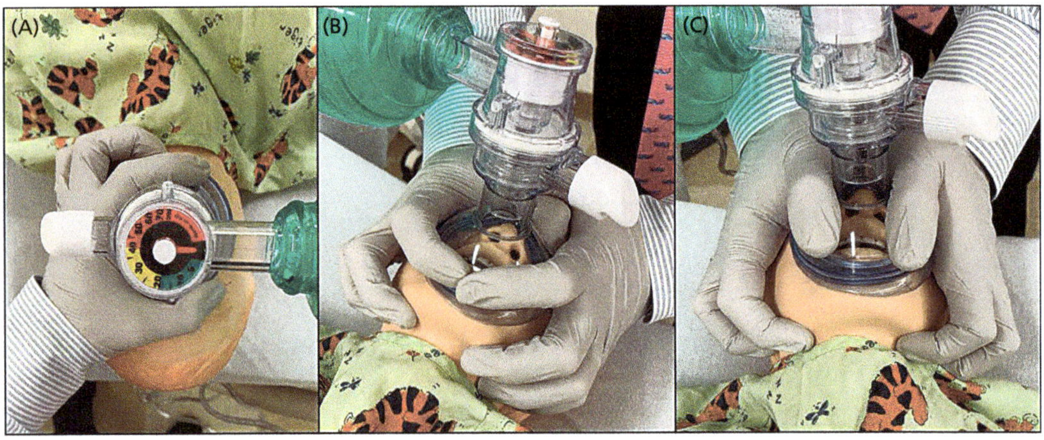

FIGURE 5.4 Hand positioning for BMV. Hand position to achieve mask seal can include a one- or two-handed "E–C" technique (A and B) or use of the thenar technique (C), which may achieve better ventilation, particularly over longer periods of time.

ED is traditionally performed using a non-rebreather mask, which can be supplemented with a nasal cannula. The nasal cannula may be preferred in infants who are preferential nasal breathers or may supplement the FiO_2 when used in conjunction with a non-rebreather mask. Either a self-inflating or a flow-inflating bag can be used to increase the delivered FiO_2 as long as providers remember that spontaneously breathing infants and young children may not have the inspiratory force to open the one-way valve in self-inflating devices and positive pressure breaths must be applied for oxygen delivery. Although flush rate oxygen delivery is effective in improving preoxygenation in adults, it is not clear if increasing flow beyond 15 liters per minute (LPM) is beneficial in younger pediatric patients given that the minute ventilation in an infant or child is a fraction of that of an adult and the proportion of room air entrained in these patients is likely very low.

Apneic oxygenation is well suited for pediatric airway management given the shorter safe apnea time. Although only limited data exist to support the use of apneic oxygenation for pediatric patients in the ED, many centers are now using it routinely. Importantly, it is unclear what flow rates would provide optimal physiological benefit without increased risk, such as distending the esophagus or filling the gastrum with air. Three currently proposed recommendations in pediatric emergency medicine are (1) 1 or 2 LPM per year of age (e.g., 2 LPM for a 1-year-old and 10 LPM for a 5-year-old); (2) 2 L/min for patients younger than age 3 years, 4 L/min for those aged 3–8 years, and 6 L/min for those older than age 8 years; or (3) 5 LPM for infants and children and 15 LPM for adolescents. Each of these approaches is deemed to be safe and likely beneficial, although further data are required to better understand optimal approaches. Anesthesia-based protocols have described flow rates of 1 L/kg/min but with a maximum of 15 LPM to maximize oxygen delivery in the youngest infants who desaturate more rapidly. Importantly, assessment and preparation for intubation (including fasting) are different in elective surgery than in pediatric emergency medicine.

Positioning is also important. As mentioned previously, aligning the external auditory meatus with the sternal notch will help avoid flexion of the airway and facilitate glottic visualization.

Rapid Sequence Intubation

Rapid sequence intubation (RSI) is the mainstay of pediatric emergent airway management. It involves the near simultaneous administration of a sedative and neuromuscular blockade. RSI provides optimum intubating conditions and results in higher intubation success rates than using sedation alone. Modifications for use in pediatric patients are addressed here.

"True" or "pure" RSI avoids positive pressure breaths after medication delivery to minimize insufflation of air into the stomach, which might increase the risk of regurgitation and aspiration. As previously reviewed, children are apt to desaturations during intubation, even with adequate pre- and apneic oxygenation; therefore, slow, gentle positive pressure ventilation after medication administration is commonly used to maintain or restore oxygenation. This approach is referred to as "modified" or "controlled" RSI and has been demonstrated to be safe in the operating room setting, as well as anecdotally through common practice in pediatric emergency medicine. Many pediatric patients will also require mask ventilation if success is not achieved on the first pass. If a nasal cannula is utilized for apneic oxygenation, this may impede an adequate mask seal. If so, the nasal cannula should be immediately removed because effective oxygenation through mask ventilation takes precedence over continued passive delivery of oxygen by nasal cannula in the apneic pediatric patient.

Weight-based dosing for sedative agents and neuromuscular blocking agents (NMBAs) is summarized in Table 5.3. Etomidate, ketamine, propofol, opioids such as fentanyl, and benzodiazepines such as midazolam are all sedative options for pediatric intubations. Based on the pharmacology and effects of these drugs, some may be more or less appropriate in given populations.

There is often a temptation to intubate pediatric patients without using NMBAs. This temptation may arise from the practice of doing so in the delivery room for depressed newborns who do not have vascular access, as well as a reluctance to relinquish spontaneous respirations based on concern for inability to successfully secure the airway in this less familiar patient population. However, data suggest that intubation success rates are higher when intubation is performed with an NMBA. In general, NMBAs should be used in emergent pediatric airway management. Situations to consider avoiding NMBAs include cases in which there exists difficulty with preintubation BMV or if there are concerning predictors of airway difficulty. Non-depolarizing muscle relaxants such as rocuronium and depolarizing agents such as succinylcholine may both be used in pediatric patients. When using higher dose rocuronium (1.2 mg/kg), onset time is essentially equivalent. The duration of action of succinylcholine is shorter than that of non-depolarizing agents, so it is sometimes used when concerns exist for a difficult airway; however, the introduction of suggammadex has made reversal of non-depolarizing agents possible as well. Some providers avoid succinylcholine based on the risk of hyperkalemia when used in patients with undiagnosed myopathy, which can be difficult to appreciate in young infants.

Controversy exists regarding the use of atropine as a premedication for pediatric patients. Bradycardia is relatively common during intubation; however, this tends to most commonly result from associated hypoxemia. The premise

TABLE 5.3 MEDICATION DOSING GUIDELINES FOR PEDIATRIC INTUBATION

Medication	Weight-Based Dosing (IV Administration)
Premedication	
Atropine	0.02 mg/kg; no minimum dose
Sedatives	
Etomidate	0.3 mg/kg
Fentanyl	1–2 μg/kg
Ketamine	1.5–2 mg/kg
Midazolam	0.3–0.4 mg/kg
Propofol	1–2 mg/kg
Neuromuscular blocking agents	
Succinylcholine	1–2 mg/kg
Rocuronium	1–1.2 mg/kg
Sugammadex	16 mg/kg
Non-depolarizing agent (. . . "onium") reversal	

IV, intravenous.

for atropine use as a premedication is to attenuate the high vagal tone common in young infants that can be triggered by the placement of the laryngoscope in the hypopharynx. Atropine is not predicted to prevent hypoxia-induced bradycardia, and the data regarding the efficacy of atropine are conflicting. PALS guidelines do not recommend routine use of atropine but call for its use as a premedication in circumstances in which there may be a higher risk of bradycardia, such as in the youngest patients (<6–12 months of age), in whom vagal-mediated bradycardia is most likely to occur.

Finally, limiting lengths of laryngoscopic attempts may be valuable. Although common practice is to continue attempts until oxygen saturation decreases below some predetermined level (often 90–92%), it has been suggested that limiting attempts by time (e.g., 30–45 seconds) may reduce the frequency of hypoxia because longer attempts may not consistently lead to improved success rates.

Videolaryngoscopy

Use of videolaryngoscopy (VL) for endotracheal intubation is increasing in pediatrics, either as a primary modality or as a rescue device. A number of the currently available videolaryngoscopes are designed for use in children, including some with a full complement of pediatric blade sizes ranging from neonatal through adolescent/adult. Much of the currently available data in children have shown that VL improves glottic visualization, although there are mixed data regarding the impact on first pass success: Some data have shown improvement in pediatric intubation performance in select age groups or with select devices, although time to success may be longer when using VL. Possible explanations for why improved view does not consistently translate to improved success include the following: (1) The longer time to intubation with VL is more significant in pediatric patients with rapid time to desaturation, (2) bulkier blades and handles result in difficulty manipulating the endotracheal tube, (3) directing pediatric-sized endotracheal tubes with malleable stylets around the tongue and into the glottis under indirect visualization can be challenging, and (4) the infrequency in performing intubation in any given pediatric age group with any device makes it more difficult to achieve and maintain procedural competence.

In addition to potential procedural benefit, VL offers other advantages. By providing a shared view of the airway anatomy and procedural progress, other clinicians can offer real-time guidance to the primary laryngoscopist. Videolaryngoscopy allows attempts to be recorded, making it a valuable tool for quality assurance and procedural teaching.

The three most commonly utilized VL devices with blade sizes that encompass all pediatric ages are briefly reviewed here. Given nuances with the use of each device, it is recommended that providers aim for comfort with one or two devices for use with children rather than attempt to master all available devices.

- C-MAC: The C-MAC laryngoscope allows either direct laryngoscopy or VL using the same device. This allows for the primary laryngoscopist to perform direct laryngoscopy or VL while a second clinician can provide guidance based on the shared screen view. The ability to look directly can limit inadvertent lip/oral trauma and can be valuable if blood or secretions obscure the video camera lens, preventing indirect viewing. The C-MAC offers a range of both Miller and Macintosh blades from size 0 to size 4. A hyperangulated "D" blade for indirect laryngoscopy only is also available in a single pediatric and adult size. When using hyperangulated blades, deliberately backing out to provide a broad, "bird's-eye" view facilitates endotracheal tube passage.
- Airtraq: The Airtraq is a single-use laryngoscope with an integrated rubber eyepiece, as well as the option to use it with a Wi-Fi camera hood. It has a guide channel to direct the endotracheal tube during insertion without direct visualization. To facilitate tube passage through the channel, the endotracheal tube should be well lubricated. The infant size 0 device can be used with size 2.5–3.5 endotracheal tubes, and the pediatric size 1 device accommodates size 3.5–5.5 endotracheal tubes. The Airtraq is designed to be inserted in the midline and requires sufficient space within the mouth and larynx to accommodate the device, usually at least 1 cm of mouth opening.

- Glidescope: The Glidescope consists of a reusable light source with disposable single-use laryngoscopy blades and an associated monitor. The Glidescope is designed to be inserted in the midline and does not require displacement of the tongue. It can only be used for indirect laryngoscopy. The tube is passed using a stylet designed to direct the tube anteriorly toward the glottic opening. There are some data indicating that for the Glidescope, providers may want to use a size smaller than that suggested by a pediatric patient's weight. As with other hyperangulated blades, backing out for a bird's-eye view may be helpful for tube passage.

Post-Intubation Management

When planning for intubation, ED providers should also consider the immediate post-intubation period. The initial and crucial step is confirmation of the appropriate placement of the endotracheal tube. Placement of the tube within the tracheobronchial tree is definitively made by documenting the presence of end-tidal CO_2; other supporting signs include mist in the tube, chest rise, and breath sounds. A chest X-ray should be obtained as soon as possible because misplacement of the endotracheal tube within the tracheobronchial tree, either too high in the trachea or within the mainstem bronchi, is common in pediatric patients, occurring in more than one-third of intubations. In addition, flexion or extension of the head in an intubated child can displace the endotracheal tube by 1 or 2 cm, which can easily result in mainstem intubation or unintentional extubation. Therefore, care should be taken to avoid head movement, even in a child in whom the endotracheal tube is well secured.

Providers should also plan to have a ventilator available as well as post-intubation sedation, which can be provided in the short term with boluses or infusions of opioids and benzodiazepines or with a propofol infusion. Careful attention must be paid to choosing age-appropriate respiratory rates and tidal volumes when programming the ventilator (see Chapter 6). Pulse oximetry, end-tidal CO_2 monitoring, and short-term measurement of blood gases should be employed to assess the adequacy of ventilation and oxygenation.

DIFFICULT AIRWAY: IDENTIFICATION AND MANAGEMENT

Definition

Although the definition of the difficult airway is not standardized in the literature, the American Society of Anesthesia (ASA) defines a difficult airway as the clinical situation in which there is difficulty with face mask ventilation of the upper airway, difficulty with tracheal intubation, or both. Difficulty with supraglottic device ventilation is also included in some definitions. Difficulty can arise from any combination of patient factors, the clinical setting, and skills of the practitioner attempting to secure the airway. Such difficulties have been shown to be common in pediatric patients, specifically those aged 1 year or younger, and can be devastating. It is also important to remember that in addition to anatomic difficulties, airway management in some patients may be physiologically challenging as well.

Predicting Difficult Airways in Pediatric Patients

Providers must take into account a number of unique considerations when confronted with difficult pediatric airways. As described previously, younger children have a short safe apnea period prior to the development of hypoxemia. Second, traditional tools used to assess the adult airway may be less applicable in pediatric patients. Predictors of difficult laryngoscopy in adults, such as the Mallampati tests and anthropomorphic measures (e.g., hyomental and thyromental distances), are poorly characterized for pediatric patients. Studies have shown that difficulty intubating is *unanticipated* in approximately 20% of pediatric intubations.

A number of anatomical abnormalities have been identified that can make airway management difficult in children. Providers should anticipate potential challenges with BMV and/or intubation in pediatric patients with the following:

- Macroglossia: A proportionately large tongue can obstruct the airway, impeding mask ventilation and preventing an adequate view of the glottic opening. This can be the result of a congenital defect (e.g., trisomy 21) or can be acquired secondary to trauma or an allergic response.

- Cervical spine abnormalities: Conditions that cause either instability or decreased mobility of the cervical spine can contribute to challenging laryngoscopy. Instability can be congenital (e.g., trisomy 21) or the result of an acute injury. Patients with possible cervical spine injury require in-line stabilization with the head and neck in a neutral position during attempted intubation, limiting the opportunity for optimizing alignment of the oropharyngeal, hypopharygeal, and laryngeal axes and achieving adequate visualization of the larynx.
- Micrognathia: Micrognathia describes an undersized mandible, which leaves little room for tongue displacement out of the oral cavity into the mandibular fossa. This can impede mask ventilation and impair the ability to obtain adequate visualization of the glottic inlet with direct laryngoscopy.
- Cleft palate: Patients with cleft palate are at risk for obstruction, and the cleft can hamper movement of the laryngoscope blade. Providers should also be aware that more than 25% of patients with cleft palate have congenital heart disease, which may have implications for their hemodynamic response to sedation and intubation.
- Supraglottic, infraglottic, or subglottic airway obstruction: Both congenital conditions resulting in airway masses (e.g., vascular and lymphatic malformations) and acutely acquired conditions causing inflammation (epiglottitis, inhalational injury, and angioedema) can compromise the perilaryngeal airway. External soft tissue pathologies, such as tumors and abscesses, can also contribute to obstruction. The result is compromise in mask ventilation, laryngoscopy, tube passage, or all three.

Approaches to the Difficult Airway

For anticipated difficult intubations in pediatrics, it is essential to plan ahead, have all equipment available, and recruit appropriate airway experts (e.g., an anesthesiologist and/or otorhinolaryngologist). Optimization of intubating conditions by ensuring adequate preoxygenation and apneic oxygenation is also critical.

Depending on the reason(s) for anticipated difficulty, certain strategies may be more or less appropriate in children. The previously described VL devices may be useful in certain pediatric patients with difficult airways. For patients with micrognathia, direct laryngoscopy with a curved Macintosh blade may be difficult because it requires compressing the tongue into a small mandibular space in order to visualize the laryngeal structures. Experience from the anesthesia literature suggests that using indirect laryngoscopy may be favorable in these patients. Hyperangulated videolaryngoscope blades are also helpful in providing a view of the glottic structures with the least amount of cervical manipulation (e.g., in trauma patients) and in improving the laryngoscopic view in patients with Cormack and Lehane grade ≥3 views by direct laryngoscopy.

The bougie is commonly used in adults to help facilitate intubation if either visualization or tube passage is difficult, and it is also an effective tool to increase first pass success when used as a primary intubation device. Although pediatric bougies exist, experience in pediatric intubations is poorly characterized. Questions have been raised regarded equivalent benefit in children because tactile stimulation (i.e., "clicks") received when the angled tip strikes the tracheal rings may be less pronounced in less mature airways. In addition, concerns have been raised regarding potential injury to glottic structures or the tracheal bronchial tree. Use of bougies may at some point match the success and safety witnessed in the adult population; however, limited data and experience to date have precluded more widespread use.

When managing a potential anatomically difficult pediatric airway, providers should consider using induction agents that allow for preservation of spontaneous respiration. This can be achieved with careful titration of propofol or ketamine without the use of neuromuscular blockade. When possible, this technique is easier to perform in the operating room with inhaled volatile anesthetics. Airway management in the operating room also allows for additional airway management strategies, including fiberoptic intubation, either in an awake patient or through a laryngeal airway, using pediatric-sized equipment that may not be available in the ED setting.

RESCUE DEVICES

Of greatest concern is the "can't intubate can't ventilate" or "can't intubate can't oxygenate" scenario, in which a patient cannot be effectively ventilated or oxygenated by face mask and tracheal intubation is unsuccessful. For example, in patients with congenital or traumatic craniofacial abnormalities, it may be both difficult to achieve an adequate seal for BMV with a face mask and difficult to perform successful intubation. Providers should ensure that all appropriate steps have been taken to maximize potential success with BMV via a face mask, including head extension, jaw thrust, assistance with mask seal through two-operator mask ventilation, suctioning and trial of an oral and/or nasal airway. If such optimization maneuvers fail and the patient cannot be ventilated, the ASA protocols call for rescue devices to sustain effective assisted ventilation until the airway can be secured.

The most common of these rescue devices is the laryngeal airway. A range of sizes and manufacturers (LMA, Ambu, Air-Q, and I-gel) of laryngeal mask airways exist, permitting their use in newborns through adults. The packaging and/or device display information on patient size and required air volume for cuff inflation so providers are not required to remember those details. Laryngeal airways are easy to place and use with low complication rates among pediatric patients. Second-generation devices that permit higher seal pressures and gastric decompression through esophageal lumens exist in a full range of pediatric sizes. Although additional supraglottic devices exist, limited data are available on their use in pediatric patients outside of the operating room setting. The laryngeal tube now comes in a range of sizes, including a size 0 that can be used in patients less than 5 kg.

In cases in which a patient cannot be successfully intubated and the use of a rescue device to maintain oxygenation and ventilation has failed, providers must resort to invasive techniques including needle or surgical cricothyroidotomy.

Physiologically Difficult Intubations

In addition to obtaining an adequate view of the glottic inlet and successfully passing an endotracheal tube through the vocal cords, intubation frequently involves sedation, paralysis, and/or mechanical ventilation. These interventions can result in physiologically challenging intubations, even in the absence of an anatomically difficult airway (see Table 5.3). Many patients intubated in the pediatric ED setting are critically ill from processes that pose unique difficulties in managing the physiologic changes of the peri-intubation period, including the following:

- Asthma: In patients with severe obstruction, air trapping results in increased intrathoracic pressure that decreases cardiac preload while simultaneously increasing afterload. Prior to induction, adequate access and fluid resuscitation should be a priority to maximize intravascular volume status and preload. In severe asthma, manipulation of the airway can increase airflow obstruction, making optimization of first pass success critically important. Ketamine is often the preferred induction agent due to its bronchodilatory effects. Propofol also produces bronchodilation, although less reliably than ketamine, and can worsen hypotension due to myocardial depression. Finally, severe airway obstruction leads to significantly prolonged expiration, which can result in breath stacking and increased lung volumes that can lead to barotrauma as well as compromised cardiac function. Patients must be ventilated at a low enough rate to accommodate this prolonged expiratory phase, with goal minute ventilation of less than 115 mL/kg.
- Congenital or acquired cardiac disease: During the peri-intubation period, patients with underlying cardiac disease are at risk for acute decompensated systolic heart failure, arrhythmias, hypotension, and, most concerning, cardiac arrest. Important considerations include pre-induction optimization, including having adequate vascular access and defibrillation equipment available. Depending on the level of concern regarding the cardiac function and the urgency of intubation, ED providers may consider moving the patient to a setting in which

extracorporeal membrane oxygenation is available. Induction agents should be carefully selected and titrated to minimize myocardial depression and vasodilation. Ketamine and fentanyl are both relied on to achieve this goal. ED providers should consider having rescue vasoactive drugs, such as epinephrine or dopamine, available. Patients presenting in pulmonary hypertensive crisis pose additional challenges requiring increased attention to minimizing pulmonary vascular resistance through ameliorating metabolic and respiratory acidosis; optimizing alveolar recruitment while minimizing mean airway pressure through controlled mask ventilation; maximizing oxygenation and using inhaled nitric oxide if available to achieve pulmonary vasodilation; and supporting right ventricular function through use of vasopressors, most commonly epinephrine or vasopressin.

- Diabetic ketoacidosis/severe metabolic acidosis: Metabolic acidosis, such as is seen with diabetic ketoacidosis or severe dehydration, poses unique peri-intubation considerations, including hypovolemia, electrolyte disturbances that predispose to arrhythmias, acidosis that compromises cardiac contractility, and the need to maintain compensatory respiratory alkalosis. Intubation may be required for airway protection if the patient is severely obtunded or unconscious, but it is avoided when possible given the risk of resulting increase in partial pressure of carbon dioxide (PCO_2) and the risk of worsening cerebral edema. Fluid resuscitation to restore circulating intravascular volume is a priority. During and after intubation, close attention should be paid to maintaining a similar PCO_2/end-tidal CO_2 to match the patients' preintubation compensatory hyperventilation.
- Sepsis/septic shock: Patients presenting with sepsis or septic shock may require endotracheal intubation to promote oxygenation and reduce the work of breathing in order to decrease metabolic demand. Such patients are often hemodynamically unstable, and ED providers should focus on providing appropriate fluid resuscitation and catecholamine support in fluid-refractory shock prior to or during intubation. Ketamine is the preferred sedative in this patient population given its hemodynamic stability and associated catecholamine release. The use of etomidate is controversial given the known inhibition on cortisol production, but without demonstrated difference in clinical outcomes. PALS and other guidelines currently suggest etomidate not be routinely used in patients with septic shock; however, many centers continue to use it based on predictable sedation with favorable hemodynamics.
- Trauma: Of particular concern are pediatric patients presenting with head trauma. The goal is to avoid worsening the cerebral insult during the intubation procedure. This entails minimizing noxious stimuli to avoid increasing intracranial pressure (ICP), maintaining cerebral perfusion pressure by ensuring normotension and normovolemia, avoiding hypoxemia during intubation attempts, and paying close attention to achieving a low-normal end-tidal CO_2. If there is clinical concern for herniation, hyperventilation is warranted. The head of the bed should be dropped from 30 degrees of elevation for as brief a time as possible. The use of lidocaine to blunt the sympathetic response to laryngoscopy is not supported as a premedication in pediatric patients. Etomidate is the favored sedative in head-injured patients in whom hypotension should be avoided. Prior concerns regarding the potential of ketamine to increase ICP have largely been dispelled, and it is also an appropriate sedative in normo- or hypotensive head-injured pediatric patients.

COMPLICATIONS

Potential complications of endotracheal intubation include dental or mucosal injury from the laryngoscope blade, vomiting with aspiration, hypoxia, barotrauma and air leak from positive pressure ventilation, hemodynamic instability from either the use of sedatives or the transition for negative to positive pressure ventilation, and, finally, arrest from either hypoxia or hemodynamic instability. The risk of complications is known to increase when intubations require additional attempts. Strategies to minimize complications include preintubation optimization with adequate fluid resuscitation and preoxygenation; maximizing first pass success by having appropriate equipment and personnel available and considering apneic oxygenation; and careful attention to post-intubation management, including prompt endotracheal tube placement confirmation, avoidance of head movement, and thoughtful titration of ventilator settings including age-appropriate respiratory rates and tidal volumes.

It is important to recognize that indirect-only VL devices pose additional increased risk of palate or airway injury if the intubator inserts the blade or the styletted endotracheal tube indirectly while looking at the screen or eyepiece. To minimize the risk, a four-step approach has been proposed: (1) Look in the mouth while inserting the laryngoscope and gently advance toward the base of the tongue, (2) look at the screen to optimize the position of the laryngoscope, (3) look back in the mouth while inserting the styletted endotracheal tube and advance as close to the tip of the laryngoscope as possible, and (4) look at the screen while guiding the endotracheal tube toward the glottic opening and into the trachea.

KEY POINTS

- Early and effective airway management is integral to the resuscitation of critically ill pediatric patients presenting for emergency care.
- Providers should adapt airway management approaches to address the anatomic and physiologic differences in pediatric patients.
- Modified RSI with the use of neuromuscular blockade with a cuffed endotracheal tube is generally recommended.
- Weight-, length-, and age-based guidelines can assist providers in selecting appropriate dosing and equipment.
- Given the growing availability of pediatric videolaryngoscopes, providers should consider the advantages and disadvantages of utilizing these new technologies.
- Emergency providers must assess for predictors of anatomically or physiologically difficult airways that may warrant a modified approach, including utilization of alternative personnel, equipment, or pharmacologic regimens.

PITFALLS

- Failing to position a patient properly makes airway management more difficult.
- Selecting inappropriately sized equipment may result in ineffective airway management, including both BMV and endotracheal intubation.
- Aggressive BMV or bag ventilation through an endotracheal tube can easily result in barotrauma and clinical deterioration.
- Relying on memory or formulas to choose equipment sizes or drug dosing may be challenging in the context of high-stress resuscitations, particularly involving critically ill pediatric patients.
- It is very common for the endotracheal tube to be inserted too deeply, resulting in an increased rate of complications such as atelectasis and hypoxemia.
- Head movement after successful intubation can result in mainstem intubation or unintentional extubation.
- Pediatric airway management skills may quickly atrophy given the relative infrequency to utilize them; therefore, providers should consider alternative strategies (e.g., procedural training in simulation or video review of intubations) to maintain exposure.

Further Reading

Eisenberg MA, Green-Hopkins I, Werner H, Nagler J. Comparison between direct and video-assisted laryngoscopy for intubations in a pediatric emergency department. *Acad Emerg Med.* 2016;23(8):870–877. doi:10.1111/acem.13015.

Fiadjoe JE, Nishisaki A, Jagannathan N, et al. Airway management complications in children with difficult tracheal intubation from the Pediatric Difficult Intubation (PeDI) registry: A prospective cohort analysis. *Lancet Respir Med.* 2016;4(1):37–48. doi:10.1016/S2213-2600(15)00508-1.

Mittiga MR, Rinderknecht AS, Kerrey BT. A modern and practical review of rapid-sequence intubation in pediatric emergencies. *Clin Pediatr Emerg Med.* 2015;16(3):172–185. doi:10.1016/J.CPEM.2015.08.001.

Pallin DJ, Dwyer RC, Walls RM, Brown CA. Techniques and trends, success rates, and adverse events in emergency department pediatric intubations: A report from the National Emergency Airway Registry. *Ann Emerg Med.* 2016;67(5):610–615e1. doi:10.1016/j.annemergmed.2015.12.006.

Silva L OJE, Cabrera D, Barrionuevo P, et al. Effectiveness of apneic oxygenation during intubation: A systematic review and meta-analysis. *Ann Emerg Med.* 2017;70(4):483–494.e11. doi:10.1016/j.annemergmed.2017.05.001.

6

Emergency Pediatric Noninvasive Ventilation and Invasive Mechanical Ventilation

GARRETT S. PACHECO

INTRODUCTION

Respiratory impairment is common in children and a primary reason for emergency department (ED) visits. Acute respiratory failure (ARF) is a frequent presentation to the ED. Typically, patients respond to simple supportive treatment, whether it is airway clearance therapy, oxygen therapy, or bronchodilators. However, a small subset of patients will require aggressive respiratory support to address their physiologic derangement. Noninvasive ventilation (NIV) strategies such as high-flow nasal oxygen (HFNO) and noninvasive positive pressure ventilation (NIPPV) are important interventions that may support a child in respiratory distress while avoiding the more invasive endotracheal intubation (ETI) procedure. It is also imperative that the emergency physician (EP) be capable of managing the mechanically ventilated pediatric patient. This chapter reviews clinical indications and settings for HFNO and NIPPV, and it discusses initiation and troubleshooting of invasive mechanical ventilation (IMV) for critically ill infants and children treated in the ED.

Comparison with Adult Physiology

Similar to ARF in adults, perturbations in airway resistance and pulmonary compliance are the primary contributors to ARF in children. Resistance is inversely proportional to the radius of the airway. Because young infants and small children have significantly smaller peripheral airways, any reduction in airway diameter can lead to four times higher airway resistance compared to that of adults. Furthermore, infants and small children have decreased functional residual capacity (FRC), increased basal oxygen consumption, and increased CO_2 production—all likely exacerbated by critical illness.

Children often manifest a prodrome of symptoms (e.g., tachypnea, agitation, retractions, head bobbing, and grunting) to prevent fatigue that leads to acute respiratory insufficiency/ARF. Pediatric patients will increase their respiratory rate (RR) to increase their minute ventilation (MV) and use their accessory muscles to increase their work of breathing before they experience ARF.

NONINVASIVE VENTILATION

Background

Noninvasive ventilation is a modality that includes HFNO and NIPPV strategies. NIPPV includes continuous positive airway pressure (CPAP) and bilevel positive airway pressure

(BiPAP). NIV significantly reduces intubation rates in pediatric patients with respiratory distress by improving gas exchange and decreasing the work of breathing. Successful NIV requires appropriate patient selection and a properly fitting interface.

High-Flow Nasal Oxygen

High-flow nasal oxygen is an effective therapy for pediatric patients with respiratory insufficiency and hypoxemia. HFNO devices deliver oxygen at rates that match or exceed patients' inspiratory flow rates (up to as high as 60 L/min in adults), resulting in higher concentration of oxygen [fraction of inspired oxygen (FiO_2)] due to limited entrainment of room air. These devices consist of an adjustable flow meter, an adjustable air–oxygen blender that can deliver an FiO_2 from 21% to 100%, a chamber for heating and humidification, a high-performance circuit, and an appropriately sized nasal cannula (neonatal, pediatric, and adult sizes are available). The flow should be adjusted based on patient age, but exact rates remain controversial. See Table 6.1 for an example flow rate guideline. The humidified air provides oxygen at optimal warmth (36°–37°C) and increases patient comfort. HFNO improves work of breathing and may also provide some positive end-expiratory pressure (PEEP), but this is variable. HFNO should remain in place for apneic oxygenation prior to intubation (see Chapter 5 on airway management). HFNO is also well tolerated by patients and has an excellent safety profile.

Noninvasive Positive Pressure Ventilation

Continuous Positive Airway Pressure

Continuous positive airway pressure provides a constant positive distending airway pressure during all phases of the respiratory cycle of a spontaneously breathing patient. CPAP can be administered through nasal masks, nasal prongs, face masks needing a tight seal to the patient's face to prevent air leaks, or the application of a helmet. The intention of CPAP is to improve the FRC, reduce the work of breathing, and improve oxygenation in patients with adequate respiratory drive, making it an ideal tool in patients with hypoxemic respiratory failure. Typical pressure is 5–10 cm H_2O.

Bilevel Positive Airway Pressure

Bilevel positive airway pressure, in contrast to CPAP, delivers pressures at two different levels. The inspiratory positive airway pressure (IPAP) and expiratory positive airway pressure (EPAP) can be synchronized to or delivered independently of spontaneous respiratory effort. The preset values are triggered by inspiratory effort or a preset backup mandatory RR. Effective ventilation will also result in improved oxygenation as the ventilation:perfusion ratio improves. The difference between IPAP and EPAP determines the tidal volume (Vt) generated. Multiple parameters are set with BiPAP: EPAP and IPAP (typically 5–10 and 8–15 cm H_2O, respectively), FiO_2, and backup ventilation rate for patients experiencing intermittent apnea or hypopnea. See Figure 6.1 for initial NIV settings. The smallest interface with the least air leak should be chosen to minimize dead space. BiPAP is the preferred modality with more significant hypoxemia or CO_2 retention because it delivers higher mean airway pressures while offloading inspiratory effort.

Both CPAP and BiPAP can be used with different interfaces, including nasal cannula, nasal mask, full face mask, or helmet. In neonates and infants, a nasal cannula (e.g., RAM Cannula) may be the best tolerated. It is

TABLE 6.1 EXAMPLE FLOW RATE FOR HIGH-FLOW NASAL OXYGEN[a]

Patient Weight (kg)	Starting Flow (L/min)	Maximum Flow (L/min)
<5	6	8
5–10	8	15
10–20	15–20	20
20–40	25–30	40
>40	25–30	40–60

[a]The nasal cannula will often determine the maximum flow rate as suggested by the manufacturer weight based formulas help determine maximum flow rate. Some recommend 2 L/kg/min for the first 10 kg and then 0.5 L/kg/min for each kg >10 kg.

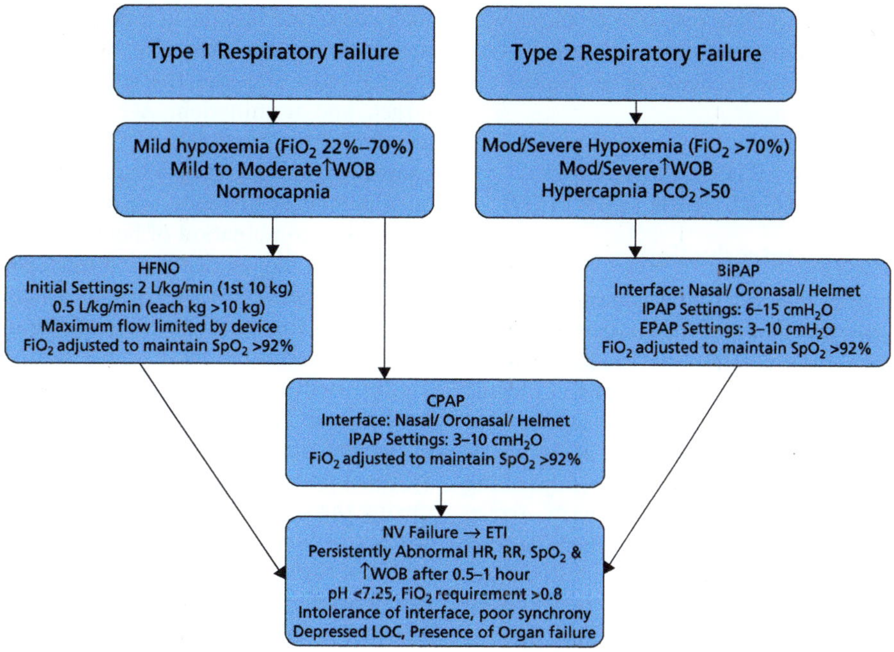

FIGURE 6.1 NIV indications and initial settings. WOB, work of breathing.

recommended that in the absence of contraindications, NIV is first-line management for pediatric respiratory distress unless in cardiorespiratory failure or other contraindication. Contraindications to the initiation of NIV are related to the absence of spontaneous respiration, compromise of airway patency, significantly depressed sensorium placing the patient at risk for regurgitation/aspiration, the inability to achieve a good interface fit, or ventilatory dyssynchrony. Most children, with appropriate coaching and provider patience during initiation, will tolerate NIV, although some require anxiolysis or sedation. Medications may facilitate NIV but should be used with caution, and patients should be vigilantly monitored (see Chapter 49). In general, respiratory support should be started low to allow the patient to acclimate and determine their tolerance to the interface, and it should be increased as tolerated.

Disposition

Most patients receiving NIV will require intensive care admission due to a tenuous respiratory status requiring frequent monitoring. Uncomplicated patients on HFNO may be managed on the hospital wards (depending on institutional protocols).

Complications

The most concerning complication of NIV is delayed intubation and failure to recognize clinical deterioration. Complications reported specifically with HFNO use are few and similar to complications reported for NIPPV. These include interface-related pressure injury, gastric insufflation leading to increased risk of abdominal distension with subsequent regurgitation and possible aspiration, air leak (e.g., pneumomediastinum, subcutaneous emphysema, and pneumothorax), eye irritation, nasal dryness/epistaxis, and inability to monitor capnography continuously.

Key Points

- NIV, including both HFNO and NIPPV, improves oxygenation, decreases work of breathing, and decreases the need for pediatric emergent intubation.
- HFNO is best applied to the patient with acute respiratory insufficiency, CPAP is indicated for hypoxemia, and BiPAP is preferred for significant hypoxemia and/or CO_2 retention.

Pitfalls

- Failure to recognize complications associated with NIV, specifically air leak.

- Failure to evaluate response to therapy within 1 hour, leading to delayed intubation and recognition of clinical deterioration.

PEDIATRIC INVASIVE MECHANICAL VENTILATION

Introduction

Knowledge of the underlying disease process as well as the trajectory of illness determine the indications for pediatric mechanical ventilation. Patients who will benefit from ETI include those with refractory respiratory failure that has not responded adequately to HFNO/NIV and those who have dynamic or impending airway obstruction, cardiopulmonary arrest, or significant disability placing them at risk for regurgitation/aspiration pneumonitis. Also, ETI should be performed for patient control to facilitate medical evaluation so that there is no delay in identifying a potentially dangerous condition or given the patient's expected clinical course. The care of the emergently ventilated pediatric patient requires understanding of respiratory mechanics and pathophysiology of cardiopulmonary disease. There is significant variability in daily practice of IMV due to a lack of evidence in this arena. Often, practice is driven by institutional expectations and those that provide definitive care in the pediatric intensive care unit.

Modes of Ventilation and Initial Settings

Three modes of standard ventilation in IMV are assist control (AC); synchronized intermittent mandatory ventilation (SIMV); and spontaneous ventilation, such as pressure support ventilation. During AC, all prescribed breaths are delivered in this volume-targeted mode during the given inspiratory time (Ti). The trigger can be the patient or the ventilator. This mode is commonly used in adult emergency medicine and has the advantages of full ventilator support for the patient with no spontaneous respiratory effort and the ability to measure mechanics. Termination, the variable that discontinues the breath given by the ventilator, occurs once the volume is achieved for the flow given over a specific time period when using AC. On the other hand, SIMV can have a pressure- or volume-targeted setting. The patient or the ventilator can initiate each supported breath. In a pressure mode, the breath terminates after a Ti. With each mode, the EP must consider the appropriate trigger, target, and termination. AC or SIMV modes of mechanical ventilation can be pressure-controlled, volume-controlled (occasionally the terminology of pressure- or volume-limited is used), or a combination of both.

There is no evidence that one particular mode is superior for applying to different disease states. Pressure control ventilation (PCV) and volume control ventilation (VCV) are two modes used primarily in pediatric emergency medicine. PCV is often selected for use in newborns and small infants. It delivers each breath at the same peak inspiratory pressure (PIP) during the set Ti, and it has a decelerating flow pattern. Advantages include improved comfort with the variable flow rates/pattern. With PCV, the dependent variable is the Vt that is determined by the independent variable PIP. PCV has a rectangular pressure curve compared with the exponential or "shark fin" pressure curve of VCV (Figure 6.2).

PCV settings that the provider must enter include an age-appropriate RR and an appropriate Ti (length of the inspiratory phase of the breathing cycle) for the patient's age and disease process (Table 6.2). PCV also requires an applied PEEP. As mentioned previously, the PIP is the maximum pressure delivered during inspiration, and it is the independent variable that determines the dependent Vt variable. Specifically, the driving pressure (ΔP = PIP − PEEP) is adjusted to achieve a Vt of 5–8 mL/kg ideal body weight (IBW), usually with a limited PIP of 30 mmHg to avoid ventilator-induced lung injury (VILI) and barotrauma. Recommendations for patients with severe respiratory failure and compromised respiratory compliance are Vts of 3–6 mL/kg IBW. This open strategy of ventilation has been found to be the only factor to reduce mortality in mechanically ventilated patients.

The provider should also enter a prescribed PEEP for IMV. Applied PEEP helps prevent alveolar collapse and atelectasis by maintaining pressure during expiration. Alveolar trauma is reduced when atelectasis is avoided. PEEP improves oxygenation by decreasing the shunt fraction and increasing FRC. PEEP can be initially set at 5–8 cm H_2O and adjusted as needed to improve mean airway pressure (P_{AW}) considering the patient's FiO_2 requirement. The

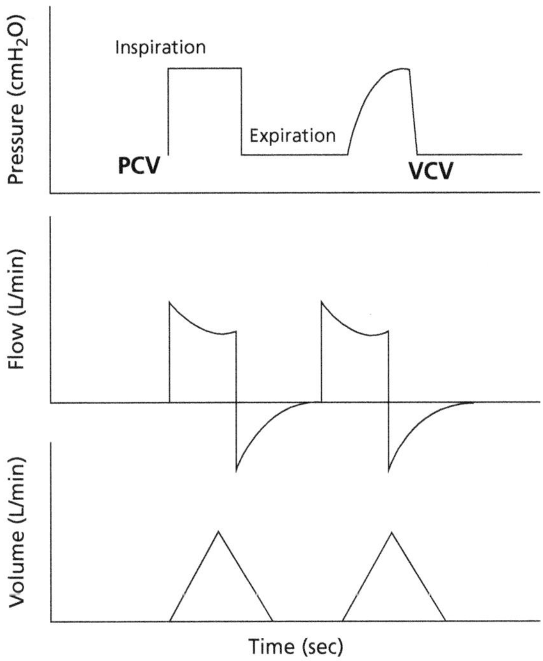

FIGURE 6.2 Ventilator waveforms.

Pediatric Acute Lung Injury and Consensus Conference recommends "moderately" elevated levels of PEEP, defined as 10–15 cm H_2O, for patients with severe pediatric acute respiratory distress syndrome (PARDS), titrated to observed oxygenation and hemodynamic response. There is no ARDSNET table equivalent in pediatric critical care to guide the EP to assign PEEP based on an FiO_2 requirement. Generally, the EP at the bedside can obtain a chest radiograph for the hypoxemic patient requiring increased FiO_2. If the radiograph demonstrates significant opacification, PEEP will likely need to be increased. High levels of PEEP (e.g., 15 cm H_2O) may be needed to maintain P_{AW}, but close consultation with the pediatric intensivist is warranted if this or more support is required by the patient. With high levels of PEEP, the EP should be cognizant of cardiopulmonary interactions and risk of hemodynamic compromise. The FiO_2 should be started at 1.0 and weaned immediately to avoid dysoxia and its associated complications. Ideally, the arterial partial pressure of oxygen should be between 60 and 80 mmHg and achieve a peripheral capillary oxygen saturation (SpO_2) >92%. In PARDS or significant hypoxemia, this may be lowered to an acceptable SpO_2 >88%.

VCV is often used for the older child. AC is included within the VCV strategies. Dual or hybrid modes exist, such as adaptive pressure ventilation, that deliver pressure-cycled breaths to the patient to achieve a prescribed Vt. This mode combines features of both PCV and VCV. It has various names on different ventilator

TABLE 6.2 INITIAL MECHANICAL VENTILATION SETTINGS

Initial Ventilator Settings	Neonate	Infant/Child	Adolescent
Respiratory rate[a]	30–40	20–35	16–20
Inspiratory time (sec)[b]	0.3–0.5	0.5–0.9	0.9–1.5

[a]The patient's minute ventilation prior to intubation should be matched, unless they have significant obstructive lung disease. In this scenario, a decreased respiratory rate would be preferred to allow for adequate exhalation.
[b]Reference starting inspiratory time. Changes may be needed to adjust desired oxygenation and ventilation.

types, such as pressure-regulated volume control (PRVC), Volume Guarantee, and Volume Control Plus. For the remainder of this chapter, it is referred to as PRVC. The advantage of this strategy is that there is still the decelerating flow pattern characteristic of the pressure-limited mode paired with a defined Vt. The preset Vt will be delivered to the patient while obtaining the lowest possible peak airway pressure (PAP). The ventilator in PRVC calculates the plateau pressure (P_{PLAT}; discussed later) and, during the next few breaths, automatically adjusts the minimal inspiratory pressure required to obtain the desired Vt. If more Vt is achieved than the preset value, the ventilator will decrease the pressure with the next breath given. This dual mode allows dynamic breath-to-breath variability in patient pulmonary compliance, providing additional patient comfort.

PCV, VCV, and PRVC modes of ventilation are often paired with the SIMV breath type, the most common setting of ventilation used in pediatrics. Once the pediatric patient's sedation is lightened or their neuromuscular blockade (NMB) is cleared, children often overbreathe the ventilator. If the initial strategy was AC/VCV, each breath could potentially be fully supported by the ventilator. As mentioned previously, in AC, each breath preset or initiated by the patient will be delivered. This can lead to respiratory alkalosis, breath stacking, and patient–ventilator dyssynchrony. SIMV provides synchronized, fully supported breaths for the set RR but often is coupled with at least partially assisted breaths for every additional breath over and above the set RR. A pressure support (PS) is usually added to partially support the breaths not fully synchronized over the applied PEEP, and this is typically set at 5–10 cm H_2O depending on the patient's respiratory effort (SIMV + PS). This PS can be adjusted to achieve a target Vt of 4–8 mL/kg of IBW. After initial settings are finalized, the patient should be assessed for ventilator synchrony, SpO_2, and continuous capnography ($ETCO_2$). An arterial/venous blood gas should be obtained, correlated with $ETCO_2$, and adjustments to the initial settings should be made if needed while the patient is in the EP's care.

Treatment

Addressing Hypercapnia

Variables that affect oxygenation and ventilation can be adjusted to achieve normoxia and normocapnia. A blood gas should be obtained within 20–30 minutes of initiating mechanical ventilation and should be completed if the patient is still in the ED at this time. By doing this, the patient will avoid prolonged periods of inadequate ventilation before transfer to their definitive care destination. Alveolar ventilation (MV − dead space ventilation) is the primary mark to regulate CO_2 clearance. A pediatric patient's $PaCO_2$ is directly proportional to their CO_2 production by the body, and it is inversely proportional to CO_2 clearance by alveolar ventilation.

Hypercapnia (i.e., increases in partial pressure of CO_2) can be addressed by either increasing the patient's RR or augmenting their Vt. If the patient is being ventilated with PCV, adjustments that can be made include increasing the RR or the ΔP. In PRVC or AC, hypercapnia can be treated by increasing the RR, or the Vt can be increased. Preferably, adjustments should be made in the RR because increases in Vt may compromise the lung protection strategy. Whenever adjustments are made in the RR, it is imperative that the Ti is also adjusted, if necessary, to ensure acceptable pulmonary mechanics. Both RR and Ti are closely correlated and cannot be judged independent from each other.

When addressing hypercapnia, if the Ti is not changed after adjusting the RR, the patient is at risk for developing dynamic hyperinflation or intrinsic/auto-PEEP. Failure to recognize this adjustment will be clinically apparent by air leak or hypotension and potential cardiac arrest. A typical respiratory cycle has an inspiratory:expiratory (I:E) ratio of 1:2 (1 second for inspiration and 2 seconds for expiration, which resembles physiologic breathing) or 1:3. This may need to be adjusted for pediatric patients with obstructive lung physiology, which would demand a prolonged expiration time (e.g., 1:4 or greater). For example, a child with a set RR of 22 breaths per minute has a respiratory cycle of 2.7 seconds (60 seconds ÷ 22 breaths per minute = 2.7 seconds). To achieve an I:E ratio of 1:2, the patient's Ti should be 0.9 seconds. The maximum Ti at this set ventilator rate is 1.3 seconds (2.7 seconds ÷ 2 = 1.3 seconds). If not set correctly, the EP may unintentionally initiate inverse ratio ventilation. For example, if the same patient has hypercapnia treated with an increase in RR to 35 breaths per minute, they would have a respiratory cycle of 1.7 seconds and a maximum Ti of 0.9 seconds. If there were no adjustment in the Ti of 0.9 seconds, the I:E ratio is 1:1, which will not allow adequate time for exhalation. With inadequate time for exhalation, there is risk for dynamic hyperinflation, which may lead to air leak disease such as pneumothorax or increased end-expiratory lung volume causing increased intrathoracic pressure leading to preload reduction with subsequent risk for hemodynamic collapse. Ensuring the flow curve returns to baseline ensures no dynamic hyperinflation and adequate time for exhalation. This can also be evaluated by performing an expiratory hold maneuver.

Although treatments for hypercapnia have been discussed previously, there are circumstances in which hypercapnia is actually desired. Permissive hypercapnia in critically ill pediatric patients targets a mild acidosis (e.g., pH 7.25–7.33) to allow ventilated patients to have lower P_{PLAT} (the pressure applied to the small airways and alveoli) and Vt in an attempt to reduce VILI. This strategy should be used with caution and is contraindicated in patients with increased intracranial pressure, sickle cell disease, myocardial dysfunction, and pulmonary hypertension. Furthermore, moderate hypercapnia can increase cardiac output and regional systemic blood flow, but at the expenditure of increased cardiac metabolism and debilitated stroke volume.

Addressing Hypoxemia

Providing adequate PEEP to maintain FRC, utilizing recruitment maneuvers to improve alveolar patency ultimately improving $P_{AW,}$ and increasing FiO_2 treat the ventilated hypoxemic patient. Ti directly affects P_{AW}, which has a powerful influence on oxygenation. A longer Ti can be used cautiously to aid in improving oxygenation if there is no significant obstructive lung disease and adequate time for exhalation is ensured.

A safe strategy for pediatric patients to boost their oxygen saturation is to increase their FiO_2. This is not the case, however, for patients with decreased pulmonary vascular resistance, which leads to a disproportionate amount of pulmonary blood flow in patients with a large ventricular septal defect, or in some patients with unrestricted single-ventricle cardiac physiology. These patients develop pulmonary overcirculation and decreased systemic cardiac output. Because excessive FiO_2 may lead to dysoxia and denitrogenation atelectasis, the minimum necessary FiO_2 should be selected to avoid these complications.

Sedation Options for the Mechanically Ventilated Child

The mechanically ventilated child will often need sedation and analgesia to tolerate this treatment. Typically, children do not receive postintubation sedation in an adequate time frame. The strategy of addressing and optimizing analgesia and then adding a sedative agent is encouraged. Patients typically receive an induction agent and often an NMB agent for tracheal intubation. These are usually medications that metabolize quickly. Soon after intubation, a child will benefit from a bolus of fentanyl or morphine if not already given during drug-assisted intubation. Once adequate analgesia is established, add a sedative for hypnosis, amnesia, and anxiolysis. Typically, fentanyl is given continuously at an initial dose of 1 μg/kg/hr, with incremental infusion changes of 0.5 μg/kg/hr. The sedative commonly selected is midazolam, which can be given continuously 0.05–0.1 mg/kg/hr or by intermittent doses depending on sedation goals. A sedation assessment tool is recommended (e.g., the State Behavioral Scale) when providing analgesia and sedation to the ventilated pediatric patient. Dexmedetomidine is another option, but its use is limited in the initial resuscitation of the ventilated pediatric patient in the ED because it only recently became generic, it often requires a loading infusion, and it does not provide analgesia. Ketamine infusion may be effective for patients with obstructive lung disease (e.g., asthma). This agent provides sedation, analgesia, amnesia, and bronchodilation. It can be given as a bolus of 1–2 mg/kg, followed by an infusion of 0.25–1 mg/kg/hr.

Prolonged use of lorazepam, another option for sedation, is discouraged due to the propylene glycol diluent used in parenteral formulations. Propylene glycol toxicity places the patient at risk for cardiac dysrhythmias, significant lactic acidosis, seizure, and multiorgan system failure. Prolonged propofol use is also discouraged in children. Although a rare event, propofol infusion syndrome (severe metabolic acidosis, multiorgan failure, and potential death) occurs more commonly in children than adults. Prolonged propofol use may also lead to hypertriglyceridemia and pancreatitis.

Propofol infusion syndrome has been reported as early as 12 hours after initiation, but it tends to occur at 48 or more hours at doses of >4 mg/kg/hr. Given the severity of this complication, many pediatric intensive care units will avoid its continued use for sedation of the intubated patient.

Prolonged paralysis with an NMB agent should not typically be started in the ED. Potential myopathy and induced paresis may occur with prolonged use of NMB. Pediatric patients who have PARDS and severe hypoxemia, ventilator dyssynchrony despite appropriate ventilatory management, and appropriate pharmacologic analgesia and sedation are a small targeted group that may benefit from NMB therapy when mechanically ventilated.

Troubleshooting Ventilator Alarms

When the ventilator alarm triggers, the EP should treat this warning as if it is announcing a code event. Increased PAP in VCV modes or reduced Vt alarm triggers in PCV modes should prompt the use of an algorithmic approach to troubleshoot the patient's respiratory mechanics. Settings should be adjusted to ensure that Vt is given while identifying the culprit for the alarm. The provider should consider and serially discard all etiologies of increased airway resistance versus decreased pulmonary compliance and keep in mind which patient pathology may be contributing to the increased PAP alarm (Table 6.3).

With worsening respiratory compliance, it should be quickly determined whether the patient is having issues with the airway or if the problem is with the lungs (alveoli). The PAP represents the amount of positive pressure required to deliver a breath through the endotracheal tube (ETT), move through the large conducting airways to get through the bronchioles, and ultimately arrive at the alveoli. The PAP includes the alveolar P_{PLAT}, which represents static pulmonary compliance (Figure 6.3). As the P_{PLAT} increases, pulmonary compliance decreases. This can be readily measured in VCV modes by performing an inspiratory hold maneuver that allows the EP to identify the pressure during a period of no airflow. An inspiratory hold maneuver can be performed in pressure modes, however, care must be taken when interpreting the measured pressure. The patient may need to be paralyzed to get the plateau pressure. Peak inspiratory pressure does not necessarily equal P_{PLAT} if resistance is high or the Ti is too short. The P_{PLAT} is helpful when deciding if the issue is in the large conducting airways or the lungs. When an inspiratory hold maneuver is performed in VCV, the difference between the PAP and

TABLE 6.3 TROUBLESHOOTING INCREASED PEAK AIRWAY PRESSURE

Etiology of Increased PAP	Treatment
Kinked or obstructed ETT	↑ Airway resistance. Reposition the child's head. Attempt to pass a suction catheter or bougie. Place a bite block. May need to ↑ sedation if patient is biting ETT.
Mucus plugging	↑ Airway resistance. Obtain an immediate CXR or perform POCUS. Attempt to suction tracheal tube and tracheal secretions. ACT with CPT or expectorants.
Asthma/bronchospasm	↑ Airway resistance. Administer bronchodilators and corticosteroids.
PARDS	↓ Pulmonary compliance. Appropriate Vt 3–6 mL/kg IBW and SpO_2 >88%.
Pneumonia	↓ Pulmonary compliance. Appropriate antibiotics. Treatment of parapneumonic effusion.
Atelectasis	↓ Pulmonary compliance. CPT.
Cardiogenic pulmonary edema	↓ Pulmonary compliance. Add inotropes, adjust PEEP, or give diuretics.
Mainstem bronchus intubation	↓ Pulmonary compliance. Pull the ETT back to appropriate depth.
Pneumothorax	↓ Pulmonary compliance. Decompress chest/finger thoracostomy/tube thoracostomy.

ACT, airway clearance therapy; CPT, chest physical therapy; CXR, chest X-ray; ETT, endotracheal tube; IBW, ideal body weight; PAP, positive airway pressure; PARDS, pediatric acute respiratory distress syndrome; PEEP, positive end expiratory pressure; POCUS, point-of-care-ultrasound; SpO_2, peripheral capillary oxygen saturation; Vt, tidal volume.

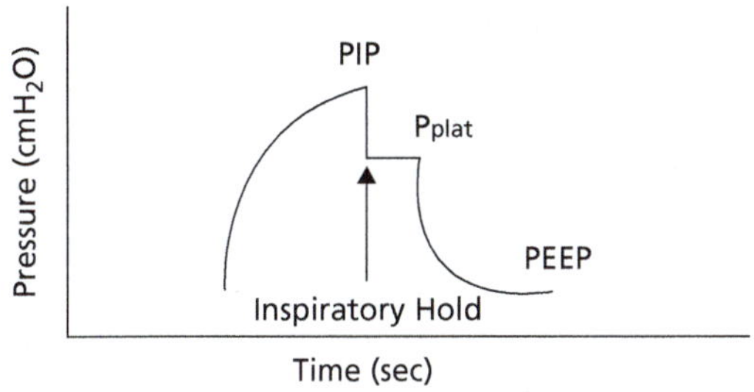

FIGURE 6.3 Inspiratory hold maneuver is performed during VCV to determine P_{PLAT}.

P_{PLAT} is normally <5 cm H_2O. If there is an increase in PAP without an increase in P_{PLAT}, there is increased airway resistance (>5 cm H_2O difference between PAP and P_{PLAT}). When the PAP is increased and there is an increase in P_{PLAT}, there is decreased pulmonary compliance (<5 cm H_2O difference between PAP and P_{PLAT}). Unfortunately, in PRVC and PCV, an inspiratory hold maneuver is difficult to interpret, making the distinction between airway resistance issues and pulmonary compliance troublesome. Both airway resistance and pulmonary compliance need to be considered and quickly eliminated as a cause of increased PAP.

Causes of increased airway resistance include mucus plugging, a narrow ETT, a kinked or obstructed tube, and bronchospasm. Once an airway resistance issue has been eliminated, the EP should test pulmonary compliance. This may be obvious based on the patient's clinical condition and reason for initial intubation. Causes of increased PAP from decreased lung compliance include mainstem bronchus intubation (a common etiology in pediatrics for increased PAP alarm), PARDS, cardiogenic pulmonary edema, atelectasis, pneumothorax, and pneumonia (Figure 6.4).

Approach to the Decompensating Ventilated Pediatric Patient

The decompensating ventilated pediatric patient should be assessed in a meticulous but rapid manner. Santanilla published an algorithmic approach that can be followed and modified to address the decompensating ventilated pediatric patient. The patient should immediately be disconnected from the ventilator, placed on 100% oxygen via BVM, and the DOPES mnemonic (discussed later) should be investigated. A rapid rush of air following disconnection of the ventilator with improvement in hemodynamics suggests the presence

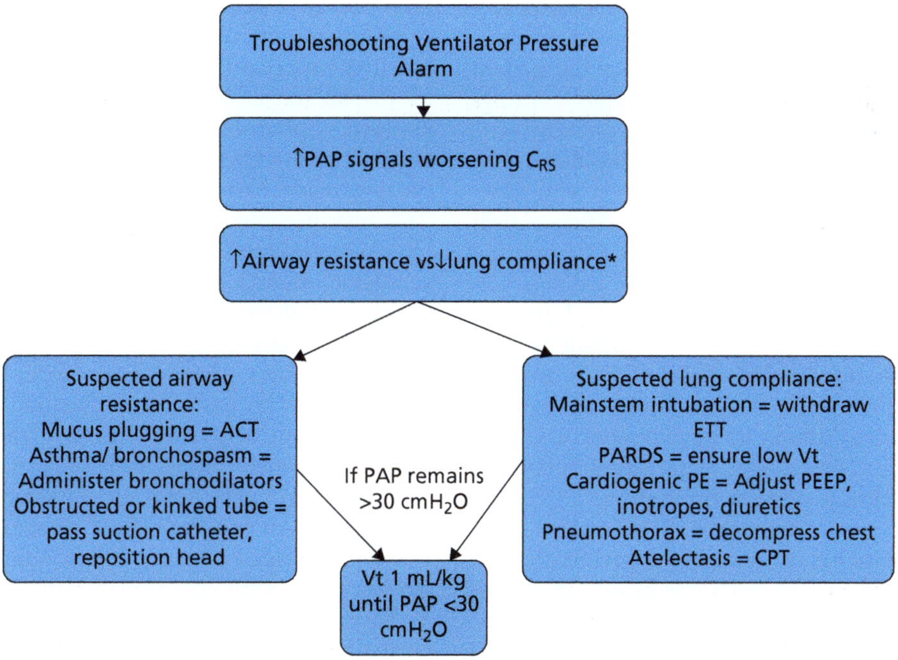

FIGURE 6.4 Troubleshooting ventilator PAP alarm. *These need to be considered in a methodical manner, and the reason for intubation should be considered immediately as a potential contributor to the ventilator alarm. If Vt and MV are inadequate for oxygenation and ventilation then higher PAP may need to be tolerated.

CRS = respiratory system compliance

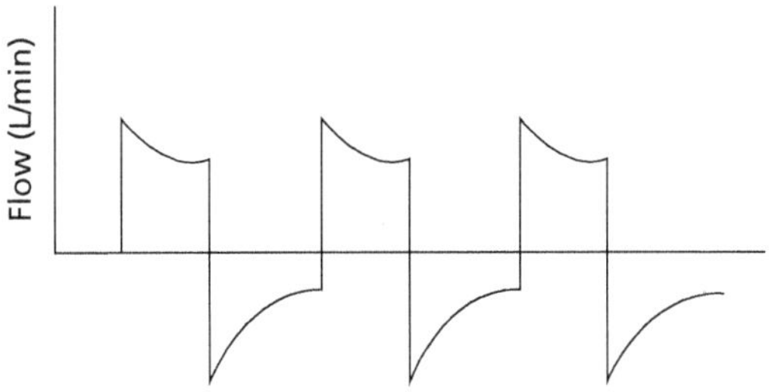

FIGURE 6.5 Flow curve not returning to baseline and development of intrinsic PEEP.

of intrinsic PEEP. The EP should determine the etiology of the dynamic hyperinflation. Is the patient overbreathing the ventilator, is the respiratory rate set too high, or do ventilator adjustments need to be made considering the patient's obstructive lung disease? The EP can lower the set RR/Ti; lower the Vt in patients with obstructive lung disease; give additional analgesic/sedative; or, if necessary, provide NMB to ensure ventilator flow-time waveforms return to baseline or perform an expiratory hold maneuver to ensure there is no intrinsic PEEP (Figure 6.5).

DOPES refers to the possibility of a *d*isplaced ETT, *o*bstructed ETT (mucus plug or kink), *p*neumothorax, *e*quipment failure, and *s*tacking/sedation. As previously mentioned, to test for equipment failure, EPs will disconnect the ventilator and manually bag the patient, assess the tubing, assess ventilator settings, and assess lung compliance manually while bagging. Sedation should be considered after all other potential issues have been addressed.

With the decompensating pediatric patient, it is necessary to determine if the ETT is still in the trachea. Given that pediatric patients have a short trachea and the ETTs placed are even shorter, small movements can result in accidental extubation. Multiple methods are used to confirm placement, including capnography, direct visualization by laryngoscopy, and passing a suction catheter or pediatric bougie/airway exchange catheter through the ETT. If the device inserted into the ETT to confirm placement does not easily pass, the patient could be biting the ETT (insert a bite block), or it could be kinked or twisted (reposition the patient's head). If there is any concern that the ETT is not in the correct location (loss of capnography or not directly visualized entering the larynx), the child may need to be reintubated. The EP should assume that this will be a difficult airway because it is likely that there is some residual edema or trauma following the unexpected extubation. Once the ETT is confirmed to be in place, and while the patient is being bagged, the patient is assessed for equal chest rise and the chest is felt for crepitus and auscultated to ensure no air leak or unequal breath sounds are present. Unequal or unilateral bronchial breath sounds may indicate migration of the ETT into the right mainstem. This complication is a common etiology of increased PAP and significant hypoxemia following intubation in children. Right mainstem intubation needs to be considered early when assessing the ventilated pediatric patient who develops unexplained hypoxemia.

After obstruction or displacement of the ETT has been ruled out, it is important to continue to identify potential etiologies for the patient's decompensation. Unequal breath sounds combined with crepitus are suggestive of pneumothorax and subcutaneous emphysema. Audible air leak is highly suggestive of a cuff leak or an inadequately sized ETT. This can be detected by auscultating over the neck. With the presence of a cuff leak, air can be easily heard escaping when a stethoscope is held against the neck. Palpating the pilot balloon may not be a sufficiently sensitive indicator. Appropriate cuff inflation can be determined by auscultation or with a manometer. The ventilator display screen will also show a discrepancy between inspiratory Vt (Vti) and expiratory Vt (Vte) (Figure 6.6). If the air leak is too large, causing inadequate inspiratory pressures, the ETT may need to be replaced. After addressing these potential issues, the settings of the ventilator should be reassessed, ventilator waveforms observed, and gas exchange reevaluated. Once stabilized and reconnected to the ventilator, the flow waveform should be scrutinized to ensure that dynamic hyperinflation is not occurring. The flow waveform should completely return to baseline to complete exhalation before the next initiated ventilator breath. An expiratory hold maneuver can also be performed to ensure there is no development of dynamic hyperinflation.

Several procedures should be undertaken, particularly if the patient's clinical status is not improving. A chest radiograph should be ordered immediately. Point-of-care ultrasound (POCUS) can be used to confirm ETT

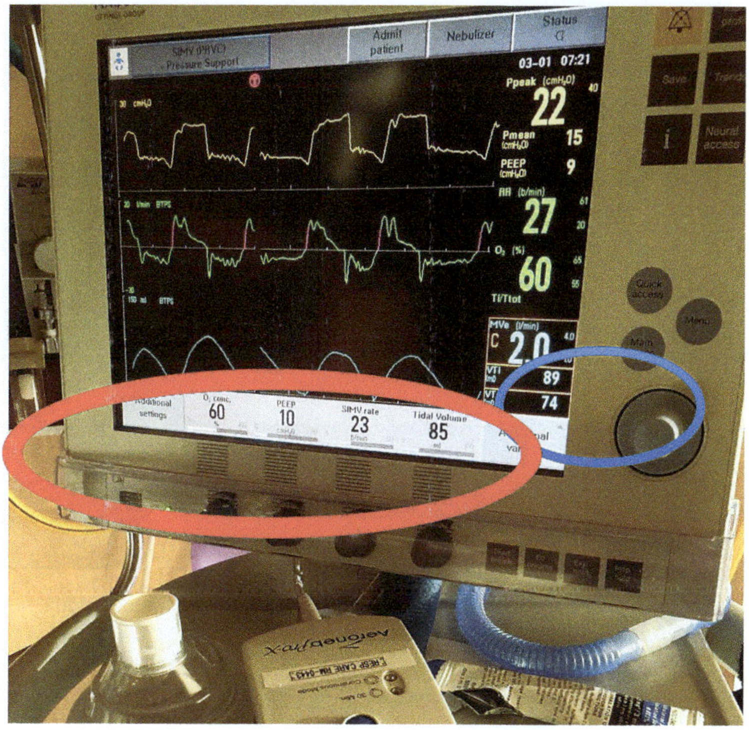

FIGURE 6.6 Mechanical ventilation display screen. In the upper left corner, the ventilator mode is listed. On the left side of the screen are the measured respiratory pressures, rates, and volumes. In this case, P_{peak} = 22 (peak airway pressure), P_{mean} = 15 (P_{AW}; mean airway pressure), PEEP = 9 (the PEEP that the patient is actually receiving, which may be more, less, or the same as the set PEEP depending on respiratory mechanics), and RR = 27 (the patient's measured respiratory rate; i.e., this patient is overbreathing the set ventilator rate). In the three small boxes, MVe = 2 L/min (minute ventilation), Vti is the inhaled tidal volume delivered by the ventilator, and Vte is the exhaled tidal volume returned to the ventilator. If there is significant discrepancy between Vti and Vte, there may be a large cuff leak or inadequately sized ETT. The bottom row of numbers circled in red are the settings chosen by the EP.

placement and to identify pneumothorax. If a pneumothorax is present, immediate needle decompression/finger thoracostomy followed by tube thoracostomy can take place. POCUS for a well-appearing lung will show normal lung sliding. In the M-mode, a seashore sign will be visible. With the presence of pneumothorax, lung sliding will be absent, and in M-mode the stratosphere sign/barcode sign will be present. If the patient stabilizes and takes asynchronous breaths with the ventilator, sedation should be optimized. This treatment should be initiated only after a full assessment for other potential adverse events.

Clinical Algorithm

See Figure 6.7 for initial ventilator settings. See Figure 6.8 for the care of the decompensating ventilated pediatric patient.

Disposition

Patients who have undergone ETI and IMV are critically ill and injured. Their care is usually transitioned to the pediatric intensive care unit or to the operating room, depending on the disease state that led to the need for IMV.

Complications

Invasive mechanical ventilation is not a natural way of breathing and is associated with several complications. There may be direct injury to the upper airways and lungs. The upper airway can be injured during laryngoscopy and tracheal intubation. Examples include dental injury and pharyngeal and laryngeal injury on a spectrum from mild edema to significant bleeding from laceration. Laryngeal injury includes minimal vocal cord damage to subluxation of the arytenoid cartilages. There is also

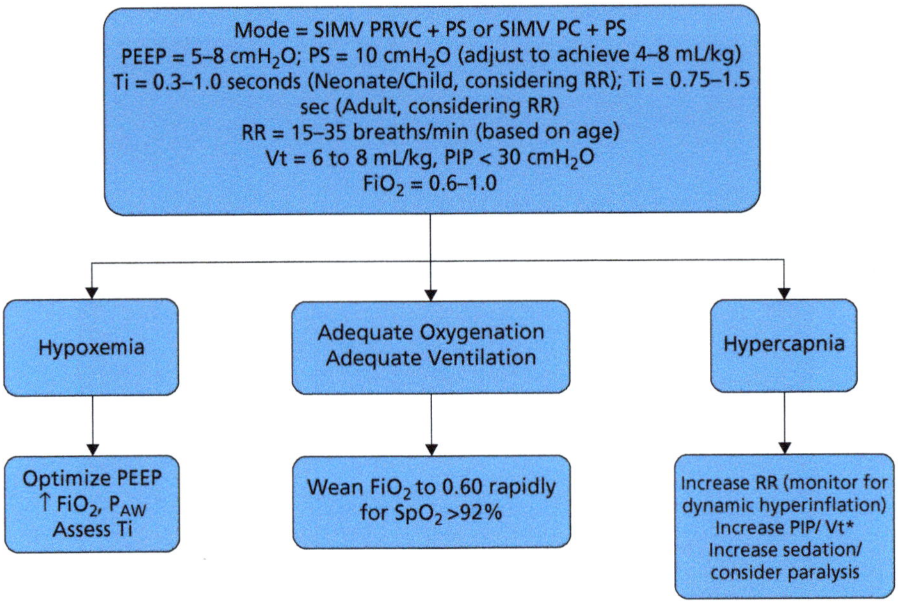

FIGURE 6.7 Initial mechanical ventilation settings, addressing hypoxemia and hypercapnia.

**If Vt is increased, take care to not sacrifice the open lung strategy.*

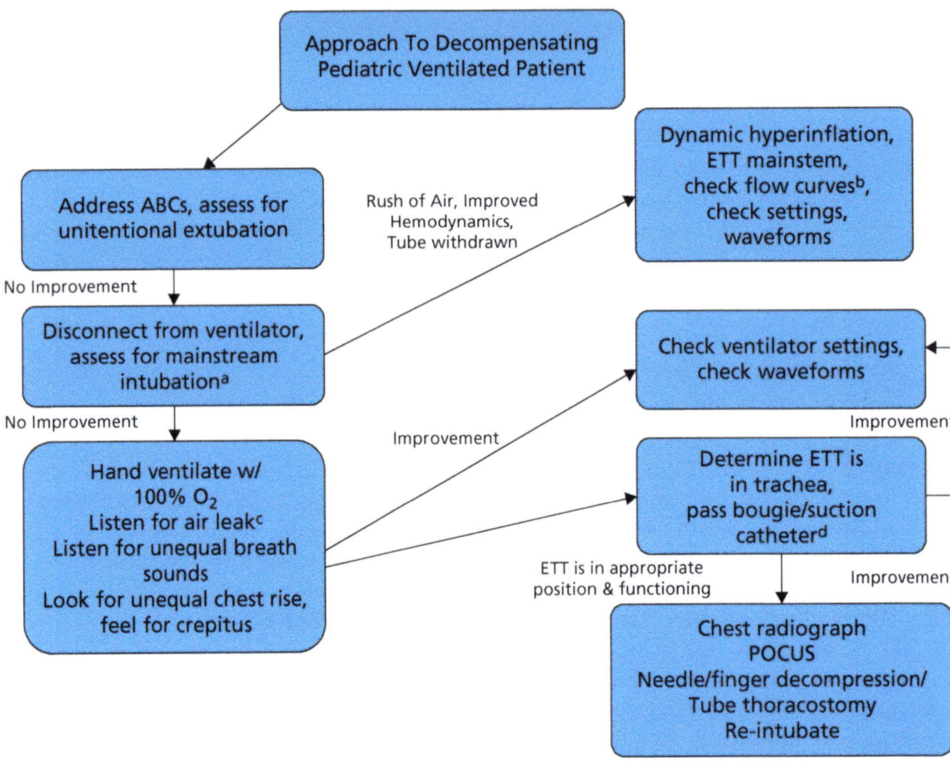

FIGURE 6.8 Approach to the decompensating pediatric mechanically ventilated patient. (a) Address right main stem intubation considering the shorter trachea leading to ETT displacement. (b) Ventilator flow waveform should return to baseline to ensure no intrinsic/auto-PEEP is developing. (c) Decompensation may be secondary to an ETT that is too small or a damaged ETT cuff. (d) The bougie or suction catheter will have hold up anywhere from 4 to 8 cm considering the short length of the trachea. Anything beyond this is suspicious for an esophageal intubation.

Source: Courtesy of ACEP. Modified from Santanilla JI, Daniel B, Yeow ME. Mechanical ventilation. *Emerg Med Clin North Am.* 2008;26(3):849–862; and Santanilla JI. The crashing ventilated patient. In: Winters ME, et al., eds. *Emergency Department Resuscitation of the Critically Ill.* 2nd ed. Dallas, TX: American College of Emergency Physicians; 2017:17–26.

a risk of subglottic injury from the tracheal tube, leading to pressure necrosis and stenosis. Continuous changes in volume and pressure lead to lower airway VILI. Macroscopic air leak (pneumothorax, pneumomediastinum, and pneumopericardium) has been reported in up to 40% of children receiving mechanical ventilation, but the rate is likely much lower. Ventilation-associated respiratory infections are also a significant problem faced in the pediatric intensive care unit and can lead to prolonged length of stay, increased duration of mechanical ventilation, and increased mortality.

Key Points

- NIV and IMV are critical for the EP to understand when taking care of critically ill children.
- Hypercapnia can be treated by changes in the RR/Ti, ΔP, or Vt.
- Hypoxemia can be treated by addressing the FiO_2 and the determinants of P_{AW}, including PEEP, Ti, or increasing the driving pressure (P_{PLAT} - PEEP).

Pitfalls

- If adjustments are made in the RR but not the Ti, dynamic hyperinflation may occur.
- Ventilator alarms should be treated like an overhead "code" alarm.
- An algorithmic systematic approach is necessary when caring for the deteriorating ventilated pediatric patient.

Further Reading

Gupta R, Rosen D. Paeditric mechanical ventilation in the intensive care unit. *BJA Educ.* 2016;16(12): 422–426.

Kesavan S, Ramachandran B. Humidified high-flow nasal cannula oxygen therapy in children: A narrative review. *J Pediatr Crit Care.* 2016;3(4): 29–34.

Kneyber MC, De Luca D, Calderini E, et al. Recommendations for mechanical ventilation of critically ill children from the Paediatric Mechanical Ventilation Consensus Conference (PEMVECC). *Intensive Care Med.* 2017;43(12):1764–1780.

Pavone M, Verrillo E, Caldarelli V, et al. Non-invasive positive pressure ventilation in children. *Early Hum Dev.* 2013;89(Suppl 3):S25–S31.

Santanilla JI, Daniel B, Yeow ME. Mechanical ventilation. *Emerg Med Clin North Am.* 2008;26(3): 849–862.

7

Neonatal Resuscitation

ANNEKA HOOFT AND SEEMA SHAH

INTRODUCTION

The majority of neonates born in the United States do not require special assistance, but approximately 10% require some intervention, and less than 1% require extensive resuscitation measures. Although the number of infants delivered in the emergency department (ED) is unknown, out-of-hospital births have been increasing; thus, pediatric emergency physicians should be prepared for the possibility of a neonatal resuscitation in the ED.

In contrast to pediatric and adult resuscitation, resuscitation of neonates requires close attention to the normal increase in oxygen saturations over time after birth. Because respiratory failure is the most common cause of arrest in the neonate, initial resuscitation measures, even for bradycardia, rely primarily on optimizing oxygenation and ventilation. Extra care must also be taken to ensure infants remain warm during the resuscitation process.

CLINICAL APPLICATION

A 28-year-old gravida 3, para 2 woman delivers an infant estimated to be 33 weeks 2 days gestation by dates and fetal ultrasound. The infant is brought emergently into the resuscitation bay.

Initial resuscitation of the neonate continues to rely on the Neonatal Resuscitation Program (NRP) algorithm (see https://www.ahajournals.org/doi/full/10.1161/circ.102.suppl_1.I-343; simplified measures are shown in Figure 7.1). Emergency departments should have quick access to neonatal resuscitation equipment, including a radiant warmer, airway equipment (neonatal bag mask, laryngoscopes, endotracheal tubes, suction, and laryngeal masks), medications, and equipment for umbilical line placement and needle thoracentesis.

Initiation of NRP requires quick assessment of heart rate (HR), color, tone, and respiratory effort. This should be done simultaneously within the first minute of life (the "golden minute"). Heart rate is typically assessed by auscultation or palpation of pulse in the umbilical stump. If the infant has an HR <100 beats per minute (bpm) or is giving poor respiratory effort after attempts to dry, stimulate, and suction the airway, then resuscitation measures should be initiated and a pulse oximeter should be placed.

Despite 30 seconds of initial attempts to dry and stimulate the baby, HR is 85 bpm and the infant has decreased tone with poor respiratory effort.

Initial Care → warm, dry, stimulate

If HR is <100 bpm → positive pressure ventilation

If HR is < 60 bpm → compressions coordinated with positive pressure ventilation (at a 3:1 ratio)

FIGURE 7.1 Key interventions in newborn resuscitation.

Positive pressure ventilation (PPV) should be provided if the HR is <100 bpm. Care should be taken to use the lowest fraction of inspired oxygen (FiO_2) necessary to maintain oxygen saturations, noting that it takes up to 10 minutes after birth, even in a normal infant, for saturations to reach >90%. Positive pressure can be provided using a self-inflating, flow-inflating, or T-piece resuscitator at a rate of approximately 40 breaths per minute, typically at a peak pressure of 20 mmHg and a positive end-expiratory pressure (PEEP) of 5 mmHg, titrating for effect. Attempts should be made to suction and reposition the infant if saturations and HR are not improving.

If HR improves but respiratory effort continues to be inadequate, the infant can be transitioned to noninvasive ventilatory support, such as nasal continuous positive airway pressure. This should also be considered for infants less than 32 weeks' gestational age and/or weighing <1.5 kg, regardless of their work of breathing, due to the likelihood of underlying lung immaturity.

For infants in severe distress and/or persistent hypoxia despite administration of PPV, intubation should be performed. If intubation cannot be performed, other airway adjuncts, such as laryngeal masks, may be used for infants older than 34 weeks or >2 kg. Although intubation for meconium aspiration is no longer routinely recommended, this may be considered if a meconium plug is likely and the infant's respiratory status is not improving with noninvasive measures. Rapid sequence intubation medications are not routinely administered to nonvigorous infants during emergent intubation in the immediate postnatal period, but they are not contraindicated.

After 30 seconds of PPV, the infant continues to look dusky with poor tone. The infant is intubated and demonstrates good chest rise and equal breath sounds. Despite these measures, HR is decreasing and is now 54 bpm.

If HR is not improving after 30 seconds of adequate ventilation with a secure airway, and begins to drop below 60 bpm, chest compressions should be initiated and epinephrine should be given. It is important to note that in the neonate, compressions should be given at a ratio of 3:1 coordinating with breaths. The two-thumb circling cardiopulmonary resuscitation (CPR) method is recommended because it has demonstrated better efficacy in comparison to the two-finger method. Epinephrine can be administered intravenously (IV) or, if IV access has not yet been established, via endotracheal tube (ETT) at a dose of 0.01 mg/kg IV or 0.1 mg/kg, respectively. Emergent umbilical venous catheter or intraosseous placement should be considered if a peripheral IV cannot be placed quickly (see Chapter 45).

Volume replacement should be considered because blood loss and trauma during birth can contribute to poor circulation. An initial 10 mL/kg bolus of crystalloid fluid should be administered, and this may be repeated as needed. Dextrose administration should also be considered for possible hypoglycemia. Naloxone is no longer routinely recommended if there is concern for opioid exposure, and instead respiratory support should be provided until the potential drug's effect has worn off.

After two rounds of epinephrine, CPR, and intubation, the infant's HR is now 110 bpm. Color is becoming pink, and the infant's tone has improved. The transport team arrives and places the infant in an isolette for transport to the nearest neonatal intensive care unit (NICU).

PITFALLS

Fluid Administration

Renal perfusion and function in the neonate do not peak until several days after birth, so constant re-evaluation should be performed during fluid administration.

After initial resuscitation, neonates should be started on an initial rate of 10% dextrose in water of 60–80 mL/kg/day to prevent fluid overload and electrolyte disturbances.

Ventilation

As with any airway, securing the neonatal airway and ensuring adequate ventilation are critical during the resuscitation process. Adjunct measures such as mask adjustment and ensuring proper size and fit and suctioning can make a considerable difference. Positioning the infant in the sniffing position, taking care not to hyperextend at the neck given the infant's more anterior trachea and relatively large head size, can also facilitate quality ventilation. A nasal or oral airway may be considered, especially in infants with congenital variations of their airway anatomy (i.e., micrognathia with Pierre-Robin sequence or macroglossia due to Beckwith-Wiedemann syndrome). For extremely premature infants with poor lung compliance, peak pressures and PEEP may need to be gradually increased to improve ventilation. Per NRP guidelines, the mnemonic MR SOPA (*m*ask, *r*eposition, *s*uction, *o*pen the mouth, *p*ressure, *a*lternative airway) can be used to help recall these strategies.

If breath sounds are unequal, or chest rise becomes extremely poor, the physician should consider needle decompression or emergent chest tube placement for possible pneumothorax.

For meconium plug syndrome or severe aspiration, a meconium aspirator can be attached to the ETT and then to suction and used to suction the trachea during intubation.

Hyperoxygenation of the neonate, especially in the first few minutes of life, should be avoided. The lowest possible FiO_2 should be used during resuscitation to maintain oxygen saturations according to the NRP guidelines for saturations by minute of life.

Intraosseous Placement

Intraosseous lines in the neonate should ideally be placed in the proximal tibia or distal femur. The lack of ossification in the proximal humerus in this age group makes this site unsuitable. Typically, the smallest sized needle should be used (the pediatric needle), and care should be taken to avoid advancing too deeply and going through the bone, especially in very small infants.

Thermoregulation

For premature infants, <32 weeks or 1.5 kg, additional measures must be taken to prevent heat loss. This can include covering the infant's body in plastic wrap (Neowrap) or utilizing a bowel bag. The goal should be normothermia, which requires continuous temperature monitoring. Hyperthermia can also be detrimental to the neonate, especially to infants who may have hypoxic ischemic encephalopathy (HIE).

Hypoxic Ischemic Encephalopathy

For term or late preterm infants with evidence of birth asphyxia during delivery, prolonged resuscitation, or neurologic depression on examination after birth, arrangements should be made for transfer to a NICU with hypothermia protocol and HIE treatment capabilities. Criteria for hypothermia protocols vary by institution, so this should be discussed with a neonatologist prior to transfer.

Further Reading

American Heart Association. Major Guidelines Changes. https://www.ahajournals.org/doi/full/10.1161/circ.102.suppl_1.I-343.

Lee JE, Lee J, Oh J, et al. Comparison of two-thumb encircling and two-finger technique during infant cardiopulmonary resuscitation with single rescuer in simulation studies: A systematic review and meta-analysis. *Medicine (Baltimore).* 2019;98(45):e17853.

Levesque BM, Burnham L, Cardoza N, et al. Improving respiratory support practices to reduce chronic lung disease in premature infants. *Pediatr Qual Saf.* 2019;4(4):e193.

Wyckoff MH, Aziz K, Escobedo MB, et al. Part 13: Neonatal resuscitation: 2015 American Heart Association guidelines update for cardiopulmonary resuscitation and emergency cardiovascular care. *Circulation.* 2015;132(18 Suppl 2):S543–S560.

8

Pediatric Resuscitation

MATTHEW MENDES AND TAYLOR MCCORMICK

INTRODUCTION

This chapter focuses on the recognition and resuscitation of critically ill children in respiratory failure, shock, and cardiopulmonary arrest (neonatal resuscitation is discussed in Chapter 7). Pediatric cardiopulmonary arrest is rare and most commonly due to respiratory failure. Studies of pediatric out-of-hospital cardiac arrest report survival rates ranging from 4% to 38% and favorable neurologic outcomes in 1–16% of children. Shockable rhythms, witnessed arrest, bystander cardiopulmonary resuscitation (CPR), and age >1 year are associated with improved survival.

HISTORY AND PHYSICAL EXAMINATION

Emergency physicians are experts at resuscitating a patient while concurrently obtaining a focused history and physical examination. Obtaining a SAMPLE history [*s*igns/symptoms, *a*llergies, *m*edications (including medications of household members), *p*ast medical and surgical history, *l*ast meal and menses, and *e*vents leading up to ED presentation] should not delay a rapid assessment and initiation of resuscitative procedures.

The Pediatric Assessment Triangle (PAT) is used to determine clinical status ("sick vs. not sick") and illness category in children (Figure 8.1). It can be performed "from the doorway" in 30–60 seconds by observation alone and can help guide triage decisions and resuscitation priorities. The three components of PAT are appearance, work of breathing, and circulation. Assess the child's appearance using the TICLS mnemonic (*t*one, *i*nteractiveness, *c*onsolability, *l*ook/gaze, and *s*peech/cry); work of breathing noting abnormal airway sounds, retractions or nasal flaring, or positioning; and

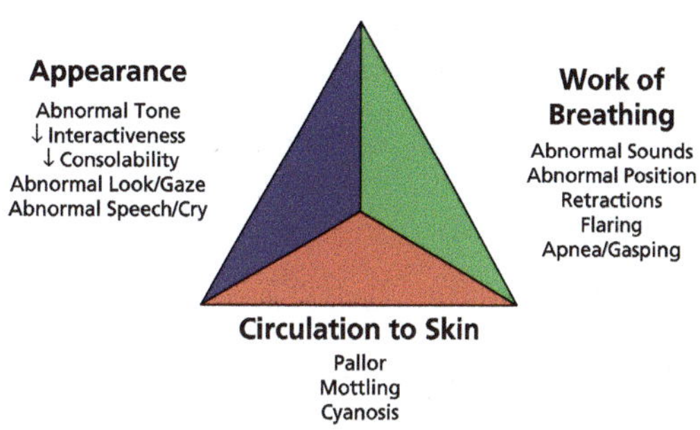

FIGURE 8.1 Pediatric Assessment Triangle.

Source: Reproduced with permission from Horeczko T, Enriquez B, McGrath NE, Gausche-Hill M, Lewis RJ. The Pediatric Assessment Triangle: Accuracy of its application by nurses in the triage of children. *J Emerg Nurs*. 2013;39(2):182–189. https://www.ncbi.nlm.nih.gov/pmc/articles/PMC4318552.

circulation to the skin, looking for pallor, mottling, or cyanosis. An abnormality of any arm of the PAT suggests a potentially unstable child and should prompt immediate assessment of the ABCDEs (airway, breathing, circulation, disability, exposure) and concurrent intervention as needed (Table 8.1; Figure 8.2). If PAT is normal, continue with a secondary assessment including a more thorough history and head-to-toe physical examination.

WORKUP

It is essential to obtain a weight in kilograms for the pediatric patient. If an actual measured weight is not possible and the parents are not able to provide a reliable estimation, estimate the patient's weight by using an age-, weight-, or length-based medication and equipment system (e.g., Luten–Broselow or Handtevy systems). Obtain a fingerstick glucose and correct hypoglycemia as soon as possible. A pregnancy test should be performed on all pubescent females.

Laboratory evaluation should be guided by the overall clinical picture. In most cases of the acutely ill or poorly perfused child, it is reasonable to obtain a complete blood count, electrolyte panel, hepatic function panel, and venous blood gas. A type and screen should be considered for patients who may require blood products. In suspected sepsis, obtain blood cultures, urinalysis and urine culture, serum lactate, and cerebrospinal fluid studies or stool studies as clinically indicated.

TABLE 8.1 SPECIAL CONSIDERATIONS FOR THE PEDIATRIC ABCDE APPROACH

	Pediatric Considerations	All Patients	Treatments
Airway	Assess for strong cry or speaking ability	Obstruction Pooling of secretions	Towel roll under shoulders, chin lift, jaw thrust Suction NPA OPA Intubation if above unsuccessful
Breathing	Grunting Stridor Stertor	Positioning Respiratory rate Lung sounds Oxygen saturation Capnography/end-tidal CO_2	Nasal cannula or NRB if SpO_2 <95% Consider heated high-flow nasal cannula Needle or tube thoracostomy for pneumothorax Albuterol for bronchospasm Racemic epinephrine for croup Intubation if above unsuccessful
Circulation	Cyanosis Mottling Delayed capillary refill Hypotension (SBP <70 + age × 2)	Pallor Cool extremities Thready peripheral pulses	Obtain IV/IO access 20 mL/kg bolus of crystalloid solution (use 10 mL/kg initially if concern for possible cardiac etiology) pRBCs Vasopressor (e.g., epinephrine or norepinephrine) if refractory to fluid
Disability	AVPU Seizure activity Movement and tone	Glucose Pupils	Suspected increased ICP: elevate head of bed 30 degrees, give hypertonic saline or mannitol, and avoid hypoxia and hypotension Correct hypoglycemia Treat seizures with benzodiazepines
Exposure	Remove hats and diapers for a full examination	Completely undress	Maintain normothermia

AVPU is a scale for level of consciousness: awake, awakens to verbal stimulation, awakens to painful stimulation, unresponsive; ICP, intracranial pressure; IO, intraosseous; IV, intravenous; NPA, nasopharyngeal airway; NRB, non-rebreather oxygen mask; OPA, oropharyngeal airway; pRBCs, packed red blood cells; SBP, systolic blood pressure; SpO_2, peripheral capillary oxygen saturation.

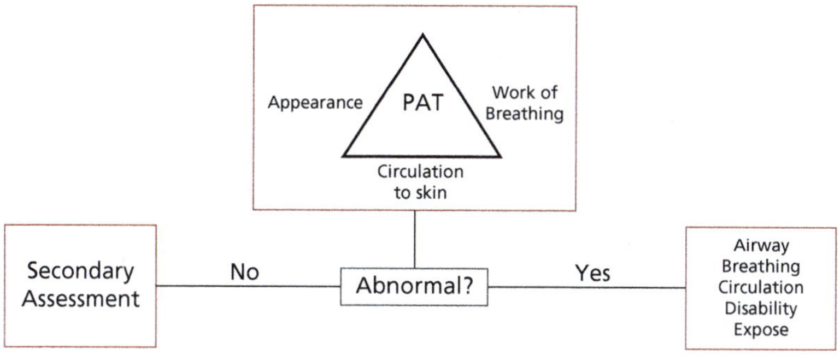

FIGURE 8.2 If there is any change in clinical status, repeat the PAT and ABCDE.

Serum troponin and brain natriuretic peptide levels help diagnose suspected congestive heart failure, myocarditis, or cardiac ischemia. Toxicologic studies should be guided by the clinical picture and index of suspicion. Coagulation studies are indicated in cases of known coagulopathy, suspected disseminated intravascular coagulation, or if the patient is on anticoagulant medications.

Clinical presentation dictates imaging and other testing, such as electrocardiogram (ECG), chest X-ray, and computed tomography scans (for specific indications, see Chapters 15, 17, 19, and 33). Bedside ultrasound may evaluate for intra-abdominal free fluid, pericardial effusion, pneumothorax, and global cardiac function.

DIFFERENTIAL DIAGNOSIS

Prompt recognition and management of impending respiratory failure and correction of the shock state can prevent cardiopulmonary arrest. Figure 8.3 utilizes the PAT to guide emergency clinicians in their differential diagnosis.

The etiology of respiratory failure can be thought of in terms of upper airways and lower airways (for a more detailed discussion on respiratory conditions, see Chapter 15). Examples of upper airway pathology are foreign body, congenital abnormalities, croup, tracheitis, epiglottitis, peritonsillar abscess, and retropharyngeal abscess. Lower airway diseases can include pneumonia, bronchiolitis, asthma, cystic fibrosis, pulmonary edema, and foreign body.

Shock occurs in four subtypes. In children, these subtypes often overlap, particularly in sepsis (see Chapter 12). Children have high sympathetic tone, which results in an ability to maintain a normal blood pressure despite significant threats such as blood loss or sepsis. Although not exhaustive, Table 8.2 provides a differential diagnosis based on the subtype of shock. The ability of healthy children to sustain a state of compensated shock (i.e., normal blood pressure) through tachycardia and vasoconstriction cannot be understated. Signs of compensated shock include elevated heart rate, cool skin, weak pulses, prolonged capillary refill, and decreased urine output. Hypotensive shock should be thought of as a sign of impending cardiopulmonary arrest.

Non-accidental trauma should be considered in any case in which the history is inconsistent with the degree of illness or pattern of injury found on examination (see Chapter 54).

TREATMENT AND PROCEDURES

Use the PAT–ABCDE approach to identify critically ill children and aggressively treat respiratory failure and shock. All critically ill children

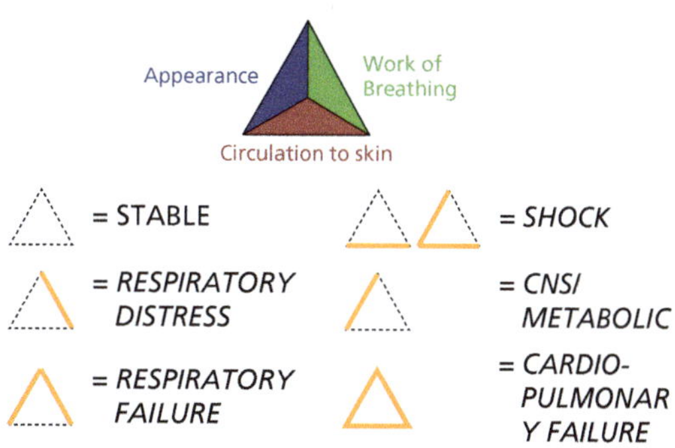

FIGURE 8.3 Pediatric Assessment Triangle: general impression.

Source: Reproduced with permission from Tim Horeczko, MD, and the Pediatric Emergency Playbook Podcast.

TABLE 8.2 SHOCK TYPES

Type	Pathophysiology	Specific Etiologies
Hypovolemic	Inadequate circulatory volume	Hemorrhage, diarrhea, decreased oral intake, diabetic ketoacidosis, third spacing (pancreatitis)
Distributive	Decreased systemic vascular resistance	Sepsis, anaphylaxis, neurogenic shock
Cardiogenic	Inadequate myocardial function	Myocarditis, arrhythmia, cardiomyopathy, congenital heart disease, drug toxicity
Obstructive	Obstructed cardiac filling and output	Tension pneumothorax, pulmonary embolism, cardiac tamponade, congenital heart disease

should have a weight documented or estimated to further guide dosing and equipment size. Patients should be placed on cardiopulmonary monitoring, and intravenous (IV) or intraosseous (IO) access should not be delayed.

Respiratory Failure

Etiologies of respiratory failure are discussed further in Chapter 15, and interventions are detailed in Chapters 5 and 6. Targeted intervention may include nebulized albuterol/ipratropium or racemic epinephrine, heated high-flow nasal cannula, continuous positive airway pressure, or bilevel positive airway support. If these noninvasive measures do not work, proceed with rapid sequence endotracheal intubation (RSI). RSI can be achieved with the induction agents etomidate or ketamine and the paralytics succinylcholine or rocuronium. The 2015 American Heart Association (AHA) Pediatric Advanced Life Support (PALS) guidelines do not recommend routine atropine pretreatment to prevent peri-intubation bradycardia but state that it may be reasonable in specific emergency intubations for which there is a higher risk of bradycardia (e.g., when giving succinylcholine for paralysis) at a dose of 0.02 mg/kg with no minimum dose.

Shock

Table 8.3 lists therapeutic interventions based on type of shock. Patients with unstable tachycardia or bradycardia should be treated according to the corresponding PALS algorithms (Figures 8.4 and 8.5).

TABLE 8.3 SIMPLIFIED TREATMENT RECOMMENDATIONS BASED ON SHOCK ETIOLOGY

Shock Type	Intervention
Hypovolemic	20 mL/kg crystalloid bolus or 10 mL/kg of pRBC bolus: Repeat either as needed
Distributive	20 mL/kg crystalloid bolus repeat two or three times If fluid refractory, start pressors Warm shock: Norepinephrine Cold shock: Epinephrine Suspected adrenal insufficiency: Hydrocortisone Anaphylaxis: Epinephrine
Cardiogenic	Tachydysrhythmia (unstable): Synchronized cardioversion Bradycardia (unstable): Epinephrine and pacing Other etiologies (e.g., CHF): Norepinephrine; add dobutamine if shock persists and inotropy is thought to be impaired
Obstructive	Tension pneumothorax: Needle decompression Pulmonary embolism: Thrombolysis Pericardial tamponade: Pericardiocentesis

CHF, congestive heart failure; pRBC, packed red blood cells.

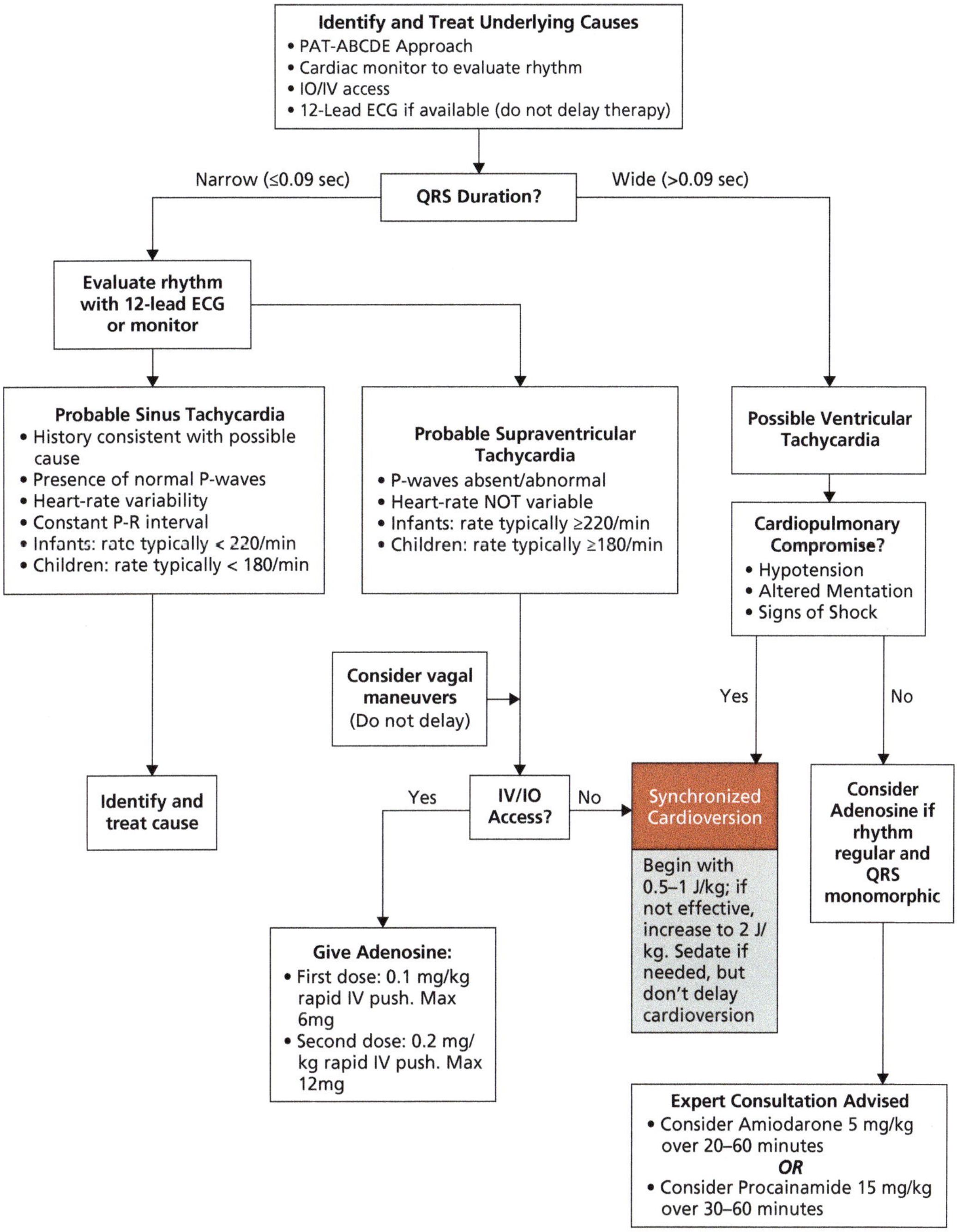

FIGURE 8.4 Pediatric tachycardia with a pulse and poor perfusion.

Cardiopulmonary Arrest

The 2018 PALS cardiac arrest algorithm is shown in Figure 8.6. Chest compressions and rescue breaths should be initiated when an unresponsive child is pulseless with absent/abnormal breathing *or* if a child's heart rate is less than 60 beats per minute with evidence of end-organ hypoperfusion (e.g., depressed mental status). Chest compressions should be performed at a rate of 100–120 compressions per minute and a depth of approximately one-third the diameter of the chest. For infants, the compressor should use two thumbs, with the hands encircling the chest; the two-finger

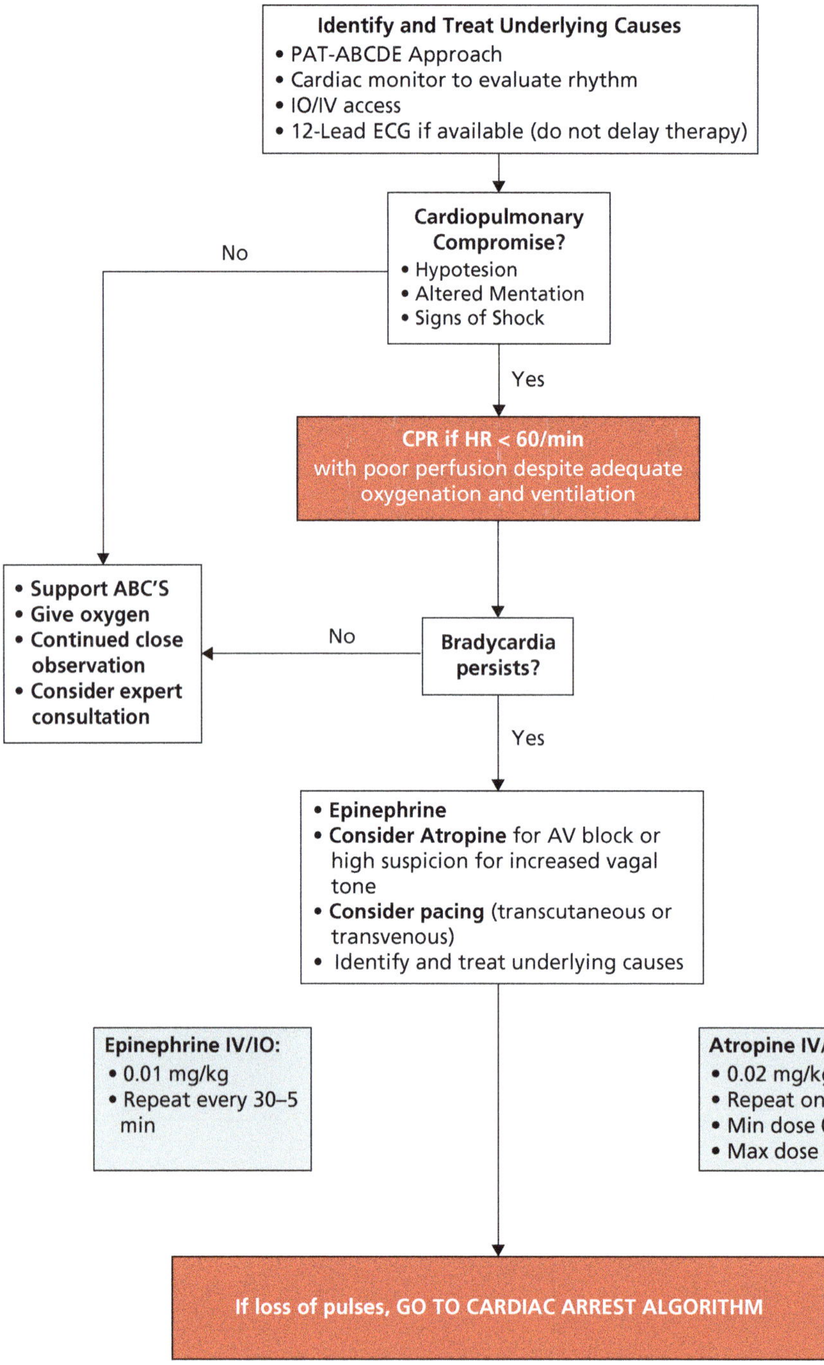

FIGURE 8.5 Pediatric bradycardia with a pulse and poor perfusion.

method is less effective. For children ≥ 1 year of age, traditional compressions should be delivered using one or two hands on the sternum, depending on the size of the child. The evidence for compression-only CPR in the pediatric population is lacking, and given the high likelihood of a respiratory etiology for cardiopulmonary arrest, the AHA's 2017 Focused Update recommends that chest compressions and ventilation should be provided at a ratio of 15:2 until definitive airway is in place. Ventilation with a bag valve mask, a

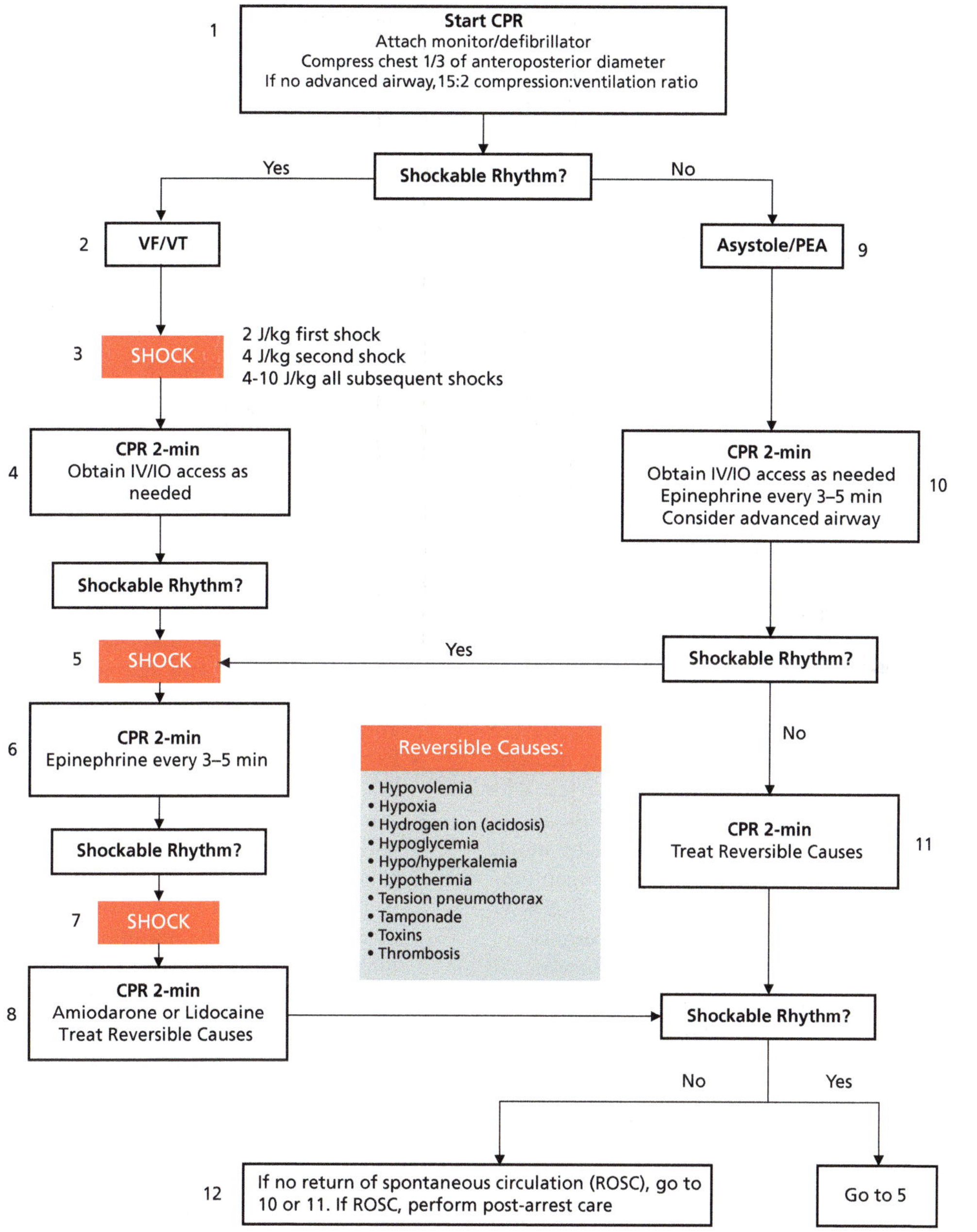

FIGURE 8.6 Pediatric cardiac arrest.

supraglottic device, or endotracheal intubation are all reasonable approaches to airway management during cardiopulmonary arrest. As with adults, high-quality, uninterrupted chest compressions and early defibrillation should be prioritized. If available, pediatric pads should be used for all children younger than age 8 years who are undergoing defibrillation. The pads can be placed in either the anteroposterior or the anterolateral position. The energy used for defibrillation should be 2 J/kg for the first attempt, 4 J/kg for the second attempt, and up to 10 J/kg for any subsequent attempts. Epinephrine may be given every 3–5 minutes for all rhythms at a dose of 0.01 mg/kg IV/IO. For ventricular fibrillation and pulseless ventricular tachycardia, amiodarone (5 mg/kg IV/IO) or lidocaine (1 mg/kg IV/IO) should be given. Other medications should be targeted toward the presumed etiology of the cardiopulmonary arrest (e.g., calcium chloride for hyperkalemia or dextrose for hypoglycemia).

Existing literature strongly supports family presence during resuscitation. Witnessing a resuscitation helps with the grieving process and is preferred by most parents. All providers should be aware when family is present, and professional behavior must be maintained. Ideally, a staff member is also available to explain specific interventions and activities to families.

Extracorporeal Membrane Oxygenation and Extracorporeal Cardiopulmonary Resuscitation

Extracorporeal membrane oxygenation and its use in prolonged CPR shows favorable outcomes for significant cardiopulmonary failure and in-hospital cardiac arrest.

Post-Arrest Care

Hyperthermia should be avoided. Therapeutic hypothermia does not impact long-term neurobehavioral outcomes. The 2019 AHA/PALS update states that targeted temperature management can be considered for cardiac arrest with continuous monitoring of the core temperature.

For intubated patients, the ventilator should be optimized to maintain a normal oxygen saturation and normal carbon dioxide levels ($PaCO_2$ of 35–45 mmHg) while avoiding hyperoxia.

Hypotension (systolic blood pressure <70 + age × 2) should be avoided with the use of norepinephrine or etiology-specific therapies, as noted in Table 8.3.

DISPOSITION

Admit all patients who are survivors of cardiopulmonary arrest, children with ongoing respiratory insufficiency/failure, and children with ongoing shock to a pediatric intensive care unit. If not available, the patient should be promptly transferred to a facility that has pediatric critical care expertise.

KEY POINTS AND PITFALLS

- The evaluation and management of critically ill children largely mirrors that of adults, with special consideration of a few key anatomic and physiologic differences.
- The use of age- or length-based medication dosing and equipment systems reduces time to medication delivery, dosing errors, and provider anxiety.
- Do not rely on hypotension to identify shock in children; tachycardia or poor perfusion may be the only clues.
- Use the PAT–ABCDE approach to prevent cardiopulmonary arrest by early recognition and aggressive treatment of respiratory failure and shock.
- Familiarize yourself with PALS bradycardia, tachycardia, and cardiac arrest algorithms, which align closely with adult resuscitation algorithms.
- If return of spontaneous circulation is achieved, avoid hypotension and hyperthermia while maintaining normal oxygen and carbon dioxide levels.
- Move quickly to intraosseous access if peripheral intravenous access is not easily obtained.
- Families should be given the opportunity to be present for their child's resuscitation.

9

Fever in the Young Infant

PAUL ISHIMINE

INTRODUCTION

Fever is the most common complaint of children who present to the emergency department (ED), but the management of the febrile child, particularly the febrile young child, remains controversial. Most febrile children have fevers caused by infection, and most commonly, these infections are self-limited viral illnesses. However, some children have serious bacterial infections (SBIs) and life-threatening viral illnesses that put these children at higher risk of adverse outcomes if these infections are not identified and managed properly.

Febrile young children can be further subdivided into two groups: febrile neonates (aged 0–28 days) and febrile young infants (aged 29—56 days). Approximately 12% of febrile neonates and young infants have SBIs (bacteremia, meningitis, urinary tract infections, pneumonia, bacterial gastroenteritis, and osteomyelitis). Emergency physicians are faced with the challenge of identifying patients with these serious infections while limiting unnecessary testing, treatment, and hospitalizations.

Comparison/Contrast with Adult Physiology

Although patients of all ages present to EDs with fever, the approach to febrile young infants warrants special consideration. Febrile young infants have immature immune systems and are frequently unable to localize signs and symptoms, thus making the identification of focal bacterial infections challenging compared with doing so in older children and adults. Typical causative pathogens and examination findings vary significantly by age.

CLASSIC CLINICAL PRESENTATION

Fever may have both infectious and noninfectious causes, but most febrile children who present to the ED have fevers arising from infections. Although there are fluctuations in the normal body temperature, fever in young children is generally accepted as a temperature of 38.0°C (100.4°F) or higher. Rectal thermometry is more accurate than oral, axillary, tympanic membrane, and temporal artery thermometry, and young infants should have their temperatures measured by this route. Salient historical points include the duration of fever, associated signs and symptoms, underlying medical conditions, maternal fever, prematurity, and exposure to ill contacts. Although the presence of hyperpyrexia (temperature ≥40°C) may be associated with increased rates of serious bacterial infection, the height of fever does not reliably distinguish serious and nonserious underlying causes of fever. Response to antipyretic medications does not distinguish between bacterial and viral causes. Neither bundling nor teething cause significant changes in body temperature. The hepatitis B vaccination is the only vaccine routinely given to children younger than age 2 months. Therefore, the patient's immunization status is not pertinent in the assessment of the febrile young child because the most common pathogens in this age group are group B streptococcus, *Escherichia coli, Staphylococcus aureus*, and *Enterococcus*, and none of these pathogens are prevented by vaccination.

The physical examination is a critical part of the assessment of the febrile young child. Most well-appearing children do not have serious bacterial infections, but the association between well appearance and absence of bacterial infection is imperfect. Conversely, ill-appearing children are more likely than well-appearing children to have serious bacterial infection. Patients with septic shock who present with abnormal mental status, weak peripheral pulses and cool extremities, hypotension, and/or delayed capillary refill frequently have underlying bacterial infections. The physical examination may reveal foci of infection, and the identification of a specific infection may decrease the need for additional testing. Generally, when a source of fever is identified by the history and examination, the clinician can take a more selective approach to diagnostic testing and antibiotic therapy. Febrile children with clinically recognizable viral conditions (e.g., croup, chickenpox, and stomatitis) have lower rates of bacteremia compared to children with no obvious source of infection. Young children who have fever without a localizing source of infection pose more of a management dilemma, and the approach to these children is discussed later.

ATYPICAL CLINICAL PRESENTATION

Patients will frequently present with a history of fever but are afebrile upon presentation to the ED. Subjective determination of fever by caretakers at home is a moderately accurate predictor of true fever. In one large study of 3,825 infants aged ≤60 days, the prevalence of SBIs in patients with fever by history alone (8.8%) was lower than the prevalence of SBIs in patients who were febrile in the ED (12.8%), but it was not low enough to obviate the need for evaluation for SBIs in these patients. A patient with a fever measured rectally at home should undergo the same evaluation as if this measurement were obtained in the ED.

DIFFERENTIAL DIAGNOSIS

Fever may have both infectious and noninfectious causes, but most febrile children who present to the ED have fevers arising from infections. Viral infections are the most common infectious causes of fever. Specific viruses range from relatively benign viruses, such as rhinovirus, to potentially life-threatening causes of infections, such as herpes simplex virus (HSV) infection. Urinary tract infections (UTIs) are the most common bacterial causes of fever; other potentially serious causes of bacterial infection include bacteremia, bacterial meningitis, pneumonia, gastroenteritis, osteomyelitis, septic arthritis, and skin and soft-tissue infections. Other causes of fever include post-immunization reactions, environmental heat illness, toxicologic, rheumatologic, and oncologic causes.

DIAGNOSTIC CONFIRMATION

Neonate

Neonates are a particularly high-risk group because of higher rates of bacteremia and meningitis compared to those of older children. Because the physical examination is limited in its ability to identify serious infections in neonates, evaluation of febrile neonates must incorporate the use of diagnostic studies. Blood, urine, and cerebrospinal fluid (CSF) cultures should be obtained in these patients. A peripheral white blood cell (WBC) count is often ordered in the evaluation of febrile neonates, but the discriminatory value of the WBC count is insufficient to differentiate between patients with SBIs and those with nonbacterial infection. Additional blood testing may be useful. Thrombocytopenia and elevated liver enzymes are associated with herpes simplex infections. Although the urinalysis is a very good test to identify UTIs, this test does not detect all cases of UTIs, so urine cultures must be ordered in all of these patients. Urine should be collected by bladder catheterization or suprapubic aspiration because bag urine specimens are associated with high rates of contamination. Because the peripheral WBC is a poor screening test for meningitis, a lumbar puncture should be performed in all febrile neonates. Chest radiographs are indicated in the presence of respiratory symptoms, and stool cultures are indicated in the presence of diarrhea.

Unlike the risk stratification rules derived for febrile young infants, no risk assessment criteria have been created and validated specifically for neonates, and attempts to extrapolate risk-stratification rules for infants to this neonatal group have been unsuccessful in identifying a subset of neonates at low risk of SBIs.

Febrile Young Infant

Febrile young infants, defined for the purposes of this chapter as children aged 29–56 days, are at high risk for bacterial infections. The most common cause of SBIs in this age group is UTIs. Young infants also develop bacteremia (most commonly from *E. coli*) and, much less frequently, bacterial meningitis.

Evaluation of these young infants has utilized various criteria to categorize patients as being at high or low risk for SBIs. Because relying solely on the clinical examination results in a substantial number of missed SBIs, laboratory testing is required for this age group. Several different sets of criteria have been derived to risk-stratify these patients (e.g., Rochester criteria, Boston criteria, and Philadelphia criteria). Although these criteria differ somewhat in the details, they have several components in common:

- Infants must be well-appearing
- No focal infection on physical examination
- Peripheral WBC count within a specified range
- Rapid urine testing without evidence of urinary tract infection

Blood and urine testing should be obtained in all patients. The results of these screening criteria help risk-stratify these young children. The need for lumbar puncture (LP) is controversial. Although the Boston and Philadelphia criteria require CSF analysis, the Rochester criteria does not mandate LP. In selected, full-term, well-appearing febrile infants, LP can be either performed or deferred, with the caveat that neither the clinical examination nor the peripheral WBC count is completely reliable in diagnosing meningitis in this age group. However, an abnormally high or low peripheral WBC count increases the concern for meningitis and thus an LP should be obtained in these children with these abnormalities if not initially obtained. Chest radiographs should be obtained in young febrile infants with signs of pulmonary disease (tachypnea ≥50 breaths/minute, rales, rhonchi, retractions, wheezing, coryza, grunting, nasal flaring, or cough). Stool studies for WBC counts and stool cultures should be ordered in patients with diarrhea.

The WBC count is considered abnormal if the count is >15,000/mm^3 or <5,000/mm^3 or if the band:neutrophil ratio is >0.2. The urine is considered abnormal if the urine dipstick is positive for nitrite or leukocyte esterase, if there are ≥5 WBCs/high power field (HPF) on microscopy, or if bacteria are seen on a gram-stained sample of uncentrifuged urine. The most common bacterial infections in this age group are UTIs; correspondingly, the most common bacterial pathogen identified in this age group is *E. coli*. If LP is performed, there should be <8 WBCs/mm^3 and no organisms on Gram stain of the CSF (although sterile CSF pleocytosis can be seen in a small percentage of febrile young infants with UTIs). If obtained, there should be <5 WBCs/HPF on the stool specimen and no evidence of pneumonia on chest X-ray.

Patients who meet low-risk criteria are typically discharged home, whereas those who fall into the high-risk category are usually started on antibiotics and admitted to the hospital. These criteria are generally very effective in identifying patients who are unlikely to have SBIs.

These risk stratification tools have had long-standing acceptance because of their high sensitivities and the universal availability of the tests for the rules, but they have been criticized for their lack of specificity and the need for LP (in the Boston and Philadelphia rules). More recent studies have focused on the use of procalcitonin to diagnose SBIs, with the hope that its use results in more accurate diagnosis of bacterial infection in these febrile young infants. The Step-by-Step approach incorporates patient appearance, urinalysis, procalcitonin, C-reactive protein, and the absolute neutrophil count (ANC) to identify patients at high, intermediate, or low risk for bacterial infection. A similar decision rule was developed by another research group, incorporating urinalysis, ANC, and procalcitonin to identify patients at low risk for bacterial infection. These rules have not been externally validated but demonstrate the promise of procalcitonin as a better screening test for bacterial infection.

Viral Testing

Rapid viral testing allows for the identification of potential sources of fever. Febrile young infants with any viral infection detected on viral testing have lower rates of SBIs compared to virus-negative patients. Specifically, the rates of SBIs in febrile young children are lower in patients who test positive with rhinovirus, respiratory syncytial virus, or influenza. Patients who were diagnosed clinically with bronchiolitis also had lower rates of SBIs compared to children without clinically diagnosed bronchiolitis. Although individual studies suggest that rapid viral testing leads to reduction in further testing, a meta-analysis of these data did not detect a difference in the rates of ancillary testing, antibiotic use, adverse events, or hospital admission in patients who underwent rapid viral testing in the ED. Febrile young infants with documented viral infections have a lower, but still substantial, risk of serious bacterial infection. Therefore, a positive viral test should not alter the ED workup in febrile neonates. Febrile young infants with positive viral tests still should undergo urine testing, and additional testing should be strongly considered.

HSV infections are a specific subset of viral infections requiring special consideration. Children with HSV infections usually present within the first 2 weeks of life, but HSV infection can be seen in infants up to age 9 weeks. Historical risk factors include primary maternal HSV infection, especially for neonates delivered vaginally; prolonged rupture of membranes; the use of fetal scalp electrodes; and seizures. Patients are at higher risk of HSV infection if they appear ill; have characteristic skin, eye, or mouth lesions; or have CSF pleocytosis. Patients with these risk factors should undergo HSV testing because delays to treatment are common.

TREATMENT

Neonatal

The baseline rate of SBIs in febrile neonates is high, and ED screening tools miss a significant number of bacterial infections. Thus, all febrile neonates should receive antibiotics. Typically, these patients are treated with third-generation cephalosporins, such as cefotaxime, 50 mg/kg intravenously (IV) (100 mg/kg if there is a concern for meningitis based on CSF results), or gentamicin, 2.5 mg/kg IV. Because of the concern of inducing unconjugated hyperbilirubinemia, ceftriaxone is not recommended for neonates who are jaundiced. Ampicillin, 50 mg/kg IV (100 mg/kg IV if there is a concern for meningitis), is recommended in the empiric treatment of these patients, although the incidence of *Listeria monocytogenes* is low. Patients who generate sufficient concern to undergo HSV testing should get empiric treatment with acyclovir (20 mg/kg IV). All febrile neonates should be hospitalized.

Young Infant

Patients who have abnormal test results or who appear to be too ill for discharge should receive empiric, broad-spectrum antibiotic therapy. Ceftriaxone, 50 mg/kg IV (100 mg/kg if meningitis is suspected), is commonly used for these patients. Additional antibiotics should be considered in select circumstances (e.g., ampicillin or vancomycin for suspected infection by *Listeria*, gram-positive cocci, or *Enterococcus*).

The role of empiric antibiotic therapy in patients who meet all risk screening criteria is controversial. Published recommendations state that parenteral antibiotics should be "considered" if an LP is performed. Ceftriaxone, 50 mg/kg IV or intramuscularly, can be given prior to discharge. Although these risk stratification algorithms perform very well, a small subset of patients with SBIs, including meningitis, will be missed, even with strict adherence to these criteria. In addition, there is some concern that performing an LP in a bacteremic patient may lead to meningitis. However, the vast majority of children who meet low-risk criteria will not benefit from empiric antibiotic therapy, and so withholding antibiotics in these low-risk patients is acceptable as well. Patients who did not undergo LP in the ED should not receive antibiotics because this will confound the evaluation for meningitis if the patients are still febrile on follow-up examination.

CLINICAL ALGORITHM

Figure 9.1 demonstrates an approach to the febrile child.

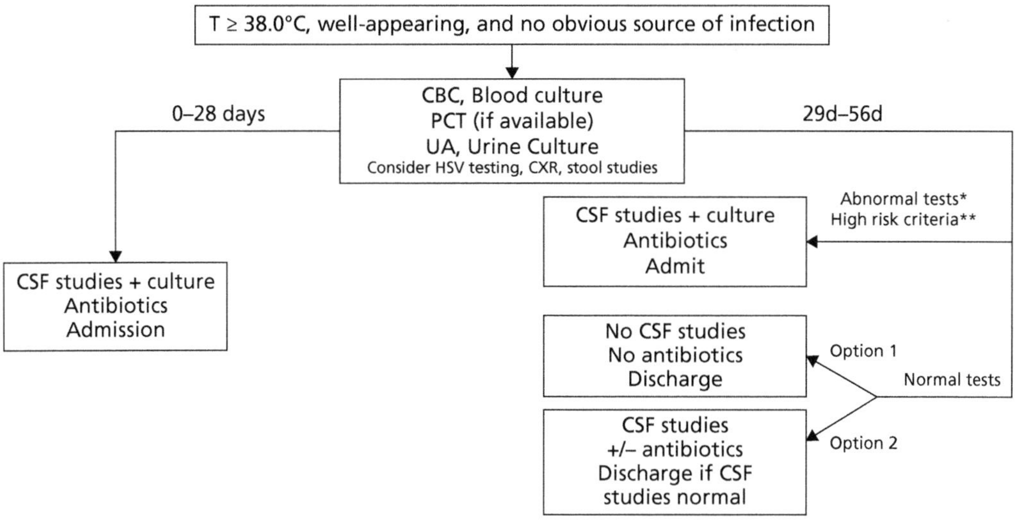

Abbreviations
CBC = Complete blood cell count
CXR = Chest X-ray
CSF = Cerebrospinal fluid
HSV = Herpes simplex virus testing
PCT = Procalcitonin
T = Temperature
UA = urinalysis

*Abnormal Test Results
CSF: ≥8 WBC/mm^3 and/or organisms on Gram stain
HSV Testing: Positive
Peripheral white blood cell count: <5000/mm^3 or >15,000/mm^3 and/or bands: neutrophil ratio > = 0.2
Procalcitonin (if available): ≥0.5 ng/mL
Urinalysis: Leukocyte esterase and/or nitrite positive and/or ≥5 white blood cells/high power field
CXR (if obtained): infiltrate
Stool (if obtained): > = 5 white blood cells/high power field

**High Risk Criteria
Antibiotics within 72 hours
Chronic medical problems
Prematurity < 37weeks gestation
Temperature ≥ 40°C

FIGURE 9.1 Approach to the febrile child aged ≤56 days.

DISPOSITION

Hospitalization is strongly recommended for all febrile neonates because the standard screening regimen still misses a substantial proportion of neonates with SBIs. Hospitalization is also generally recommended for febrile young infants with abnormal screening studies, with the exception of some patients who only have an abnormal urinalysis. Although there is considerable practice variation, recent studies suggest that selected patients in this age group with UTIs are at low risk for adverse sequelae, including meningitis, and may be treated on an outpatient basis.

Most febrile young infants who are otherwise healthy and born at full-term, well-appearing, and who have normal results on screening evaluation can be managed on an outpatient basis. If the caretakers have a working phone and can obtain follow-up within 24 hours, if they have a method of immediately accessing health care if there is a change in the patient's condition, and if the primary care physician understands and agrees with this plan of care, then the patient may be discharged home.

COMPLICATIONS

Untreated bacterial infections can lead to significant sequelae, including septic shock, brain injury, multiorgan dysfunction, and death. Although febrile seizures are common complications of fever in older children, a seizure associated with fever in an infant younger than age 6 months is, by definition, not a simple febrile seizure and thus requires appropriate diagnostic evaluation and testing.

KEY POINTS

- The febrile neonate (aged 0–28 days) is at high risk for serious infection, even with a benign examination and normal screening laboratory results. These patients all need blood, urine, and CSF cultures. Selected neonates will need HSV testing, as well as chest X-rays and stool cultures.
- All febrile neonates should receive empiric antibiotic coverage. Patients thought to be at risk for HSV infection should receive acyclovir as well.
- All febrile neonates should be admitted.
- Febrile young infants (aged 29—56 days) can be stratified into high- and low-risk categorizes based on results of diagnostic tests. These patients need complete blood counts, blood cultures, urinalyses, and urine cultures. An LP with CSF analysis can be considered. When clinically indicated, chest radiographs and stool studies should be obtained as well.
- If test findings are abnormal, these patients should receive ceftriaxone and should be admitted to the hospital. Discharge may be considered for a well-appearing young infant with an uncomplicated UTI.
- If the initial laboratory results are normal, a patient can be discharged if follow-up within 24 hours can be ensured. A dose of intramuscular ceftriaxone can be considered in patients who have undergone blood, urine, and CSF testing prior to ED discharge.

PITFALLS

- Relying solely on the examination and not performing laboratory testing in febrile neonates and young infants
- Not administering antibiotics and admitting all febrile neonates, regardless of test results
- Not ensuring timely follow-up for febrile young infants who are discharged home

Further Reading

Cruz AT, Freedman SB, Kulik DM, et al. Herpes simplex virus infection in infants undergoing meningitis evaluation. *Pediatrics.* 2018;141(2):e20171688.

Gomez B, Mintegi S, Bressan S, Da Dalt L, Gervaix A, Lacroix L. Validation of the "Step-by-Step" approach in the management of young febrile infants. *Pediatrics.* 2016;138(2):e20154381.

Krief WI, Levine DA, Platt SL, et al. Influenza virus infection and the risk of serious bacterial infections in young febrile infants. *Pediatrics.* 2009;124:30–39.

Kuppermann N, Dayan PS, Levine DA, et al. A clinical prediction rule to identify febrile infants 60 days and younger at low risk for serious bacterial infections. *JAMA Pediatrics.* 2019;173:342–351.

Levine DA, Platt SL, Dayan PS, et al. Risk of serious bacterial infection in young febrile infants with respiratory syncytial virus infections. *Pediatrics.* 2004;113:1728–1734.

Mace SE, Gemme SR, Valente JH, et al. Clinical policy for well-appearing infants and children younger than 2 years of age presenting to the emergency department with fever. *Ann Emerg Med.* 2016;67:625–39.e13.

Mahajan P, Browne LR, Levine DA, et al. Risk of bacterial coinfections in febrile infants 60 days old and younger with documented viral infections. *J Pediatr.* 2018;203:86–91.e2.

Mintegi S, Gomez B, Carro A, Diaz H, Benito J. Invasive bacterial infections in young afebrile infants with a history of fever. *Arch Dis Child.* 2018;103:665–669.

Mintegi S, Gomez B, Martinez-Virumbrales L, Morientes O, Benito J. Outpatient management of selected young febrile infants without antibiotics. *Arch Dis Child.* 2017;102:244–249.

Nigrovic LE, Mahajan PV, Blumberg SM, et al. The Yale Observation Scale score and the risk of serious bacterial infections in febrile infants. *Pediatrics.* 2017;140:e20170695.

Powell EC, Mahajan PV, Roosevelt G, et al. Epidemiology of bacteremia in febrile infants aged 60 days and younger. *Ann Emerg Med.* 2018;71:211–216.

Ramgopal S, Janofsky S, Zuckerbraun NS, et al. Risk of serious bacterial infection in infants aged ≤60 days presenting to emergency departments with a history of fever only. *J Pediatr.* 2019;204:191–195.

Rogers AJ, Kuppermann N, Anders J, et al. Practice variation in the evaluation and disposition of febrile infants ≤60 days of age. *J Emerg Med.* 2019;56:583–591.

Rosenfeld-Yehoshua N, Barkan S, Abu-Kishk I, Booch M, Suhami R, Kozer E. Hyperpyrexia and high fever as a predictor for serious bacterial infection (SBI) in children: A systematic review. *Eur J Pediatr.* 2018;177:337–344.

Schnadower D, Kuppermann N, Macias CG, et al. Outpatient management of young febrile infants with urinary tract infections. *Pediatr Emerg Care.* 2014;30:591–597.

Thomson J, Cruz AT, Nigrovic LE, et al. Concomitant bacterial meningitis in infants with urinary tract infection. *Pediatr Infect Dis J.* 2017;36:908–910.

Tzimenatos L, Mahajan P, Dayan PS, et al. Accuracy of the urinalysis for urinary tract infections in febrile infants 60 days and younger. *Pediatrics.* 2018;141(2):e20173068.

Velasco R, Benito H, Mozun R, Trujillo JE, Merino PA, Mintegi S. Febrile young infants with altered urinalysis at low risk for invasive bacterial infection: A Spanish Pediatric Emergency Research Network's study. *Pediatr Infect Dis J.* 2015;34:17–21.

Woll C, Neuman MI, Pruitt CM, et al. Epidemiology and etiology of invasive bacterial infection in infants ≤60 days old treated in emergency departments. *J Pediatr.* 2018;200:210-7.e1.

10

Evaluation of the Extended Fever

SHARON E. MACE

INCIDENCE OF FEVER

Of all emergency department (ED) visits for pediatric patients annually, fever is the most frequent complaint. Fever accounts for 15% of all pediatric ED visits and 30% of all pediatric outpatient visits.

DEFINITIONS

Definitions of fever vary. Unfortunately, what constitutes a fever and the various definitions related to fever are not uniformly agreed upon. Traditionally, normal body temperature has been defined as 37°C (98.6°F) based on an adult study of axillary temperatures in the 19th century in which 38°C (100.4°F) was the upper limit of normal. This is the cutoff [e.g., a rectal temperature of 38°C (100.4°F)] when considering a serious bacterial infection (SBI). Yet for a persistent fever or fever of unknown origin (FUO), the cutoff value has been defined as a temperature >38.3°C (>101°F).

Fever without a source (FWS), also referred to a fever without a focus, is an acute fever of ≤1 week duration without localizing signs. It is diagnosed if, after a careful history and physical examination, a specific etiology of the fever cannot be identified.

The original definition of FUO in adults was a fever >38.3°C (>101°F) on several occasions, persisting for ≥3 weeks despite at least 1 week's investigation in hospital or, more recently, after a reasonable outpatient or inpatient evaluation or after history, physical examination, and some preliminary studies for infectious, autoimmune, or neoplastic etiologies fail to determine a diagnosis. Controversy remains regarding the definition of FUO in children, but it has more recently suggested to be ≥8 days duration.

For all these definitions, the common denominator is that the cutoff temperature is generally >38.3°C (>101°F) and there is no etiology even after a history, physical examination, and some diagnostic testing or evaluation has been done, although the required fever duration varies. The timeline of 7–10 days is generally used in pediatrics because most viral illnesses in children last <7–10 days, and any duration longer than that often portends a more serious etiology for the fever. Setting an exact time cutoff is difficult because there are no explicit criteria. However, because FWS is ≤7 days, perhaps a practical definition of FUO in pediatrics is a fever lasting ≥8 days in a child or infant for whom an evaluation including a detailed and thorough history and physical examination combined with an initial diagnostic workup (e.g., appropriate laboratory and radiology studies) have not yielded an etiology for the fever (Box 10.1).

Persistent fever or FUO must not be confused with a "pseudo FUO," in which one febrile illness follows another but there are different etiologies for the two (or more) respective febrile illnesses. Often, the first of these sequential febrile illnesses is viral with

BOX 10.1
STUDIES OFTEN INCLUDED IN THE INITIAL EVALUATION OF A FEVER OF UNKNOWN ORIGIN

Laboratory Tests

Hematology tests
- CBC: leukocyte count and differential, hemoglobin/hematocrit, platelet count

Metabolic tests
- Glucose, renal function tests: BUN, creatinine
- Electrolytes: sodium, potassium, chloride, CO_2, calcium, magnesium
- Liver function tests: total bilirubin, alkaline phosphatase, ALT (also known as SGPT), AST (also known as SGOT), albumin, total protein

Inflammatory markers
- ESR, CRP level

Urine
- Urinalysis

Tuberculosis tests
- TST or IGRA; if aged <5 years, TST, not IGRA, should be performed

Other tests
- Lactate dehydrogenase
- Creatine kinase
- Protein electrophoresis

Depending on history and physical examination
- If infection is considered: blood cultures, urine cultures
- If autoimmune disorder is suspected: anti-nuclear antibodies, rheumatoid factor

Radiology Studies

- Chest X-ray
- Abdominal ultrasound; if ultrasound is not helpful, consider abdominal CT scan

ALT, alanine aminotransferase; AST, aspartate aminotransferase; BUN, blood urea nitrogen; CBC, complete blood count; CRP, C-reactive protein; CT, computed tomography; ESR, erythrocyte sedimentation rate; IGRA, interferon-γ release assay; SGOT, serum glutamic oxaloacetic transaminase; SGPT, serum glutamic pyruvic transaminase; TST, tuberculin skin test.

nonspecific symptoms associated with the fever, so a specific diagnosis is not made.

HYPERTHERMIA

Fever is an elevated body temperature that is one component of the body's physiologic response to a pathogen. Fever is an increased body temperature with an *increased* hypothalamic set point. Fever should be differentiated from hyperthermia. Hyperthermia is an increased body temperature that ensues with a normal hypothalamic thermoregulatory set point resulting from an abnormal equilibrium or homeostasis in which the body's heat production is greater than the body's ability to dissipate heat. Hyperthermia generally is due to environmental heat exposure (heat illness) or drugs that disrupt normal thermoregulation in the central nervous system (CNS), the periphery, or both. Heat illness refers to the range of disorders caused by environmental exposure to heat and ranges from heat cramps to heatstroke, which is the most severe case of heat illness.

PATHOPHYSIOLOGY OF FEVER

Fever, a physiologic defensive response by the body (or the host) to the invasion of microorganisms coordinated by the thermoregulatory region of the brain located primarily in the anterior hypothalamus and the preoptic area, results in an elevation of the core body temperature above normal. Neuroendocrine, hepatic, and hematopoietic changes, and alterations in the components of the plasma, occur in addition to fever.

What Is the Normal Temperature?

Traditionally, the normal body temperature has been defined as 37°C (98.6°F) based on a 19th-century study of multiple axillary temperature measurements in approximately 25,000 healthy adults. A study from the late 20th century confirmed the diurnal variation in temperature and found a mean oral temperature in healthy adults to be 36.8°C (98.2°F), with the upper limit of the normal oral temperature range in healthy adults aged 40 years or younger being 37.2°C (98.9°F) at 6 a.m. an 37.7°C (99.9°F) at 4 p.m.

At any given point in time, the body has many different temperatures depending on the body part or site of measurement. The body can be grouped into two compartments: the core and the shell. The core includes the thoracic viscera, the brain, and the arterial and central venous blood. The shell insulates the core of the body from the environment and consists primarily of the skin but also the subcutaneous fat and bones. Tissues nearer the body surface generally have lower temperatures than deeper tissues. During shock and extreme environmental conditions, these differences in body temperature based on location in the body tend to be greater. Body organs with higher metabolic rates have higher temperatures than organs with lower metabolic rates. Organs with higher metabolic rates can have a temperature 1.3°C (2.3°F) higher than that of arterial blood.

Site of Anatomic Measurement of Temperature

Traditionally, rectal temperatures have been considered the most accurate and practical or easiest method for measuring core temperature. In general, rectal temperatures are 0.4°C (0.8°F) higher than simultaneous oral and 0.8°C (1.6°F) higher than simultaneous tympanic membrane temperatures.

Variations in Body Temperature

Body temperature varies according to age, gender, time of day, location or site of body where temperature is measured, and other factors.

Body temperature follows the normal circadian rhythm, associated with the sleep–wake cycle. Body temperature is lowest in the early morning hours between 2 and 8 a.m. (nadir at approximately 6 a.m.) and highest in the afternoon between 4 and 9 p.m. (peak between 4 and 6 p.m.). The variation may be as great a 1°C (1.8°F). Newborns up to age 8 weeks are an exception to this circadian rhythm, having hourly variations in their body temperature. The adult circadian rhythm variation in temperature is present by age 10 weeks. Mean rectal temperatures vary based on age and are higher in infants and young children than in older children.

Temperature Measurement

Evaluation for a persistent fever or FUO can be time-consuming and expensive, and some testing may be uncomfortable and/or frightening for a young child. Thus, there should be documentation of a fever prior to embarking on an extensive evaluation.

First, determine if there really is a fever. Ask, "How did you take the temperature?" Did the parent touch the child and conclude the child felt warm and thus had a fever? A parent's tactile perception of fever may be fairly accurate and should not be discounted. In addition, documentation of a fever at home should be considered valid even if the temperature in the ED is normal.

Devices for Measuring Temperature

Digital thermometers are most commonly used. However, in general, they are less accurate in infants and young children and are more apt to underestimate body temperature. Forehead thermometers, which may be infrared contact or noncontact devices, measure the amount of heat produced by the temporal arteries. There is much variation between temporal artery and rectal temperature measurements. Therefore, the following thermometers should not be used when making clinical decisions, such as whether to initiate a "septic" workup or evaluation for a SBI: infrared tympanic membrane, temporal artery, and infrared, liquid crystal thermometers.

Anatomic Site of Temperature Measurement

Considerable differences in temperature can exist depending on the anatomic site at which the temperature is taken.

Rectal

For measuring body temperature, rectal temperatures are considered more accurate (i.e., closest to core body temperature) than temperatures at other sites, including axillary, oral, skin, and tympanic sites. Rectal temperatures are the gold standard for measurement of core temperature and are recommended if the temperature measurement has implications for care, such as whether to initiate a "septic" workup or evaluation for an SBI in infants and young children. According to the American Academy of Pediatrics, oral thermometry is preferred for children aged 4 years or older, and rectal thermometry is preferred for younger children, especially infants younger than age 1 year. In neutropenic or immunocompromised patients, rectal temperatures are contraindicated because bacterial systemic seeding may occur.

Oral

Oral temperatures are also deemed to be accurate. Oral temperatures are usually obtained in older children and adolescents who are able to cooperate. Oral temperatures are generally 0.4–0.6°C (0.7–1.0°F) lower than rectal readings. Accurate oral temperatures may be difficult to obtain in children younger than age 5 years or uncooperative patients. Recent per os intake of cold or hot liquids and tachypnea may affect the oral temperature.

Axillary

Axillary temperatures can be used in patients unable to cooperate and in neutropenic patients who cannot use an oral thermometer and in whom rectal temperatures are contraindicated. Axillary temperatures are lower than rectal temperatures. In older children, axillary temperatures may be ≥0.5°–0.6°C (0.92°–1°F) lower than rectal temperatures.

Tympanic

Infrared tympanic membrane thermometry measures the heat production by the tympanic membrane. Although easy to obtain and less traumatic than rectal measurements, these devices are less accurate and should not be used for clinical management decisions.

Skin

Like tympanic thermometry, skin (e.g., forehead) measurements are quicker and less traumatic than rectal temperatures and can be used for screening, but they cannot replace rectal temperature measurements. Vascular changes (e.g., shock) and sweating may affect forehead temperature measurement.

ETIOLOGIES FOR PERSISTENT FEVER OR FEVER OF UNKNOWN ORIGIN

In pediatric patients, unexplained fever, especially that lasting <8 days, is most commonly due to a viral illness. The majority of these shorter episodes of unexplained fever, including FWS, resolve spontaneously, or signs and/or symptoms will develop, thus allowing for recognition of a given illness. The failure to attain a diagnosis in FUO patients is thought to be higher now than in the past (i.e., before the 1990s) for many reasons, including improved diagnostic techniques (e.g., computed tomography and magnetic resonance imaging) and the fact that patients with fever seek medical care (or are brought by their families) for their fever much earlier than in the past.

Etiology of Fever of Unknown Origin by Category

The etiology of FUO is generally grouped into five categories: infections, neoplasms, noninfectious inflammatory diseases (connective tissue disorders), other or miscellaneous, and undiagnosed. In children, infections are the number one etiology for a FUO.

Viral infections, urinary tract infections, osteomyelitis, cat scratch fever (Bartonellosis), and tuberculosis are some of the most common infectious etiologies. The majority of FUOs are due to unusual manifestations of common diseases/disorders rather than due to a rare disease/disorder.

Infectious diseases are subdivided into systemic and localized infections (Box 10.2). The most frequent etiologies for localized infections tend to be common pediatric infections, whereas the systemic infections tend to be less common .

Almost any malignancy can cause a fever. Leukemia and lymphoma are the most frequent malignancies responsible for pediatric FUO, although solid tumors can also be the underlying reason for pediatric FUO (Box 10.3).

Rheumatologic disorders or connective tissue diseases are a significant cause of FUO in children, with juvenile idiopathic arthritis (previously termed juvenile rheumatoid arthritis) being the most common. Systemic lupus erythematous may also cause FUO.

BOX 10.2

ETIOLOGY OF FEVER OF UNKNOWN ORIGIN: INFECTIONS

Localized infectious diseases
- Upper respiratory tract infections, including tonsillitis/pharyngitis
- Localized ear, nose, and throat infections: otitis media, sinusitis, mastoiditis
- Urinary tract infections and pyelonephritis
- Joint/bone infections: osteomyelitis, septic arthritis
- Undiagnosed abscesses: most commonly abdominal abscesses, including hepatic abscesses, pelvic abscesses, perinephric abscesses, subdiaphragmatic abscesses
- Sexually transmitted diseases
- Endocarditis: uncommon, but consider if history of heart disease, especially valvular heart disease

Systemic infectious diseases
- Viruses
  - Infectious mononucleosis: Epstein–Barr virus
  - Hepatitis viruses
  - Cytomegalovirus
  - Adenoviruses
  - Arboviruses such as arthropod-borne encephalitis, including West Nile virus, St. Louis encephalitis
  - Herpes viruses
  - HIV (less common)
- Bacteria
  - Cat scratch fever (Bartonellosis)
  - Salmonellosis
  - Tuberculosis
  - Brucellosis
  - Tuleremia
  - Spirochetes: leptospirosis
  - Chlamydophila: lymphogranuloma venereum
  - Chlamydophila: psittacosis (parrot fever)
- Other infectious agents
  - *Rickettsia*: Rocky Mountain spotted fever
  - Parasites: malaria, toxoplasmosis

Vasculitis is another noninfectious disease that can cause FUO. Polyarteritis arteritis nodosa is in this grouping. Kawasaki disease is also generally placed in the vasculitis category. In young children, especially those younger than age <1 year, Kawasaki disease should be in the differential of FUO. All infants with an unexplained fever lasting ≥7 days should have laboratory evaluation for Kawasaki (see Chapter 23 on dermatologic emergencies).

Inflammatory bowel disease, especially Crohn's disease and, less frequently, ulcerative colitis, can present with fever and a paucity of gastrointestinal complaints and should be in the differential of pediatric FUO.

CNS dysfunction that can occur with severe brain damage or various CNS diseases may result in abnormal thermoregulation with an elevated body temperature.

Drugs—whether prescription, over-the-counter, illicit or illegal, vitamins, herbal supplements, or anesthetics—can be the underlying cause of a pediatric FUO. Generally, when the drug is stopped, the fever dissipates in 2 or 3 days, but it may take 1 or more weeks before the fever disappears.

Another cause of pediatric FUO is a factitious fever, which refers to a false report of a fever or manipulation of body temperature (e.g., by placing the thermometer into a hot liquid) by

BOX 10.3

ETIOLOGY OF FEVER OF UNKNOWN ORIGIN: NONINFECTIOUS[A]

Noninfectious inflammatory diseases
- Connective tissue diseases (rheumatologic disorders)
  - Juvenile idiopathic arthritis (most common in this category; >90% of FUOs in this category in multiple series of FUOs)
  - Systemic lupus erythematosus
- Vasculitis
  - Kawasaki disease, including incomplete forms, especially in those younger than age 5 years
  - Polyarteritis nodosa

Neoplasms (malignancies)
- Leukemia
- Lymphoma
- Hodgkin's lymphoma
- Solid tumors

Gastrointestinal
- Inflammatory bowel disease: ulcerative colitis, Crohn's disease, other colitis (drug-induced, pseudomembranous), etc.

Central nervous system disorders
- Central nervous system lesions/diseases: severe brain damage, tumor, central diabetes insipidus

Periodic fevers, including familial Mediterranean fever

Drug-related fevers: should be considered with almost any drug—prescription drugs, illegal or illicit drugs, over-the-counter drugs, herbal supplements, vitamins, anesthetics; by any route of administration—intravenous, intramuscular, intranasal, oral, rectal, topical; also includes serum sickness

Factitious fever includes Munchausen syndrome

Rare, often inherited disorders: immunodeficiencies, cyclic neutropenia, hemophagocytic lymphohistiocytosis, endocrine—thyrotoxicosis, nephrogenic diabetes insipidus, infantile cortical hyperostosis (Caffey disease), familial dysautonomia (Riley–Day syndrome), Kikuchi (Kikuchi–Fujimoto) disease

[a]For the etiology of FUO, key items are mentioned. This is a comprehensive but not all-inclusive list.
FUO, fever of unknown origin.

a parent or caregiver. Munchausen's syndrome (also known as Munchausen syndrome by proxy) occurs when an individual, usually the parent or caregiver, fabricates the symptoms and signs of a child's illness. In cases in which Munchausen syndrome involves a fever, the parent or caregiver may inject the child with infectious and/or foreign substances to cause the fever.

A number of uncommon disorders can lead to FUO. Diabetes insipidus, whether central or nephrogenic, can lead to FUO. Endocrine disease, specifically thyrotoxicosis, is in the differential of a pediatric FUO. Multiple, usually inherited, rare disorders may be responsible for a pediatric FUO. These include periodic fevers (e.g., familial Mediterranean fever), some immunoglobulin deficiencies, cyclic neutropenia (also known as cyclic hematopoiesis), hemophagocytic lymphohistiocytosis, infantile cortical hyperostosis (Caffey disease), familial dysautonomia, and Kikuchi disease (also referred to as Kikuchi–Fujimoto disease).

Evaluation of the Child or Infant with a Fever of Unknown Origin

Hospitalization may be indicated for the pediatric patient with an FUO if the child or infant has a toxic appearance or looks acutely ill, has unstable vital signs, is showing signs of clinical deterioration, has worsening or progressive symptoms, or has significant associated signs or symptoms in addition to the fever (e.g., petechiae or a new murmur); if there is concern for child maltreatment (as with neglect or Munchausen syndrome); if it is necessary to observe the child or infant in a supervised or controlled environment; or if there is a need for studies/procedures best coordinated in an inpatient setting.

First, does the fever meet the criteria for an FUO? What is the pattern, height, and duration of the fever? History is of paramount importance. Has there been an association with the outdoors (as with Rocky Mountain spotted fever, Lyme disease, or tularemia) or animals (as with cat scratch fever or reptiles associated with *Salmonella*, psittacosis, or brucellosis) or recent travel (e.g., to areas endemic with malaria, chikungunya, or tuberculosis). Is there the possibility of an inherited disorder (e.g., Mediterranean or Middle Eastern descent for familial Mediterranean fever, Jewish descent with familial dysautonomia, or Kikuchi disease with young Asian females)? Dietary history might reveal contaminated food, such as poultry or eggs with *Salmonella* and ingestion of game meat (e.g., venison) with toxoplasmosis. Leptospirosis follows exposure to a contaminated environment in a tropical climate such as after swimming in contaminated water, with the portal of entry through mucous membranes, conjunctiva, or non-intact skin (e.g., skin with abrasions or cuts). Is the patient taking any drugs? Is there any weight loss as might occur with malignancy, diabetes mellitus or insipidus, inflammatory bowel disease, or other systemic conditions?

Physical examination may reveal a source of infection. In infants and young children, is there tenderness over a bone or joint suggesting osteomyelitis or a septic joint or infantile cortical hyperostosis? Is there a new murmur as with endocarditis? Is there hepatomegaly or right upper quadrant tenderness as might occur with a liver abscess? Splenomegaly could be a clue to Epstein–Barr virus infection. The presence of a rash may be helpful. Petechiae can occur with endocarditis, meningococcemia, bacteremia, as well as viral and rickettsial infections. Is there the classic rash of lupus or Lyme disease? Examination of the head, eyes, ears, nose, and throat may suggest a local infection from pharyngitis, sinusitis, or mastoiditis. Lymphadenopathy may be a clue to neoplastic disease, an infection, or an inherited disorder. Is there conjunctivitis or oral mucosal changes characteristic of Kawasaki disease? Does the genitourinary examination suggest a sexually transmitted disease (genital lesions, ulcers or rashes, or discharge)? Is there abdominal tenderness or a perianal fistula as might occur with an inflammatory bowel disease? Are there signs of dehydration as might occur with diabetes mellitus or insipidus? Is the neurologic examinations indicative of CNS dysfunction, resulting in disordered thermoregulation? Is there any muscle tenderness, which may occur with trichinellosis, vasculitis (e.g., polyarteritis nodosa), rheumatologic disorders (e.g., dermatomyositis), and some arbovirus infections? Are the deep tendon reflexes (DTRs) abnormal? Hyperreflexia may occur with hyperthyroidism, whereas absent or hypoactive DTRs occur with familial dysautonomia.

Laboratory and ancillary studies should be directed by the history and physical examination findings. The following laboratory tests are commonly performed: glucose, renal function tests (blood urea nitrogen and creatinine), liver function tests, electrolytes (which may all be included in a complete metabolic profile), complete blood count/differential, smear, urinalysis, and acute phase reactants—erythrocyte sedimentation rate, C-reactive protein, and cultures (blood, urine, and stool). Radiology studies such as chest radiograph are also commonly performed. If there is right upper quadrant (RUQ) tenderness and/or hepatomegaly, an ultrasound of the RUQ may be indicated (see Table 10.1). Medications should be discontinued, if possible, to assess for the possibility of drug-related fever. Other studies are guided by history and physical examination.

TREATMENT

Fever is part of an overall physiologic response to an infection. Fever is part of the body's inflammatory defensive response to invading pathogens. Whether fever in the previously healthy individual needs to be treated has been questioned. Whether fever is beneficial or harmful has been debated. Fever is part of the inflammatory response, and it may inhibit the growth and reproduction of some microorganisms (e.g., bacteria and viruses). However, at higher temperatures (~40°C or higher), these positive effects are lessened or lost or may have a negative impact. Some studies indicate that fever may impair immunologic response. Moreover, whether animal and/or in vitro studies on fever are applicable to humans is unknown.

The answer to the question, "Is fever is beneficial or harmful, and should we treat fever with antipyretics?" may be "It depends." The previously healthy child with fever from a mild viral illness is very different from the critically ill patient or the patient with a traumatic brain injury; thus, management of fever may likely differ depending on the clinical scenario.

Fever does have some negative effects. Fever makes individuals uncomfortable. Fever increases the metabolic rate, oxygen consumption, carbon dioxide production, and demands on the cardiac and pulmonary systems. In individuals with limited or no cardiac or pulmonary reserve, these increased demands can be harmful and counter the immunologic benefits of fever. In individuals with inherited metabolic and mitochondrial disorders, any catabolic stress should be avoided, and infections and fever should be treated. Fever in the presence of traumatic brain injury, subarachnoid hemorrhage, and stroke is associated with worse neurologic outcomes.

Who Should Receive Antipyretic Treatment for Fever?

Fever phobia is the term used to describe the misconceptions and anxiety about fever. Antipyretic therapy does not prevent the recurrence of febrile seizures. Except at high temperatures, fever, by itself, is not dangerous. Side effects during and after a febrile illness are generally not related to the fever but, rather, to the febrile illness or are caused by the antipyretic drug. However, a recent meta-analysis found that there are no data indicating that antipyretic use prolongs illness in children. It may also be useful to treat a child or infant with an antipyretic to determine whether the child's condition or activity level was related to the underlying illness or to the fever, although response to an antipyretic with a decrease in the temperature by itself does not predict the underlying severity of the disease.

The recommendations are that fever should be treated in individuals with limited cardiopulmonary reserve; those with inherited mitochondrial or metabolic disorders; those with underlying neurologic disorders; those in shock; those with burns; postoperative patients; those recovering from cardiac arrest; those with significant head trauma, subarachnoid hemorrhage, stroke (because of the increased metabolic rates with fever), and high fever (≥40°C); and for symptomatic treatment in those who are uncomfortable from the fever.

What Should the Treatment Be for Fever?

Because of the association with aspirin and Reyes syndrome, aspirin should be avoided for the treatment of fever. Acetaminophen is administered in a dose of 10–15 mg/kg (maximum of 1 g/dose) every 4–6 hours, with a maximum of five doses in a 24-hour period, 75 mg/kg/day up to a maximum of 4 g. In appropriate doses, acetaminophen is safe. However, if any skin reactions occur, acetaminophen should be stopped because Stevens–Johnson syndrome and toxic epidermal necrolysis can occur, although these side effects are rare. Ibuprofen is given in a dose of 10 mg/kg, with a maximum of 600 mg/dose up to a daily maximum of 40 mg/kg up to 2.4 g/day. Ibuprofen should not be used in children younger than age 6 months due to diminished renal clearance and increased risk of bleeding. When taken with food and in appropriate doses, ibuprofen is generally safe, although gastritis, gastrointestinal bleeding, and kidney injury have been reported.

FEVER PEARLS

- Do not use tympanic or skin temperatures when deciding whether or not to initiate a fever workup for SBI in infants and young children.
- Do not take rectal temperatures in neutropenic or immunocompromised patients.
- Do not dismiss parental tactile assessment of fever because a parent's tactile assessment of fever has a similar sensitivity and specificity as those of axillary and tympanic thermometry.
- Do not use alcohol (in a sponge bath or applied directly to the skin) to decrease body temperature.

KEY POINTS

- Oral and axillary temperatures are generally lower than rectal temperatures.
- Oral thermometry is preferred for children older than age 4 years, and rectal thermometry is preferred in younger children, especially infants younger than age 1 year (according to the American Academy of Pediatrics).
- Body temperature varies according to many factors, including age, gender, location/site of measurement, activity,

postprandial, pregnancy, environment, bundling, climate, and season.
- By itself, fever is not harmful (except for high temperatures in pathological states).
- Fever is only one component of the body's physiologic/immunologic response to an invading microbial organism.
- In both fever and hyperthermia, there is an increase in body temperature. Fever occurs with an increase in the normal hypothalamic set point, whereas hyperthermia occurs with a normal hypothalamic set point.
- There are five main categories of FUO: infections, noninfectious inflammatory diseases (rheumatologic or connective tissue disorders), malignancies, other or miscellaneous, and undiagnosed.
- In pediatric patients, FUO is due to infections (systemic or localized; (~50%), noninfectious etiology (~25%), or is undiagnosed or unexplained (~25%), with bacterial infections accounting for approximately half of the infections. In adults, neoplasms account for approximately 50% of FUOs.
- Most FUOs are due to atypical or unusual presentations of common disorders rather than a rare disease.

PITFALLS

Failure to treat fever in appropriate patients, including:

- Those with limited cardiopulmonary reserve
- Mitochondrial or metabolic disorders
- Shock
- Postoperative patients
- Post-cardiac arrest patients
- Neurologic disorders
- Stroke
- Traumatic brain injury
- Subarachnoid hemorrhage
- High fever and those uncomfortable from the fever

Further Reading

Hara M, Takao S. Five-year study of viral etiology and features of febrile respiratory tract infections with prolonged fever in Japanese pediatric outpatients. *Pediatr Infect Dis J.* 2017;36(12):e358–e360.

Long SS. Diagnosis and management of undifferentiated fever in children. *J Infection.* 2016;72:S68–S76.

Mace SE, Gemmes SR, Valente JH, et al. Clinical policy for well-appearing infants and children younger than 2 years of age presenting to the emergency department with fever. *Ann Emerg Med.* 2016;67(5):625–639.

Purssell E, While AE. Does the use of antipyretics in children who have acute infections prolong febrile illness? A systematic review and meta-analysis. *J Pediatr.* 2013;163(3):822–827.e1–2.

Wright WF. Fever of unknown origin. In: Bennett JE, Dolin R, Blaser MJ, et al. eds. *Mandell, Douglas, and Bennett's Principles and Practice of Infectious Diseases.* 9th ed, Philadelphia, PA: Elsevier; 2020:721–731.

11

Common Infections in Children

SOLOMON BEHAR

UPPER RESPIRATORY INFECTIONS

Background

Viral upper respiratory infections (URIs) are the second most common reason, after fever, that a child is brought to medical attention, representing 7.7% of pediatric emergency department (ED) visits. They are caused by a wide variety of viruses, including (but not limited to) rhinovirus, parainfluenza, influenza, respiratory syncytial virus, adenovirus, influenza, and coronavirus. Patients may present at any age and present with cough, congestion and/or rhinorrhea, along with fever of any height early on in the illness. Typically, the fever defervesces after the first few days of illness, whereas the cough and nasal symptoms often persist for days to weeks. Infants are obligate nose breathers and may present with poor feeding and, in extreme cases, dehydration or, rarely, cyanosis while feeding if nasal obstruction is severe.

Differential Diagnosis

Differential diagnosis includes viral URI, infectious pneumonia, aspiration pneumonia, otitis media, sinus infections, bronchiolitis, asthma exacerbations, congestive heart failure, foreign body aspiration, nasal foreign body, gastroesophageal reflux, and congenital airway anomalies.

Diagnostic Confirmation

The diagnosis of viral URI is clinical, often aided by the absence of features of lower airway disease (clear bilateral breath sounds, normal pulse oximetry, and the absence of wheezing). When acute otitis media is present, they are almost universally preceded by a viral URI. Radiography is unnecessary unless there is diagnostic uncertainty or concern for lower airway disease or foreign body aspiration. Data are mixed regarding the use of viral rapid respiratory polymerase chain reaction (PCR) testing. Viral PCR array testing may help diagnose specific viruses causing URIs, but it is expensive and time-consuming. However, some overall cost reduction, decreased use of chest X-rays (CXRs), and more judicious use of antibiotics may be afforded by rapid viral respiratory testing. During influenza season, rapid viral PCR testing affords more accurate use of anti-influenza medication. Viral respiratory PCR tests may remain positive for many weeks after initial infection, reflecting past infections instead of the current illness, which may confuse the clinical picture.

Treatment

Treatment is largely supportive, with nasal saline and suction using bulb syringes or a handheld parent-controlled suction device. Over-the-counter cough suppressants are ineffective and potentially dangerous in younger children and should be avoided. Children older than age 1 year may try honey as needed for cough suppression, and this may be as effective as dextromethorphan and better than placebo or diphenhydramine. Use of honey has not been studied in children aged 1 to 2 years, although it is reasonable to use it for this age group. Antibiotics are not indicated except in cases in which a URI has progressed into AOM or there is suspicion for bacterial sinusitis. (See Chapter 39 for further discussion on sinus infections.)

Disposition

Most children with URIs may be sent home with supportive care and instructions to return if they develop respiratory distress, cyanosis, apnea, or prolonged fevers (>5 days).

Complications

Most viral URIs are self-limited and benign. URIs can lead to development of AOM and its sequelae and sinus infections. A viral URI is a common prodrome to more severe infections, such as bacterial meningitis and pneumonia. Rarely, systemic sequelae may occur, including myopericarditis (discussed later) and delayed neurologic conditions (see Chapter 20 on neurologic emergencies).

Key Points

Viral URI is one of the most common diagnoses seen in the pediatric ED. The vast majority of these will be self-limited illness not requiring testing, imaging, or antibiotics.

Pitfalls

Consider retained nasal foreign body if you see unilateral rhinorrhea, especially if it is foul smelling and in a child in the toddler age range. Assess for a history of foreign body aspiration in the afebrile young child with abrupt-onset cough. Sinus infection may be considered in the setting of (1) prolonged rhinorrhea (>10 days), (2) severe purulent rhinorrhea with fever for more than 3 consecutive days, or (3) a worsening of thick rhinorrhea after initial improvement ("re-sickening"). Always examine the tympanic membranes in the setting of fever and URI because AOM can develop following URI. Nasopharyngitis is the usual prodrome of bacterial meningitis, so make sure to clinically evaluate for this condition. Pulse oximetry in children with viral URIs should be normal; if it is low, you should suspect lower airway disease instead of a simple URI (see Chapter 15 for further discussion on respiratory infections).

ACUTE GASTROENTERITIS

Background

Acute gastroenteritis (AGE) is a common intestinal ailment in children of all ages presenting with vomiting, diarrhea, abdominal pain, and +/- fevers. Most viral causes of AGE present with nonbloody, nonbilious vomiting and watery, nonbloody diarrhea. Since the advent of the rotavirus vaccine, ED and inpatient hospitalizations for rotavirus AGE have plummeted, while norovirus is now the most common viral cause of AGE in children in the United States. Among children younger than age 5 years, norovirus and rotavirus have similar incidences, and they are still the most commonly detected pathogens seen in AGE. Chronic diarrhea (lasting >14 day) can be infectious, but noninfectious etiologies such as milk protein allergy or other food-induced allergy should be considered. in children younger than age 2 years with chronic diarrhea. *Clostridium dificile* testing should only be performed in infants if they have evidence of pseudomembranous colitis, toxic megacolon, or if they have clinically significant diarrhea and other causes of diarrhea have been excluded. This is because up to 40% of infants (<1 year of age) are colonized with this bacteria, and the results of this assay will be difficult to interpret if it comes back positive. The decision on whether to treat for *C. dificile* in infancy should be made in consultation with an infectious disease or gastroenterology specialist.

Differential Diagnosis

Vomiting and diarrhea can be presenting symptoms of a variety of viral, bacterial, or parasitic infections. Food-borne illness, zoonoses, malabsorptive processes [e.g., exocrine pancreas dysfunction, celiac disease, and inflammatory bowel disease (IBD)], paraneoplastic processes such as a VIPoma (vasoactive intestinal peptide) seen in neuroblastoma, antibiotic-associated diarrhea, and post-antibiotic *C. dificile*-associated colitis are other considerations. Primary immune deficiency may present with chronic diarrhea, fungal infections, and failure to thrive.

Diagnostic Confirmation

Viral AGE is usually a clinical diagnosis. When stools are bloody or if presentation is severe, stool studies may be sent. Newer stool PCR assays allow for timely diagnosis to be made, although most viral and many bacterial causes are self-limited conditions and the cost-effectiveness of these assays has not been established.

Stool cultures are still done in many institutions, but they are limited in utility given long turnaround times. Sending stool for ova and parasites can be helpful in cases with a history of travel, well water, outdoor swimming, camping, or other outdoor exposure. Giardia and cryptosporidiosis can be detected with enzyme immunoassays or direct fluorescent antibody testing in those at risk.

Treatment

Oral hydration with a balanced electrolyte solution is the cornerstone of therapy in acute AGE. No liquids or foods are contraindicated in AGE. However, lactose-containing rehydration liquids (cow's milk products, most standard formulas for infants, and breastmilk) may be difficult to absorb in acute AGE because the inner lining of the small intestine villi containing the lactase enzyme is sloughed off during acute AGE. Younger infants (<6 months old) should continue to breastfeed ad libitum through the illness. For prolonged diarrheal symptoms, a temporary trial of lactose-free formula may be helpful, especially if gassiness and bloating are an ongoing problem.

If the child exhibits signs of mild to moderate dehydration and is unable to tolerate an oral challenge, intravenous (IV) or subcutaneous (also called "hypodermoclysis") rehydration should be instituted, along with correction of electrolyte abnormalities. This is done by placing a butterfly needle in the subcutaneous tissue located between the shoulder blades and instilling 150 units of recombinant hyaluronidase enzyme to break up the connective tissue to allow for absorption of the IV fluids into the subcutaneous space, where it will be absorbed into the venous system. Hypodermoclysis should not be used in cases of hypovolemic shock; instead, intraosseous or central line venous access should be obtained to rapidly rehydrate the patient. Oral antiemetics such as ondansetron (0.15 mg/kg IV, PO, or oral dissolving tablet) is safe and effective in reducing the need for IV fluids. A limited number of doses (1- or 2-day supply) may be prescribe for use at home in children older than age 2 years. For severe dehydration or hypovolemic shock, isotonic fluid resuscitation with boluses of 20 cc/kg should be rapidly given, with reassessment of the child's hemodynamic status between boluses. Check electrolytes and renal and liver function in cases of hypovolemic shock. In bacterial causes of AGE, treatment should be guided by specific pathogen. The American Academy of Pediatrics' (AAP) *Red Book Report of the Committee on Infectious Disease* (https://redbook.solutions.aap.org/book.aspx?bookid=2205) provides periodically updated recommendations for therapies based on specific pathogen. Parasitic causes may be suggested by a travel history to areas of endemic disease or a history of outdoor camping and outdoor water exposures. Giardia infections are treated with nitazoxanide or tinidazole for 1–3 days. Most Cryptosporidial infections are self-resolving, but for severe illness, a course of nitazoxanide (100 mg PO BID ×3 days for children aged 1–3 years and 200 mg PO BID ×3 days for children aged 4–11 year) can be used. Treatment of initial cases of nonsevere *C. dificile* infection in children infected with *C. dificile* should be with oral vancomycin 7.5 mg/kg/dose TID or QID or metronidazole 10 mg/kg/dose QID for 10 days. In more severe illness, oral or rectally administered vancomycin is preferred over metronidazole. Recurrent episodes of *C. dificile* may be treated with a longer course of vancomycin orally or alternative regimens of oral rifaxamin or fecal transplant in consultation with a pediatric infectious disease or pediatric gastrointestinal specialist.

Disposition

Children who are clinically well hydrated without ongoing losses may be discharged home with or without antiemetics and oral rehydration. Moderate to severely dehydrated children and those with rapid ongoing losses should be IV hydrated with consideration of hospital admission for continued IV hydration if losses persist or if there is more than moderate dehydration.

Complications

Dehydration and Hypovolemic Shock

When a child's losses exceed intake and end organs become underperfused, hypovolemic shock may occur. Elevated heart rate and decreased urine output are the early signs of mild to moderate hypovolemia. Severe dehydration may lead to altered mental status, cool extremities, end organ damage, and eventually hypotension and cardiovascular collapse. Blood pressure in children does not drop until very late in the course of hypovolemic shock.

Hemolytic Uremic Syndrome

The combination of thrombocytopenia, acute kidney injury, hypertension, and a microangiopathic hemolytic anemia is seen in diarrhea-associated hemolytic uremic syndrome (HUS). This feared complication arises due to a shiga toxin from *Escherichia coli* strain O157:H7. The risk of HUS is thought to be elevated after antibiotic treatment of these infections, thus the recommendation not to empirically treat suspected bacterial diarrhea until the pathogen is known (and is not a toxin-producing strain of *E. coli*).

Key Points

Most cases of AGE in children are self-limited illness that can be managed with supportive care. Antiemetics facilitate oral rehydration. Treat more severe cases with IV fluid rehydration. Do not empirically treat suspected bacterial diarrhea with antibiotics given the risk of HUS with certain strains of *E. coli* (O157:H7).

Pitfalls

Be wary of diagnosing the child with vomiting only (without diarrhea) of having AGE. Many serious illnesses can present with vomiting only—for example, obstructive gastrointestinal (GI) illness such as intussusception, appendicitis, intracranial pathology, new-onset diabetes mellitus, and urinary tract infection/pyelonephritis.

If the stool pathogen is the O157:H7 *E. coli* strain (a shiga toxin-producing strain), consider consultation with an infectious disease specialist to help make the decision whether or not treating with antibiotics is indicated, given the historical association of this infection with the development of HUS in children. In general, antibiotics are avoided in this specific clinical scenario.

High concentrations of sugar in rehydration drinks (e.g., sports drinks or apple juice) may prolong diarrhea through an osmotic gradient set up in the gut pulling water into the intestinal lumen. One well-done study supports mixing one-half water and one-half apple juice to avoid this problem if the child is unwilling to take a standard balanced electrolyte solution. Probiotics do not appear to shorten the course of diarrhea in viral AGE, although there is mixed evidence to support its use in antibiotic-associated diarrhea.

VIRAL EXANTHEMS

Background

Rashes with fevers in children are a combination that makes many non-pediatric clinicians concerned, yet there are typical patterns of certain viral exanthems. Being able to distinguish the viral exanthema from a potentially serious bacterial cause of a rash is crucial.

Differential Diagnosis

The differential diagnosis of viral exanthems includes drug rash, scarlet fever, contact dermatitis, drug allergy, Kawasaki disease, serum sickness, vasculitis, and erythema multiforme.

Diagnostic Confirmation

Most viral exanthems are associated with fever and a variable number of other systemic symptoms. Some have a typical clinical appearance, seasonality, and time course. Although viral rashes are too numerous to discuss them all, a few deserve to be discussed individually. Measles rash is classically described as blanching, red clusters of papules that start on the head and face ("like cracking an egg on the head") and spread caudally and distally. Measles is typified by the three C's of cough, coryza, and conjunctivitis. Koplik spots may be seen prior to the rash on the buccal mucosal surface early in the course but are only present for 1–3 days and so may not be present by the time the pathognomonic rash appears. As one of the most contagious (and vaccine-preventable) viruses, cases of measles should be reported to the public health department.

Roseola is caused by human herpesvirus-6 (HHV-6) and usually occurs in older infants who present with high fevers (usually >39°C). After the third day of fever, it deverfesces and a fine red maculopapular rash appears all over the body, sparing the palms and soles, and the child returns to their well state. HHV-6 is often associated with febrile seizures. Varicella (chicken pox) is a vaccine-preventable disease. The first dose of vaccine is given at 12 months, so occasionally wild-type disease is seen in younger infants. It typically starts with fevers and a pruritic vesicular rash on the face/scalp and trunk before spreading to the rest of the body (Figure 11.1). Lesions may appear at different stages of healing, which is a helpful clinical clue to the diagnosis. Parvovirus, also known as fifth disease or "slapped cheek" disease, is a common childhood exanthem that starts with low-grade fevers, runny nose, and headache; after 1 or 2 days, patients develop a bright red macular rash over both cheeks (Figure 11.2). This is usually followed by a lacy, blanching rash over the body (sparing the palms and soles) and myalgias. Epstein–Barr virus (EBV) infection may cause a variety of rashes, including Gianotti–Crosti syndrome, or papular acrodermatitis. As the name implies, this unique-appearing rash occurs in the extremities and is more pronounced over the extensor joints over the elbows and knees, buttocks, and face. The rash mostly spares the trunk, palms, and soles. The rash consists of flat-topped pink papules and can sometimes appear vesicular. Gianotti–Crosti syndrome can also be precipitated with hepatitis B and a variety of other viral infections. Hand–foot–mouth disease (HFMD) is caused by coxsackie virus and features papules or vesicles on the palmar and plantar surfaces along with fever and oral ulcers.

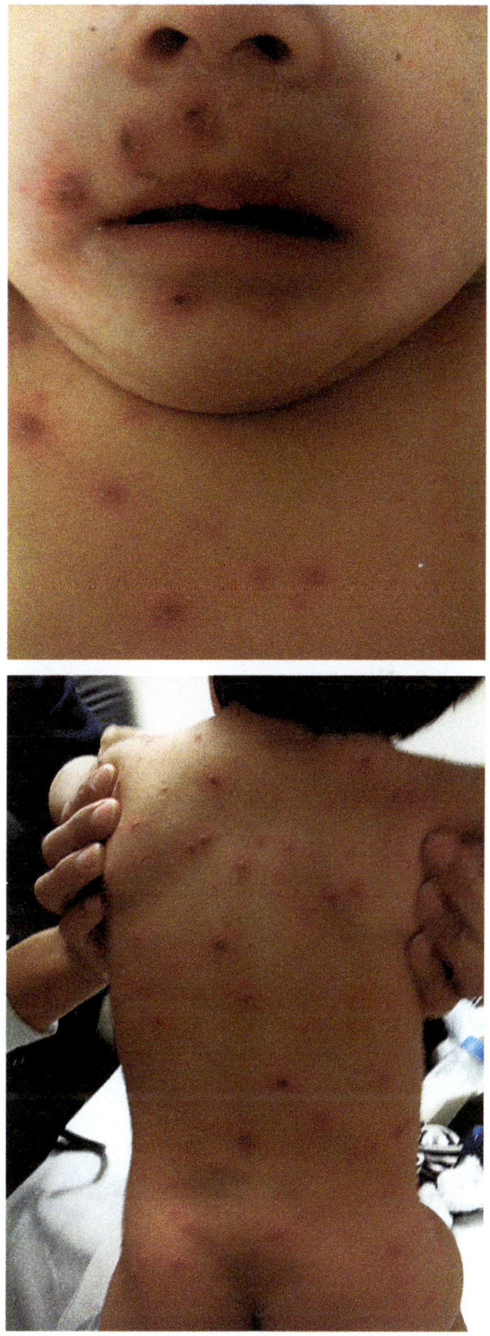

FIGURE 11.1 Chicken pox in an 11-month-old who had not yet been vaccinated. Note the vesicles in different stages of healing.

Treatment

Treatment of viral exanthems is largely supportive, with oral antihistamines (diphenhydramine 0.5–1 mg/kg/dose, maximum 50 mg every 6 hours) given to aid with pruritus, although they should be used with caution in children younger than age 1 year due to concern for respiratory depression, especially in the setting of concurrent respiratory illness. It is not necessary to apply topical agents for most viral rashes, although some clinicians will recommend topical calamine lotion to relive the itch associated with primary varicella (chicken pox). Immune-competent patients with varicella do not routinely need to receive antiviral medications, unless the course is complicated.

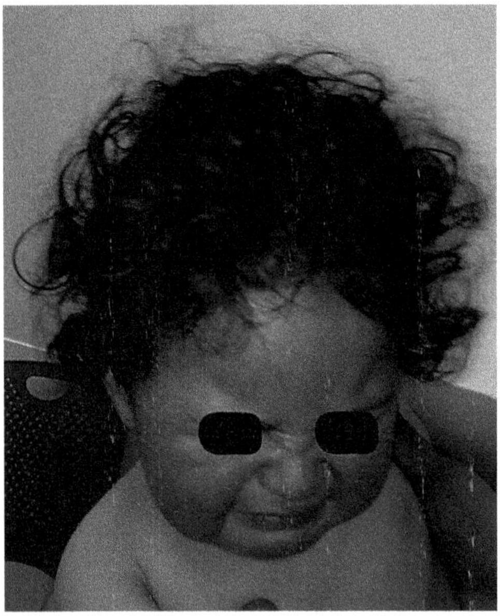

FIGURE 11.2 Typical "slapped cheek" appearance of parvovirus infection in an infant.

Disposition

Most patients with viral exanthems may be discharged home. Patients who are exhibiting dehydration or central nervous system (CNS), pulmonary, hematologic, or cardiac complications of the inciting virus may need to be hospitalized.

Complications

Varicella infection can be complicated by bacterial skin infections, pneumonia, or cerebellitis. Varicella infection may also precede an erythema multiforme rash typically presenting with targetoid lesions starting in the extremities and possibly involving not more than one mucous membrane site. Involvement of eyes and multiple mucous membrane sites should alert the clinician to the possibility of a more serious rash, such as Stevens–Johnson syndrome [SJS; if <10% body surface area (BSA) involved], toxic epidermal necrolysis (TEN; if >30% BSA involved), or an overlap syndrome of SJS/TEN (if 10–30% BSA involved). Parvovirus has been associated with CNS complications such as meningitis, peripheral neuropathy, and stroke. Parvovirus B19 infection may precipitate an aplastic crisis in children with sickle cell disease or other hemolytic structural red blood cell problem. Parvovirus infection may also cause fetal hydrops from fetal anemia and sometimes fetal demise, so patients with this infection should avoid contact with pregnant women who are parvovirus non-immune.

Key Points

Viral exanthems mostly are a self-limited process only requiring supportive care. Infections such as measles require notification of the public health department, and measures must be taken to prevent the spread of this agent to susceptible patients [especially unvaccinated children (children <12 months old and those who opt out or delay vaccinations)]. Ensure through careful history and physical examination (and sometimes laboratory work) that your patient does not have one of the more severe cutaneous adverse reactions, such as SJS, TEN, or drug rash with eosinophilia and systemic signs (DRESS) syndrome.

Pitfalls

Always include examination of the eyes and mucous membranes (both oral and genitourinary areas) to not miss a subtle finding of SJS or TEN. Review medications to ensure that the rash you are evaluating is not a drug-related reaction.

LYMPHADENITIS AND LYMPHADENOPATHY EVALUATION

Background

Swollen lymph nodes can be a distressing symptom for families, with concerns for malignancy at the forefront of their concerns. Most lymphadenopathy is cervical in location and develops in response to local infectious or inflammatory processes, but occasionally it can be a sign of systemic illness or malignancy. Exposure to kittens (for cat scratch disease) or a person with active tuberculosis (TB) or travel to a TB endemic area should be ascertained. Location (unilateral cervical, bilateral cervical, or diffuse lymphadenopathy), number (single or multiple nodes), temperature, color, presence or absence of pain, presence of systemic "B" symptoms (night sweats and weight loss), presence of hepatosplenomegaly, and mobility of the lymph node all are important historical and physical findings to ascertain to lead you to the proper diagnosis.

Differential Diagnosis

Reactive lymphadenopathy (to local nearby infections), bacterial lymphadenitis, abscess (including a necrotizing lymphadenitis eponymously called Kicuchi syndrome), infected congenital remnants (e.g., branchial cleft cysts, thryoglossal duct cysts, and lymphangiomas), Kawasaki disease, lymphoma, TB, atypical mycobacteria, HIV, cat scratch disease, group A *Streptococcus* (GAS), EBV, cytomegalovirus, and a variety of other infectious agents all may cause localized cervical lymphadenopathy. Inguinal regional lymphadenopathy may be related to sexually transmitted infections [e.g., herpes simplex virus (HSV), syphilis, and lymphogranuloma venereum] or nearby skin or follicular infections. Generalized lymphadenopathy may be a symptom of systemic infectious disease (e.g., HIV, EBV, or TB), malignancy, or autoimmune disease. Swollen or painful joints, weakness, or rash with lymphadenopathy suggests the possibility of underlying rheumatologic disease. Rarely, systemic lymphadenopathy can be associated with metabolic diseases such as Niemann–Pick or Gaucher's disease when seen in the presence of hepatosplenomegaly. Some antiseizure medications can be associated with widespread lymphadenopathy as part of a drug hypersensitivity syndrome.

Diagnostic Confirmation

Often, diagnoses of reactive lymphadenopathy and bacterial lymphadenitis are made clinically. Reactive cervical lymphadenopathy may occur in response to viral and bacterial infections of the head and neck (e.g., otitis media, pharyngitis, and dental infections commonly). Preauricular lymph nodes are commonly seen in scalp infections, including tinea capitis. Typically, reactive nodes are bilateral, small, warm, mobile, and without overlying skin changes.

GAS pharyngitis-associated cervical lymphadenopathy should be suspected in a school-age child (5–15 years) with tender, enlarged, bilateral cervical lymphadenopathy with fevers, enlarged and/or exudative tonsils, along with the absence of a prominent cough or rhinorrhea. Rapid tests from throat swabs are both sensitive and specific. EBV-associated cervical lymphadenopathy tends to be located posteriorly compared with GAS, which tends to be anteriorly located (Figure 11.3).

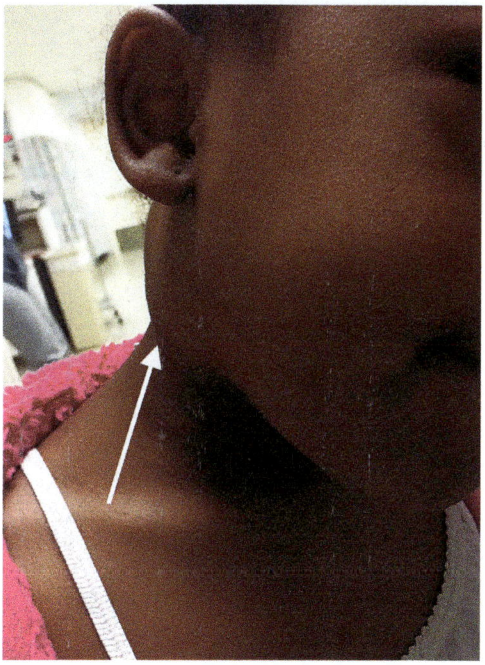

FIGURE 11.3 Six-year-old girl with prominent bilateral posterior cervical lymphadenopathy associated with EBV infection.

Malignancy may be suggested by any combination of the following: the presence of a cold, firm, matted, fixed, or rapidly growing nodes; and the presence of lymph nodes with "B" symptoms (weight loss, fevers, and night sweats). Supraclavicular lymphadenopathy is especially concerning for lymphoma. Diagnosis is made from excisional biopsy of the node.

Check a CXR in patients with risk factors for or clinical suspicion of TB (to rule out pulmonary TB) and in cases of suspected malignancy to rule out a mediastinal mass, most often associated with a Hodgkin's lymphoma (Figure 11.4) and less commonly with T cell leukemia.

Unilateral cervical lymphadenopathy along with prolonged fevers lasting more than 5 days, nonpurulent conjunctivitis, extremity edema or peeling, rash, and mucous membrane changes (cracked lips or strawberry tongue) should arouse suspicion for Kawasaki disease. Criteria for the diagnosis of complete and incomplete Kawasaki disease are provided in Chapter 24.

Labs may occasionally help when you are uncertain of the diagnosis. They should include a complete blood count with differential and lactate dehydrogenase. When clinically

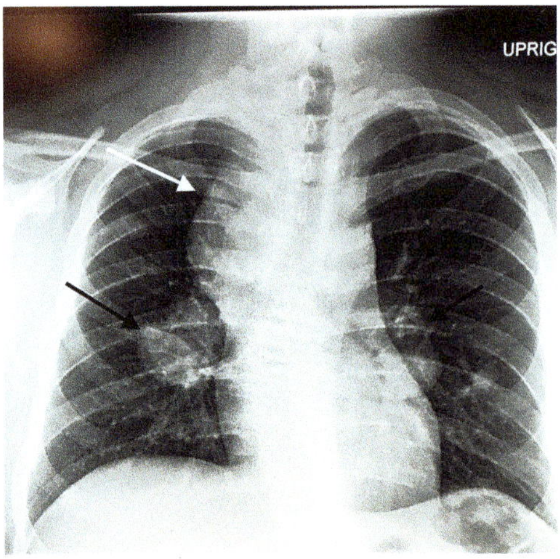

FIGURE 11.4 Mediastinal mass (white arrow) and perihilar lymphadenopathy (black arrows) in a 15-year-old with supraclavicular lymphadenopathy, prolonged fevers, and weight loss. Final diagnosis on biopsy was lymphoma.

indicated, GAS, EBV titers (younger children) or a Monospot (to detect heterophile antibody) test for EBV (in children >9 years old), purified protein derivative testing, and *Bartonella* titers for cat scratch disease may be done. Inflammatory markers (erythrocyte sedimentation rate and C-reactive protein), liver function tests (searching for hypoalbuminemia and transaminitis), and urinalysis [searching for white blood cells without bacteria ("sterile pyuria")] may aid the diagnosis of Kawasaki disease.

Ultrasound is the initial imaging modality of choice in children and may be helpful in differentiating between infectious, reactive, and malignant lymphadenopathy. Computed tomography and magnetic resonance imaging are sometimes employed when diagnostic uncertainty remains or if surgical planning is necessary. Biopsy of a lymph node is usually reserved for cases with suspicion of malignancy, lymphadenopathy present for more than 1 month without cause not improving after a trial of antibiotics, lymphadenopathy increasing in size over 2 weeks or large size (>2 cm), or lymphadenopathy associated with an abnormal CXR.

Treatment

Treatment depends on the underlying cause. Bacterial lymphadenitis is usually caused by staphylococcus (all ages), streptococcal species (including group B strep in neonates), or anaerobes (older children and teens), and it is treated using oral cephalexin or clindamycin. Atypical mycobacteria infections present as a slow-growing "cold" neck mass in a 1- to 5-year-old child. The cervical mass often has an area that darkens to a violaceous color before a sinus tract appears. It is treated with complete surgical resection with the addition of a macrolide [clarithromycin and one or two anti-mycobacterial medications (ethambutol and rifampin) should be given in consultation with an infectious disease specialist] for cases with incomplete surgical resection or recurrence. Cat scratch disease-related lymphadenopathy is usually treated with a macrolide such as azithromycin. Malignancy requires specific chemotherapy after consultation with an oncology specialist. A less common cause of enlarged cervical lymph nodes is periodic fever, aphthous ulcers, pharyngitis, and cervical adenopathy (PFAPA). Children, typically aged 2–5 years, present with cervical bilateral adenopathy, oral ulcers, recurrent sore throat, and fevers. Tonsillectomy is thought to be curative of this otherwise self-limited condition of unknown etiology.

Clinical Algorithm

Figure 11.5 provides an algorithm for generalized versus localized lymphadenopathy. An algorithm for cervical lymphadenopathy is shown in Figure 11.6.

Disposition

Most lymphadenopathies require parental reassurance and no further intervention. Children with simple bacterial lymphadenitis may be sent home on oral antibiotics (cephalexin 50 mg/kg/day divided TID or QID or clindamycin 30 mg/kg/day divided TID ×10 days), although if they have failed a course, they may need to be admitted for IV antibiotics. Reactive nodes usually will self-resolve, although if associated with GAS infection, oral penicillin or amoxicillin may be used [for antibiotic regimens, see the section titled "Pharyngitis (Streptococcal and Viral)"]. Lymphadenopathy associated with malignancy will require admission for further workup, whereas rheumatology-associated lymphadenopathy is usually worked up as an outpatient if there are no emergent comorbidities, such as cerebritis, nephritis, elevated

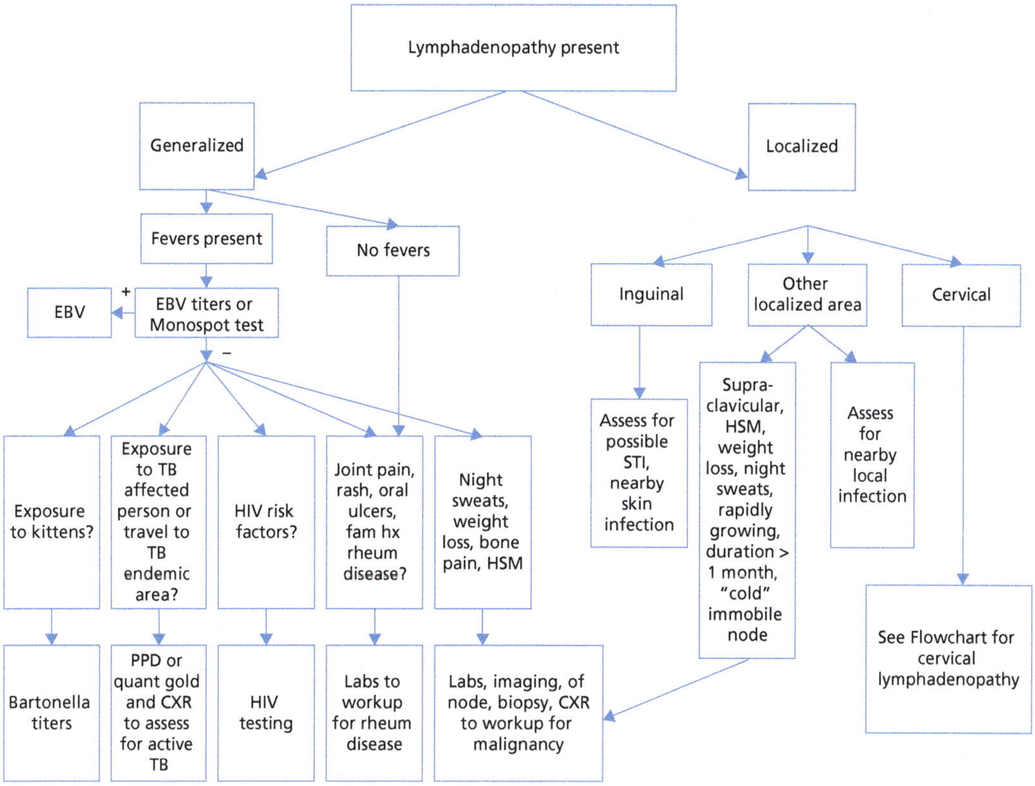

FIGURE 11.5 Evaluation of lymphadenopathy.

blood pressure (stage 2 hypertension), or acute or chronic kidney injury/insufficiency.

Complications

Bacterial lymphadenitis may progress to an abscess requiring surgical incision and drainage.

Key Points

Cervical lymphadenopathy is extremely common in children and most often associated with viral and bacterial infections of the head and neck, such as bacterial or viral pharyngitis. These reactive nodes most often have a benign course, especially when bilateral. Unilateral cervical lymphadenopathy may represent a reactive node or a primary infection of the node, with staphylococci, streptococci, anaerobes, bartonella, and mycobacteria as leading causes. Concern for malignancy should be considered if the patient has longstanding (>1 month), hard, "cold" nodes, especially in the setting of hepatosplenomegaly, or "B symptoms" such as prolonged fevers, night sweats, or weight loss. Rheumatologic disease associated lymphadenopathy is often associated with joint pain/swelling, weakness, or rashes.

Pitfalls

Missing a malignancy or mediastinal mass associated with lymphoma is a potentially life-threatening situation. Generalized lymphadenopathy or persistent cervical lymphadenopathy may be a symptom of HIV infection. Remember to look at medication lists because some anti-seizure medications can lead to generalized lymphadenopathy.

HAND–FOOT–MOUTH AND HERPANGINA

Background

Coxsackie and enteroviral infections may lead to a clinically recognizable pattern of physical findings, such as HFMD and herpangina, that can occur in children of any age but tend to have the most impact on infants and toddlers. The incubation period for these infections is 3–6 days, and they are usually spread by respiratory and orofecal routes or via fomites.

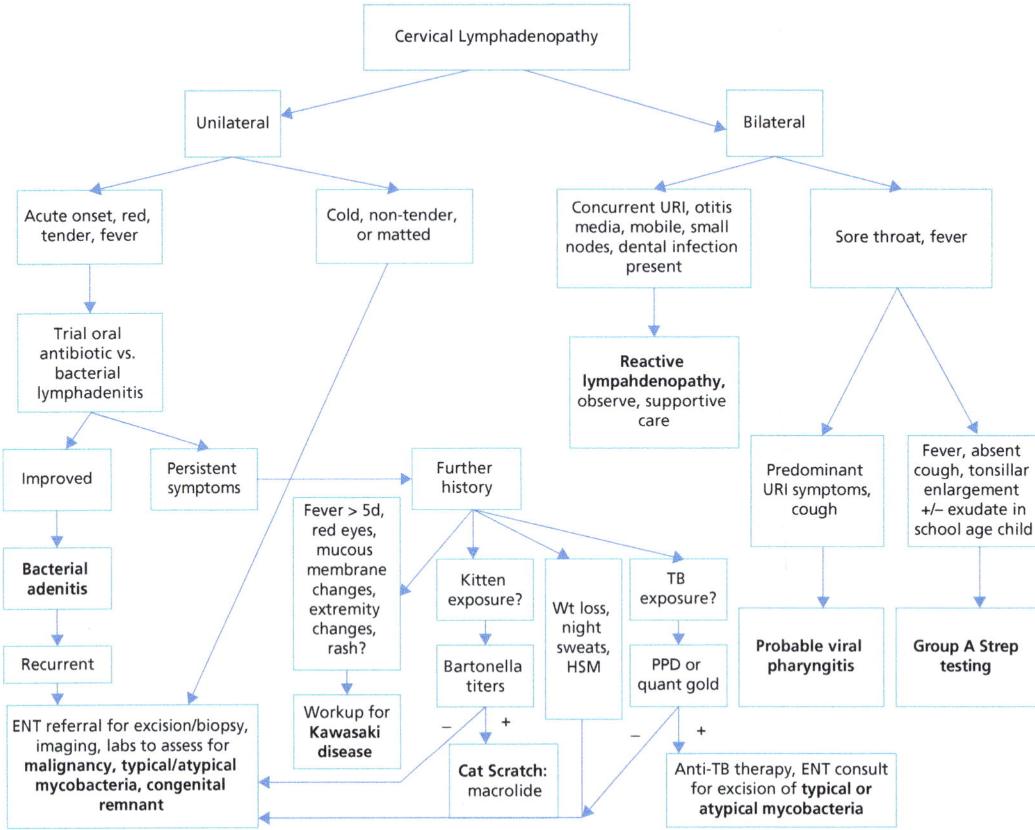

FIGURE 11.6 Evaluation of cervical lymphadenopathy.

Differential Diagnosis

The differential diagnosis of HFMD and herpangina infections includes HSV gingivostomatitis, Bechet's disease, Reiter's syndrome, oral ulcers associated with IBD, streptococcal pharyngitis, viral pharyngitis (with EBV, adenovirus, and influenza being common causes), aphthous ulcers, and a variety of conditions associated with viral exanthems.

Diagnosis

Most cases of HFMD and herpangina are identifiable by simple history and physical examination. Typical findings include punched-out ulcerations over the tonsillar pillars, tongue, and (rarely) uvula; and a rash (macules, papules, or vesicles) that clusters over the palms, soles, and diaper areas (Figure 11.7). Less specific manifestations include fevers, vomiting/diarrhea, and cough/rhinorrhea. Herpangina is clinically similar to HFMD with regard to the oral lesions and systemic symptoms, but it lacks the exanthem on the palms, soles, and diaper area (Figures 11.8 and 11.9). If there is clinical uncertainty, the virus can be detected from stool or throat swabs. The virus can also be detected from urine, blood, or cerebrospinal fluid (CSF) if these sites are infected. In addition, a PCR assay is available for CSF

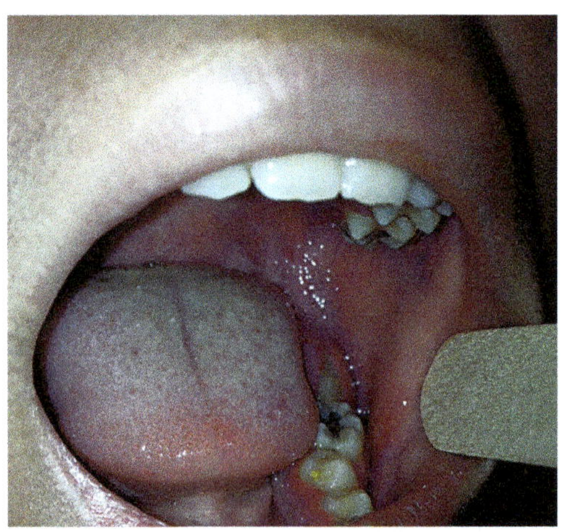

FIGURE 11.7 Oral lesion on buccal mucosa associated with coxsackie virus-related HFMD. Most commonly, ulcers appear on the posterior tonsillar pillars, but they can also be present on the tongue and buccal mucosa.

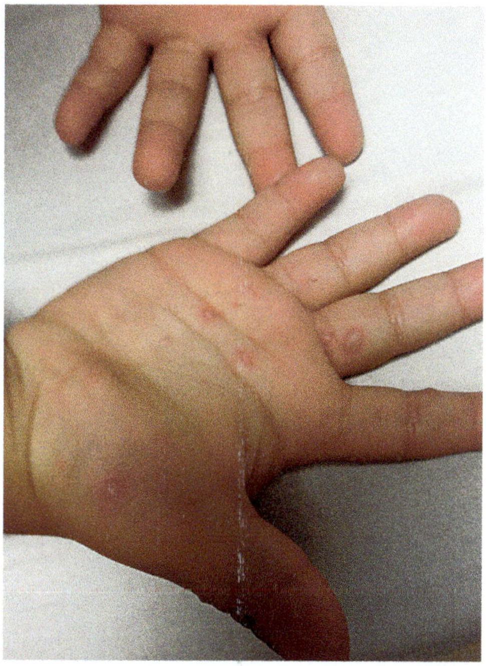

FIGURE 11.8 Typical lesions on the palms of coxsackie virus-related HFMD. Lesions can be popular, macular, or vesicular.

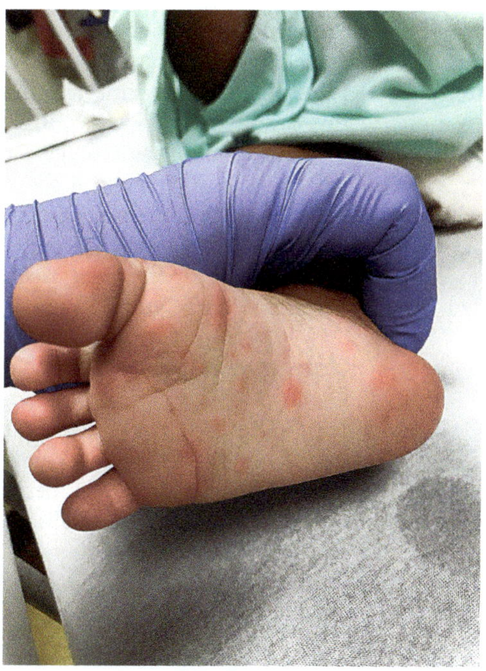

FIGURE 11.9 Typical lesions on the soles of coxsackie virus-related HFMD. Lesions can be popular, macular, or vesicular.

specimens; the assay has rapid turnaround but does not detect specific serotypes of virus.

Treatment

Treatment is mostly supportive with hydration and pain control with nonsteroidal anti-inflammatory drugs (NSAIDs) and/or acetaminophen. Some clinicians prescribe "magic mouthwash"—a 1:1:1 mixture of diphenhydramine, aluminum hydroxide, and 1% lidocaine—for oral ulcer pain relief in a swish and spit manner. For infants, many leave out the lidocaine component due to concern for lidocaine toxicity from swallowed magic mouthwash. Liquid sucralfate is beneficial to treat pain from oral ulcerative conditions and mucositis, and although not studied specifically in HFMD or HSV gingivostomatitis, it potentially might help reduce pain by same mechanism that helps patients with peptic ulcers. The addition of honey to a course of acyclovir shortened duration of time of oral HSV lesions, decreased drooling, and improved ability of children to eat and drink sooner compared with acyclovir alone. Use of honey should be avoided in children younger than age 1 year due to risk of infantile botulism. Viscous lidocaine has historically been used for relief of oral pain associated with oral ulcers, but it did not improve oral intake in one ED study (performed on patents with HSV gingivostomatitis lesions), and it has the potential for toxicity. Gentian violet has also historically been prescribed by pediatricians for oral pain relief, although there is not much evidence to support its use. Intravenous immunoglobulin (IVIG) has been used for the potential life-threatening complication of myopericarditis without much evidence to support its use.

Disposition

Most patients have a self-limited course and may be discharged home unless they are exhibiting signs of dehydration.

Complications

Due to throat pain and unwillingness of the child to take adequate liquids, dehydration is the most common complication of HFMD and herpangina. Myopericarditis is a dreaded (but rare) complication of coxsackie-associated HFMD/herpangina. It may present as respiratory distress, poor feeding, cyanosis, chest pain, or lethargy/weakness. Physical findings may include tachycardia out of proportion to fever, hypotension, peripheral edema, hepatosplenomegaly, or an S_3 heart sound. Electrocardiogram is abnormal in most with myopericarditis, with findings of sinus tachycardia, ST elevations or depression, low-voltage QRS waves, or inverted T waves in lateral leads (V5/V6). Labs may reveal elevated brain natriuretic peptide and troponin, although if normal, this does not rule out the condition. CXR often shows cardiomegaly with pulmonary edema. Coxsackie and enteroviral infections are well-known causes of viral meningitis, and patients will present with typical findings of nuchal rigidity, headaches, vomiting, and photophobia. Treatment is largely supportive. In children with underlying eczema, patches of eczema may become invaded by coxsackie virus leading to "eczema coxsackium," a version of HFMD that may be confused with bullous impetigo, eczema herpeticum, vasculitis, or primary bullous disease. Although usually only a cosmetic concern, children with HFMD may develop nail peeling (onychomadesis) weeks to months after coxsackie infection.

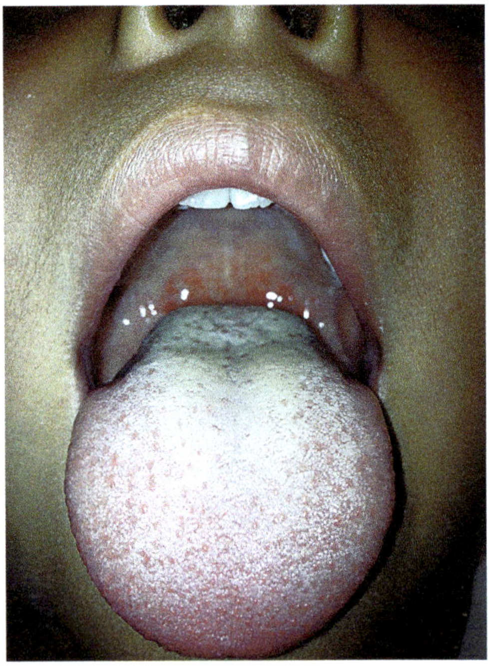

FIGURE 11.10 Palatal petechiae in a young child with GAS pharyngitis.

Key Points

Coxsackie infections usually lead to a self-limited disease of fevers; oral ulcerations; and sometime rash over the palms, soles, and groin area. Rare serious complications of dehydration, myopericarditis, and aseptic meningitis may occur.

Pitfalls

Remember to instruct patients with coxsackie infection not only about the potential for dehydration but also about symptoms associated with the more sinister complications, such as cardiac, pulmonary, and CNS complications.

PHARYNGITIS (STREPTOCOCCAL AND VIRAL)

Background

Sore throat and fever are common presenting symptoms in the pediatric ED, and although most causes of sore throat are benign, being able to differentiate viral from bacterial pharyngitis from deep space neck infections is crucial. GAS pharyngitis tends to affect children aged 5–15 years at its peak, and it is associated with fevers, palatal petechiae (Figure 11.10), tender anterior cervical lymphadenopathy, and absent to minimal cough/rhinorrhea. Headache and abdominal pain are common complaints associated with GAS infections. The presence of palatal petechiae, exudate, or tonsillar enlargement is not a reliable way to differentiate viral from bacterial pharyngitis; both viral and bacterial pharyngitis can lead to this same clinical appearance. In children younger than age 2 or 3 years, GAS pharyngitis is rare, and it should only be considered if there is a close sick contact with known GAS infection or the patient has a scarlatiniform (sandpapery) rash associated with GAS scarlet fever (Figure 11.11).

Differential Diagnosis

Differential diagnosis of sore throat includes viral pharyngitis (EBV, adenovirus, influenza, and many others), bacterial pharyngitis, PFAPA syndrome, herpangina/HFMD, herpes gingivostomatitis, retropharyngeal abscess, peritonsillar and parapharyngeal abscess, foreign body ingestion (e.g., batteries and fish bones), and caustic ingestions.

Diagnosis

Throat culture and rapid GAS tests can identify GAS pharyngitis, although up to 25% of

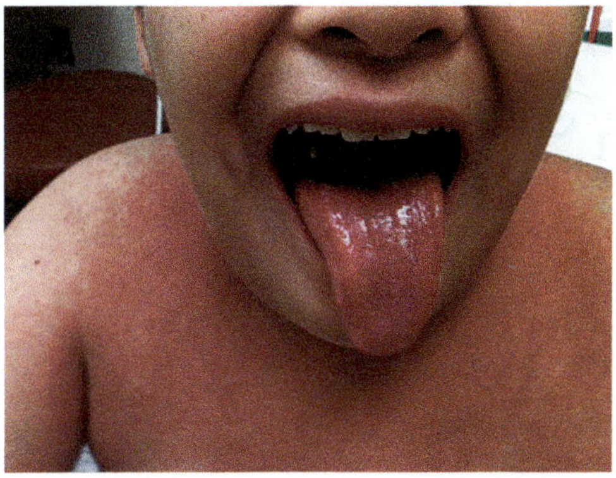

FIGURE 11.11 Scarlatinform rash in a child with GAS scarlet fever. The rash appears like red, raised goose bumps that are rough to the touch.

school-age children may be colonized with GAS. Rapid strep assays have high specificity but variable sensitivity, so if a rapid test is positive, do not send a throat culture to confirm the diagnosis of GAS infection. In older children, heterophile antibody testing (Monospot) is a reasonable test to diagnose EBV infection. EBV titers are the most reliable way to diagnose EBV infection in younger children, especially those younger than age 4 years, because they have low rates of production of heterophile antibody in response to EBV infection. Centor criteria are unreliable for GAS prediction in children.

Treatment

Group A streptococcus pharyngitis is treated using penicillin-based antibiotic (penicillin VK or amoxicillin). Once-daily dosing of penicillin VK or amoxicillin (50 mg/kg, maximum of 1,000–1,200 mg daily for 10 days) may also be used. In younger children, amoxicillin may be preferable due to better palatability compared with penicillin VK. If compliance is a concern, a single intramuscular (IM) injection of a long-acting depot penicillin [penicillin G benzathine (Bicillin) 600,000 units IM ×1 if <27 kg, 1.2 million units IM if >27 kg] may be used. Penicillin-allergic patients may be treated using a macrolide antibiotic (azithromycin 12 mg/kg day 1, followed by 6 mg/kg ×4 more). If treatment is with erythromycin or clarithromycin, it should be done for 10 days, but these have a higher incidence of GI side effects compared with azithromycin. To decrease unnecessary antibiotic use, treatment may be delayed until culture results, although ideally treatment is started before 9 days of symptoms to prevent the development of acute rheumatic fever. There is controversy regarding treatment of non-GAS bacterial pharyngitis. It may be prudent to treat with antibiotics if symptoms persist for a prolonged period of time, but there is no risk of **acute** rheumatic fever (ARF) or glomerulonephritis with this type of infection, so it is not necessary to treat with antibiotics. Patients may return to school or day care within 12 hours after treatment is initiated, as long as they are afebrile and clinically improved, because the bacteria is eradicated soon after starting antibacterial therapy. Treatment of viral pharyngitis is largely supportive with pain control using over-the-counter pain medicine (NSAIDs and/or acetaminophen) and encouragement of hydration.

Disposition

Unless there are signs of severe dehydration, respiratory compromise from enlarged tonsils, acute rheumatic fever, or abscess formation, most patients with pharyngitis may be discharged home with oral pain medications and instructions to hydrate, in addition to appropriate antibiotics if GAS is identified.

Complications

Dehydration from severe throat pain is the most common complication of pharyngitis. Spread of pharyngitis to nearby structures can lead to abscess of the retropharyngeal, peritonsillar, and parapharyngeal spaces. GAS throat infections can rarely be complicated by ARF. Although rare in the United States, ARF is common in Africa, Asia, and Australia/Oceania. Post-strep reactive arthritis, glomerulonephritis, and toxic shock syndrome may rarely occur. There is currently controversy regarding the existence of the condition described as pediatric autoimmune neuropsychiatric disorders associated with streptococcal infection (PANDAS). This is a group of poorly understood acute neurologic changes (e.g., sudden-onset behavior changes, motor tics, and varied neuropsychiatric disturbances) that are proposed to take place after GAS infection. Currently, the AAP does not recommend antibiotic prophylaxis, IVIG, or plasmapheresis for suspected PANDAS. EBV-related pharyngitis can be complicated by splenic enlargement and rupture, encephalitis, transverse myelitis, myocarditis, hemolysis, and hemophagocytosis.

Key Points

Avoid strep testing in low-risk populations presenting with sore throat: the very young (<3 years old) and those with prominent cough and rhinorrhea (more likely viral etiology). Treat GAS pharyngitis to minimize risk of suppurative and nonsuppurative complications. Always provide pain relief to ensure all patients with pharyngitis stay well hydrated. Use EBV titers instead of heterophile antibody testing to diagnose children younger than age 4 years with EBV infection.

Pitfalls

Empiric treatment of a sore throat caused by EBV with penicillin antibiotics frequently results in the development of a rash 7–14 days after antibiotic exposure that is not IgE mediated but is often misinterpreted as an allergy to penicillin.

HERPES SIMPLEX VIRUS GINGIVOSTOMATITIS

Background

Painful oral lesions are a common occurrence in toddler-age children. HSV gingivostomatitis is a clinically recognizable entity of fevers, poor oral intake/drooling, and typical-appearing lesions in and around the oral cavity.

Differential Diagnosis

The differential diagnosis includes coxsackie-associated herpangina, Bechet's disease, PFAPA, Reiter's syndrome, oral ulcers associated with IBD, streptococcal pharyngitis, viral pharyngitis, aphthous ulcers, and a variety of conditions associated with viral exanthems.

Diagnosis

Herpes simplex virus gingivostomatitis is a clinically identifiable condition commonly affecting the toddler-age group (although any age can be affected). It features high fevers; yellow plaques on the tongue and anterior mouth, often with friable, hyperemic gingiva that easily bleed; perioral vesicles; and often halitosis (Figure 11.12). If there is clinical uncertainty, lesions can be swabbed and sent for HSV PCR testing. The presence of vesicular lesion on a finger ("herpetic whitlow"; Figure 11.13) or perioral vesicles can aid in the diagnosis of HSV gingivostomatitis.

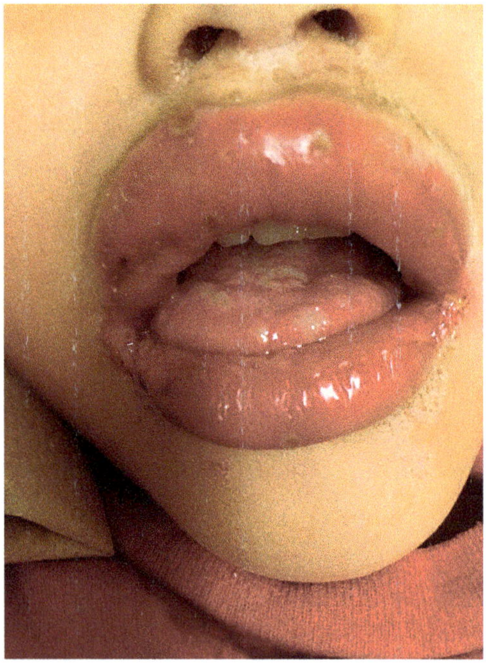

FIGURE 11.12 Severe HSV gingivostomatitis in a toddler. Note the vesicles at the vermillion border, yellow plaque on the tongue, and hyperemic swollen gingiva.

Treatment

Treatment is largely supportive with over-the-counter pain medications (NSAIDs and acetaminophen) for pain and hydration with cold, non-acidic liquids. Frozen balanced electrolyte solution popsicles are a good way to numb the painful oral lesions and hydrate the patient. Acyclovir is not routinely used in immunocompetent patients, but it may be considered in the immune-suppressed patient. Antiviral medications, if used, should ideally be given within the first 48 hours of development of lesions to have the most efficacy.

Disposition

If well hydrated and no eye lesions, most patients may be discharged home with instructions to hydrate and control pain. Children who are clinically dehydrated and not tolerating oral liquids may need to be admitted for IV rehydration. Immune-competent children do not routinely need therapy with acyclovir, although there is limited evidence that severe

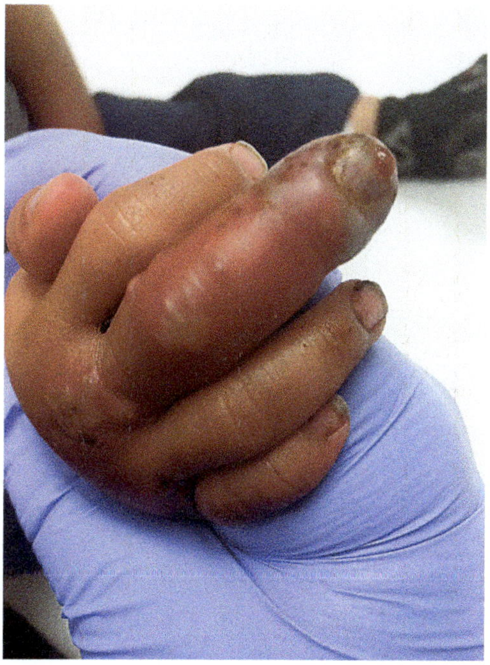

FIGURE 11.13 Herpetic whitlow in a 9-month-old. Note the vesicles near the distal tip of the finger and confluence of vesicles in the more proximal portion, which can be confused for an abscess.

cases may be shortened if started within 48 hours of first onset of symptoms.

Complications

Dehydration is the most common complication of HSV gingivostomatitis.

HSV ocular keratitis can present as a red, painful eye with typical fluorescein appearance (dendrites—a spidery pattern). Herpes keratitis can lead to permanent vision impairment and should be emergently referred to see an ophthalmologist as soon as possible for evaluation and treatment with topical acyclovir. Bell's palsy has been described as a complication of HSV gingivostomatitis. Rare cases of acute disseminated encephalomyelitis, a condition presenting with cranial nerve palsies, headaches, vomiting, weakness, and confusion, have been associated with HSV gingivostomatitis. HSV infections can precede serious skin conditions such as SJS.

Key Points

Herpes simplex virus gingivostomatitis is usually a self-limited viral illness with oral lesions, poor oral intake, and typical-appearing oral lesions. Antivirals are usually not needed, and pain control is the mainstay of therapy to avoid dehydration.

Pitfall

Not recognizing HSV keratitis in the patient with HSV gingivostomatitis and red eye can lead to permanent visual impairment.

Further Reading

Abdel-Naby Awad OG, Hamad AH. Honey can help in herpes simplex gingivostomatitis in children: Prospective randomized double blind placebo controlled clinical trial. *Am J Otolaryngol.* 2018;39(6):759–763.

Chen CK, Wu SH, Huang YC. Herpetic gingivostomatitis with severe hepatitis in a previously healthy child. *J Microbiol Immunol Infect.* 2012;45(4):324–325.

Johnston BC, Goldenberg JZ, Parkin PC. Probiotics and the prevention of antibiotic-associated diarrhea in infants and children. *JAMA.* 2016;316(14): 1484–1485.

Marshall-Andon T, Heinz P. How to use...the Monospot and other heterophile antibody tests. *Arch Dis Child Educ Pract Ed.* 2017;102(4):188–193.

Stone RC, Micali GA, Schwartz RA. Roseola infantum and its causal human herpesviruses. *Int J Dermatol.* 2014;53(4):397–403.

12

Pediatric Sepsis

ANGELICA W. DESPAIN AND IOANNIS KOUTROULIS

INTRODUCTION

Sepsis is a leading cause of morbidity and mortality in the United States, with a mortality rate of 8–21%. Associated prolonged pediatric intensive care unit (PICU) and overall hospital length of stays incur significant cost. The treatment for severe sepsis and shock is timely fluid resuscitation, antibiotic administration, vasoactive agents if needed, and support of affected organs. The Surviving Sepsis Campaign recommends antibiotics within 1 hour of recognition of sepsis ("golden hour") and timely fluid administration of isotonic fluids for best outcomes. Pediatric hospitals in the United States have largely adapted highly sensitive sepsis recognition screening tools in efforts to never miss a case of sepsis. Even so, the recognition of sepsis in a pediatric patient can be challenging due to lack of reliable diagnostic tests and evolving definitions.

The 2016 Sepsis-3 Consensus emphasized that sepsis is characterized by the presence of life-threatening organ dysfunction as a result of a dysregulated host response to infection. However, the Sepsis-3 Consensus did not include pediatric guidelines. Scoring systems to predict mortality, such as the Pediatric Sequential Organ Failure Assessment (pSOFA) score, Pediatric Logistic Organ Dysfunction (PELOD) score, and Pediatric Multiorgan Dysfunction Score (P-MODS), have been validated in the intensive care setting but are not as useful in the emergency room setting. Early goal-directed therapy developed more than a decade ago that focused on manipulation of cardiac preload, afterload, and contractility in septic shock has not been shown to decrease mortality. The survival for pediatric sepsis has steadily improved, although incidence is increasing. Bundled care, established protocols, and timely resuscitative efforts improve morbidity and mortality in sepsis.

Comparison/Contrast with Adult Physiology

The presentation of shock differs significantly in children compared to adults, and this difference both impacts the recognition of shock in children and changes management with regard to vasopressor choice. Adults typically develop warm shock, whereas pediatric patients usually develop cold shock. Children have a high sympathetic tone and little variation in stroke volume, rendering norepinephrine less effective in management of shock. In pediatrics, culture-negative shock and viral shock account for 30–75% of sepsis cases. Children with a complex medical history are more likely to become septic and have worse outcomes. Similar to adults, rapid intravenous (IV) fluid resuscitation is important for the management of pediatric sepsis in developed nations.

CLASSIC CLINICAL PRESENTATION

The most common causes of sepsis in a previously healthy child are pneumonia, urinary tract infections, invasive skin and soft tissue infections, and bronchiolitis. Risk factors for sepsis include age younger than 60 days, static encephalopathy, cancer and bone marrow transplant history, central or indwelling lines, medically complex history, or any condition that predisposes to a weakened immune response. Smaller children will often present obtunded and in decompensated shock. Older children may present with more subtle signs. Hypotension is not required for the diagnosis of sepsis in children. Tachycardia is often the initial sign of sepsis and is the most sensitive indicator of a septic process. Sepsis should be considered with tachycardia, hypotension, temperature instability, tachypnea, or hypopnea.

ATYPICAL CLINICAL PRESENTATION

Septic neonates are a special category because presentation and findings are variable and the absence of fever does not indicate that the patient is not septic. They can be hyperthermic, hypothermic, or even normothermic. They may present with jaundice, irritability, lethargy, or decreased oral intake. Symptoms of sepsis in this age group can mimic those of congenital heart disease (see Chapter 2).

DIFFERENTIAL DIAGNOSES

The following types of shock present similarly to sepsis and septic shock:

- Distributive shock: Distributive shock caused by anaphylaxis can be misleading. Children may have fever, altered mental status, hypotension, rash, vomiting, diarrhea, and/or respiratory distress.
- Hypovolemic shock: Hypovolemic shock may occur with severe dehydration secondary to acute gastroenteritis and can present with fever, tachycardia, vomiting, diarrhea, and hypotension.
- Cardiogenic shock: Cardiogenic shock can present with vomiting, lethargy, and hypotension. Sepsis also causes myocardial dysfunction, which contributes to diagnostic uncertainty. A gentle fluid bolus (10 mL/kg) may be given even if cardiogenic shock is suspected because ill patients are frequently volume depleted regardless of etiology. Reassess after each bolus for overall clinical appearance, pulmonary edema, and a palpable liver edge.

Depending on age, the differential diagnoses for sepsis can be broad. In infants and young children, consider the following:

- Cardiac etiology (congenital heart disease, arrhythmias, and myocarditis): Undiagnosed critical coarctation of the aortic presents similar to fluid-resistant shock with poor perfusion. Infants with ventricular septal defects may present with tachypnea and tachycardia due to congestive heart failure.
- Metabolic (hypoglycemia and inborn errors of metabolism): Metabolic abnormalities often present with lethargy or altered mental status.
- Other (toxic exposure, non-accidental trauma, and environmental exposure): Hemodynamic abnormalities may occur from unrecognized hemorrhage or toxic ingestions.

DIAGNOSTIC CONFIRMATION

The definition of sepsis is constantly evolving. Current recommendations are to use the 2005 Goldstein definitions for pediatric sepsis (Table 12.1). The 2016 Sepsis-3 Consensus definitions for sepsis and septic shock apply only in adults; these guidelines did not include pediatric recommendations (Table 12.2). The diagnosis can be subtle and often made clinically in the absence of strict consensus criteria. Sepsis causes temperature instability, hypotension, tachycardia, and altered mental status, resulting in organ dysfunction, shock, and possibly death. The diagnosis of sepsis is time sensitive; delay in fluid resuscitation and time to antibiotics are associated with increased mortality in pediatric sepsis. Maintain a high clinical suspicion for sepsis in any ill-appearing patient.

Many institutions employ a highly sensitive electronic screening tool at triage to aid nurses

TABLE 12.1 GOLDSTEIN 2005 DEFINITIONS FOR PEDIATRIC SIRS, SEPSIS, SEVERE SEPSIS, AND SEPTIC SHOCK[a]

SIRS	The presence of at least two of four criteria, one of which must be abnormal temperature or leukocyte count: Core temperature of >38.5°C or <36°C Tachycardia (HR >2 SD above normal for age) or, for children <1 year old, bradycardia (HR <10th percentile for age) Tachypnea (RR >2 SD above normal for age) Leukocyte count elevated or depressed for age or >10% bands
Sepsis	SIRS in the presence of a suspected or known invasive infection
Severe sepsis	Sepsis with one of the following: Cardiovascular organ dysfunction Acute respiratory distress syndrome Two or more other organ dysfunctions
Septic shock	Sepsis and cardiovascular organ dysfunction

[a]See Table 12.2 for updated Sepsis-3 definitions in adults, in which SIRS and severe sepsis are no longer used.
HR, heart rate; RR, respiratory rate; SD, standard deviation; SIRS, systemic inflammatory response syndrome.

and clinicians in early identification (Table 12.3). Tools include screening for abnormal vital signs, history of hyper-/hypothermia or concern for infection, mental status and perfusion, and history of any high-risk conditions (cancer, immunocompromised, and indwelling central line). A positive screen prompts immediate clinician assessment. Many screening tools use systemic inflammatory response syndrome (SIRS) criteria to screen for sepsis; however, SIRS is common in many febrile children. Using SIRS alone is unreliable and results in overtriggering as a screening tool, which leads to alert fatigue.

CLINICAL ALGORITHM

Figure 12.1 presents an algorithm for the management of suspected severe sepsis in pediatric patients.

TREATMENT

Treatment of pediatric sepsis should be protocolized to achieve best outcomes. Bundled care improves morbidity and mortality by significantly reducing time to receipt of time-sensitive interventions and decreasing treatment variation. The Surviving Sepsis Campaign recommends the "Hour-1" bundle, which involves starting fluid resuscitation, obtaining blood cultures and lactate, administering antibiotics, and starting vasoactive agents if needed within the first hour of suspected sepsis. Many institutions have electronic order sets that are tailored to pediatric sepsis patients. These will have prechecked laboratory studies, IV/intraosseous (IO) placement orders, fluid options, recommended antibiotics for different age groups and populations, stress dose steroids, vasoactive infusions, imaging orders, and recommended

TABLE 12.2 SEPSIS-3 DEFINITIONS FOR SEPSIS, ORGAN DYSFUNCTION, AND SEPTIC SHOCK[a]

Sepsis	The presence of life-threatening organ dysfunction as a result of a dysregulated host response to infection
Organ dysfunction	Acute rise in the SOFA score of ≥2 points from up to 48 hours before the infection to 24 hours after the infection and received antimicrobial therapy
Severe sepsis	No longer used
Septic shock	Sepsis in which a vasoactive infusion is used to maintain MAP ≥65 mmHg and a maximum serum lactate level >2 mmol/L (18 mg/dL)

[a]The 2016 Sepsis-3 guidelines apply to adults only. The cutoffs for lactate and SBP are for adult patients. Currently, there are no official updated pediatric sepsis definitions.
MAP, mean arterial pressure; SOFA, Sequential Organ Failure Assessment.

TABLE 12.3 TRIAGE SCREENING TOOL AT CHILDREN'S NATIONAL HOSPITAL[A]

Points		Patient Vital Signs or Examination Abnormalities								
		Age <1 month	Age ≥1 to 2 months	Age 3–11 months	Age 1 year	Age 2–3 years	Age 4–5 years	Age 6–9 years	Age 10–13 years	Age >13 years
☐	Temperature (°C)	<36 or >38		<36 or >38.5						
☐	Systolic blood pressure (mmHg)	<60	<70	<70	<70+(age ×2)	<70+(age ×2)	<70+(age ×2)	<70+(age ×2)	<90	<90
☐	Heart rate (beats per minute)	>205	>205	>190	>190	>140	>140	>140	>100	>100
☐	Respiratory rate (breaths per minute)	>60	>60	>60	>40	>40	>34	>30	>30	>16
☐	Capillary refill time	<1 second (flash) or ≥3 seconds								
☐	Mental status	Irritability, confusion, inappropriate crying or drowsiness, poor interaction with parents, lethargy, decreased arousability, obtunded								
☐	Pulses	Decreased/weak or bounding								
☐	Skin	Petechiae below the nipple, any purpura, mottled and cool, flushed, ruddy, erythroderma other than on face								
☐	High-risk condition	Malignancy, sickle cell disease, central or indwelling line/catheter, bone marrow or solid organ transplant, severe intellectual disability or otherwise unable to evaluate patient's mental status, immunodeficiency or immunosuppression, asplenia								

[a]For a screen ≥3 points, clinician is notified to assess patient.
Source: Adapted from the tool developed for the Pediatric Septic Shock Collaborative sponsored by the American Academy of Pediatrics.

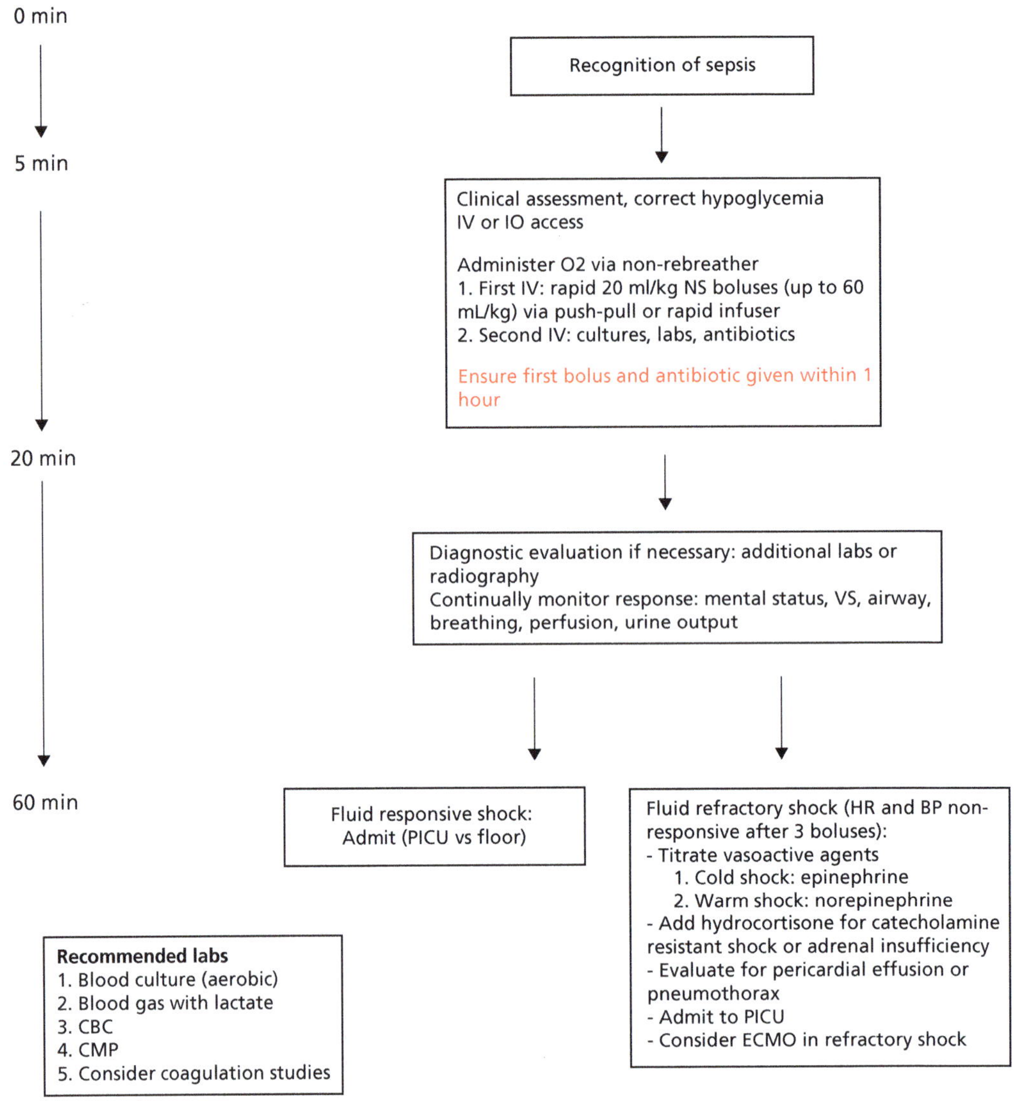

FIGURE 12.1 Algorithm for management of suspected severe sepsis in pediatric patients.

rapid sequence intubation medications. A pre-checked electronic order improves efficiency and accuracy of orders.

Initial Response to Septic Shock

Place the patient on a continuous monitor. Initiate Pediatric Advanced Life Support assessment and intervention as needed (see Chapter 8). Septic shock patients should be placed on 100% oxygen via a non-rebreather. Although the patient's saturation may be normal, tissues in sepsis have increased oxygen demand, worsened oxygen extraction, and altered oxygen metabolism. Escalate to high-flow nasal cannula, continuous positive airway pressure, bilevel positive airway pressure, or intubation as needed to achieve adequate oxygenation and ventilation. A child who is obtunded, nonresponsive, or not protecting his airway requires a definitive airway. Avoid etomidate in rapid sequence intubation because it may suppress adrenal function. If mechanical ventilation is required, cardiovascular instability during intubation is less likely after fluid and cardiovascular resuscitation.

Access

Obtaining vascular access and labs is often difficult in children, especially in cases of sepsis and septic shock. Escalate early if unable to achieve

TABLE 12.4 IV ACCESS ESCALATION PLAN

Minutes	Access Procedure
0–5	First peripheral IV largest gauge and as proximally located as possible IO immediately in severely ill or obtunded patients
5–10	Second peripheral IV attempt
After 10	If no access IO US-guided IV IV team External jugular

IO, intraosseous; IV, intravenous; US, ultrasound.

access (Table 12.4) because access is the major barrier to delivering time-sensitive treatment in sepsis care. Consider IO placement early if patients are severely ill, after two failed attempts, or if access is not obtained within 10 minutes of assessment. Two access points with the largest bore IVs possible as proximal as possible is recommended. Prioritizing fluid resuscitation in pediatric shock leads to improved outcomes; therefore, secure the first vascular access point quickly and use it for fluid resuscitation. The second access point can be done more meticulously and used for obtaining cultures, labs, and administering antibiotics. Providers from other departments who are skilled in difficult pediatric access may be utilized, such as the hospital's IV team, those in the neonatal ICU or PICU, and the peripherally inserted central catheter line team. Intraosseous access is preferred if peripheral access is difficult, but ultrasound-guided lines and external jugular lines may also be considered. A central line may be indicated for continued resuscitation but should not be the initial access due to relative increased difficulty of placement in children. Providers often delay resuscitation and definitive therapy when attempting central access. Intramuscular antibiotics should be given if an IV is delayed.

Fluid Resuscitation and Vasoactive Agents

Children usually exhibit large fluid deficits and require 40–60 mL/kg of initial fluid resuscitation with balanced solutions. Fluid boluses should be 20 mL/kg and given push–pull or using a pressure bag. Reassess after each bolus for need for more boluses (i.e., hypotension, tachycardia, delayed or flash capillary refill). If rales or hepatomegaly develops and hypotension persists, start vasoactive agents and hold fluid resuscitation. If after three 20 mL/kg boluses the patient is still hypotensive, consider fluid-refractory shock and initiate vasoactive agents.

In contrast to adults, children typically present with cold shock and require different vasoactive agents compared to warm shock that occurs more commonly in adults (Table 12.5). Patients with cold shock will have evidence

TABLE 12.5 REFRACTORY SHOCK AND VASOACTIVE AGENTS

	Physical Examination	Vasoactive Agent Choice
Cold shock	Evidence of vasoconstriction (mottled, cool, or clammy extremities) Capillary refill >3 seconds Diminished peripheral pulses	Begin epinephrine at 0.1 µg/kg/min (maximum 1 µg/kg/min)
Warm shock	Evidence of vasodilation (warm, flushed extremities) Brisk capillary refill Bounding peripheral pulses Wide pulse pressure	Begin norepinephrine at 0.1 µg/kg/min (maximum 2 µg/kg/min)

Start a second agent and steroids if epinephrine or norepinephrine is running at ≥0.3 µg/kg/min and desired effect is not achieved.

Dopamine is no longer considered first-line treatment for pediatric fluid refractory shock. Dopamine can be used as a second agent.

Milrinone is the ionotropic agent of choice for decompensated heart failure and frequently used in cold shock with poor cardiac function (with concomitant epinephrine). Milrinone may cause/exacerbate hypotension.

of vasoconstriction on physical examination, including mottled, cool, or clammy extremities; delayed capillary refill; and diminished peripheral pulses. Patients with warm shock will have evidence of vasodilation on examination, including warm, flushed extremities; brisk capillary refill; bounding peripheral pulses; and wide pulse pressures. Epinephrine is first line for cold shock and norepinephrine is first line for warm shock. Consider starting a second agent and steroids if epinephrine or norepinephrine is running at ≥0.3 μg/kg/min and desired effect is not achieved (e.g., if using epinephrine, add norepinephrine or dopamine). Dopamine is no longer considered first-line treatment in pediatric shock, although it can be used as a second agent. Milrinone is the inotropic agent of choice for decompensated heart failure. It increases contractility and reduces afterload without significantly increasing myocardial consumption. Vasoactive agents can be given peripherally until central venous access is obtained.

There are no formal prospective studies to indicate superiority of lactated Ringer's (LR) or normal saline (NS) boluses in pediatric sepsis or septic shock. NS is currently used in most cases of pediatric septic shock, although there are concerns that 0.9% NS contains supraphysiologic amounts of chloride and can worsen systemic inflammation and acidosis. In adults, buffered crystalloids, including LR, have demonstrated a 1–4% absolute mortality reduction and lower odds of dialysis compared to NS in observational and nonrandomized interventional studies. Retrospective studies in pediatrics examining any use of LR in resuscitation showed that LR was not associated with improved outcomes in pediatric sepsis. The use of albumin does not improve mortality in patients with sepsis.

Labs

If the clinical picture permits, draw blood cultures prior to antibiotic administration. Because anaerobic bacteremia is less common in pediatrics, prioritize aerobic blood cultures. The blood culture is usually negative in pediatric sepsis due to viral causes of sepsis and low bacterial load that cannot be detected by culture. Between 30%-75% of children with sepsis will have no infectious etiology identified. There is utility in obtaining a complete blood count (CBC) and lactate. CBC may reveal leukocytosis or leukopenia for age and bandemia. Check a blood gas with lactate. Lactate will be elevated if there are issues with end organ perfusion or function. An initial lactate >36 mg/dL is indicative of three times higher odds of mortality at 30 days compared to initial lactate levels <36 mg/dL. Liver function tests are often elevated in sepsis due to liver dysfunction and in neonates with systemic herpes infection. There are no current guidelines for the use of biomarkers in pediatric sepsis, and commonly used erythrocyte sedimentation rate and C-reactive protein offer little diagnostic value. An elevated procalcitonin (PCT) level > 0.5 ng/mL indicates a likely bacterial etiology for sepsis; however, one should not wait for PCT results to administer empiric antibiotics.

Antibiotic Therapy

Antibiotics should be tailored to the suspected infection. If unknown/undifferentiated or significantly ill, broad-spectrum coverage should be initiated and adjusted to culture results. Local resistance patterns vary and a local antibiogram should be followed. Empiric antibiotics vary by age and patient risk factors (Table 12.6). Infants younger than age 3 months are at risk for group B *Streptococcus, Listeria monocytogenes, Escherichia coli,* and herpes simplex viruses. Methicillin-resistant *Staphylococcus aureus* is also increasing in relative incidence. Neonates are also at higher risk for intracranial infections; therefore, antibiotic choice and dosing should be adequate to penetrate into the central nervous system. Herpes simplex encephalitis most commonly presents in young neonates. Add acyclovir in ill-appearing infants. Under- or unvaccinated children are at higher risk for sepsis and should be evaluated and treated more aggressively. Consider intramuscular antibiotics if IV or IO access cannot be achieved.

Steroids

Administer hydrocortisone in cases of fluid refractory, catecholamine-resistant shock and suspected or known adrenal insufficiency. Children with chronic steroid use will need stress-dose steroids.

Reassessment

The initial therapeutic end point of resuscitative efforts includes capillary refill ≤2 seconds,

TABLE 12.6 ANTIBIOTIC GUIDE BASED ON PATIENT HISTORY

Patient History	Antibiotic Choices	Additional Considerations
Previously healthy with community acquired infection	Ceftriaxone	Broaden with vancomycin Add clindamycin if suspect toxin-mediated syndrome
Neonate	Ampicillin and gentamicin (cefotaxime instead of gentamicin if high suspicion for meningitis for central nervous system penetration)	Consider acyclovir especially if ill-appearing
Suspected intra-abdominal source of infection	Piperacillin/tazobactam and vancomycin *Or* Ceftriaxone, metronidazole, and vancomycin	
Immunocompromised patient, history of cancer, chronic medical conditions, recent hospitalization, resides in a long-term care facility, indwelling central line	Cefepime and vancomycin	Consider antifungal coverage

normal blood pressure for age, normal pulses, warm extremities, urine output >1 mL/kg/hr, and baseline mental status. Continued monitoring and reassessment should occur, including documentation of mental status, vital signs, respiratory effort, capillary refill, and urine output. Mental status may be waxing and waning. Progression of illness may require a definitive airway. Initial fluid-responsive shock may quickly require vasoactive infusions.

DISPOSITION

All patients with suspicion of sepsis should be admitted. Ward admission may be reasonable if the patient has stabilized with appropriate therapy. Septic shock requires intensive monitoring and most commonly requires PICU admission. All children with persistent altered mental status, hemodynamic instability with or without need for vasoactive agents, and noninvasive or invasive respiratory support should be admitted to the PICU for continuous monitoring.

Children with shock who are initially treated at facilities without the capability of further treating these children in case end organ dysfunction persists should be immediately transported to an appropriate facility once stabilized. Using specialized pediatric transport teams is associated with improved patient outcomes. Call for transport early on during resuscitative efforts.

COMPLICATIONS

Pediatric sepsis is associated with high morbidity and mortality. Approximately 5,000 children die annually from septic shock in the United States. Every organ system is affected by sepsis, including the circulatory, pulmonary, central nervous, renal, and digestive system.

Circulatory dysfunction, usually manifesting as hypotension, is caused by mediator release to promote vasodilation in an attempt to match oxygen availability to changing tissue oxygen metabolism. Hypotension is also caused by increased endothelial permeability, reduced vascular tone, and increased capillary pressure causing third spacing. Myocardial function is depressed in sepsis, making it more difficult to maintain necessary blood pressure for end organ perfusion in the setting of vasodilation. Lungs are injured due to increased permeability causing pulmonary edema, which in turn creates ventilation–perfusion mismatch leading to hypoxemia. Hypoxemic injury ultimately results in acute respiratory distress syndrome.

Central nervous system complications occur frequently in septic patients, most commonly altered mental status (encephalopathy). The gastrointestinal tract shunts blood away during sepsis. In addition, the gastrointestinal tract's normal barrier function may be depressed, which allows translocation of bacteria and endotoxin into the systemic circulation, thereby worsening the dysregulated host response. Sepsis often results in acute renal injury. Poor perfusion and hypoxemia cause acute tubular necrosis, prompting the need for dialysis in 16–31% of cases. There is an increase in mortality for patients who develop renal failure—50% compared to 2–6% for those without renal failure.

KEY POINTS

- Pediatric sepsis can be subtle and does not require hypotension for diagnosis.
- Cold shock is more common in children, which makes epinephrine the first-line vasopressor agent.
- Bundled pediatric care improves morbidity, mortality, and outcomes in sepsis.
- Administer one to three 20 mL/kg boluses within the first 15 minutes and parenteral antibiotics within 60 minutes.
- If IV placement is not achieved within 10 minutes of initial assessment, consider placing an IO line in patients with septic shock.
- Fluid resuscitate with first IV; use second IV for cultures, labs, and antibiotics.
- Septic neonates are a special category with findings such as jaundice, irritability, lethargy, hyper- or hypothermia, or even normothermia.

PITFALLS

- Failure to recognize sepsis in a patient without hypotension or altered mental status
- Failure to obtain rapid access and administer fluids in a septic patient
- Failure to administer antibiotics quickly
- Failure to utilize appropriate vasopressors when indicated (epinephrine rather than norepinephrine in cold shock)

References

Balamuth F, Weiss SL, Neuman MI, et al. Pediatric severe sepsis in US children's hospitals. *Pediatr Crit Care Med.* 2014;15(9):798–805.

Cruz AT, Perry AM, Williams EA, et al. Implementation of goal-directed therapy for children with suspected sepsis in the emergency department. *Pediatrics.* 2011;127(3):e758–e766.

Dellinger RP, Levy MM, Rhodes A, et al. Surviving Sepsis Campaign: International guidelines for management of severe sepsis and septic shock: 2012. *Crit Care Med.* 2013;41(2):580–637.

Singer M, Deutschman CS, Seymour CW, et al. The Third International Consensus Definitions for Sepsis and Septic Shock (Sepsis-3). *JAMA.* 2016;315(8):801–810.

Weiss SL, Keele L, Balamuth F, et al. Crystalloid fluid choice and clinical outcomes in pediatric sepsis: A matched retrospective cohort study. *J Pediatr.* 2017;182:304–310.

13

Selected Infectious Disease Emergencies

SCOTT KOBNER AND EMILY ROSE

MENINGITIS

Background

Meningitis is an inflammation of the meninges that typically occurs in response to an infectious process, which can quickly lead to devastating neurological morbidity and high mortality rate if not identified and treated expediently. Untreated bacterial meningitis has nearly a 100% mortality rate. Even in children who are rapidly diagnosed and given appropriate therapy, neurological sequelae are common—especially in cases of bacterial meningitis. Secondary to successful vaccination programs, the incidence of *Haemophilus influenzae* type b (Hib), *Streptococcus pneumoniae*, and *Neisseria meningitidis* has significantly decreased. The highest incidence of bacterial meningitis remains in children younger than age 2 months, but the median age has shifted from younger than age 5 years to mid-adulthood in the current vaccination era. Currently, *S. pneumoniae* and *N. meningitidis* are the most common causes of bacterial meningitis in children older than age 1 month.

Risk factors include prenatal herpes simplex virus (HSV) or untreated group B *Streptococcus* in young infants, lack of immunizations in children older than age 2 months, communal living environment (e.g., a dormitory residence for college-age patients), or recent exposure.

Classic Presentation

The presenting signs of meningitis vary based on the age of the child and the etiology of meningeal inflammation. Meningitis may be acute and fulminant or more slowly progressive over several days. Upper respiratory symptoms frequently, and gastrointestinal symptoms occasionally, precede meningeal signs. Classic symptoms include fever, headaches, photophobia, nausea, vomiting, irritability, confusion, and lethargy.

Febrile neonates (<28 days) should be considered to have meningitis until proven otherwise because signs and symptoms in this age group are less reliable. Patients may present with seizures but typically have additional symptoms, such as preceding altered mental status, meningeal signs, or rash. It is extremely uncommon for bacterial meningitis to present with seizure in isolation of other symptoms or physical examination findings.

Children with bacterial meningitis are typically ill/toxic appearing. On physical examination, signs of meningeal irritation are less reliable in infants and may not occur or only be present late in the infection. Nuchal rigidity and signs of meningeal irritation (Kernig's or Brudzinksi's signs) become more reliable with age. Signs of increased interaction pressure may also be present on examination, such as papilledema or bulging fontanelle in infants. Cutaneous findings, such as petechiae and purpura, may be seen in cases of bacterial meningitis, most notably in cases of *N. meningitidis*.

The signs and symptoms of viral meningitis are similar to but less severe than those of bacterial meningitis. Enterovirus infection is the most common etiology of viral meningitis.

Diagnostic Confirmation

The gold standard confirmatory test for suspected cases of meningitis is lumbar puncture (LP) with cerebrospinal fluid (CSF) analysis.

CSF analysis can rapidly differentiate broad categories of meningitis by utilizing typical fluid patterns for various infectious processes (Table 13.1). However, these patterns are incompletely sensitive and specific, and they cannot entirely exclude infection. Rapid polymerase chain reaction (PCR) analysis may also assist with specific diagnosis. CSF culture typically confirms diagnosis, but results are typically delayed 1or 2 days, which limits emergent utility.

Additional laboratory tests to obtain include complete blood count (CBC), basic metabolic panel (BMP), liver function tests (LFTs), blood glucose, urinalysis, prothrombin time/partial thromboplastin time, and blood cultures. Additional serologic tests, such as HIV, HSV, measles, mumps, rubella, Epstein–Barr virus (EBV), varicella zoster virus, syphilis studies, or Lyme studies, may be useful with associated encephalitis.

Rapid neuroaxial imaging should be considered in all patients with acute altered mental status to exclude alternative etiology or to evaluate contraindications to LP. Head computed tomography (CT) is only necessary prior to LP in patients with signs or symptoms of increased intracranial pressure, which include depressed mental status, papilledema, known space-occupying lesion, history of trauma, and known CSF shunt or hydrocephalus, or those with focal neurologic symptoms.

Treatment

Antibiotic therapy should be initiated immediately in suspected bacterial meningitis. Ideally, CSF samples and blood cultures should be procured prior to initiation of therapy; but antibiotic administration should not be delayed for imaging or a contraindication to LP. Given the difficulty of clinically distinguishing bacterial from viral meningitis, antimicrobial therapy should be initiated until the etiology has clearly been differentiated. Specific empiric antibiotic and antiviral therapy varies by age because suspected pathogens are more likely in certain groups (Box 13.1). These therapies can then be tailored as more clinical data become available.

For many viral etiologies, specific antimicrobial treatment is not available. Acyclovir should be considered in all neonates (see Chapter 2 on the crashing neonate), particularly with CSF pleocytosis and in all children with associated encephalitis. Acyclovir should also be given in suspected HSV infections and in varicella. Ganciclovir may improve outcomes in cytomegalovirus (CMV) infection. Influenza may be treated with oseltamivir or zanamivir.

In addition to the previously mentioned therapies, all patients should receive routine

TABLE 13.1 SIMPLIFIED CEREBROSPINAL FLUID FINDINGS IN CENTRAL NERVOUS SYSTEM INFECTIONS

Condition	Glucose	WBC Count	Protein	Opening Pressure
Bacterial meningitis	Low	Elevated. Neutrophil predominance.	Elevated	Elevated
Viral meningitis	Normal	Normal, mildly elevated. Lymphocytic predominance.	Normal, mildly elevated	Normal
Fungal/TB	Normal or mildly low	Normal, mildly elevated. May be eosinophilic.	Elevated	Normal to elevated
Encephalitis	Normal or low	Normal, mildly elevated. Lymphocytic predominance.	Elevated	Normal

WBC, white blood cell.

BOX 13.1
ANTIMICROBIALS FOR THE TREATMENT OF MENINGITIS

Empiric antimicrobials for neonatal meningitis

Cefotaxime 100–200 mg/kg div q6–8h *or* gentamicin 2.5 mg/kg q8–12h *and* ampicillin 50–200 mg/kg IV div q6h.

Vancomycin 15 mg/kg IV q8–24h (adjust based on serum levels); dose should be given in cases of prior neonatal intensive care unit stay, suspicion for resistant organisms, and abnormal CSF results.

Acyclovir 20 mg/kg q8h should be considered in a neonate with a vesicular rash, a maternal history of herpes, or abnormal CSF, particularly within the first 2–3 weeks of life.

Empiric antimicrobials for suspected meningitis in children ≥1 month of age

Cefotaxime 150 mg/kg div q8h *or* ceftriaxone 100 mg/kg q12–24h *plus* vancomycin 15 mg/kg (maximum 1 g) IV q6–8h; adjust dose based on serum levels.

Antimicrobials for special circumstances

Cancer and neutropenia: gentamicin 7.5 mg/kg per day IV in 3 divided doses, or amikacin 15–22.5 mg/kg per day IV in 3 divided doses (maximum 1.5 g/day) should be added.

T-cell Disorders: high-dose ampicillin (300 to 400 mg/kg IV per day (maximum 10 to 12 g/day) in 4 or 6 divided doses should be added.

Extended-spectrum beta-lactamase (ESBL)-producing organism suspected: 40 mg/kg/dose every 8 hours (maximum 2,000 mg/dose).

CSF, cerebrospinal fluid; IV, intravenously.

supportive care and be closely monitored for seizure activity. Seizures can be managed with typical antiepileptic strategies (see Chapter 20 on neurologic emergencies).

The use of dexamethasone to prevent neurologic sequela remains controversial. The best available evidence only supports the use of appropriately timed steroids (given before or at the same time as initial empiric antibiotics), only in cases of meningitis caused by Hib. Steroids should not be given to patients with non-gram-negative, aseptic, or nonbacterial meningitis or if they are younger than age 6 weeks.

Disposition

All patients with suspect meningitis require admission. Level of care depends on clinical scenario; all patients with high suspicion of disease require intensive care.

Complications

Complications of bacterial meningitis include hearing loss, intellectual disabilities, movement disorders, and seizure disorders. Most patients with viral meningitis recover without complications.

Key Points

- Meningitis is a life-threatening disease process that requires prompt recognition and treatment.
- Bacterial meningitis has an untreated mortality rate approaching 100%.
- Do not delay empiric antibiotic and antiviral therapy (where appropriate) for LP or CT.
- All patients with suspected meningitis require hospital admission.

Pitfalls

- Failure to consider meningitis in a patient with altered mental status
- Delaying empiric therapy if LP is contraindicated or CT is required

ENCEPHALITIS

Background

Encephalitis is an inflammation of the brain parenchyma that presents clinically with neurologic dysfunction. Most commonly, this inflammation is the result of an infectious process, but many rheumatologic and immunologic phenomena produce similar clinical manifestations of disease. Encephalitis can be clinically challenging to diagnose because significant overlap syndromes exist—inflammation is not always limited to brain parenchyma and may involve the meninges or other structures (meningoencephalitis). Infectious pediatric encephalitis is predominately viral in etiology and is relatively uncommon: The incidence of disease is 3–13 per 100,000 children per year. Encephalitis predominantly affects younger children, with the highest incidence in infants. See Chapter 20 on neurologic emergencies for more information on other causes of encephalitis in children.

Classic Presentation

The signs and symptoms of viral encephalitis vary broadly, and symptoms will largely depend on the area and location of involved brain. Presenting features include fever, seizures (especially focal seizure activity), focal neurologic signs, and decreased level of consciousness.

In neonates and infants, signs and symptoms are largely nonspecific and include irritability, poor feeding, and lethargy. Notably, fever is a variable finding in this age group, and the absence of fever may cause diagnostic error. A history of preceding viral illness may be present. Because HSV encephalitis is a devastating infection, this diagnosis should always be considered, particularly in neonates younger than age 3 weeks. Vesicular rash and fever only occur in the minority of patients.

As children become older, signs and symptoms become even broader and at times localized to the area of the brain that is infected. Patients can present with movement disorders, ataxia, localized neurologic signs and deficits, confusion, or changes in behavior. Psychiatric symptoms can also predominate, ranging from affective disorders personality changes or even frank psychosis. New, sudden onset of psychiatric symptoms should trigger consideration of encephalitis as an underlying etiology.

In the most severe cases of encephalitis, disease progression is often acute and may present with diffuse cerebral edema or status epilepticus.

Atypical Presentation

Less common etiologies of infectious encephalitis can lead to atypical presentations of disease and may prompt alternative therapies or public health interventions. A detailed travel history should be obtained to assess for etiologies that may be endemic to various regions (e.g., Lyme disease and West Nile virus). A history of possible exposure to pathogens or pathogen carriers may also enlighten the clinical to an underlying cause (e.g., tuberculosis exposure, high-risk sexual practices, and encounters with livestock). Finally, an understanding of a patient's immune status is essential: Lack of vaccinations exposes patients to measles virus encephalitis, and immunodeficiencies such as HIV increase the likelihood that fungal or parasitic infections are present. Fungal and parasitic pathogens in particular may present with a subacute time course, making diagnosis even more challenging on an initial encounter.

The majority of cases of infectious encephalitis are caused by viruses, of which enteroviruses and Herpesviridae (e.g., EBV, CMV, and HSV) are the most common pathogens. Exanthems may be associated with specific etiologies, such as a vesicular rash in HSV, oral/palm/sole ulcerations of hand–foot–mouth disease with coxsackie virus, a maculopapular rash with West Nile virus, and lesions on wrist/ankles that progress to palms/soles in Rocky Mountain spotted fever (see Chapter 23 on dermatological emergencies).

Diagnostic Confirmation

Encephalitis is a clinical diagnosis, and in the emergent setting, no diagnostic test can reliably exclude the presence of infectious encephalitis. Clinical criteria may facilitate diagnosis (see Table 13.1).

All patients should also undergo emergent neuroaxial imaging. Magnetic resonance imaging (MRI) is the imaging study of choice because it has superior diagnostic sensitivity; however, noncontrast CT may be indicated to exclude contraindications to LP or other emergent alternative diagnoses.

Evaluation of patients with suspected encephalitis should have a similar diagnostic workup as the evaluation of meningitis, including an LP and CSF analysis. CSF analysis includes cell count and differential, glucose, protein, gram stain, culture, and PCR analysis. If available, it may be useful to order specific CSF antibody or antigen titers or to freeze additional CSF samples to facilitate diagnosis in the inpatient setting.

CSF studies may appear similar to those seen in viral meningitis if a viral etiology is present. Classically, a lymphocytic pleocytosis is observed; however, early in the course of disease, studies may reflect a granulocytic pleocytosis. Significant red blood cells or xanthochromia is suggestive of HSV infection. Normal CSF findings can be observed in up to 5% of cases of encephalitis.

PCR studies may identify etiology and direct targeted therapies.

In addition to LP, patients should also undergo evaluation for other etiologies of altered mental status, including blood cultures, CBC, BMP, LFTs, and HIV serologies, in addition to metabolic and toxicological studies.

Treatment

Initial treatment of suspected encephalitis includes stabilization of the airway as indicated and ensuring adequate perfusion. Empiric acyclovir therapy should be initiated in most cases until HSV infection is excluded. Empiric antibiotic therapy (vancomycin and a third-generation cephalosporin such as ceftriaxone or cefotaxime) is typically also indicated until bacterial infection is excluded.

Tick-borne illnesses such as rickettsial and ehrlichial infections should also be considered (see Chapter 23). If there is a clinical concern that patients may have Rocky Mountain spotted fever, Q fever, ehrlichiosis, or anaplasmosis, empiric treatment with doxycycline 2.2 mg/kg (maximum 100 mg) BID PO or intravenously (IV) is indicated and improves outcomes.

In addition to antimicrobial agents, supportive care is the mainstay of emergency therapy. Seizure activity should be actively treated (see Chapter 20). Currently, there is no role for adjunctive therapies such as steroids, plasmapheresis, or IV immunoglobulin for infectious encephalitis.

Disposition

All patients with suspected encephalitis should be admitted. Most require intensive care during initial evaluation and management.

Complications

The sequelae of infectious encephalitis vary with etiology. Mortality rate is 7% overall, but it can be as high as 20–30% with HSV infection. Poor outcome is associated with coma, seizures, or focal neurologic deficits. Approximately 50% of patients with infectious encephalitis recover without neurological sequelae, whereas the other 50% suffer from a wide array of neurologic problems ranging from focal motor dysfunction to developmental delays, behavioral disorders, and seizure disorders. Nearly all HSV encephalitis survivors have neurologic deficits.

Key Points

- Encephalitis is a life-threatening disease with significant morbidity and mortality.
- All cases of encephalitis should be initially treated with acyclovir.
- Consider specific etiologies based on clinical data, and provide additional empiric therapies on this basis.
- All patients with suspected encephalitis require admission.

Pitfalls

- Failure to consider encephalitis with a new-onset psychiatric disorder
- Failure to administer acyclovir

RETROPHARYNGEAL ABSCESS

Background

Retropharyngeal abscess (RPA) is a potentially life-threatening airway emergency secondary to an infection of the retropharyngeal soft tissue space. The retropharyngeal soft tissue is a potential space between the posterior pharyngeal wall and prevertebral fascia with the potential to extend into the mediastinum or occlude the airway. This space is rich in lymph tissue, which drains the commonly infected structures of the head. An abscess may develop from contiguous spread, hematogenous seeding, or direct posterior oropharyngeal trauma. These lymphatic tissues are prominent in young children but atrophy before puberty. RPAs most commonly occur in children aged 2–4 years.

Classic Presentation

Presenting symptoms include fever, odynophagia, dysphasia, drooling, torticollis, dysphonia, and trismus. Severe inflammation of the retropharyngeal space that begins to occlude the airway may also cause significant respiratory distress, including tachypnea and stridor. Patients with RPA are often reluctant to extend the neck and unwilling to look side to side. Neck stiffness may mimic the nuchal rigidity of meningitis.

Atypical Presentation

Although the retropharyngeal lymphatics regress before puberty, RPA may develop in older children and adults. Direct posterior oropharyngeal trauma is typically the inciting event.

In delayed presentations or rapidly necrotizing infections, RPAs may present as fulminant airway obstruction or mediastinitis.

Differential Diagnosis

Other causes of upper airway obstruction and infection include epiglottis, peritonsillar abscess, bacterial tracheitis, anterior cervical lymphadenitis, pharyngitis, malignancies, and traumatic injury. Meningitis and discitis may also present with neck pain.

Diagnostic Confirmation

Neck CT with IV contrast is the most commonly used modality for diagnosis of RPA. CT can differentiate an abscess from cellulitis or simple edema and evaluate airway involvement. MRI may be alternatively used if available.

Lateral radiographs of the neck have been historically used to assess the size of the prevertebral space as a surrogate marker for RPAs. In settings in which CT is not available, this may be a useful adjunct; but suggestive radiographs alone are not definitive for diagnosis or management.

Treatment

Management is dictated by the clinical status of the patient, the size of the abscess, and the degree of airway obstruction. In patients with symptoms of impending airway obstruction, aggressive and definitive management of the airway is the most important aspect of emergency management. However, intubation may be complicated by distorted anatomy and may lead to abscess rupture, so early otolaryngology consultation is advised.

Some retropharyngeal infections respond to IV antibiotics and do not require surgical intervention. Imaging features suggestive of abscess (and more likely to require surgical drainage) include lesions larger than 2.5 cm, rim enhancement, and scalloping of the abscess wall. Empiric antibiotic therapy should target typical aerodigestive tract flora. Options include ampicillin–sulbactam 50 mg/kg q6h or clindamycin 15 mg/kg q8h. Vancomycin should be added with significant toxicity or if methicillin-resistant *Staphylococcus aureus* infection is suspected.

Disposition

All patients with retropharyngeal infections should be admitted for IV antibiotics. Immediate surgical intervention may be warranted with airway compromise. Intensive care may be required with significant toxicity or potential airway compromise.

Complications

Complications from RPAs arise from extension of the infection into surrounding structures or airway obstruction. RPAs can extend both down into the mediastinum and also laterally into the vasculature of the neck, causing a septic thrombophlebitis. When an RPA ruptures—due to either internal pressure or external manipulation—aspiration pneumonia can result. Airway obstruction, respiratory failure, sepsis, and death are potential complications of untreated RPA.

Key Points

- Retropharyngeal infections are deep space neck infections that typically affect children aged 2–4 years.
- Airway compromise and significant extension are potential complications.
- Difficulty extending the neck or looking laterally are classic physical examination findings.
- CT of the neck with IV contrast is the diagnostic study of choice.

Pitfalls

- Failure to obtain imaging in suspected cases
- Failure to anticipate airway compromise

CAT SCRATCH DISEASE

Background

Cat scratch disease (CSD) is an infectious lymphadenopathy caused by *Bartonella henselae* after exposure to cats or cat fleas. It is most commonly a self-limited disease found in younger children, but it can have rare, life-threatening complications, including central nervous system (CNS) involvement. This disease is typically diagnosed based on history and physical examination.

Transmission typically occurs via a scratch or bite from a cat infected with *B. henselae* or from exposure to carrier fleas. Infection may also occur via contact with cat saliva to broken skin or mucosal surfaces.

Classic Presentation

The majority of children present with cutaneous symptoms at the site of inoculation, followed later (2 weeks) by regional lymphadenopathy proximal to the inoculation site.

Local cutaneous changes develop over the inoculation site several days after transmission; these may be erythematous, papular, or vesicular. Weeks later, proximal, tender lymphadenopathy develops. This most commonly involves lymph nodes of the upper extremities, axilla, and neck. Lymph nodes are typically tender with overlying erythema and may be suppurative. They are most commonly 1–5 cm but may be up to 10 cm. Single lesions or regional lymphadenopathy may be present. However, diffuse lymphadenopathy is atypical and should prompt the consideration of alternative diagnoses. Fever may or may not be present at the time of presentation.

Atypical Presentation

Cat scratch disease has several known, potentially life-threatening, atypical presentations. The most consequential is CNS infection, which can manifest as encephalopathy, transverse myelitis, or cerebral vasculitis. Presenting features include focal neurologic deficits, seizures, and confusion.

CSD may also present with ocular manifestations. The spectrum of disease encompasses neuroretinitis (with acute vision loss from optic nerve edema) to more localized infections of the eye. Parinaud oculoglandular syndrome typically occurs after inoculation of a cat bite/lick near the eye. It presents with regional lymphadenopathy (preauricular, submandibular, or cervical lymph nodes) and infection of the epithelial surfaces of the eye (conjunctiva), eyelid, or surrounding skin. Unilateral injection, tearing, foreign body sensation is common. Serous or even purulent ocular discharge may be present.

Visceral CSD infection may occur, and it is an important consideration in the evaluation of a fever of unknown origin (see Chapter 10 on the evaluation of the extended fever). Patients with visceral disease usually have necrotizing granulomas of the liver and/or spleen, resulting in hepatosplenomegaly, fever, and weight loss.

Musculoskeletal symptoms such as myalgias, arthritis/arthralgias, and boney involvement may also occur.

Differential Diagnosis

Lymphadenitis may occur with localized bacterial infection, mycobacterium infections, viral syndromes, and other rare causes of bacterial lymphadenitis such as tularemia. Malignancy, particularly lymphoma, should also be considered with lymphadenopathy and systemic symptoms.

Diagnostic Confirmation

The diagnosis of CSD is made based on history and examination findings for cutaneous disease. Although serologic testing does exist, it is not sensitive, and immunologic studies can be falsely negative throughout the course of illness. Culture data are also difficult to obtain because *Bartonella* requires a protracted incubation period and special culture medium.

Treatment

Antibiotic treatment is indicated for all cases of suspected CSD, even though many cases are self-limited and resolve without treatment. For cutaneous disease with lymphadenitis, initial therapy is a 5-day course of azithromycin. Alternatively, 7–10 days of rifampin or trimethroprim–sulfamethoxazole may be used as initial therapy. More significant disease or treatment nonresponse should be treated with an additional agent (most commonly rifampin).

Visceral disease should be treated initially with a combination of azithromycin and rifampin. When neurologic involvement is present, doxycycline plus rifampin is the preferred treatment regimen. If vision-threatening infections are present, doxycycline should be given even if patients are younger than age 8 years.

Disposition

Patients may be discharged with uncomplicated cutaneous CSD. Patients with visceral, ocular, or CNS manifestations of disease frequently require admission and IV antibiotics.

Complications

Most CSD resolves without sequelae. Untreated lymphadenopathy often resolves after several months. Disseminated infections are more severe with immunocompromise or concomitant HIV. Long-term sequelae are more common in ocular or CNS involvement and include permanent neurologic deficits.

Key Points

- CSD is a bacterial infection caused by *B. henselae* after exposure to cats or cat fleas.
- CSD most commonly presents as a localized cutaneous lesion followed by proximal lymphadenitis approximately 2 weeks after inoculation.
- Atypical and more severe visceral, ocular, and CNS manifestations of disease may occur.
- Initial treatment is 5 days of azithromycin.

Pitfalls

- Failure to recognize atypical presentations of CSD and initiate appropriate treatment
- Failure to initiate doxycycline in severe infections

14

Vaccine-Preventable Disease

LOREN G. YAMAMOTO

Vaccines are the most cost-effective strategy to prevent these diseases and their complications. Many adults have no experience with many of these diseases because many have become very uncommon. Because many parents have refused vaccines for their children, epidemics of vaccine-preventable diseases have occurred and will continue to occur. These epidemics can affect immunocompromised individuals and children who are too young for vaccines (e.g., a measles epidemic can expose infants to measles before they can be vaccinated). Table 14.1 summarizes some key clinical features of vaccine-preventable diseases.

Herd immunity offers some degree of protection against an epidemic in susceptible (nonvaccinated) individuals if the vaccination rate is high enough. However, this protection is incomplete because of frequent and rapid international travel through concentrated points of entry such as airports, cruise ships, theme parks, sports events, concerts, shopping centers, schools, mass transit systems, hotels, and restaurants.

Immunization recommendations in the United States are established by the Advisory Committee on Immunization Practices of the Centers for Disease Control and Prevention (CDC) and the Committee on Infectious Disease (also known as the Red Book Committee) of the American Academy of Pediatrics.

DTAP AND TDAP

The DtaP and TdaP vaccines provide protection against diphtheria, tetanus, and pertussis. The new "acellular" ("a") pertussis vaccination has less adverse effects but a shorter duration of immunity. The diphtheria component is a toxoid (denatured diphtheria toxin) that results in an immune response against the diphtheria toxin rendering it inactive. DTaP and DT have a higher potency diphtheria toxoid component and are for children younger than age 7 years. After this age, TdaP and Td with the lower potency diphtheria toxoid are used instead.

Diphtheria

Diphtheria is due to an infection with *Corynebacterium diphtheria*, which produces an exotoxin that inhibits protein synthesis and causes local tissue necrosis, resulting in severe nasopharyngitis (a thick gray membrane visible over the pharynx), airway symptoms known as membranous croup, cervical lymphadenitis (known as "bull neck"), myocarditis, and cranial/peripheral neuropathy. Treatment consists of antibiotics (erythromycin and penicillin) and diphtheria antitoxin.

TABLE 14.1 SUMMARY OF CLINICAL PRESENTATION AND TREATMENT OF VACCINE-PREVENTABLE DISEASES

Vaccine	Disease Entity	Virulent Agent	Vaccine Immunizing Strategy	Clinical Disease Manifestations	Virulence Factor	Incubation Period	Dominant Transmission Mode	Confirmatory Testing	Antimicrobials	Likely to Encounter in U.S.
DTaP	Diphtheria	Bacteria, toxin	Toxoid	Severe pharyngitis, menbranous nasopharyngitis/croup, skin lesions, cervical lymphadenitis (bull neck), myocarditis, cranial/peripheral neuropathy	Exotoxin inhibits protein synthesis and causes local tissue necrosis	2–5 days (range 1–10 days)	airborne respiratory droplets, direct contact	culture, MALDI-TOF*	diphtheria antitoxin, erythromycin, penicillin	No
	Tetanus	Toxin, bacteria	Toxoid	Generalized tetanus presents with trismus (masseter spasm, "lock jaw"), followed by stiffness, risus sardonicus (sardonic smile), opisthotonos (extreme body hyperextension), airway obstruction, seizures. Neonatal tetanus manifested by difficulty feeding, diminished movement, stiffness.	Tetanus neurotoxin (tetanospasmin)	2–14 days (range 2–21 days)	direct wound inoculation or newborn (umbilical stump) contamination.	unreliable	tetanus antitoxin, IVIG, metronidazole, penicillin, tetanus toxoid (prophylaxis)	No
	Pertussis	Bacteria, toxin	Acellular bacterial antigens	Pertussis (also known as "whooping cough"). Classic stages: 1) catarrhal, 2) paryoxysmal cough, 3) convalescent.	Pertussis toxin, other toxins	7–10 days (range 5–21 days)	respiratory droplets	rapid respiratory panel testing, PCR, serology, culture	azithromycin, (alternative trimethoprim/ sulfamethoxazole)	Yes

IPV	Polio	Virus	Inactivated virus	Most often non-symptomatic. 25% have low grade fever and sore throat. 1%-5% have viral meningitis. <1% develop paralytic poliomyelitis. Vaccine associated paralytic poliomyelitis (VAPP) occurred in rare cases of live attenuated oral poliovirus (OPV) vaccine. VAPP cases no longer occur with IPV vaccine.	virus	3–6 days for non-paralytic polio, but 7–21 days for paralytic polio (range 3–35 days)	fecal-oral, contact with respiratory secretions	viral culture (to cell media) from pharynx and stool	none	No
HepB	Hepatitis B	Virus	Inactivated virus	hepatitis (often asymptomatic), liver failure, chronic hepatitis, cirrhosis, hepatocellular carcinoma	virus	60–180 days	blood and body fluids are highest risk, other transmission routes possible.	serology	HBIG (prophylaxis only), interferon and necleoside/ nucleotide inhibitors for chronic hepatis B	Yes
HepA	Hepatitis A	Virus	Inactivated virus	acute hepatitis (frequently asymptomatic), liver failure is rare	virus	15–19 days (range up to 50 days)	fecal-oral, food/ water borne	serology	gamma globulin (prophylaxis only)	Yes
Rotavirus	Rotavirus	Virus	Live attenuated virus	Rotavirus gastroenteritis, dehydration	virus	less than 2 days (range 1– 7 days)	fecal-oral, direct contact, fomites	rapid stool testing	none	Yes
Varicella (monovalent or part of combined MMRV)	Varicella	Virus	Live attenuated virus	Cutaneous varicella (chickenpox), cerebelar ataxia, encephalitis, pneumonia, disseminated varicella, zoster (shingles)	virus	14–16 days (range 10–21 days)	direct contact with skin lesions	PCR, direct fluorescent antibody, serology. Tzank smear is non-specific.	acyclovir, varicella/ zoster immune globulin	Yes

(*continued*)

TABLE 14.1 CONTINUED

Vaccine	Disease Entity	Virulent Agent	Vaccine Immunizing Strategy	Clinical Disease Manifestations	Virulence Factor	Incubation Period	Dominant Transmission Mode	Confirmatory Testing	Antimicrobials	Likely to Encounter in U.S.
MMR	Measles	Virus	Live attenuated virus	Rubeola (measles), exanthem/enanthem, pneumonia, acute encephalitis, subacute sclerosing panencephalitis (SSPE), blindness	virus	8–12 days to onset of symptoms	direct contact with droplets or by airborne spread	serology, reverse transcriptase PCR	ribavirin (limited), IVIG (limited)	Yes
	Mumps	Virus	Live attenuated virus	Parotitis, orchitis, oophritis	virus	16–18 days (range 12–25 days)	contact with respiratory droplets or saliva	serology	none	Yes
	Rubella	Virus	Live attenuated virus	German measles, exathem, congenital rubella syndrome	virus		direct or droplet contact from nasopharyngeal secretions	serology	none	Yes
Hib	Haemophilus influenza type b	Bacteria	Polysaccharide capsule antigens	Meningitis, sepsis, epiglottitis, septic arthritis, cellulitis, pneumonia	polysaccharide capsule	not known, probably highly variable	inhalation of respiratory droplets or direct contact with respiratory secretions	NAAT**, gram stain, culture	cefotaxime (or ceftriaxone), see text. rifampin for susceptible child contact prophylaxis only	Yes
PCV-13	Pneumococcus	Bacteria	Polysaccharide capsule antigens	Sepsis, meningitis, pneumonia, otitis media, sinusitis	polysaccharide capsule	highly variable but as short as 1–3 days	respiratory droplets, high nasapharyngeal carrier rate	NAAT**, gram stain, culture	high dose amoxicillin (outpatient), cefotaxime (or ceftriaxone) plus vancomycin (for invasive disease), see text	Yes

Meningococcus	Menincococcus	Bacteria	Polysaccharide antigens	Sepsis, meningitis	polysaccharide capsule	1–10 days	contact with respiratory droplets, requires close contact	NAAT**, gram stain, culture, MALDI-TOF*	cefotaxime (or ceftriaxone), see text. child/adult susceptible contact prophylaxis options, see text.	Yes
Influenza	Influenza	Virus	Inactivated virus; live attenuated intranasal version available	Pneumonia, respiratory failure.	virus	1–4 days	direct contact and respiratory droplets from coughing/sneezing	rapid testing, PCR	oseltamivir, see text	Yes
Palivizumab	RSV	Virus	Passive monoclonal antibody	bronchiolitis in low risk patients; severe pneumonia and respiratory failure in high risk patients. Palivizumab is only used for high risk patients.	virus	4–6 days (range 2–8 days)	direct or close contactwith respiratory droplets	rapid viral testing	ribavirin	Yes
Available vaccines not used routinely in the U.S.										
Rabies	Rabies	Virus	Inactivated virus	Encephalitis, death	virus	1–3 months	bite from a rabid mammal or close contact with a rabid bat	reverse transcriptase PCR	no treatment available; for post exposure prophylaxis, administer rabies immune globulin (RIG) into the bite wound and rabies vaccine at a separate site.	No

(*continued*)

TABLE 14.1 CONTINUED

Vaccine	Disease Entity	Virulent Agent	Vaccine Immunizing Strategy	Clinical Disease Manifestations	Virulence Factor	Incubation Period	Dominant Transmission Mode	Confirmatory Testing	Antimicrobials	Likely to Encounter in U.S.
BCG	Tuberculosis	Bacteria	Live attenuated mycobacterium	Tuberculosis (TB), meningitis, osteomyelitis, many other manifestations. Atypical mycobacteria can cause similar disease	mycobacteria	Ranges from very short to very long	inhalation of airborne mucus droplet nuclei	tuberculin skin testing, interferon gamma release assay (IGRA)	extensive list of anti-TB drugs	Yes
Typhoid	Typhoid fever	S. typhi	live oral attenuated or intramuscular polysaccharide vaccine	enteric fever (typhoid fever): fever, bacteremia, abdominal pain, hepatosplenomegaly, headache, lethargy, "rose spots," shock, and occasionally myocarditis	bacteria	7–14 days (range 3–60 days)	fecal-oral, direct contact, food/water borne	culture, immunoassay, PCR	azithromycin, third generation cephalosporin, fluoroquinolone	Yes

*MALDI-TOF (matrix-assisted laser desorption/ionization time of flight mass spectroscopy) applied to colonies yielding a mass spectroscopy profile that identifies the organism and its subtype.

Tetanus

Tetanus is due to an infection with *Clostridium tetani*, which is an anaerobic organism that can infect contaminated wounds. The infection itself is noninvasive; however, the organism produces the neurotoxin tetanospasmin (tetanus toxin), resulting in a syndrome called "locked jaw." Penetrating wounds are at higher risk than superficial wounds. Treatment consists of antibiotics (metronidazole and penicillin), wound debridement, and tetanus immune globulin (TIG). The active vaccine is a toxoid directed at the tetanus toxin. It is very effective at preventing tetanus, but it does not prevent colonization with *Cl. tetani* organisms. Tetanus toxoid booster immunization is commonly of interest for patients in the emergency department (ED) presenting with penetrating wounds. The current recommendation is to administer a tetanus toxoid booster for nonminor contaminated wounds if the patient's most recent tetanus booster was more than 5 years ago. This largely applies to patients aged 9–12 years because most children have had a DTaP series with their last dose at age 4 or 5 years and their next TdaP dose is administered at approximately age 11 or 12 years. Plain tetanus toxoid is no longer available, and TdaP has largely replaced Td for routine tetanus prophylaxis. TIG prophylaxis is recommended for tetanus-prone wounds if the patient has had no primary immunizing series or if the patient has significant risk factors (for specific recommendations, see Chapter 26 on wound care).

Pertussis

Pertussis (also known as "whooping cough") is due to an infection with *Bordetella pertussis*, which produces several toxins, of which pertussis toxin is the major virulence factor. Three stages are classically described. First, the catarrhal stage begins 3–12 days following exposure (1 or 2 weeks' duration) and manifests with cold symptoms. Second, the paroxysmal stage (2–6 weeks' duration) is characterized by severe cough in paroxysms. Classically, these are series of uninterrupted coughs during the same exhalation, with eyes bulging/watering and tongue protruding, followed by a noisy coarse inhalation (the "whooping" sound). Infants often turn red during these episodes and are sometimes cyanotic. Third, the convalescent stage (≥2 weeks' duration) is characterized by gradual recovery. Young infants (aged <3 months) can have atypical courses with less coughing and noisy breathing. Apnea is sometimes present in young infants and may be the only presenting sign (see Chapter 3 on brief resolved unexplained events). Rapid testing can be helpful in distinguishing pertussis from other respiratory illnesses when the symptoms are early and not as severe. Direct fluorescent antibody testing is no longer performed routinely. Culture is too slow to be helpful in the ED. Rapid testing for pertussis is available in most EDs, with a result time of 2 hours or less. Comprehensive respiratory pathogen testing can identify other respiratory viruses and mycoplasma as alternate diagnoses. Older children, adolescents, and adults can have atypical courses, but the dominant feature is severe coughing with a prolonged course. Fever is often absent in pertussis. High-risk infants should be hospitalized for supportive care because of higher complication rates of apnea, respiratory failure, pulmonary hypertension, bacterial pneumonia, brain hypoxia, and hemorrhage. Antibiotic treatment with azithromycin is recommended, but it does not affect the clinical course if started during the paroxysmal stage. Azithromycin does shorten the period of contagiousness, and it reduces the symptoms if administered during the catarrhal stage or as post-exposure prophylaxis. Consider azithromycin's effect on prolonging the QT interval and its association with hypertrophic pyloric stenosis.

Pertussis immunity derived from natural disease or immunization is not lifelong. Immunization with DTaP vaccine might result in shorter immunity duration compared to the older whole cell DTP vaccine. Pregnant mothers are immunized with TdaP between 27 and 36 weeks' gestation. This provides the newborn with passive immunity, and it reduces the risk that the mother can expose the child during infancy. Most adults (young and old) are not routinely immunized with TdaP. Because their immunity has waned, a large reservoir of susceptible individuals exists. The only adults who have some immunity are mothers immunized during pregnancy, health care workers receiving routine TdaP immunization, and patients with a wound given TdaP for tetanus prophylaxis. Hence, herd immunity does not apply to pertussis because the immunity rate of the population is very low.

POLIO

The inactivated polio virus (IPV) vaccine immunizes recipients against polio. Wild poliovirus strain types 1–3 initially formed the basis for trivalent oral poliovirus (OPV) vaccine. Because poliovirus type 2 has been eradicated from the globe as of 1999 and no cases of poliovirus type 3 have been identified worldwide since 2012, it is likely that only poliovirus type 1 remains. Wild poliovirus infection in susceptible children is most often nonsymptomatic, but approximately 25% have low-grade fever and sore throat, 1–5% have viral meningitis sometimes associated with paresthesias, and less than 1% develop asymmetric acute flaccid paralysis, known as paralytic poliomyelitis. The overall risk for paralytic poliomyelitis following wild polio infection is 1 in 1,000 susceptible infants and 1 in 100 susceptible adolescents. Cranial nerve involvement is known as bulbar poliomyelitis. Paralysis of the diaphragm and intercostal muscles can lead to hypoventilation requiring assisted ventilation. The CSF findings are consistent with viral meningitis. Poliovirus is in the enterovirus genus; thus, enteroviral PCR testing will be positive but not specifically diagnostic for poliovirus. Paralytic poliomyelitis can rarely be caused by OPV vaccine (live attenuated) known as vaccine-associated paralytic poliomyelitis (VAPP). The last non-imported US case of wild polio occurred in 1979. From 1979 to 2000, 6–8 persons developed VAPP in the United States annually. OPV was switched to sequential IPV/OPV in 1997 and then completely to IPV in 2000, which has eliminated VAPP cases. IPV is still trivalent. Bivalent OPV is still used in other countries. It is extremely unlikely that any clinician in the United States will encounter a new case of polio, although acute flaccid myelitis clinically presents similarly to polio (see Chapter 20 on neurologic emergencies).

HEPATITIS B

Hepatitis B vaccine immunizes recipients against hepatitis B. Some patients develop acute or subacute hepatitis with anorexia, nausea, malaise, and/or jaundice. Fewer patients develop fulminant hepatitis. Hepatitis B serology clinically measures the presence of antigen or antibody to the surface antigen (HBsAg and anti-HBs), the envelope antigen (HBeAg and anti-HBe), or antibody to the core antigen (anti-HBc). The core antigen can only be detected in liver specimens (not in the blood). Generally, the antigen and related antibody should not be positive in the same serum sample at the same time. A patient with a positive HBsAg has active hepatitis B and is contagious. A patient with a positive anti-HBs is immune against hepatitis B, either through immunization or through recovery from acute/subacute infection with hepatitis B virus. Some patients develop chronic hepatitis B, defined as persistence of HBsAg or HBeAg for more than 6 months. Transmission of hepatitis B is greatest via exposure to infected blood or body fluids. Newborn infants with perinatally acquired hepatitis B virus infections have a much higher risk of developing chronic infection. Hepatitis B serology is routinely obtained on pregnant mothers. It is recommended that all newborn infants be given hepatitis B vaccine routinely to prevent perinatal transmission. Infants of HBsAg-positive mothers are given concurrent passive immunity with hepatitis B-specific immune globulin. Patients who develop chronic hepatitis B are at risk for cirrhosis and hepatocellular carcinoma. Treatment options for chronic hepatitis B include interferon and nucleoside/nucleotide analogs (e.g., lamivudine, adefovir, entacavir, and tenofovir).

Hepatitis A vaccine is routinely administered to children, but most adults are not immunized and remain susceptible. Hepatitis A infection results in acute hepatitis. Jaundice is often lacking. Adolescents, adults, and immunocompromised children are more likely to be symptomatic with fever, anorexia, nausea, malaise, vomiting, and jaundice for 1 or 2 weeks. Full recovery occurs most of the time. Acute liver failure is rare. Transmission is fecal–oral. Epidemics are often associated with foods such as uncooked shellfish, frozen berries, and raw vegetables. Post-exposure prophylaxis with intramuscular γ-globulin (for infants and those older than age 40 years) or hepatitis A vaccine (aged 12 months to 40 years) is available.

ROTAVIRUS

Rotavirus vaccine protects against rotavirus gastroenteritis. The estimated annual incidence of rotavirus worldwide is more than 100 million cases in children younger than age 5 years, resulting in 500,000 deaths per year. In the United States, it is estimated that rotavirus causes 2 million cases of diarrhea and 20–40 deaths per year. The greatest risk is in infants; therefore, this vaccine has most of its efficacy during infancy. There are rotavirus serogroups, subgroups, and serotypes. In the United States, two rotavirus vaccines—one pentavalent and the other monovalent—are available, both of which are live attenuated viruses administered orally; there is no recommendation of one over the other. Recipients of this vaccine have a slight risk of developing intussusception estimated at 1 excess case in 20,000–100,000 vaccinated infants. It is estimated that rotavirus vaccine has reduced hospitalizations for rotavirus in the United States by 75% or more (>40,000 fewer hospitalizations per year nationwide). Furthermore, there were 60,000 fewer annual ED visits and 260,000 fewer annual outpatient office visits nationwide. Rotavirus spreads by the fecal–oral route, but because it can survive in the environment for weeks to months and has been found on toys and hard surfaces in child care centers, these function as fomites that can transmit disease by hand-to-mouth contact. Rotavirus can be confirmed by rapid fecal testing; however, because there is no specific antiviral treatment for rotavirus, the value of confirmatory testing is marginal. Norwalk virus, other calciviruses, and astrovirus are frequent causes of gastroenteritis, which similarly have no specific antiviral treatment. Most of the treatment is focused on hydration and oral intake optimization. (For management of pediatric dehydration, see Chapter 21 on fluid and electrolyte emergencies.)

VARICELLA

Varicella vaccine provides protection against primary varicella (chicken pox). The virus known as varicella zoster virus (VZV) is a member of the herpesviridae family, and like its other family members, it establishes lifelong latency in sensory dorsal root, cranial nerve, and autonomic ganglia, emerging periodically as zoster (shingles) most often in a cutaneous dermatome. The vaccine is a live attenuated virus that can be given as a monovalent vaccine or as part of the combined quadrivalent measles–mumps–rubella–varicella (MMRV) vaccine. Prior to varicella vaccine, nearly everyone acquired varicella during childhood. A few who escaped this eventually were exposed to varicella during adolescence and adulthood, which was typically associated with more severe varicella infections. Common complications of varicella include secondary bacterial infection of skin lesions, usually impetigo with *Staphylococcus aureus* and *Streptococcus pyogenes* (group A streptococcus). Some patients can present with a febrile erythroderma. Although most of these are due to scarlet fever, an occasional patient can present with early toxic shock syndrome, which can be visually indistinguishable. Treating the patient with antibiotics and monitoring the patient's status in the ED for several hours can help determine if the patient is stable or is developing signs of early shock. Cerebellar ataxia occurs in 1 in 4,000 cases. Patients have cerebellar signs, but they usually resolve. More concerning complications include encephalitis, varicella pneumonia (higher risk in patients on previous corticosteroids during the incubation period), and Reye syndrome associated with salicylate use.

Varicella is highly contagious to susceptible individuals, including infants and immunocompromised patients. The early stages of varicella can be recognized by the initial skin lesions that usually appear in the mid-torso (sometimes the face/scalp) as tiny vesicles over an irregular pink oval lesion that resemble dew drops on a pink rose petal. The only other entity that mimics this is the vesicle-like lesions of severe enteroviral hand–foot–mouth disease, but these lesions more commonly appear in the groin, lower abdomen, or lower extremities, and upon close examination, the "vesicle" is larger and extremely shallow, unlike the true hemispherical shape of early varicella vesicles, which are clearly fluid-filled (like dew drops on a rose petal). Later presentations demonstrate more extensive lesions in different stages of development. Zoster lesions typically appear more numerous in a shorter period of time. Patients often experience pain or pruritus prior to the onset of the lesions. They exhibit herpetic clustering, and some of these lesions are vesicular, but their major characteristic is that they occupy a classic dermatome. Whereas torso lesions are easily recognizable as a dermatome, facial zoster can appear in a V1, V2, or V3 dermatome, and sacral or anal lesions can be difficult to recognize as a dermatome. Herd immunity does not protect susceptible individuals because zoster can expose susceptible individuals at any time. Zoster can occur in vaccinated individuals, but the risk of zoster is higher in those who have had wild varicella.

It is reasonable to treat patients with varicella or zoster with acyclovir because the treatment is not likely to cause adverse effects. Some patients develop more severe varicella infections, and acyclovir treatment might prevent some of these. Exposure prophylaxis options include varicella zoster immune globulin, intravenous immunoglobulin (IVIG), acyclovir, or varicella vaccine. Newborn perinatal exposure is particularly high risk.

MEASLES–MUMPS–RUBELLA VACCINE

The MMR vaccine provides protection against measles, mumps, and rubella. The combined MMRV vaccine adds varicella protection. All of these are highly contagious, but measles is the most serious acute infection, and rubella is the most serious congenital infection. Parental refusal of MMR vaccine leads to susceptibility to these entities and the potential for epidemics of these diseases. Although antiviral treatment for varicella is available, no such agents exist for measles, mumps, and rubella.

Measles

Measles (rubeola) is a serious and highly contagious disease. Initial symptoms include fever, conjunctivitis, oral mucosal erythema (red tongue and lips), coryza/cough, Koplik spots, and morbilliform rash. Most clinicians have seen cases of roseola and Kawasaki disease but not a case of measles. The measles rash (exanthema) looks like that of roseola (morbilliform); the high fever and the appearance of the eyes and mouth (enanthem) resemble those seen in Kawasaki disease. In addition, patients have severe nasal congestion (coryza) and coughing. The coryza/cough helps distinguish measles from Kawasaki disease. Koplik spots are pinpoint white or yellow spots overlying the reddened oral mucosa, gingiva, or conjunctiva (classically described as grains of sand in a red sea) that are pathognomonic for measles. Patients with measles are almost always non-immunized, and they often contract measles in the midst of a known epidemic. The source index case could easily come through an international port of entry where large numbers of people congregate in crowded conditions. Patients with measles are contagious for approximately 4 days before the onset of the rash. The rash begins on the face and proceeds downward and outward over 3 days. Lab confirmation will likely be slow, so a clinical diagnosis must be made. In conjunction with a known epidemic, this should not be difficult in most instances. No specific treatments for measles exist, although ribavirin and IVIG have been used for some high-risk patients. Low levels of vitamin A are associated with higher morbidity and mortality, so treatment with vitamin A is indicated for all patients with measles. Measles was ubiquitous in the pre-vaccine era and most patients recovered spontaneously, with a mortality rate of approximately 1%. Mortality rates are currently much lower with improved nutrition and medical care. The decision to hospitalize a patient with measles is based on clinical risk, immunocompetence, social factors affecting clinical risk, and community contagious considerations. Complications include pneumonia, acute encephalitis, subacute sclerosing panencephalitis, and blindness.

Mumps

Mumps is a self-limited illness most often occurring in children. The most common and characteristic finding of mumps is salivary parotid swelling. Patients often present with chief complaints of neck swelling and pain or facial swelling. Parotitis can be distinguished from lymphadenitis clinically by palpating the upslope of the angle of the mandible. The inflamed parotid generally will overlie this and obscure its palpation. In more uncertain cases, ultrasound can identify the swollen structure as the parotid or lymph nodes, and it can also identify the presence of an abscess in most instances. Most patients are not very ill and do not require hospitalization. Because orchitis can occur (more commonly after puberty), the testicles should be examined, but sterility only rarely occurs. Mumps outbreaks are relatively common because two MMR vaccines provide only 88% efficacy in preventing mumps. A third MMR vaccine is recommended in the midst of a mumps epidemic.

Rubella

Rubella (also known as German measles and 3-day measles) is a relatively mild exanthem of childhood, although its symptoms are more severe in adults. Its most important clinical consequence is congenital rubella. Susceptible pregnant mothers who are exposed to rubella develop a viremia, and if this occurs during the first or second trimesters, the virus spreads to the fetus, resulting in miscarriage or congenital rubella syndrome, the most common manifestations of which include cataracts, microphthalmos, congenital glaucoma, patent ductus arteriosus, peripheral pulmonic stenosis, sensorineural hearing impairment, microcephaly, cognitive delay, intrauterine growth retardation, pneumonitis, bone disease, hepatosplenomegaly, thrombocytopenia, and blueberry muffin rash.

HAEMOPHILUS INFLUENZAE TYPE B, PNEUMOCOCCAL, AND MENINGOCOCCAL VACCINES

Haemophilus influenzae type b (Hib) vaccine, pneumococcal conjugate vaccine (PCV), and meningococcal vaccine all utilize the polysaccharide capsule virulence factor of the organism to confer immunity to vaccine recipients. Polysaccharide capsules are virulence factors that make these organisms more invasive by shielding the organism from immune system recognition, opsonization, and phagocytosis. Without the capsule, these organisms are much less invasive and typically cause more minor disease. For example, Hib causes sepsis and meningitis, whereas nontypable (not encapsulated) *H. influenzae* more typically causes otitis media and sinusitis. Similarly, encapsulated pneumococci cause pneumonia and meningitis, whereas nonencapsulated pneumococci more typically cause otitis media and sinusitis. Encapsulated versions of these three organisms are inherently invasive. Patients can present acutely or insidiously with meningitis and sepsis. Patients with asplenia (sickle cell disease), immunodeficiency, nephrotic syndrome, and other chronic disease are at higher risk for invasive disease with these encapsulated organisms.

When sepsis or meningitis with Hib, pneumococcus, meningococcus, or other invasive organism is suspected, ideally obtain an immediate blood culture, perform an immediate lumbar puncture (LP), and immediately administer high doses (anti-meningitis levels) of cefotaxime (or ceftriaxone) and vancomycin. The cefotaxime/ceftriaxone will cover HiB, meningococcus, and most pneumococci, but vancomycin is necessary to cover resistant pneumococci. Add pseudomonas coverage if indicated. Do not delay the administration of antibiotics. Obtaining a blood culture, LP, or IV access might prove to be difficult, slow, or harm the unstable patient, in which case anything that delays antibiotic administration can justifiably be deferred (or done later) so that administering antibiotics can occur as soon as possible (intramuscular or intraosseous administration is acceptable if IV access is delayed or difficult). Brain imaging, if indicated, should be done after antibiotic administration initiation. Dexamethasone is beneficial for children with Hib meningitis if administered before or concurrently with the first antibiotic dose. Dexamethasone recommendations for pneumococcal and meningococcal meningitis are less clear. Because the organism cannot be confirmed until much later, administer dexamethasone (0.15 mg/kg) immediately if bacterial meningitis is suspected. Subsequent doses can be guided by forthcoming definitive laboratory testing results and organism identification via nucleic acid amplification testing (NAAT) and culture. Gram stain can be helpful, but it can be misleading as well. NAAT is preferred. Follow the sepsis protocol in place at your institution.

Haemophilus Influenzae Type B

Hib vaccine is a dramatic success story. Hib used to be the most common cause of pediatric bacterial meningitis and sepsis until Hib vaccine was introduced. During the pre-Hib vaccine era, it was common for multiple Hib meningitis patients to be managed on the inpatient service of a children's hospital. In addition, Hib caused less common but still serious invasive infections, such as epiglottitis, septic arthritis, cellulitis, and pneumonia. Cellulitis with a violaceous hue in the cheek region (buccal cellulitis) was classically due to invasive Hib, and it should be treated as possible sepsis. Hib vaccine has reduced the occurrence of invasive Hib disease by 99%. Although Hib can cause otitis media and sinusitis, these entities are more commonly caused by the less virulent nontypable *H. influenzae*, which are largely unaffected by this vaccine. Rifampin prophylaxis is a consideration for susceptible contacts.

Pneumococcus

Pneumococcal conjugate vaccine provides protection against invasive *Streptococcus pneumonia* (pneumococcus) infections. PCV7 (7 serotypes) was introduced in 2000. This resulted in substantial reductions in the rates of invasive pneumococcal disease by 99% for the PCV7 serotypes and by 76% overall in children younger than age 5 years. More recently, PCV13 (13 serotypes) has replaced PCV7, which has resulted in further reductions in invasive pneumococcal disease, noninvasive pneumococcal disease, and nasopharyngeal colonization rates. There are more than 90 known serotypes of pneumococci, but PCV7 and PCV13 have targeted the more common serotypes associated with invasive pneumococcal disease. Pneumococcus is commonly carried in the nasopharynx and is a common cause of otitis media and sinusitis. Some pneumococci produce penicillin-binding proteins that result in resistance to penicillin; however, because this is not an enzyme phenomenon, this resistance mechanism can be overwhelmed with high-dose amoxicillin in the 80 to 100 mg/kg/day range. For invasive pneumococcal disease that includes significant pneumonia, sepsis, and suspected meningitis, administer cefotaxime and vancomycin as described previously. In the current era of Hib vaccine, pneumococcus is the leading cause of bacterial meningitis in young children (other than neonates). PPSV23 (polyvalent pneumococcal vaccine, 23 serotypes) is licensed for use in adults and children older than age 2 years; however, it does not induce immunologic memory or boosting with subsequent doses in children, and it does not reduce the nasopharynx pneumococcal colonization rates in children.

Meningococcus

Meningococcal conjugate vaccine (MCV) provides protection against infections due to *Neisseria meningitidis* (meningococcus), which is an invasive organism causing sepsis and meningitis, resulting in a 15% mortality rate. It is currently the leading cause of bacterial meningitis in older children, yet most meningococcal infections occur in infants and young children. MCV is currently quadrivalent, covering the A, C, W, and Y serotypes (MenACWY). A separate MCV provides protection against the B serotype (MenB). There are 13 known serotypes. The routine administration age for meningococcal vaccines is currently 11 years, but these vaccines are licensed to be administered as early as age 8 weeks for high-risk patients (e.g., those with asplenia or immunodeficiency). If it is immunogenic at a young age for these patients, in the future routine MCV might be initiated for all infants, which could further reduce rates of meningococcemia and meningococcal meningitis. Sequelae include hearing loss, neurologic disability, digit or limb amputation, cognitive delay, and behavioral problems. Most cases are sporadic, but small outbreaks can occur. Because meningococcus can affect adults, antibiotic prophylaxis for close contacts should be initiated promptly, even for contacts who have received MCV because the vaccine is not 100% effective. Antibiotic prophylaxis options are ceftriaxone, rifampin, ciprofloxacin, or azithromycin. Health care personnel need not receive antibiotic prophylaxis unless they have had exposure to respiratory secretions during mouth-to-mouth resuscitation, intubation, or suctioning.

INFLUENZA

Influenza vaccine targets the dominant strains of influenza that are anticipated to arise in the community. Influenza types A–D exist. Influenza D is recently detected in animals only. Influenza C occurs sporadically with mild disease. Influenza B types are more stable, with only slight varying strains. Influenza A exhibits extensive variation, which is dominated by the hemagglutinin (HA) and neuraminidase (NA) proteins on the virus surface. "H2N3" refers to an influenza A strain that has the type 2 HA and the type 3 NA. Additional influenza A antigenic variation occurs via antigenic drift and antigenic shift. These create uncertainty and challenges in predicting the vaccine components for the upcoming influenza season. Influenza is an RNA virus, and point mutations can occur during viral replication creating new influenza strains of the same HA type, known as antigenic drift. Influenza A's RNA segments can also undergo reassortment, known as antigenic shift, when two different strains of influenza affect a host at the same time or by direct adaptation of a nonhuman (avian, swine, etc.) influenza virus to humans. This antigenic shift is more dramatic and can result in a human influenza strain for which most people have little or no immunity. Coupled with high virulence and characteristics that facilitate person-to-person contagiousness, this causes influenza "pandemics." Very large numbers of patients worldwide are affected by the newly emerged "novel" influenza A virus (an antigenic type that human immune systems have not encountered). The 1918 pandemic killed an estimated 50 million people worldwide.

Influenza is a respiratory illness almost always causing a high fever and varying degrees of respiratory symptoms. Headaches, myalgia, vomiting, and diarrhea can occur. Pneumonia can result either primarily from influenza virus or from a secondary bacterial etiology. Immunocompromised patients or those with significant underlying cardiopulmonary or other chronic diseases are at higher risk of severe complications from influenza. Rapid influenza testing is available, but the CDC reports that its sensitivity is 50–70% (i.e., the test missed 30–50% of the influenza cases). Clearly, not all tests are the same. One commercial test had a demonstrated sensitivity of 77%. PCR testing has greater sensitivity, but currently its turnaround time is not fast enough for routine ED use. Clinicians must use their judgment in how to use these tests in conjunction with clinical risk/benefit assessments to determine treatment with oseltamivir. With time, the tests are expected to become more accurate and faster. Although oseltamivir dominates influenza treatment in children, other anti-influenza agents exist and more are expected in the future. Exposure prophylaxis with oseltamivir or influenza vaccines are available options.

Palivizumab is a monoclonal antibody that provides passive immunity against respiratory syncytial virus (RSV). Immunity against RSV is of short duration; therefore, the potential reservoir of susceptible hosts is extremely large, and because RSV is highly contagious, infants exposed to the community will very likely be exposed to RSV. Although RSV causes bronchiolitis in most infants, premature infants and other young infants with severe systemic or cardiopulmonary disease are at high risk for respiratory failure and apnea. High-risk infants are given monthly injections of palivizumab during the RSV season (maximum of five doses). Ribavirin has in vitro activity against RSV, but it has significant toxicity and its clinical benefit is unclear.

Other vaccines are available but are not routinely administered in the United States, including those for rabies, bacille Calmette–Guérin (BCG), typhoid, cholera, yellow fever, Japanese encephalitis, and smallpox. Some of these could benefit travelers or those in high-risk professions.

RABIES

Rabies is transmitted through the bite of a rabid mammal or via aerosol exposure of a rabid nearby bat. Cats and dogs are the most common transmitters of rabies, but because pets can be vaccinated against rabies, bites from known vaccinated animals pose no rabies risk. Bites from cats and dogs with unknown rabies vaccination status, ferrets, bats, skunks, raccoons, foxes, woodchucks, and most carnivores, or contact with or close bat exposure without a bite, have some risk. Livestock, rodents (mice, rats, hamsters, guinea pigs, etc.), and rabbits are unlikely to carry rabies. For bites and exposures placing patients at risk, administer rabies immune globulin into the wound site and begin active immunization with killed rabies vaccine. Encephalitic rabies begins with fever, sore throat, malaise, headache, nausea, vomiting, and weakness. This is followed by encephalopathy, agitation, depressed mentation, hydrophobia (agitation and fear when offered a drink) and aerophobia (agitation when fanning air on the face), choking, and aspiration. Seizures are rare, but dyskinesia and myoclonus can appear seizure-like. Death soon follows.

BCG vaccine contains a live attenuated strain of *Mycobacterium bovis*. It is used in other countries for protection against tuberculosis (TB; *Mycobacterium tuberculosis*) and is usually administered as a single dose in infancy. BCG efficacy is demonstrated in most but not all trials. Its main benefit appears to be preventing life-threatening forms of TB in infants and young children. Newer vaccines are in development. Rather than using BCG vaccine, the approach used in the United States is to screen and treat skin test converters. Recipients of BCG vaccine will often have positive tuberculin skin tests (TSTs), but these could also be due to TB exposure. When uncertain, an interferon-γ release assay (IGRA) can be run to more accurately assess for TB exposure because this test does not react with BCG vaccine. IGRA tests include QuantiFERON-TB Gold and T-SPOT.TB. Patients with a positive TST or IGRA should have a chest radiograph. A known TB contact with an infant should raise the suspicion of TB meningitis, which has a very short incubation period (compared to the extremely long incubation period for other manifestations of TB). The topic of TB is extensive and beyond the scope of this chapter.

Typhoid vaccine protects against infections with *Salmonella enterica* (serovar Typhi), which causes enteric fever known as typhoid fever, characterized by fever, bacteremia, abdominal pain, hepatosplenomegaly, headache, lethargy, "rose spots," shock, and occasionally myocarditis. Typhoid fever is uncommon in the United States but is highly endemic in many other countries. There are several typhoid vaccine options, including an oral live attenuated vaccine (four doses) and a single-dose intramuscular polysaccharide vaccine.

The other remaining vaccines are interesting, but clinicians are not likely to encounter disease entities related to them in the United States.

Further Reading

American Academy of Pediatrics. Committee on Infectious Diseases (COID). https://www.aap.org/en-us/about-the-aap/Committees-Councils-Sections/Pages/Committee-on-Infectious-Diseases.aspx.

Centers for Disease Control and Prevention. Advisory Committee on Immunization Practices (ACIP). https://www.cdc.gov/vaccines/acip/index.html.

Centers for Disease Control and Prevention. Travelers' Health.https://wwwnc.cdc.gov/travel/destinations/list.

Kimberlin DW, Brady MT, Jackson MA, Long SS; Committee on Infectious Disease. eds. *Red Book: 2019–2021 Report of the Committee on Infectious Diseases*. 31st ed. Itasca, IL: American Academy of Pediatrics; 2018.

Kliegman RM, St. Geme JW, Blum NJ, et al. eds. *Nelson Textbook of Pediatrics*. 21st ed. Philadelphia, PA: Elsevier; 2020.

15

Pediatric Respiratory Emergencies

EMILY ROSE

INTRODUCTION

Respiratory emergencies are common in children, and emergency providers must anticipate respiratory compromise and intervene early. Signs of respiratory distress may initially be subtle. Up to 95% of all cases of cardiac arrest in children are of respiratory etiology.

Comparison with Adult Physiology

Children are uniquely predisposed to respiratory failure for several reasons. They have a higher resting metabolic rate with relatively increased oxygen demand. This translates specifically to a shorter safe apneic time. For example, a healthy young adult may have a safe apneic time of 6–8 minutes (after preoxygenation). In contrast, an infant will desaturate after approximately 1 or 2 minutes of apnea. In addition, children have anatomic differences that predispose them to obstruction. Infants are "obligate nose breathers," and nasal obstruction can cause significant respiratory difficulty and decreased ability to maintain adequate hydration. Mechanical obstruction can more easily occur due to a child's relatively large head and more easily compressible airway. Young children also have a smaller airway caliber, which is prone to significant relative obstruction with edema or infections.

Overall, there is significant overlap and some inherent difficulty distinguishing the clinical and radiologic features of bronchiolitis, reactive airway disease, and pneumonia, particularly in young children.

CROUP

Background

Croup (laryngotracheobronchitis) is the most common infectious cause of upper airway distress and obstruction in children. More than 90% of all cases of stridor in children are caused by croup. It occurs most commonly in those aged 6 months to 3 years but can occur in young infancy through school age. Parainfluenza is the most common etiology, but other causes include respiratory syncytial virus, influenza, and rhinoviruses; even measles can manifest as croup.

Inflammation of the submucosal tissues of the subglottic space occurs in croup. Edematous, inflamed mucosa and exudate can expand into the airway lumen and cause stridor and obstruction. The cricoid cartilage forms a complete cartilaginous (nonexpanding) ring in this part of the trachea that contributes to the pathophysiology and potential complications in croup.

Classic Clinical Presentation

The typical case of croup involves a young child with a 1- to 3-day prodrome of mild fever and nonspecific/mild upper respiratory infection symptoms. This is followed by a fairly abrupt onset of barky cough, hoarse voice, and high-pitched inspiratory stridor. A barky cough is the predominant presentation in infants and young children. Hoarseness predominates in older children. The barky cough typically lasts 3 days. Other symptoms typically resolve in 4–7 days.

Croup is classified as mild, moderate, or severe (see Figure 15.1). A child with mild croup is minimally distressed but may have a notable seal-like cough or stridor with agitation. Moderate croup involves increased work of breathing (retractions, tachypnea, and tachycardia), audible stridor at rest, and worsening stridor with agitation. Approximately 85% of croup is mild; severe croup is rare and accounts for less than 1% of cases. A child with significant respiratory distress has severe croup that may be associated with altered mental status. A lack of stridor may occur with severe respiratory obstruction due to limited air movement.

Atypical Clinical Presentation

A small subset of children will have involvement of the lower airway with concomitant bronchoconstriction (but this usually suggests another disease). Hypoxia is rare in croup, and its presence may indicate lower airway involvement, another disease process, or rarely occur in severe croup with significant airway obstruction.

Mild croup may only have faint stridor with agitation, mild hoarseness, and/or intermittent barky cough.

Spasmodic or atypical croup does not have diagnostic consensus and is a heterogeneous group of conditions that typically occur in older children. There is significant association with allergy, atopy, airway hyperreactivity, asthma, and gastroesophageal reflux. Airway lesions and/or subglottic stenosis may contribute to symptoms. These patients typically

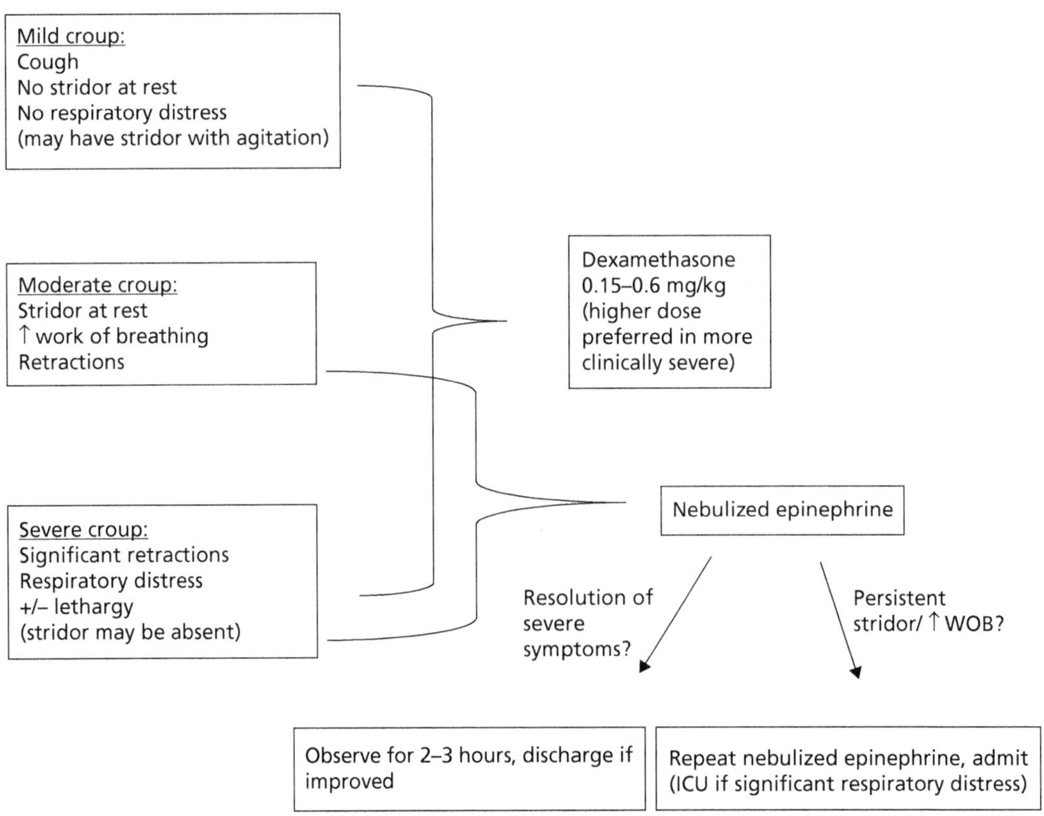

FIGURE 15.1 Simplified croup algorithm. WOB, work of breathing.

present with recurrent episodes of croup-like symptoms well into the school age.

Differential Diagnosis

Table 15.1 presents a simplified clinical approach to the differential diagnosis of upper airway symptoms in children.

Diagnostic Confirmation

Croup is diagnosed clinically by the symptoms and time course detailed previously. No confirmatory diagnostic testing is required. Many viruses can cause the disease process, and radiographs are neither sensitive nor specific. The classic chest X-ray (CXR) finding "steeple sign" of a tapered, narrowing of the subglottic trachea can be seen in children without the disease and is typically not clinically useful.

Treatment

All children with croup should be given a one-time dose of glucocorticoids. Steroids improve symptoms, reduce the need for aerosolized epinephrine, decrease admission rates, as well as decrease both emergency department (ED) and hospitalization length of stay. Dexamethasone is the preferred glucocorticoid. Oral dexamethasone was originally studied at a dose of 0.6 mg/kg, but a dose as low as 0.15 mg/kg has been shown to be as effective. There is evidence that a dose of 0.6 mg/kg may be better in more severe cases. The recommended maximum dose given ranges from 10 to 16 mg. The intravenous (IV) form of dexamethasone may be given orally (with flavored syrup). This form has much smaller total volume than the commercially available oral concentration. Severe cases should receive intramuscular (IM)/IV dosing. Inhaled budesonide (2 mg/dose) may be used, but it is likely less effective than PO/IM/IV dexamethasone and is more expensive. Prednisolone may perform similarly in milder cases of croup, but dexamethasone is preferred due to its longer duration of action in a one-time dose.

Aerosolized epinephrine should be given with increased work of breathing, stridor at rest, and/or if severe croup is suspected. Epinephrine reverses edema and alleviates symptoms via subglottic mucosal vasoconstriction. Racemic epinephrine is equally effective as regular ("crash cart" or L-) epinephrine. It typically works quickly (<10 minutes), with a duration of approximately 2 hours. Patients should be observed in the ED after epinephrine administration (for 2 or 3 hours) to evaluate for return of severe symptoms. Repeat dosing may be given as symptoms indicate. Nebulized epinephrine dosing is 0.5 mL/kg (maximum 5 mL) or 0.5 mL of 2.25% racemic epinephrine given via nebulizer over 15 minutes.

Severe croup with signs of impending airway obstruction, respiratory failure, altered mental status, and/or hypoxia unresponsive to treatment requires intubation. An endotracheal tube at least a half size smaller than calculated for age may be necessary to pass through the edematous tissue.

Clinical Algorithm

Figure 15.1 presents a simplified treatment algorithm of croup.

TABLE 15.1 SIMPLIFIED DIFFERENTIAL DIAGNOSIS OF UPPER AIRWAY SYMPTOMS

Condition	Distinguishing Features
Anaphylaxis	Abrupt onset, associated trigger, other organ system involvement
Croup	URI symptoms, acute onset of barky cough, stridor, no distinct positional preference
Bacterial tracheitis	Fever, toxicity, prolongation of symptoms, lack of response to croup treatment
Epiglottitis	Drooling a predominant symptom, patient desire to remain sitting, muffled voice (but hoarseness typically absent), cough absent, anxiety
Retropharyngeal abscess	Fever, toxicity, torticollis, neck pain/stiffness, ± drooling, ± muffled voice
Foreign body aspiration	History of choking episode, absence of URI symptoms or hoarseness, ± drooling
Peritonsillar abscess	Sore throat, trismus, muffled voice, pharyngeal erythema and edema, uvular deviation

URI, upper respiratory tract infection.

Disposition

Most patients can be safely discharged home after a one-time dose of dexamethasone. Patients given epinephrine should be observed in the ED for at least 2 hours and evaluated for return of stridor at rest or increased work of breathing.

Admission should be considered for patients with severe croup, persistent respiratory distress/failure despite treatment, hypoxia, significant dehydration/PO intolerance, poor social circumstances, or complex past medical history with ongoing morbidity (prematurity or pulmonary or cardiac disease).

Return instructions for parents include dehydration prevention and rehydration techniques (see Chapter 21 for specific instructions), signs of worsening respiratory distress including sings of retractions, increased work of breathing, and inability to tolerate liquids.

Complications

The most serious complication is complete airway obstruction, failure, and arrest. Fortunately, this is extremely rare.

Bacterial Tracheitis

Bacterial tracheitis is a significant cause of airway obstruction and is more likely than croup alone or epiglottitis to cause airway obstruction. Severe inflammation of the tracheal epithelium occurs with thick secretions. Pseudomembranes may form and slough into the airway. Microabscesses may form within the trachea wall.

Bacterial tracheitis should be considered particularly in the child with croup-like symptoms who has more prolonged duration of symptoms, if the child appears toxic, or if the child is not very responsive to either steroid or nebulized epinephrine treatment. The majority of patients with bacterial tracheitis require intubation for airway support. Bronchoscopy (with debridement) is diagnostic and therapeutic. Broad antibiotic coverage with anti-staphylococcal agents (e.g., vancomycin and clindamycin) plus a third-generation cephalosporin (e.g., cefotaxime and ceftriaxone) is recommended.

Key Points

- Croup is a common childhood illness and presentation of respiratory distress.
- Croup should be treated with 0.15–0.6 mg/kg (maximum 16 mg) of dexamethasone in a one-time dose.
- Nebulized epinephrine should be given for stridor at rest, significant retractions, or increased work of breathing.
- Patients should be observed for 2 or 3 hours after nebulized epinephrine to evaluate for return of respiratory distress.

Pitfalls

- Failure to administer nebulized epinephrine in the patient with stridor at rest or significant respiratory distress
- Failure to observe patient for return of distress after administration of nebulized epinephrine
- Failure to consider bacterial tracheitis in the patient who is not responsive to treatment
- Failure to consider the diagnosis of severe croup due to absence of stridor in the significantly obstructed patient
- Failure to have a smaller endotracheal tube available and ready if intubation is required

BRONCHIOLITIS

Background

Bronchiolitis is a seasonal clinical syndrome that occurs in children younger than age 2 years. Outbreaks occur annually from October to May, with peaks in January and February. The viruses that cause bronchiolitis are highly contagious and spread via large droplets. Approximately one-third of children contract bronchiolitis in the first year of life, and 90% by age 2 years. Many viruses can cause the clinical presentation, including respiratory syncytial virus (RSV; ~70% of cases), parainfluenza, adenovirus, rhinovirus, and influenza. Many children (up to one-third of those hospitalized) have co-infection with more than one virus. The co-infection of RSV with rhinovirus may be the most severe phenotype.

The viral infection of the bronchioles induces necrosis of the respiratory epithelium, which causes mucosal edema. This inflammation causes obstruction in the relatively small airways of infants and toddlers. Cellular debris can obstruct bronchioles and cause partial lobar collapse. In severe cases, viral-induced pneumonia can develop with lung necrosis and permanent scarring.

Classic Clinical Presentation

The classic bronchiolitis clinical presentation is an infant or toddler with initial symptoms of a runny nose on days 1 or 2. The significance of symptoms varies and correlates with age, the severity of infection, and patient comorbidities. Lower respiratory tract signs and symptoms begin on days 2 or 3 of illness. Concomitant fever often occurs with associated irritability, malaise, and anorexia. Many infants have decreased oral intake secondary to nasal obstruction and difficulty breathing. Tachypnea, retractions, nasal flaring, and increased work of breathing are common. Wheezing or rales are commonly present on examination. Peak severity of symptoms occurs on approximately days 3–5 and then gradually resolves. The average length of cough is 2 weeks.

Atypical Clinical Presentation

Apnea may precede infectious symptoms, particularly in the neonate and ex-premature young infant. A prolonged course may occur in young infants and in those with comorbid conditions.

Differential Diagnosis

Table 15.2 presents a simplified differential diagnosis of lower airway symptoms in children.

Diagnostic Confirmation

Bronchiolitis is a clinical diagnosis. No laboratory or radiologic confirmation is required. The American Academy of Pediatrics (AAP) recommends against obtaining a routine CXR. Chest imaging may be normal, demonstrate hyperaeration, show viral patterns of infection such as peribronchiolar cuffing, or show overt consolidation. Consolidation occurs in approximately 25% of cases and typically represents atelectasis rather than bacterial superinfection.

Fever is common with bronchiolitis. Neonates and young infants may have concomitant serious bacterial infections with clinical bronchiolitis. See Chapter 9 regarding the management of the young infant with fever.

Treatment

The cornerstone of management for acute bronchiolitis is suctioning and respiratory support as indicated. No medical therapies have been proven to significantly impact clinical course. Hydration status should be assessed and dehydration treated as needed.

Virtually all patients with bronchiolitis benefit from suctioning. Nasal suctioning should be encouraged, particularly prior to feeding. There are many commercially available suctioning devices that facilitate nasal suctioning at home. Deeper suctioning can clinically improve symptoms, but aggressive deep suctioning may induce further edema and exacerbate symptoms.

Respiratory support may be required, particularly in young infants and in those with severe disease. Positive pressure may decrease work of breathing, improve gas exchange, and decrease the need for endotracheal intubation. Supplemental oxygen is recommended with saturation <90%. There is emerging evidence to support administration of home oxygen for those with oxygen saturations <90%, but there is a significant bounce-back rate with these patients. The AAP recommendations state that currently there is not enough evidence to support

TABLE 15.2 SIMPLIFIED DIFFERENTIAL DIAGNOSIS OF LOWER AIRWAY SYMPTOMS

Condition	Distinguishing Features
Bronchiolitis	<2 years, seasonal symptoms, rales/wheezing with copious rhinorrhea
Asthma	Expiratory and/or inspiratory wheezing, prolonged expiration, recurrent symptoms with triggers
Congestive heart failure	Wheezing, shortness of breath, cardiomegaly, pulmonary congestion, hepatomegaly, decreased exercise tolerance, difficulty feeding and associated failure to thrive (infancy)
Myocarditis	Similar to CHF, often preceding URI, elevated troponin
Pneumonia	Fever, focal crackles, consolidation on imaging
Malignancy	Symptoms depend on etiology but include chest pain, pleural effusion, mediastinal mass, weight loss, rash, fatigue, fever, hepatosplenomegaly, lymphadenopathy

CHF, congestive heart failure; URI, upper respiratory tract infection.

routine home oxygen. Heated, humidified nasal cannula oxygen administration improves clinical symptoms of respiratory distress. Positive pressure ventilation with noninvasive measures may help with those in more significant distress (see Chapter 6). Intubation may be required in severe cases and in those with apnea.

Dehydration should be managed appropriately (see Chapter 21). Intravenous fluids may be required if significant dehydration is present and the child is not tolerating liquids due to respiratory distress.

Beta-agonists have not been proven to impact disease resolution, hospitalization rates, or length of stay. They may improve clinical scores acutely, but the AAP recommends against their routine use due to the lack of impact on disease course. The AAP concludes that the cost and potential risk of their use outweigh the benefit.

Nebulized hypertonic saline increases mucociliary clearance. It has been demonstrated to be safe and effective at improving symptoms after 24 hours of use. It has not been shown to decrease rate of hospital admission but has been shown to decrease hospital length of stay. The AAP recommends against the use in the emergency department setting but states that it may be administered to hospitalized patients.

Steroids should not be used in the treatment of bronchiolitis because they have not been shown to impact clinical course or admission rates. In addition, steroid use may prolong viral shedding.

A bacterial superinfection of the lungs is extremely rare in bronchiolitis, and antibiotics are not indicated.

Nebulized epinephrine has not been proven to impact clinical course, and one study demonstrated an increased length of stay when nebulized epinephrine was used on a fixed schedule.

Clinical Algorithm

Figure 15.2 presents a simplified bronchiolitis algorithm.

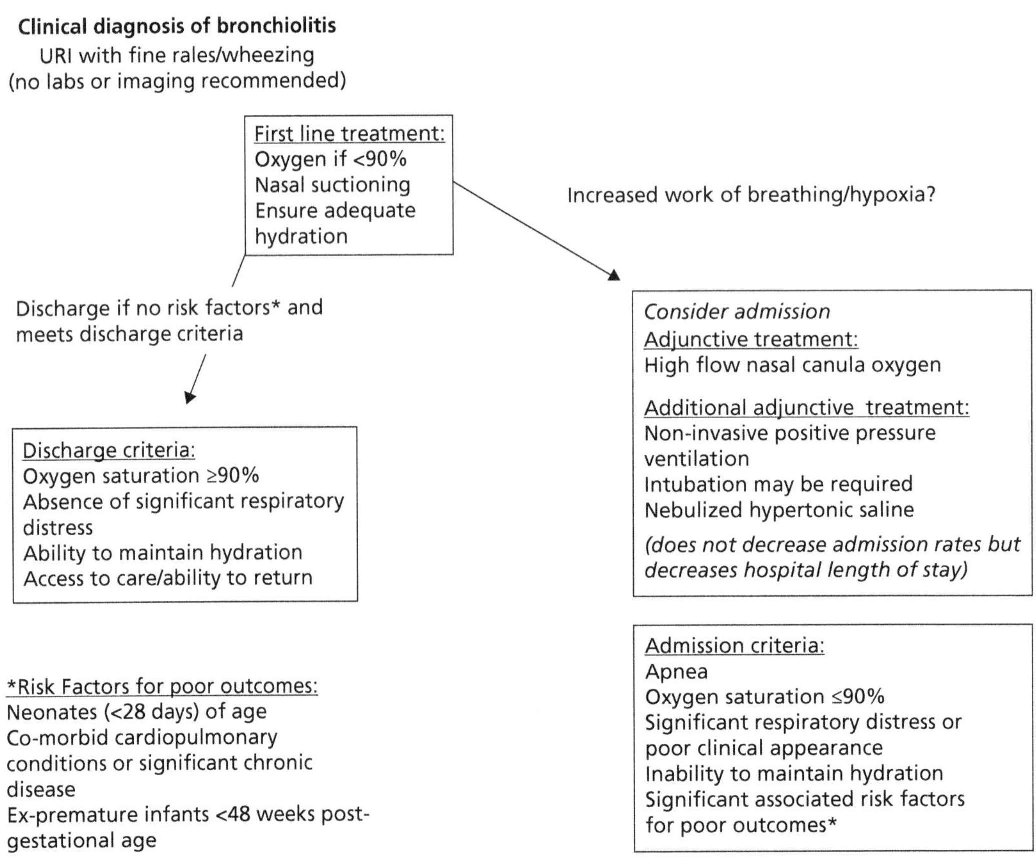

FIGURE 15.2 Simplified bronchiolitis algorithm.

Disposition

Bronchiolitis is a significant cause of both morbidity and mortality in children, so disposition should be carefully considered, particularly in the neonate, premature infant <48 weeks' gestational age, and those with comorbidities. However, most children will meet criteria to be discharged and can be sent home to a safe environment in which care and return instructions can be followed. Close follow-up is recommended for those with significant symptoms, particularly if seen early in their disease course, prior to peak severity.

Patient who are well appearing, well hydrated/able to tolerate feeds, with no apnea, and not in respiratory distress with an oxygen saturation >90% can be discharged home. Caregivers should monitor for signs of respiratory distress and diminishing ability to tolerate liquids. Any episodes of apnea should prompt emergency department evaluation and admission is recommended.

Admission indications include apnea, significant respiratory distress not responsive to suctioning, oxygen saturation <90%, tachypnea >60–80 breaths per minute, inability to tolerate liquids, or significant underlying cardiopulmonary or neurologic disease. A low threshold for admission should be maintained in the neonate, premature infant <48 weeks' gestational age, those with comorbidities, and those with unstable social situations. In addition, length of symptoms may assist in disposition decision. A patient on day 1 or 2 of illness is likely to worsen and increase in clinical severity. In contrast, a patient on day 4 or 5 of illness is typically less likely to progress.

Complications

Apnea occurs in approximately 5% of patients hospitalized for bronchiolitis. Risk factors for apnea include the neonate; prematurity with a gestation age <48 weeks; and comorbidities including respiratory, cardiac, and neurologic disorders and immunocompromise. There is no increased risk of apnea with RSV compared to other viral etiologies of bronchiolitis.

Key Points

- Bronchiolitis is a viral-induced clinical syndrome that occurs in children younger than age 2 years seasonally (October–April, with the peak in January and February).
- The diagnosis of bronchiolitis is clinical. No viral testing or imaging are required.
- Risk factors for complications include <1 month of age, prematurity with a gestational age <48 weeks, and comorbidities.
- Treatment is suctioning, respiratory support, and oxygen if needed.
- Admission should be considered for apneic episodes, hypoxia, respiratory distress, and PO intolerance. A low threshold for admission should be maintained for the neonate and those with comorbidities.
- Children who are well appearing and well hydrated/tolerating orals with oxygen saturation >90% can be discharged home with good parental instructions.

Pitfalls

- Failure to admit an at-risk infant with apnea
- Failure to consider social situation and hydration status in disposition decision-making
- Failure to anticipate disease worsening if patient seen prior to day 3 of illness
- Failure to detail care and return instructions to caregivers

PNEUMONIA

Background

Pneumonia is a common cause of hospital admission for children and a significant cause of death in young children in developing countries. Approximately three-fourths of all deaths from pneumonia are of bacterial etiology. Overall, 60–90% of pediatric pneumonia is of viral etiology. The epidemiology of pneumonia is impacted by age and vaccination status (although there is some herd immunity protection). The bacterial etiologies of neonatal pneumonia are the same as in sepsis/meningitis (see Chapter 9). Viruses are the most common cause of pneumonia, particularly in older infants, toddlers, and young children. Lobar pneumonia/"typical pneumonia" is most commonly caused by *Streptococcus pneumoniae* in all ages (although incidence has decreased since the introduction of Prevnar vaccination). Atypical infection due to mycoplasma is more common in children older than age

5 years, although the relative prevalence is increasing in those younger than age 5 years with improved vaccination coverage. Several recent studies have demonstrated that the true prevalence of various etiologies of community-acquired pneumonia in children is unknown, and the incidence of bacterial pneumonia is likely even lower than previously thought.

Complicating diagnostic confidence is the fact that the clinical presentations of bronchiolitis, reactive airway disease, and pneumonia in the young child can look quite similar and be difficult to reliably distinguish. There are no radiographic or laboratory features that are usually indicated or that can confirm diagnosis.

Classic Clinical Presentation

Bacterial Pneumonia (Most Common *Streptococcus pneumoniae*; Less Common *Staphylococcal aureus* Group A Streptococcus)

Children with pneumonia typically present with worsening clinical condition, severe symptoms, moderate to severe respiratory distress, prolonged fever, or development of a new fever after initial upper respiratory symptoms. Classic symptoms of pneumonia include cough, tachypnea, retractions, and fever. However, these symptoms are neither sensitive nor specific to differentiate the etiology (typical/atypical bacteria or viral) of pneumonia. Lack of tachypnea and hypoxia may be the best clinical clue to exclude pneumonia. In general, longer symptom duration correlates with increased likelihood of pneumonia. However, a prolonged cough (≥4 weeks) is unlikely to be caused by an acute bacterial pneumonia.

Most children with bacterial pneumonia appear clinically ill and have moderate to significant fever. Onset of symptoms is fairly abrupt. Focal chest pain and sepsis are much more common with typical bacterial pneumonia than other etiologies. Grunting is a sign of impending respiratory failure associated with significant airway disease. It is more common with severe pneumonia than other etiologies of respiratory distress.

Physical examination findings of pneumonia include focal crackles and signs of consolidated lung parenchyma (decreased breath sounds, dullness to percussion, and/or abnormal transmission of sounds). Wheezing is characteristic of bronchiolitis and asthma but may also be present in viral pneumonia and atypical bacterial pneumonia.

Atypical Bacterial Pneumonia (*Mycoplasma mycoplasma* and *Chlamydia trachomatis*)

Patients with atypical bacterial pneumonia often present with nonspecific viral-type symptoms such as fever, myalgias, headache, and sore throat, with gradually worsening cough that persists despite improvement of other symptoms. Mycoplasma has many extrapulmonary systemic symptoms, including dermatologic, gastrointestinal, neurologic, cardiac, and hematologic manifestations.

Patients are relatively well appearing. Diffuse wheezing or crackles are often present on physical examination. Radiography is often more impressive than the clinical appearance of disease.

Viral Pneumonia

Patients with viral pneumonia often have associated or preceding upper respiratory symptoms. Viruses are the most common etiology of pneumonia, particularly in older infants and toddlers.

Atypical Clinical Presentation

Community acquired methicillin-resistant *Staphylococcus aureus* can cause a particularly severe necrotizing pneumonia, frequently with empyema. It may cause severe disease, complicating influenza infection.

Consider the possibility of an aspirated lower airway foreign body with recurrent lobar pneumonia in the same location if the child is otherwise healthy. Bronchoscopy is diagnostic and should be considered because children can have retained aspirated lower airway foreign bodies for weeks or years (see Chapter 16).

Infants younger than age 1 year may develop afebrile pneumonia of infancy. Patients typically have rhinorrhea, tachypnea, and staccato cough. Inspiratory crackles are often noted on examination, and a CXR demonstrates a diffuse interstitial pattern. *Chlamydia trachomatis* is the most common etiology, but many others may cause this, including cytomegalovirus and ureaplasma. Patients may have a history of conjunctivitis at 5–14 days of life (although many do not).

Fungal pneumonia (e.g., coccidioidomycosis and histoplasmosis) may occur in endemic areas, particularly in those with immunocompromise.

Rarely, *Bordetella pertussis* may cause severe pneumonia. The patient may have characteristic persistent cough with intermittent whoop and/or known infectious exposure (although frequently unidentified). Fever may or may not be present.

Differential Diagnosis

See Table 15.2 for a simplified differential diagnosis of lower airway symptoms in children.

Diagnostic Confirmation

Chest X-ray is not required for the diagnosis of uncomplicated community-acquired pneumonia (CAP) in the well-appearing child. Laboratory evaluation and blood cultures are not recommended for patients with CAP amenable to outpatient therapy.

Imaging is indicated if the diagnosis is inconclusive, if severe disease is present, if the patient has recurrent or worsening symptoms, or if the patient will be hospitalized. A lateral CXR generally does not change management if imaging is read by a radiologist. However, it may improve diagnostic accuracy in non-radiology-trained provider readings.

Atypical bacteria and viruses more commonly spread along the bronchial tree and typically present with a bronchopneumonic pattern on CXR. However, typical bacterial infections may also cause this pattern. In addition, pulmonary consolidation (of typical bacterial infection) in young children can often appear spherical (so-called "round pneumonia").

Cavitations, pleural effusions, and necrotizing processes are typically of bacterial etiology. Mediastinal and hilar adenopathy are associated with mycobacterial and fungal etiology. Chlamydia often causes hyperinflation with an interstitial pattern.

See Chapter 17 for further details regarding interpreting a pediatric CXR.

Laboratory markers (e.g., white blood cells, c-reactive protein, erythrocyte sedimentation rate, and procalcitonin) are neither sensitive nor specific to confirm or exclude bacterial pneumonia. Low procalcitonin (PCT) may help exclude bacterial pneumonia, but predictive thresholds have not been established in children. PCT levels typically rise after 4 hours of a bacterial infection, peak at 6–8 hours, and remain high for 48 hours. PCT levels do not significantly increase with viral or other inflammatory processes. Hyponatremia occurs in approximately one-third of children hospitalized with pneumonia. Its presence is associated with increased length of stay and complications. Blood cultures do not typically change management in outpatient CAP but may be somewhat useful in hospitalized patients. Sputum culture is very difficult to obtain in young children, and nasopharyngeal swabs do not typically yield clinically relevant results.

Moderate to significant pleural effusions should have diagnostic thoracentesis to tailor therapy and assist in resolution.

Treatment

The treatment of pneumonia is based on the age of the patient, likely underlying etiology, and whether the pneumonia is community acquired or health care associated.

Neonate

See Chapter 9 for management of neonatal fever. Cephalosporins are typically used, with the addition of vancomycin if there is suspicion for resistant organism. The most likely bacterial culprit in afebrile atypical pneumonia in young infants is *Chlamydia trachomatis*, which is treated with azithromycin. *Bordetella pertussis* may also rarely cause severe pneumonia and is also treated with azithromycin.

Toddler

Viral pneumonia is the most common etiology in this age group. It is treated with supportive care.

Streptococcus pneumoniae is the most common etiology of bacterial pneumonia in children. Lobar pneumonia is treated with amoxicillin to cover similar microbes that cause otitis media; a higher dose of 90 mg/kg/day is recommended. Duration of therapy is 7–10 days. Inpatient treatment is with ceftriaxone; azithromycin is added if atypical infection is suspected. Atypical pneumonia (including neonatal chlamydia) is treated with macrolides for 5 days.

Symptoms should improve within 48–72 hours of treatment. In patients with failure to improve with antibiotics, consider resistant *Streptococcus pneumoniae* or atypical bacterial coverage. In addition, consider underlying medical conditions or the possibility of a retained aspirated foreign body.

Further diagnostic testing, such as diagnostic bronchoscopy with bronchoalveolar lavage, may be required in those with worsening symptoms despite maximal therapy.

Disposition

There are no well-validated, clinically useful severity scores for pneumonia in children to guide treatment and disposition. Pneumonia severity is clinically assessed by the patient's overall appearance and age-appropriate behavior. The presence of hypoxemia and respiratory distress indicates severe disease.

Indications for admission include severe disease (respiratory distress and hypoxia); complications including pleural effusion and empyema; hemodynamic instability; immunocompromise; comorbidities; and young age (the exact age cutoff remains controversial).

Follow-up is recommended within 24–48 hours for outpatient treatment; phone follow-up is acceptable. Follow-up imaging is not indicated in uncomplicated cases.

Complications

Complications of pneumonia include sepsis, respiratory distress/failure, treatment failure, and pleural effusion or empyema. Pleural effusion/empyema presents with significant chest pain and frequently with splinting. Dullness to percussion, distant breath sounds, and a pleural friction rub may be heard. Death from bacterial pneumonia is the most common cause of infectious pediatric death worldwide, but it is less common in industrialized nations.

Key Points

- The etiology of pneumonia in children varies by age.
- Most pneumonia in young children is viral in etiology.
- Radiographic findings are poor indicators of etiology of pneumonia and cannot be relied on entirely for diagnosis.

Pitfalls

- Failure to consider underlying etiology of recurrent pneumonia including malignancy, immunocompromised state, or retained aspirated foreign body
- Failure to consider the clinical setting (age, appearance of the child, and pretest probability of infectious etiology) when treating a child

ASTHMA

Background

Asthma is the most prevalent chronic disease of childhood in resource-rich countries. It remains a significant public health problem. There are significant racial and socioeconomic disparities in incidence, treatment, and outcomes. Exacerbations occur more commonly in African American children, those who are poor, and those who live in rural areas. In addition, African American children are 500 times more likely to die of an asthma exacerbation compared to white children.

Asthma is a lower airway disease with pathologic bronchoconstriction, bronchial hyperresponsiveness, and mucosal edema/inflammation. Acute asthma exacerbations involve bronchospasm, increased secretions, focal inflammatory response, and air trapping. Asthma is an obstructive process in which patients can inhale but cannot completely exhale.

Status asthmaticus is the most common medical emergency in children. The death rate of asthma remains alarmingly high for a disease that can be managed effectively with preventative therapy. Risk factors for fatal asthma include prior intensive care unit (ICU) admission, prior intubation, rapid deterioration (or persistent worsening despite home treatment), poor adherence to prescribed medication, food allergies, and respiratory deterioration despite effective treatment. However, it is important to note that up to one-third of children who die of asthma were not previously classified as being at risk for fatal asthma. This has important implications when educating parents regarding preventative therapy and the importance of having rescue medications available.

Classic Clinical Presentation

Approximately 80% of asthmatics present prior to age 5 years. The most common symptoms include coughing and wheezing. Patients frequently have a recurrent, seasonal/situational, and/or nocturnal cough. Cough is frequently the sole presentation of asthma in children and may occur without wheezing. Chest pain/

pressure/tightness and shortness of breath are also common symptoms.

Asthma frequently occurs with concomitant atopy. These patients typically have additional allergic symptoms, such as rhinitis, conjunctivitis, and/or eczema with seasonal flares.

Viral upper respiratory infections are the most common trigger of asthma exacerbations for patients of all ages. Other sources of exacerbations include weather changes, seasonal changes (tree pollination in spring, grasses in summer, and weeds in fall) and other allergens (insect and pet exposures, dust, and molds), tobacco smoke, stress, and chemical irritants (e.g., perfumes and cleaning sprays).

There is no consistently utilized asthma score to determine clinical severity. The scores that are simpler and have more objective data tend to perform with better interrater reliability. Measurements include respiratory rate, the presence of retractions, hypoxia, wheezing, and degree of prolongation of expiration.

Moderate to severe asthma exacerbations have inspiratory to expiratory ratios ≥1:2 and accessory muscle use. Severe asthma is associated with oxygen requirement and significant work of breathing. Inspiratory wheezing only is associated with less severe disease. Inspiratory and expiratory wheezing demonstrates more significant disease. Severe disease may also present with limited air movement, and wheezing may not be initially heard despite significant involvement. Minimal or absent air entry portends critical disease. Severe exacerbations may also have restlessness/lethargy, extreme tachypnea and tachycardia, significant accessory muscle use, and oxygen saturation <92%; peak expiratory flow rate (if obtained) is <40% predicted.

Atypical Clinical Presentation

The first symptom in reactive airway disease is often cough. Wheezing may be absent or only present after a trial of bronchodilators. Cough variant bronchoconstriction tends to be especially worse at night.

Exercise-induced bronchospasm may occur in up to 90% of children with asthma. These patients describe shortness of breath, chest tightness, and cough triggered by exertion.

Differential Diagnosis

Cardiac disease in children often presents with respiratory symptoms that are often initially misdiagnosed as asthma. Acute myocarditis is often treated as asthma exacerbation prior to worsening clinical course. Bronchiolitis is difficult to clinically distinguish by physical examination alone. It has been documented that patients with intrabronchial foreign bodies improve with inhaled corticosteroids/asthma treatment.

Diagnostic Confirmation

Asthma is frequently suspected based on history and physical examination. Spirometry measurements (forced vital capacity and forced expiratory volume in 1 second) are the confirmatory diagnostic measurements of choice for asthma in children. These measurements are typically performed in an outpatient clinic setting and cannot be obtained in children younger than age 5 years. There is significant debate regarding how to classify and diagnose infants and young children with recurrent wheezing. A trial of medication (and symptom response) is typically used to diagnose in young children. Most virus-induced wheezing resolves by age 5 years. It is unclear what percentage of these patients have mild asthma.

Peak expiratory flow measurements are more variable and effort dependent compared to spirometry. There is also variability in ideal reference values, thus limiting diagnostic utility of measurements for asthma. The ideal peak flow is based on a patient's height and weight. Peak flows may be used to monitor medication response but are often of limited usefulness in the emergent setting. Young children (<5 years old) are not able to perform peak flows, and these are often not reliable even in older children. Up to two-thirds of children older than age 5 years are not able to complete peak expiratory flow rate evaluation during an asthma exacerbation.

Few validated or objective measures are available to assess disease severity. Clinicians are inaccurate and inconsistent even when grading the same patient. Scores with fewer and more objective measurements may perform better. In addition, scoring may be of limited usefulness because any moderate to severe exacerbation has the potential to progress to a severe or life-threatening episode.

CXR typically is not indicated unless severe symptoms are present. It may be considered in a patient with new-onset wheezing that clinically appear to have bronchiolitis or an underlying condition is suspected (such as congestive heart failure (CHF), lesions such as right-sided aortic arch, mediastinal mass, or foreign body aspiration).

CXR rarely reveals pneumonia or other unsuspected diagnoses. Laboratory values are of limited usefulness in the ED care of severe asthma unless an additional underlying condition is suspected.

Treatment

The goals of acute treatment are to resolve hypoxemia, relieve airflow obstruction, and decrease acute airway inflammation. Preventative therapy goals are to improve the patient's acute lung function and decrease permanent lung remodeling. Implementing a clinical pathway in the ED improves care, decreases time to appropriate medication administration, decreases unnecessary imaging, and reduces admission rates.

Short-Acting β-Agonists

Short-acting β-agonists (SABA; e.g., albuterol) are the primary therapy for asthma. Nebulized therapy requires approximately 10 minutes, and only approximately 10% of the drug is delivered to the small airways. Aerosolized therapy does not require precise coordination of breathing efforts and can be given concomitantly with oxygen and anticholinergic therapy.

Metered dose inhalers (MDIs) with holding chambers (spacers) are equivalent to nebulizer delivery. MDI use decreases ED length of stay and causes less tachycardia and tremor in patients.

The benefit of spacers is that they hold a reservoir of medication that is available to be inhaled. Precise coordination of breathing is not required. Children should spray (actuation) and then take five to eight breaths. This decreases deposition into the oropharynx (and systemic absorption). Spacer mouthpieces are preferred (because they decrease nasal administration), but face mask-equipped spacers are available for infants and children not able to use the mouthpiece.

The speed of MDI actuation is approximately 60 mph; a spacer decreases medication deposition to the pharynx by approximately half. Optimum dosing for MDI therapy is also not well established. In the ED, 5 mg nebulized albuterol is equivalent to approximately eight MDI puffs.

The specific SABA medication dosing guidelines vary, and there remains some controversy regarding both nebulized and MDI therapy. Nebulized albuterol dosing is frequently given as 0.15 mg/kg, with a maximum dose of 5 mg. Young children have low deposition of medication in the lungs, and so weight-based dosing in young children may undertreat patients. For this reason, a minimal dose of 2.5 mg nebulized albuterol should be used for young children (exact age/weight recommendations vary from infancy to children <30 kg). Patients who require frequent therapy or do not improve after several treatments should have continuous nebulization administered. Continuous albuterol maximum dosing recommendations also vary. Commonly recommended dosing is 10 mg/hr for children 5–10 kg, 15 mg/hr for those 10–20 kg, and 20 mg/hr for those >20 kg.

Maximum recommended dosing varies from 10 to 30 mg/hr. Many national association guidelines recommend a maximum SABA dose of 10 mg/hr. There is evidence that dosing higher than official asthma guideline recommendations (e.g., albuterol 25 mg/hr) provides greater bronchodilation. In addition, many pediatric emergency medicine and pediatric ICU protocols utilize much higher SABA dosing (up to 50–100 mg/hr). Some experts theorize that higher than recommended SABA dosing may contribute to cardiac arrhythmias and deaths in asthma, but definitive evidence is lacking.

Corticosteroids

Early steroid therapy is important to impact acute disease course and decrease hospitalization rate. The number needed to treat with steroids in the first hour to prevent one admission is six. Steroids are indicated for moderate and severe exacerbations. Critically ill patients should receive IV steroids at a dose of 2 mg/kg (range, 1–4 mg/kg) of methylprednisolone (maximum 60–125 mg) if too ill to swallow, if gastric absorption is thought to be impaired, or if they are at risk for vomiting. Less severe cases may have oral prednisone/prednisolone or dexamethasone. Prednisone/prednisolone dosing is 1 mg/kg/day (maximum 60 mg), and dexamethasone dosing is 0.6 mg/kg (maximum 16 mg; 18 mg maximum if single dose). Patients tend to have more vomiting with prednisolone compared to dexamethasone. Approximately 1 mg of dexamethasone is equivalent to 5 mg of prednisolone. Dexamethasone has roughly 80% oral bioavailability, so the oral form is preferred to the more painful IM/IV administration. As with croup, in the ED, the IV solution may be given orally for a decreased total solution volume.

Anticholinergics

Ipratropium bromide is an inhaled anticholinergic agent. Anticholinergic therapy works synergistically with β-agonists by decreasing bronchomotor tone and decreasing mucosal edema and secretions. There is limited systemic absorption and so the complication rate is minimal. Dosing is 250 µg/dose for patients <20 kg and 500 µg/dose for patients >20 kg. There does not seem to be a benefit of more than three doses in 24 hours or use beyond the ED setting.

Ipratropium bromide is available as an MDI. However, this route is relatively expensive compared to the nebulized form, so most hospitals utilize the nebulized form for better cost-effective therapy.

Adjunctive Therapies

Intravenous fluids should be administered in severe disease to manage concomitant dehydration due to decreased PO intake and increased losses with work of breathing.

Magnesium provides smooth muscle relaxation with resultant bronchodilation. Magnesium also inhibits degranulation of mast cells. It has been demonstrated to decrease hospital admission rates in children and improve short-term lung function. Dosing is 25–75 mg/kg (maximum 2 g) IV over 20–30 minutes. Side effects include flushing, hypotension, nausea/vomiting, respiratory depression, and loss of deep tendon reflexes. It should not be used routinely in mild exacerbations but is beneficial and safe in severe patients. Magnesium should be administered slowly (over 20 minutes) and with IV fluids to decrease the incidence of hypotension.

Parental β_2-agonists are indicated with persistent symptoms despite the previously discussed therapy. Terbutaline (a selective β_2-agonist) or epinephrine (a nonselective agent but commonly used due to availability and nursing comfort) may be used.

Terbutaline IV can be given as 10 µg/kg IV loading dose over 10 minutes followed by an infusion of 0.1–10 µg/kg/min). Alternatively, it may be started at 0.1 µg/kg/min and increased in 0.1–1 µg/kg/min increments every 30 minutes to a maximum dose of 10 µg/kg/min.

Epinephrine may be administered initially IM (0.01 mg/kg, maximum 0.5 mg). Alternatively, a 0.15-mg dose may be given for a younger child and 0.3-mg dose to a child >35 kg in an emergent setting with severe respiratory distress.

Ketamine promotes bronchodilation but also increases secretion, which may further complicate disease course. Due to its bronchodilatory effects, it is the induction agent of choice for asthma. It may also be used as a drip in severe disease.

The data are conflicting for heliox, and its use is not routinely recommended. It has not been demonstrated to impact clinical outcomes such as admission rate, length of stay, and intubation rate for mild to moderate exacerbations. There may be a role for heliox in severe exacerbations.

Noninvasive positive pressure ventilation (NIPPV, see Chapter 6) assists with the work of ventilation. It increases functional residual capacity and compliance and decreases fatigue. However, it also has potential negative hemodynamic effects, increases air trapping, and elevates intrathoracic pressure. Elevated intrathoracic pressure impacts cardiac function by decreasing venous return. NIPPV should be utilized in the patient who is fatiguing to help stave off intubation, but it should not be used in cases of mild or moderate exacerbation. High-flow nasal cannula therapy may also be utilized to support respiratory effort.

Intubation may be required in cases of severe asthma, but it should be used with caution and reserved for patients with continued progression toward respiratory failure despite maximal medical therapy. It is important to remember that intubation is not a definitive therapy and has the significant risk of barotrauma. NPPV may avoid the need for intubation by easing the work of breathing while awaiting the maximal therapeutic effects of medical intervention.

If intubation is required, ventilation settings should be lung protective to minimize complications and the risk of barotrauma. No specific mode of ventilation (pressure or volume controlled) has been demonstrated to be superior. See Chapter 6 for further recommendations regarding ventilation management. The respiratory rate should be low and expiration time adequate to promote exhalation (e.g., inspiration:expiration ratio of 1:4 or 1:5). Plateau pressure should be <30 cm H_2O. Accept hypercapnia as a result of these settings because a patient will handle acidosis better than complications of barotrauma. Patients have auto-positive end-expiratory pressure (PEEP); asthmatics are less responsive to adding PEEP than are non-asthmatics.

ASTHMA DEATH

The breath stacking that occurs from obstruction in asthma results an increased intrathoracic pressure. This increased pressure results in decreased venous return. In a cardiopulmonary arrest, there are four common treatment recommendations that are based on the pathophysiology of asthma but are not necessarily evidence-based. A trial of apnea decreases breath stacking and minimizes the increased thoracic pressure. An IV fluids bolus may improve venous return. Manual pressure may be administered externally to the chest to assist in exhalation. Finally, all cases of cardiopulmonary arrest in asthma should have at least a needle thoracostomy if not a finger or tube thoracostomy placed to treat a potential unrecognized or untreated pneumothorax.

Asthma is a reversible condition, and extracorporeal membrane oxygenation (ECMO) should be considered early in severe, refractory status asthmaticus.

Simplified Treatment Summary

Mild to Moderate Asthma

All patients with an asthma exacerbation should receive SABA therapy in the ED. If several treatments are required, the addition of inhaled ipratropium bromide (up to three doses) improves symptoms. Most patients should receive corticosteroids. Dexamethasone (one or two doses) is better tolerated.

Moderate to Severe Asthma

SABA and anticholinergic agents should be administered with consideration of continuous nebulized therapy. All patients should receive corticosteroids within the first hour of ED arrival. Intravenous access with fluids and magnesium should be given in patients with severe disease or persistent symptoms after 1 or 2 hours of treatment. Additional adjunctive therapies may be utilized early with severe disease or with persistent symptoms after treatment.

Outpatient prescription of inhaled corticosteroids should be considered after discharge.

Disposition

Pulse oximetry <92–94% one hour after treatment is predictive of need for hospitalization. Children with persistent signs/symptoms after 1 or 2 hours of treatment likely would benefit from admission.

Children sustaining clinical improvement after 60 minutes from the last SABA treatment may be discharged. SABA should be weaned over the next 3–7 days. Controller medications should be continued.

After discharge for an acute asthma exacerbation, albuterol MDI administration guidelines for every 4 hours are as follows: younger than age 5 years, two puffs; aged 5–12 years, four puffs; older than age 12 years, six puffs.

Steroid dosing at discharge is commonly given as 1 mg/kg (maximum 60 mg/day) of prednisone or prednisolone one or two times per day. The half-life of dexamethasone is approximately double that of prednisone, and it typically lasts up to 72 hours after the first dose. Oral dexamethasone 0.6 mg/kg (maximum 16 mg) given twice (on day 1 and day 2 or 3) is as effective as a 5-day course of oral prednisone and has fewer side effects. Two-day dexamethasone has been demonstrated to be superior to 5-day prednisone/prednisolone in cost-effectiveness, palatability, and patient compliance. A one-time dexamethasone dose appears to be equivalent to a 3-day course of prednisone. A longer steroid course (7–14 days) may be required in severe cases or with frequent exacerbations.

Prescription of an inhaled corticosteroid should be considered at discharge for preventative therapy. Inhaled corticosteroids are not as effective as oral steroids for severe exacerbations, and they should be used as adjunctive therapy and not as a substitute. Preventative education and ensuring proper follow-up and medication refills are also important upon ED discharge.

Complications

Common adverse effects of β-agonist medication include tremulousness, agitation, and a sense of jitteriness. Hypokalemia is also common. The clinical significance of this is controversial. Hypokalemia is transient and resolves after SABA cessation but may result in muscular weakness, and patients may appear more ill as a result. Some experts argue that higher dosing of SABA may induce cardiac arrhythmias.

Hypoxemia may ensue after treatment initiation due to a ventilation–perfusion mismatch.

Patients are at significant risk for barotrauma. Unrecognized and/or untreated pneumothorax may be a cause of death in acute asthma exacerbations.

Severe obstruction may result in death despite maximal therapy.

Key Points

- Asthma is an important public health problem and a common chronic disease of childhood.
- The mainstay of treatment is short-acting β-agonists.
- Inhaled anticholinergic therapy improves lung function in moderate exacerbations.
- Early corticosteroid therapy decreases symptoms and admission rates in asthma exacerbations.

Pitfalls

- Failure to aggressively treat acute asthma exacerbations
- Failure to administer corticosteroids early in the ED course
- Failure to educate patients and families about the asthma treatment and risk of death
- Failure to perform needle or tube thoracostomy in an asthmatic cardiopulmonary arrest
- Failure to consider ECMO therapy in a patient with refractory status asthmaticus

ANAPHYLAXIS

Background

Anaphylaxis is a potentially fatal disorder with a rapid onset of symptoms after exposure. It is a systemic reaction involving vasodilation and multiple organ systems. The major pathophysiology involves activation of systemic IgE production.

BOX 15.1

COMMON ALLERGENS IN CHILDREN

Food:[a] peanuts, tree nuts, fish, shellfish, cow's milk, soy, egg, sesame
Medications
Insect venom
Latex

[a]Most common anaphylactic trigger in children

The most common triggers include food, drugs, and insect venom (Box 15.1). Overall, food is the most common cause of anaphylaxis in children. Ingestion is the most typical cause, but inhalation of aerosolized food particles may also induce anaphylaxis.

Asthma is a risk factor for severe anaphylaxis. Risk factors for fatal food-induced anaphylaxis include concomitant asthma, adolescence, peanut or tree nut allergy, and delayed access to epinephrine autoinjectors.

Classic Clinical Presentation

The diagnosis of anaphylaxis is made clinically based on history of exposure and acute symptoms. Confirmatory laboratory testing is not typically emergently available.

Symptoms of anaphylaxis are typically rapid in onset. Food-related anaphylaxis typically presents within 30 minutes of ingestion. Parental medication and insect stings can induce anaphylaxis within seconds to minutes. Untreated, death can occur within minutes.

The skin is involved in the majority of cases of anaphylaxis but may not be involved in up to 20% of cases. Many organ systems can be affected, including the skin, the upper and lower respiratory system, the gastrointestinal system, and the cardiovascular system (Boxes 15.2 and 15.3).

Atypical Clinical Presentation

Anaphylaxis is underrecognized and undertreated. More subtle cases and those without cutaneous or respiratory symptoms are more commonly missed.

Most cases present within 1 hour of exposure to the trigger, although symptoms can be delayed for more than 10 hours.

BOX 15.2

SYMPTOMS OF ANAPHYLAXIS INVOLVING VARIOUS ORGAN SYSTEMS

Skin: warmth, pruritis, urticaria, facial erythema/flushing, angioedema
Oral: pruritis or edema of lips/tongue/palate
Respiratory system: rhinitis, hoarseness, laryngeal edema, stridor, dyspnea, cough, wheeze
Gastrointestinal system: abdominal pain/cramping, vomiting, diarrhea
Cardiovascular system: dizziness, hypotension, syncope, shock. Cardiovascular symptoms occur less commonly in adults than in children, perhaps due to a higher underlying sympathetic tone.
Neurologic: anxiety, sense of impending doom, seizure, headache, behavioral changes (particularly in young, preverbal children)
Ocular: periorbital erythema/edema/pruritis, conjunctival injection, tearing

Diagnostic Confirmation

Anaphylaxis is a clinical diagnosis typically made without confirmatory testing.

Treatment

Epinephrine is the only first-line treatment for anaphylaxis and should be given immediately if anaphylaxis is clinically the most likely diagnosis. Epinephrine effectively treats all of the signs and symptoms of anaphylaxis and stabilizes mast cells to prevent further histamine release. The initial administration is an IM injection in the lateral thigh. The IM dose is 0.01 mg/kg (maximum 0.5 mg) of the 1:1,000 concentration. This dose may be repeated in 5 minutes. There are no contraindications to epinephrine administration.

Early use of epinephrine improves outcomes and decreases repeat use and ED length of stay. In addition, there is evidence that early epinephrine use decreases rebound anaphylaxis or "biphasic reactions."

If symptoms persistent despite multiple IM doses, then an IV epinephrine infusion is indicated. Intravenous epinephrine should be administered with the 1:10,000 concentration at a dose of 0.1 μg/kg/min (up to 1 μg/kg/min in children). The drip should be titrated to effect, increasing at a rate of 0.05 μg/kg/min until blood pressure, mentation, and perfusion improve.

The trigger should be removed if possible. Nebulized epinephrine may be used as adjunctive therapy. β-Agonists (SABAs) should be administered with wheezing. Oxygen administration should be given as needed, and IV fluids should be given to support hypotension due to systemic vasodilation.

BOX 15.3

NATIONAL INSTITUTE OF ALLERGY AND INFECTIOUS DISEASES AND FOOD ALLERGY AND ANAPHYLAXIS NETWORK CRITERIA FOR ANAPHYLAXIS

The diagnosis of anaphylaxis is likely when any one of the following three criteria are fulfilled:

1. Acute onset of an illness with involvement of the skin, mucosal tissue, or both and at least one of the following: respiratory compromise and cardiovascular compromise
2. Two or more of the following that occur rapidly after exposure to a likely allergen
   a. Involvement of the skin or mucosal tissue (hives, pruritis/flushing or angioedema)
   b. Respiratory symptoms/compromise (dyspnea, wheezing, stridor, hypoxia)
   c. Hypotension/cardiovascular compromise
   d. Persistent gastrointestinal symptoms
3. Hypotension after exposure to a known allergen

Young children aged <2 years provide additional diagnostic difficulty because they are unable to describe subjective features of anaphylaxis. The incidence of anaphylaxis in this population is likely underdiagnosed.

Antihistamines and corticosteroids are adjunctive therapies (not primary therapy). There is no direct evidence that histamine blockers are beneficial in anaphylaxis. Histamine H_1 and H_2 blockers can reduce urticaria but do not treat anaphylaxis. Their use should be considered adjuvant therapy only to minimize discomfort rather than treatment of anaphylaxis. Corticosteroids act too slowly to effectively treat acute anaphylaxis. There is also no evidence that steroids decrease biphasic reactions.

Disposition

Current guidelines recommend observing patients for 4 hours after treatment due to risk of biphasic reactions. Risk factors for biphasic reactions include delayed epinephrine administration, repeat dosing requirements, bronchodilator requirements, and wide pulse pressure upon presentation.

Patients with respiratory compromise should be monitored for recurrent symptoms. Recommendations vary from 4 for 8 hours. If hypotension was a presenting symptom, monitoring should be extended to 12–24 hours.

Higher risk presentations include those with prior protracted episodes or biphasic reactions, episodes that require two or more doses of epinephrine, significant laryngeal or bronchial involvement on presentation, hypotension, and refractory symptoms. History of asthma should trigger more conservative observation.

All patients with anaphylaxis should be prescribed an epinephrine autoinjector (with appropriate teaching) prior to discharge. The dose is 0.15 mg (children <30 kg); 0.3-mg autoinjectors are prescribed for children >30 kg.

Complications

Fatal anaphylaxis occurs in approximately 1% of cases in industrialized nations. Most biphasic reactions occur within 8 hours of the first episode, but delays up to 72 hours have been reported. The incidence varies from 1% to 20% of all anaphylaxis cases. Biphasic reactions tend to be associated with more severe initial presentations and delay in epinephrine administration. There is limited evidence regarding how to prevent biphasic reactions. Early epinephrine administration is the only medical therapy that has some evidence to support a decreased incidence in biphasic reactions. Corticosteroids have not been proved to decrease incidence. However, they are commonly given for 48–72 hours after anaphylaxis and continue to be recommended by experts.

Key Points

- Anaphylaxis is frequently underrecognized and undertreated.
- Food allergies are the most common cause of anaphylaxis in children.
- Symptoms of anaphylaxis commonly involve the skin, respiratory system, gastrointestinal system, and cardiovascular system.
- Epinephrine is the treatment of choice for acute anaphylaxis.

Pitfalls

- Failure to use epinephrine in suspected cases of anaphylaxis
- Failure to not consider anaphylaxis in cases without respiratory or dermatologic findings
- Failure to prescribe an epinephrine autoinjector prior to discharge

EPIGLOTTIS

Background

The incidence of this feared pediatric entity has significantly decreased since vaccination implementation of *Haemophilus influenzae* type b (Hib) in the 1980s. Currently, infectious epiglottitis is relatively more common in older children. Hib is still the most common overall infectious etiology, but many other bacterial strains may cause epiglottitis (other *Haemophilus* strains, staph, and strep). Hib infections may rarely occur in fully immunized patients. Atypical infections may occur in the immunocompromised, and noninfectious causes may rarely occur from thermal burns or irritant injuries.

Classic Clinical Presentation

Bacterial epiglottitis is notoriously acute in onset. Symptoms include rapid progression of high fever, intense focal sore throat, and toxic appearance. Children appear anxious, with classic positioning to maintain airway patency. A sniffing/tripoding position is common, with mandible protrusion and neck extension. Drooling is common due to the inability to swallow secretions. This presentation has been described as the three hallmark D's: dysphagia, drooling, and distress.

Infectious epiglottitis caused by bacteria other than Hib both tends to have a slower onset in symptoms and is less likely to cause airway compromise.

Atypical Clinical Presentation

Less commonly, young patients may present predominantly with altered mental status. Older patients with epiglottitis are less likely to have dramatic airway obstruction. A larger airway diameter is protective against severe disease, and more significant swelling is required to produce airway obstruction. Patients often complain of significant focal sore throat (frequently out of proportion to physical findings) and may have anterior neck tenderness to palpation.

Differential Diagnosis

Croup is a common mimic and often the initial misdiagnosis. Epiglottitis is often distinguished by the absence of cough and the predominant symptoms of refusal to swallow, dysphagia, and drooling. Patients with epiglottitis also have a strong preference to remain sitting.

Diagnostic Confirmation

A lateral neck radiograph may be obtained to help confirm the diagnosis. However, the classic "thumbprint" sign of an enlarged epiglottis is only present in approximately 30% of patients. Observation, reassessment, and laryngoscopic evaluation should be considered based on patient age, clinical severity, and likelihood of Hib infection (considering vaccination status and exposure risk).

Treatment

Bacterial epiglottis is a rare and severe airway emergency, and difficulty should be anticipated. It is much better to be overprepared than have unexpected difficulty in securing the airway.

In the young child, emergent securing of the airway takes precedence over diagnostic evaluation. Ideally, these patients should be transported to an operative setting in which a definitive airway can be placed with multiple difficult airway algorithm tools available as backup, including endoscopic intubation and surgical intervention.

Older children and adolescents have much lower risk of respiratory failure. Intravenous antibiotics and admission to a monitored setting are reasonable. Immediate airway intervention is not mandated unless the clinical picture dictates as such.

Children requiring intubation typically remain intubated for approximately 3–5 days with IV antibiotics (second- or third-generation cephalosporin and possibly an anti-staphylococcal agent such as vancomycin).

Epiglottitis due to thermal burns does not benefit from antibiotics. Steroids have not been demonstrated to be of benefit in epiglottitis of any etiology.

Disposition

All cases of suspected epiglottis should be admitted to a monitored setting.

Complications

The mortality rate of acute bacterial epiglottitis is 1–3%. Most deaths are due to airway compromise and typically occur early in disease presentation (typically in route or immediately after hospital arrival). Epiglottic abscess or secondary infection may complicate disease. Associated systemic toxicity/sepsis from Hib or other bacterial infection may also occur.

Key Points

- Epiglottitis is a life-threatening condition due to potential airway obstruction.
- Young children are particularly at risk for airway compromise due to a narrow-caliber airway.
- Hib remains the most common etiology of infectious epiglottitis, but the incidence has significantly decreased due to widespread vaccination.

Pitfalls

- Failure to consider the diagnosis of epiglottitis despite normal imaging; plain radiographs are insensitive to make this diagnosis
- Failure to secure the airway prior to diagnostic evaluation, particularly in the young child and/or in the patient with signs of clinical compromise
- Failure to anticipate a difficult airway
- Failure to prepare multiple advanced airway interventions

16

Airway Foreign Bodies

C. ANTHONEY LIM, RACHEL WHITNEY, AND JEREMY M. ROSE

INTRODUCTION

The presentation of an airway foreign body can range from benign to truly life-threatening. Respiratory tract obstruction from an airway or esophageal foreign body is relatively rare but remains a leading cause of morbidity and mortality among children. Up to half of patients with a confirmed foreign body do not have a history suggestive of aspiration, and 20% of children are misdiagnosed and improperly treated for a month or more before diagnosis. A high index of suspicion and thorough physical examination skills are necessary in the initial evaluation of these patients.

There are limited epidemiological data on the morbidity and mortality of airway foreign bodies. The most recent update from the Centers for Disease Control and Prevention in 2001 cited an estimated 17,537 children aged 0–14 years visited the emergency department for choking; 1,844 of these were hospitalized. A mortality rate of 2.75% has been documented for pediatric patients admitted with the diagnosis of aspirated foreign body. The majority of airway foreign bodies occur in children younger than age 4 years, with a slight male predominance. Foods such as hard candy, seeds, and nuts are the most frequently retrieved objects from the respiratory tract, followed by nonorganic objects such as small toy parts, beads, and rocks.

Due to a combination of developmental and anatomic factors, children are especially at risk for foreign body aspiration and its complications. Molars are used to crush and grind food prior to swallowing; prior to the eruption of primary molars in children younger than age 3 years, the lack of these teeth may increase the risk of aspiration because it is more difficult to appropriately reduce the size of food boluses by chewing. It is for this reason that hard foods such as carrots and nuts are generally not recommended in this age group. Developmentally, hand–mouth exploration of their environment is a common activity for children, which also increases the risk of aspiration in this age group.

The management of foreign bodies in a pediatric airway should take multiple factors into consideration, including the presence of respiratory distress, the potential location and type of foreign body, the ability to visualize and reach it, and the child's compliance with removal.

NASAL FOREIGN BODY

See Chapter 46 on foreign body removal.

HYPOPHARYNGEAL FOREIGN BODY

The hypopharynx is the short anatomical area extending from the epiglottis to just below where the trachea and esophagus separate into distinct tracts. The larynx is the first part of the trachea. Retained hypopharyngeal foreign bodies are rare but precarious and require immediate recognition to avoid worsening obstruction. The most common retained foreign bodies in this area are bony portions of fish or chicken or a large/partially masticated food bolus.

Other objects such as coins, batteries, and small toys may also be ingested by young children during oral environmental exploration.

Presentation

Children typically will present acutely due to the dysphagia caused by the lodged foreign body. Bloody secretions may be present secondary to removal attempts or associated retching. Frank hematemesis is concerning for potential catastrophe caused by a button battery eroding through the esophageal mucosa or a full-thickness penetration of an object in the esophagus. Prior to arrival, there may have been some attempts at manual removal or drinking water or swallowing other food in the hopes of dislodging the object.

Prior to arrival, parents often encourage drinking water or swallowing food in an attempt to dislodge foreign bodies associated with food. Manual removal attempts may occur with both food and foreign object aspiration. Frequently, foreign object aspiration occurs and is witnessed as choking episodes followed by dysphagia and/or drooling resulting from the child's inability to swallow their own saliva.

Anatomical Considerations

The location of the foreign body may be determined by the location of pain. Anatomically, foreign bodies often get lodged around the tonsillar pillars and aryepiglottic folds. Congenital abnormalities such as vascular rings or a right-sided aortic arch may create a narrowing in the esophagus and lead to potential points of obstruction. The upper aerodigestive tract contains sensory innervation; patients can often localize their pain to the area where the foreign body is located. The lower esophagus below the hypopharynx contains visceral innervation; thus, discomfort is often reported as vague, nonlocalized chest or throat pain.

Diagnosis

In patients in whom a hypopharynx/upper aerodigestive foreign body is suspected, information regarding the approximate timing of the event and type of foreign body should be obtained.

Direct visualization may be possible using a tongue depressor and otoscope light, or a laryngoscope may be utilized to identify and localize the foreign body if it is located around the area of the tonsils. If unsuccessful and the patient is cooperative, a nasal fiberoptic scope may be utilized to visualize the hypopharynx to the area of the vocal cords for foreign objects. Topical benzocaine spray can make visualization much more comfortable for the patient.

Imaging techniques are varied and depend on the index of suspicion that a foreign body remains in situ. Among patients in whom a large radio-opaque foreign body is suspected, anterior–posterior and lateral radiographs of the neck soft tissues may demonstrate the object in the hypopharynx to thoracic inlet. Note that the orientation of a discoid object may suggest its location; due to the shape of the cartilaginous rings in the upper airway, coins will appear edge-on in anterior–posterior views, whereas they will appear face-on if they are in the esophagus.

Smaller foreign bodies such as fish bones may not be easily identified using a simple radiograph. Among children with a high suspicion of a small, retained foreign body, ultrasound, noncontrast computed tomography, or magnetic resonance imaging of the neck may be useful in identifying the type and location of the object. Complicating diagnostic certainly, an abrasion to the mucosa can cause a persistent foreign body sensation even if the offending object has been swallowed or spit up.

Management

For children with uncontrolled hematemesis with high suspicion of esophageal perforation from a sharp foreign body or erosion from button battery, immediately secure the airway and consult the ear, nose, and throat and/or thoracic surgery department. Similarly, patients with stridor, drooling, tripoding, or other signs of respiratory distress should be kept calm, and surgical consultations should be obtained and the child taken to an operating room for foreign body removal. It is important to note that large objects that are lodged in the esophagus may compress the airway and cause obstruction.

If the foreign body is visualized and graspable, attempts may be made at removal using alligator forceps or similar instruments. In the absence of airway compromise, children may be provided pain control with nonsteroidal anti-inflammatory drugs, benzocaine spray, or viscous lidocaine. If nonvisualized, there is a moderate or low suspicion of a retained foreign body, and the patient is tolerating adequate PO, a plain radiograph may be obtained and, if negative, the patient sent home with pain control and instructed to return for more advanced imaging if symptoms persist.

Disposition

Patients presenting with airway symptoms, in which there is a history or concern for significant bleeding, or with deep neck space infections arising from retained foreign bodies should be admitted for further observation and management. Complications of hypopharyngeal and upper aerodigestive tract foreign bodies include perforation, associated bleeding, and deep neck space infections, which may lead to mediastinitis.

Key Points

- The hypopharynx is the anatomic area directly superior to the division of the trachea and the esophagus. Foreign bodies lodged in this area have a high risk of aspiration and upper airway obstruction.
- Fiberoptic scope or other advanced imaging, such as computed tomography, may be needed for diagnosis.
- Subspecialty consultation is needed for removal, and any signs of respiratory distress constitute an emergent intervention.

Pitfall

- A child with a retained hypopharyngeal foreign body who is maintaining an open airway should be left until appropriate difficult airway escalation setup can be obtained (including subspecialty consultation and potential operative intervention as indicated).

UPPER AIRWAY FOREIGN BODY

Upper airway foreign bodies are among the immediate life-threatening conditions. Foreign body aspiration strikes abruptly, afflicts mostly previously healthy children, and, if unsuccessfully treated, imparts a 45% mortality rate, leaving another 30% of children with permanent disabilities resulting from hypoxic ischemic encephalopathy. Younger children with oral exploration activity are most at risk for upper airway aspiration. The provision of developmentally inappropriate foods, lack of molars to crush hard foods, or the disorganized oromotor process in children with neurodevelopmental delay can increase the chances of aspiration.

Presentation

The initial presentation will depend on the location and whether the obstruction is partial or complete. Patients may begin with coughing in an attempt to dislodge the object, develop stridor, or rapidly progress to respiratory failure.

Following dislodgement of foreign bodies, children may rarely present with a postobstructive pulmonary edema (POPE), which is a form of acute interstitial pulmonary edema resulting from negative inspiratory pressure against an obstructed airway.

Anatomical Considerations

Children aged 2–4 years are far more likely to have foreign bodies removed from the larynx and trachea, whereas children aged 5 or 6 years are more likely to have foreign bodies in the bronchus or lower airways.

Diagnosis

Diagnostic evaluation can be challenging, particularly if the choking event is unwitnessed or if it is unclear if an object was involved in the choking episode. Choking or coughing episodes have a reported sensitivity of 80–82% and a specificity of 34% for foreign body aspiration. The type of object causing the obstruction, the duration of the choking episode, attempts at removal, and patient status are important points of information to gather. The diagnosis of foreign body aspiration should always be considered, particularly in children with out-of-hospital cardiac arrest or those with difficult ventilation—especially due to oromotor neurodevelopmental delay or tracheostomy tubes.

Management

Awake, alert children often expel an acute foreign body through coughing. Among children, post-tussive emesis can occur as a result. Parents may still seek care as a result of the episode or if there is suspicion that the entire foreign body was not expelled. During a coughing episode following a suspected foreign body aspiration, closely monitor the child and prepare for back blows or a Heimlich maneuver if the coughing ceases or respiratory distress worsens. Objects may move within the airway due to coughing and cause varying levels of obstruction.

Should this occur, the next approach is to promote a forceful exhalation from the lungs in an attempt to eject the foreign body and relieve the obstruction. In children younger than age 1 year, this is achieved through back blows and chest thrusts; for children older than age 1 year, the Heimlich maneuver is utilized. For infants, in a seated position, lay the child prone along the length of the forearm, supporting the head and neck with the hand. With the head placed lower than the chest, deliver five forceful back blows to the area between the infant's shoulder blades. Immediately following, transfer the infant to the other forearm, turning the infant supine. Using two fingers from the initially supporting hand, provide five chest thrusts to the area of the breastbone at the nipple line, again with the infant's head placed lower than the chest. Continue to repeat the maneuvers until the obstruction is relieved or the patient loses consciousness.

Among unconscious patients suspected of having a foreign body obstructing the upper airway, the initial approach is for direct laryngoscopy and, if the object is visualized, removal using McGill forceps.

If mechanical removal attempts are unsuccessful, or if the object is not visualized and there remains a high suspicion for an upper airway obstruction from a foreign body, the next step is to convert a laryngeal or tracheal obstruction into a unilateral pulmonary main stem obstruction in order to ventilate one lung. This temporizing method will then allow mobilization of operating room resources to definitively alleviate the obstruction. Use a bag valve mask to provide positive pressure, intubate with the appropriately sized endotracheal tube and ventilate, or employ a bougie stylet to force the object distally to relieve the midline obstruction.

If the patient remains difficult to oxygenate and ventilate, a surgical cricothyroidotomy is indicated in children aged 8 years or older, and a needle cricothyroidotomy and jet insufflation are indicated for children younger than age 8 years. Rapid initiation of extracorporeal membrane oxygenation should be considered for children who fail all of the previously discussed approaches.

Disposition

In minor choking episodes in which the object is expelled by initial cough, discharge may occur if the assessment is normal. Most significant choking episodes involving the upper airway and trachea require admission and monitoring for signs of POPE. For all children suspected of upper airway obstruction, soft tissue neck and chest radiographs should be obtained to evaluate for signs of lower airway obstruction as well as POPE. Initial radiographs demonstrating new infiltrates may indicate developing interstitial alveolar edema. If children develop signs of respiratory distress during their period of observation, repeat chest radiographs should be obtained. Positive pressure respiratory support, judicious intravenous hydration, and, in some cases, antidiuretics are utilized to treat POPE.

Anticipatory guidance should be provided to all families presenting with children following choking episodes. Avoidance of age-inappropriate foods, use of toys meeting Consumer Product Safety Commission standards, and education regarding supervision and first aid should be provided.

Complications

Significantly high mortality and morbidity rates are associated with upper airway foreign bodies. Children surviving severe episodes often develop the sequelae of hypoxic–ischemic static encephalopathy.

Airway, thoracic, and abdominal trauma may result from attempts at removal of the foreign object. Laryngotracheal injury, pneumothorax and pneumomediastinum, POPE, rib fractures, and solid and hollow organ injury have been reported in children.

Key Points

- Upper airway obstruction is associated with extremely high morbidity and mortality.
- Allow a choking person to cough in an attempt to dislodge a foreign body.
- Rapidly progress through back blows/ Heimlich maneuver, direct visualization and removal, or distal displacement with bag valve mask, intubation, or bougie in patients with a complete upper airway obstruction.
- Following the resolution of a significant upper airway obstruction, monitor children for signs of POPE.

Pitfall

- Failure to consider postobstructive sequelae after successful foreign body dislodgement

LOWER AIRWAY FOREIGN BODY

Aspiration of foreign bodies may have a wide range of presentations and present insidiously or acutely and dramatically. Aspirated foreign bodies lodge in the trachea in 5–15% of cases and are managed in a similar manner as upper airway foreign bodies. Up to 95% of aspirated foreign bodies lodge distal to the carina. Thirty to forty percent lodge in the main stem bronchi, where there is an equal prevalence in laterality among otherwise healthy children. Literature suggesting that aspiration occurs more frequently on the right side predominantly examined children with neuromuscular disorders that were baseline recumbent. Foreign bodies come to rest in the lobar bronchi in 5–15% of cases.

Presentation

The majority of aspiration episodes are witnessed because children at highest risk are often in the age range requiring continuous supervision. There should be a high index of suspicion for an aspirated foreign body when a history is elicited of acute onset of cough paroxysm with persistent respiratory symptoms that began while eating or during exploratory activities. Children aged 12–36 months, as well as children with neurodevelopmental delays and persistent oromotor behaviors, are most commonly affected.

Up to 20–30% of patients with lower airway foreign body aspiration present more than 1 week after the event. The smaller and more commonly organic objects implicated may elicit a less dramatic cough paroxysm or are completely unwitnessed.

Among children with aspirated foreign bodies, the most common physical examination finding is tachypnea, followed by unilateral wheezing or crackles on focal lung examination. Children with recurrent pneumonias localizing to the same area without interval clearing of the chest radiograph should be evaluated for an aspirated foreign body.

Diagnosis

As with every potential airway foreign body, the history plays a significant role in the diagnostic workup. A concerning history and physical examination demonstrating focal wheezing or change in oxygenation should trigger definitive treatment. However, many aspirated foreign bodies may have an equivocal history, physical examination, or both. If aspiration is suspected, various diagnostic techniques are available with variable sensitivity. Choice of modality will depend on the acuity of the presentation and the level of suspicion following history and physical examination.

Chest radiographs can be obtained rapidly and relatively easily. They can be obtained in a portable manner in children who are too unstable to leave the emergency department. In addition, it is an initial diagnostic tool for children with low to moderate suspicion. A four-view series may be obtained to further evaluate for an aspirated foreign body, including anterior–posterior, lateral, and inspiratory–expiratory or bilateral decubitus views. Because younger children suspected of foreign body aspiration cannot follow instructions for inspiratory–expiratory views, decubitus views imitate forced expiration of the dependent lung and may uncover air trapping if present. However, the presence of air trapping is neither sensitive nor specific for foreign body aspiration.

Approximately 26% of foreign bodies are radiolucent. Obstruction is often inferred from signs of air trapping, which manifests as unilateral hyperinflation or atelectasis. Atelectasis is often assumed to be an infectious infiltrate, and children are treated with antibiotics. The lack of resolution of these focal findings on a radiograph in 4–6 weeks following antibiotic course should prompt the suspicion of a potential foreign body. Organic foreign bodies can serve as a nidus for infection, making the patient's initial presentation indistinguishable from a bacterial pneumonia. Overall, the sensitivity radiographs in detecting aspirated foreign bodies is 63%, and the specificity is 79%.

New low-dose computed tomography protocols are also available and have the advantage of identifying the exact location of airway obstructions. Their disadvantage is the still relatively high dose of ionizing radiation compared to that used with other methods, but their use may avoid the need to undergo general anesthesia and bronchoscopy.

Bronchoscopy is a simultaneously diagnostic and therapeutic intervention for aspirated foreign bodies. General anesthesia and skilled personnel are required to perform bronchoscopy.

Management and Disposition

The management and disposition of children suspected of foreign body aspiration depend on the severity of symptoms and the level of suspicion elicited from the history and physical examination.

Those considered high risk include children presenting with a concerning history and those who are noted to be symptomatic by parents or providers, have a suggestive physical examination, have a strongly suggestive radiography, and/or are in extremis. These patients should have emergent consultation for bronchoscopy and admission.

Those with moderate risk may present with a questionable history or no witnessed episode suggestive of aspiration, are asymptomatic and have no focal findings on physical examination, and have negative radiographs. These patients may be discharged with specific return instructions and have follow-up with the primary care provider or pulmonologist. Should further symptoms develop, they can be subsequently scheduled for advanced radiographic studies or a bronchoscopy.

For children who present with a history providing low suspicion for aspiration, are asymptomatic with a normal physical examination, and have a negative radiograph, discharge home with anticipatory guidance and routine pediatric follow-up are indicated. Parents should be informed that should the child develop respiratory symptoms or illnesses in the coming weeks, they should inform their physician of the significant history because it may prompt evaluation that otherwise would not occur without a suspicion for aspiration.

Complications

The most severe complication of foreign bodies is respiratory failure, which may occur in tracheal or main stem obstructions. Pneumonitis and other local reactions may occur around aspirated objects, typically organic material, and lead to recurrent pneumonia.

Key Points

- Suspect foreign body aspiration in children with recurrent lobar pneumonias and in those in whom infiltrates on chest radiographs do not resolve 4–6 weeks after treatment.
- Bilateral decubitus films may demonstrate hyperinflation in the setting of foreign body aspiration but are incompletely sensitive.
- A majority of children present immediately after a witnessed choking episode, but many may present more than 1 week after the event.

PITFALLS

- Failure to consider the possibility of an aspirated foreign body in a patient with remote history of a choking episode
- Failure to consider the possibility of an aspirated foreign body in a patient with known choking episode but normal imaging and physical examination

Further Reading

Oncel M, Sunam GS, Ceran S. Tracheobronchial aspiration of foreign bodies and rigid bronchoscopy in children. *Pediatr Int*. 2012;54(4):532–535.

Orji FT, Akpeh JO. Tracheobronchial foreign body aspiration in children: How reliable are clinical and radiological signs in the diagnosis? *Clin Otolaryngol*. 2010;35(6):479–485.

Pan H, Lu Y, Shi L, Pan X, Li L, Wu Z. Similarities and differences in aspirated tracheobronchial foreign bodies in patients under the age of 3 years. *Int J Pediatr Otorhinolaryngol*. 2012;76(6):911–914.

Pinto A, Muzj C, Gagliardi N, et al. Role of imaging in the assessment of impacted foreign bodies in the hypopharynx and cervical esophagus. *Semin Ultrasound CT MR*. 2012;33(5):463–470.

Sink JR, Kitsko DJ, Georg MW, Winger DG, Simons JP. Predictors of foreign body aspiration in children. *Otolaryngol Head Neck Surg*. 2016;155(3):501–507.

17

The Pediatric Chest X-Ray

LOREN G. YAMAMOTO

INTRODUCTION

The pediatric chest X-ray (CXR) provides a wealth of useful information. In most instances, clinicians are seeking more definitive information regarding the lungs; however, the CXR provides information about the airway, heart, aorta, vena cava, pulmonary vessels, mediastinum, indwelling devices, bones (ribs, spine, clavicle, and upper extremities), soft tissue, gastrointestinal tract, liver, spleen, diaphragm, etc. These findings can be subtle or obvious, but difficult to notice. "Tunnel vision" permits the human brain to focus on areas of interest, only to miss other important findings. Examine the CXR in Figure 17.1, which was obtained for respiratory symptoms.

X-RAY DENSITIES

Standard X-rays classically describe five radiographic densities (metallic, calcific/bone, soft tissue/water, fat, and air), yet the human eye can discern more than 200 shades of gray and the hardware/software of the imaging devices and displays can adjust brightness and contrast factors to optimize visualization of even more densities. For example, denser parts of the bone appear whiter than other parts of the bone even though both of these are "bone density." Similarly, densities combine to create intermediate densities, which is why lung parenchyma appears to be denser (whiter) than air but less dense (blacker) than the soft tissue of the chest wall. Structures reveal themselves when different X-ray densities overlie or are adjacent to each other. The trachea is visible over the spinous processes and mediastinum because it is filled with air. "Air bronchograms" occur because the underlying lung tissue has greater water content, such as in neonatal respiratory distress syndrome or pulmonary consolidation, as opposed to the fairly low water content of normal lung tissue.

OBTAINING A CHEST X-RAY

A CXR can be obtained in a cooperative older child in the usual adult manner, while standing with arms upright and inhaling and then holding their breath. The lungs must be fully inflated to confirm normality or disease as accurately as possible. Because infants cannot do this, most facilities utilize an adjustable restraining device to hold the chest and upper extremities pointing upward. This almost always results in a crying child, during which the X-ray technician must time the image acquisition when the child is maximally inhaling. This device will be unpopular with parents; thus, it is advisable to counsel parents

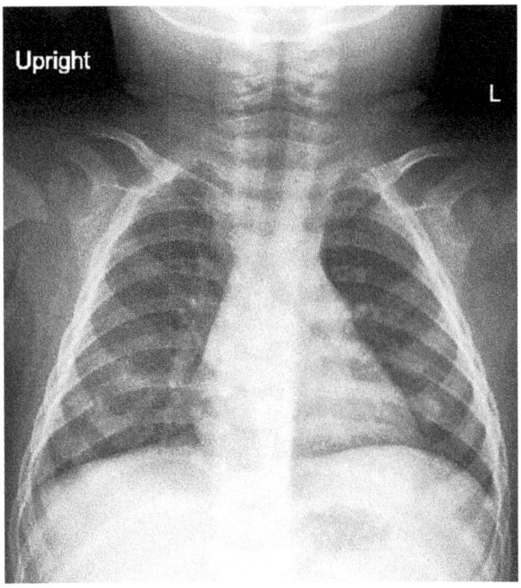

FIGURE 17.1 "Tunnel vision" focuses attention on the heart and lungs. Significant abnormalities can be missed in other parts of the CXR. In this case, examine ribs 4–6 on the right, which are fractured at the anterolateral region. Ribs 3 and 7 might be fractured as well. Rib 4 on the left is also fractured. Although these rib fractures are obvious upon inspection, it might be difficult to notice this if attention is focused on the heart and lungs.

Source: Copyright and courtesy of Paul Eakin, 2019.

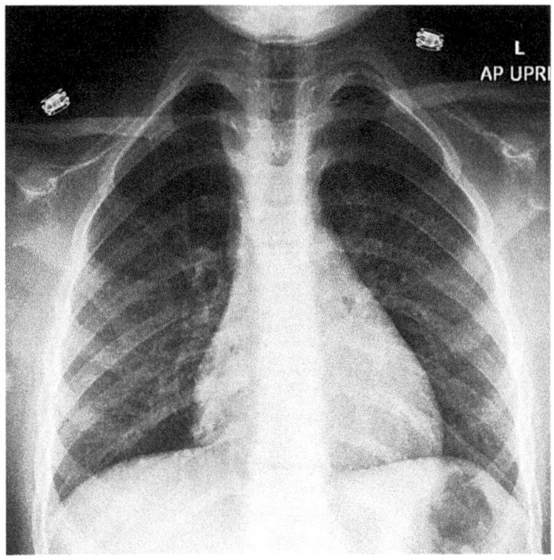

FIGURE 17.2 This is a CXR of of a 6-year-old taken from the AP direction. The pulmonary markings are slightly increased. The cardiac silhouette looks slightly larger than it should be, but this is a consequence of the AP view compared to the PA view, which typically has a smaller cardiac silhouette.

Source: Copyright Loren Yamamoto, 2019.

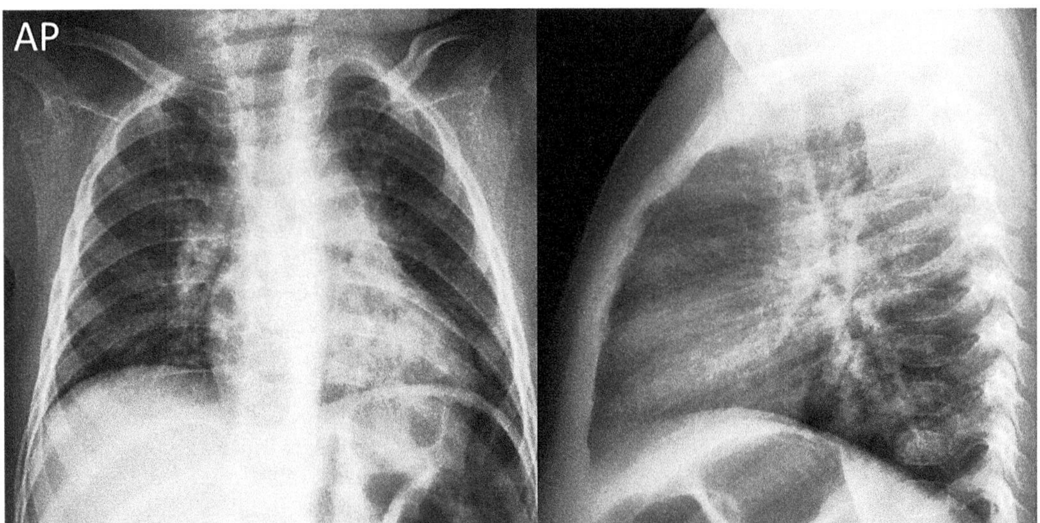

FIGURE 17.3 This is a CXR of a 13-month-old. There are patchy infiltrates. The AP view is rotated. Note that the medial ends of the clavicles are not symmetric about the vertebral column. Counting the posterior ribs, the diaphragm encounters the 9th posterior rib. It is preferable to have approximately 10 posterior ribs of lung expansion. The limited inspiration further accentuates the infiltrates. It also makes the cardiac silhouette appear larger than it is in reality. In addition, this is an AP view (rather than a PA view), which makes the cardiac silhouette appear larger. Thus, there are two factors associated with this AP view that make the cardiac silhouette appear to be larger than it is in reality. The lateral view should show the vertebral bodies becoming blacker as they proceed from T1 to T12. Note that in the lower portion of the lungs, the last full vertebral body visible above the diaphragm appears to be whiter than the vertebral body above it. This is due to an overlying infiltrate.

Source: Copyright Loren Yamamoto, 2019.

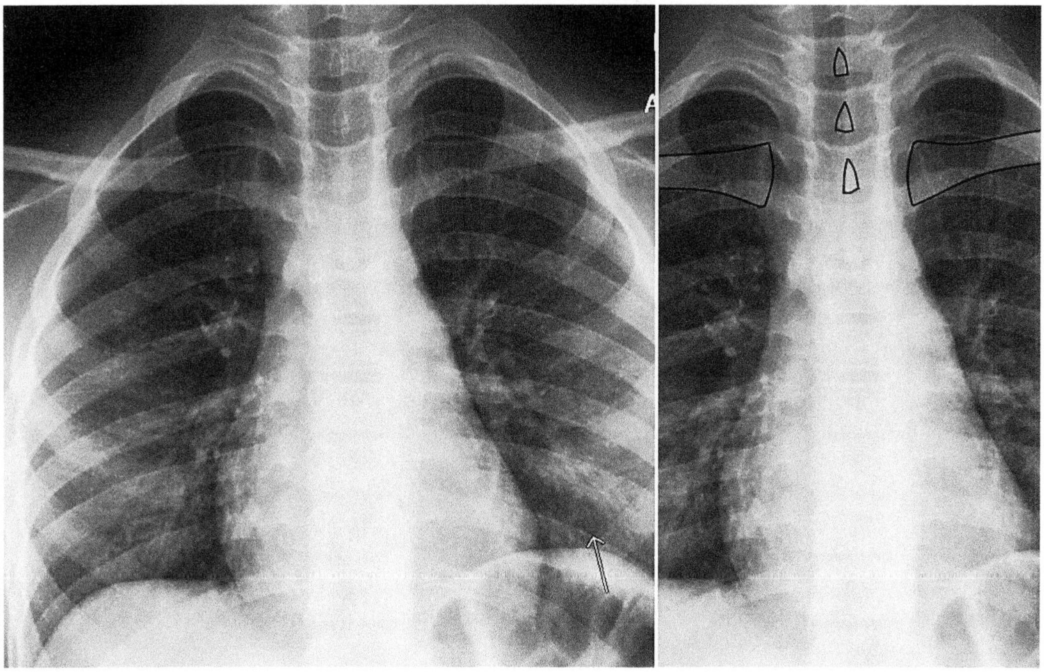

FIGURE 17.4 This is a CXR of a 7-year-old. The arrow points to a left lower lobe infiltrate. Examine the degree of rotation. The insert on the right outlines the clavicles and the spinous processes (triangles) as they overlie the vertebrae. Note that the medial ends of the clavicles are slightly asymmetric around the spine. The spinous process appears to be fairly symmetric within the vertebral bodies. The right border of the heart appears to be slightly prominent because of the slight degree of rotation.

Source: Copyright Loren Yamamoto, 2019.

about this device before they get to the X-ray department. Two views are obtained for most routine CXRs. The posterior–anterior (PA) view is obtained with the X-ray recording plate (or "film" in the past) anterior to the patient. The X-ray source is posterior to the patient. The X-rays travel from the patient's posterior to the patient's anterior, hence the term "PA" view. Because the X-ray beam is not perfectly parallel, structures farther from the X-ray recording plate appear relatively larger compared to structures closer to the X-ray recording plate. For this reason, it is often not highly accurate to measure structures on a CXR. For example, it is not possible to measure the diameter of an esophageal coin to identify the type of coin. It will frequently measure as a nickel but turns out to be a penny. For patients who are unstable or cannot be placed in a restraining device, a portable anterior–posterior (AP) CXR is obtained at the bedside, with the X-ray recording plate placed under the patient's back and the X-ray source anterior to the patient. The main difference between a PA and an AP CXR is that the heart looks larger on an AP

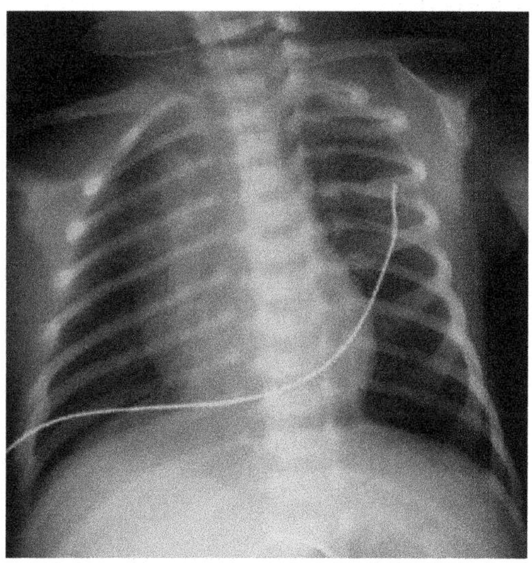

FIGURE 17.5 This is a CXR of a newborn. The view is very rotated, which makes the heart appear to be located on the right. However, this is simply due to rotational artifact. Note that the medial ends of the clavicles are not centered around the spine. Also, the vertebral bodies do not appear to be symmetric in appearance because the spine is rotated as well.

Source: Copyright Loren Yamamoto, 2019.

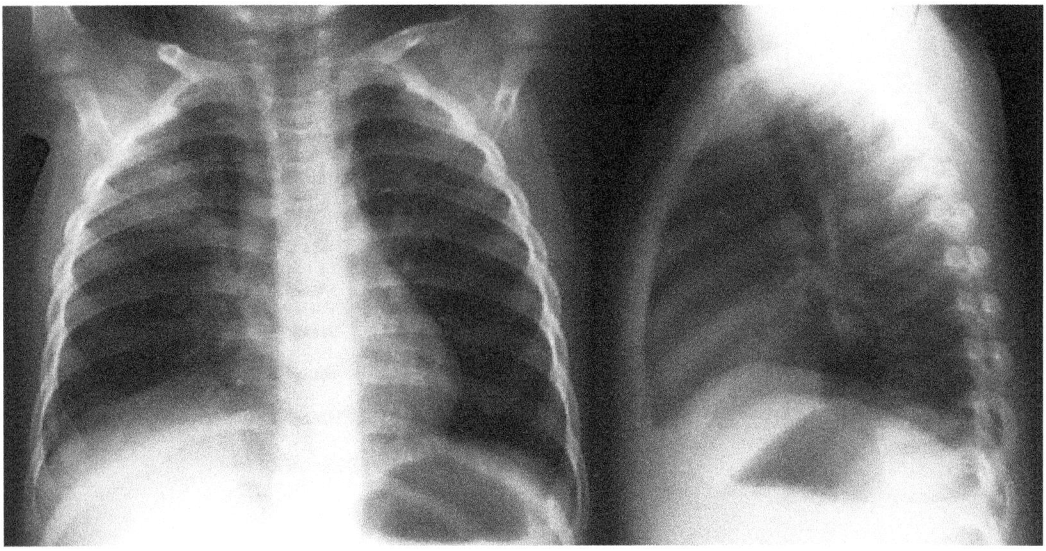

FIGURE 17.6 This is a CXR of a 15-month-old. There is a density in the right upper lobe. This is not due to the scapula because the other side does not have this appearance. This is a patchy area of consolidation in the posterior portion of the right upper lobe (pneumonia).

Source: Copyright Loren Yamamoto, https://www.hawaii.edu/medicine/pediatrics/pemxray/v4c05.html.

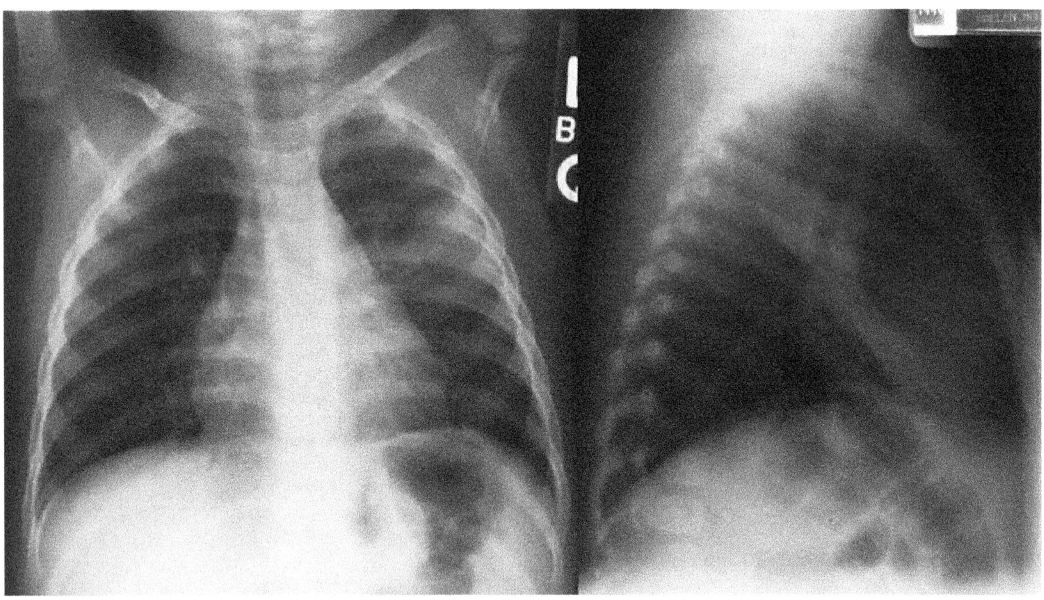

FIGURE 17.7 The PA view of this 14-month-old demonstrates haziness in the left upper lobe (pneumonia). The lateral view demonstrates a triangular density in the upper lung and a flat density positioned obliquely over the heart (atelectasis). The lower density over the heart is a consolidation of the lingula. Note that the PA view does not demonstrate any densities on the right in the area of the right middle lobe.

Source: Copyright Loren Yamamoto, https://www.hawaii.edu/medicine/pediatrics/pemxray/v4c05.html.

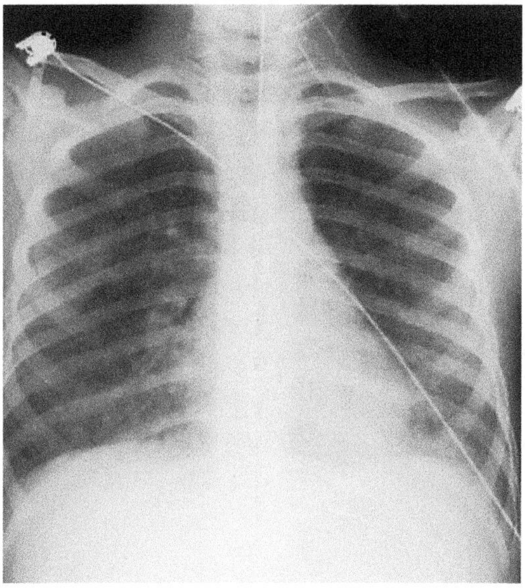

FIGURE 17.8 This is a CXR of an 11-month-old female who experienced a near-drowning episode in a bathtub resulting in pulmonary edema. In cardiogenic pulmonary edema, the cardiac silhouette is generally enlarged.

Source: Copyright Loren Yamamoto, https://www.hawaii.edu/medicine/pediatrics/pemxray/v5c15.html.

CXR because the heart is closer to the X-ray source and farther from the X-ray recording plate (Figure 17.2). A lateral view is obtained with most PA CXR views but not with portable CXRs. A cross-table lateral view can be obtained with a portable CXR, but usually it must be specifically requested. In the interpretation of the CXR, the clinician must know if the CXR was obtained PA or AP.

Ideally, the lungs should be expanded to include 10 posterior ribs. Less of an inspiratory effort will result in less air in the lungs and artifact widening (enlarging) of the cardiac silhouette (Figure 17.3). Detection of infiltrates and atelectasis is maximized when the normal lung tissue contains as much air as possible.

The CXR can sometimes be rotated slightly because it is not always possible to obtain a perfectly PA or AP view (Figures 17.3–17.5). Rotated CXRs will expose more or less of the right or left hilum, giving it the appearance of an infiltrate. The left lateral boarder of the heart could give the appearance of cardiomegaly if it is displaced laterally due to the rotation. The degree of rotation can be determined

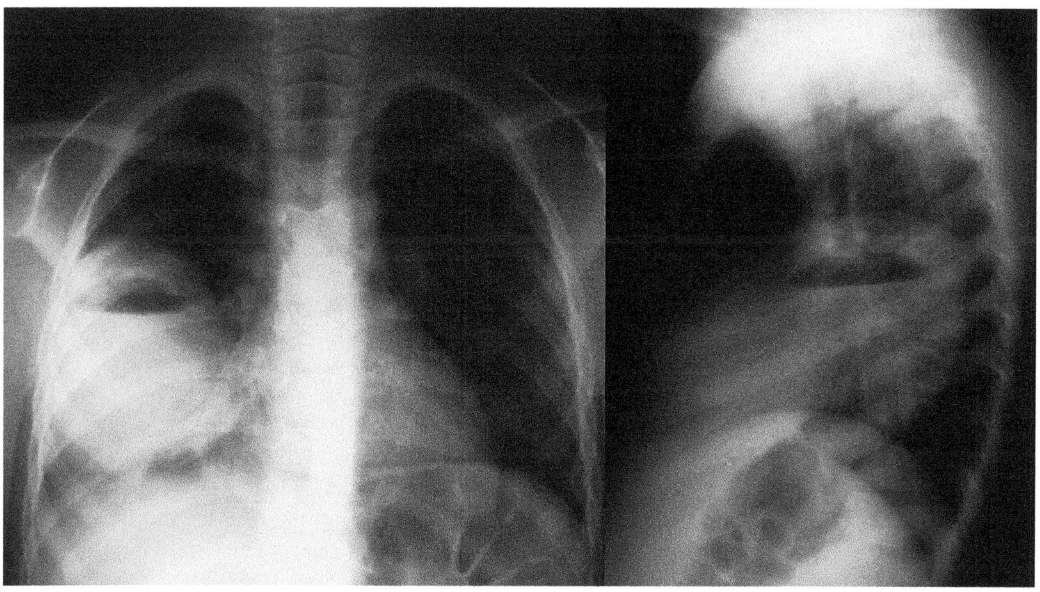

FIGURE 17.9 This is a CXR of a 5-year-old. The PA view shows a right-sided circular density with an air-fluid level. The lateral view shows the same mass with an air-fluid level. A CT scan confirmed this to be a thick-walled abscess. Culture grew nontypable *Haemophilus influenza.*

Source: Copyright Loren Yamamoto, https://www.hawaii.edu/medicine/pediatrics/pemxray/v7c03.html.

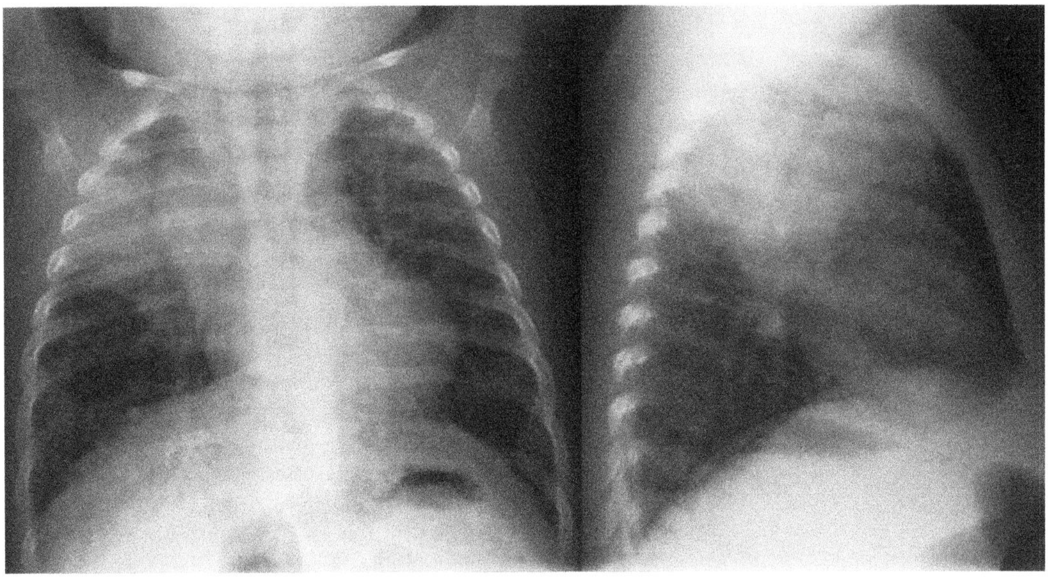

FIGURE 17.10 This is a CXR of a 7-month-old with military tuberculosis. There are multiple small nodules throughout the lungs bilaterally. There is a focal consolidation in the right upper lobe.

Source: Copyright Loren Yamamoto, https://www.hawaii.edu/medicine/pediatrics/pemxray/v4c06.html.

by examining the clavicles and the symmetry of the vertebrae. The medial ends of the clavicles should be symmetric about the spine. The spinous processes should be centered within the vertebrae.

RADIATION EXPOSURE

Parents will frequently ask if the radiation exposure from a CXR is dangerous. It is preferable to avoid all radiation exposure, but in general, the radiation exposure from a CXR is small—approximately 0.02–0.1 mSv. Compare this to the radiation exposure during a flight from New York to London at 0.05–0.1 mSv. Using the low end of the radiation exposure range, parents can be told that radiation exposure from taking their child on a round-trip transatlantic (or transcontinental) flight is the equivalent of the child receiving approximately three or four CXRs.

PATHOLOGY VISIBLE ON CHEST X-RAY

In conjunction with clinical history and examination findings, examine the lungs for radiographic evidence of pneumonia (Figure 17.6), atelectasis (Figure 17.7), pulmonary edema (Figure 17.8), lung abscess (Figure 17.9), tuberculosis (Figure 17.10), pleural effusion/empyema (Figure 17.11), bronchial foreign bodies (Figure 17.12), lobar emphysema (Figure 17.13), pneumothorax (Figure 17.14), respiratory distress syndrome (of prematurity) (Figure 17.15), pulmonary interstitial emphysema (Figure

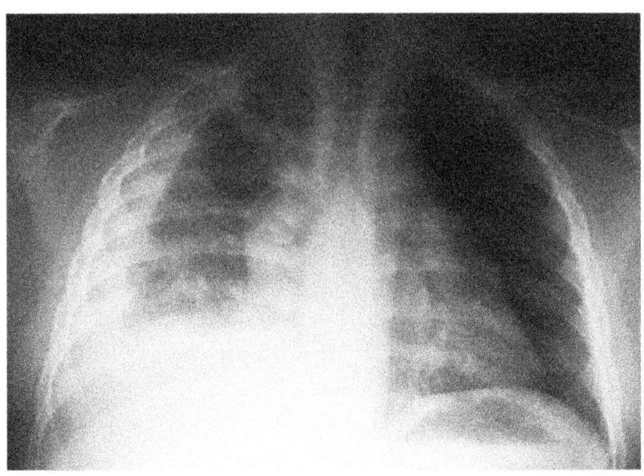

FIGURE 17.11 This is a CXR of a 6-year-old presenting with tachypnea and abdominal pain. A computed tomography scan of the abdomen showed right-sided infiltrates and a small pleural effusion in the upper abdomen (lower chest). Due to worsening clinical status, this CXR was performed a few hours after the CT scan. This CXR now shows a large right-sided pleural effusion that turned out to be an empyema associated with a *Staphylococcus aureus* pneumonia.

Source: Copyright Loren Yamamoto, https://www.hawaii.edu/medicine/pediatrics/pemxray/v2c05.html.

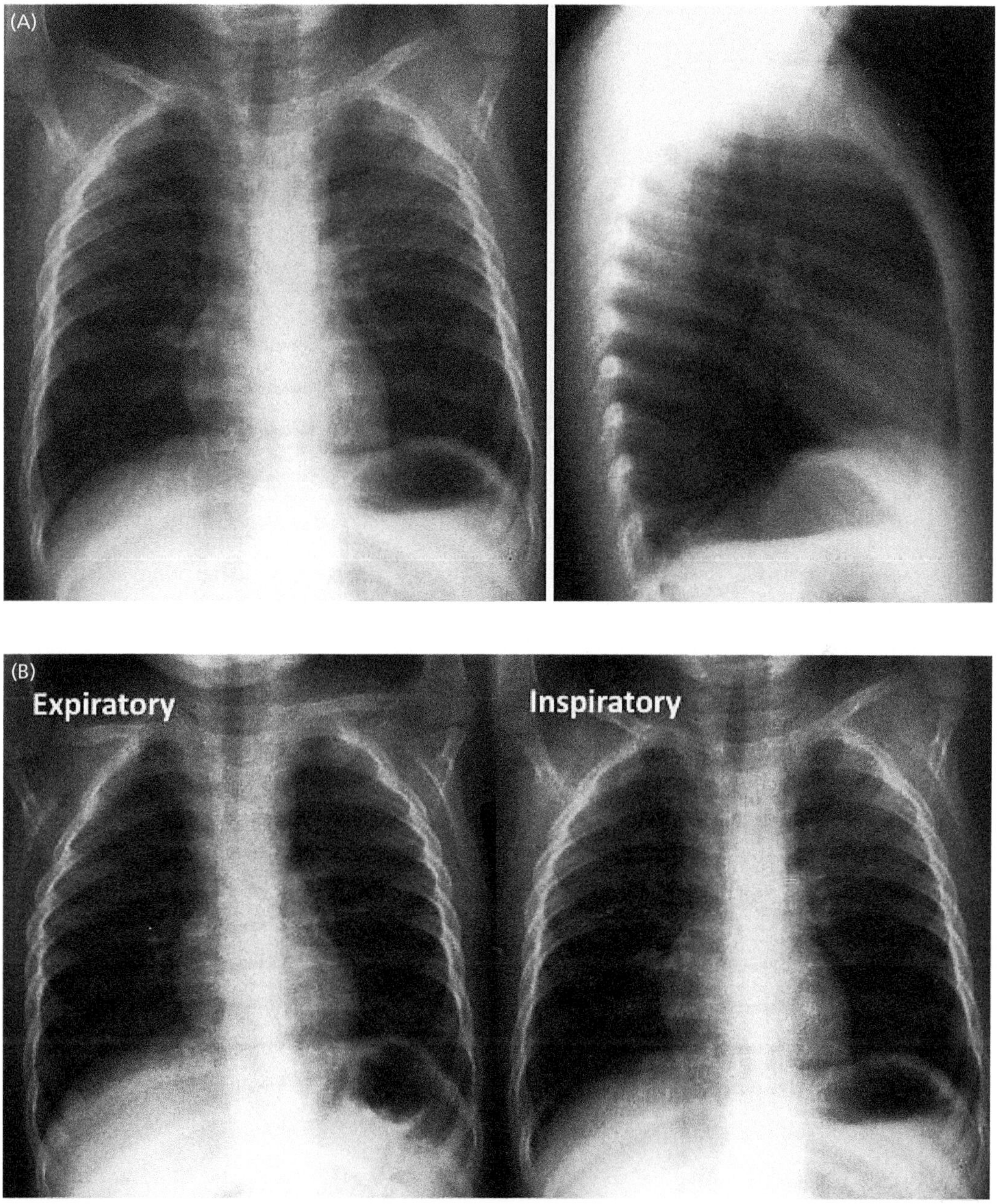

FIGURE 17.12 (A) This is a CXR of a 17-month-old who presented with noisy and abnormal breathing after choking on a chocolate and almond candy bar.

(B) An expiratory view on the left looks almost the same as the inspiratory view. This suggests that there is bilateral air trapping preventing both lungs from deflating during exhalation. This could also occur from poor timing by the X-ray technician. In other words, the "expiratory" view could have been taken during inspiration.

(C) Bilateral decubitus views were obtained on this patient which demonstrate that the dependent side does not compress, indicating that air trapping is present on the dependent side. These views are highly suggestive of bilateral bronchial foreign bodies with air trapping.

Source: Copyright Loren Yamamoto, https://www.hawaii.edu/medicine/pediatrics/pemxray/v1c08.html.

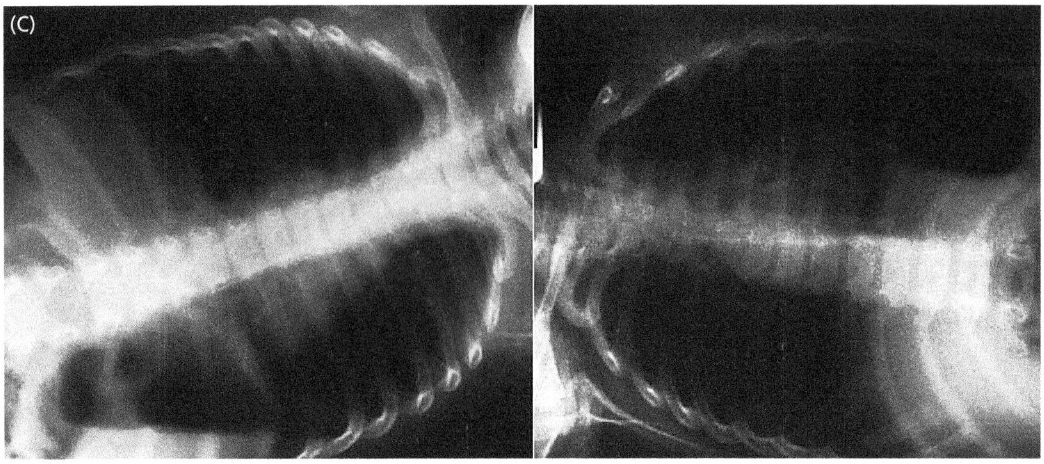

FIGURE 17.12 Continued

17.16), chronic lung disease (Figure 17.17), diaphragmatic hernia (Figure 17.18), pulmonary perfusion, and congenital pulmonary vascular anomalies (Figure 17.19). If clinically suspected, a small pneumothorax can be difficult to identify. Obtaining an expiratory view increases the radiographic density of the lungs so that the sliver of pleural air can be more visible (see Figure 17.14). Bedside ultrasound is more effective at identifying small pneumothoraces; however, a CXR is still useful to determine the size of the pneumothorax. If clinically suspected, a bronchial foreign body can cause bilateral or unilateral air trapping that can be difficult to see on an inspiratory CXR. Obtaining an expiratory view or lateral

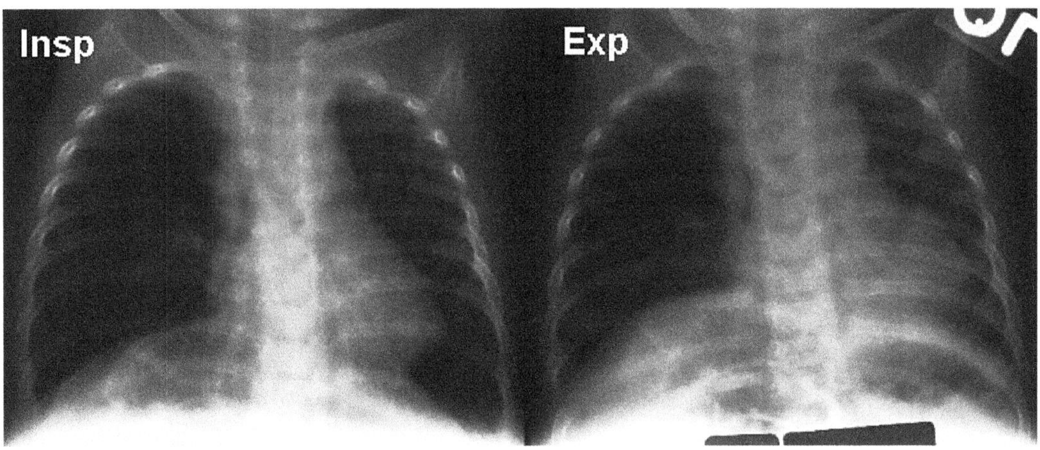

FIGURE 17.13 Posterior–anterior inspiratory and expiratory views of a 4-month-old are shown. The inspiratory view demonstrates hyperexpansion of the right hemithorax. The right hemithorax is blacker than the left. The right hemithorax is also larger than it should be. Lung markings are evident throughout both lungs, making this incompatible with a pneumothorax. The expiratory view shows satisfactory emptying of the left lung but persistent hyperexpansion of the right lung. The diagnosis of foreign body is considered, but the typical age group for a bronchial foreign body is 2 years or older. This child's past history is significant for complaints of abnormal breathing. Closer examination of the radiographs on the right shows a density in the upper medial hemithorax (small density compressed against the upper mediastinum). This is probably a compressed right upper lobe. An obstruction in the intermediate right bronchus is suspected. This child was ultimately found to have a congenital lobar emphysema of the right middle lobe.

Source: Copyright Loren Yamamoto, https://www.hawaii.edu/medicine/pediatrics/pemxray/v4c05.html.

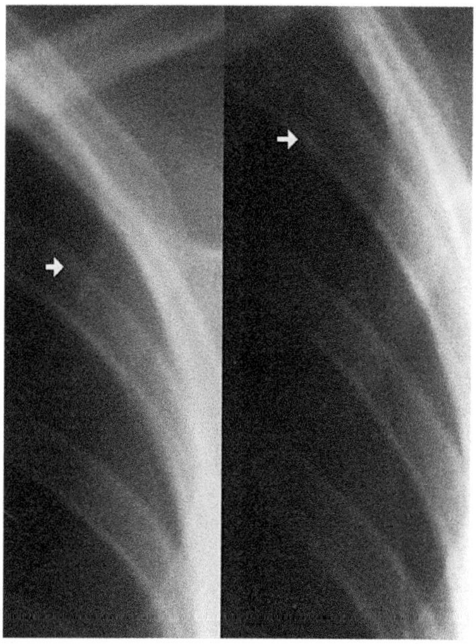

FIGURE 17.14 This is a CXR of a 15-year-old presenting with chest pain after lifting his mother. This is a focused view of the left upper thorax. The arrows point to the edge of the lung. The image on the left is the inspiratory view. The image on the right is an expiratory view. The pneumothorax is small. It was difficult to view. With an expiratory view, the lung compresses and appears to be denser while the pneumothorax remains lucent, such that the lung and the pneumothorax are easier to identify.

Source: Copyright Loren Yamamoto, https://www.hawaii.edu/medicine/pediatrics/pemxray/v3c13.html.

decubitus views can better confirm air trapping because air trapping will prevent the lung from deflating; an expiratory view will resemble an inspiratory view (see Figure 17.12B), or the lateral decubitus view will fail to show the heart moving downward with gravity compressing the affected lung (see Figure 17.12C). The lateral view of the CXR shows portions of the lung that are behind the heart and difficult to assess. The lung tissue overlying the vertebral bodies should become more lucent (blacker) proceeding inferiorly. Figure 17.20 shows a CXR in which this is not the case.

In conjunction with clinical history and examination findings, examine the heart for radiographic evidence of cardiomegaly (Figure 17.21), congestive heart failure (Figure 17.22), congenital heart disease (Figure 17.23), myocarditis (Figures 17.24 and 17.25), pericarditis (no example shown, but will resemble cardiomegaly), and pneumopericardium

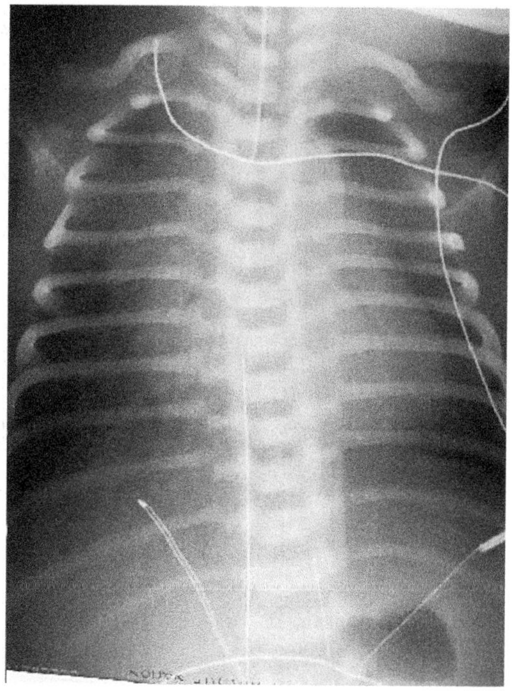

FIGURE 17.15 This is a CXR of a premature neonate showing the ground glass appearance of the lungs in neonatal respiratory distress syndrome. An endotracheal tube is in place. Electrocardiogram monitoring and temperature probe wires are visible. Umbilical arterial and venous lines are visible on the CXR.

Source: Copyright Loren Yamamoto, https://www.hawaii.edu/medicine/pediatrics/neoxray/neoxray.html.

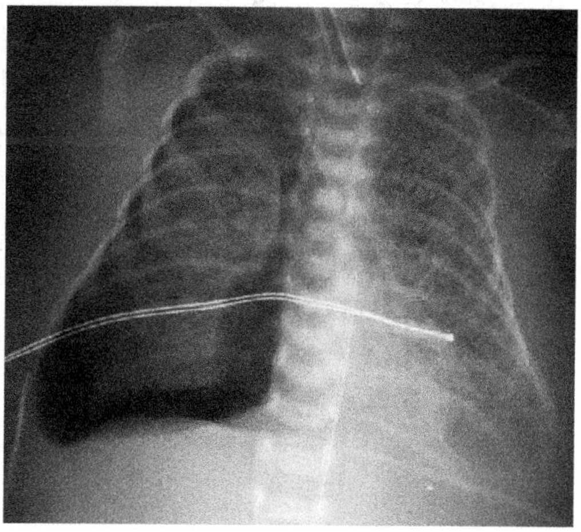

FIGURE 17.16 This is a CXR of a premature infant with neonatal respiratory distress syndrome. The CXR shows the development of pulmonary interstitial emphysema in which air dissects through the lung parenchyma, which is sometimes a precursor to a pneumothorax, as has occurred on the right.

Source: Copyright Loren Yamamoto, https://www.hawaii.edu/medicine/pediatrics/neoxray/neoxray.html.

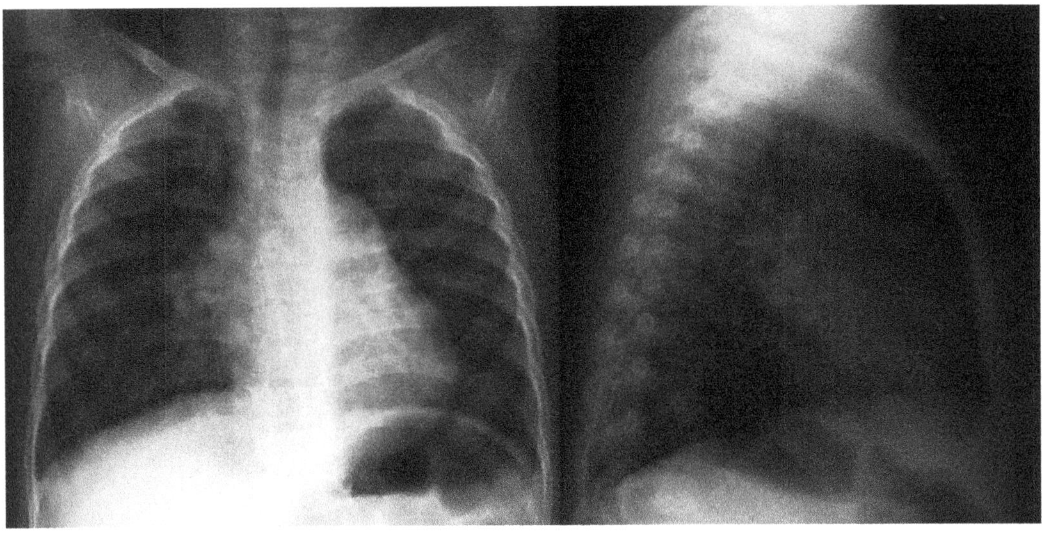

FIGURE 17.17 This is a CXR of a 14-month-old with a history of prematurity and chronic lung disease. The pulmonary outflow tract is prominent. The central markings are accentuated and fluffy, more so on the right. This is evident on the PA view. However, the lateral view also demonstrates increased markings and fluffiness around the hilum. These findings are consistent with chronic lung disease and possibly suggestive of pulmonary hypertension.

Source: Copyright Loren Yamamoto, https://www.hawaii.edu/medicine/pediatrics/pemxray/v4c05.html.

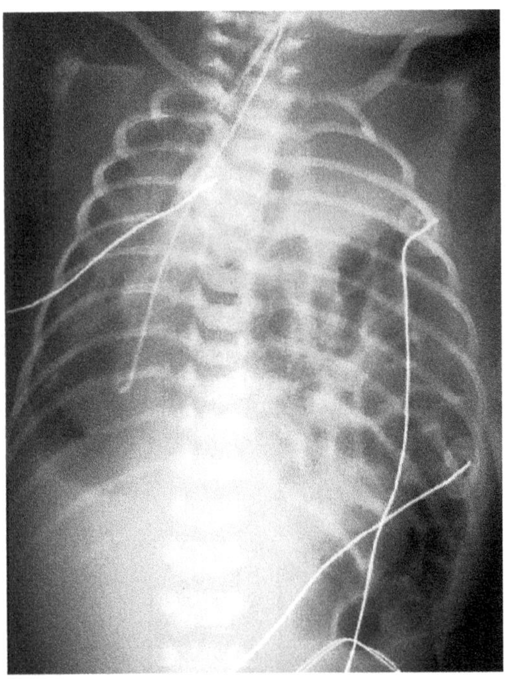

FIGURE 17.18 Bowel contents have herniated into the left hemithorax through a diaphragmatic hernia. The bowel has compressed the left lung and displaced the mediastinum to the right, compressing the right lung as well.

Source: Copyright Loren Yamamoto, https://www.hawaii.edu/medicine/pediatrics/neoxray/neoxray.html.

(Figure 17.26). The cardiac silhouette could be enlarged due to causes of artifact, including a suboptimal inspiration or an AP view (instead of a PA view). If the cardiac silhouette is truly enlarged, this could represent a pericardial effusion or congestive heart failure. A pericardial effusion can be confirmed on a bedside ultrasound. Congestive heart failure can be confirmed by echocardiographic measures of contractility, chamber sizes, and valvular function. Serum chemistry markers of congestive heart failure can confirm this as well.

Examine the aorta for radiographic evidence of aortic dissection and aortic arch direction. An aortic dissection can only be identified or ruled out with a vascular study of the aorta. Computed tomography aortography is commonly employed. In many patients with an aortic dissection, the mediastinum in the area of the aortic arch might appear to be widened (Figure 17.27). In nearly everyone, the aortic arch courses over the left main stem bronchus (a left-sided aortic arch). This causes the distal trachea to bend very slightly to the right (Figure 17.28). This might be difficult to notice in most patients. In rare instances, the patient has a vascular ring associated with a right-sided aortic arch (Figure 17.29) or a double aortic arch (Figure 17.30). It might

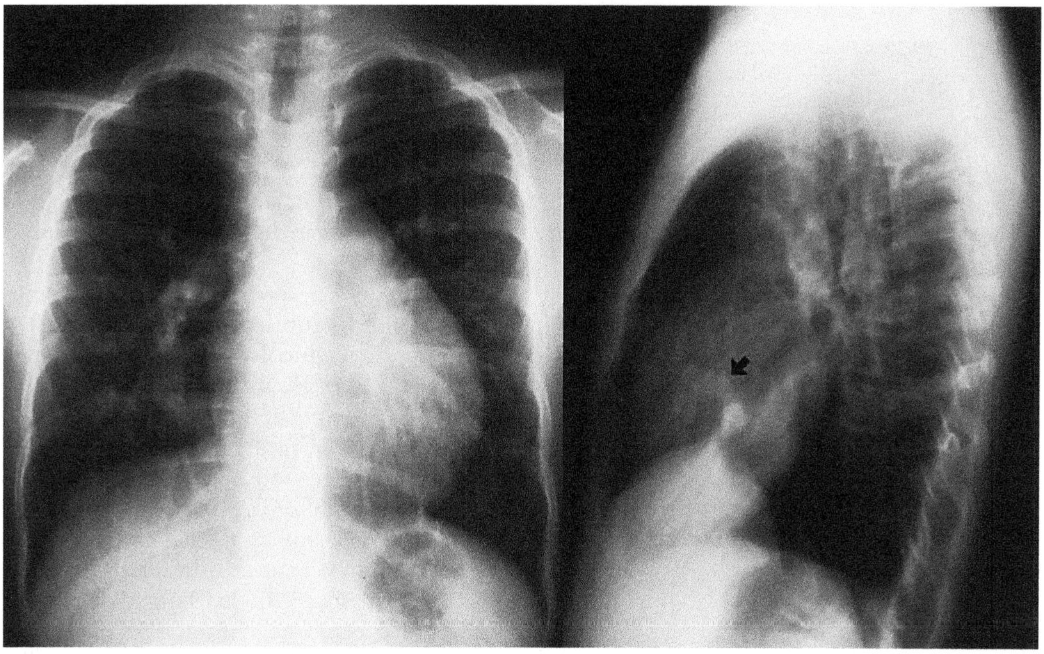

FIGURE 17.19 This is a CXR of an 11-year-old who presents with hemoptysis. She has a history of frequent respiratory infections and poor weight gain. This CXR demonstrates slight cardiomegaly. The right lung is smaller than the left lung. The lateral view shows an odd shape of the diaphragm and a curvilinear density (arrow), which might be a "scimitar" of Scimitar syndrome. Further evaluation of this patient confirms a hypoplastic right lung, an atrial septal defect, and an anomalous blood supply of the right lower lung coming from the aorta instead of the pulmonary artery and draining into a systemic vein instead of a pulmonary vein. Other syndromes of pulmonary vascular anomalies include pulmonary sequestration and venolobar syndrome.

Source: Copyright Loren Yamamoto, https://www.hawaii.edu/medicine/pediatrics/pemxray/v5c13.html.

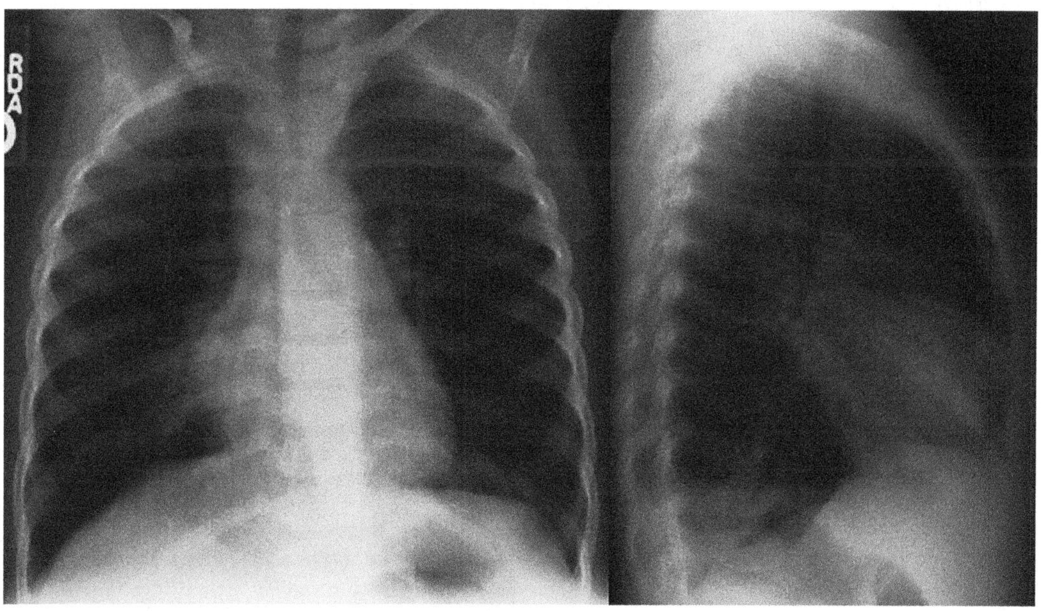

FIGURE 17.20 This is a CXR of a 15-month-old with fever, coughing, and tachypnea. The lateral view shows the increasing lucency of the vertebral bodies proceeding inferiorly, except at the bottom, where the vertebral bodies appear whiter because of overlying infiltrates.

Source: Copyright Loren Yamamoto, https://www.hawaii.edu/medicine/pediatrics/pemxray/v3c20.html.

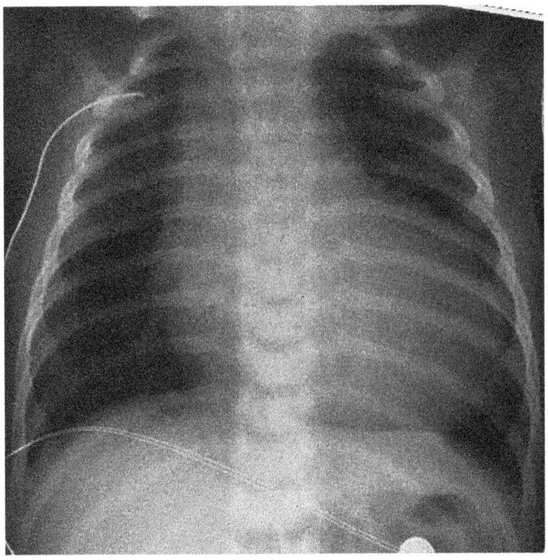

FIGURE 17.21 This is a CXR of a 7-week-old presenting with wheezing, coughing, and vomiting. Cardiomegaly is evident. Coarctation of the aorta was confirmed on further investigation.

Source: Copyright Loren Yamamoto, https://www.hawaii.edu/medicine/pediatrics/pemxray/v2c06.html.

be possible to note that the distal trachea bends very slightly to the left. In conjunction with clinical findings of dysphagia or airway symptoms, this radiographic finding might be indicative of a right-sided aortic arch and a vascular ring, or the tracheal air shadow might be narrower due to extrinsic compression (Figure 17.31).

Examine the mediastinum for thymus enlargement (Figures 17.32 and 17.33), thymic absence (Figure 17.34), mediastinal mass (Figure 17.35), right ventricular enlargement (Figure 17.36), pneumomediastinum (Figure 17.37), and esophageal coins (Figure 17.38). In older children and adults, the thymus is largely not visible. The PA/AP view shows a configuration similar to that of adults. The lateral view shows lung tissue in the anterior mediastinum space. If this lung tissue is not visible, this could be indicative of a mediastinal mass or right ventricular enlargement. The thymus is large in newborns. On the PA/AP view, the mediastinum can be very large

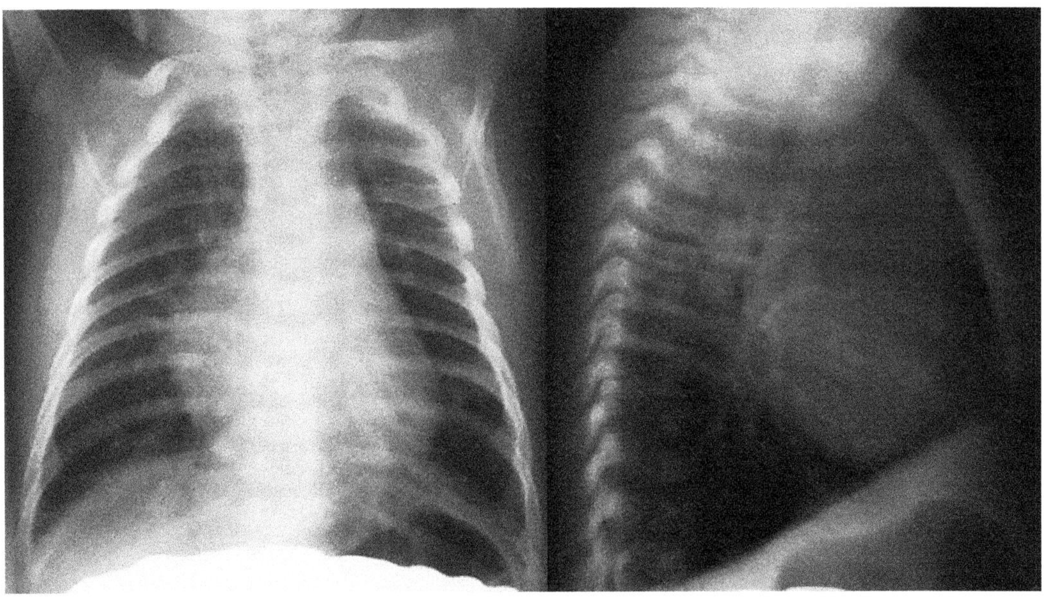

FIGURE 17.22 This is a CXR of a 2-month-old presenting with noisy, rapid breathing and confirmed wheezing. The CXR shows slight cardiomegaly with increased lung markings. In conjunction with cardiomegaly, this is more likely to be pulmonary vascular congestion rather than infiltrates. Echocardiogram confirmed congestive heart failure with an atrial septal defect, a membranous structure within the left atrium (functionally three atrial chambers, known as cor triatriatum), right atrial enlargement, and right ventricular dilation.

Source: Copyright Loren Yamamoto, https://www.hawaii.edu/medicine/pediatrics/pemxray/v4c03.html.

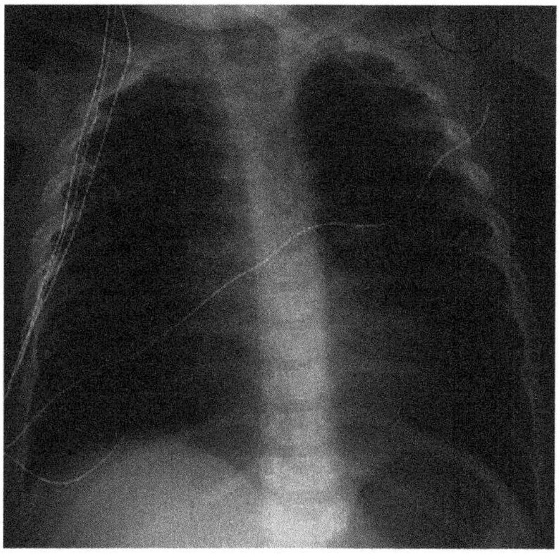

FIGURE 17.23 This is a CXR of a 16-month-old with respiratory symptoms and wheezing on examination. His oxygen saturation is noted to be 78% in room air. He is placed on oxygen, and his oxygen saturation decreased to the 50% range when crying, returning to the 70% range when more calm. The CXR shows cardiomegaly. This is not very obvious at first because the CXR is rotated so that much of the heart appears to be in the right hemithorax. If the CXR is more centered, the apex of the heart would be far to the left. It is actually "boot-shaped." The lungs appear blacker than they should be. Although this could be due to exposure artifact and contrast/brightness adjustment, in conjunction with hypoxemia that does not respond to oxygen, the hyperlucent lungs are more likely to be due to pulmonary vascular hypoperfusion. Further evaluation confirmed that this patient had a previously undiagnosed tetralogy of Fallot (right ventricular hypertrophy, pulmonic stenosis, ventricular septal defect, and aortic override). The boot-shaped heart occurs because the left atrium is smaller than it should be due to the pulmonic stenosis and poor filling of the left atrium from the pulmonary veins in conjunction with the right ventricular hypertrophy.

Source: Copyright Loren Yamamoto, https://www.hawaii.edu/medicine/pediatrics/pemxray/v2c03.html.

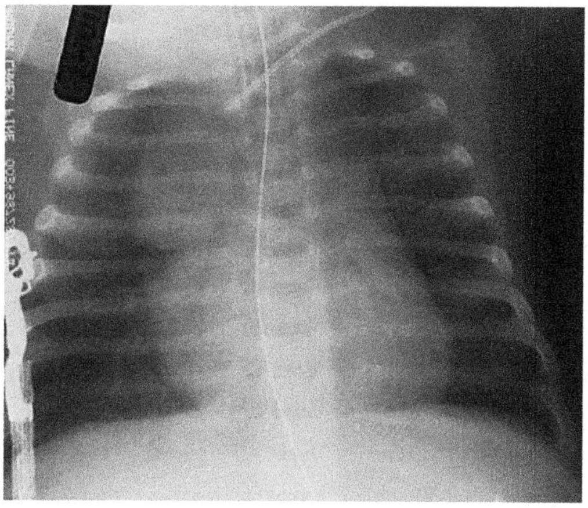

FIGURE 17.24 This is a CXR of a 2-month-old presenting to the emergency department in cardiac arrest. He has a history of a conjunctival injection and chapped lips. There is no history of rash. He developed a slight fever on the day of presentation. This CXR, which was obtained following intubation, shows cardiomegaly and a slight increase in the central pulmonary markings. Because this is an AP CXR and there is ongoing cardiac arrest and chest compressions, the cardiomegaly could be an artifact of these factors. However, on autopsy, the cardiac findings demonstrated myocarditis due to Kawasaki disease.

Source: Copyright Loren Yamamoto, https://www.hawaii.edu/medicine/pediatrics/pemxray/v3c01.html.

because of a normal thymus. The lateral view should show soft tissue and not lung tissue in the anterior mediastinum. Thymic aplasia in a newborn lacks the normal large thymic presence. Pneumomediastinum typically shows air densities around the trachea, subcutaneous emphysema in the soft tissue of the neck, and vertical air densities in the mediastinum.

Examine the bones for clavicle fractures, rib fractures (see Figure 17.1), cervical spine fractures, thoracic spine fractures (Figure 17.39), discitis (Figure 17.40), osteopenia, osteomalacia, and osteogenesis imperfecta (Figure 17.41).

Examine the abdomen and the neck. Although this might not be the clinical reason for obtaining the CXR, pathology in these areas could be serious. For example, hepatomegaly, splenomegaly, air under the diaphragm, a foreign body in the neck, subcutaneous air in the neck, or a vertebral anomaly could be visible on the CXR.

CXRs are often obtained for the placement of indwelling devices such as endotracheal tubes and vascular access lines. If placement is suboptimal, adjust the position of the device and either document this in the patient's chart

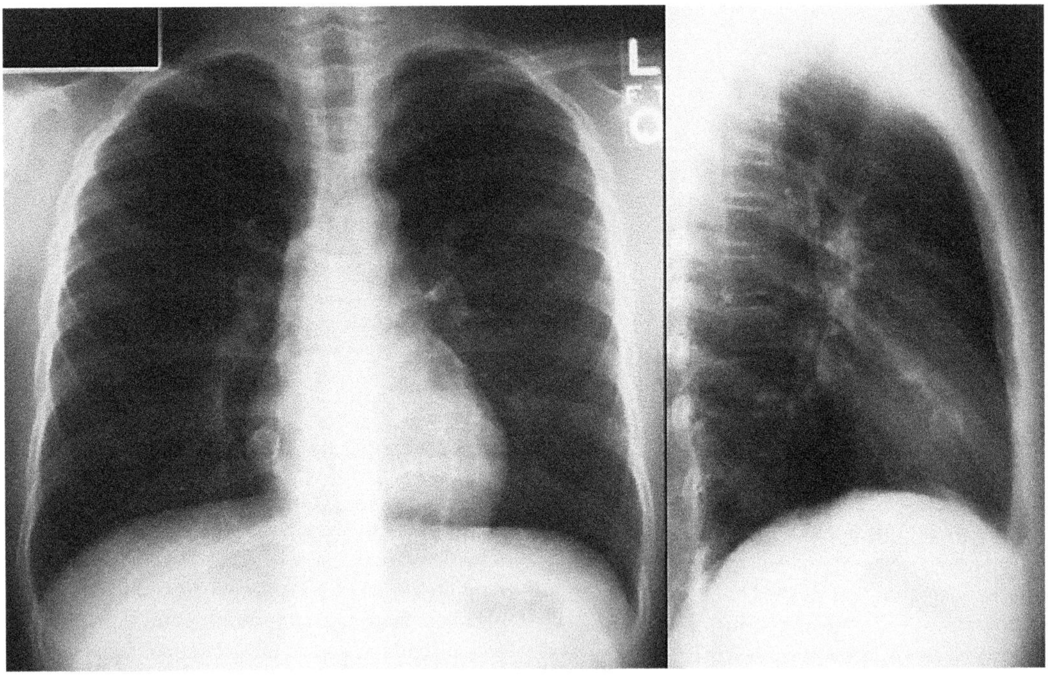

FIGURE 17.25 This is a CXR of a 12-year-old visiting from Asia presenting with respiratory symptoms suggestive of possible pneumonia. The CXR shows no infiltrates; however, spherical calcifications are noted over his heart, especially on the lateral view. This patient had untreated Kawasaki disease and secondary coronary aneurysms that have calcified.

Source: Copyright Loren Yamamoto, https://www.hawaii.edu/medicine/pediatrics/pemxray/v4c04.html.

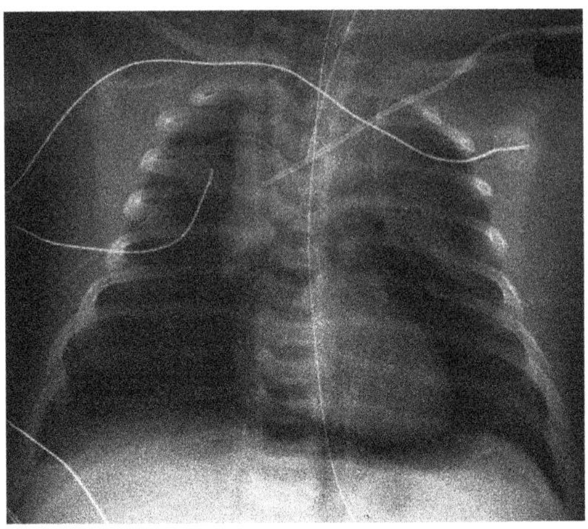

FIGURE 17.26 This is a CXR of a 5-week-old in the intensive care unit who develops acute deterioration thought to be due to a tension pneumothorax. The CXR shows a visible lucency surrounding the heart and accentuation of the inferior margins of the thymus (bilateral sail signs) due to a pneumopericardium.

Source: Copyright Loren Yamamoto, https://www.hawaii.edu/medicine/pediatrics/pemxray/v3c20.html.

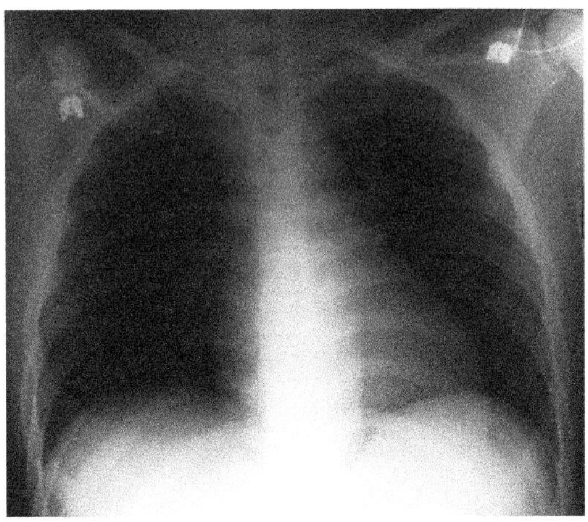

FIGURE 17.27 This is a CXR of a 14-year-old presenting with severe back and abdominal pain radiating into his throat that he describes as "pressure" pain. There is a family history of aortic dissection in a sibling. This CXR is suspicious for widening of the aortic shadow. The distal trachea is excessively deviated to the right. Computed tomography aortography confirmed an aortic dissection.

Source: Copyright Loren Yamamoto, https://www.hawaii.edu/medicine/pediatrics/pemxray/v3c12.html.

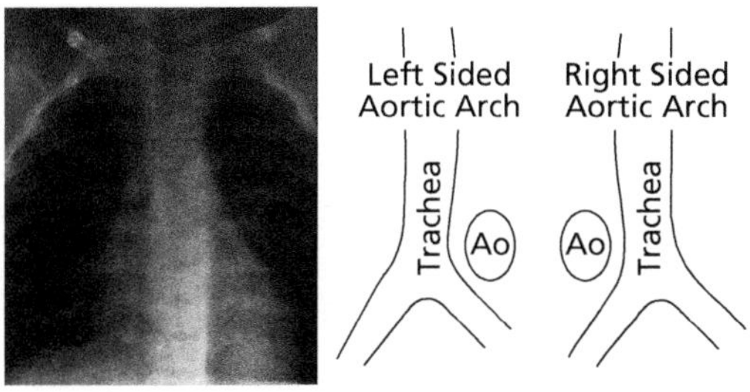

FIGURE 17.28 The CXR shows the distal tracheal bending slightly to the right. This is typically the normal configuration seen with a left-sided aortic arch [the aorta (Ao) courses over the left main stem bronchus]. If the trachea bends toward the left, this could indicate the presence of a right-sided aortic arch.

Source: Copyright Loren Yamamoto, https://www.hawaii.edu/medicine/pediatrics/pemxray/v4c05.html and https://www.hawaii.edu/medicine/pediatrics/pemxray/v6c19.html.

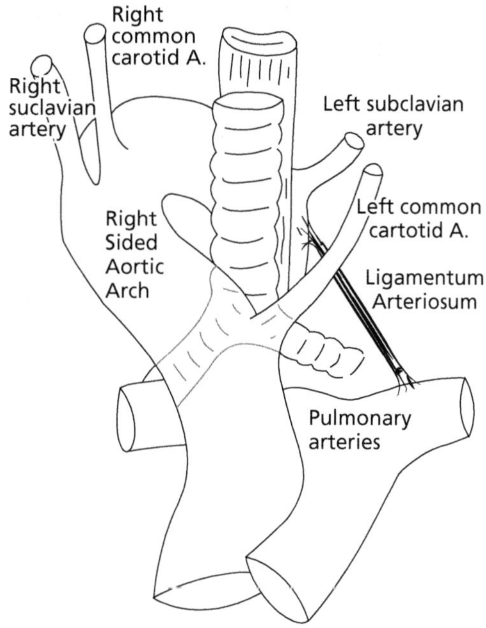

FIGURE 17.29 This is a vascular ring with a right-sided aortic arch. The "ring" around the esophagus and trachea is completed with the ligmentum arteriosum. This type of vascular ring might be visible on CXR if the distal trachea bends to the left.

Source: Copyright Loren Yamamoto, https://www.hawaii.edu/medicine/pediatrics/pemxray/v6c19.html.

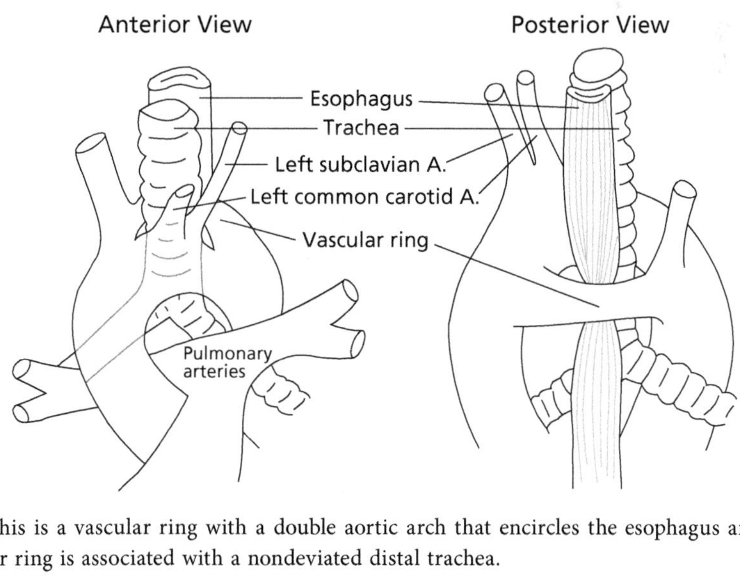

FIGURE 17.30 This is a vascular ring with a double aortic arch that encircles the esophagus and trachea. This type of vascular ring is associated with a nondeviated distal trachea.

Source: Copyright Loren Yamamoto, https://www.hawaii.edu/medicine/pediatrics/pemxray/v6c19.html.

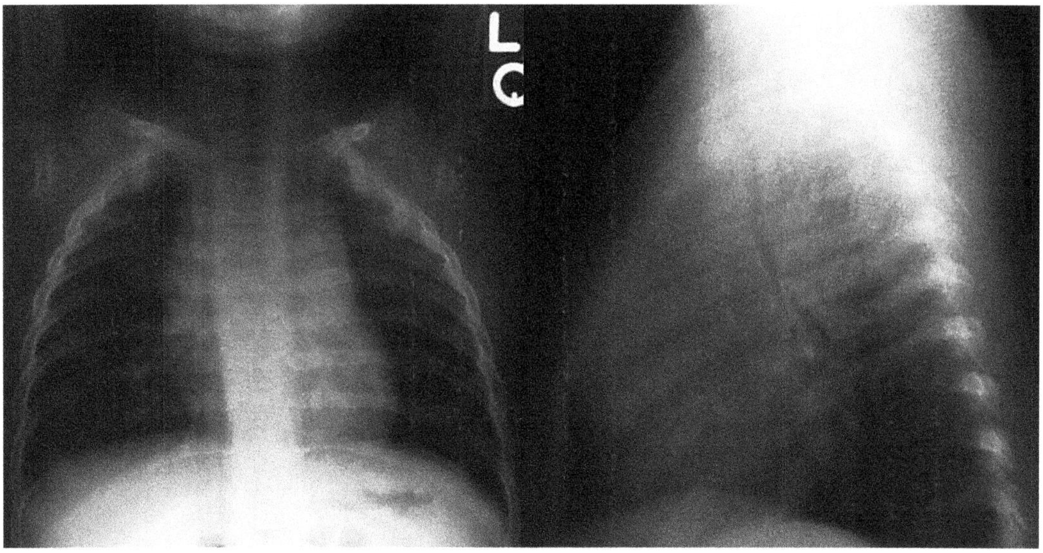

FIGURE 17.31 This is a CXR of a 6-month-old with several episodes of wheezing and difficulty breathing. His lungs appear to be clear. His distal trachea is not deviated. The lateral view shows this tracheal air column, which is very thin and perhaps deviated, suggesting that it is being compressed. An esophagram demonstrates extrinsic compression of the esophagus. An echocardiogram confirms a vascular ring.

Source: Copyright Loren Yamamoto, https://www.hawaii.edu/medicine/pediatrics/pemxray/v6c19.html.

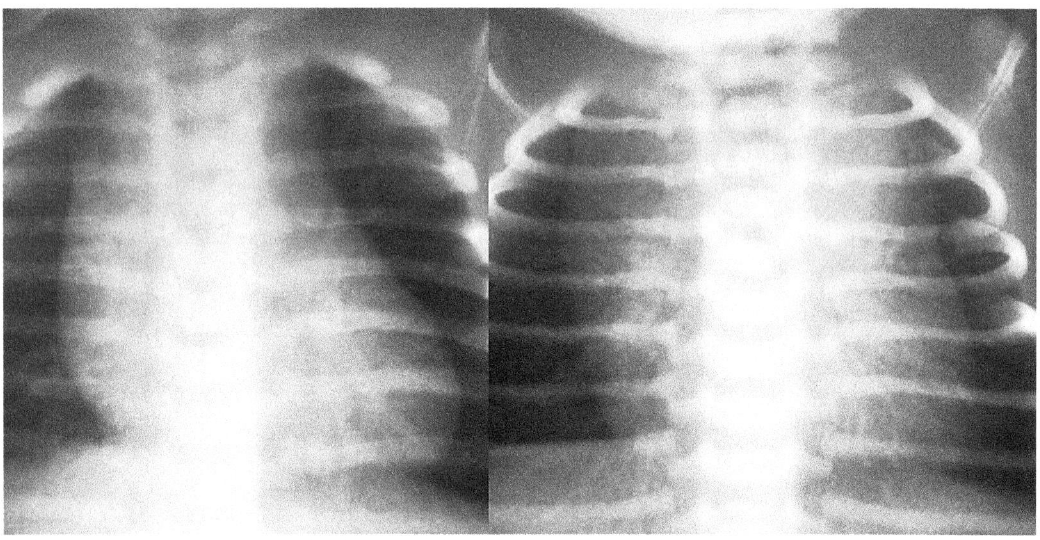

FIGURE 17.32 Both of these CXRs are from newborns. The left image shows moderate widening of the mediastinum due to the normally enlarged thymus of newborns. The right image shows a larger thymus, but this is still normal for newborns.

Source: Copyright Loren Yamamoto, https://www.hawaii.edu/medicine/pediatrics/pemxray/v2c02.html.

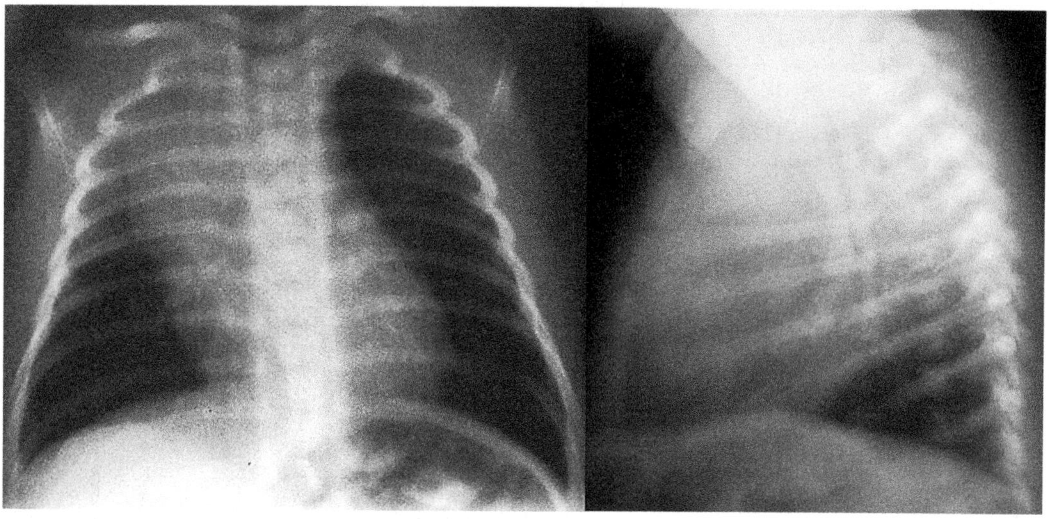

FIGURE 17.33 This is CXR of a 6-week-old. The normal thymus can be asymmetric as in this CXR. Rotation exaggerates this asymmetry. In this case, the right thymus partially obscures the right upper lobe infiltrate. Note that the right upper lobe lung tissue adjacent to the thymus is clearly denser than the lung tissue inferior to it.

Source: Copyright Loren Yamamoto, https://www.hawaii.edu/medicine/pediatrics/pemxray/v3c20.html.

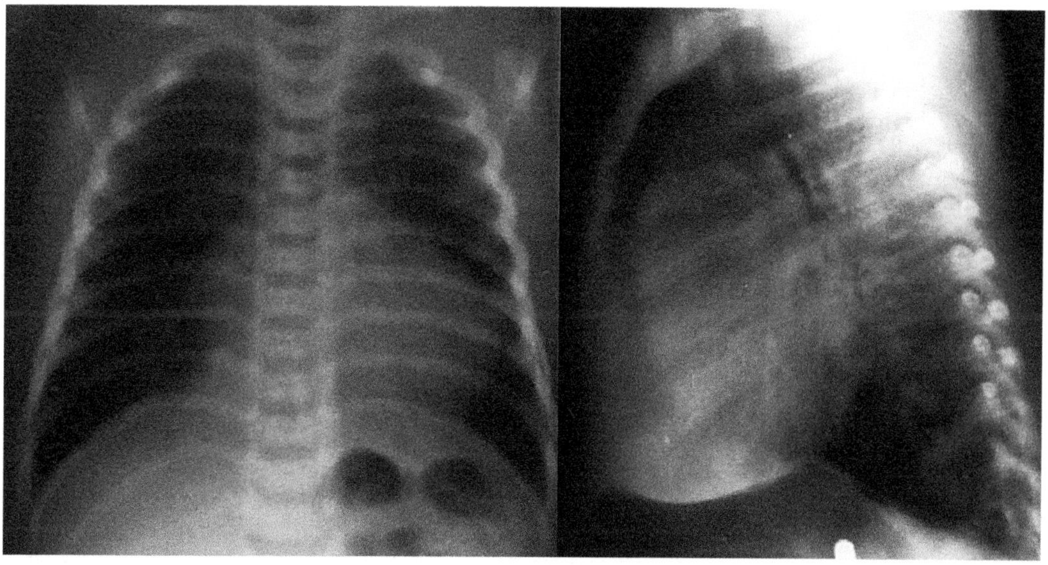

FIGURE 17.34 This is a CXR of a newborn with a ventricular septal defect. The CXR shows cardiomegaly. Because this is a newborn, the AP view should show a more prominent thymic shadow, but this is lacking. The lateral view should show the normal obliteration of the lung tissue in the anterior mediastinum. In the lateral view, lung tissue is clearly present, confirming that the thymus is absent or very small. This patient has DiGeorge syndrome (ventricular septal defect, thymic aplasia, and parathyroid aplasia).

Source: Copyright Loren Yamamoto, https://www.hawaii.edu/medicine/pediatrics/pemxray/v2c02.html.

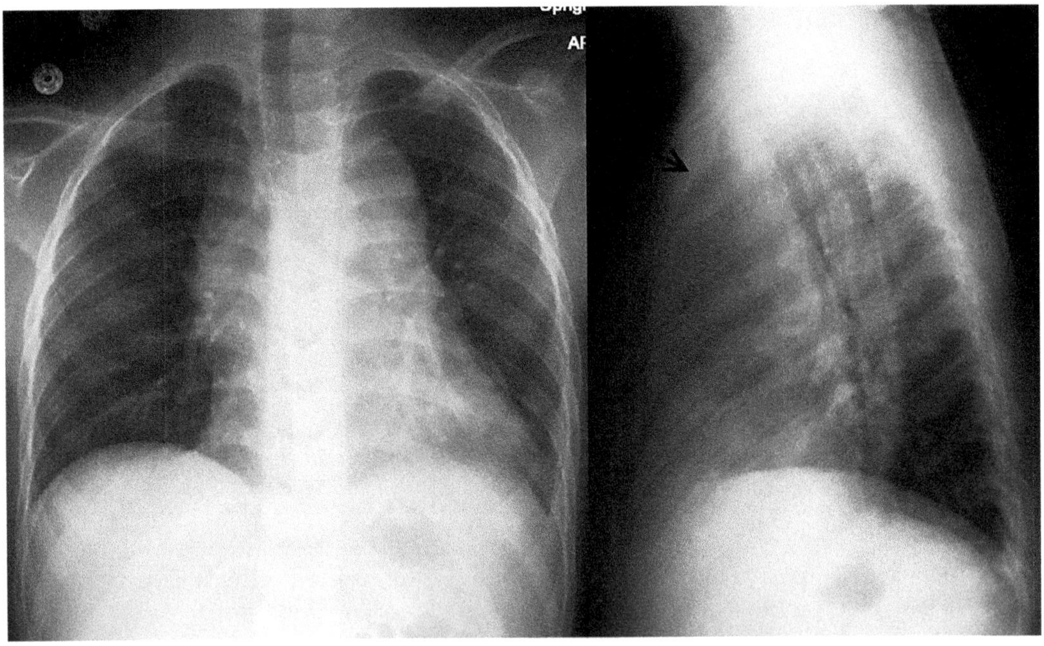

FIGURE 17.35 This is a CXR of an 8-year-old. The CXR shows a widened mediastinum on the AP view. The lateral view shows soft tissue density in the anterior mediastinum (arrow) that is due to the mass occupying the mediastinum. This area is normally filled with lung tissue except in infants, in whom it can still be occupied by the thymus.

Source: Copyright and courtesy of Paul Eakin, 2019.

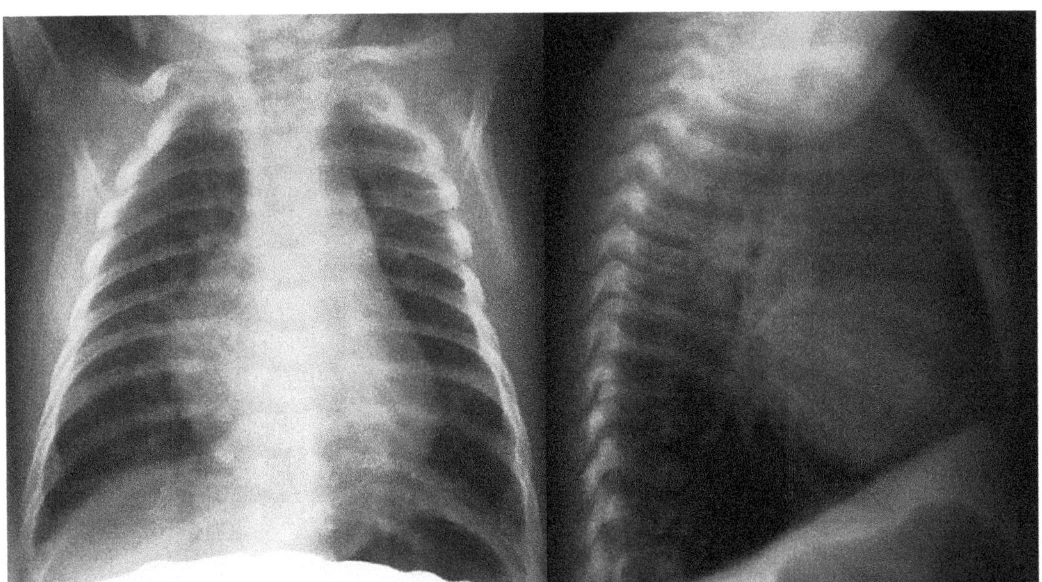

FIGURE 17.36 This is a CXR of a 2-month-old (same image as that shown in Figure 17.22, cor triatriatum). The right ventricle is enlarged. The CXR is rotated so that the right heart boarder extends into the right hemithorax, making it appear extra large. The lateral view shows obliteration of the normal lung tissue in the anterior mediastinum. Because the child is only 2 months old, this could be the normal thymus, but the PA view shows minimal widening of the thymic shadow, suggesting that the obliteration of the lung tissue in the anterior mediastinum is more likely due to right ventricular enlargement. Because the right ventricle is anatomically anterior, enlargement of the right ventricle is often best seen on the lateral view.

Source: Copyright Loren Yamamoto, https://www.hawaii.edu/medicine/pediatrics/pemxray/v4c03.html.

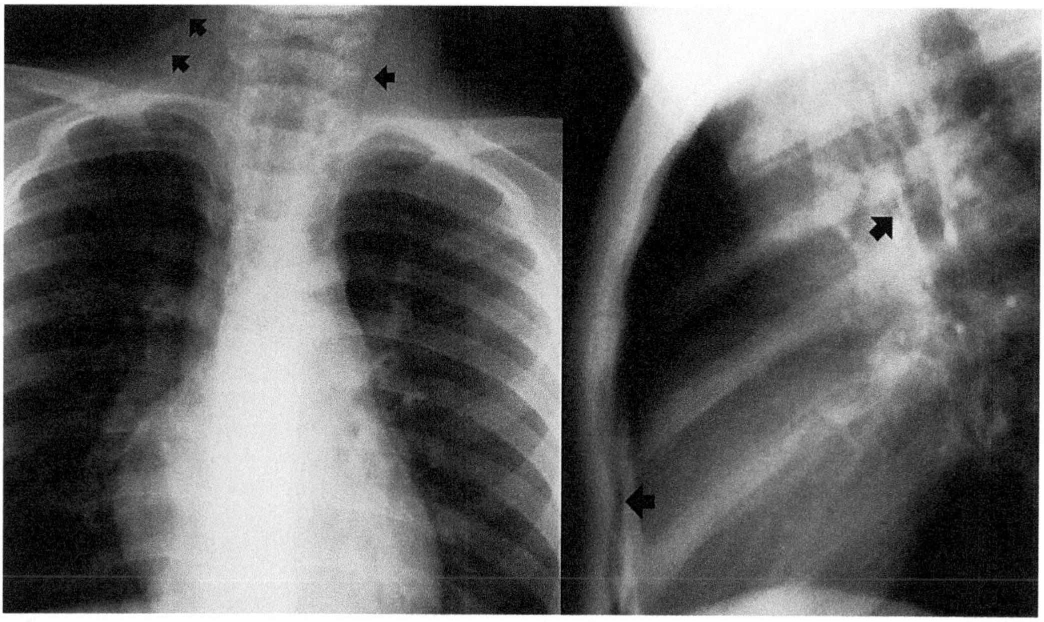

FIGURE 17.37 This is a CXR of a 6-year-old presenting with chest pain and difficulty breathing. A pneumomediastinum is the likely etiology. (Left) The arrows in the PA view point at air dissecting (subcutaneous emphysema) in the neck. (Right) The arrows in the lateral view point at air dissecting anteriorly and around the trachea (air density outside the tracheal air column).

Source: Copyright Loren Yamamoto, https://www.hawaii.edu/medicine/pediatrics/pemxray/v6c12.html.

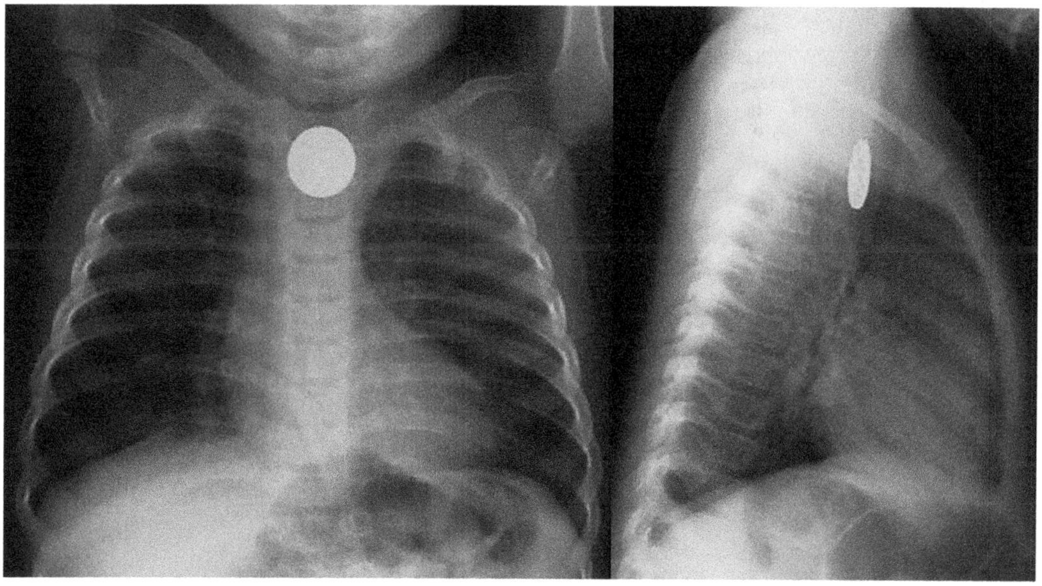

FIGURE 17.38 This is a CXR of a 15-month-old presenting with a choking episode. The CXR shows an esophageal coin. Some practitioners recommend that a lateral view be obtained routinely to confirm that the coin is in the esophagus and not the trachea. However, most coins are too large to fit in the trachea, so this recommendation it not truly justified in cases in which a coin is involved. In this case, the tracheal air column is thinner than it should be, suggesting external compression of the trachea. Further evaluation of this patient identified a vascular ring in addition to the esophageal coin.

Source: Copyright Loren Yamamoto, https://www.hawaii.edu/medicine/pediatrics/pemxray/v6c20.html.

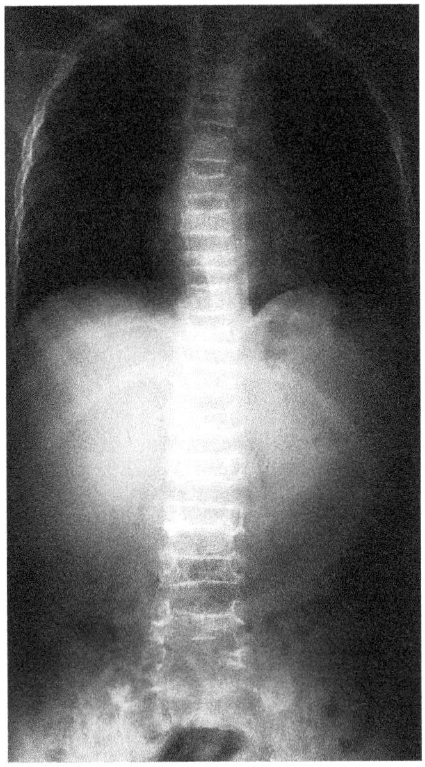

FIGURE 17.39 This is a CXR of an 8-year-old presenting with abdominal pain. The thoracic and lumbar vertebral bodies are compressed (compression fractures). She was subsequently diagnosed with leukemia.

Source: Copyright Loren Yamamoto, https://www.hawaii.edu/medicine/pediatrics/pemxray/v1c04.html.

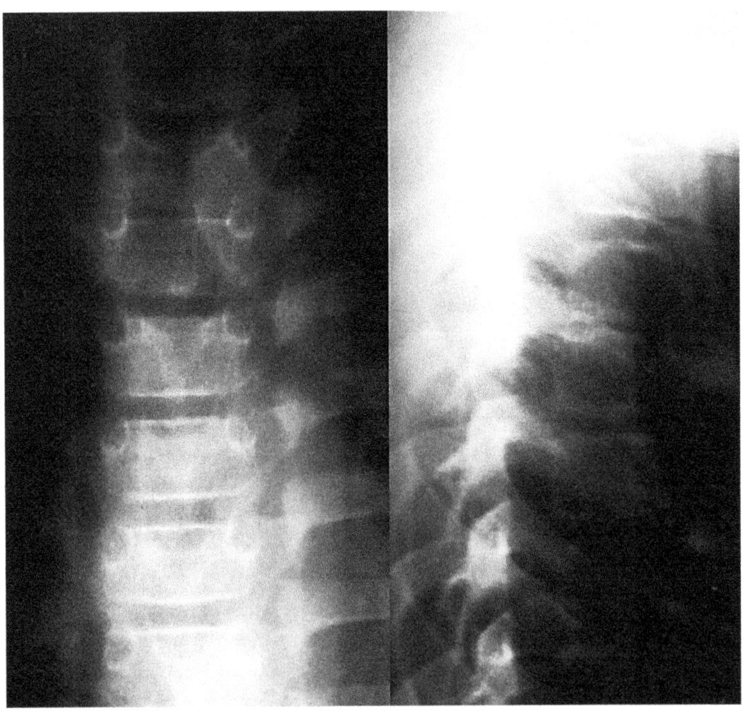

FIGURE 17.40 This is an X-ray of an 8-year-old presenting with fever. Upper back tenderness is noted over the thoracic spine. This X-ray shows narrowing of the intervertebral disc space indicative of discitis.

Source: Copyright Loren Yamamoto, https://www.hawaii.edu/medicine/pediatrics/pemxray/v7c01.html.

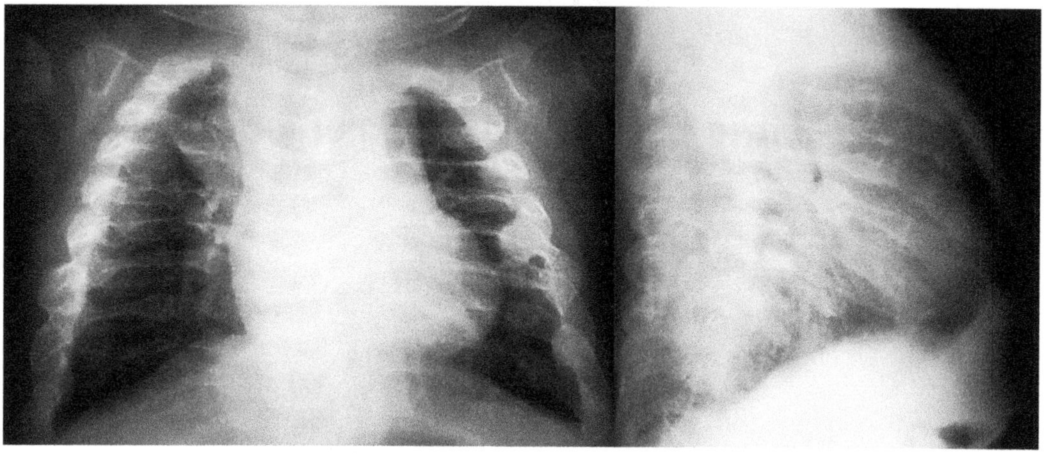

FIGURE 17.41 This is a CXR of a 3-month-old presenting with respiratory distress and a known diagnosis of osteogenesis imperfecta. This CXR demonstrates scoliosis, osteopenia, and multiple healing rib fractures (callus bulbs on the ribs).

Source: Copyright Loren Yamamoto, https://www.hawaii.edu/medicine/pediatrics/pemxray/v6c03.html.

or obtain another CXR to confirm proper placement. Other pathology on the CXR could be missed because the focus is limited to the indwelling device.

Avoid pitfalls by understanding the human nature factors that permit us to limit our examination of the CXR. One method is to serially examine the heart, lungs, aorta, mediastinum, bones, neck, and abdomen. Another suggestion is to examine the periphery of the image at some point during the CXR review.

18

Pediatric Cardiovascular Emergencies

JERRI A. ROSE

INTRODUCTION

Cardiovascular disease is relatively uncommon in children, but a delay in diagnosis can have devastating consequences. Although pediatric cardiac emergencies may arise from a wide spectrum of pathophysiologic states and manifest with a variety of clinical presentations, the common denominator is compromised cardiac output. Cardiovascular disease in infants and children may arise from structural lesions, conduction abnormalities, and acquired illnesses. A challenge for emergency medicine providers is to promptly identify children with cardiac disease, even when their chief complaints are not obviously "cardiac" in nature. Physicians should consider heart disease when evaluating children presenting with common, nonspecific symptoms, including lethargy, poor feeding, respiratory distress, wheezing, and abdominal pain. Rapid recognition, stabilization, and restoration of cardiac output in children presenting with cardiovascular emergencies are paramount.

Comparison with Adult Physiology

In contrast to the adult patient population, most cases of cardiac arrest in children arise from respiratory failure rather than a primary cardiac etiology. However, decreased cardiac output from cardiovascular disease may certainly progress to cardiac arrest in children if not promptly recognized and managed appropriately. Children generally have robust vascular compensatory mechanisms and are often able to maintain a relatively normal blood pressure despite significantly compromised cardiac output. Hypotension is often a late (and ominous) finding in children with shock. Tachycardia is an extremely important sign that can indicate developing shock (including cardiogenic shock) in children, and it should always be noted and carefully evaluated. Children have a higher resting metabolic rate with increased oxygen demands compared to adults. As a result, they may decompensate more rapidly in the setting of compromised cardiac output.

CONGENITAL HEART DISEASE

Background

Congenital heart disease (CHD) is the most common type of birth defect in newborns. Approximately 25% of newborns with CHD will require surgical (or catheter-based) intervention in the first year of life, and nearly half of deaths from CHD occur during infancy. Although many newborns with critical CHD are identified prenatally or soon after birth, others do not present until following discharge from their birth hospitalization.

CHD encompasses a wide spectrum of structural abnormalities; clinical presentations for specific forms of CHD may also be variable. In the emergency department (ED) setting, it is not essential to know the exact anatomical defect when a child with CHD presents; rather, the focus should be on the cardiac physiology and on restoring cardiac output.

Structural CHD can be divided into two major categories: cyanotic CHD and ductal-dependent CHD. Cyanotic CHD includes lesions that allow circulation of deoxygenated blood in the systemic circulation via intracardiac or extracardiac shunting.

Ductal-depending congenital heart lesions depend on a patent ductus arteriosus (PDA) to supply pulmonary or systemic blood flow or to allow for adequate mixing between parallel circulations. Many (but not all) forms of cyanotic CHD are also ductal-dependent. One of the more common non-cyanotic ductal-dependent lesions that may present following the initial newborn hospitalization is critical coarctation of the aorta.

Classic Clinical Presentation

Closure of the PDA within the first few days of life can result in acute clinical decompensation in infants with ductal-dependent cardiac lesions. Life-threatening clinical manifestations may include severe metabolic acidosis, cardiogenic shock, pulmonary edema, cardiac arrest, seizures, and decreased end-organ perfusion. A cardiac etiology should be suspected in newborns presenting with cyanosis and/or shock that fails to improve or worsens with volume resuscitation.

Newborns with critical CHD may present with cyanosis, signs of congestive heart failure (CHF), and poor perfusion (including weak lower extremity pulses). Signs of CHF in a newborn include tachypnea, labored breathing, tachycardia, and hepatomegaly. These infants may have wheezing or crackles on examination due to pulmonary vascular overload. Caregivers may report a history of nonspecific symptoms, including poor feeding, excessive sweating with feeding, irritability, and decreased activity.

Infants with CHD lesions that depend on a PDA to support flow to the systemic circulation or the pulmonary circulation will present with shock or cyanosis, respectively, when the PDA begins to close. CHD lesions that involve shunting of blood to the pulmonary circulation present with symptoms of pulmonary overcirculation as the pulmonary vascular resistance decreases.

Weaker or absent femoral pulses in a lethargic, poorly perfused child with normal or strong radial pulses should raise concern for critical coarctation of the aorta.

Atypical Clinical Presentation

Children with noncritical CHD lesions (including atrial septal defects, ventricular septal defects, and aortic and pulmonic valve stenosis) may present beyond the newborn period with characteristic heart murmurs that are detected on physical examination. Depending on the nature of the CHD lesion and pathophysiology, older children with CHD may present with signs of CHF (including tachypnea, dyspnea, poor feeding, sweating during feeds, decreased activity level, and failure to thrive).

Differential Diagnosis

Table 18.1 presents a simplified clinical approach to the differential diagnosis of CHD in children.

CONGESTIVE HEART FAILURE

Diagnostic Confirmation

In infants and children with suspected CHD, the following studies are useful in confirming the diagnosis and also in differentiating between cardiac and other disorders:

Four-extremity blood pressure (BP) measurements: BPs ≥10 mmHg higher in the arms than legs should raise concern for critical ductal-dependent CHD lesion, classically aortic coarctation (or other aortic arch obstruction).

Pulse oximetry: Pre- and postductal pulse oximetry measurements should be obtained to assess for cyanosis and differential cyanosis in children with suspected CHD.

Chest radiography: Chest X-rays help differentiate between cardiac and pulmonary pathology and are indicated in infants with cyanosis and/or significant respiratory symptoms. In children

TABLE 18.1 CLINICAL APPROACH TO THE DIFFERENTIAL DIAGNOSIS OF CONGENITAL HEART DISEASE IN CHILDREN

Condition	Distinguishing Features
Sepsis	Associated fever and/or hypothermia; hepatomegaly not typically present; generally responsive to fluid administration; no differential between upper and lower extremity pulses
Pulmonary disorders (including respiratory infections, respiratory distress syndrome, pneumothorax, congenital airway and/or lung disorders)	Associated cough and wheeze with pulmonary infections; focal findings (crackles/wheeze) and/or asymmetric breath sounds; stridor/upper airway noise with airway abnormalities; generally improves with oxygen administration; murmur absent
Inborn errors of metabolism	Onset often more gradual; vomiting/feeding intolerance may be associated; metabolic acidosis, hypoglycemia, and/or hyperammonemia are laboratory hallmarks; signs of CHF not present
Hypoglycemia	Generalized lethargy; CHF signs not expected; improves promptly with glucose administration
Hemoglobin abnormalities (e.g., methemoglobinemia, polycythemia)	CHF signs not associated; more chronic presentation if congenital; methemoglobinemia may be associated with toxic exposures or acute diarrheal illnesses in children
Benign acrocyanosis	Infant appears well with normal pulses and perfusion, bluish coloration of hands and feet, perioral area with pink mucous membranes, and normal central perfusion; resolves in first few days of life

CHF, congestive heart failure.

with CHD, radiographic findings may include cardiomegaly, abnormal cardiac silhouette, and/or abnormal pulmonary vascular markings. Chest radiographs can aid in identifying noncardiac causes of cyanosis and respiratory distress, such as pneumonia, pneumothorax, pulmonary malformations, diaphragmatic hernia, pleural effusions, and airway disease.

Electrocardiogram (ECG): An ECG should be obtained in children with suspected CHD. Although findings may be normal in some children with CHD, some lesions are associated with specific ECG patterns.

Echocardiography: An echocardiogram will provide a definitive diagnosis of CHD, with specific information on a child's cardiac anatomy and function. An echocardiogram should be obtained (in consultation with a pediatric cardiology) in children with signs or symptoms concerning for critical CHD.

Treatment

In ill children with suspected critical CHD, the main goals of treatment are to provide basic life support and to restore compromised cardiac output in order to ensure adequate end-organ perfusion.

Although immediate stabilization of the airway, breathing, and circulation are the first steps in managing all children presenting in shock, initiating infusion of prostaglandin (PGE_1) to re-establish patency of the ductus arteriosus is an essential life-saving measure in infants with critical ductal-dependent CHD lesions. Intravenous (or intraosseous) infusion of PGE_1 should be rapidly initiated at a dose of 0.05–0.1 μg/kg/min and titrated until femoral pulses are palpable and/or oxygenation and perfusion improve. Clinical improvement should be noted within 30 minutes with prostaglandin infusion in children with critical ductal-dependent lesions.

Endotracheal intubation and mechanical ventilation can significantly decrease cardiac demands and protect against apnea, which is a known side effect of PGE_1. Hypotension, rash, and fever are also known side effects of PGE_1.

Cautious fluid resuscitation to increase preload may be beneficial in some children with CHD, but those with severe CHF and pulmonary overload may worsen clinically with fluid administration. Inotropic support with agents such as dopamine, epinephrine, norepinephrine, and/or milrinone may be indicated for some children with cardiogenic shock due to CHD.

Emergent consultation with a pediatric cardiologist should be obtained as early as possible for infants and children with suspected critical CHD. Once stabilized, these patients should be admitted (or transferred) to a center with pediatric cardiology, surgical, and critical care expertise.

Disposition

All critically ill children with confirmed or suspected CHD should be admitted to a center with pediatric cardiology, surgical, and critical care expertise once initial stabilization has been completed.

Clinically stable and asymptomatic children with murmurs that raise suspicion for CHD lesions that are *not* ductal-dependent may be referred for evaluation by a pediatric cardiologist on an outpatient basis.

Complications

Life-threatening complications of critical CHD include cardiogenic shock, severe metabolic acidosis, pulmonary edema, seizures, decreased end-organ perfusion, and cardiac arrest. Promptly recognizing and restoring compromised cardiac output in infants and children with critical CHD lesions can help prevent these complications from occurring.

Key Points

- CHD should be considered in any neonate presenting with acute decompensation and/or signs of shock.
- Evaluate femoral pulses in all newborns and infants to aid detection of aortic coarctation.
- Consider a cardiogenic etiology in children presenting with shock who fail to improve or clinically worsen with fluid resuscitation.
- Pediatric patients with cardiac disease may present with nonspecific symptoms, including decreased activity, irritability, poor feeding, failure to thrive, labored breathing, and gastrointestinal complaints.
- Persistent tachycardia is an extremely important sign that can indicate developing shock (including cardiogenic shock) in children, and it should always be noted and carefully evaluated.

Pitfalls

- Failure to consider CHD as a potential etiology in infants with nonspecific symptoms, including poor feeding, sweating, irritability, poor weight gain, and decreased activity level
- Failure to promptly initiate prostaglandin (PGE_1) infusion as a life-saving measure in children with critical ductal-dependent CHD lesions
- Failure to carefully monitor clinical response to fluid resuscitation in an infant or child presenting with shock
- Failure to obtain early emergent pediatric cardiology consultation in ill children with suspected CHD
- Failure to recognize that apnea and hypotension are known side effects of PGE_1 infusion

ACQUIRED HEART DISEASE (PERICARDITIS, MYOCARDITIS, AND ENDOCARDITIS)

Background

Acquired heart disease can be a challenge to diagnose in children because symptoms can be very nonspecific and mimic those related to much more common pediatric conditions. Pericarditis, myocarditis, and endocarditis are three types of acquired heart disease in children that are reviewed here.

Myocarditis is an acute inflammatory disorder of the myocardium that can result in variable degrees of myocardial dysfunction. Viral infections (particularly with enteroviruses and adenovirus) are the primary etiology of myocarditis in North America and Western Europe. Rheumatic carditis, Chagas disease (*Typanosoma cruzi*), and bacterial infections are etiologies of pediatric myocarditis that are more commonly seen in developing countries. Less commonly, myocarditis may arise from autoimmune disorders, exposure to medications or toxins, vasculitic processes, and other infectious etiologies including mycobacteria and fungi. Due to the vague and nonspecific associated symptoms, the diagnosis of myocarditis is often missed during a child's initial presentation.

Pericarditis is inflammation of the pericardial layers overlying the heart. After musculoskeletal chest wall pain, pericarditis is the second most commonly identified cardiac cause of chest pain in children. There are many potential etiologies of pericarditis. Overall, viral or postviral etiologies are the most common cause of pericarditis in children in North America and Europe. Viral infections that are commonly associated with pericarditis in children include coxsackie virus, echovirus, adenovirus, and influenza. Bacterial causes may include *Staphylococcus aureus, Streptococcus pneumoniae, Haemophilus influenzae, Neisseria meningitis,* and tuberculosis. Although most viral or idiopathic cases of pericarditis are not life-threatening, bacterial pericarditis is a serious disorder and may be life-threatening.

Endocarditis is an infection—typically bacterial—of the endocardium that usually involves the cardiac valves. This disease is rare in children compared to adults. Historically, most cases of pediatric endocarditis involved children with rheumatic heart disease. It is now seen most often in children with CHD, including those with prosthetic heart valves, indwelling central venous catheters, or other intracardiac devices. Endocarditis can cause significant morbidity and mortality, and prompt recognition and appropriate management are essential. Seeding of bacteria causing endocarditis can arise due to dental caries; skin infections; and manipulation of the airway, gastrointestinal tract, or genitourinary tract. Endocardial injury, from either turbulent blood flow or an indwelling device, can create a locus for bacteria to adhere.

Classic Clinical Presentation

Myocarditis

Children with myocarditis often present with vague, nonspecific symptoms that can easily be misattributed to other more common childhood illnesses: fever, decreased activity, poor feeding, irritability, vomiting, diaphoresis, labored breathing, and pallor.

A history of a preceding or current viral upper respiratory or gastrointestinal illness within the past 10–14 days is commonly present in children with myocarditis.

Older children with myocarditis may complain of (or display) fatigue, shortness of breath, chest pain, nausea, anorexia, abdominal pain, and/or palpitations.

Physical examination findings may include tachycardia, signs of respiratory distress, a gallop rhythm on cardiac examination, and hepatomegaly. Tachycardia that seems out of proportion to the overall clinical appearance of a child should lead clinicians to consider myocarditis as a potential diagnosis.

In adolescents, myocarditis may resemble an acute coronary syndrome. These patients present with chest pain, ECG changes indicative of ischemia, and elevated troponin levels.

Boys with Duchenne muscular dystrophy (DMD) are especially susceptible to developing myocarditis. Clinicians should have a high index of suspicion of myocarditis and evaluate accordingly in patients with DMD presenting with chest pain or other signs of myocarditis.

Pericarditis

Children with pericarditis classically present with sharp chest pain that improves with sitting up and learning forward and worsens with inspiration, coughing, and/or lying down. Many present with associated fever. A history of a current or recent viral illness is also common.

Although physical examination findings may be normal in a number of children with pericarditis, a classic finding is a pericardial friction rub on auscultation. The sound of a pericardial friction rub has been described as scratchy or "creaking leather," which may become louder when the child is sitting or with inspiration. Children with pericardial effusions from pericarditis may have muffled heart sounds, which may impair auscultation of the classic pericardial friction rub. Tachycardia is frequently noted in children with pericarditis.

Endocarditis

Infectious endocarditis may be classified as acute or subacute, with the subacute form presenting more commonly. Children with subacute endocarditis typically present with persistent fever (often low grade), with associated myalgias, chills, malaise, and fatigue.

Physical examination findings in children with endocarditis may include a new murmur, signs of congestive heart failure (from insufficiency of the cardiac valves), petechiae, or new neurologic findings. The classic findings of Roth spots, Janeway lesions, and Osler nodes are seen much more commonly in adult patients than in children.

Atypical Clinical Presentation

Myocarditis

Children with fulminant forms of myocarditis may present in frank cardiogenic shock. These children will appear very ill on presentation, with poorly perfused extremities, weak peripheral pulses, a gallop cardiac rhythm, hepatomegaly, and possibly signs of pulmonary overload (rales and dyspnea).

Life-threatening arrhythmias and conduction abnormalities may also occur in children with myocarditis. These may include atrioventricular block and ventricular arrhythmias.

Although these cases are rare, myocarditis may cause sudden death in pediatric patients.

Pericarditis

Children with severe cases of pericarditis may develop large pericardial effusions and even manifest with signs of cardiac tamponade. These patients may present with muffled heart sounds, neck vein distention, decreased peripheral pulses during inspiration, pulsus paradoxus, hypotension, anxiety, and severe discomfort when lying down. Fortunately, most cases of pericarditis in children are not this severe.

Although pericarditis often affects previously healthy children, an effusion may develop due to postpericardiotomy syndrome in children with a recent history of cardiac surgery.

Endocarditis

Acute infectious endocarditis is seen less commonly than the subacute form. Children with acute endocarditis present with high fevers and signs of sepsis.

Involvement of other organs can result from septic emboli and/or from an immune-mediated response (e.g., the development of glomerulonephritis) in children with endocarditis.

Differential Diagnosis

Table 18.2 presents a simplified clinical approach to the differential diagnosis of acquired heart disease in children.

TABLE 18.2 CLINICAL APPROACH TO THE DIFFERENTIAL DIAGNOSIS OF ACQUIRED HEART DISEASE IN CHILDREN

Condition	Distinguishing Features
Sepsis	Hepatomegaly, pulmonary venous congestion, other CHF signs not typically present; poor perfusion often improves with fluid resuscitation (while fluids may worsen clinical status in children with acquired heart disease)
Pulmonary disorders (including respiratory infections, respiratory distress syndrome, pneumothorax, congenital airway and/or lung disorders)	Associated cough, wheeze, focal crackles more typical with pulmonary infections; abnormal findings on cardiac auscultation (new murmur, friction rub) not consistent with pulmonary disorders
Musculoskeletal chest wall pain	Often reproducible with palpation of anterior chest wall; chest pain worsens with cough and/or deep inspiration and improves with learning forward in children with pericarditis
Nonspecific viral syndromes	Fever, malaise, cough, congestion, GI symptoms very common; signs of CHF and abnormalities on cardiac auscultation (murmur, friction rub) not consistent with common viral illness; tachycardia out of proportion to clinical appearance of child should raise suspicion for myocarditis; endocarditis should be suspected in children with underlying risk factors (i.e., structural CHD, indwelling central venous catheters, intracardiac devices)

CHD, congenital heart disease; CHF, congestive heart failure; GI, gastrointestinal.

Diagnostic Confirmation

Myocarditis

The initial diagnostic evaluation of children suspected to have myocarditis based on history and physical examination should include cardiac enzymes, ECG, chest radiography, and echocardiography (in consultation with a pediatric cardiologist).

Elevated cardiac enzymes will help confirm cardiac inflammation and injury. Troponin I and T levels are more frequently elevated than creatine kinase muscle–brain levels in children with acute myocarditis. Normal cardiac enzyme levels do not completely exclude myocarditis.

Electrocardiogram abnormalities are commonly found in children with myocarditis. Nonspecific findings—including sinus tachycardia, low QRS voltages, ST- and T-wave abnormalities, and prolongation of the QT interval—may be noted. Arrhythmias may also be present.

Chest radiography in children with myocarditis may reveal cardiomegaly, pulmonary venous congestion, pulmonary edema, and pleural effusions, depending on the severity of the disease.

Echocardiography is useful in evaluating for dilatation of the heart chambers, measuring systolic and diastolic function, and detecting the presence of a pericardial effusion in children with suspected myocarditis. This study can also help rule out other causes of cardiac pathology. An echocardiogram should be obtained in children with suspected myocarditis (in consultation with a pediatric cardiologist).

Cardiac magnetic resonance imaging (MRI) is becoming a more commonly used tool for assessing children with myocarditis. Endomyocardial biopsy is considered the gold standard for confirming the diagnosis. These studies would not be part of the initial ED evaluation of children with suspected myocarditis.

Pericarditis

Electrocardiography and chest radiography can be useful in the initial evaluation of children with suspected pericarditis. Classic ECG findings that support the diagnosis of pericarditis include diffuse ST segment elevations and low-voltage QRS complexes. ECG findings are dynamic. T wave inversion frequently follows the ST elevation phase.

Cardiomegaly is a classic finding on chest radiography in children with pericarditis, particularly with associated pericardial effusion. However, the cardiac silhouette and pulmonary vascular markings may appear normal in a child with pericarditis.

Echocardiography is a useful study for evaluating children with suspected pericarditis. An echocardiogram can confirm the presence and size of a pericardial effusion; it can also help differentiate pericarditis from myocarditis.

Endocarditis

Obtaining blood cultures prior to antibiotics and echocardiogram are essential for the diagnosis (and treatment) of bacterial endocarditis. Children who are acutely ill should have three blood cultures drawn from separate sites during the first hour prior to antibiotic administration. Children who are less acutely ill may have their initial set of three blood cultures drawn over a more prolonged (i.e., 24-hour) time frame.

Other laboratory findings that may help support the diagnosis of endocarditis include elevated acute-phase reactants (erythrocyte sedimentation rate and/or C-reactive protein), leukocytosis, anemia, and/or hematuria.

Treatment

Management of all children with acquired heart disorders includes supporting the ABCs (airway, breathing, and circulation), treating congestive heart failure and arrhythmias, and rapidly restoring cardiac output in patients presenting in cardiogenic shock. Emergent pediatric cardiology consultation should be obtained in ill children with acquired heart disease.

Myocarditis

Specific treatment for myocarditis depends on the suspected underlying cause and clinical presentation. Some cases may resolve spontaneously. In ill children with myocarditis, aggressive support of the ABCs is paramount. Children with severe cardiac dysfunction due to myocarditis may require intubation, mechanical ventilation, and hemodynamic support with vasopressors, inotropes, and intravenous diuretics. Children presenting with life-threatening arrhythmias should be treated according to current Pediatric Advanced Life Support (PALS) algorithms (see Chapter 8 on pediatric resuscitation).

Children with refractory cardiogenic shock from myocarditis may require extracorporeal membrane oxygenation (ECMO) or a ventricular assist device (VAD).

Pericarditis

Nonsteroidal anti-inflammatory drugs (NSAIDs) such as ibuprofen and naproxen are the recommended therapy for acute pericarditis in children.

Corticosteroids are not routinely recommended for the treatment of children with pericarditis. Previous studies have demonstrated an association between corticosteroid use and an increased risk of recurrence in children and adults with pericarditis.

Children with severe cases of pericarditis involving large pericardial effusions may require pericardiocentesis, which can be both therapeutic and diagnostic.

Endocarditis

Broad-spectrum intravenous antibiotics with coverage for streptococci and staphylococcal organisms (including methicillin-resistant *Staphylococcus aureus*), as well as gram-negative bacteria, should be initiated in the ED for ill children with suspected endocarditis. For more well-appearing children, antibiotic administration can be delayed until a causative organism can be determined.

Pediatric cardiology consultation should be obtained for all children with suspected bacterial endocarditis; these patients should be hospitalized for further evaluation and treatment. Operative management may be necessary for children with large cardiac vegetations at risk of embolizing as well as for children with significant cardiac valvular insufficiency or concern for intracardiac abscess.

Disposition

Myocarditis

Pediatric cardiology consultation should be obtained early in children with suspected myocarditis. Children suspected to have this disorder should not be discharged home until this diagnosis (along with other potentially life-threatening disorders) has been excluded.

Once stabilized, children with myocarditis should be transferred to a center with pediatric cardiology and critical care expertise, along with ECMO, VAD implantation, and/or heart transplant capabilities by a pediatric critical care transport team.

Pericarditis

Well-appearing children with uncomplicated pericarditis (i.e., clinically stable without any pericardial effusion and/or cardiac dysfunction) may be able to be discharged home with NSAID therapy and close follow-up with their primary physician, along with a pediatric cardiologist.

Children with confirmed or suspected pericarditis who are ill-appearing, who have significant pericardial effusions, and/or who are suspected to have a life-threatening underlying etiology (including bacterial pericarditis) should be admitted to a center with pediatric cardiology and pediatric critical care support available.

Endocarditis

Emergent pediatric cardiology consultation should be obtained in children with suspected bacterial endocarditis; these patients should be hospitalized for further evaluation and treatment.

Complications

Myocarditis

Life-threatening complications of myocarditis in children may include CHF, cardiogenic shock, ventricular arrhythmias, heart block, multisystem organ dysfunction, and cardiac arrest. In rare cases, sudden cardiac death in children may arise from myocarditis.

Pericarditis

The space between the two pericardial layers normally contains less than 20–30 mL of serous fluid. Rapid accumulation of additional fluid in the pericardial space secondary to pericarditis could potentially lead to cardiac tamponade. Fortunately, this complication is quite rare in children.

Although most cases of viral, postviral, or idiopathic pericarditis in children are not life-threatening, bacterial pericarditis is often serious and may become life-threatening. Bacterial pericarditis is more common in children younger than age 2 years.

Endocarditis

Potential life-threatening complications of endocarditis in children include cardiac valvular insufficiency with resultant CHF, cardiac arrhythmias, embolization of bacterial vegetations to other organs (including the lungs and brain), development of intracardiac abscesses, and sepsis. The mortality rate of endocarditis ranges from 4% to 24%.

Key Points

- Maintaining a high index of suspicion for acquired cardiac diseases in children is critical because these diagnoses may easily be missed. These disorders are relatively uncommon in pediatrics, and early symptoms may be overlooked or misattributed to those of more common pediatric conditions (including uncomplicated viral infections).
- One of the most common signs of myocarditis in children is unexplained tachycardia. Clinicians should consider myocarditis as a potential diagnosis in a child with tachycardia that seems out of proportion to the child's clinical appearance.
- Children with pericarditis classically present with sharp chest pain that improves with sitting up and leaning forward and worsens with inspiration, coughing, and/or lying down. Many have associated fever.
- NSAIDs are a mainstay in treating acute pericarditis in children.
- Infectious endocarditis is seen most commonly in children with underlying structural heart disease and/or indwelling central venous catheters or intracardiac devices. The diagnosis should be suspected when these at-risk patients present with unexplained fever, myalgias, new murmur, and elevated inflammatory markers.
- Obtaining blood cultures prior to antibiotics and echocardiogram are essential for the diagnosis (and management) of bacterial endocarditis.

Pitfalls

- Failure to consider acquired heart diseases as a diagnosis in children presenting with nonspecific symptoms, particularly in those children with unexplained tachycardia
- Failure to obtain early pediatric cardiology consultation for a child with suspected acquired heart disease
- Failure to admit/transfer children with confirmed or suspected myocarditis to a center with ECMO, VAD implantation, and/or heart transplant capabilities (along with pediatric cardiology and critical care support)
- Failure to obtain a set of blood cultures prior to antibiotic administration in children with suspected endocarditis
- Failure to initiate broad-spectrum parenteral antibiotics (after obtaining blood cultures) in ill-appearing children with suspected or confirmed endocarditis

ARRHYTHMIAS IN THE PEDIATRIC PATIENT

Background

Disorders of heart rate and rhythm are relatively rare in children. Arrhythmias may affect healthy children as well as those with underlying cardiac disease. Pediatric arrhythmias may be congenital or acquired and involve a fast or slow heart rate. Although cardiac arrhythmias may be well tolerated by many children, persistent arrhythmias may lead to CHF, decreased cardiac output, and cardiac arrest. Some cardiac channelopathies, including long QT syndrome, may present with sudden cardiac death as the first symptom in pediatric patients.

The most common type of abnormal tachycardia encountered in the pediatric population is supraventricular tachycardia.

Pediatric arrhythmias that arise from structural heart lesions typically have a worse prognosis than those occurring in children with structurally normal hearts. Furthermore, children with underlying structural heart disease generally do not tolerate arrhythmias as well as otherwise healthy children.

Classic Clinical Presentation

The clinical presentation of pediatric arrhythmias will vary depending on the type of heart rate and rhythm involved, the patient's age, how long the patient has been in the abnormal rhythm, and whether the patient has associated conditions such as structural heart disease.

Infants and small children with arrhythmias may present with increased fussiness, decreased activity level, poor feeding, pallor/poor color, vomiting, wheezing, tachypnea, and increased work of breathing.

Older children and adolescents with tachycardia may report that their heart is suddenly "fluttering" or beating fast. Older children may have symptoms of fatigue, dizziness, lightheadedness, anxiety, chest pain, abdominal pain, vomiting, and shortness of breath.

Pediatric patients with symptomatic bradycardia may present with symptoms including weakness, fatigue, irritability, pallor, and syncope (or near syncope).

Atypical Clinical Presentation

Clinically unstable children with arrhythmias may present with signs of decreased cardiac output, including dizziness, fatigue, diaphoresis, tachypnea, syncope, and even sudden death.

Some infants and children with stable arrhythmias may be asymptomatic. In these patients, an abnormal heart rate and rhythm may be detected during routine health maintenance visits or during evaluations for other illnesses or injuries.

Differential Diagnosis

Pediatric dysrhythmias may occur in healthy children as well as in those with underlying heart disease.

Although dysrhythmias may arise from congenital or acquired heart disease in children, they may also be triggered by noncardiac causes. Possible triggers include hypoxia, electrolyte disturbances, exposure to toxins, and infectious/inflammatory diseases. Exposure to cardioactive agents, including digoxin, antiarrhythmics, tricyclic depressants, illicit drugs, and over-the-counter cold medications, should also be considered.

Table 18.3 presents key features of specific types of arrhythmias that may be seen in pediatric patients.

Diagnostic Confirmation

An ECG is the gold standard for diagnosing and categorizing arrhythmias in pediatric patients.

Treatment

The primary goal in treating children with cardiac arrhythmias is rapidly identifying and correcting unstable arrhythmias while simultaneously documenting the rhythm on ECG. A secondary goal is to identify children at risk for sudden cardiac death and referring them to a pediatric cardiologist for further evaluation and definitive management.

The emergency management of dysrhythmias depends on three factors: heart rate, QRS width, and the patient's level of clinical stability. Management should be based on interpretation of a 12- or 15-lead ECG; single-lead rhythm strips obtained from cardiac monitors can often be misleading.

Many children tolerate cardiac rhythm disturbances well from a clinical standpoint, which allows for time to accurately identify the specific underlying dysrhythmia and even to obtain emergent pediatric cardiology consultation in many cases.

The recommended management for specific pediatric arrhythmias is summarized as follows:

Sinus tachycardia: Treatment should focus on identifying and addressing the underlying condition.

Supraventricular tachycardia (SVT): For stable children with SVT, vagal maneuvers can be attempted to convert the arrhythmia. Techniques include applying a bag of ice and water over the nose and eyes for 15- to 30-second intervals, having the child blow into an occluded straw or syringe with plunger, and placing infants in a knees-to-chest position.

If vagal maneuvers are unsuccessful in converting SVT in stable patients, adenosine 0.1 mg/kg intravenously (IV) should be administered via rapid push through a large-bore IV, followed rapidly by a saline flush. If the initial dose of 0.1 mg/kg (maximum 6 mg) adenosine is ineffective, repeat doses of 0.2 mg/kg (12 mg one time maximum, up to three times) are recommended.

Adenosine will be unsuccessful in converting SVT to sinus rhythm in approximately 15% of children with SVT. For these children, pediatric cardiology should be consulted emergently for recommendations regarding administration of alternative antiarrhythmic agents (options include digoxin, propranolol, esmolol, amiodarone, and procainamide).

TABLE 18.3 KEY FEATURES OF SPECIFIC TYPES OF ARRHYTHMIAS IN PEDIATRIC PATIENTS

Arrhythmia Type	Distinguishing Features
	Fast Heart Rate
Sinus tachycardia	HR higher than normal for patient's age. Extremely common. May arise from fever, dehydration, pain, anxiety. May be associated with more serious conditions—anemia, sepsis, hypoxia, hyperthyroidism, toxic ingestion.
Supraventricular tachycardia	Most common childhood dysrhythmia. Narrow complex tachycardia. Features: abrupt onset with HR >220 bpm (infants) or HR >180 bpm (children and adolescents), absence of normal P waves, little rate variation. Approximately half of cases present within the first year of life.
Atrial flutter and fibrillation	Rare in children. Occurs most often in patients with congenital heart disease, rheumatic fever, or dilated cardiomyopathy. Children with associated accessory pathway or hypertrophic cardiomyopathy are at risk for sudden death. Features: irregularly irregular, narrow QRS rhythm.
PVCs	Rare in infants and young children. Unifocal PVCs begin manifesting in healthy children as adolescents. Patients are often asymptomatic with normal exams and ECGs. PVCs that diminish during exercise or stress are benign. Some patients with PVCs and associated cardiac disease, syncope, or exercise-induced PVCs may require therapy.
VT	Rare in children. Can be confused with other forms of tachycardia. Features: wide QRS complexes, atrioventricular dissociation with P wave and QRS independence. Narrow complexes can be noted in infants with VT. Idiopathic VT can occur in asymptomatic children without structural cardiac disease. Recurrent exercise-induced syncope may result from VT in children.
Ventricular fibrillation	Rare but life-threatening. Hallmark is chaotic irregular and ineffective ventricular contractions. ECG reveals rapid HR and QRS complexes with varying sizes and configurations. Causes may include postoperative complications following structural heart disease repair, severe hypoxemia, hyperkalemia, medications, myocarditis, and myocardial infarction.
	Slow Heart Rate
Sinus bradycardia	Can be normal in well-conditioned athletes, but may indicate serious underlying disease. Serious underlying causes include hypoxia, hypoglycemia, hypothyroidism, hypo- or hyperkalemia, increased intracranial pressure, medication/toxin exposure, cardiac tamponade, pulmonary thrombosis, and tension pneumothorax. Often an ominous sign of serious illness in infants, requiring rapid evaluation and treatment.
Atrioventricular blocks	May be congenital or acquired. Acquired heart block may result from myocarditis, endocarditis, rheumatic heart disease, cardiomyopathy, Lyme carditis, tumors, medications, and illicit drugs. Postoperative heart blocks may arise following cardiac surgery. Symptoms are dependent on HR and degree of block.

bpm, beats per minute; ECG, electrocardiogram; HR, heart rate; PVCs, premature ventricular contractions; VT, ventricular tachycardia.

Hemodynamically unstable children with SVT should be treated with synchronized cardioversion, 0.5–1 J/kg, increasing to 2 J/kg as needed.

Atrial flutter and fibrillation: Unstable patients should be cardioverted with 0.5–1 J/kg. Cardiology should be consulted for guidance related to drug therapy and indications for pacing.

Ventricular tachycardia: Unstable children with wide-complex tachycardia should undergo synchronous cardioversion with 0.5–1 J/kg.

For cases of shock-resistant ventricular tachycardia, either amiodarone or lidocaine may be given.

For children with stable ventricular tachycardia, amiodarone 5 mg/kg over 1 hour or lidocaine 1 mg/kg bolus followed by infusion, is recommended.

Ventricular fibrillation: For children with unwitnessed arrests, high-quality cardiopulmonary resuscitation (CPR) should be administered prior to defibrillation.

The 2015 American Heart Association's PALS guidelines recommend that pediatric patients with ventricular fibrillation and pulseless ventricular tachycardia receive immediate chest compressions and defibrillation within less than 3 minutes.

Defibrillation should initial be administered at 2 J/kg, followed by 4 J/kg for subsequent shocks.

CPR should be immediately resumed following defibrillation, and it should not be interrupted for a pulse/rhythm check until after five cycles of CPR or 2 minutes.

Either amiodarone or lidocaine may be used for children with refractory ventricular defibrillation.

For children with torsades de pointes, magnesium sulfate should be administered at a dose of 25–50 mg/kg (maximum 2 g).

Sinus bradycardia: If an underlying condition (e.g., hypoxia) is suspected as the cause of sinus bradycardia, aggressive treatment of this condition often improves the heart rate.

If the cause of sinus bradycardia is uncertain and the child's level of ventilation and oxygenation is adequate, chest compressions should be started and epinephrine administered.

Epinephrine dosing for sinus bradycardia is 0.01 mg/kg IV/intraosseous of 1:10,000 solution.

Some children with symptomatic bradycardia may require cardiac pacing.

Atropine 0.02 mg/kg (minimum dose 0.1 mg) is indicated only for children with vagally mediated bradycardia or first- and second-degree heart blocks.

Pediatric patients who are well perfused with asymptomatic bradycardia do not require emergent treatment.

Atrioventricular blocks: Cardiac pacing may be required for some children with symptomatic bradycardia due to atrioventricular blocks.

Recent advances have improved the long-term management of arrhythmias in the pediatric population. Ablation of aberrant conduction pathways via cardiac catheterization can cure most tachyarrhythmias and can be performed safely in small children. When indicated, implantable pacemakers and defibrillators can be used even in infants and young children. Furthermore, many diseases that put patients at risk for sudden cardiac death may now be diagnosed through genetic testing, enabling preventive management.

Disposition

In general, pediatric patients presenting to the ED with new-onset arrhythmias should be hospitalized and evaluated emergently by a pediatric cardiologist for an underlying accessory pathway or other structural heart disease.

Complications

Although cardiac arrhythmias may be well tolerated by many children, persistent arrhythmias may lead to CHF, decreased cardiac output, and cardiac arrest.

Some cardiac channelopathies, including long QT syndrome, may present with sudden cardiac death as the first symptom in pediatric patients.

Due to potential risk for stroke, immediate cardioversion should be avoided in patients who have been in atrial fibrillation for 48 hours or more.

Adenosine is generally a safe drug, but it can have adverse side effects. Physicians should always be well-prepared for the possible need for defibrillation, external pacing, or advanced airway management when giving adenosine.

Adenosine is contraindicated in children with Wolff–Parkinson–White syndrome who present in atrial fibrillation (wide-complex irregular tachycardia). Use of adenosine in these patients could lead to ventricular fibrillation and death.

Sedating agitated children with bradycardia may trigger cardiac arrest.

Key Points

- Any child presenting with a heart rate that is outside the normal range for the patient's age and clinical setting should be quickly assessed for a potential arrhythmia.
- Emergency management of dysrhythmias depends on heart rate, QRS width, and the patient's level of clinical stability. Management should be based on interpretation of a 12- or 15-lead ECG.
- The most common type of abnormal tachycardia encountered in the pediatric population is SVT.
- Sinus bradycardia in infants and young children is often an indicator of serious underlying disease and should be aggressively evaluated and treated.

Pitfalls

- Failure to recognize and address sinus bradycardia as a sign of serious illness in infants and young children
- Failure to rapidly evaluate full vital signs and perfusion in any child presenting with a heart rate out of the normal range for age and clinical situation
- Failure to obtain pediatric cardiology consultation early on in children presenting with arrhythmias
- Administering adenosine to patients with a wide-complex irregular rhythm (which may result in ventricular fibrillation and death)
- Administering sedative agents to children with agitation due to underlying sinus bradycardia or other arrhythmias
- Failure to recognize that QRS complexes may appear narrow in infants with ventricular tachycardia
- Failure to provide high-quality CPR prior to defibrillation in pediatric patients with ventricular fibrillation

PEDIATRIC CHEST PAIN

Background

Chest pain is a common chief complaint among children presenting for emergency care. Although chest pain can be quite worrisome to children and their caregivers, it is rarely life-threatening in pediatric patients. Whereas chest pain in adults raises concern for coronary ischemia and can often be life-threatening, the vast majority of children and adolescents presenting with chest pain do not have cardiac pathology.

A wide range of etiologies can cause chest pain in children, including disorders affecting the respiratory, cardiovascular, gastrointestinal, musculoskeletal, neurologic, and psychiatric systems. In many children presenting with chest pain, no specific organic or psychiatric cause can be identified.

Classic Clinical Presentation

Most chest pain in children without history of significant trauma is caused by acute respiratory illnesses, minor musculoskeletal injury or strain, anxiety, or inflammation. Most pediatric patients with chest pain are well-appearing and present without signs or symptoms of cardiorespiratory distress. In many cases, the chest pain has resolved by the time of the ED evaluation.

Children with nonspecific, idiopathic chest wall pain—one of the most common causes of chest pain in children—typically describe occasional episodes of sharp chest pain lasting for a few seconds to minutes, with or without exercise and with no other associated symptoms. These children are typically well-appearing with normal physical examination findings and pain that is not reproducible with palpation of the chest wall.

Key clinical characteristics of other etiologies of chest pain in children are summarized in Table 18.4.

Atypical Clinical Presentation

Cardiac ischemia is extremely rare in pediatrics, but it can present with persistent substernal crushing chest pain with or without radiation, diaphoresis, nausea, shortness of breath, and/or syncope. Affected children are typically in significant distress and will have abnormal physical examination findings, including diaphoresis, pallor, heart murmur, gallop rhythm, and decreased peripheral perfusion. Children with a history of Kawasaki disease (KD) may develop myocardial ischemia/infarction due to a thrombosed coronary artery aneurysm, which may arise as a sequelae of KD.

Although infants are unable to verbalize chest pain, those with coronary ischemia due to conditions such as anomalous origin of the left coronary artery from the pulmonary artery present with persistent crying, irritability, drawing their knees to their abdomens after feeding, diaphoresis, pallor, and signs of cardiogenic shock. These infants can be misdiagnosed as having colic.

Differential Diagnosis

Table 18.4 presents a simplified clinical approach to the broad differential diagnosis of chest pain in children without history of significant traumatic injury.

Diagnostic Confirmation

Most cases of pediatric chest pain can be differentiated through a careful, comprehensive medical history and physical examination alone. For all children with chest pain, history obtained should include a detailed description of the pain and any associated symptoms, past medical and surgical history, family history, any history of genetic disorders, history of trauma, exposure to drugs/toxins, and social history (including recent psychological stressors). Diagnostic testing is not required for many children presenting with chest pain.

Well-appearing children who have a history and physical examination consistent with nonspecific idiopathic or benign musculoskeletal chest pain do not require any additional diagnostic evaluation or referral.

The diagnostic evaluation for children presenting with chest pain should be individualized, based on their presenting and past medical history, physical examination findings, and associated symptoms.

Chest radiography may be helpful in identifying pulmonary and cardiac processes including cardiomegaly, bony lesions, pneumothorax, radiopaque airway foreign bodies, abnormalities of the lung parenchyma or pleura, and mediastinal masses in children with presentations concerning for such disorders.

Electrocardiography can aid in the evaluation for arrhythmias, heart block, signs of cardiac ischemia, pericarditis, and cardiac chamber hypertrophy in children suspected to have a cardiac cause for their chest pain. Not all children presenting with chest pain require an ECG; however, ECG is generally recommended for children with chest pain if cardiac disease is being considered as a possibility. Studies support that most cases of cardiac-related chest pain can be identified based on history, past medical history, concerning family history, physical examination, and an ECG.

Studies other than ECGs and chest radiography are rarely indicated in pediatric patients with chest pain. Laboratory studies such as troponin are seldom helpful. Obtaining troponin levels may be useful in children suspected to have myocarditis, pericarditis, or acute myocardial infarction based on history of ECG abnormalities.

Toxicology screens may be useful in cases involving suspected (or reported) exposure to illicit drugs, such as cocaine and amphetamines.

Emergency consultation with a pediatric cardiologist for suspected cardiac conditions such as myocarditis, pericarditis, acute myocardial infarction, and left ventricular outflow tract obstruction or significant ECG abnormalities may be required to facilitate a more extensive cardiac workup, including echocardiography.

Treatment

Reassurance, non-opioid analgesics, rest, or any combination of these three interventions is the recommended treatment for the majority of children with benign noncardiac chest pain. NSAIDs such as ibuprofen and acetaminophen administered for a few days to 1 week often relieve the pain and inflammation associated with musculoskeletal-related chest pain.

For children with chest pain arising from specific pulmonary, gastrointestinal, cardiac, psychogenic, and miscellaneous causes, management should focus on treating the underlying disorder. For example, appropriate antibiotic therapy should be initiated in patients with pneumonia. In children with pain due to gastroesophageal reflux disease, a trial of antacids followed by initiation of an H_2 receptor antagonist or protein pump inhibitor may help improve symptoms.

In some cases, outpatient referral to an appropriate subspecialist for ongoing treatment may be indicated. For example, children with recurrent episodes of psychogenic chest pain may benefit from long-term follow-up with a mental health professional.

TABLE 18.4 CLINICAL APPROACH TO THE BROAD DIFFERENTIAL DIAGNOSIS OF CHEST PAIN IN CHILDREN WITHOUT HISTORY OF SIGNIFICANT TRAUMATIC INJURY

Condition	Distinguishing Features
	Musculoskeletal Causes
Costochondritis	Unilateral sharp, stabbing pain along the upper costochondral joints. Usually worsened by deep breathing. Palpation over affected area can reproduce pain. Generally self-limited; intermittent exacerbations can occur in adolescents.
Tietze syndrome	Benign inflammatory condition involving isolated swelling of a costochondral, costosternal, or sternoclavicular joint seen in adolescents/young adults. Usually involves single joint. Signs of inflammation (warmth, swelling, and tenderness) may be present on exam. May be associated with upper respiratory infection/coughing.
Nonspecific (idiopathic) chest wall pain	Common cause of pediatric chest pain. Sharp pain lasting seconds to minutes, localizing to midsternal area or under breasts. Signs of inflammation typically absent on exam. May be worsened by deep breathing or manual pressure on sternum or ribs.
Slipping rib syndrome	Relatively rare. Intense pain in lower chest or upper abdomen due to hypermobility trauma of anterior aspect of 8th, 9th, and 10th ribs (which lack direct attachment to sternum). Pain reproduced by "hooking maneuver" (placing fingers under inferior rib margin and pulling rib edge outward and upward). Patients may report a popping or clicking sensation followed by pain.
Minor trauma and muscle strain	Common in active children. Localized pain and tenderness, often exacerbated by motion of affected areas. Erythema, swelling, and bruising may be present over chest wall.
Xiphodynia (hypersensitive xiphoid syndrome)	Localized discomfort over xiphoid process. Can be worsened by eating heavy meal, coughing, and bending or rotating motions. Palpation of xiphoid causes dull pain. Underlying cause unknown.
	Pulmonary and Airway-Related Causes
Asthma	Associated cough (classically worse at night), wheezing, and family history of atopy. Chest tightness, dyspnea, wheeze (may be exercise-induced in some children).
Pulmonary infections (bronchitis, pneumonia, pleurisy, empyema, pleural effusion, lung abscess)	Often associated with fever, malaise, cough, congestion. Tachypnea, tachycardia, respiratory distress, and hypoxia may be noted in severe cases. Physical exam may reveal focal pulmonary findings (crackles, rhonchi, decreased breath sounds).
Aspirated pulmonary foreign body	Choking history may be present. Chest pain may be associated with cough, decreased breath sounds, unilateral wheeze, and fever.
Pneumothorax	May occur spontaneously or secondary to trauma. Acute onset of unrelenting, pleuritic chest pain. Decreased breath sounds on affected side, respiratory distress in patients with moderate to large pneumothoraces.
Pulmonary embolism	Rare in children, associated with underlying risk factors. Intense pleuritic chest pain, often with associated hypoxia, hemoptysis, and respiratory distress.
Acute chest syndrome	Suspect in patients with sickle cell disease and chest pain. Focal pulmonary findings, hypoxia, and respiratory distress may be present.
	Gastrointestinal Causes
Gastroesophageal reflux disease	Chest pain typically burning in quality, worse in recumbent position, related to eating. Examination may be positive for epigastric tenderness.
Esophageal spasm or strictures	May be associated with difficulty swallowing.
Peptic ulcer disease/gastritis	Epigastric tenderness may be present. Pain often burning in quality.

TABLE 18.4 CONTINUED

Condition	Distinguishing Features
Esophageal foreign body	May be associated with drooling, dysphagia, and odynophagia. History of choking or foreign body ingestion may be present.
	Miscellaneous Noncardiac Causes
Psychiatric: anxiety, hyperventilation, conversion disorder	Triggered by recent stressors. May be accompanied by symptoms of difficulty breathing, dizziness, and paresthesias. Common cause of chest pain in adolescents.
Precordial catch syndrome ("Texidor's twinge")	Affects healthy adolescents. Acute sharp, well-localized pain of short duration (few seconds). Has been associated with poor posture. Position change (sitting up) may relieve pain. Physical exam typically normal.
Breast-related conditions: physiologic (menstrual or pregnancy-related), mastitis, fibrocystic disease, breast lesions/ tumors, gynecomastia	Unilateral or bilateral chest pain. Pain localized to breasts. Breast tenderness, erythema, and/or other lesions may be present on physical exam.
Mediastinal mass	Suspect with chest pain, pressure, and dyspnea that worsens in supine position.
	Cardiac Causes
Inflammatory disorders: pericarditis, myocarditis	Stabbing chest pain that improves with sitting up and learning forward with pericarditis. Friction rub, fever, distant heart sounds, and respiratory distress may be present in pericarditis. Myocarditis patients may have chest pain and fatigue with associated fever, dyspnea, tachycardia, and signs of cardiogenic shock.
Increased myocardial demand or decreased oxygen supply: cardiomyopathy, left ventricular outflow tract obstruction, arrhythmias	Chest pain may manifest or worsen with exercise. Fatigue may be reported. Some children may present with syncope or sudden cardiac death. Palpitations may be associated in children with arrhythmias. Systolic murmur that intensifies with standing or Valsalva in those with hypertrophic cardiomyopathy.
Coronary artery abnormalities: congenital and acquired	Chest pain associated with exertion may be an initial symptom. Pain may be described as a squeezing, tightness, pressure, constriction, burning, or fullness. Infants with coronary insufficiency may present with crying, irritability, poor feeding, and findings of shock.
Drug-induced cardiac chest pain: cocaine, amphetamine, etc.	Patients may have associated confusion, combativeness, and mydriasis with marked tachycardia and hypertension.
Aortic dissection	Extremely rare in children. Suspect in pediatric patients with Marfan syndrome and other underlying connective tissue disorders. Sudden onset of severe, tearing chest pain with radiation to the back.
Pain related to cardiac devices/stents	Consider in children with history of intracardiac devices and stents.
Pulmonary hypertension	May present with chest pain associated with fatigue and exertion dyspnea or syncope.

Most children who require referral to a pediatric cardiologist for further evaluation and management should be advised to avoid strenuous physical activity until they have undergone further cardiology evaluation and are "cleared."

Clinical Algorithm

Because pediatric chest pain can arise from a wide spectrum of etiologies (with many cases being idiopathic), a single clinical algorithm cannot be applied to managing all children presenting with this symptom. A careful, comprehensive history and physical examination are always the first steps in evaluating chest pain in any child.

Disposition

Most well-appearing children with noncardiac chest pain can be discharged home to follow-up with their primary physicians and appropriate specialists, following careful evaluation in the ED to exclude life-threatening pathology and determine an underlying cause.

In general, children who present to the ED with chest pain and associated cardiorespiratory distress require immediate stabilization and should not be discharged until the underlying cause of their pain can be identified and treated.

Chest pain that is acute in onset, crushing in nature with or without radiation to the left arm or neck, awakens a child at night, or is associated with exertion, syncope, fever, fatigue, dyspnea, decreased exercise tolerance, or palpitations is concerning and warrants a more extensive evaluation. Emergent pediatric consultation should be obtained for these children; patients with these "red flag" symptoms may require hospitalization until serious underlying cardiac and/or pulmonary pathology can be excluded.

Indications to refer a child or adolescent with chest pain to a pediatric cardiologist include abnormal cardiac findings; exertional chest pain; chest pain associated with syncope; chest pain with palpitations; ECG abnormalities; positive family history for arrhythmias, sudden cardiac death, or genetic disorders; past history of cardiac surgery or interventions (including cardiac transplant); history of KD; and first-degree relatives with familial hypercholesterolemia.

Complications

In children with chest pain due to underlying cardiac disorders, life-threatening complications that may arise include arrhythmias, CHF, pulmonary hypertension, cariogenic shock, and sudden cardiac death. The risk of these complications depends on the patient's underlying cardiac pathology.

Children with chest pain due to underlying pulmonary infections may develop complications including severe respiratory distress with progression to respiratory failure, hypoxemia, significant pulmonary effusions, empyema, and sepsis.

For children with chest pain due to an underlying pneumothorax, there is a risk of progression to tension pneumothorax, which could ultimately result in obstructive shock and cardiopulmonary arrest.

Children with drug-induced chest pain secondary to cocaine or amphetamine exposure are also at risk for development of hypertensive emergencies, malignant hyperthermia, and life-threatening central nervous system complications including seizures and stroke.

Potential complications in children with chest pain due to serious underlying gastrointestinal pathology, such as peptic ulcer disease or cholecystitis, may include intestinal perforation, gastrointestinal bleeding, peritonitis, and sepsis.

Key Points

- Few cases of pediatric chest pain (<1%) arise from a cardiac cause.
- Most chest pain in children without a history of significant trauma is idiopathic or musculoskeletal in nature. Other common causes include acute respiratory illnesses, anxiety, and gastroesophageal reflux.
- Providing education and reassurance for children and families about the benign nature of pediatric chest pain is extremely important.
- Although chest pain in children is generally benign, pediatric chest pain associated with cardiorespiratory distress requires immediate attention.
- Any child with a clinical history or examination findings concerning for cardiac-related chest pain should be promptly evaluated by a pediatric cardiologist.

Pitfalls

- Failure to complete a careful, comprehensive history and physical examination in all children presenting with chest pain
- Failure to refer children with chest pain who have risk factors or clinical findings concerning for a cardiac cause to a pediatric cardiologist
- Obtaining unnecessary diagnostic tests in children with presentations consistent with benign noncardiac chest pain

SYNCOPE

Background

Syncope is a sudden, transient loss of consciousness and postural muscle tone that reverses without intervention. Its pathophysiologic mechanism involves a temporary decrease in cerebral blood flow or glucose supply, which the brain constantly depends on to function normally.

Up to 3% of all ED visits in the pediatric population are for syncope. Approximately 15–25% of children and adolescents will experience at least one episode before adulthood. The incidence peaks in the late teen years and occurs more commonly in females. The causes of syncope range from completely benign to life-threatening.

Although cardiac causes for syncope are relatively common in adults, most syncope in children and adolescents is benign and not due to cardiac pathology. The etiologies of syncope can be classified into several broad categories, including autonomic-mediated (reflex syncope), situational, cardiac, neurologic, psychogenic, metabolic, toxicologic, and miscellaneous. Autonomic-mediated reflex syncope accounts for approximately 75% of all pediatric syncope cases.

When evaluating a child with syncope in the ED, the main goal is to determine whether serious conditions are present or whether symptoms are due to a more benign cause.

Classic Clinical Presentation

A classic clinical presentation for pediatric syncope involves a healthy adolescent who feels lightheaded or dizzy for a brief time while standing and "passes out" for less than 1 minute, with a rapid return to his or her neurologic baseline. This is a classic presentation for vasovagal syncope, which accounts for more than half of pediatric syncope cases seen in the ED.

Atypical Clinical Presentation

Most cases of syncope in children are not related to underlying cardiac pathology. However, syncope that occurs suddenly without warning—including episodes without any presyncopal prodrome—should be assumed to be due to cardiac pathology until proven otherwise. Syncope that occurs while a child is actively exercising or that is preceded by severe chest pain or palpitations is also concerning for a cardiac etiology. Any child who becomes pulseless during syncope and/or requires CPR or defibrillation should undergo an extensive evaluation for cardiac pathology.

Differential Diagnosis

Table 18.5 presents a simplified clinical approach to the broad differential diagnosis of syncope in children.

Diagnostic Confirmation

The combination of a careful history, physical examination, and ECG will identify cardiac causes of syncope in the majority of affected children, with high sensitivity. ECG is highly useful in diagnosing cardiac causes of syncope and is generally indicated in all children presenting with syncope or a similar event. A 12- or 15-lead ECG will provide information about heart rhythm, atrioventricular conduction, and the presence of ischemic changes.

Screening blood tests in pediatric patients with syncope are generally not indicated, unless they are obtained to confirm a specific diagnosis that is clinically suspected based on history and physical examination findings. Testing for hypoglycemia, anemia, pregnancy, drug exposure, and elevated carboxyhemoglobin levels may be indicated in specific clinical scenarios, but it is certainly not recommended in all patients. Cardiac enzymes are routinely recommended in pediatric patients with syncope, but they may be useful in children with suspected myocarditis or cardiac ischemia.

Echocardiography is generally indicated only in pediatric patients with clinically suspected cardiac disease or exercise-induced syncope. This test is not routinely indicated in most children with syncope.

Ambulatory ECG (Holter) monitoring may be helpful in children with a history suggestive of a cardiac arrhythmia who have normal ECGs in the ED.

Neuroimaging studies (computed tomography of the head and/or MRI of the brain) are generally not needed as part of the evaluation of pediatric patients with syncope, unless there is a particular concern for intracranial pathology based on history and physical examination.

An electroencephalogram may be useful in patients suspected of having a seizure as a cause of their syncope. For patients who have returned

TABLE 18.5 CLINICAL APPROACH TO THE BROAD DIFFERENTIAL DIAGNOSIS OF SYNCOPE IN CHILDREN

Condition	Distinguishing Features
Autonomic-Mediated Causes (i.e., "reflex syncope")	
Vasovagal syncope	Most common etiology of syncope in children; often preceded by brief prodrome (dizziness, feeling warm, nausea, vision changes, palpitations) followed by syncopal event lasting <1 minute. Often associated with standing or change in position (i.e., lying to sitting, sitting to standing).
Postural orthostatic tachycardia syndrome	Involves HR increase of >30 beats per minute, without hypotension within 10 minutes of standing upright. Patients can have presyncope or syncope. Associated with chronic fatigue, gastrointestinal problems, headaches, poor sleep, difficulty concentrating, and decreased exercise tolerance. Substantial psychological influence to symptoms in some patients.
Orthostatic hypotension	Decrease in systolic BP >20 mmHg or diastolic BP >10 mmHg within minutes of assuming upright position. Can occur with prolonged bed rest or prolonged standing, or in patients with chronic medical conditions. Can be related to dehydration, acute or chronic illness, pregnancy, medications, and autonomic dysfunction.
Situational syncope	Similar presentation and mechanism as vasovagal syncope but has specific trigger. Triggers may include seeing blood, pain, fear, coughing, hair brushing, micturition, and other emotional triggers.
Cardiac Causes	
Structural heart disease (including hypertrophic cardiomyopathy, severe aortic or pulmonic stenosis, coronary artery anomalies, primary pulmonary hypertension) Myocardial dysfunction (including dilated cardiomyopathy, myocarditis) Arrhythmias (including atrioventricular block, sinus node dysfunction, supraventricular tachycardia, ventricular tachycardia, long QT syndrome, Wolff–Parkinson–White syndrome, Brugada syndrome, arrhythmogenic cardiomyopathy)	Syncope results from inadequate cerebral perfusion due to failure of heart as a pump. Frequently occurs without warning signs (i.e., no presyncopal prodrome). Should be suspected in cases of syncope occurring during exercise. May also present with syncope following chest pain, rapid heart rate, and/or palpitations.
Neurologic Causes	
Seizure	Patients may have sustained tonic–clonic movements with a subsequent period of confusion/postictal state. Loss of bowel or bladder control may occur (but is not typically seen in vasovagal syncope).
Complex migraine syndrome	Patient may have previous history of migraines. Typically associated with headache and nausea. Children with basilar migraine syndrome may have loss of consciousness, ataxia, or vertigo.
Intracranial mass or bleed	May be associated with severe headache, vomiting, change in mental status, and neurologic abnormalities on exam.

TABLE 18.5 CONTINUED

Condition	Distinguishing Features
	Psychogenic Causes
Psychogenic syncope (non-epileptogenic seizures, conversion disorder, "fainting spells")	Episodes typically occur in the presence of witnesses or at specific times (e.g., before school). Frequently associated with emotionally charged settings. Episodes may be prolonged (up to 1 hour or more). Some children may have underlying history of emotional, physical, or sexual abuse.
	Miscellaneous Causes
Eating disorders (anorexia)	May result in syncope associated with combination of bradycardia, hypovolemia, and hypoglycemia. History of recent weight loss, food restriction, and/or binging and purging behaviors may be present.
Breath-holding spells	Typically occur in younger children (6–24 months) and are triggered by emotional upset (pain, anger, or fear). Patients typically hold breath until syncope occurs, with return to normal consciousness and respiratory pattern within seconds. Children may appear cyanotic or pale during episodes.
Toxin-related	May be associated with intentional or inadvertent exposure to a wide variety of substances, including alcohol, drugs, and carbon monoxide. Associated symptoms vary depending on specific toxic exposure involved.
Hypoglycemia	Patients often feel weak, hungry, sweaty, or confused prior to syncope.
Anemia	Syncope may be associated with pallor, history of blood loss, and tachycardia
Hyperventilation	Usually associated with emotional stress. Patients may have associated chest tightness, dyspnea, lightheadedness, and visual disturbances.
Heat-related syncope	Typically presents after completing a vigorous workout or race, generally with exposure to heat. Patients may be hyperthermic on presentation.
Anaphylaxis	History of exposure to allergen may be present. Associated symptoms may include flushing, urticaria, itching, cough, wheeze, angioedema, and gastrointestinal symptoms.
Pregnancy	Suspect in adolescent females with pregnancy-related symptoms (amenorrhea, nausea, breast enlargement/tenderness, etc.).

BP, blood pressure; HR, heart rate.

to their neurologic baseline in the ED, this study can be obtained on an outpatient basis.

Treatment

Appropriate treatment of pediatric syncope requires identification and management of the underlying etiology.

For children and adolescents with vasovagal syncope, recommended management consists of nonpharmacologic measures including increased water and salt intake, avoidance of caffeine, routine exercise, and performing techniques to mechanically increase blood return to the heart (i.e., contracting the extremity muscles, toes raises, leg crossing, and keeping knees slightly bent while standing).

Clinical Algorithm

Figure 18.1 provides a clinical algorithm to guide the evaluation and management of

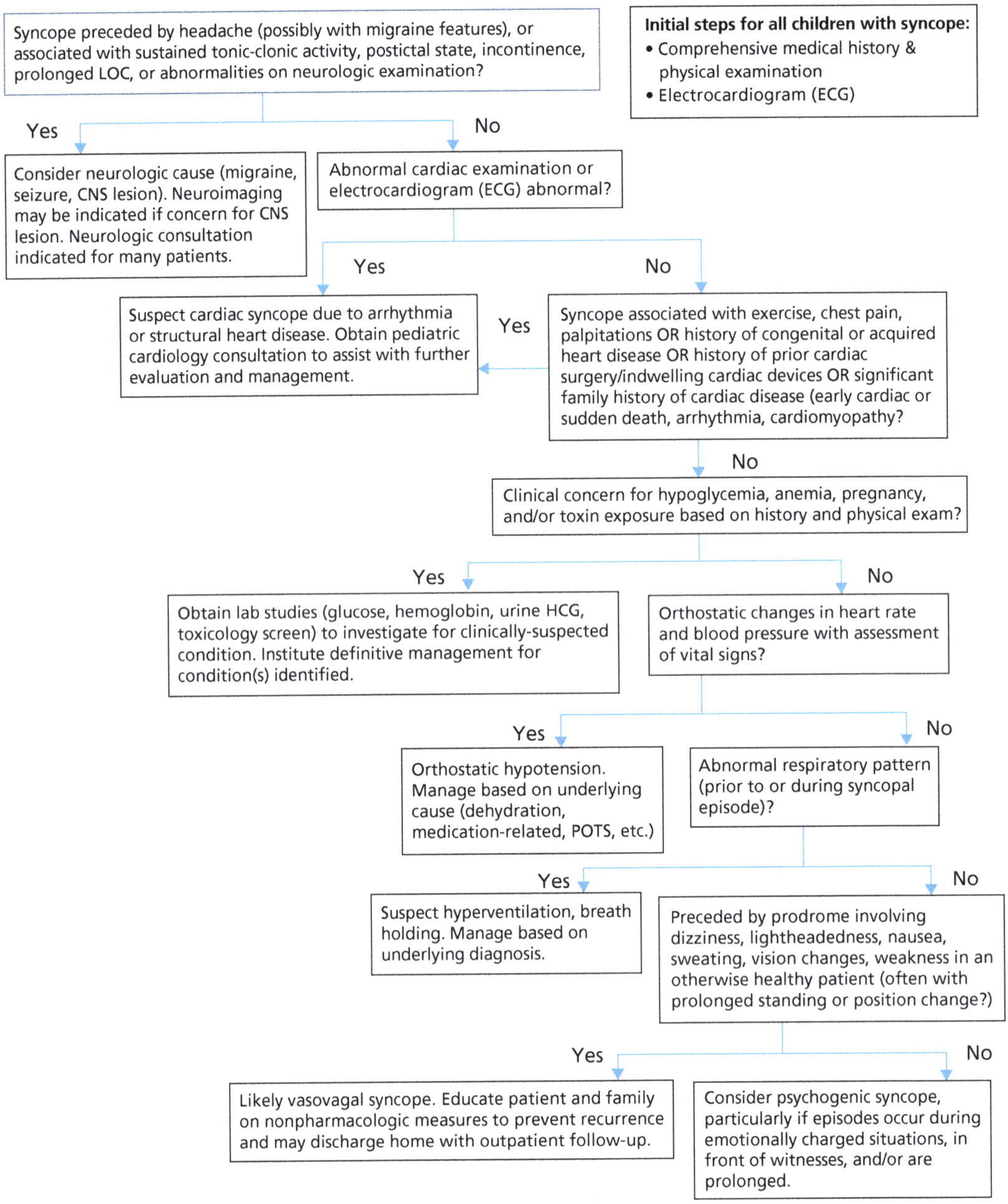

FIGURE 18.1 Clinical algorithm to guide the evaluation and management of children with syncope. CNS, central nervous system; HCG, human chorionic gonadotropin; LOC, loss of consciousness; POTS, postural orthostatic tachycardia syndrome.

pediatric patients presenting to the ED with syncope.

Disposition

The majority of pediatric patients with syncope who have returned to their neurologic baselines and have no red flags for cardiac syncope can be discharged home, with outpatient follow-up by their primary care physicians.

Children suspected to have a cardiac etiology for their syncope based on history, physical examination, or ECG findings should be either evaluated in the ED by a pediatric cardiologist or referred urgently for outpatient evaluation. These children should be instructed to avoid strenuous activity until cleared by a pediatric cardiologist.

Any patient with syncope who required CPR or defibrillation (either in or outside the hospital setting) should be thoroughly evaluated by a pediatric cardiologist before discharge from the ED or hospital.

Children with suspected seizure activity as the cause of syncope (who have fully returned to their neurologic baseline) should be referred for follow-up with a pediatric neurologist. Children and adolescents with psychogenic syncope may need to be referred for outpatient follow-up with a mental health professional.

Most pediatric patients with syncope do not require hospitalization. However, admission to the hospital for further evaluation and management is indicated for children with the following characteristics:

- Evidence of serious cardiovascular disease (i.e., heart failure, arrhythmia, heart block, or persistent symptomatic bradycardia)
- Persistent alteration in mental status and/or other abnormal neurologic findings
- Hypotension with continued postural syncope that does not resolve with fluid therapy
- Concern for other life-threatening etiologies of syncope requiring immediate management, such as severe anemia and carbon monoxide toxicity

Complications

Although cardiac-related syncope in children is rare, some children with underlying cardiac conditions, such as hypertrophic cardiomyopathy and long QT syndrome, may present with sudden cardiovascular collapse. Longer episodes of cardiac syncope can result in sudden death or neurologic sequelae from prolonged cerebral hypoperfusion.

Key Points

- Syncope is quite common and typically benign in the pediatric patient population.
- Patients with syncope occurring during active exercise, sudden syncope occurring without warning, and syncope following severe chest pain and/or rapid palpitations may have underlying cardiac pathology and should be further evaluated for cardiac disease.
- Although most causes of syncope can be determined through a careful history and physical examination, ECG is also useful in the evaluation of pediatric patients with syncope to help rule out cardiac etiologies.
- Blood testing and neuroimaging studies are generally not necessary for evaluating pediatric patients with syncope.
- The primary therapies for autonomic (vasovagal) syncope are conservative measures including increasing fluid and salt intake, avoiding caffeine, routine exercise, and purposeful muscle movements in the arms and legs to mechanically increase blood return to the heart.

Pitfalls

- Failure to refer children with syncope and clinical or ECG findings suggestive of cardiac disease to a pediatric cardiologist for a more in-depth evaluation
- Routinely obtaining neuroimaging studies in pediatric patients with syncope
- Failure to educate pediatric patients with vasovagal syncope and their families about nonpharmacologic measures to help prevent further episodes of syncope
- Failure to consider syncope (and potential underlying life-threatening arrhythmia or conduction abnormality) in a patient presenting with "new-onset seizure"

ELECTROCARDIOGRAMS IN CHILDREN

Background

There are a number of nuances to ECGs in children that arise from physiologic age-specific changes in the cardiovascular system that occur as a child matures from infancy to adulthood. For example, fetal circulation relies primarily on the right side of the heart; at birth, the right ventricle is larger and thicker than the left ventricle in healthy neonates. During infancy, the left ventricle gradually enlarges so that it becomes twice as thick as the right ventricle by 6 months. By adolescence, the left ventricle becomes at least 2.5 times as thick as the right. These changes—part of normal physiologic development—lead to variations in what is "normal" to find on ECGs in children, which can complicate the interpretation of pediatric ECGs in the ED.

Clinical Application

Common indications for obtaining ECGs in children include chest pain, suspected arrhythmia, syncope, seizure, toxic exposures/ingestion, electrical burns, electrolyte abnormalities, known history of cardiac abnormality, and abnormal physical examination findings (i.e., cardiac gallop, murmur, signs of CHF, or clinical findings concerning for KD).

ECGs can alert physicians to cardiac conduction and/or structural cardiac defects in pediatric patients, as well as to indications of myocardial and pericardial diseases.

Although ECGs are often obtained to investigate for myocardial ischemia/infarction in the adult population, ischemic changes are extremely rare in the pediatric population and findings will differ from those typically seen in adults.

Key Points

- Age and chamber force differences may complicate the interpretation of pediatric ECGs, but keeping a few basic principles in mind can be helpful. Physicians should utilize a systematic technique for interpreting pediatric ECGs, just as they do when interpreting adult ECG studies. When analyzing pediatric ECGs, however, it is often necessary to consult a pediatric handbook because ECG normal ranges can vary greatly by age.
- The software used by some ECG machines for electronic interpretation is calibrated with adult values; therefore, the machine interpretation can often be inaccurate for pediatric ECGs.
- An important difference between adult and pediatric ECGs is the need for placement of an additional lead, V4R, in young children (younger than age 5 years). This additional lead is necessary because neonates and young children physiologically have a right axis deviation, which may obscure the typical findings of right-sided heart disease. The addition of the V4R (and sometimes V3R) lead helps increase the sensitivity of the ECG in detecting right atrial or ventricular hypertrophy in children with suspected CHD.
- A normal ECG in a neonate and infant will reveal right axis deviation, tall R waves in the right precordial leads (V1–V3), and upright T waves in the right precordial leads (V1–V3).
- In healthy neonates, a decrease in pulmonary vascular resistance and an increase in systemic vascular resistance occur after birth with the first few breaths. These changes will result in the left ventricle becoming larger and thicker than the right ventricle within the first few weeks of life. During the first week of life, the upright T waves in V1–V3 on a neonatal ECG will become inverted, which results in a typical "juvenile T wave inversion pattern" that may persist into adolescence. As a child ages, the T waves will first become upright in V3 and then in V2.
- Cardiac conduction intervals (PR interval and QRS duration) are shorter in children than in adults due to children's smaller cardiac size. Normal values for these intervals vary depending on a child's age.
- Resting heart rates are much faster in infants and small children, decreasing as they grow older. A healthy newborn, for example, generally has a normal resting heart rate of 110–150 beats per minute.
- In pediatric patients, the calculated QT interval (QTc) may normally be up to 490 msec in infants (younger than age 6 months), whereas the QTc in infants and children older than age 6 months should not be longer than 440 msec.
- The following ECG findings, which would generally be considered abnormal in an adult patient, are often completely normal in children:
  - Heart rate >100 beats per minute
  - Rightward QRS axis > +90°
  - Inversion of T waves in V1–V3 (juvenile T-wave pattern)
  - Dominant R wave in V1
  - RSR′ pattern in V1
  - Marked sinus arrhythmia
  - Short PR interval (<120 msec) and QRS duration (<80 msec)
  - Slightly peaked P waves (<3 mm in height is normal in infants aged 6 months or younger)
  - Longer QTc interval (≤490 msec) in infants aged 6 months or younger
  - Q waves in the inferior and left precordial leads

- Elevated J points in adolescents, which is indicative of early repolarization (but may be challenging to differentiate from ST segment elevation)

Pitfalls

- Failure to consult a pediatric reference to determine age-specific ECG norms for a pediatric patient because normal ranges for cardiac conduction intervals, axis, wave voltages/amplitude, and heart rate can vary significantly by age
- Failure to recognize sinus bradycardia, which is often an ominous sign, in sick infants and children
- Failure to obtain pediatric cardiology consultation for children with abnormal ECG findings

19

Pediatric Neurovascular Emergencies

ELLEN DUNCAN AND EMILY ROSE

PEDIATRIC STROKE

Stroke is a leading cause of childhood mortality. Moreover, stroke survivors are at risk for persistent neurological deficits, seizures, and stroke recurrence. Up to two-thirds of children will exhibit persistent neurological deficits after a stroke. Delay in diagnosis is common in children. Stroke is a true neurological emergency, but many strokes in children are not diagnosed until more than 24 hours after symptom onset.

Comparison with Adult Stroke

There are significant differences between children and adults with respect to the etiology, risk factors, and pathophysiology of stroke. While atherosclerosis is the major contributor to adult stroke, it plays almost no role in pediatric stroke.

ISCHEMIC STROKE

Acute ischemic stroke (AIS) accounts for 50% of strokes seen in pediatric patients. Ischemia is related to arteriopathy (from infection, systemic disease, or trauma) in half of all cases. Other causes include cardiac defects, prothrombotic states (as seen in systemic disorders such as sickle cell disease and lupus), sepsis, and genetic abnormalities. Mortality is approximately 10% in AIS.

Classic Clinical Presentation

Children with AIS typically present with sudden onset of symptoms. Children, particularly infants, are more likely than adults to present with altered mental status and seizures. Focal neurologic deficits may be subtle, and may include hemiplegia, unilateral weakness, sensory disturbances, dysarthria, aphasia, dysphagia, and vision changes. Presenting symptoms may include acute changes in mood or behavior.

Atypical Clinical Presentation

Patients with cervical artery dissection may present with neck pain, and those with carotid dissection may present with Horner's syndrome (triad of miosis, ptosis, and anhidrosis).

Diagnostic Confirmation

All patients presenting to the emergency department with focal neurological deficits, altered mental status, seizure, or behavioral changes should undergo a detailed neurological examination, and a stroke diagnosis should be considered. Implementation of a stroke protocol increases the likelihood of identifying pediatric stroke and facilitates diagnosis and more rapid intervention. The National Institutes of Health Pediatric NIH Stroke Scale is helpful for

TABLE 19.1 PEDIATRIC STROKE MIMICS

Peripheral neurologic causes	Intracranial lesions
Bell's palsy	Mass
Myasthenia gravis	ADEM
Guillain–Barré syndrome	Post-infectious cerebellitis
Migraine	Infection
Seizures	Meningitis
Todd's palsy	Encephalitis
Syncope	Brain abscess
Conversion disorder	Metabolic derangements
Other psychogenic causes	Toxins
Non-accidental trauma	TBI

ADEM, acute disseminated encephalomyelitis; TBI, traumatic brain injury.

making the diagnosis (see http://www.mdcalc.com/pediatric-nih-stroke-scale-nihss).

Laboratory studies (glucose, electrolytes, complete blood count, and coagulation studies) should be obtained. Magnetic resonance imaging (MRI) is the most valuable imaging modality in cases of pediatric stroke (especially with neck angiography) because it is more sensitive for acute ischemia, better able to evaluate the posterior fossa, and more effective at determining the etiology of stroke or differentiating stroke from its mimics (Table 19.1). Alternatively, a noncontrast computed tomography (CT; and CT angiography if hemorrhage is present) may be obtained if MRI is not emergently available.

Migraine is a common stroke mimic and may be difficult to differentiate from stroke. Headache is common in both conditions. However, the neurological deficit most commonly seen in migraine is focal numbness. Visual symptoms and vomiting are also frequently present in migraine. Neurologic symptoms of migraines typically resolve in less than 30 minutes. In contrast, patients with AIS may experience acute focal weakness, speech changes, ataxia, and/or seizures. Migraines are more likely to affect older children.

Treatment

Initial management should prioritize stabilization of any life-threatening respiratory or hemodynamic abnormalities.

There are few data on the specific treatment of ischemic stroke in pediatric patients, and most of the current management regimen is extrapolated from treatment of adult stroke. Accepted treatments include anticoagulants such as low-molecular-weight heparin or unfractionated heparin, as well as antiplatelet agents such as aspirin. Revascularization is used in conjunction with aspirin in patients with Moyamoya disease. Because of a lack of data on both safety and efficacy in children, thrombolytics are not currently the standard of care in the hyperacute period of pediatric stroke. Mechanical thrombectomy may be performed in some cases; however, the literature on children is limited.

HEMORRHAGIC STROKE

In children, unlike adults, hemorrhagic stroke accounts for half of all strokes, and mortality is higher (25% vs. 10% for AIS; Table 19.2).

Classic Clinical Presentation

Children with hemorrhagic stroke often present with headache as well as signs and symptoms of increased intracranial pressure (ICP).

Treatment

Hemorrhagic stroke commonly leads to increased ICP. Treatment includes efforts to reduce ICP while maintaining cerebral perfusion pressure in order to prevent herniation. The head of the patient's bed should be elevated to 30 degrees. Other important measures

TABLE 19.2 HEMORRHAGIC STROKE: COMMON ETIOLOGIES AND RISK FACTORS

Vascular anomalies	Oncologic processes
Arteriovenous malformation	Intracranial tumor
Cavernous malformation	Leukemia
Aneurysm	Hematologic abnormalities
Hereditary hemorrhagic telangiectasia	Sickle cell disease
Collagen vascular diseases	Thrombocytopenia
Ehler–Danlos syndrome	Hemophilia
Marfan syndrome	Disseminated intravascular coagulation
	Liver failure

include avoiding hypoxemia, hypoglycemia, and hypotension. Hyperosmotic agents (mannitol and hypertonic saline) may be used to temporarily lower ICP. Targeted treatment of bleeding abnormalities (e.g. platelets, fresh frozen plasma, and clotting factor) may be indicated. Neurosurgical intervention may be necessary to control bleeding or relieve ICP.

CEREBRAL SINUS VENOUS THROMBOSIS

Background

Cerebral sinus venous thrombosis (CSVT) is a rare but important cause of stroke in children, and can lead to ischemia or hemorrhagic transformation. It is important to note that the ischemia may not follow a classic arterial pattern. CSVT may be associated with surgical procedures; head infections such as mastoiditis, otitis media, and sinusitis; prothrombic states; anemia; and dehydration. Underlying medical issues such as congenital heart disease, nephrotic syndrome, lupus, and malignancy may also predispose to this condition.

Classic Clinical Presentation

Cerebral sinus venous thrombosis generally presents with neurologic symptoms such as altered mental status, seizures, and focal neurologic deficits. It may lead to signs and symptoms of increased ICP, including headache, papilledema, isolated cranial nerve palsy, and encephalopathy. However, it may also present with nonfocal neurologic signs and symptoms, which can impede diagnosis. Neonates most frequently develop seizures, whereas older children are more likely to have focal or diffuse neurologic signs and symptoms.

Treatment

Management of CSVT involves treatment of the underlying cause, often in conjunction with antibiotics, as well as anticoagulation with unfractionated heparin (UFH) or low-molecular-weight heparin (LMWH). Surgical intervention is rarely required.

STROKE ASSOCIATED WITH SICKLE CELL DISEASE

The pediatric sickle cell population is at particular risk of stroke because of red blood cell dysmorphology. Ischemic strokes are most common, although hemorrhagic stroke and cerebral venous thrombosis may occur as well. A reticulocyte count, percentage hemoglobin S, and type and crossmatch should be performed in addition to the labs detailed previously.

Treatment

The primary goal of treatment in stroke due to sickle cell disease is to decrease the amount of hemoglobin S to less than 30% of total hemoglobin. The ideal treatment is exchange transfusion, but simple transfusion can initially be performed as a temporizing measure if the hemoglobin is less than 9 g/dL. Aspirin is also commonly given.

NEONATAL STROKE

Neonatal stroke, which is caused by cerebral injury between 20 weeks of fetal life and 28 days of postnatal life, may be ischemic or hemorrhagic, or it may be related to cerebral sinus venous thrombosis. It can be caused by intrauterine factors, delivery, and congenital abnormalities such as congenital heart disease.

Seizure is the most common presentation of neonatal stroke. Other presenting symptoms include altered mental status (lethargy/irritability), vomiting, and apnea. Focal neurological deficits, bulging fontanelle, abnormal tone, and increased head circumference may be seen on examination.

Disposition

All patients with possible diagnosis of stroke should be admitted to the hospital for treatment. Intensive care is required for acute symptoms, particularly in the case of children with potential to decompensate or require respiratory or hemodynamic intervention.

Key Points

- Pediatric stroke is a leading cause of childhood mortality.
- Diagnostic delay is common.
- A detailed neurologic examination should be performed on every child with altered mental status, seizure, or behavioral changes.
- Point-of-care glucose is an important first step in evaluation.
- MRI is the preferred imaging option to evaluate stroke.

- Thrombolytics are not routinely recommended for AIS in children younger than age 12 years.

Pitfalls

- Failure to consider the diagnosis of stroke in a child with altered mental status, focal neurological deficit, seizure, or behavioral changes
- Failure to perform a detailed neurological examination on a child with neurological symptoms

VENOUS THROMBOEMBOLISM

Background

Venous thromboembolism (VTE) most commonly refers to deep vein thrombosis (DVT) and pulmonary embolism (PE), although it can occur anywhere in the vascular system, including the renal and portal circulation systems. Virchow's triad of stasis, endothelial injury, and hypercoagulability are the primary risk factors for VTE. VTE is significantly less common in children than in adults. Compared with adults, children have less chronic disease that damages vascular endothelium and fewer acquired prothrombotic risk factors. Furthermore, children generate less thrombin and have better inhibition, so clots are less likely to form.

Nearly all children with VTE have at least one risk factor, and many have more than one (Table 19.3). The most common risk factor is indwelling central venous catheter (CVC).

Classical Clinical Presentation

Presentation of VTE depends on the location as well as the size of the thrombus. VTEs may be asymptomatic, or they may cause local or extensive symptoms.

When symptomatic, patients with CVC-associated VTE may have swelling and discoloration of the affected limb. More extensive VTEs can lead to superior vena cava syndrome, pulmonary embolism, and chylothorax.

Because of their association with CVCs, DVTs occur more commonly in the upper extremities of children than in adults. Pain, associated swelling, and discoloration of the affected limb may occur.

The presentation of pulmonary embolism is similar in children and in adults, but the incidence is significantly lower in children. In addition, children typically have better physiologic reserve, and even significant PEs found incidentally on imaging may be clinically silent or minimally symptomatic. Classic symptoms include chest pain, dyspnea, tachypnea, cough, and hypoxia.

Differential Diagnosis

Table 19.4 presents the differential diagnosis for VTE.

Diagnostic Confirmation

Ultrasonography is both sensitive and specific for the diagnosis of extremity DVT. CT pulmonary angiography is the test of choice for suspect PE. However, because of the significant associated radiation of CT, it should be performed only in children with significant risk factors and a high pretest probability/clinical suspicion (rather than searching for the quite rare "occult PE" in a child).

TABLE 19.3 RISK FACTORS FOR VENOUS THROMBOEMBOLISM

Central venous catheter	Infection
Peripherally inserted central catheter	Trauma
Thrombophilia	Nephrotic syndrome
Factor V Leiden	Autoimmune disease
Protein C or S deficiency	Inflammatory bowel disease
Antithrombin deficiency	Systemic lupus erythematosus
Increased lipoprotein(a) levels	Medications (e.g., oral contraceptive pills)

TABLE 19.4 DIFFERENTIAL DIAGNOSIS FOR VENOUS THROMBOEMBOLISM

Symptom	Other Causes
Extremity skin changes	Cellulitis, superficial thrombophlebitis
Extremity swelling	Lymphangitis, lymphatic blockage
Extremity pain	Musculoskeletal injury
Chest pain, dyspnea, hypoxia	Cardiac disease, arrhythmia, pneumothorax, foreign body, acute chest, cardiac tamponade, pneumonia

Treatment

Anticoagulants such as UFH, LMWH, and vitamin K antagonists such as warfarin are mainstays of therapy. Thrombolytics are not routinely used unless occlusion is so extensive that it threatens the viability of organs or extremities.

Treatment is aimed not only at addressing an existing thrombus and preventing extension, but also at preventing recurrence and reducing complications. Patients are often maintained on anticoagulant therapy, and underlying issues need to be addressed. Patients with unprovoked VTE require longer treatment. This may include the removal of a CVC, if possible, as well as discontinuation of medications such as oral contraceptive pills.

VTE prophylaxis includes both mechanical means, such as compression boots, and pharmacologic prophylaxis.

Disposition

Patients with VTE usually require close monitoring. Stable patients on appropriate therapy may be discharged with close follow-up. However, most patients with VTE have significant associated comorbidities and require admission for monitoring. Intensive care may be required for significant PEs or associated complications.

Complications

Rare complications of DVTs include ischemia and compartment syndrome. Propagation may occur to the lungs and cause PE. Large PEs may result in cardiovascular collapse and death. Anticoagulant therapy may also result in bleeding, which is rarely life-threatening.

Key Points

- Virtually all VTEs in children occur with risk factors, frequently more than one.
- Indwelling CVCs are the most significant risk factor for VTE in children.
- Although VTE is rare in children, it can cause significant morbidity and mortality.

Pitfall

- Do not search for an occult PE in a child without risk factors.

HYPERTENSIVE EMERGENCY

Hypertension in children may be primary or secondary (due to an underlying etiology that requires identification and intervention). Common etiologies of secondary hypertension are listed in Table 19.5.

TABLE 19.5 SECONDARY HYPERTENSIVE ETIOLOGIES BY AGE

Age Group	Etiologies
Infant	Renovascular disease Congenital renal anomalies Coarctation of the aorta Congenital adrenal hyperplasia Bronchopulmonary dysplasia
Child	Glomerulonephritis Renovascular disease Endocrine abnormalities
Adolescent	Renal parenchymal disease Toxicologic causes Serotonin syndrome

An accurate blood pressure reading is best obtained with ideal positioning and appropriately sized cuff. The patient should be seated with the arm at the level of the heart (the reading can be falsely elevated if the arm is lower than the heart). The bladder length should be 80% of the patient's arm circumference, and the width of the cuff should be at least 40% of the patient's arm circumference.

Classical Clinical Presentation

Hypertensive emergency is defined as acute severe hypertension with target organ damage or life-threatening features. Hypertensive encephalopathy (presenting with altered mental status and/or seizures) is the most common hypertensive emergency in children. Signs and symptoms of target organ damage are listed in Table 19.6.

TABLE 19.6 SIGNS AND SYMPTOMS OF TARGET ORGAN DAMAGE

Organ System	Symptoms
Central nervous system	Headache, altered mental status, seizures
Eye	Papilledema, retinal hemorrhage, retinal exudates
Heart	Left ventricular heart failure
Kidney	Glomerulonephritis (hematuria, proteinuria), acute kidney injury

Reversible posterior leukoencephalopathy syndrome (RPLS), also called posterior reversible encephalopathy syndrome (PRES), is an emergent condition that can occur in patients with hypertensive encephalopathy as well as in patients in kidney failure, those with systemic diseases such as systemic lupus erythematosus, and those with eclampsia. This condition is characterized by white matter changes in the posterior hemispheres and by headache, altered level of consciousness, visual changes, and seizures. Treatment of hypertension-related RPLS involves emergent management of hypertension as well as seizure intervention (see Chapter 20 on neurologic emergencies).

Diagnostic Confirmation

Hypertensive emergencies should be identified clinically based on specific symptomatology and examination findings. Additional confirmatory diagnostic tests include laboratory studies (e.g., basic metabolic panel, urinalysis, and complete blood count) to evaluate for kidney function and the presence of hemolysis. Electrocardiography should be performed to evaluate for signs of heart strain; chest X-ray may reveal cardiomegaly or signs of congenital abnormalities; and head imaging (CT or MRI) may be required with altered mental status, focal deficits, or seizures. Four limb blood pressures may help confirm suspected coarctation.

Treatment

Anti-hypertensive medications should be initiated in symptomatic patients. The most commonly used medications in hypertensive emergency are intravenous labetalol and nicardipine; see Table 19.7 for anti-hypertensive agents. The goal is to reduce the patient's blood pressure to below the 95th percentile (the appropriate number varies by age and can be found in many online and app-based resources). Hypertension-related seizures should also be treated with anticonvulsants (see Chapter 20 on neurologic emergencies).

Although emergent management is indicated in symptomatic patients, it is imperative to note that aggressively lowering blood pressure can be dangerous. Cerebral perfusion must be maintained; ischemia may be induced if long-standing hypertension or conditions with elevated ICP are treated aggressively. (See Chapter 44 on obstetrical emergencies for management of pre-eclampsia/eclampsia.)

Disposition

Patients with hypertensive emergency should be admitted to the hospital, in most cases to the intensive care unit, particularly if they are on intravenous infusions. Further management should be based on underlying etiology and associated symptoms.

Management of Non-Emergency Hypertension

Patients with asymptomatic hypertension are commonly seen in the pediatric emergency department. These patients should have good follow-up to manage

TABLE 19.7 ANTI-HYPERTENSIVE AGENTS FOR HYPERTENSIVE EMERGENCIES IN CHILDREN

Agent	Classification	Dosing	Comments
Labetalol	α- and β-adrenergic blocker	Bolus: 0.2–1 mg/kg/dose, up to 40 mg/dose Infusion: 0.25–3 mg/kg/hr IV	Contraindicated in asthma, heart failure, diabetes May cause hyperkalemia and hypoglycemia
Nicardipine	Calcium channel blocker	Bolus: 30 μg/kg to 2 mg/dose Infusion: 0.5–4 μg/kg/min IV	May cause reflex tachycardia
Hydralazine	Direct vasodilator	0.2–0.6 mg/kg maximum single dose 20 mg IV or IM	May cause reflex tachycardia, fluid retention, or headaches
Esmolol	β_1-Adrenergic blocker	100–500 μg/kg/min, up to 1,000 μg/kg/min	Very short-acting May cause bradycardia Contraindicated in asthma and heart failure

IV, intravenously; IM, intramuscularly.

hypertension, both to reduce risk of target organ damage in childhood and to reduce risks of hypertension and vascular disease in adulthood.

Key Points

- Assess for target organ damage in all hypertensive patients.
- Hypertensive encephalopathy is the most common hypertensive emergency in children.
- Titratable intravenous therapy (most commonly labetalol and nicardipine) should be judiciously administered and titrated to symptoms and target blood pressure of 95th percentile for age.

Pitfalls

- Failure to recognize hypertensive emergency and initiate treatment in children.
- Failure to consider secondary hypertension and underlying cause.

Further Reading

Buckowski A, Rose E. Pediatric stroke: Diagnosis and management in the emergency department. *Pediatr Emerg Med Pract.* 2019;16(11):1–20. PMID 31647863

20

Neurologic Emergencies

MOLLY HARTRICH AND EMILY ROSE

SEIZURE

Background/Epidemiology

Children have a lower seizure threshold and seize more commonly than adults. The majority of seizures in children are febrile seizures. Up to 5% of children have febrile seizures, with peak incidence at approximately 18 months.

Classic Clinical Presentation

The classic presentation of seizure in children depends on category of seizure. In generalized seizure activity, both cerebral hemispheres are involved. The following are types of generalized seizures:

- Absence seizures in which children may have a "blank stare" with reduced awareness and responsiveness lasting seconds.
- Tonic–clonic seizures have two phases. They typically begin with an alteration in consciousness, after which muscles stiffen. The clonic phase typically involves jerking and twitching of all limbs. Seizure activity may be tonic without a clonic phase or clonic without a tonic phase. Simple febrile seizures are often generalized tonic–clonic seizures.
- Myoclonic seizures result in a sudden jerk of a part of the body.
- Atonic seizures are also known as drop seizures, akinetic seizures, or drop attacks. During these seizures, there is a partial or complete loss of muscle tone.

A partial seizure is an electrical disturbance that is limited to one hemisphere:

- Simple partial seizures may involve sensory, motor, psychic, or autonomic disturbances during which normal consciousness is maintained.
- Complex partial seizures involve motor, sensory, psychic, or autonomic disturbances during which there is an altered level of consciousness.
- Partial seizures with secondary generalization occur when the electrical disturbance that was initially limited to one area of the brain spreads to both hemispheres, resulting in tonic–clonic seizures and loss of consciousness.

Seizures may be provoked as a result of head trauma, fever, toxins, hypoglycemia, or electrolyte abnormalities. They may also be unprovoked as a result of brain malformation, disturbance of neuronal migration, or a genetic syndrome, or they may be cryptogenic.

Differential Diagnosis and Seizure Mimics

Seizure mimics vary by age group. In infancy and young childhood, gastroesophageal reflux, breath-holding spells, normal neonatal reflexes, and jitteriness as well as migratory myoclonic movements or sleep myoclonus are self-limited and benign. Most seizure mimics are due to benign causes, but there are more concerning causes. For example, hyperekplexia is a profound startle in infants to any sudden touch or sound that may render the child apneic. Children with opsoclonus–myoclonus–ataxia may have neuroblastoma.

As children age, the differential diagnosis of seizure activity becomes similar to that of adults:

- Syncope
- Migraine variants
- Myoclonic jerks
- Movement disorders/tics
- Sleep disorder: night terrors and narcolepsy
- Cataplexy
- Psychogenic nonepileptic seizure

Life-threatening causes of seizure activity in children are also broad and include the following:

- Electrolyte derangements
- Infection
- Inborn errors of metabolism
- Trauma and non-accidental trauma
- Infection
- Withdrawal syndromes
- Hypoxemia
- Ruptured arteriovenous malformation
- Brain tumor
- Hypertensive encephalopathy
- Eclampsia
- Cryptogenic
- Toxic ingestions

Seizure Variants

Neonatal seizures can be difficult to distinguish because they are frequently subtle and tonic–clonic movements are not commonly seen. Rather, neonates may exhibit generalized fragmented clonic movements; focal clonic activity; myoclonic jerks; tonic extensions; or automatisms such as bicycling movements with their legs, lip smacking, and ocular movements.

The following are the most common causes of neonatal seizure:

- Hypoxic–ischemic encephalopathy (usually within 48 hours)
- Intracranial hemorrhage (10% of neonatal seizures)
  - Birth trauma
  - Preterm infants
- Congenital intracranial anomalies
- Benign familial neonatal seizures
- Non-accidental trauma
- Metabolic disturbances
  - Formula mishaps and inborn errors of metabolism causing hypernatremia or hyponatremia
  - Hypoglycemia
  - Hypocalcemia
  - Hypomagnesemia
  - Pyridoxine deficiency
- Infection
  - Herpes simplex encephalitis particularly in neonates with focal seizure activity

Investigation and Diagnosis

A full septic workup should be initiated for neonates with seizure, particularly those with fever or hypothermia. Additional testing with early point-of-care glucose, electrolytes including magnesium and calcium levels, complete blood count, blood and urine cultures, toxicology screen, and cerebrospinal fluid (CSF) analysis should be part of the initial workup. If inborn errors of metabolism are suspected, serum studies for amino acids, pyruvate, ammonia, and urine organic acids may be added. Extra red and green top tubes can also be set aside for the pediatric geneticist. [See Chapter 2 on the crashing neonate for further details on inborn errors of metabolism (IEM) diagnosis.]

Ultrasound (US), computed tomography (CT), and magnetic resonance imaging (MRI) have utility in the workup of a neonate with seizure activity. US can detect abnormalities in ventricular size, either due to hydrocephalus with or without ventricular hemorrhage or due to hypoxemic injury and edema, as well as intraparenchymal hemorrhage, but it lacks sufficient sensitivity. MRI is the diagnostic imaging method of choice and is most sensitive to detect cerebral dysgenesis.

Treatment

Because the etiology of neonatal seizure is usually secondary to an underlying infection or metabolic or structural abnormality, seizure activity is usually not responsive to conventional therapies. When sepsis is suspected, early antimicrobials are important, as is treating any underlying electrolyte or metabolic derangement.

Phenobarbital is the first-line antiepileptic in neonates, followed by fosphenytoin or phenytoin. Pyridoxine 100 mg intravenously (IV) should be given if the first phenobarbital does not stop the initial seizure (for treatment of pyridoxine deficiency IEM). Levetiracetam, Ativan, lidocaine, and midazolam are second-line alternatives, although they are not as thoroughly studied.

Disposition

All neonates with seizures should be admitted for further evaluation and treatment. Aside from a few benign genetic neonatal epilepsies that are diagnoses of exclusion, most neonatal seizures are secondary to a provoking factor.

FEBRILE SEIZURE

Simple febrile seizures occur in neurologically normal children aged 6 months to 5 years. The seizure duration is less than 15 minutes, and there is no focality. There should be no recurrence within 24 hours. A complex febrile seizure does not meet criteria for simple febrile seizure by duration, frequency, patient population, or semiology. Approximately one-third of febrile seizures are classified as complex.

Investigation and Diagnostics

For children who meet criteria for simple febrile seizure, minimal testing is required in those who are well-appearing and have returned to neurologic baseline. A point-of-care glucose should be obtained. Additional testing is guided by clinical appearance of the child (see Chapter 9 on fever). In well-appearing, fully immunized children with simple febrile seizure, lumbar puncture is not recommended by recent American Academy of Pediatrics guidelines.

In contrast to simple febrile seizure, the heterogeneity of complex febrile seizures limits its definitive management guidelines. Although isolated seizure without additional findings is an uncommon presentation for meningitis, a thorough neurological examination and mental status assessment should be performed in all patients with seizure. Complex febrile seizures with focal seizures are at increased risk of intracranial pathology or infection. Any child with a focal neurologic deficit, persistent altered mental status, or febrile status epilepticus should be considered higher risk, and imaging and lumbar puncture should be considered.

Treatment

Treatment of febrile seizures is based on the following three principles:

1. Acute seizure management: Cessation of seizure activity and providing necessary respiratory and hemodynamic support are acute management priorities.
2. Diagnose and management of cause of fever: In a resolved simple seizure, there are no additional evaluation requirements.
3. Anticipatory guidance for parents and families can be the most important portion of the treatment algorithm in a child with a simple febrile seizure. Parental/provider fear of the witnessed seizure requires significant and detailed reassurance. Education should include emphasis on the excellent overall prognosis and low likelihood of long-term sequelae. Approximately one-third to one-half of all simple febrile seizures recur, and recurrence is more likely in those younger than age 18 months and those with a family history of febrile seizure, shorter duration of fever prior to seizing, or lower temperature at onset of seizure. The risk for epilepsy for a child after febrile seizure is similar to that for the general population at approximately 1%, which may assuage fears about chronic seizure disorder or brain injury caused by seizure.

Disposition

Most children with a simple febrile seizure who have a normal mental status, normal neurologic examination that is appropriate for age and development, and no known central nervous system (CNS) disease can be safely discharged home with personal medical doctor follow-up within 1 week. No outpatient imaging is indicated.

Complex febrile seizures may be observed if well-appearing. Persistent altered mental status or focal neurological deficits should trigger further evaluation.

FIRST-TIME SEIZURE IN AFEBRILE PATIENT

Children have a lower seizure threshold than adults. By age 14 years, approximately1% of children in the United States have had one afebrile seizure, with incidence highest in children younger than age 3 years. Seventy percent of first-time, unprovoked seizures are idiopathic, and recurrence rate varies between 14% and 65%. The vast majority (nearly 90%) of recurrent seizures occur within 2 years.

Investigation and Diagnostics

Laboratory studies and imaging are not routinely indicated in a well-appearing child with a normal neurologic examination. Electrolyte studies should be obtained in children younger than age 6 months and those with prolonged seizures, history of diabetes or other metabolic abnormality, dehydration, history of excess free water intake (i.e., formula mishaps), persistent altered level of consciousness, or developmental status at which a normal neurologic status is unable to be obtained. Pregnancy testing should be performed in all pubescent females because eclampsia may present with seizure. An electrocardiogram (ECG) should strongly be considered in all patients to evaluate for life-threatening arrhythmias because syncope with clonic movements may be mistaken as seizure activity (even by medical personnel).

Imaging should be considered for high-risk features such as focal activity, persistent altered mental status, or underlying medical conditions including sickle cell disease, bleeding diatheses, cerebral vascular disorders, malignancy, HIV/AIDS, or associated trauma.

Treatment

Outpatient antiepileptic medications are not recommended after an initial afebrile seizure and are typically started after a second seizure.

Disposition

Well-appearing children with a normal neurological examination may be discharged home with outpatient follow-up. Outpatient electroencephalogram (EEG) is recommended for all first-time unprovoked seizures.

BREAKTHROUGH SEIZURE IN PATIENT WITH KNOWN SEIZURE DISORDER

Investigation and Diagnostics

Breakthrough seizures may occur secondary to acute infection (which may lower the seizure threshold), growth of child [resulting in subtherapeutic dosages of antiepileptic drugs (AEDs)], medication noncompliance, disruption in sleep/stress, among many other causes. Thorough history and physical examination with detailed neurologic assessment should be performed.

Routine laboratory testing in a well-appearing child who is at neurologic baseline is of little utility outside of checking levels for antiepileptic medications. Low levels or toxic levels may lead to increased seizures.

Children with recurrent seizures who present to the emergency department (ED) without new neurologic abnormalities or evidence of trauma do not necessitate neurologic imaging.

Treatment

Acute seizure termination and respiratory support are the management priorities.

If the patient's home medication level is subtherapeutic, a bolus dose can be given, and a dose increase may be recommended in conjunction with the patient's pediatric neurologist.

Disposition

Patients who have returned to their neurologic baseline and have no evidence of infection, toxic ingestion, or other reversible cause for breakthrough seizure that would necessitate hospitalization can be discharged home with parents and close pediatric neurologist follow-up.

SEIZURES DUE TO TOXIC INGESTIONS

Benzodiazepines are the first-line medication for seizure in presumed toxic ingestion; however, phenytoin and fosphenytoin should be avoided. Seizures that are toxin mediated may be due to sodium channel blockade, and phenytoin/fosphenytoin may exacerbate the underlying condition.

The following are important toxins associated with seizures:

- Antidepressants
  - Bupropion has significant potential to produce seizure in overdose. Management is supportive, but patients may require intubation.
- Antihistamines with anticholinergic properties
- Anticonvulsants in overdose may induce seizure activity. In addition, children who are chronically dependent on or abusing benzodiazepines may have withdrawal seizures.
- Isoniazid [isonicotinic acid hydrazide (INH)] in overdose can rapidly produce seizures or even death. Doses >30 mg/kg produce seizures, and doses 80–150 mg/kg can rapidly lead to death. In a known quantity of overdose in adults and adolescents, a 1:1 ratio of pyridoxine to ingested INH should be administered. In unknown dose, 5 g of pyridoxine can be administered empirically in adolescents and repeated if seizures continue. In younger children, a dose of 70–300 mg/kg can be given. Benzodiazepines may have a synergistic effect with the pyridoxine in seizure termination and should also be given.
- Baclofen, an antispasmodic frequently used in children with spasticity such as cerebral palsy, can cause seizure in overdose and when discontinued too rapidly.

STATUS EPILEPTICUS

Status epilepticus (SE) is the most common serious neurological emergency in children. A treatment algorithm should be initiated promptly because seizure termination becomes more difficult the longer a seizure is sustained. See Figure 20.1. Although the traditional definition of SE was seizure activity for 20–30 minutes, the current recommendation is to initiate an SE treatment algorithm within 5 minutes of seizure to decrease morbidity and improve the likelihood of successful termination. Permanent neurologic sequelae may occur after 30 minutes of tonic–clonic SE.

Approximately 10% of children with new-onset pediatric seizure present to the ED in SE. Up to 25% cases of SE are attributed to febrile seizures (although SE only occurs in ~5% of febrile seizures overall).

After a prolonged period of convulsive seizures, the significant physical manifestations of the child's seizure activity may diminish to become so subtle or even nonconvulsive so that differentiating between a postictal state and nonconvulsive SE (NCSE) may be nearly impossible by physical examination alone. NCSE may account for 25% of all cases of SE, and 25% of all cases of convulsive SE devolve into subtle or "burnt out" generalized SE or NCSE.

After 20–30 minutes of seizure activity, 10–25% of cases of SE become refractory, and breathing often becomes irregular, frequently necessitating intubation and mechanical ventilation.

Investigation and Diagnostics

Because of the risk of decompensation in children with SE, simultaneous evaluation and treatment are imperative with a focus on general supportive care and evaluation and management of the patient's airway, breathing, and circulation (ABC). Management of the ABCs are paramount while simultaneously working to terminate the seizure and for the prevention of seizure recurrence, treatment of the precipitating cause, and treatment of potential complications.

When a child with epilepsy on an AED develops SE, AED levels should be obtained because low or toxic levels may precipitate SE. Toxicology studies and metabolic studies for inborn errors of metabolism should be considered in children with SE when there are clinical indicators for concern or when the initial evaluation reveals no etiology.

An EEG should be considered in a child with SE. This is helpful in determining subclinical or nonconvulsive SE as well as determining

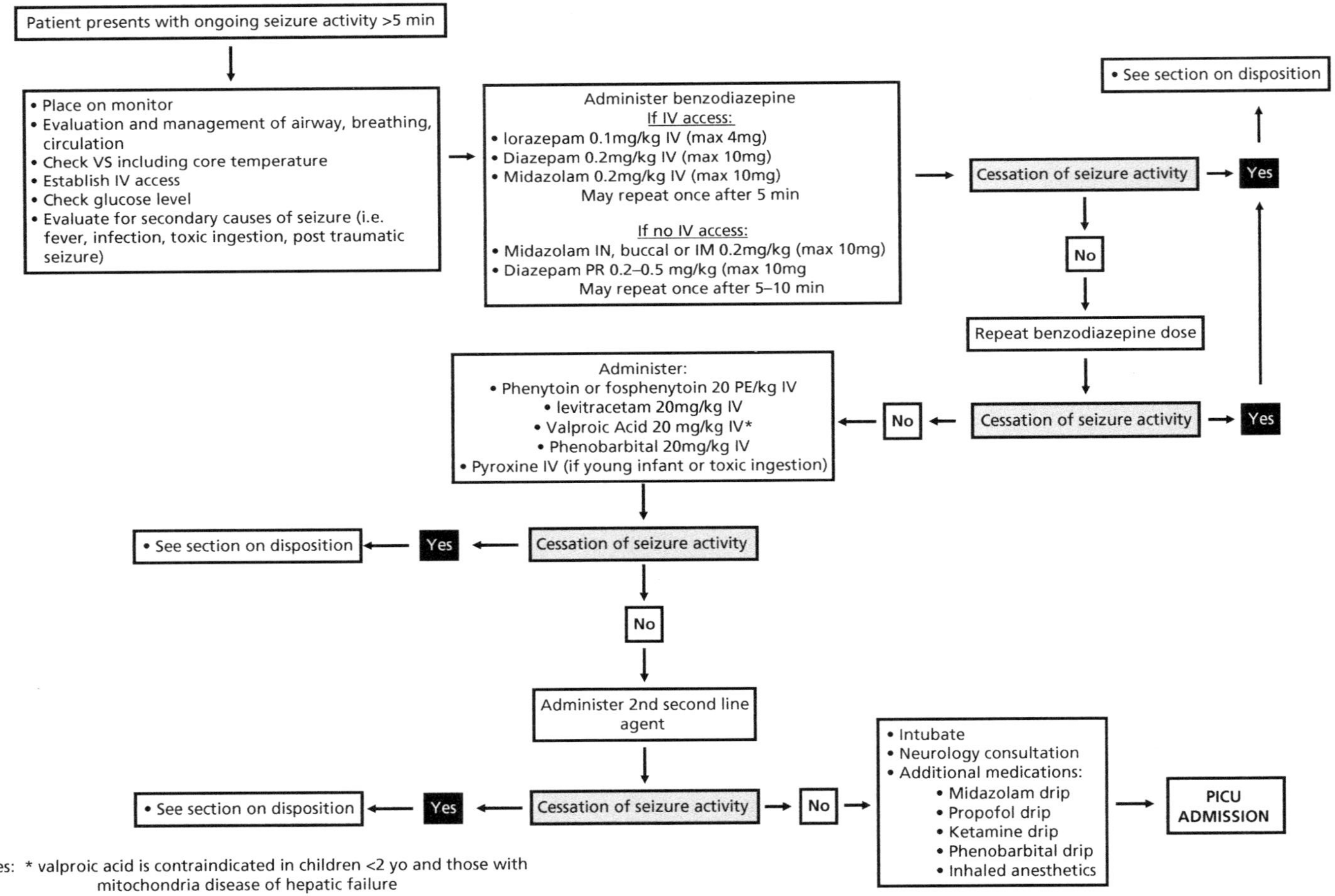

Notes: * valproic acid is contraindicated in children <2 yo and those with mitochondria disease of hepatic failure

FIGURE 20.1 Treatment algorithm for the management of status epilepticus.

whether there are focal or generalized epileptiform abnormalities that may guide further testing for the etiology of SE. Finally, EEG is helpful when there is a suspicion of pseudostatus epilepticus (nonepileptic SE).

Neuroimaging may be considered after the child with SE has been stabilized if there are clinical indications or if the etiology is unknown.

Evaluation for pregnancy should occur in pubescent females to rule out eclampsia as the etiology.

Treatment

Termination of seizure activity should initially be managed with benzodiazepines (Table 20.1).

Many children may need respiratory support with bagging during an active seizure or immediately after cessation. Children who are not able to protect their own airway and those who are hypoxic, apneic, or who generally have disordered control of breathing necessitate intubation. Care should be taken to monitor hemodynamics of children with SE, especially those receiving multiple AEDs because a number of AEDs have a side effect of hypotension.

Disposition

Most children with SE require hospital admission. Those with persistent seizures, altered mental status, or respiratory failure require intensive care management.

Complications of SE involve many organ systems and include cardiopulmonary failure, metabolic abnormalities, and permanent neurological sequelae.

Pitfalls

- Failure to utilize alternative formulations [intramuscular (IM), intranasal, buccal, or intraosseous] in an actively seizing child without IV access.
- Failure to recognize patients on ketogenic diets. Many medications and fluids have glucose, which can disrupt treatment. Children on ketotic diets will also have lower baseline glucose levels (50–75 mg/dL). These children are also at risk for hypoglycemia and should be treated at glucose levels of 45 mg/dL, being mindful that breaking the ketotic cycle can worsen seizure.
- Do not use sodium channel blocking agents such as carbamazepine, gabapentin, lamotrigine, and phenytoin in children with Dravet's syndrome. The first-line treatment for this complex seizure disorder is usually valproic acid (VPA). However, VPA is generally not prescribed to children younger than age 2 years unless at the discretion of the child's primary neurologist due to concerns for liver toxicity.
- Check any antiepileptic level that is measurable in your laboratory. Breakthrough seizures may be due to subtherapeutic and supratherapeutic toxicity.

TABLE 20.1 BENZODIAZEPINE DOSING FOR INITIAL SEIZURE MANAGEMENT

Drug	Route	Dose
Diazepam	IV	0.1–0.3 mg/kg, max 10 mg
	Rectal	Age 2–6 years: 0.5 mg/kg
		Age 6–12 years: 0.3 mg/kg
		Age >12 years: 0.2 mg/kg
Midazolam	IN	0.2 mg/kg, max 10 mg
	IM	0.1–0.2 mg/kg, max 10 mg
Lorazepam[a]	IV	0.1–0.2 mg/kg, max 10 mg
	IN	0.1 mg/kg

[a]IM lorazepam has inconsistent absorption and should not be used for seizure termination.

IN, intranasal; IM, intramuscular; IV, intravenous.

MOTOR DYSFUNCTION/ WEAKNESS SYNDROMES

Distinguishing features of weakness syndromes are presented in Table 20.2.

Guillain–Barré Syndrome

Guillain–Barré syndrome (GBS) is an autoimmune polyneuropathy that is usually triggered by an antecedent infection in which autoantibodies are produced that attack peripheral nerve components. Approximately two-thirds of patients have preceding respiratory or gastrointestinal infection. *Campylobacter* is the most common culprit, but Epstein–Barr virus, cytomegalovirus, influenza-like illnesses, *Mycoplasma pneumoniae*, and HIV have also been indicated. GBS may also occur after surgery, vaccination, trauma, or bone marrow transplantation. GBS is the most common cause of flaccid paralysis in children in the post-polio era.

Classic Clinical Presentation

Classically, patients will have pain and paresthesia in the fingers and toes that ascends symmetrically in a matter of hours to days and may affect the respiratory muscles, requiring mechanical ventilation. Areflexia is common. The most common presenting chief complaints in children with GBS are gait instability, neuropathic pain, and inability to walk. In half of children with GBS, there is a component of autonomic dysfunction with cardiac dysrhythmias, hypotension and hypertension, ileus, diaphoresis, and bladder dysfunction.

Atypical/Nonclassic Clinical Presentations

Guillain–Barré syndrome is a heterogeneous group of diseases, the most common of which is acute inflammatory demyelinating polyneuropathy (AIDP). AIDP affects up to 90% of children with GBS and has the classic presentation of ascending flaccid paralysis with paresthesias.

Acute motor axonal neuropathy (AMAN) is a purely motor neuropathy most commonly associated with *Campylobacter* infection. Rates of mechanical ventilation are higher with AMAN.

Miller Fisher syndrome is characterized by ophthalmoplegia, ataxia, and muscle weakness.

Many other GBS variants affect localized areas including cranial nerves, encephalopathies, pure sensory, proximal upper body/ neck involvement, and isolated autonomic dysfunction.

Mimics and Other Polyneuropathies

Severe vitamin B_1 deficiency, acute arsenic poisoning, *n*-hexane neurotoxicity (in glue sniffing neuropathy), vasculitis, Lyme disease, tick paralysis, porphyria, sarcoidosis, leptomeningeal disease, paraneoplastic disease, and critical illness may present with similar symptoms as GBS. Spinal cord disorders may also mimic GBS, and patients may have decreased deep tendon reflexes as well. Severe low back pain is often seen in GBS, as well as in spinal cord compression syndromes such as spinal epidural abscess or cauda equina syndrome. Neuromuscular junction disorders such as botulism and myasthenia gravis (MG) also present with weakness but do not have a sensory component. Acute polymyositis, acute rhabdomyolysis, and other myelopathies are also mimics.

Investigation and Diagnosis

Diagnosis is made clinically, but electrodiagnostic studies, CSF analysis, MRI, and serum

TABLE 20.2 DISTINGUISHING FEATURES OF WEAKNESS SYNDROMES

	Neuropathy	Myopathy	Neuromuscular Junction	Myelopathy
Distribution of weakness	Distal > proximal	Proximal > distal	Diffuse	Variable, usually symmetric
Reflexes	Decreased	Normal to decreased	Normal	Increased
Sensory involvement	Yes	No	No	Yes, often specific level
Tone	Normal or decreased	Normal	Normal	Increased
Pain	Often	Variable, usually none	None	Yes, often back pain
Bowel/bladder dysfunction	Normal	Normal	Normal	Present

immunoglobulin G (IgG) analysis support diagnosis. CSF will frequently yield high protein (>45 mg/dL) and normal white blood cell count. Concurrent HIV infection or other viral infection causing flaccid paralysis, such as West Nile virus, poliovirus, enterovirus 71, or Lyme disease, should be on the differential when sending CSF studies. A clinically important pitfall on CSF analysis is that it is frequently normal early in the disease. Only 50% of patients will have elevated protein levels after 1 week of symptoms and 75% will have elevated levels after 3 weeks of illness, so the clinician should not be dissuaded of the diagnosis if protein is not elevated.

Treatment

Mainstays of treatment for GBS are plasmapheresis and intravenous immunoglobulin (IVIG). Neither is more efficacious, and using two treatments simultaneously is not more efficacious than using one alone. Steroids do not appear to be helpful in hastening recovery and should not be initiated in the ED.

Disposition

Most patients will require an intensive care unit (ICU) level of care with continuous cardiac and respiratory monitoring until disease progression ceases and clinical improvement occurs.

Pitfalls

- Early in the disease course, symptoms may be very atypical of classic GBS.
- CSF studies should not be relied on early in the disease course because these studies may be falsely negative
- Muscle weakness may be proximal early in disease course, and reflexes may be preserved early.

Myasthenia Gravis

Myasthenia gravis is an autoimmune disorder in which autoantibodies directed at the acetylcholine receptor on the post-synaptic membrane are attacked, which results in inhibition of neuromuscular transmission at the post-synaptic membrane. Subtypes are juvenile, congenital, and transient neonatal. The earlier a diagnosis is made, the better the prognosis.

Differential Diagnosis

The differential diagnosis includes botulism; GBS (especially the Miller Fisher variant); Lambert–Eaton syndrome; hypermagnesemia; tick paralysis; brainstem tumors or mass lesions near the orbit, cavernous sinus, or sella turcica; brainstem encephalitis; multiple sclerosis; acute spinal cord compression with extremity weakness, with facial muscles spared in this case; organophosphate toxicity; and ingestion of other drugs known to worsen MG (including many antibiotics).

Myasthenia Gravis Subtypes in Children

Transient neonatal MG occurs in 10–20% of infants born to mothers with MG and is more common in mothers with active disease. Symptoms usually arise within a few hours of birth but can present as late as 3 days of life. In the rare occurrence an infant of an undiagnosed mother presents with symptoms of respiratory failure, bulbar weakness, hypotonia, ptosis, or ophthalmoplegia, treatment is supportive and further testing may be performed as an inpatient. More than 90% of infants recover by age 2 months.

Congenital MG is clinically indistinguishable from other forms, but the workup is often negative and traditional treatments are ineffective.

Juvenile MG is clinically identical to adult MG but is rare. There are two main forms: ocular and generalized. In ocular MG, isolated ptosis and diplopia occur without other generalized involvement. In generalized MG, generalized weakness may be the presenting symptom, or it may begin with ocular symptoms and progress to generalized within 1 year. Children with prepubertal onset tend to have more ocular and mild generalized MG and will more likely go into remission, whereas the postpubertal onset is most similar to adult-onset MG.

Investigation and Diagnostics

Diagnostic confirmation was historically performed with the "tensilon test" using edrophonium (now controversial due to medication side effects). Neostigmine is sometimes alternatively used. Onset of action is within 15 minutes, and the effects last 1 hour. An easy and safe test in the ED in a patient who presents with ptosis is the ice test (cold decreases acetylcholine degradation). An ice bag is applied to the affected eyelid for 2–5 minutes. An improvement in ptosis of >2 mm is considered a positive test. The definitive neurodiagnostic study in suspected MG is repetitive nerve stimulation.

Treatment

Treatment consists of anticholinesterase medications, the mainstay of which is pyridostigmine bromide. Immunosuppressive agents such as prednisone, azathioprine, tacrolimus, cyclophosphamide, and rituximab may be added to pyridostigmine nonresponders.

Thymectomy is best done during the early course of disease. Plasmapheresis or IVIG is used in myasthenic crisis.

The treatment algorithm for myasthenic crisis begins with stabilization of a critically ill patient. Precipitating infections should be treated, and causative medications should be withdrawn.

Myasthenic crisis is an exacerbation of symptoms that typically requires ventilatory assistance. Adults and children with MG who are in crisis will have bulbar weakness, dysphagia, dysphonia, and risk of choking and aspiration necessitating mechanical ventilation. In one-third to one-half of cases, no precipitating cause for crisis is found, but infection, particularly respiratory illness, is often a precipitating factor. Pregnancy, childbirth, surgery, emotional stress, sleep deprivation, certain medications, and changes in immunomodulating medications can precipitate myasthenic crisis. Often, there is a progressive generalized muscle weakness that leads to respiratory failure; however, patients may present with sudden respiratory failure without preceding generalized weakness.

Ventilatory support is the management priority for patients in myasthenic crisis. Noninvasive positive pressure ventilation may preclude the need for endotracheal intubation. Assessment of respiratory function during an acute exacerbation may be challenging in children.

One suggested assessment in children who are able to count is to have them try to count to 30 in one breath. Those who cannot count to 20 are likely to have significant impairment of their respiratory muscles. Other bedside tests that may be helpful in the clinical assessment are forced vital capacity (FVC) and negative inspiratory force (NIF), both of which respiratory therapists may assist in obtaining. Normal FVC is >60 mL/kg, and intubation should be considered below 15–20 mL/kg. A normal NIF is >70 cm H_2O, and a worrisome NIF is <30 cm H_2O.

Neuromuscular blocking agents in children with myasthenic crisis are safe; however, dosages must be adjusted. Given the decreased density of Ach receptors at the motor end plate, two to four times the usual dose of succinylcholine is recommended. In contrast, nondepolarizing agents such as rocuronium have significantly enhanced activity and prolonged duration of action. One-half the normal dose should be given with nondepolarizing agents.

Cholinergic crisis may be precipitated by excessive cholinergic medications causing weakness. This is very difficult to decipher from a myasthenic crisis but should be suspected in patients taking high doses of pyridostigmine. Symptoms of cholinergic crisis are similar to the muscarinic effects of cholinergic toxicity: excessive secretions, lacrimation, perspiration, vomiting, and diarrhea, as well as bradycardia and bronchorrhea. Nicotinic effects include muscle weakness and fasciculations.

Disposition

Disposition is based on the clinical condition. Children in myasthenic crisis require ICU-level care; however, many children with MG are able to be discharged from the ED with outpatient follow-up. Factors include the rate of neurologic decline or change based on treatments and the presence or absence of concerning examination features such as bulbar weakness, dysphagia, or respiratory compromise. In mild flares such as worsening ptosis or diplopia, an increase in the dose of anticholinergic medications or initiation of steroids may be sufficient for the patient to be discharged with close outpatient follow-up after discussion with a pediatric neurologist.

Pitfalls

- Be cautious when initiating new medications in patients with MG, and check potential interactions.
- Assessment of respiratory status is paramount in any patient with MG who presents with intermittent worsening of symptoms.

Infantile Botulism

Infantile botulism is a flaccid paralysis caused by colonization of the intestinal tract by *Clostridium botulinum*. Colonization causes botulinum neurotoxin to be released and blocks presynaptic cholinergic neurotransmission, which affects smooth and skeletal muscle. Infantile botulism is seen predominantly in children up to age 1 year and is the most common form of botulism in the United States. Approximately 95% of cases occur in the first 6 months of life, with the median age of occurrence of 3 to 4 months. Sources of *C. botulinum* spores include disrupted soil that is brought into the home due to parental occupations or from the surrounding environment and also consumption of honey and corn syrup.

Investigations and Diagnostics

The diagnosis of infant botulism is clinical. Toxin and organisms may be isolated from stool, but this can take up to 4 days. Constipation is the most common initial sign, but this is often overlooked. The first signs of weakness involve muscles innervated by cranial nerves. Bulbar symptoms such as weak cry, poor suck and feeding, ptosis, and poor head control are followed by symmetric descending weakness involving the trunk and then extremities and, finally, the diaphragm, causing respiratory failure. Infants with botulism will also have decreased tone, reflexes, and autonomic dysfunction leading to tachycardia, hypertension, hypotension, urinary retention, and constipation.

Course

Weakness and paralysis progress for 1 or 2 weeks after onset of symptoms and may remain at that nadir for an additional 1–3 weeks before showing signs of improvement. The majority of children require intubation.

Treatment

The treatment for infant botulism is botulism immune globulin (BabyBIG), which binds circulating toxin. BabyBIG decreases duration of symptoms, length of mechanical ventilation, and hospitalization.

The store of BabyBIG for the United States is maintained by the California Department of Public Health via the Infant Botulism Treatment and Prevention Program (IBTPP). To obtain BabyBIG for a patient with suspected infant botulism (anywhere in the United States), the physician must contact the on-call physicians at IBTPP at (510) 231-7600 (24/7/365).

There is no role for antibiotics in this disease.

Disposition

All infants with suspected botulism should be admitted to a critical care setting. Prognosis is usually good with appropriate supportive care and antitoxin. Recovery is usually complete; however, it may be prolonged, up to 1 year.

Pitfalls

- Failure to recognize bulbar palsies in children
- Failure to consider botulism in infants with neuromuscular weakness and poor tone

Transverse Myelitis

Transverse myelitis is a rare, acquired neuro-immune disorder that affects both children and young adults. Acute transverse myelitis (ATM) presents with rapid onset of weakness, sensory changes, and autonomic dysfunction including bowel and bladder dysfunction. Symptoms can vary widely, but most patients will have collections of symptoms with weakness, sensory changes, and sphincter dysfunction, rather than isolated symptoms at onset. Symptom nadir can be rapidly progressive in hours to as long as 20 days. There is frequently a spinal cord level below which patients have sensory loss. The thoracic spine is the most common site involved.

Investigations and Diagnosis

Symptoms of weakness, sensory dysfunction, or autonomic instability generate a large differential diagnosis. See Box 20.1 for ATM diagnostic criteria.

Diagnostic certainty of ATM is often elucidated over time, after hospital admission. However, initiation of the workup (particularly exclusion of surgical emergencies) must be initiated in the ED. Transfer to specialty centers is often required.

Initial evaluation with MRI of the entire spine with and without gadolinium is necessary to rule out a compressive pathology that necessitates immediate surgical decompression. Brain MRI evaluates for alternative diagnoses (e.g., multiple sclerosis and acute demyelinating encephalomyelitis). Management is based on whether acute inflammation is suspected based on labs, CSF, and MRI findings.

BOX 20.1
DIAGNOSTIC CRITERIA FOR TRANSVERSE MYELITIS

Sensory, motor, or autonomic dysfunction attributable to the spinal cord
Bilateral signs and/or symptoms
Clearly defined sensory level
No evidence of compressive cord lesion
Inflammation defined by cerebrospinal fluid pleocytosis or elevated IgG index or gadolinium enhancement
Progression to nadir between 4 hours and 21 days

IgG, immunoglobulin G.
Source: Adapted from Krishnan C, Greenberg B. Transverse Myelitis. UpToDate. www.uptodate.com. Published 2016. Accessed June 16, 2019.

Treatment

High-dose IV steroids have been the mainstay of treatment for ATM. Adolescent patients may receive adult dosing, which is 1,000 mg of methylprednisolone daily or 200 mg of dexamethasone daily for 3–5 days. In younger children, 30 mg/kg/day of methylprednisolone is appropriate. Plasmapheresis may be considered if there is no clinical response, if there is worsening within the first 24–48 hours after initiation of steroids, or if there is significant motor dysfunction. Definitive airway management may be required if the cervical spine is involved.

Approximately one-third of patients recover with little or no sequelae, one-third are left with a moderate degree of permanent disability, and one-third have severe disabilities. Rapid progression of symptoms, back pain, and spinal shock portend poor prognosis.

Disposition

Children with suspected TM should be admitted with frequent neurologic checks. ICU is required with cervical spine involvement.

Pitfalls

- Failure to rule out compressive pathology that requires surgical decompression
- Failure to rule out other life-threatening pathology, such as meningitis and spinal cord ischemia
- Negative MRI in up to 40% of ATM cases

Periodic Paralysis

Periodic paralysis may be seen in hypokalemia and hyperkalemia, and it may be seen with and without concurrent thyroid dysfunction. Most forms of periodic paralysis in children have a family history of the disease.

Differential Diagnosis

- Guillain–Barré syndrome
- Transverse myelitis
- Myasthenia gravis
- Toxins such as ciguatera and tetrodotoxin
- Acute disseminated encephalomyelitis
- Porphyria

Hypokalemic periodic paralysis is the most common form of periodic paralysis. It is due to defects in muscle calcium and sodium channels and is associated with profound weakness that comes on after certain triggers, namely intense exercise and heavy carbohydrate meals, but can also be triggered by cold temperatures, emotional stress, menses, and pregnancy. Typically, the patient will notice weakness upon waking from sleep. Weakness begins in the proximal lower extremities and moves distally before affecting the upper extremities. Weakness progresses until flaccid paralysis with areflexia but with retained sensation. Cranial nerves and respiratory function are rarely affected. Mental status is preserved.

Diagnosis

Patients may have a serum potassium level <2 and may be initially identified with hypokalemia during an attack. Although the serum potassium levels are low, total body potassium is usually normal due to the shift of potassium into inexcitable muscle cells.

Treatment and Disposition

Patients may be repleted with 1 or 2 mEq/kg/dose every 30 minutes. Intravenous potassium should be avoided because total body potassium is normal. An ECG and continuous cardiac monitoring and neurological checks should be performed during repletion.

Thyrotoxic periodic paralysis is associated with hypokalemia, and treatment rests on correcting thyroid function before potassium repletion.

Acute Flaccid Myelitis

Acute flaccid myelitis (AMF) is a type of acute flaccid paralysis, of which poliovirus is the most well-known. Since 2012, there has been an epidemic of a polio-like AMF associated with enterovirus D68. AMF occurs as an acute viral infection that attacks the spinal cord and brainstem gray matter. Cranial nerves may also be affected. Acute flaccid paralysis is broadly defined by the World Health Organization as a sudden onset of paralysis/weakness in any part of the body of a child younger than age 15 years.

An antecedent illness commonly precedes the onset of weakness by 5–10 days. Weakness usually develops over 2–4 days. Pain, paresthesia, and hyperesthesia of the affected limbs are often present. Patients have hyporeflexia. Bulbar symptoms such as dysphagia, dyspnea, dysarthria, and pooling of secretions may also be seen.

Differential Diagnosis

- Acute myelopathy
  - Transverse myelitis
  - Cord compression (paraspinal or epidural abscess, tumor, hematoma)
- Poliomyelitis vaccine-associated paralytic poliomyelitis
- Non-polio enteroviruses
- Other viruses (Japanese encephalitis virus, West Nile virus, European tick-borne encephalitis virus, etc.)
- Polyradiculoneuropathy
  - Guillain–Barré syndrome
  - Peripheral neuropathy
- Infection-related: diphtheria, tick bite paralysis, Lyme disease, relapsing fever
- Chemicals (lead, arsenic, thallium)
- Medications (colchicine, aminoglycosides)
- Neuromuscular junction
  - Myasthenia gravis
  - Botulinum toxin
  - Tetanus toxin A
- Animal toxins (snake venom, dart-poison frog, puffer fish tetrodotoxin)
- Organophosphate poisoning
- Muscle disorders
- Polymyositis myositis (viral)
- Hypokalemic periodic paralysis

Investigations and Diagnostics

Diagnosis of AFM includes the presence of acute focal limb weakness and MRI evidence of predominantly gray matter lesion(s) spanning one or more spinal cord segments. CSF may have an elevated white blood cell count with lymphocytic predominance.

Treatment and Disposition

Because AFM occurs due to direct viral attack of the spinal cord, immunosuppression should be avoided. Care is supportive. There are no current established treatment regimens. Most children will have some recovery, but they will also have some persistent and possibly permanent weakness.

ALTERED LEVEL OF CONSCIOUSNESS

Consciousness is a state of awareness of both one's self and the environment. In contrast, coma is a state of unconsciousness in which an individual is not responsive to any stimuli, even painful ones. Between these extremes are a number of altered levels of consciousness (ALOCs), including the following:

- Confusion, during which there is a loss of clear thinking and difficulty following commands.
- Disorientation often accompanies confusion. Usually, a loss of orientation to time occurs first, followed by loss of orientation to place and then disorientation to self.
- Delirium is associated with confused and disorganized or disconnected ideas.
- Lethargy is a state of extreme drowsiness. A lethargic child can be aroused with moderate stimulus.
- Stupor is diminished responsiveness.

There are both medical and structural causes for ALOC, and although these disorders can occur at any age, there are certain pediatric age groups for which some of these conditions are more common.

Clinical Presentation

The presentation of altered mental status in children is as varied as the etiologies that cause this pathologic state. For example, a child may present with ALOC in subclinical SE due to brain tumor, hyponatremia, or cerebral edema from diabetic ketoacidosis (DKA). A child who has altered respiratory function may have accidentally ingested opiate medication or have a structural lesion in the pons or medulla. A broad differential for children with ALOC must be maintained no matter the dominant clinical features of the presentation.

Differential Diagnosis

The etiology of ALOC falls into two general categories: structural and metabolic. Structural causes involve pathology of the brain parenchyma. They may be focal (e.g., intracerebral tumor or brain abscess) or diffuse (e.g., trauma with corresponding diffuse cerebral edema). Metabolic causes include underlying infectious, toxic, or metabolic derangements such as DKA, anoxia, or opiate intoxication or overdose.

Helpful mnemonics to ensure a broad differential are AEIOU TIPS and MOVESTUPID. They are both fairly comprehensive and are helpful in the acute setting to ensure clinicians explore the most life-threatening causes of ALOC in children.

A	Alcohol, acidosis
E	Epilepsy
I	Insulin
O	Overdose
U	Uremia
T	Trauma
I	Infection
P	Psychosis
S	Stroke
M	Metabolic: inborn errors of metabolism
O	Oxygen insufficiency: hypoxia due to cardiopulmonary etiology, hypercarbia, carbon monoxide poisoning
V	Vascular/cardiac causes: cerebrovascular accident, vasculitis (SLE, MI), ventriculoperitoneal shunt malfunction
E	Endocrine/electrolyte: DKA, hypoglycemia, electrolyte abnormalities
S	Seizure/sepsis/shock
T	Tumor/trauma/temperature/toxins
U	Uremia
P	Psychiatric/porphyria
I	Infection/intussusception
D	Drugs/drama

A systems-based review is discussed next.

Toxicologic

Altered level of consciousness due to toxicologic exposure is secondary to either direct neurologic effect of the poisoning or a pathologic process due to the effect of the toxin, such as hypoglycemia in sulfonylurea ingestion or hepatic encephalopathy from acetaminophen toxicity. Also consider carbon monoxide poisoning, accidental or intentional ingestion, psychotropic medications, methemoglobinemia, and substance use disorder and overdose. See Chapter 50 on toxicologic emergencies for further details.

Trauma

Head trauma may have associated intracranial hemorrhage, diffuse axonal injury, diffuse cerebral edema, anoxic brain injury, non-accidental trauma, and concussion. These children have a variety of presentations that may be related to the etiology of symptoms and include ALOC, headache, irritability, apnea, ataxia, and focal neurologic deficits.

Neurologic

The evaluation and management of neurologic emergencies seizure, complicated migraine, encephalopathy leading to ALOC are discussed elsewhere in this chapter. Ischemic and hemorrhagic stroke are discussed in Chapter 21, and CSF shunt malfunction is discussed in Chapter 49.

Cardiac

Syncope with associated concerning cardiac etiology or arrhythmia-induced hypoxia or hypoperfusion may have associated ALOC (see Chapter 18 on cardiac emergencies).

Children with essential hypertension or hypertension due to another disease process (malignancy, renal disease, lupus, or sickle cell disease) may develop a hypertensive emergency such as posterior reversible encephalopathy with altered mental status as a sign of end-organ damage. See Chapter 19 on neurovascular emergencies.

Pulmonary

Any child with evidence of hypoxia or hypercarbia may be altered, but elucidating the cause of these metabolic derangements is key to management. Children with chronic lung conditions such as cystic fibrosis may be chronically hypoxic and hypercarbic and present altered, particularly in exacerbations of disease. Other children who are hypoventilating or present with late-stage disease in croup, bronchiolitis, or asthma may become hypercarbic and develop somnolence due to carbon dioxide narcosis.

Endocrine

- Hypoglycemic states
  - Hypoglycemia is a dangerous metabolic derangement with a multitude of etiologies, including infectious, toxicologic, oncologic, adrenal insufficiency, and malnutrition.
  - Drugs such as sulfonylureas and β-blockers can induce hypoglycemia in children even with one pill in exploratory ingestion (see Chapter 50). Children exhibit tremor, diaphoresis, weakness, pallor, and autonomic changes in addition to ALOC with confusion, seizure, or coma. Children may also be hypothermic in hypoglycemic states in which glucose is <55 mg/dL and sepsis may be an underlying cause.
- Hyperglycemic states (See chapter 30)
  - DKA
  - Hyperosmolar hyperglycemic state is relatively more common with epidemic obesity and the rise of type 2 diabetes mellitus.
- Thyroid emergencies (See chapter 30)
  - Hashimoto encephalopathy
  - Thyrotoxicosis
  - Myxedema coma

Gastrointestinal

- Intussusception frequently presents with lethargy.
- Lethargy and altered mental status in intussusception are seen more frequently in infants and young children. They are hypothesized to be secondary to release of endogenous opioids or endotoxins from the ischemic bowel.
- Other acute abdominal catastrophe such as malrotation with midgut volvulus.

Renal, genetic, and metabolic

- Electrolyte derangements (see Chapter 21)
- Hyper/hyponatremia
- Uremic encephalopathy
  - Hemolytic uremic syndrome
- Hepatic encephalopathy → hyperammonemia
  - Inborn errors of metabolism
  - Valproic acid toxicity
- Dehydration

Hematologic/oncologic

- CNS tumor (see Chapter 29 for additional details on CNS malignancies)
- Headache, seizure, altered mental status
- Hyperleukocytosis in acute lymphoblastic leukemia or acute myeloid leukemia
- Tumor lysis syndrome
- Severe anemia → sleepiness, irritability
- Iatrogenic causes due to medications given during disease process → benzodiazepines, opiates, antihistamines, or antiemetic medications with anticholinergic properties

Infectious

- Meningitis
- Encephalitis
- Tick-borne disease
- Intracranial abscess
- Sepsis

Special cases/environmental

- Shock (distributive, cardiogenic, hypovolemic, obstructive)
- Hyperthermia
- Hypothermia
- Porphyria
- Noninfectious encephalitis
- Psychiatric
- Thiamine deficiency
- Wernicke encephalopathy

Diagnostic Confirmation and Treatment

The history and physical examination are paramount to discovering etiology for undifferentiated ALOC in a child. Damage to the brainstem produces a depressed level of consciousness as well as loss of the vestibulo-occular reflex and pupillary light reflexes. However, if these cranial nerve functions are preserved, the dysfunction most likely lies within the cerebral cortex either as a localized lesion above the level of the brainstem or due to global cerebral dysfunction.

The pupillary reflex is generally resistant to metabolic insults, so assessing pupillary response to light is a critically important element when differentiating etiology of ALOC. Although certain metabolic or toxicologic insults may cause miosis, pupils should be reactive and equal. If pupils are unequal and sluggishly reactive, there should be concern for a lesion causing compression on the brainstem, such as an expanding temporal epidural hematoma causing uncal herniation.

Other physical examination findings, such as change in respiratory pattern, motor abnormalities (asymmetric movement or posturing), organomegaly in undiagnosed cardiac disease, acute hepatitis or metabolic disorder causing hepatic encephalopathy, may additionally narrow etiology in a child with undifferentiated ALOC. Specific skin findings, such as petechiae, vesicles, or the distribution and initial location of rash, can further narrow down particularly infectious causes of ALOC in children.

In addition, important historical factors, such as timing of onset of ALOC, should be elucidated. Gradual onset of symptoms over days or several hours suggests metabolic, infectious, or toxic insult. Rapid change in consciousness may reflect CNS hemorrhage such as ruptured aneurysm or arteriovenous malformation or obstructive hydrocephalus.

Imaging and treatment should be based on suspected etiology. However, if etiology is unclear, a broad workup should be undertaken focusing on resuscitation should the patient's ABC be unstable.

HEADACHE

The majority of childhood headaches are cause by a primary headache disorder, such as migraine, tension, or cluster headaches; however, secondary causes of headache must always be considered. Secondary headache disorders are due to an identifiable cause, such as a structural, metabolic, neoplastic, vascular, traumatic, infectious, or other identifiable cause.

Classification of Pediatric Headache

Primary headache syndromes are those that cannot be attributed to another cause and include tension-type headache, migraine headache, and cluster headache.

Migraine headache in children differs from migraine in adults. Childhood migraine tends to be bilateral and often lasts for a shorter duration. Family history of migraine, particularly in first-degree relative, is seen in >70% of childhood migraine sufferers.

Migraine is seen with and without aura. Migraine with aura is accompanied by transient neurologic symptoms that often precede the headache but may accompany the headache or occur after resolution, and most often resolve within 60 minutes of onset. The aura may be visual, sensory, verbal, or a combination of these.

The onset of migraine aura symptoms typically occurs over a longer period of time than the symptoms of stroke or seizure, and the symptoms are completely reversible. Children with neurologic symptoms that are prolonged, not completely reversible, and not related to headache should have the appropriate evaluations to rule out stroke, seizure, or other serious pathology.

Specific Headache Types

Table 20.3 describes rare forms of migraine headache.

Migraine triggers include stress, anxiety, light, menses, trauma, inadequate sleep or poor sleep quality, high altitude, infection, foods (e.g., cheese, chocolate, tea, coffee, colas, citrus fruits, cured meats, foods with monosodium glutamate, wine and beer, and artificial sweeteners), and medications (oral contraceptives, selective serotonin reuptake inhibitors, ondansetron, phosphodiesterase inhibitors, etc.).

Tension-type headaches are similar in onset to migraine headaches but are thought to be less debilitating. Tension headaches may last from 1 hour to several days, are often described as a band-like sensation around the head, and may be associated with neck and shoulder pain. Tension headaches may be episodic, occurring <15 days per month, or chronic, occurring ≥15 days per month. Triggers are similar to those for migraine.

Cluster headaches are attacks of severe, unilateral pain that last between 15 minutes and 3 hours and occur in clusters up to eight times per day. The pain is the most severe and debilitating of all primary headache syndromes. Typically, pain is orbital and associated with ipsilateral lacrimation, conjunctival injection, ptosis, miosis, eyelid edema, as well as nasal congestion, rhinorrhea, and sweating.

Migraine, tension, and cluster-type headaches comprise the majority of primary headache syndromes in children. Other causes of headache are known as secondary headaches and range from non-life-threatening causes,

TABLE 20.3 RARE FORMS OF MIGRAINE HEADACHE

Form	Characteristics
Familial hemiplegic migraine	Abrupt onset of hemiparesis, often followed by headache. Genetically heterogeneous autosomal dominant disorder often associated with episodic ataxia and generalized epilepsy.
Basilar artery migraine	More common in girls. At least two of dysarthria, tinnitus, hyperacusis, diplopia, decreased consciousness, vertigo, ataxia, visual disturbances in both hemifields, bilateral sensory problems.
Ophthalmoplegic migraine	Two or more headache episodes with paresis of cranial nerves III, IV, and/or VI. Must exclude posterior fossa, parasellar, or orbital fissure lesion.
Retinal migraine	Characterized by sudden, monocular blackouts or bright, blind episodes—before, during, or after headache. Time frame is brief from seconds to 1 hour.
Alice in Wonderland syndrome	Characterized by unusual visual illusions and spatial distortions that precede headaches.
Acute confusional migraine	Characterized by agitation, lethargy, and impaired sensorium. Focal neurologic deficits such as aphasia, anisocoria, and memory problems may also be seen. Typically lasts 4–24 hours.
Migraine equivalents	Periodic paroxysmal syndromes without associated headache: cyclic vomiting. Abdominal migraine (often precursor to more typical type migraine), benign paroxysmal vertigo, benign paroxysmal torticollis.

Source: Adapted from Alfonzo MJ, Bechtel K, Babineau S. Management of Headache in the Pediatric Emergency Department. *Pediatr Emerg Med Pract.* 2013;10(1):1–25.

such as the headache associated with sinus disease or ocular muscle strain, to more serious causes, such as headache due to meningitis, aneurysm, or carbon monoxide poisoning.

Red flags for potential secondary headache include the following:

- Progressive headache patterns—becoming more severe and/or frequent
- Change in headache character
- Increased headache with straining, coughing, sneezing, and Valsalva maneuver
- Sudden onset or severe onset of headaches (<6 months' duration)
- Systemic symptoms such as fever, weight loss, rash, and joint pain
- Patients in special risk groups: immune compromised, hypercoagulable state, neurocutaneous disorders, sickle cell disease, and malignancy
- Neurologic signs or symptoms, abnormal neurologic examination, papilledema, ALOC, abnormal eye movements, ataxia or other gait abnormalities, seizures, and visual field defects
- Sleep-related headache, headache upon waking or headache always present in the morning, or vomiting with headache upon waking
- Post-traumatic headache
- Occipital headache
- Poor response to therapy
- Increased intracranial pressure

Increased Intracranial Pressure

Headaches due to increased intracranial pressure may be caused by space-occupying lesions, hemorrhage, or other causes of impeded CSF flow. These headaches are progressive, associated with night-time awakening, and are worse with Valsalva or exertion. Children with increased intracranial pressure are prone to persistent vomiting, personality change, and lethargy. Papilledema and ophthalmoplegia are common.

Idiopathic intracranial hypertension, also known as pseudotumor cerebri, is associated with poorly characterized pain, sometimes with nausea and vomiting. Transient vision changes or diplopia may occur, and there is a risk of permanent vision loss.

Infection

Stiff neck and photophobia are common in CNS infections and necessitate a full septic workup with lumbar puncture, particularly with associated fever and ALOC (see Chapter 13). Children with viral, bacterial, or autoimmune encephalitis often have headache associated with other psychiatric and behavioral symptoms.

Vascular Disorders

Arteriovenous malformations, aneurysms, venous sinus thrombosis, cervical artery dissection, stroke, and posterior reversible encephalopathy are rare causes of headache in children. The thunderclap headache—sudden onset and maximal at onset, lasting approximately 5 minutes before pain decreases—is cause for concern and is described in spontaneous intracranial hemorrhage of ruptured aneurysms, ruptured arteriovenous malformation, and cervical artery dissection. Children with cervical artery dissection often present with ipsilateral neck pain and/or pain around the orbit, mandible, or ear. Focal neurologic deficits may also be present.

Children who present with sudden-onset headache with focal neurologic findings and/or depressed level of consciousness warrant immediate evaluation and stabilization, including emergent imaging such as CT angiography of the head and neck.

Another uncommon but notable vascular cause for headache in children is cerebral venous sinus thrombosis (CVST). Children with CVST may present with a combination of headache, focal neurologic deficits, seizure, decreased level of consciousness, and papilledema. Most children who have CVST have a risk factor for this condition, such as head and neck infection, prothrombotic state, or recent head trauma.

Common presenting symptoms are related to the structures that pass through the cavernous sinus. Limitations of extraocular movement, particularly with regard to central nerve VI, are common. Periorbital edema, chemosis, and proptosis may also be seen. Diagnosis is made using CT venogram or MRI venography with contrast.

Structural Disorders and Tumors

Parental fear of a brain tumor often triggers evaluation for headache. Tumors are uncommon, and the vast majority of patients with tumor have focal neurological findings present on examination. Often, these children will also show signs of increased intercranial hypertension, such as persistent and progressive headache, nocturnal awakenings, morning headache with or without vomiting, and increased headache with Valsalva or cough (see Chapter 29).

Post Traumatic Headache

See Chapter 32 for further discussion/recommendations regarding post-traumatic headache.

Diagnostic Confirmation

One of the most important elements in diagnosis is an appropriate history and thorough physical examination with a complete neurological assessment including evaluation for papilledema and visual field deficits. Bedside US to evaluate for optic nerve dilation may also be an additional data point of evaluation.

The following are imaging recommendations for primary headaches:

- Imaging is *not* indicated for
  - Typical migraine with or without aura
  - Common migraine of >6 months' duration with a positive family history
  - Nonprogressive migraine headache
- MRI, when readily available, is recommended to rule out structural lesions in certain primary headaches, including
  - Migraine with neurologic deficit (first presentation)
  - Ophthalmologic migraine with unilateral ptosis or complete third nerve palsy
  - Basilar artery migraine syndrome
  - Acute confusional migraine syndrome that persists
  - Progressive chronic headache
  - Hemiplegic migraine
  - Seizures and postictal headache

The following are imaging recommendations for secondary headaches:

- MRI is recommended for
  - Neurologic signs of symptoms of increased intracranial pressure
  - Intracranial hemorrhage (with MR angiography)
  - Encephalitis
  - Brain abscess (MRI is the study of choice)

- CT of the head without contrast is recommended for
  - Sudden severe headaches (thunderclap)
  - Exclusion of impending herniation prior to lumbar puncture (most commonly with altered mental status in suspected acute bacterial meningitis)
  - Subdural empyema or other intracerebral complications of sinusitis or mastoiditis
  - Trauma
  - Concerning cases in which urgent MRI is not available
- CT angiography is recommended for
  - Subarachnoid hemorrhage
  - Infarction
  - Arterial dissection
  - Aneurysm
- MR angiography is less sensitive but may be an adequate substitute for CT angiography.
- CT venography or MR venography is recommended for venous sinus thrombosis.

Finally, if there is suspicion for a serious infectious cause of headache or if headache is thought to be due to increased intercranial pressure or subarachnoid hemorrhage, after neuroimaging is normal, lumbar puncture should be performed with or without opening pressures as appropriate.

Treatment

Management of headache due to secondary cause is based on etiology.

Management of Primary Headache Syndromes

Although primary headache syndromes are not life-threatening, they do cause significant dysfunction for the child and family. Early treatment of the primary headache episode is most likely to be effective. Decreasing stimulation in the examination room by closing the door or curtain and turning off the lights may help those experiencing photophobia and phonophobia. Abortive analgesics such as ibuprofen (10 mg/kg) and acetaminophen (15 mg/kg) are effective. These should be given orally if the patient is tolerating fluids. If the patient is not tolerating fluids, ketorolac IV or IM (0.5 mg/kg, maximum 30 mg) or IV acetaminophen (IV dose equivalent to PO dose), if available, may be used.

Because dehydration may cause or exacerbate headaches, IV hydration may be considered, particularly if the patient has associated vomiting. Antiemetic medications such as prochlorperazine (0.15 mg/kg, maximum 10 mg) and metoclopramide (0.1 mg/kg, maximum 10 mg) are effective in treating migraine headache. There is a minor risk of akathisia or dystonia using these medications, and diphenhydramine (1 or 2 mg/kg, maximum 50 mg) may be used should these arise. In addition, small doses of caffeine, such as a limited amount of coffee, tea, or soda, may be effective when combined with nonsteroidal anti-inflammatory drugs (NSAIDs) or acetaminophen.

If NSAIDs and acetaminophen are not effective, triptans may be effective in children older than age 6 years. Dihydroergotamine is sometimes used in refractory cases. Opiates, barbiturates, and benzodiazepines are never indicated for headache treatment.

Treatment for cluster headaches is 100% oxygen via high flow at 15 L/min. In addition, triptans may be used.

Psychiatric and somatic comorbid conditions may contribute to increased headache symptoms. Discussing sleep hygiene, healthy diet, exercise, stress reduction, and hydration, as well as expectations and goals for treatment, provides an important contribution to headache remission.

Preventative medications initiated by specialists for chronic headaches include tricyclic antidepressants; antiepileptics; antihypertensives; and supplements such as magnesium, riboflavin, and coenzyme Q10.

Disposition

Most children who present with primary or secondary headache not due to a serious or life-threatening cause can be treated and safely discharged home with primary care follow-up if symptoms improve and they have a normal neurologic examination. Children who have a serious cause for headache, such as meningitis, intracranial bleeding, and mass lesion, should be admitted or stabilized and transferred to a center with appropriate specialty services. Patients who have pain due to a primary headache syndrome may be admitted when symptoms are refractory, such as with status migranosis or analgesic rebound headaches.

Children with abnormal neurologic examinations and who have headaches that are worse in severity or are of unclear etiology should be admitted or transferred for further evaluation and treatment. It may be necessary to consult pediatric neurology or another appropriate service (trauma surgery or neurosurgery) while in the ED if the headache is due to a serious secondary cause.

Complications and Pitfalls

- Failure to perform complete, age-appropriate neurologic examination with failure to capture abnormal neurological signs.
- Failure to rule out serious etiologies of focal neurologic deficit, attributing it instead to atypical migraine. For example, atypical migraine with hemiplegia or ophthalmoplegia is a diagnosis of exclusion.
- Failure to start antibiotics immediately on a child with concern for intracranial infection. Do not delay antibiotics in a child with suspected meningitis for the lumbar puncture. Cultures, gram stain, and especially antigen testing will, in most cases, remain positive for hours after antibiotics have been started.
- CT imaging children with headache more frequently than is necessary, or who do not meet criteria to image, is a waste of ED resources and exposes them to unnecessary radiation.
- In children with concerning cause of headache, such as trauma and evidence of increased intracranial pressure, CT should be the initial imaging modality, even if MRI is available.

Children with primary headache syndromes are more likely to have behavioral disturbances and struggle with relationships at home and at school. They have increased rates of depression, learning difficulties, and other somatic symptoms, similar to other children with chronic diseases.

ENCEPHALITIS

Encephalitis, meningoencephalitis, and encephalomyelitis are typically due to direct invasion of the brain and/or surrounding structures (meninges and spinal cord, respectively) by an infectious agent. Encephalitis is inflammation of the brain that can be caused by infectious (bacteria, virus, fungus, and parasite) agents but also can be due to paraneoplastic, acute or chronic disease, and autoimmune processes. Anti-*N*-methyl-D-aspartate (NMDA) receptor encephalitis, acute demyelinating encephalomyelitis (ADEM), and acute cerebellar ataxia (ACA) are the most common parainfectious and autoimmune causes of encephalitis in children.

Acute Demyelinating Encephalomyelitis

Acute demyelinating encephalomyelitis is an acute demyelinating illness that occurs in children (and, rarely, adults). ADEM arises due to immune dysregulation in a genetically susceptible host after an environmental insult or preceding illness.

A preceding infection is common. Multiple different viruses, bacteria, and even (although much less common) vaccines have been implicated.

Clinical Features

Most commonly, a febrile upper respiratory illness precedes neurologic symptoms by 1–4 weeks. Patients may present with fever, headache, and meningismus at the time of onset. Encephalopathy, if not present at the time of onset, often progresses rapidly along with other neurologic symptoms, with maximum neurologic dysfunction reaching a nadir at 4–7 days. Neurologic complaints include weakness and acute hemiparesis, ataxia, cranial neuropathies including optic neuritis, spinal cord dysfunction, sensory changes, and ALOC. The ALOC can range from irritability and confusion to frank coma. Seizures may occur. Children who have cervical spinal cord myelitis may have respiratory failure if lesions extend into the brainstem.

Diagnosis

MRI is the imaging modality of choice and can show diffuse areas of demyelination. Lumbar puncture (LP) may be indicated. Preceding imaging should be perform prior to LP with altered mental status or signs of increased intracranial pressure. CSF may be normal or have mild protein elevation; 2/3 have pleocytosis with lymphocyte predominance.

Treatment

The mainstay of treatment for ADEM is immunosuppression with high-dose glucocorticoids. This is often given in conjunctive with antimicrobial medications until diagnosis is confirmed. Methylprednisolone (10–30 mg/kg/day, 1,000 mg maximum) or dexamethasone (1 mg/kg/day) followed by a 4- to 6-week taper are used. Plasmapheresis and IVIG are also adjunctive therapy.

Disposition and Clinical Course

Complete resolution of symptoms occurs in most patients, but all patients should be admitted because neurologic symptoms often progress after initial presentation (and last ~2–4 weeks).

Acute Cerebellar Ataxia

Acute cerebellar ataxia is a syndrome that occurs in previously healthy children most commonly after infection or vaccination. It is the most common cause of ataxia in childhood and is seen predominantly in children younger than age 6 years. The pathogenesis is likely autoimmune.

Clinical Features

Children with ACA appear otherwise well but have a rather abrupt onset of gait ataxia that is typically seen within 2 weeks of illness or vaccination. Gait is typically wide based, unsteady, and lurching or staggering. During the next few days, gait ataxia progresses to the trunk and limbs. Dysmetria and dysdiadokinesia may be present. Children may have difficulties maintaining posture while seated. Nystagmus and tremor are present in some children. Speech disturbances as well as vomiting may also be seen, and headache can be part of the presentation in older children.

Meningismus, fever, and seizures should not be seen in the presentation of acute cerebellar ataxia. When evaluating abnormal eye movements, while end gaze nystagmus may be normal, opsoclonus and multifocal myoclonus are typical of opsoclonus–myoclonus syndrome and are associated with neuroblastoma. There should not be asymmetric neurologic deficits, sensory deficits, weakness, or areflexia because these are indicative of a more insidious process. If present, these symptoms should prompt additional workup.

Differential Diagnosis

Life-threatening conditions associated with ataxia in children include tumor, hemorrhage, stroke, and infection. Approximately half of brain tumors in children are infratentorial. Ataxia in these cases is slow and progressive in onset, and symptoms of increased intracranial pressure are often present.

Ataxia from posterior fossa intracranial hemorrhage is rapid in onset with associated ALOC or headache.

Ataxia from infection typically has associated fever, altered mental status, or meningismus. Most cases of cerebellar abscess are otogenic. Signs and symptoms of increased intracranial pressure are likely to accompany a posterior fossa abscess.

Stroke and cervical artery dissection are extremely rare in children. Ataxia may be seen in ischemia in the basilar or vertebral artery distribution. Children at higher risk for stroke are those with sickle cell disease and those with hypercoagulable conditions. Dissection is most often due to direct trauma (including posterior oropharyngeal trauma).

The following are other causes for ataxia in children:

- ADEM
- Guillain–Barré syndrome
- Miller Fisher syndrome
- Toxic ingestions
- Labyrinthitis
- Migraine syndromes
- Opsoclonus myoclonus syndrome suggestive of neuroblastoma
- Tick paralysis
- Inborn errors of metabolism
- Degenerative genetic conditions
- Congenital anomalies of the posterior fossa

Diagnosis

Diagnosis is clinical and based on exclusion of more serious etiologies on history and physical examination. MRI and neurologic consultation may be considered if the diagnosis is unclear.

Treatment and Disposition

Acute cerebellar ataxia generally resolves in 2 or 3 weeks without specific therapy. Most children have complete resolution of symptoms, but approximately 10% of children have residual neurologic sequelae.

Anti-NMDA Receptor Encephalitis

Anti-NDMA receptor encephalitis is a relatively recently discovered (1997) condition associated with acute psychiatric symptoms. Associated tumors are common (particularly ovarian teratomas).

Clinical Features

Typically, there is a prodrome of fever, headache, and viral-like syndrome prior to psychiatric symptoms. Prominent psychiatric symptoms include anxiety, agitation, bizarre behavior, hallucinations, delusions, and disorganized thinking. Seizures, mental status changes, and autonomic instability may occur with progression (and mechanical ventilation may be required).

Diagnosis

The definitive diagnosis of anti-NMDA receptor encephalitis is confirmed by the detection of IgG antibodies to the GluN1 (also known as NR1) subunit of the NMDA receptor in serum or CSF. CSF antibodies are always present at initial presentation. In two-thirds of cases, MRI is normal, but it can also show transient abnormalities in cortical and subcortical areas.

Treatment and Disposition

All patients should be admitted. The mainstay of treatment is immune suppression using glucocorticoids, IVIG, and plasmapheresis. Tumor resection is frequently definitive therapy. The majority of patients have good outcomes with treatment, but residual symptoms may persist, and death may uncommonly occur.

Further Reading

Press CA, Lindsay A, Stence NV, Fenton LZ, Bernard TJ, Mirsky DM. Cavernous sinus thrombosis in children: Imaging characteristics and clinical outcomes. *Stroke*. 2015;46(9):2657–2660.

Raucci U, Della Vecchia N, Ossella C, et al. Management of childhood headache in the emergency department: Review of the literature. *Front Neurol*. 2019;10:886.

Santillanes G, Luc Q. Emergency department management of seizures in pediatric patients. *Pediatr Emerg Med Pract*. 2015;12(3):1–25; quiz 26–27.

Song JL, Wang VJ, Vazquez MN. Altered level of consciousness: Evidence-based management in the emergency department [Digest]. *Pediatr Emerg Med Pract*. 2017;14(1 Suppl Points & Pearls):S1–S2.

Tavasoli A, Tabrizi A. Acute transverse myelitis in children, literature review. *Iran J Child Neurol*. 2018;12(2):7–16.

Trinka E, Cock H, Hesdorffer D, et al. A definition and classification of status epilepticus: Report of the ILAE Task Force on classification of status epilepticus. *Epilepsia*. 2015;56(10):1515–1523.

21

Fluid and Electrolyte Emergencies

AMEER P. MODY

INTRODUCTION

Fluid and electrolyte emergencies are a common presenting complaint in the emergency department (ED). Dehydration emergencies can occur as a complicating factor of another illness or due to vomiting and/or diarrhea. This chapter focuses on the identification and management of common fluid and electrolyte emergencies, specifically dehydration, hypoglycemia, hyponatremia, and hypernatremia.

DEHYDRATION

Dehydration is common in children. Infants and young children are unable to independently respond to their own thirst drives, more commonly have vomiting as a component of their illness, are more susceptible to insensible losses, and have less physiologic reserve, all creating higher risk to develop dehydration. In the developing world, dehydration, particularly from infectious diarrheal illnesses, is still a significant cause of child mortality. Elsewhere, dehydration is much less likely to be a cause of death, but it is a very common reason for ED visits and admissions to the hospital.

For infants and children, the diagnosis and degree of dehydration are reliant on historical and physical examination findings. Number of days of illness, mental status, frequency of vomiting or diarrhea, oral intake, and urine output all should be queried. Examination should include age-specific vital signs, mental status, presence of a sunken fontanelle in a young infant, presence of sunken eyes, dryness of mucous membranes, presence of tears, capillary refill time, and skin turgor. For neonates in the first few weeks of life, comparing the birth weight to the current weight can be helpful in assessing hydration status. Although all these findings are necessary to gauge hydration status, the individual sensitivity of each factor in determining the degree of dehydration has not been well established. Of importance to the emergency physician is that the clinical findings of dehydration do not occur in a vacuum—for example, a patient with parental concern of decreased wet diapers who has normal mental status, moist mucous membranes, and is active is not likely significantly dehydrated. A holistic appraisal of the patient's status will determine the degree of dehydration and treatment options. A child may be mildly dehydrated with a pertinent history but no clinical signs, whereas a child with severe dehydration will have multiple physical findings and possibly symptoms of hypovolemic shock.

Diagnostic Confirmation

Laboratory testing is not required to make the diagnosis of dehydration, but it can be of value in specific situations. In a patient whose history suggests mild or minimal dehydration but physical signs suggest a greater severity of illness, hypoglycemia may be the cause. Infants and young children are more susceptible to low blood sugar with limited glycogen stores. Hypoglycemia may cause listlessness, irritability, or tachycardia that may be confused with signs of dehydration. If symptoms have been long-standing or if free water has been utilized for attempted rehydration at home or the child is with special needs requiring feeds given through a gastrostomy tube, the likelihood of abnormal electrolytes such as sodium increases significantly. As a general rule, patients with classic histories that are supported by physical examination findings, no chronic medical problems, and no worse than moderate dehydration do not require routine laboratory testing. Electrolytes and glucose should be considered in patients who fall outside these parameters. There are no clear established parameters correlating a specific laboratory value with degree of dehydration; however, serum bicarbonate <17 mEq/L is associated with >5% dehydration.

Treatment

The primary goals of treating dehydration in the ED are to replace the fluid deficit, compensate for anticipated losses, facilitate oral rehydration, and minimize invasive treatment methodologies. Patients with severe dehydration, signs of shock, and/or altered mental status require rapid initial correction of hypovolemia ideally through intravenous (IV) routes. Fluid resuscitation should not be delayed if IV access is not readily available or delayed. Alternative routes including intraosseous access, nasogastric tube, subcutaneous fluid administration, or oral rehydration can all be considered even while IV access is attempted.

Intravenous

For severely dehydrated patients, the initial IV fluid administration should be given at a volume of 20 cc/kg body weight over 20–30 minutes. A good rule of thumb regarding the rate of fluid repletion is that it should mimic the history of dehydration: Patients who histories suggest rapid dehydration (a few days of illness) should be rapidly rehydrated, whereas patients who have developed dehydration over a longer time course (several days to weeks) should be more gently rehydrated. Repeat boluses of fluid at a volume of 20 cc/kg should be administered after repeat examination for clinical response to therapy, often with total volumes of 60 cc/kg or more given for rapid fluid resuscitation.

Initial fluid bolus should be given with isotonic crystalloid fluid, most commonly 0.9% normal saline solution. Hypotonic or hypertonic fluids should not be given in the initial phase of emergent rehydration outside of specific clinical scenarios. Normal saline is readily available and of reasonable cost, but it can lead to a relative metabolic acidosis if given in large amounts. The large chloride load results in bicarbonate moving intracellularly, resulting in a net metabolic acidosis. Alternative solutions are available to mitigate this effect, including Ringer's lactate (Hartmann's) solution or Plasma-Lyte 148. These balanced solutions have a similar amount of sodium but significantly less chloride, closer matching serum plasma composition. No large multicenter trials have demonstrated absolute superiority of these solutions, and normal saline use continues to be ubiquitous; however, these solutions are safe, efficacious, and gaining more widespread appeal.

Oral Rehydration Therapy

Oral rehydration therapy (ORT) is the mainstay of treatment for up to moderate (and potentially severe) clinical dehydration. ORT provides value in both the acute and subacute treatment phases of dehydration management, facilitating both ED and home treatment. Patients should typically receive 50–100 cc/kg of oral rehydration solution (ORS) during the first 4 hours of the initial phase to replace losses. Fluids should initially be administered in small aliquots (e.g., 5 mL utilizing a syringe or teaspoon every few minutes), with slowly increasing amounts as tolerated toward the total volume goal. Subsequent episodes of emesis or diarrhea should be replaced with 5–10 cc/kg of volume.

The following is the ORT fluid replacement plan:

Initial deficit replacement: 50–100 cc/kg of ORS by mouth over 4 hours

Ongoing loss replacement: an additional 5–10 cc/kg per diarrheal stool or emesis

The initial phase of ORT does not need to be completed in the ED, however, the ability to adhere to treatment and teaching of ORT should be established prior to discharge.

There are different formulations of ORS that vary the quantity of sugar and electrolytes to enhance intestinal absorption, replace gastrointestinal (GI) losses, and enhance palatability. The original World Health Organization (WHO) electrolyte solution was created to combat cholera epidemics in the developing world and to treat severe dehydration in malnourished patients. The solution, which can be handmade, contains the ideal mix of sugar and salt to enhance intestinal absorption of water. Commercially available ORS in the United States typical has a higher sugar content than the WHO-recommended formula for reasons of palatability. In general, because the degree of dehydration and underlying nutritional status of patients from developed countries are better, the commercially available products are proven, acceptable products for oral rehydration for most patients. Juices and sodas should definitely be avoided as ORT options because their significant sugar content can exacerbate osmotic diarrhea and worsen hydration status.

Antiemetics, specifically ondansetron, can be a valuable adjunct in ORT. Ondansetron is a serotonin 5-HT_3 antagonist that suppresses the central nervous system vomiting reflex. It has been established to be safe and effective in reducing ED vomiting, ED IV fluid utilization, and decreasing hospitalization rate. As opposed to other typical antiemetics such as diphenhydramine, promethazine, or prochlorperazine, ondansetron does not cause drowsiness (interfering with ORT) and is safe to use in infants. Ondansetron has a safe side effect profile but has been shown to slightly increase the number of days of diarrheal illness in patients with gastroenteritis. It has also been shown to increase the QT interval but not to a clinically significant degree (but it should be avoided in patients with a known history of prolonged QT). Currently, only the Canadian Pediatric Society recommends routine use of ondansetron in its clinical management guidelines; however, many of the other governing bodies have not updated their guidelines since ondansetron became widely available. The recommended dose of ondansetron is 0.15 mg/kg PO (or IV), but an easier and safe dosing regimen is 2 mg for those who weigh 8–20 kg, 4 mg for those who weigh 20–60 kg, and 8 mg for those who weigh >60 kg. A short-course, as-needed prescription for ondansetron may greatly facilitate outpatient ORT.

Nasogastric and Subcutaneous

Alternative routes to oral or IV hydration include both nasogastric and subcutaneous fluid administration in the ED. The nasogastric route has been demonstrated to be both efficient and efficacious in treating ED dehydration. It may be of great use when IV access has been difficult to obtain, in toddlers with significant gingivostomatitis preventing oral intake, or in infants with tachypnea and respiratory distress from illnesses such as bronchiolitis. Utilization of a topical anesthetic such as viscous lidocaine jelly can ease the discomfort caused by nasogastric tube insertion.

Recombinant human hyaluronidase, which has recently become available, greatly enhances the ability for fluids to become absorbed from the subcutaneous tissue. The most commonly utilized site is the upper back between the scapula. The skin is cleaned in a similar manner to an IV start, then it is pinched, and a 22- or 24-gauge angiocatheter or butterfly needle is inserted into the subcutaneous tissue. A total of 150 units (1 mL) of recombinant hyaluronidase is given, followed by 20 cc/kg of normal saline.

Next Steps

After completion of the initial phase of hydration and repletion of fluid deficit, treatment should focus on maintenance of euvolemia; replacement of ongoing losses; and treatment of underlying illness, if applicable. For patients with dehydration due to gastroenteritis or other self-limited viral phenomena, the focus should be on refeeding as soon as possible. Breastfed infants should continue breastfeeding throughout the rehydration phase, utilizing ORS as a supplement. If patients are able to tolerate ORS for 12–24 hours without vomiting, a slow, deliberate advance to normal, age-appropriate diet is recommended (avoiding fried or sugary foods). Whole milk or formula can be given without dilution. If vomiting resumes, utilization of ORS for 12–24 hours should resume.

For patients requiring prolonged IV fluids or in whom the disease process requires continued IV fluid administration (e.g., pneumonia and appendicitis), the maintenance rate required to preserve euvolemia follows the 4, 2, 1 rule to calculate the hourly rate:

- 4 cc/kg for the first 10 kg of weight (0–10 kg)
- 2 cc/kg for the next 10 kg of weight (10–20 kg)
- 1 cc/kg for every 1 kg of weight thereafter

For example, a 35-kg child would receive 75 cc/hr (40 + 20 + 15) of maintenance fluids.

Similar to the discussion regarding the choice of initial fluid, the choice of appropriate maintenance fluids has undergone some evolution. Maintenance fluids should contain dextrose, particularly if the patient will not be taking any oral nutrition. A 5% dextrose-containing fluid is appropriate for most healthy patients older than age 6 weeks. Infants younger than age 6 weeks and patients with underlying metabolic disease may require higher concentrations of dextrose to compensate for increased metabolic demands. Hypotonic maintenance fluids (half normal or quarter normal saline) should be avoided because they have been shown to prolong hospitalization and lead to iatrogenic hyponatremia in pediatric patients. The latest American Academy of Pediatrics guidelines recommend patients older than age 28 days receive isotonic maintenance IV fluids.

HYPOGLYCEMIA

Hypoglycemia symptoms can mimic those of dehydration in infants and young children. Serum blood glucose should be assessed in all patients with altered mental status, more than moderate dehydration, a history of metabolic disorder, and in patients with cachexia. The typical high-concentration dextrose solution utilized for adults with hypoglycemia—for example, 25% and 50% dextrose—should be avoided in pediatric patients because of potential causticity to small peripheral veins. A 5% or 10% dextrose solution can be administered safely through a peripheral vein at a dose utilizing a simple rule of thumb: The volume multiplied by the concentration of dextrose should equal 50, meaning 10 cc/kg of D5, 5 cc/kg of D10, and 2 cc/kg of D25 (if given through a central line) for the correct initial dose to treat hypoglycemia. Awake hypoglycemic patients can also be treated with oral dextrose:

% Dextrose solution available (5, 10) × [volume to be administered] = 50

HYPONATREMIC DEHYDRATION

Hyponatremia may occur as a complicating factor in dehydration from unbalanced GI losses, renal loss, third space loss such as ascites or burns, or iatrogenically from administration of hypotonic fluids. Hyponatremia may be insidious, causing minimal symptoms until a threshold is met, or acute, causing rapid symptomatology. Most symptoms are central nervous system or musculoskeletal system related, including headache, vomiting, weakness, or altered sensorium. Signs include hypothermia, diminished reflexes, or seizures.

Often, the initial ED management of hyponatremic dehydration will be the same as that for isonatremic dehydration. The utilization of normal saline for fluid resuscitation is an appropriate choice because the 154 mEq/L of sodium will treat both the hyponatremia and dehydration at least marginally. For patients with seizure or altered mental status (with determined hyponatremia), hypertonic saline should be utilized. Three percent normal saline contains 513 mEq/L of sodium and should be administered at a bolus dose of 3–5 mL/kg. A potential substitute for hypertonic saline solution, if not readily available, is sodium bicarbonate from the emergency crash cart; it contains 595 mEq/L and can be given at a dose of 1 or 2 mL/kg.

Once seizing has abated and mental status has improved, the correction of hyponatremia should occur more deliberately over time. Overly rapid correction of hyponatremia may result in neurologic injury from central pontine myelinolysis. Serum sodium should be monitored frequently with a goal of raising the level from 8 to 12 mEq/L in 24 hours. Another good guideline for the rate of correction is that it should follow the rate of decompensation: Rapid hyponatremia can be corrected more rapidly.

HYPERNATREMIC DEHYDRATION

Hypernatremic dehydration can be the result of free water loss greater than sodium loss from diarrhea or heat stroke, pure water depletion from diabetes insipidus, or from inappropriately prepared formula in infants. The excess of extracellular sodium results in cellular shrinkage, causing neurologic symptoms including irritability, lethargy, or seizures. The classic sign of decreased skin turgor and doughy appearance is present in severe hypernatremia.

For acutely symptomatic patients with hypernatremic dehydration, normal saline is again an acceptable first-line treatment because the patient will likely have a serum sodium >154 mEq/L. As soon as stabilization has occurred, care should be taken to slowly correct the serum sodium over 48–72 hours at a rate no faster than 0.5 mEq/hr to avoid neurologic injury from fluid shifts.

KEY POINTS

- Dehydration is a clinical diagnosis, with degree of dehydration based on a holistic appraisal of multiple factors.
- ORT should be the first line of treatment for patients with mild and moderate dehydration. Ondansetron can be a useful adjunct in ORT.
- Intravenous, intraosseous, nasogastric, and subcutaneous are all potential other methods of emergent rehydration. Isotonic fluids (0.9% normal saline or equivalent) are the first-line therapy.
- Labs are not routinely required but are indicated in patients with moderate to severe dehydration, histories that do not correlate with physical examination findings, and multiple chronic medical problems.
- The pace of correction for isotonic, hyponatremic, and hypernatremic dehydration should align with the duration of illness. Long-standing symptoms should be correctly slowly; hyperacute dehydration should be correctly rapidly.

Further Reading

Feld LG, Neuspiel DR, Foster BA, et al. Clinical practice guideline: Maintenance intravenous fluids in children. *Pediatrics.* 2018;142(6):e20183083.

Powers KS. Dehydration: Isonatremic, hyponatremic, and hypernatremic recognition and management. *Pediatr Rev.* 2015;36(7):274–285.

Santillanes G, Rose E. Evaluation and management of dehydration in children. *Emerg Med Clin North Am.* 2018;36:259–273.

22

Common Pediatric Dermatologic Conditions

JULIE FURMICK AND DALE WOOLRIDGE

INTRODUCTION

Rash and skin complaints comprise a common pediatric chief complaint and among the top 20 reasons patients present to the emergency department. For this reason, it is important for emergency physicians to be able to distinguish life-threatening rashes from those that are benign. This chapter reviewed several rashes, including eczema, erythema multiforme (EM), Henoch–Schonlein purpura (HSP), scabies, tinea infections, urticaria, impetigo, and ecthyma. Clinical descriptions of the rash and supplemental photographs are utilized. Atypical presentations, diagnostic algorithms, treatment modalities, and disposition are also reviewed. By applying the principles discussed in this chapter, one should be able to diagnose and treat these common pediatric rashes simply and effectively.

ECZEMA

Background

Eczema is a broad term used for a variety of disease states that cause the skin to become erythematous, inflamed, and pruritic. There are several different types of eczema, including contact dermatitis, nummular eczema, dyshidrotic eczema, and seborrheic dermatitis, but the most common form is atopic dermatitis (AD). AD affects more than 10% of children, with a higher prevalence in African Americans. Pathophysiology is multifactorial, including a dysregulated immune response, skin barrier abnormalities, as well as genetic and environmental factors.

Classic Clinical Presentation

Classically, AD presents within the first year of life, with 90% of cases being evident by age 5 years. Presentation depends on the age of the patient. In infants and toddlers (aged <2 years), AD presents as dry, scaly, erythematous papules localized to the face and scalp. As it progresses, it can involve the trunk and extensor surfaces. The diaper area is typically spared. In severe cases, vesicles form, leading to serous exudates with crusting. In childhood eczema, typically defined as that occurring from age 2 years until puberty, the rash tends to involve the flexor surfaces, particularly the antecubital and popliteal fossae. The rash can also be seen in other creases, such as the neck, wrist, ankles, and gluteal folds. The rash is often poorly demarcated, and as it becomes more chronic, hyper- or hypopigmentation can be seen, as well as lichenification of the skin with nodular formation. After puberty, AD involves

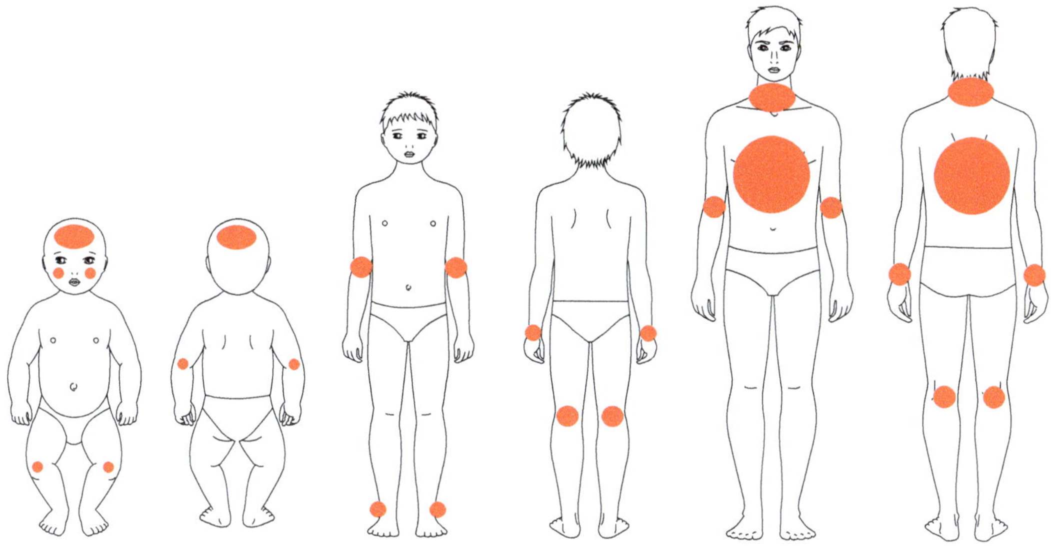

FIGURE 22.1 Common distributions patterns of AD based on age. (Left) Infantile AD (aged <2 years) most commonly involves the cheeks, scalp, elbows, and knees. (Middle) Childhood AD (aged 2 years to puberty) typically involves antecubital, popliteal fossa, wrists, and ankles. (Right) Adult-onset AD tends to involves antecubital, popliteal fossa, nape of the neck, and trunk.

Source: Atopic Dermatitis. Overview 2018 [cited 2019 Jan 30]; Available from: https://www.aad.org/public/diseases/eczema/atopic-dermatitis - symptoms

the face, trunk, nape of the neck, as well as the dorsal surfaces of the hands and feet. The antecubital and popliteal fossae are often involved. Figure 22.1 outlines the distribution of AD based on age. Independent of age, the hallmark sign of AD is severe pruritus, and most patients have severe xerosis (dry skin). The constant itching and scratching cycle affects quality of life, sleep, and increases the risk of secondary infection.

Atypical Clinical Presentation

There are no pathognomonic lesions characteristic of AD, and the lesions of AD vary based on skin tone. Dark-skinned individuals tend to have more papular or follicular lesions, as well as hyper- and hypopigmentation. Perifollicular accentuations and alopecia are also possible with AD.

Although AD is the most common type of eczema, other types include contact dermatitis, nummular eczema, dyshidrotic eczema, and seborrheic dermatitis. Contact dermatitis refers to any dermatitis that results from direct contact with an irritant. This can be a result of an allergic reaction or direct irritation of the skin from the foreign substance. Nummular eczema is rare in children but presents as small, round, coin-shaped pruritic lesions that can occur after minor trauma such as an insect bite or abrasion. Dyshidrotic eczema occurs on the palmar and plantar surface of the hands and feet, respectively. It is characterized by intensely pruritic vesicular lesions that erupt, leaving dry, cracked, painful lesions. Seborrheic dermatitis is characterized by scaling, erythema, and pruritus occurring most frequently on the scalp of young infants.

Differential Diagnosis

The differential diagnosis for AD includes scabies, seborrheic dermatitis, contact dermatitis, ichthyosis, and psoriasis. More obscure diagnoses, including Wiskott–Aldrich syndrome, Langerhans histiocytosis, and celiac disease, can present with a similar rash as that seen in AD but often have other systemic signs and symptoms. These should be considered when a patient has failure to thrive, severe recurrent infections, or fails to respond to appropriate therapy.

Diagnostic Confirmation

Atopic dermatitis is a clinical diagnosis; however, in 2013 the American Academy of Dermatology developed guidelines outlining essential, important, and associated factors to aid in the diagnosis. Patients must have all essential features, including pruritus, eczema, chronic or relapsing history, typical morphology, and age-specific patterns (see Figure 22.1); also included are facial, neck, and extensor involvement in infants and children; current or previous flexural lesions in any age group; and spares of the groin or axillary regions. Some important features that are seen in most cases of AD are early age of onset, personal or family history of AD, atopic history, immunoglobulin E (IgE) reactivity, and xerosis (dry skin). The following associated features are included in the guidelines to aid in the diagnosis but alone are too nonspecific: atypical vascular response, keratosis pilaris, pityriasis alba, hyperlinear palms, ocular or periorbital changes, perifollicular accentuation, lichenification, and prurigo lesions. Last, several ailments must be ruled out prior to establishing the diagnosis of AD, including scabies, seborrheic dermatitis, contact dermatitis, cutaneous T cell lymphoma, psoriasis, photosensitivity dermatoses, immune deficiency disease, and erythroderma.

Treatment

Atopic dermatitis is a chronic disease process characterized by relapsing and remitting flares. A holistic approach to management should be taken with these patients. This includes patient education, trigger avoidance, and regimented adherence to the treatment plan. Parental anticipatory guidance to daily management should include bathing in warm water with a mild or non-soap cleanser; there are no specific recommendations on the frequency of bathing for patients with AD. Adding agents such as oils or emollients to the bath water is not currently recommended. Hydration with emollients should occur after bathing, with frequent reapplication (at least twice daily). The type of emollient chosen is based on patient preference, but they should be free of preservatives, additives, perfumes, or fragrances and be affordable.

Acute exacerbations are often managed with topical corticosteroids (TCSs). Potency and frequency of the application depend on the severity and location on the body. Low- and medium-potency (1–2.5% hydrocortisone and 0.1% triamcinolone, respectively) TCSs are the recommended first-line agents in acute flares. Only low-potency steroids should be used on the face and intertriginous areas because these areas have inherent increased absorption and are at increased the risk of side effects. The quantity of TCSs should be based on an adult fingertip unit (the amount from the distal interphalangeal joint to the fingertip, or ~0.5 g, being applied over an area equal to two adult palms), and the treatment should be applied twice a day for up to 3 days past the point of flare resolution. Other treatment modalities include wet wrap therapy, topical calcineurin inhibitors such as 0.1% pimecrolimus cream and 0.03% tacrolimus ointment, and topical phosphodiesterase-4 inhibitors. However, these are second-line agents often used for refractory disease states and should be prescribed by a practitioner trained in their use.

Clinical Algorithm

The clinical algorithm for AD is provided in Figure 22.1.

Disposition

The majority of AD is managed on an outpatient basis. There are a few situations in which children may require inpatient management, such as when children have severe bacterial or viral superinfections and have failed outpatient treatment. Often, patients with eczema herpeticum present with systemic illness requiring intravenous (IV) antivirals, pain control, and hospital admission. In rare cases, some bacterial superinfections can disseminate, leading to bacteremia and sepsis. These patients should be admitted or transferred if pediatric services are not immediately available.

Return precautions should include persistent fevers, rapidly progressive erythema and induration, purulent drainage, yellow crusting, or other signs of secondary infection. Follow-up with a specialist should be considered when flare has not resolved within 7 days despite treatment adherence or if the patient develops contact dermatitis from standard treatment regimen.

Complications

The most widely reported comorbidity of AD is sleep loss from severe pruritus. Recent studies suggest that up to 60% of children with AD have reported sleep disturbances. Poor sleep has been linked to poor performance in school, as well as social and emotional dysfunction. There is an increased prevalence of psychiatric disorders in those with AD, including attention-deficit/hyperactivity disorder, anxiety, and depression. These patients often have increased rates of *Staphylococcus aureus* and group A streptococcus colonization, as well as subsequent superinfections. Frequently, *Staph* and *Strep* superinfections present with localized honey-crusted, exudative lesions. There have been case reports of systemic complications, including bacteremia, endocarditis, and osteomyelitis. Viral infections, such as eczema herpeticum, have been known to disseminate in those with AD, causing severe or even fatal infections. Eczema herpeticum results from a superinfection of eczema lesions with herpes simplex virus (HSV-1 or HSV-2) and most often presents as a vesicular rash. In severe cases, patients can develop lymphadenopathy, malaise, keratoconjunctivitis, and multiorgan dysfunction. Eczema also increases the risk of common viral infections such as eczema coxsackium and molluscum contagiosum, although little is known about their infectious complications.

Rarely, contact dermatitis from topical therapy can develop and present as worsening rash despite adequate treatment. If this occurs, the patient should be referred to a specialist for patch testing and further management.

Key Points

- Eczema is a broad term used for a variety of disease states that cause the skin to become erythematous, inflamed, and pruritic.
- Atopic dermatitis is the most common type of eczema; often, the terms AD and eczema are used interchangeably. The hallmark presentation of AD is a pruritic relapsing, remitting eczematous rash with associated xerosis, erythema, pigmentation abnormalities, and, in some cases, lichenification.
- Uncontrolled AD can affect the social, emotional, and physical well-being of the patient.
- Treatment of AD includes trigger avoidance, regular bathing, and regimented emollient application. Topical corticosteroids are first-line treatment for acute exacerbations.

Pitfalls

- The location and characteristics of AD can vary based on age and race.
- These patients are at increased risk for secondary skin infections that have the potential to disseminate.
- In rare cases, TCSs can cause a contact dermatitis; this should be included in the differential diagnosis for eczema that worsens in the setting of appropriate therapy and medication adherence.

ERYTHEMA MULTIFORME

Background

Erythema multiforme is an immune-mediated process presenting with rash and occasional mucous membrane involvement. For a long time, EM was considered part of a spectrum of disorders that included EM, Stevens–Johnson syndrome (SJS), and toxic epidermal necrolysis (TEN), in which the severity of disease progressed respectively. This classification system is outdated, and recent studies classify EM as a separate disorder from SJS/TEN.

Classic Clinical Presentation

Classically, EM presents as a self-limited fixed, targetoid rash distributed peripherally with predilection for extensor surfaces. The eruption tends to spread centripetally, with the characteristics of the rash varying. Early skin eruptions are erythematous, circular papules with well-defined borders often confused with urticaria or an insect sting. As the rash progresses, the papules enlarge, but are typically <3 cm in diameter, and evolve to have three concentric rings of color with a central dusky appearance. Figure 22.2 demonstrates the classic presentation of EM. There is mucosal involvement in up to 60% of patients, and the presence of mucosal lesions separates EM major from EM minor; in the latter, mucosal surfaces are spared. The oral mucosa is the most frequently affected mucosal surface.

More than 90% of EM cases are associated with infection; with the largest proportion of EM occurring 1–3 weeks after HSV infection. Another predominate infectious source is *Mycoplasma pneumoniae*, which has also been associated with cases of SJS. EM has also been linked to medications (including β-lactam

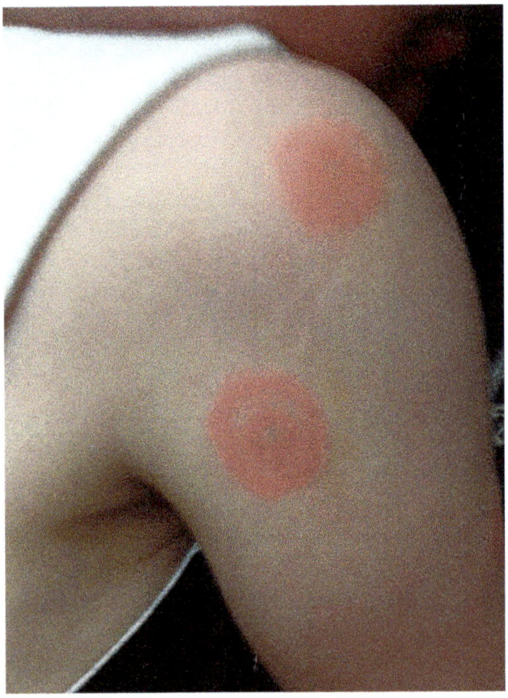

FIGURE 22.2 The classical fixed, targetoid rash seen with erythema multiforme. Note the three concentric rings of color with a central dusky appearance.

Source: Surtie F, Rehman HU. Target (iris) lesion of erythema multiforme. *Imaging J Clin Med Sci.* 2014;1(2):012. Open access publication.

antibiotics, sulfonamides, and nonsteroidal anti-inflammatory drugs), autoimmune disease, and malignancy.

Atypical Clinical Presentation

Erythema multiforme can present with atypical lesions that are raised, <3 cm in diameter, round with poorly defined edges, and have only two zones of color. Less commonly, EM can become recurrent or even persistent. Recurrent EM likely has a genetic predisposition and occurs sporadically throughout years, with the oral mucosa frequently involved. Figure 22.3 shows a young boy who presented with a rash several days after starting amoxicillin; this is an atypical pattern of EM because most lesions only have two rings of color.

Differential Diagnosis

Several rashes present in a similar manner as EM, including urticaria multiforme, serum sickness, Kawasaki disease, Henoch–Schonlein purpura, systemic lupus erythematosus (SLE), SJS, and other nonspecific drug rashes. These rashes, as well as their differentiating factors, are reviewed in Table 22.1.

Diagnostic Confirmation

There are no laboratory findings specific to the diagnosis EM. However, as with any inflammatory state, erythrocyte sedimentation rate and C-reactive protein may be elevated. In some severe cases, the patient may have a leukocytosis if the inciting factor is infectious. Titers for the most common infectious causes, such as HSV and *Mycoplasma*, can be helpful. Final diagnosis is often confirmed with

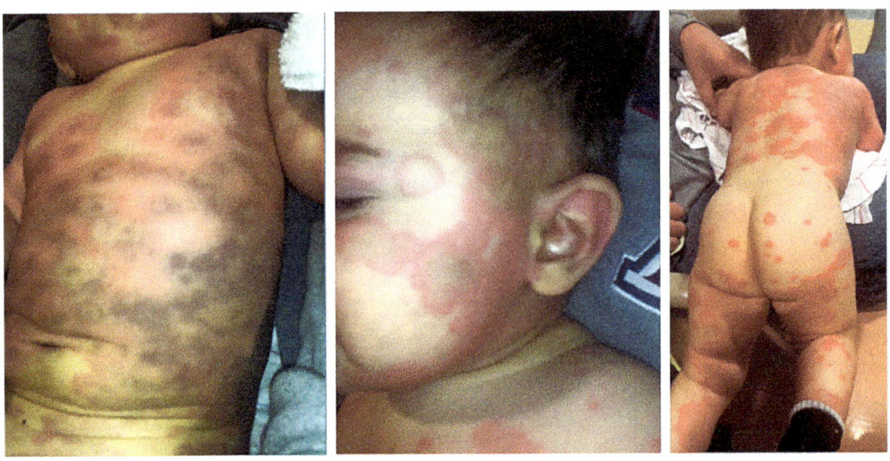

FIGURE 22.3 Atypical presentation of erythema multiforme on a young child recently treated with antibiotics. Diffuse distribution of rash with concentric circles that have both two and three rings of color can be seen in atypical presentations.

TABLE 22.1 DIFFERENTIAL DIAGNOSIS OF ERYTHEMA MULTIFORME AND ASSOCIATED DIFFERENTIATING FACTORS

Rash	Clinical Characteristics
Erythema multiforme	Fixed circular, erythematous papules with two or three rings of color and dusky central appearance. Peripheral distribution with predilection for extensor surfaces. Mucosal erosions and blisters common. Pruritic with occasional low-grade fever. No dermatographism.
Urticaria multiforme	Transient, circular, erythematous wheals with dusky, ecchymotic centers. Diffuse distribution. Some oral edema but no blisters. Lasts <2 weeks. Pruritic with occasional low-grade fever. Dermatographism is common.
Serum sickness	Fixed, circular, erythematous wheal with central clearing. Diffuse distribution. Some oral edema but no blisters. Lasts 1–6 weeks. High fever and joint pain. No dermatographism.
Kawasaki disease	Fixed erythematous macules with occasional targetoid lesions. Diffuse distribution. Mucosal lesions seen in 96% of patients. Associated desquamation, conjunctivitis, lymphadenopathy, and high fevers. No dermatographism.
Henoch–Schonlein purpura	Fixed, palpable purpura with petechiae. Occasional erythematous macules and wheals. Diffuse distribution. No mucosal involvement. Associated joint and abdominal pain. No fevers. No dermatographism.
Systemic lupus erythematosus	Lupus can have several different types of skin eruptions, including erythema multiforme-like lesions; however, these patients often have systemic symptoms such as joint pain, fevers, and abnormal labs.
Stevens–Johnson syndrome	Fixed erythematous macules with blistering and skin sloughing. <10% of body surface area affected, but distribution can be diffuse. Ocular and mucosal involvement is common. High fevers. No dermatographism.
Fixed drug rash	Fixed, erythematous plaques with central bullae and necrosis. Fewer lesions compared to erythema multiforme and rare mucosal involvement. Occurs within hours of taking offending medication.

tissue biopsy. Often, HSV DNA via polymerase chain reaction (PCR) can be detected within the lesion and can help differentiate between HSV and drug-induced EM. Box 22.1 reviews the diagnostic criteria that can aid in the diagnosis of EM.

Treatment

Treatment for EM is supportive. The lesions are pruritic, so management includes topical steroids and oral antihistamines. For patients who have limited oral involvement, treatment includes medicated mouthwashes and analgesics

BOX 22.1

DIAGNOSTIC CRITERIA FOR ERYTHEMA MULTIFORME

Lesions are <3 cm in diameter, round, and regular, with a well-defined border.

Typical lesions have least three different zones of color (two concentric rings around a dark central disk with one ring consisting of palpable edema).

Raised atypical targets: palpable lesions, reminiscent of erythema multiforme but with only two zones and/or a poorly defined border.

Less than 10% body surface area.

Source: Adapted from Siedner-Weintraub Y, Gross I, David A, Reif S, Molho-Pessach V. Paediatric erythema multiforme: Epidemiological, clinical and laboratory characteristics. *Acta Derm Venereol.* 2017;97(4):489–492. This is an open access publication.

for pain, in combination with a soft or liquid diet. For patients who have extensive oral mucosal involvement, PO intake might be affected. Hydration status should be closely monitored in this patient population, and systemic steroids are recommended [e.g., prednisone (1 or 2 mg/kg/day, maximum 60 mg/day with dosage tapered over 2–4 weeks)]. This is thought to decrease duration and severity of illness, but there is little evidence to support this recommendation. Ophthalmology consultation is also highly recommended in cases of ocular involvement. Most important, discontinuation of inciting factors is essential. If EM is thought to be drug induced, all offending medications started within the past 2 months should be stopped. Infections should be treated once confirmed positive; however, in the case of HSV-associated EM, there is little evidence that anti-HSV medication alters the course of the disease.

Disposition

Most classic cases of EM are self-limited and can be treated symptomatically in the emergency department. In minor cases, the patient can be discharged home with supportive care as outlined previously. However, in severe cases in which patients have extensive lesions, oral involvement, and/or ocular involvement, patients might require admission. These patients often need parenteral hydration and pain control. Ophthalmology consult is warranted in cases of severe ocular involvement. For those who can be discharged, return precautions should include signs of dehydration, decreased oral intake, significant progression of disease to involve a large body surface area, or signs of secondary infection. Outpatient follow-up with a primary physician is recommended to ensure lesions resolve in a timely manner. In cases of recurrent or persistent EM, follow-up with a dermatologist can be helpful.

Complications

Patients with extensive skin involvement are at risk for bacterial superinfections. Disseminated infection may occur without appropriate treatment. In cases of severe disease with ocular involvement, patients might have keratitis, conjunctival involvement, uveitis, or vision changes. In cases associated with *M. pneumoniae*, these patients might have respiratory distress, cough, low-grade fever, and shortness of breath. Skin lesions associated with EM do not cause scarring. However, some patients may have areas of hyperpigmentation that persists several months after disease resolution but fades with time.

Key Points

- EM is an immune-mediated process presenting with targetoid rash and occasional mucosal involvement.
- EM is a separate disorder from SJS/TEN and should not be considered part of this spectrum.
- More than 90% of cases are thought to be linked to preceding infection.
- In most minor cases, treatment is supportive. Offending drugs should be stopped, and patients should be treated for inciting infections. In severe cases, patients might require IV hydration, pain control, and treatment for infections.

Pitfalls

- Complications can include secondary infections, dehydration, and vision loss in those with severe ocular involvement.
- These patients are at increased risk for secondary skin infections that have the potential to disseminate.

HENOCH–SCHONLEIN PURPURA

Background

Henoch–Schonlein purpura is an immune-mediated vasculitis that primarily affects the small vessels in the skin, gastrointestinal (GI) tract, joints, and renal system, leading to a characteristic constellation of symptoms. It is the most common vasculitis seen in childhood. Caucasian children are most commonly affected, with a mean age of onset of 6 years and 90% of all cases occurring before age 10 years. Pathogenesis is thought to be driven by IgA deposits within the walls of these small vessels, leading to a characteristic leukocytoclastic vasculitis (LCV).

Classic Clinical Presentation

Classically, HSP presents with a rash, arthralgias, and abdominal pain. Rash occurs in all patients at some point during their clinical course; up to 80% of patients have arthralgias, 75% of patients have vague complaints of abdominal pain, and 50% of patients will have nonspecific pitting edema. The characteristics

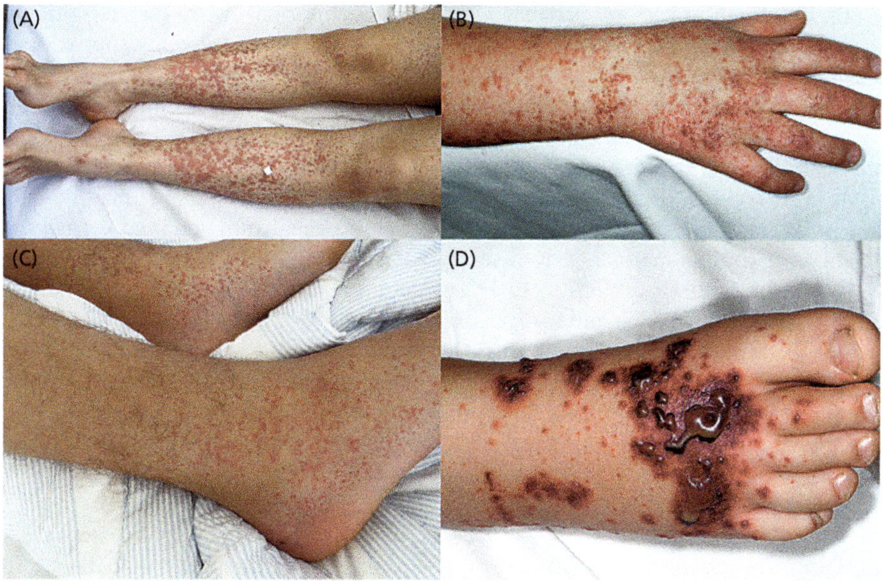

FIGURE 22.4 (A–C) Classical skin lesions of Henoch–Schönlein purpura, with palpable purpura on the extremities. (D) Bullous lesions of the lower extremities in a patient with Henoch–Schönlein purpura.

Source: Hetland LE, Susrud KS, Lindahl KH, Bygum A. Henoch–Schönlein purpura: A literature review. *Acta Derm Venereol.* 2017;97:1160–1166. Open access publication.

of the rash vary, but most frequently patients will have palpable purpura, petechiae, and edema in dependent areas. The majority of patients have the rash at presentation, but the order of presenting symptoms varies and HSP should be included in the differential diagnosis of a child who presents with diffuse arthralgias and/or abdominal pain. These arthralgias most commonly affect large joints such as the knees and ankles and can affect ambulation. Approximately 50% of patients diagnosed with HSP will have varying degrees of renal involvement from mild hematuria to severe, progressive glomerulonephritis (GN). Adults can be affected by HSP as well but are less likely to have joint involvement and abdominal complaints compared to the pediatric population. Figure 22.4 demonstrates the clinical variability seen in patients with HSP.

Atypical Clinical Presentation

Typically, patients present with a rash followed by arthralgias and abdominal pain; however, when rash is not the first symptom, diagnosis can be delayed. Joint pain can be the presenting symptoms in up to 25% of patients, preceding the rash by up to 1 week. Gastrointestinal symptoms including dull, periumbilical pain, nausea, vomiting, or hemocult-positive stools can occur in 75% of patients, with abdominal pain being the presenting symptom in 15% of patients. Renal involvement of some type occurs in roughly half of patients; however, it is very uncommon for this to be the presenting symptom because nephritic and nephrotic syndromes are often delayed weeks to months after the presenting rash. Atypically, the rash can present with vesicles and bullae in addition to palpable purpura.

Differential Diagnosis

Differential diagnosis can vary based on the order of presenting symptoms. In the 25% of patients in whom arthralgias proceed the rash, rheumatological diseases such as SLE and juvenile idiopathic arthritis (JIA) should be included in the differential diagnosis. However, JIA is less likely in this situation because the diagnostic criteria for JIA include 6 weeks of joint pain, in which time HSP would become evident. SLE and JIA also have associated rashes, although these rashes are often phenotypically different than HSP. Septic joint or transient synovitis may also be considered, but these cases often present with isolated joint involvement in which HSP is oligoarticular. In adults and adolescents, differential diagnosis of joint pain and rash should include disseminated gonococcal disease. In the small subset of patients who present with abdominal pain first, differential diagnosis often includes more common causes of periumbilical pain, such as viral gastroenteritis, constipation, early appendicitis, urinary tract infection, or intussusception.

HSP is a vasculitis; therefore, other vasculitides, such as hypersensitivity vasculitis, can present in a similar manner. Any disease process that reduces clotting ability, such as immune thrombocytopenia purpura, can also present with petechiae and bruising. The rash associated with meningococcemia can be similar in appearance to that of HSP; however, these patients are often very ill appearing, with hemodynamic instability differing drastically from the presentation of HSP.

Diagnostic Confirmation

In 2010, the European League Against Rheumatism and Pediatric Rheumatology International Trials Organization published diagnostic criteria for HSP that are shown in Box 22.2. The sensitivity and specificity of these classification criteria are high at 100% and 87%, respectively, when applied to children. No specific laboratory test can be used to diagnose HSP, and in most cases, all labs obtained will be normal with the exception of IgA, which can be elevated in approximately 50% of patients. Laboratory evaluation may help differentiate HSP from other conditions if the presentation is unclear. Complete blood count may be obtained to rule out platelet abnormalities, basic metabolic panel may be obtained to evaluate renal function, and urinalysis may be performed to evaluate for hematuria and proteinuria. In those with severe abdominal pain, imaging should be obtained because HSP has been associated with bowel perforation, infarction, and ileoileal intussusception. Abdominal ultrasound is the initial study of choice in children with severe abdominal pain.

BOX 22.2

DIAGNOSTIC CRITERIA FOR HENOCH–SCHONLEIN PURPURA

Mandatory criteria for HSP
- Palpable purpura or petechiae
- *and* one of the following
- Diffuse abdominal pain
  - LCV with predominant IgA deposits on skin biopsy
  - Acute arthritis or arthralgias in any joint
  - Renal involvement as evidenced by proteinuria and/or hematuria

Mandatory criteria
- Palpable purpura or petechiae
- *and* one of the following
  - Diffuse abdominal pain
  - LCV with predominant IgA deposits on skin biopsy
  - Acute arthritis or arthralgias in any joint
  - Renal involvement as evidenced by proteinuria and/or hematuria

LCV, leukocytoclastic vasculitis.

Treatment

Henoch–Schonlein purpura resolves spontaneously in the majority of patients; therefore, treatment is mainly supportive. For those with severe arthralgias, over-the-counter analgesic medications are recommended. Ranitidine and other H_2 blockers are helpful in those with mild GI complaints. Steroids use remains controversial. Multiple studies have demonstrated no long-term benefit in reducing the risk of developing renal complications or minimizing skin manifestations in HSP patients treated with corticosteroids. However, there is evidence that corticosteroids might augment the progression of renal disease in those with renal involvement at the time of presentation. There is also ample evidence suggesting decreased joint and abdominal complaints with steroid administration. Other treatment options include immunosuppression cell cycle inhibitors, such as cyclosporine A and mycophenolate mofetil; intravenous immunoglobulin; or plasmapheresis for those with severe renal involvement.

Clinical Algorithm

The most common severe complication of HSP is progressive renal disease. The initial workup for any patient with HSP, assuming the patient is well appearing and hemodynamically stable at the time of presentation, is a screening blood pressure and urinalysis. If these are both normal, additional labs are not warranted, and the patient can be discharged with supportive care and close primary care follow-up. If the patient has hypertension, proteinuria, or hematuria, a renal function panel is recommended to examine the degree of renal involvement. If this is normal, the patient can be discharged only if close pediatric nephrology follow-up can be arranged as an outpatient before discharge. If blood urea nitrogen or serum creatinine are abnormal or follow-up is not available, the patient should be admitted to a pediatric center in which subspecialists are available.

After discharge, surveillance for renal involvement must be ongoing. Roughly 90% of patients with HSP nephritis will develop urinary abnormalities within the first 4 weeks of disease onset, and nephritis rarely precedes the rash. Urinalysis should be done weekly while the disease state is ongoing and monthly thereafter for the following 6 months. If, after 6 months, the urinalysis remains normal, the patient is unlikely to develop renal complications. If the patient develops hematuria, proteinuria, or hypertension at any time, follow-up with a nephrologist should be arranged.

Disposition

Most patients with HSP can be managed on an outpatient basis with supportive treatment. Some patients with severe pain might require admission for pain control. In those with abdominal pain out of proportion to examination findings or with concerning physical examination findings, consider admission for further imaging or serial abdominal examination. Those with hematuria or proteinuria with a normal serum creatinine require close, expedited follow-up with a pediatric nephrologist. This can be arranged as outpatient follow-up but should be confirmed before discharge from the emergency department. If outpatient follow-up is unavailable or the patient has an abnormal creatine, admission to a pediatric hospital with the appropriate subspecialties is strongly encouraged.

The importance of follow-up should be emphasized to parents. Renal complications such as hypertension, hematuria, proteinuria, or acute renal failure have been reported up to 10 years after initial presentation, so regular follow-up is extremely important. The rash may get worse before getting better; return precautions should include signs of secondary infections or systemic symptoms such as fever, severe edema, or severe, unresolving abdominal pain.

Complications

There are several rare but serious complications of HSP. HSP is a small vessel vasculitis and therefore can affect all small vessels in the body. There have been case reports of neurological involvement including seizures, ataxia, and encephalopathy. Pleural effusions, myocarditis, and respiratory failure have also been documented. Abdominal complications include intussusception, bowel wall necrosis, and perforation.

Key Points

- HSP presents with a rash, arthralgias, and abdominal pain with rash occurring 100% of patients, although this is not always the present on initial presentation.
- The rash is described as palpable purpura, petechiae, and edema in dependent areas, but in some cases, bullous lesions can form.
- If HSP is suspected, urinalysis must be checked to ensure there is no renal involvement. If the patient has hypertension, proteinuria, or hematuria serum, creatinine should be obtained.
- Treatment is supportive with pain control. Steroids decrease the severity of joint or abdominal pain but have no effect on rash or the development of renal involvement.

Pitfall

- Complications include progressive renal disease, intussusception, bowel wall necrosis, perforation, and, in rare cases, seizures.

SCABIES

Background

Scabies is a very common parasitic infection of the skin by the *Sarcoptes scabiei* var. *hominis* mite. The female mite burrows into the epidermis and lays eggs. Most of the symptoms of scabies are secondary to a type IV hypersensitivity reaction to the feces of the mite. Scabies can affect people of all races, sex, and age, as well as social status. However, those at the extremes of age and immunocompromised individuals are at higher risk. The role of poor hygiene in the development of scabies is overestimated; there is a stronger correlation with overcrowding, such as in nursing homes, prisons, day care centers, and refugee camps. Another common misconception is that scabies is spread from animals to people; this is not the case. Animals can get scabies, causing a syndrome commonly known as mange, but this type of mite cannot survive or reproduce in human skin. Crusted (Norwegian) scabies is a severe clinical variant of scabies that occurs in the immunocompromised or extremes of age. Both types of scabies are discussed in this section, with differences highlighted.

Classic Clinical Presentation

The clinical characteristics of scabies vary according to age. Classically, patients will have a papular, erythematous, pruritic rash with nodules, burrow marks, and vesicles. Burrow marks are from the mite tunneling within the skin and look like hypopigmented or skin-colored lines. These are most prominent at the interdigital folds of the fingers, the buttocks, the flexor surfaces of the wrist and elbows, and the intertriginous areas such as inguinal folds or axilla. Nodules are significantly more common in those younger than age 2 years, and vesicles are seen more frequently in those older than age 15 years. Burrows, pruritus, and blisters are seen equally in adults and children. Location of infection can vary with age; infants are more likely to have head, neck, face, and scalp involvement, whereas upper extremities and genital involvement is seen more commonly in adults. Intense nightly pruritus is characteristic of scabies and can greatly affect quality of life if left untreated. Figure 22.5 demonstrates the clinical variability seen with scabies.

Atypical Clinical Presentation

Crusted scabies can present differently than traditional scabies and is associated with an extremely high mite burden of potentially millions of mites per body. It can be seen in anyone but is more common in those with HIV and other immunocompromising conditions, those on long-term topical steroids, and those with neuropathy or dementia. Lesions are erythematous, scaly, and hyperkeratotic. Often, more than 90% of patients' body surface area is involved, including the scalp, face, and nails. These patients can have pruritus

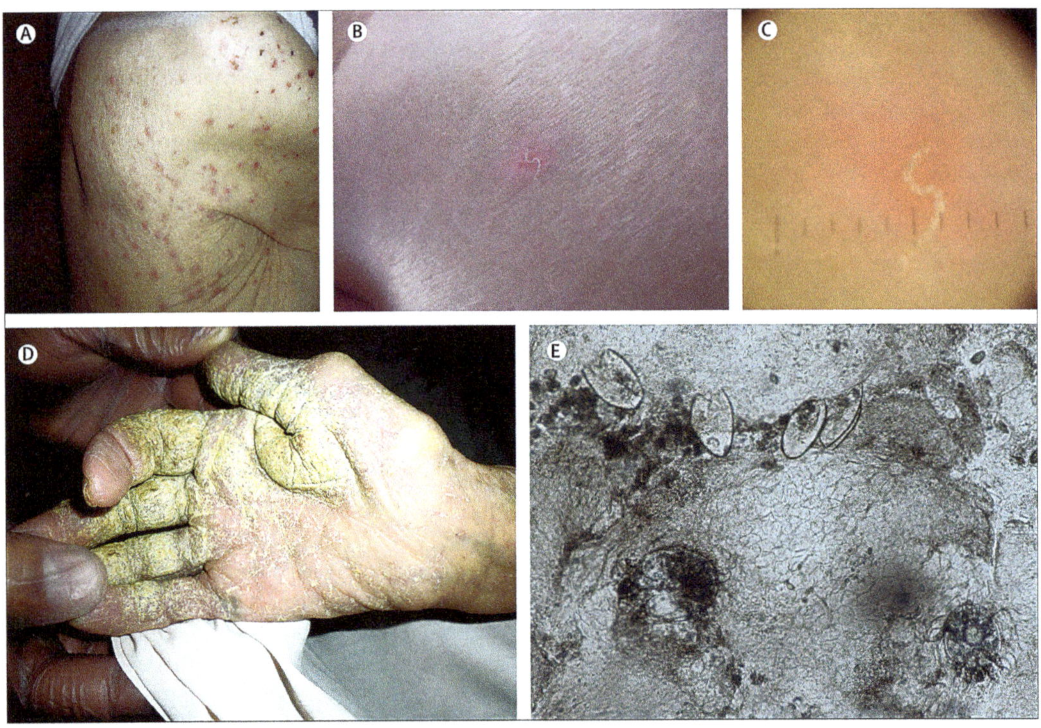

FIGURE 22.5 Papules (A) and burrows (B) in a patient with scabies. Burrows under dermatoscopy (C), hyperkeratotic skin (D), and *Sarcoptes scabiei* mites and eggs under ×10 microscopy (E).

Source: Cassell JA, Middleton J, Nalabanda A, et al. Scabies outbreaks in ten care homes for elderly people: A prospective study of clinical features, epidemiology, and treatment outcomes. *Lancet Infect Dis*. 2018;18(8):894–902. doi:10.1016/s1473-3099(18)30347-5. Open access publication.

or pain, depending on the degree of the skin breakdown. This form of scabies is highly contagious, spreading through direct and indirect contact. This can cause large-scale outbreaks in overcrowded facilities if left untreated.

Differential Diagnosis

Scabies is very similar in appearance to several different rashes, often leading to a misdiagnosis or delay in treatment. Other rashes to rule out before making the diagnosis of scabies include atopic and contact dermatitis, impetigo, or folliculitis. Papular urticaria from fleas or bedbugs should also be considered. The differential diagnosis for crusted scabies is different from that for classic scabies. The diffuse erythroderma associated with crusted scabies can cause it to be misdiagnosed as crusted psoriasis or hyperkeratotic eczema, contact dermatitis, ichthyosis, or adverse drug reaction.

Diagnostic Confirmation

Scabies is a clinical diagnosis, and there are no formal diagnostic criteria for diagnosing scabies. A history of diffuse itching, visible lesions in at least two typical locations of scabies, or a household member with a history of itching had 100% sensitivity and 97% specificity in sub-Saharan Africa; however, the prevalence there is as high as 13%. Such data are lacking in areas of lower prevalence, such as the United States.

When the diagnosis by history and physical is unclear, some bedside tests are available to help aid the diagnosis. Examining skin scrapings for the mite, egg, or mite feces under a microscope can be done by covering a scalpel with oil and scraping laterally across multiple burrows, papules, or vesicles. The scrapings are then placed on a slide and examined under a light microscope with 200× magnification. However, this method is operator dependent with little sensitivity because scabies is associated with a very low mite burden of approximately 10–15 mites per body. Two other simple methods of detection are the burrow ink test and the adhesive tape test. The burrow ink test involves using a fountain pen to gently cover a suspicious lesion with ink. Excess ink is removed with an alcohol swab, leaving visible a wavy ink-filled line where the mite has tunneled into the skin. The adhesive tape test is completed by firmly placing the adhesive side of a piece of tape to a suspicious skin lesion, pulling it off, and transferring it directly to a microscope. Although these methods can be helpful, their sensitivity and specificity are unknown. Handheld magnification devices such as dermoscopy or videography can also be used if available; however, these require specialized training. Currently, there are no laboratory tests used to diagnose scabies; there is a PCR method for detecting *S. scabiei* DNA in skin scrapings and enzyme-linked immunosorbent assay antibody testing, but these have limited availability and are expensive.

Treatment

Scabies is primarily spread through prolonged, direct skin-to-skin contact, with an incubation period of 4–6 weeks. Even those without the rash can be infectious and spread the infection to others. Thus, it is recommended to treat the patient, any sexual contacts, and all household contacts even if they are asymptomatic. Permethrin 5% cream is the first-line therapy and works to kill the mite as well as the eggs. Lindane is no longer recommended because permethrin is more effective and less toxic. In older children and adults, permethrin cream should be applied from the neck down, left on for 8 hours, and then washed off. In infants and toddlers, the cream should be applied in the same manner, but the head and neck should be included, sparing the eyes. This treatment should be repeated in 1 week. In those who cannot tolerate topical agents, a single dose of ivermectin (200 μg/kg) is safe for the treatment of scabies; however, permethrin has a higher cure rate. Crusted scabies should be treated with permethrin daily for 7 days and then twice a week until cured, in combination with oral ivermectin. Despite effective treatment, symptoms including the rash can last for up to 1 month after treatment. These symptoms should be treated symptomatically with pain control and antihistamines.

Although uncommon, scabies can spread through fomites such as clothing, bedding, towels, and stuffed animals. These items can be decontaminated by washing them in hot water and drying them on the hot cycle; dry cleaning is also effective. Mites can only live for approximately 72 hours away from human skin; therefore, if washing the item is not an option, removing it from any bodily contact and storing in a sealed plastic bag for this amount of time would also suffice.

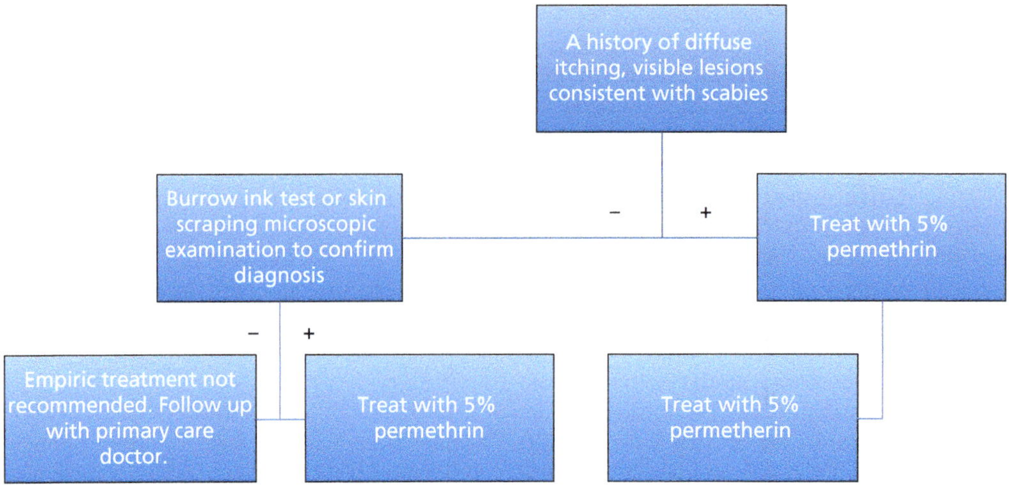

FIGURE 22.6 Clinical algorithm that can be used in the diagnosis of scabies.

Clinical Algorithm

If the patient has a history consistent with scabies, including diffuse pruritus or a household member with diffuse itching, and has a rash consistent with scabies (e.g., papules, nodules, burrow marks, and vesicles), treatment should be initiated. The patient, any sexual contacts, and all household members should be treated independent of their symptoms. If the patient has no history of pruritus, no family member with these symptoms, and the rash is not consistent with scabies, bedside testing such as skin scrapings or the burrow ink test can be completed if scabies is in the differential diagnosis. If this is negative, empiric treatment is not recommended, and the patient should follow up with their primary care doctor for further management outside of symptomatic treatement. This treatment algorithm is outlined in Figure 22.6.

Disposition

Most patients with scabies can be managed with outpatient treatment. Treatment is supportive with antihistamines and analgesia as needed, in addition to 5% permethrin cream. Those with severe bacterial or viral superinfections who have failed outpatient treatment may require admission for antibiotics or pain control. Assess hydration status to ensure the patient does not require IV fluids prior to determining disposition. The patient should be sent home with treatment for themselves and all household contacts. Instructions should be given for washing all bedding, clothes, and towels in hot water and drying on high heat. Follow-up should be arranged with a primary care doctor after treatment is complete to ensure the patient does not need additional treatments doses. For those with crusted scabies, follow-up with dermatology should be arranged given the extensive nature of the illness. Return precautions should be given for signs of secondary infections and dehydration after treatment.

Complications

The intense pruritic nature of this infection leads to scratching and increases the risk of a secondary bacterial infection and sores. There is a link between secondary infection of scabies with *Streptococcus pyogenes* and post-streptococcal GN. The itching is worse at night, so a patient's quality of sleep can be greatly affected. The scabies mite is not known to transmit infection such as those seen with ticks or mosquitoes. Dehydration should be assessed carefully in children because discomfort can lead to decreased oral intake.

Key Points

- Scabies is a very common parasitic infection causes by the *S. scabiei* var. *hominis* mite that leads to papular, erythematous, pruritic rash with nodules, burrow marks, and vesicles.
- Scabies is spread through prolonged, direct skin-to-skin contact as well as contact with infected fomites, with an incubation period of 4–6 weeks.

- Permethrin 5% cream is the first-line therapy.
- The intense pruritic nature of this infection leads to scratching and increases the risk of a secondary bacterial infection.

Pitfall

- Failure to consider scabies in any pruritic rash

TINEA INFECTIONS

Background

Dermatophytosis is a general term used to describe a fungal infection of keratinized tissues such as hair, skin, and nails. This might be referred to as ringworm by the general public. The name of the infection reflects its involved location: Tinea capitis involves the scalp; tinea barbae infects the beard; tinea manus involves the hands; tinea cruris infects the groin; tinea pedis infects the foot; and tinea unguium, also known as onychomycosis, affects the nails. The most common cutaneous fungal infection in children is tinea capitis, mostly affecting children aged 3–7 years and uncommon after puberty. Transmission is thought to occur through close contact with infected individuals or animals. Neonatal infections have been documented from skin-to-skin contact between infants and infected mothers. Risk factors for infection include immunosuppression, diabetes, the use of broad-spectrum antibiotics or corticosteroids, and a humid environment.

Classic Clinical Presentation

Independent of the location, cutaneous fungal infections involving the skin will present as pruritic, mildly erythematous, dry, scaly papules. The lesion spreads outward to form an annular plaque with central hypopigmentation and pustules. Figure 22.7 demonstrates the classical presentation of tinea corporis. Tinea pedis, also known as athlete's foot, involves the interdigital spaces and can ulcerate and fissure or become hyperkeratotic. Tinea cruris presents as unilateral scaling of the inguinal fold; the hair follicles are usually not involved. Tinea capitis and barbae are cutaneous fungal infections impacting the skin and hair follicles. Classically, presentation is often in the form of a diffuse scaly-like lesion that can initially look like dandruff. This progresses to small, erythematous circular patches of alopecia with multiple hairs broken off at the follicular level. These broken hairs can be used as a key feature to differentiate tinea infections from other forms of alopecia because they appear as small black dots within the area of alopecia that would otherwise be smooth. Figure 22.8 demonstrates tinea capitis without (Figure 22.8A) and with alopecia (Figure 22.8B). Last, tinea unguium is rare in children but presents with thickening of the nails and yellowish discoloration.

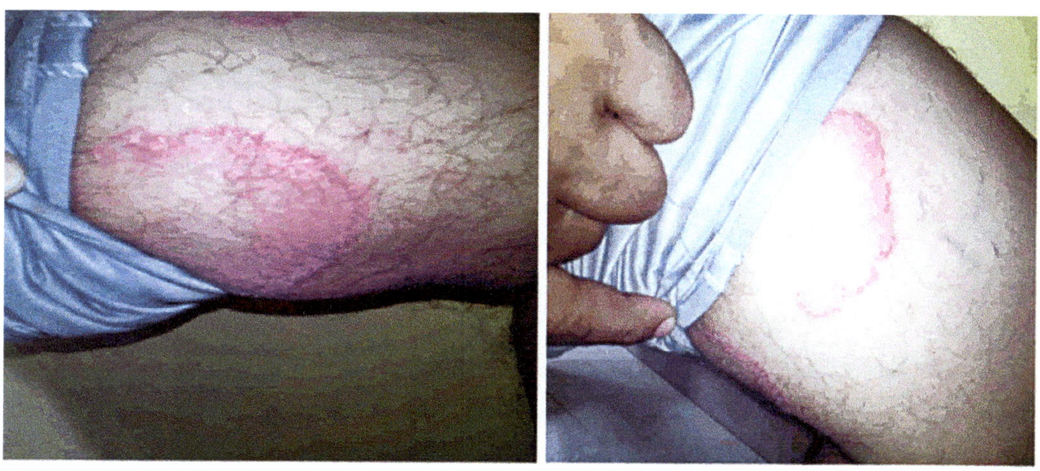

FIGURE 22.7 Classic clinical representation of tinea corporis.

Source: Metri K. Clinical image of tinea corporis. *Interdiscip J Microinflammation*. 2014;1:I102. doi:10.4172/2381-8727.1000I102. Open access publication.

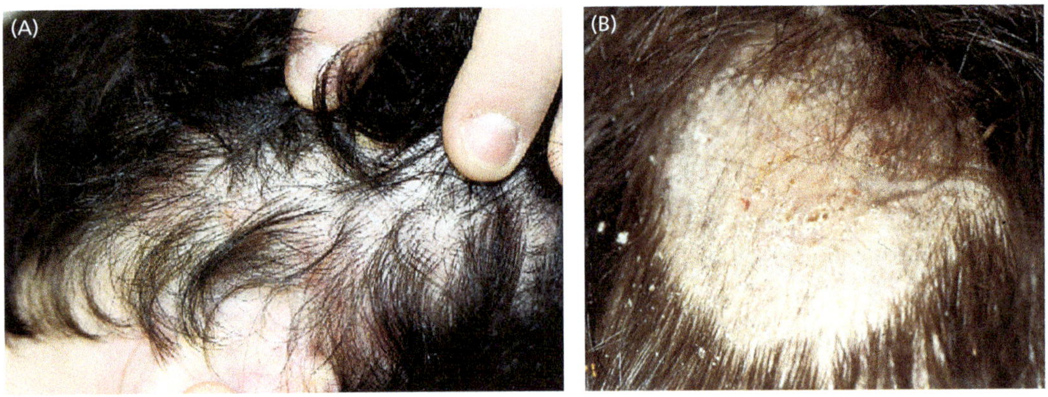

FIGURE 22.8 Tinea capitis without (A) and with (B) associated alopecia.

Sources: A, Kurian A, Haber RM. Tinea corporis gladiatorum presenting as a Majocchi granuloma. *ISRN Dermatol.* 2011;2011:1–3. doi:10.5402/2011/767589. Open access publication. B, Grimalt R. Management of tinea capitis in childhood. *Clin Cosmet Investig Dermatol.* 2010;89. doi:10.2147/ccid.s7992. Open access publication.

Atypical Clinical Presentation

Atypically, in severe cases of tinea corporis, Majocchi granuloma can develop. This occurs when the dermatophyte follows the hair follicle down to the level of the dermis, leading to follicular-based nodules or pustules. This is most common with *Trichophyton rubrum* infections, particularly when the patient has been misdiagnosed and pretreated with corticosteroids. Figure 22.9 demonstrates a Majocchi granuloma. Similarly, in severe cases of tinea capitis, patients can develop kerions. These are erythematous, localized, raised, circular lesions that are thought to result from an aggressive immune response to the infective agent rather than the infection itself. These lesions appear pustular and crusted. Kerions are occasionally associated with systemic symptoms such as pain, fever, and lymphadenopathy. If left untreated, they can cause scarring. Figure 22.10 shows a kerion.

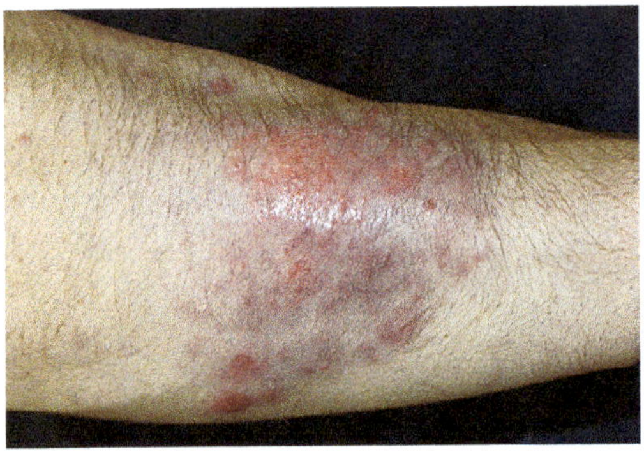

FIGURE 22.9 Majocchi granuloma from tinea corporis gladiatorum.

Source: Kurian A, Haber RM. Tinea corporis gladiatorum presenting as a Majocchi granuloma. *ISRN Dermatol.* 2011;2011: 1–3. doi:10.5402/2011/767589. Open access publication.

Another atypical presentation of tinea infections is tinea incognito, in which there is a decrease in the local inflammatory response normally seen in cutaneous fungal infections after the infection has been mistreated with topical steroids. This improves the classic superficial characteristics seen with fungal infections, giving the false impression that the rash has improved. However, the rash will return when the steroids are discontinued, often appearing darker and larger with diffuse scaling.

Differential Diagnosis

Differential diagnosis depends on the location of infection. Table 22.2 outlines the differential diagnosis based on location of the infection.

Diagnostic Confirmation

Diagnosis of cutaneous fungal infections can be made by history and physical examination. However, if diagnosis is still questionable, a skin sample can be obtained by gently scraping the edge of the lesion with the blunt side of a scalpel. Material should be placed in 10–20% potassium hydroxide and then examined under a microscope for branching hyphae. Skin scrapings can also be cultured, but this process

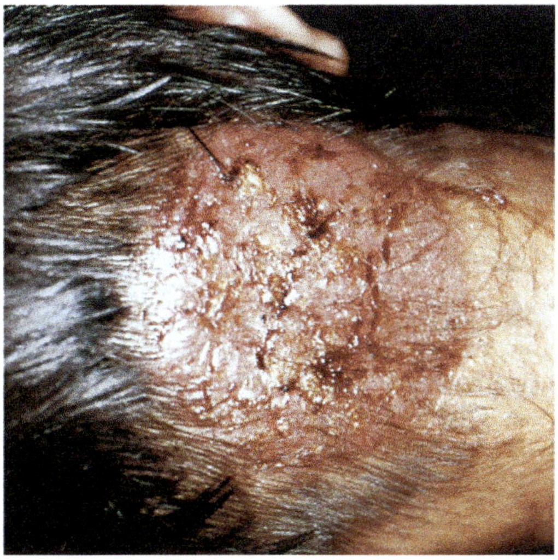

FIGURE 22.10 Kerion.

Source: Grimalt R. Management of tinea capitis in childhood. *Clin Cosmet Investig Dermatol.* 2010;89. doi:10.2147/ccid.s7992. Open access publication.

takes several weeks. Wood's lamp examination can be used to aid in the diagnosis of fungal infections involving hair, such as tinea capitis, because this will cause the hair to fluoresces a blue-green color. Dermatophyosis of the skin does not fluoresce, with the exception of tinea versicolor.

Treatment

Any fungal infections involving the hair follicle or nail bed cannot be treated with topical agents. For tinea capitis, oral griseofulvin at a dose of 10–25 mg/kg is recommended for 12 weeks. There is no requirement for blood tests before or during administration of this medication in otherwise healthy children. Reassessment of the patient's symptoms should be done monthly and at the conclusion of treatment to ensure treatment does not need to be extended. Other treatment options include terbinafine; however, hepatotoxicity is a known complication, and liver function tests are required before beginning the medication and monthly thereafter until treatment is finished. Fluconazole and itraconazole also carry a risk of hepatotoxicity. Adjunctive treatment with antifungal shampoo such as ketoconazole or selenium sulfide is recommended two or three times a week.

For infections involving the skin only, such as in cases of tinea cruris, corporis, manus, or pedis, topical antifungals are recommended. First-line treatment options include imidazoles such as chlormidazole, clotrimazole,

TABLE 22.2 DIFFERENTIAL DIAGNOSIS FOR CUTANEOUS FUNGAL INFECTIONS BASED

Infection	Differential Diagnosis
Tinea barbae	Folliculitis, furuncle, contact dermatitis
Tinea cruris	Erythrasma, candidal infection
Tinea pedis	Dyshidrotic eczema, contact dermatitis, psoriasis, candidal infection
Tinea unguium	Bacterial paronychia, nail psoriasis
Tinea corporis	Granuloma annulare, atopic dermatitis, nummular dermatitis, pityriasis rosea, fixed drug reaction or erythema migrans
Tinea capitis	Seborrhea dermatitis, dandruff, atopic dermatitis, alopecia areata

miconazole, econazole, and ketoconazole. These all have broad antifungal activity, some antibacterial activity, and systemic absorption is negligible even after prolonged exposure. Cream should be applied to infected skin and surrounding normal skin up to 2 cm from the edge of the lesion. Treatment should continue for 1 week longer than clinical cure.

Disposition

Most patients diagnosed with cutaneous fungal infections can be treated in an outpatient setting and discharged from the emergency department. Oral or topical medication should be prescribed depending on the site of infection, and patients should be encouraged to follow up with their primary care doctor because response to treatment should be monitored on a monthly basis. The patient may need monthly blood work to assess liver function, depending on the medication used. In cases of tinea capitis, barbae, or unguium, treatment might need to be extended beyond 12 weeks in refractory cases. As with any skin infection, patients with extensive skin involvement or pruritus are at risk for bacterial superinfections such as impetigo or abscesses. Depending on the severity of the superinfection, the patient may require admission to the hospital for IV antibiotics, although this is rare.

Complications

One well-known complication of antifungal medications is an interface dermatitis reaction. This is a secondary inflammatory reaction that occurs soon after starting antifungal agents. This rash can vary in appearance from a widespread vesicular rash to a localized maculopapular eruption. The underlying infection must be treated, so once allergic reaction is ruled out, continuation of antifungal medication is recommended. Symptoms can be treated with oral or topical antihistamines.

Key Points

- The most common cutaneous fungal infection in children is tinea capitis.
- For infections involving the skin, only topical antifungals, such as clotrimazole or miconazole, are recommended for 1 week longer than clinical cure.
- For tinea capitis, treatment is oral griseofulvin at a dose of 10–25 mg/kg for 12 weeks.

Pitfalls

- Atypical presentation of tinea includes tinea incognito, in which there is a decrease in the local inflammatory response normally seen in cutaneous fungal infection after the infection was treated with topical steroids.
- One well-known complication of antifungal medications is an interface dermatitis reaction. This is a secondary inflammatory reaction from the dermatophyte that occurs soon after starting an antifungal agent. Antifungals should be continued through this reaction.

URTICARIA

Background

Urticaria, also known as hives, is a rash with associated edema caused by histamine release from mast cells. The rash is typically described as pruritic, blanching, erythematous wheals that vary in size. The lesions are migratory and transient, which is a key feature used to differentiate it from other similar rashes. Concurrent angioedema occurs in 50% of cases, and the lifetime prevalence of urticaria is approximately 25%, although the exact prevalence in the pediatric population is unknown. Urticaria can be categorized into acute and chronic subtypes depending on how long the symptoms are present. In acute urticaria, symptoms last less than 6 weeks; chronic urticaria lasts more than 6 weeks and is episodic over weeks to months. Causes of urticaria include infections, drug and food hypersensitivities, and autoimmune reactions. The most common foods implicated in this type of reaction are shown in Box 22.3.

BOX 22.3

MOST COMMON FOODS IMPLICATED IN ALLERGIC URTICARIA

Eggs
Milk
Soy
Peanut
Wheat
Seafood

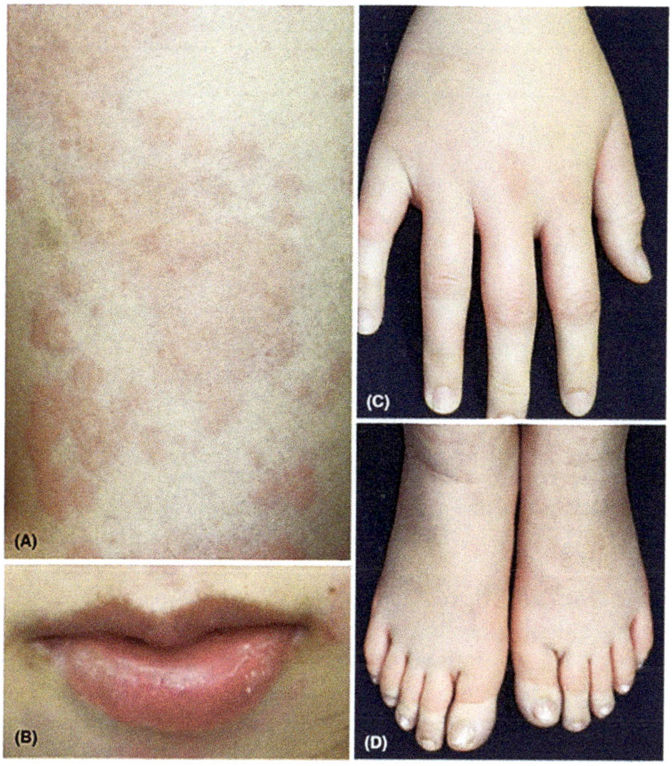

FIGURE 22.11 Clinical features of urticaria (A, C, and D) and angioedema (B).
Source: J Cutan Immunol Allergy. 2018;1(3):119–120. doi:10.1002/cia2.12024. Open access publication.

Classic Clinical Presentation

Acute urticaria is the most common subtype in children. It is described as blanching, erythematous, pruritic wheals that resolve without scaring, with only 5% of children experience symptoms after 15 days. The development of urticaria is a type 1 hypersensitivity reaction in which allergen-specific IgE is produced after contact with a particular agent. Upon further contact, the allergen bound to IgE cross-links IgE receptors on the surface of mast cells, leading to symptoms. Figure 22.11 shows typical urticarial lesions and angioedema.

Atypical Clinical Presentation

Urticaria multiforme is a subtype of acute urticaria that presents with erythematous wheals with dusky, ecchymotic centers. This can often be confused with EM. Chronic urticaria is less common than acute urticaria and is diagnosed when symptoms last longer than 6 weeks. Physical triggers are the most common precipitating factors in chronic urticaria. Subtypes of physical urticaria are detailed in Table 22.3.

Differential Diagnosis

Urticaria can mimic other disease processes such as EM or fixed drug reactions. Urticarial lesions are migratory, whereas EM and drug reactions are fixed. Urticarial vasculitis is a small vessel vasculitis that can be confused with chronic urticaria; biopsy is often required to differentiate them. Autoimmune processes such as celiac disease, thyroid disease, JIA, SLE, and type 1 diabetes mellitus have all been linked to childhood urticaria and should be ruled out in patients with refractory chronic urticaria, particularly those with a positive family history of such. Urticaria can occur with angioedema or separately. It is important to differentiate isolated urticaria from urticaria in the setting of anaphylaxis. Anaphylaxis is defined as a life-threatening reaction that often involves edema, urticaria, and, in severe cases, hypotension and shock. This is defined

TABLE 22.3 PHYSICAL URTICARIA SUBTYPES

Subtype	Characteristics
Cholinergic	Urticaria caused by an increase in core body temperature after exercise, stress, hot water, or certain foods
Demographic	Urticaria caused by stroking or scratching the skin
Aquagenic	Urticaria that occurs after skin comes in contact with water, regardless of temperature; most commonly seen in women
Cold	Cold air, wind, or water
Solar	Urticaria from sunlight or ultraviolet light exposure
Exercise	Exercise-induced anaphylaxis or urticaria
Sensation (vibration or pressure)	Urticaria in response to vibration or vertical pressure

as the involvement of two organ systems such as the skin, GI tract, angioedema, hypotension, or hypotonia.

Diagnostic Confirmation

There is limited utility to laboratory testing in the setting of acute urticaria. A thorough history and physical examination should be completed, and anaphylaxis must be ruled out. If an allergen clearly elicited the reaction, avoidance should be recommended, and the patient should be sent to an allergy specialist. Allergy testing may be warranted as an outpatient. Those with chronic urticaria should be referred to a specialist for further workup and ongoing management.

Treatment

Acute urticaria is treated symptomatically with antihistamines. Second-generation antihistamines, such as loratadine and cetirizine, are effective against urticarial reactions and often less sedating than first-generation medications such as diphenhydramine. These medications can be used together when presentation is severe. Histamine H_2 receptor antagonists such as famotidine and ranitidine can also be of some added benefit. Leukotriene inhibitors such as montelukast can also be helpful in refractory cases. Corticosteroids can be used, but only when the patient has failed the previously discussed regimen or there is significant associated angioedema; symptoms can reoccur when steroids are discontinued, and prolonged courses of systemic steroids should be avoided. An attempt should be made to identify the offending agent and subsequently avoid it, although this can sometimes be difficult.

If the patient is deemed to have anaphylaxis, an intramuscular (IM) dose of epinephrine should be given immediately. Histamine H_1 and H_2 receptor antagonists, such as diphenhydramine and ranitidine or famotidine, respectively, should be given. Corticosteroids can be used, but there is little evidence that steroids affect clinical outcome. H_1 and H_2 blockers, cyclosporine, and corticosteroids have all been used in the treatment of chronic urticaria, but such treatment should occur under the direction of a specialist. The dosing regimens for the previously mentioned medications are provided in Table 22.4. In those with vomiting, with the exception of IM epinephrine, IV formulations are best.

Disposition

If anaphylaxis has been ruled out and presentation is consistent with acute urticaria without significant angioedema, the patient can be treated symptomatically with antihistamines and discharged home. Follow-up with primary care doctor should be arranged if symptoms persist and progress into chronic urticaria. Subspecialist follow-up should be arranged for these patients or those who warrant further testing. Thorough history and physical examination should be completed, and if a trigger is identified, the patient should be counseled on avoidance. If there are concerns for an allergic reaction or anaphylaxis, the patient should be discharged with an epinephrine autoinjector and taught how to use it. Urticarial lesions will wax and wane over several days, with most cases dissipating by 15 days. Before discharge, parents should be counseled that hives might return as antihistamines wear off

TABLE 22.4 MEDIATION INFORMATION FOR TREATMENT OF ALLERGIC REACTION

Mediation	Route of Administration	Dose	Frequency
Epinephrine	IM	1:1,000 dilution 0.01 mg/kg (maximum 0.3 mg) <30 kg = 0.15 >30 kg = 0.30 autoinjectors	Every 5 minutes until symptoms resolve
Diphenhydramine	IV or PO	1 mg/kg	Every 6 hours
Ranitidine	IV or PO	1–2 mg/kg	Every 12 hours
Famotidine	IV or PO	PO: 0.5 mg/kg/dose; maximum dose 40 mg/dose IV: 0.25 mg/kg/dose; maximum dose 20 mg/dose	Every 12 hours
Cetirizine	PO only	2–6 years old: 2.5 mg >6 years old: 5–10 mg	Daily
Loratadine	PO only	2–6 years old: 5 mg >6 years old: 10 mg	Daily
Dexamethasone	IV or PO	0.6 mg/kg; maximum dose 16 mg	Every 8 hours
Prednisone or prednisolone	PO only	0.5–1 mg/kg; maximum dose 60 mg	Daily

IM, intramuscular; IV, intravenous; PO, per os.

and, in the absence of respiratory symptoms or symptoms concerning for anaphylaxis, this alone is not a reason to return to the emergency department. Return precautions should include vomiting, inability to tolerate oral intake, shortness of breath, trouble breathing, or worsening angioedema.

Typically, if the patient was treated for anaphylaxis and required two or more doses of epinephrine, admission is recommended. If isolated angioedema is noted but there is no respiratory compromise and the patient can tolerate oral intake, the patient can be discharged home with strict return precautions.

Complications

The most dangerous complication of urticaria is when there is failure to recognize the rash as part of acute anaphylaxis. This is a potentially life-threatening situation that requires rapid diagnosis and treatment. Other potential complications include progression to chronic urticaria, which is benign but can affect quality of life if symptoms are severe and frequent. Secondary bacterial infection is also a potential complication, especially when symptoms of pruritus are difficult to control.

Key Points

- Urticaria, also known as hives, is a rash described as pruritic, blanching, erythematous wheals that vary in size.
- Urticaria multiforme is a subtype of acute urticaria that presents with erythematous wheals with dusky, ecchymotic centers.
- Acute urticaria is treated symptomatically with antihistamines. Corticosteroids can be used, but only when the patient has failed all other treatment options.

Pitfall

- The most dangerous complication of urticaria is when there is failure recognize the rash as part of acute anaphylaxis. This is a potentially life-threatening situation that requires rapid diagnosis and treatment.

IMPETIGO AND ECTHYMA

Background

Impetigo is the most common skin infection affecting children aged 2–5 years and can be classified into bullous or nonbullous subtypes. The most common pathogens responsible for impetigo include *Staphylococcus aureus* and β-hemolytic *Streptococcus pyogenes*. Openly exposed skin, such as on the face and extremities, is most commonly affected. Patients with immunosuppressive states, poor hygiene, or disruptions of the skin such as eczema are at higher risk of this type of infection.

Classic Clinical Presentation

As mentioned previously, impetigo can present as bullous or nonbullous subtypes, with the latter being more common, comprising 70% of cases. Nonbullous impetigo can be further subdivided into primary and secondary forms. This subdivision simply refers to the condition of skin before infection. Primary nonbullous impetigo refers to infection of intact, healthy skin, whereas secondary nonbullous impetigo refers to the infection of a break in the skin such as those caused by rashes, insect bites, or trauma. Nonbullous impetigo starts as erythematous papular lesions that progress into fluid-filled vesicles and subsequent painful erosions with honey-colored crusting. If untreated, both subtypes of impetigo will self-resolve in 2 or 3 weeks without scarring. Some patients may have regional lymphadenopathy, but otherwise, systemic symptoms are rare. Bullous impetigo typically presents as large, flaccid bullae that rupture and leak infectious serous fluid. When the bullae rupture, patients are left with an erythematous base surrounded by thin brown crust and scales. This type of infection is exclusively caused by *Staphylococcus aureus* and is a common cause of ulcerative rash in the diaper region of infants.

Atypical Clinical Presentation

Ecthyma is a type of impetigo that erodes into the dermis, causing crusted, ulcer formation. Typically, this is caused by the same *Streptococcus pyogenes* and *Staphylococcus aureus* species that cause impetigo. This can happen in patients of all ages; however, the extremes of age are more often affected. Other risk factors for the development of ecthyma include an immunosuppressive state and impetigo that goes untreated. Complications are similar to those of impetigo, and treatment includes topical antibiotics for limited disease or oral antibiotics for those with complicated presentations.

A severe type of ecthyma is called ecthyma gangrenosum. This is a cutaneous manifestation of *Pseudomonas aeruginosa* septicemia. Those who are immunosuppressed, particularly those who are neutropenic, are at high risk of invasive *P. aeruginosa* infections and such manifestations. These lesions are described as ulcerative with a black, necrotic eschar or crust surrounded by an erythematous ring that occur primarily in the gluteal and perineal regions as well as on the extremities. The mortality rate for such an infection is as high as 55%, so early recognition and prompt aggressive antibiotic management are vital. Often, surgical excision is needed because this is a type of necrotizing soft tissue infection.

Differential Diagnosis

Several rashes should be included in the differential diagnosis of impetigo. For bullous impetigo, other bullous rashes such as bullous erythema multiforme and bullous pemphigoid should be considered. For nonbullous impetigo, atopic dermatitis, contact dermatitis, HSV, and scabies should be considered.

Diagnostic Confirmation

Impetigo is a clinical diagnosis. Skin swabs are not recommended because they do not differentiate between bacterial infection and colonization; however, if treatment fails, culture of bullous fluid can be helpful for pathogen differentiation. Serologic testing for streptococcal antibodies does not help in the diagnosis of impetigo.

Treatment

First-line treatment for impetigo includes topical antibiotic such as mupirocin 2% cream or ointment. This should be applied twice a day for 7 days. Other topical agents have been approved by the US Food and Drug Administration for the treatment of impetigo, including retapamulin; however, mupirocin is available in a generic form and is much less costly. There have been cases of mupirocin-resistant impetigo, which demonstrates the importance of follow-up with the primary doctor after discharge from the emergency department to ensure improvement with treatment. It is important to note that topical regimens should only be used in cases of nonbullous impetigo with a limited distribution; if the patient has multiple large bullae or widespread disease with large body surface area involvement, systemic antibiotics should be used. If systemic treatment is indicated, amoxicillin/clavulanate or cephalosporins have been shown to be effective, but local antibiogram should be examined secondary to resistant patterns. Oral clindamycin should be considered if methicillin-resistant *Staphylococcus aureus* is a concern; however, this should not be first-line treatment because this increases the patient's risk of developing *Clostridium difficile* colitis. Oral penicillin, macrolides, or erythromycin should not be used secondary to growing resistance patterns. Topical disinfectants are not recommended as treatment alone.

Disposition

Most cases of isolated, limited impetigo can be treated on an outpatient basis with topical antibiotics. However, oral antibiotics may be indicated for severe disease covering a large body surface area. If the patient appears septic, unstable, or there is concern for disseminated disease, such as exotoxin-mediated staphylococcal scalded skin syndrome or toxic shock syndrome, the patient should be admitted to the pediatric hospital for IV antibiotics, resuscitation, or hydration if needed. Dermatologists or infectious disease specialists should be consulted if the patient is not improving despite appropriate antibiotics or if the diagnosis is unclear. If a patient is treated and discharged from the emergency department, they should be encouraged to follow up with their pediatrician soon thereafter to ensure compliance and improvement with the prescribed regimen. Patients should be encouraged to practice good hand hygiene because this is a very contagious condition. Return precautions should include worsening disease despite appropriate treatment, persistent fevers, dehydration, and inability to tolerate oral intake.

Complications

There are a few rare complications of impetigo that involve the spread of infection to surrounding structures. The surrounding skin may become infected, leading to cellulitis, or the infection may spread to nearby joints, causing osteomyelitis or septic arthritis. There have also been documented cases of lymphadenitis or septicemia secondary to disseminated infection. Streptococcal infections can lead to toxic shock syndrome or post-streptococcal GN; however, there is no evidence that treating impetigo with antibiotics decreases the risk of post-streptococcal GN. Rheumatic fever is not a complication of impetigo. Staphylococcal infections can lead to staphylococcal scalded skin syndrome.

Key Points

- Impetigo can present as bullous or nonbullous subtypes. Nonbullous impetigo starts as erythematous papular lesions that progress to fluid-filled vesicles and subsequent painful erosions with honey-colored crusting. Bullous impetigo typically presents as large, flaccid bullae that rupture and leak infectious serous fluid. When the bullae rupture, patients are left with an erythematous base surrounded by thin brown crust and scales.
- Diagnosis is clinical, and treatment for limited infections is topical antibiotics and improved hygiene. If the infection is severe or involves a large surface area, oral antibiotics should be used.

Pitfalls

- Infection of the surrounding skin may lead to cellulitis, osteomyelitis, or septic arthritis.
- Staphylococcal infections can lead to staphylococcal scalded skin syndrome.
- Streptococcal infections can lead to toxic shock syndrome or post-streptococcal GN; however, there is no evidence that treating impetigo with antibiotics decreases the risk of this development.

Further Reading

American Academy of Dermatology
Stanford University
VisualDx

23

Dermatologic Emergencies

ERICA KIEMELE AND EMILY ROSE

INTRODUCTION

Rashes are common in the pediatric population. Most are benign and self-limited. However, there are several rashes that require rapid recognition and intervention. This chapter discusses Kawasaki disease (KD), omphalitis, staphylococcal scalded skin syndrome (SSSS), Stevens–Johnson syndrome/toxic epidermal necrolysis (SJS/TEN), necrotizing fasciitis, meningococcemia, and Rocky Mountain spotted fever (RMSF). Key features of presentation as well as atypical presentations are highlighted, with emphasis on diagnostic and management pearls.

KAWASAKI DISEASE

Background

Kawasaki disease (previously called mucocutaneous lymph node syndrome) was first described in 1967 in Japanese literature from 50 cases seen in the 1960s. It is a self-limited vasculitis, with predisposition to medium-sized arteries, particularly the coronary arteries. The cause of the disease is unknown, but it has some predilections, including children older than age 3 months and younger than 5 years, higher relative risk in those of Asian descent, and is more common in winter and early spring. Left untreated/undiagnosed, coronary artery aneurysms will develop in 20–25% of cases. KD may also rarely occur in adults, particularly in patients with HIV.

Classic Clinical Presentation

Fever is the most consistent manifestation of KD. It is typically at least 38.5°C (101.3°F) and only mildly responsive to antipyretic agents. KD diagnosis is based on the presence of fever for ≥5 days (particularly >39°C) and four of five clinical criteria shown in Box 23.1. Not all criteria may be present at the same time, and there is no typical order of appearance of features. The rash usually appears within the first few days of fever and can appear in many different forms. Perineal erythema and desquamation frequently occur early. The rash commonly is a nonspecific and diffuse maculopapular that may look similar to erythema multiforme or scarlatiniform. Rarely, bullae, petechiae, or vesicles may be present. Periungual desquamation and Beau's lines may be seen on fingers and toes during convalescence (>7days after symptom onset). Inflammation at the site of bacille Calmette–Guérin inoculation is pathognomonic for KD. Arthritis is not in the diagnostic criteria for KD but is frequently present. Nausea, vomiting, and abdominal pain may also occur in KD.

Atypical Presentation

Atypical/incomplete KD may occur and is more common in infants. This diagnosis may be made in patients who meet clinical criteria but have had a fever for <5 days or in a child with fever for 5–7 days or longer but without sufficient diagnostic clinical criteria. This diagnosis

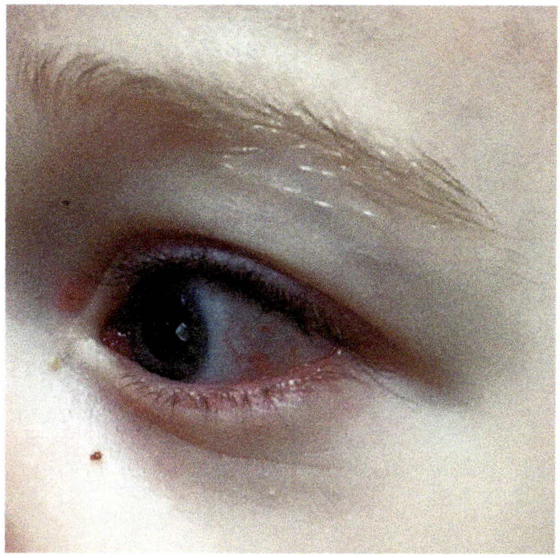

FIGURE 23.1 Conjunctival injection with limbic sparing in a patient with Kawasaki disease.
Source: Photo courtesy of Michael Stoner.

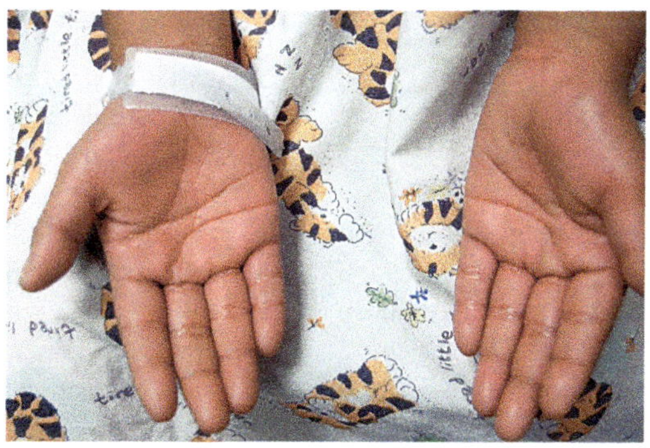

FIGURE 23.2 Palmar erythema in a patient with Kawasaki disease.
Source: Photo courtesy of Seema Shah.

BOX 23.1
DIAGNOSTIC CRITERIA FOR KAWASAKI DISEASE

Fever ≥5 days
Four out of five of the following criteria
Polymorphous rash (occurs in 70–90% of patients)
Bilateral nonexudative conjunctival injection (occurs in >75% of patients), typically perilimbic sparing (Figure 23.1); uveitis occurs in 70% of patients with ocular symptoms; photophobia common
Mucosal membrane changes (occur in 90% of patients; strawberry tongue, fissured lips, injected pharynx)
Extremity changes [occur in 50–85% of patients; peripheral edema, erythema of soles and palms (Figure 23.2), followed by periungual desquamation]
Cervical lymphadenopathy (occurs in 25–70% of patients; usually unilateral, >1.5 cm; least consistent feature)

BOX 23.2

DETERMINATION OF TREATMENT FOR SUSPECTED INCOMPLETE KAWASAKI DISEASE

Fever ≤5 days and two or three clinical criteria (see Table 23.1) or infant with fever ≥7 days without a source
Consider treatment if
- CRP ≥3.0 mg/dL and/or ESR ≥540 mm/hr
- Three or more of the following laboratory findings
  - Sterile pyuria, urine ≥10 WBCs/HPF
  - WBCs ≥16,000 mm^3
  - Elevated ALT
  - Age-specific anemia
  - Platelet count ≥450,000/μL, >7th day of fever
  - Albumin ≤3.0 g/dL

Or abnormal echocardiogram

ALT, alanine aminotransferase; CRP, C-reactive protein; ESR, erythrocyte sedimentation rate; HPF, high power field; WBCs, white blood cells.

should particularly be suspected in infants with fever for ≥7 days without a source. The decision to treat these patients is based on laboratory and imaging findings (Box 23.2). Platelet count typically does not increase until the second week of illness. The degree of thrombocytosis may correlate with the risk of coronary artery changes. Pyuria occurs from urethra sloughing and may not be present in urine obtained from a catheterized specimen. The white cells are not detected by leukocyte esterase, so a microscopic urinalysis should be obtained.

Differential Diagnosis

The clinical features of KD are nonspecific, and many viral illnesses have overlapping features with KD. Additionally, a concomitant active infection may occur with KD, confounding the diagnosis. Table 23.1 discusses common KD mimics. A clinician may also mistakenly interpret features of KD as a source of infection rather than connecting the findings to KD (such as diagnosing urinary tract infection with sterile pyuria or lymphangitis with cervical lymphadenopathy).

Diagnostic Confirmation

Although there is not one specific test for confirmed diagnosis, the previously discussed criteria for complete and incomplete KD along with an echocardiogram are the mainstay.

Treatment

The treatment of KD includes intravenous immunoglobulin (IVIG) to prevent coronary artery aneurysm development and aspirin for inhibition of platelet aggregation. Early IVIG administration

TABLE 23.1 DIFFERENTIAL DIAGNOSIS OF KAWASAKI DISEASE BASED ON CLINICAL FINDINGS

Fever	Rash	Red Eyes	Mucosal Membrane Changes	Extremity Changes	Cervical Lymphadenopathy
Rheumatic fever	Drug reaction	Uveitis	HSV	Scarlet fever	Cat scratch disease
Viral myocarditis	Vaccine reaction	SJS	Coxsackie virus	TSS	Tuleremia
Juvenile rheumatoid arthritis	Measles	Bacterial vs. viral vs. allergic conjunctivitis	Measles	Drug reactions	EBV, CMV
Polyarteritis nodosa	Leptospirosis	Measles	SJS	Enterovirus	Toxoplasmosis
	Scarlet fever				Group B strep, Staph A infection
	Rickettsial infections				

CMV, cytomegalovirus; EBV, Epstein–Barr virus; HSV, herpes simplex virus; SJS, Stevens–Johnson syndrome; TSS, toxic shock syndrome.

(within 10 days) significantly decreases the incidence of coronary artery aneurysm development (from ~25% to <5%). Aspirin itself has not been shown to impact development or regression of coronary artery aneurysms. The recommended IVIG dose is 2 g/kg given over 10–12 hours as soon as diagnosis is made. High-dose aspirin is given at 80–100 mg/kg daily over four doses until fever defervescence. The dose is then decreased to 3–5 mg/kg for 4–6 weeks or until inflammatory markers have normalized and no coronary artery damage or further damage is noted. Some patients have a persistent or recrudescent fever (>36 hours and <7 day). Also, some patients, particularly those of Japanese descent, may be at risk for IVIG resistance and may require additional therapy. In these patients, IVIG or IVIG + prednisolone (2 mg/kg in three divided doses per day until afebrile, and then prednisone oral until inflammatory markers normalize with a taper) should be repeated. More novel treatments, such as cyclosporine, have shown promise in refractory cases. Other treatments, such as tumor necrosis factor (TNF)-α inhibitor and the monoclonal antibody infliximab, may also benefit in resistant cases, but the evidence is limited.

Disposition

Patient with suspected KD should be admitted to a telemetry ward for cardiac monitoring. An echocardiogram should be obtained to evaluate for coronary artery involvement and determine the patient's *z* scores (luminal abnormalities measurements). Aspirin and IVIG should be administered early and evaluated for response. Once afebrile and symptoms improve, the risk stratification based on *z* scores (initial maximal coronary size score) from transthoracic echocardiography will guide the recommended follow-up intervals. *Z* scores can be obtained from various published regression analysis, but most pediatric institutions may have their own set based on specific patient data. Most patients are followed for repeat imaging at 4–6-weeks. However, with medium and large aneurysms, repeat imaging is performed at 3, 6, and 9 weeks (Box 23.3).

Complications

If untreated, patients have a 20–25% risk of developing coronary artery aneurysms. Approximately 30% of patients have coronary artery dilation at presentation. Aneurysms typically develop after 10 days of symptoms. Other areas of the heart may also be involved, and patients may develop pancarditis. Cardiac inflammation increases the risk of serious sequelae such as thrombosis, myocardial infarction, ventricular tachycardia, and valvular abnormalities. Cardiac risk is the highest in the first year of diagnosis. Most aneurysms with a *z* score <6 fully regress over time, but cardiac risk remains due to ongoing active arterial inflammation. Based on many case studies during the past 60 years, patients with large aneurysms (*z* score >8) may have a long-term risk for a cardiac event of up to 73%.

Vascular sequelae can affect any organ system. Gallbladder hydrops, hepatic dysfunction, multisystem organ dysfunction, and shock are less common complications.

BOX 23.3

AMERICAN HEART ASSOCIATION 2017 GUIDELINES RECOMMENDED *Z* SCORE CLASSIFICATION[A]

No involvement: <2
Dilation only: 2 to <2.5
Small aneurysm: ≥2.5 to <5
Medium aneurism: ≥5 to <10, and absolute dimension <8 mm
Large aneurysm: ≥10, or absolute dimension ≥8 mm

[a]Where *z* = 0 is the median size of coronary arteries.

Key Points

- KD predominantly affects children younger than age 5 years and of Asian descent, but it can occur at any age, including rarely in adults.
- Classic KD is diagnosed by fever >5 days and four out of five clinical criteria.
- Incomplete KD may occur when patients do not meet either the length of fever criteria or the number of clinical criteria. These patients are at similar risk for complications and should be treated as having KD.
- All infants with a fever for ≥7 days without a source should be risk stratified for KD.
- Patients with KD should be admitted and treatment initiated to reduce complications.
- An echocardiogram evaluates for cardiac complications.
- Administer IVIG 2 g/kg to decrease coronary artery aneurysm development.
- Aspirin is given at 50–100 mg/kg over four doses until fever defervescence.

Pitfalls

- Infants often present with atypical disease, and KD is underrecognized/underdiagnosed.
- Patients can have both KD and another illness simultaneously.
- Prompt diagnosis and intervention result in a decreased incidence of coronary artery aneurysms and sequelae.

OMPHALITIS

Background

Omphalitis is an infection of the umbilical stump that carries significant morbidity and potential mortality for neonates. The umbilical stump typically falls off after 5–15 days of life. The stump's devitalized tissue can be colonized by skin and enteric bacteria, providing an opportunity for bacteria to enter the bloodstream via thrombosed blood vessels, which can lead to systemic infection. Omphalitis is common in developing countries, with an incidence for deliveries at hospitals of 8% and that for deliveries at home as high as 22%. In developed countries, the incidence ranges from 0.2% to 0.7%. Systemic infection can progress swiftly and has an estimated mortality of 7–15%. Necrotizing fasciitis carries a mortality rate of up to 85%. Box 23.4 presents risk factors for developing omphalitis.

Omphalitis is a polymicrobial infection; the main organisms include *Staphylococcus aureus, Streptococcus pyogenes, Escherichia coli, Klebsiella pneumoniae,* and *Proteus mirabilis.* Anaerobes such as *Bacteroides fragilis, Clostridium tetani,* and *Clostridium perfringens* may also be involved, particularly with a history of chorioamnionitis. Chlorhexidine application decreases the incidence of omphalitis in low-resource countries. Current guidelines recommend dry cord care in routine aseptic deliveries due to the low incidence and unclear safety profile and potential for selecting for resistant organisms.

BOX 23.4

RISK FACTORS FOR DEVELOPING OMPHALITIS

Prolonged rupture of membranes
Maternal infection (chorioamnionitis)
Low birth weight
Umbilical catheterization
Home birth
Poor cord care
Prolonged labor
Immune system abnormalities (defects in leukocyte adhesion and others)

Classic Clinical Presentation

Omphalitis typically presents at approximately 3 days of age. The presentation has four grades of severity:

1. Funisitis (inflammation of the external surface of the cord only, often related to chorioamnionitis): The cord can have a foul smell, be wet, and there may be umbilical drainage but no surrounding cellulitis.
2. Omphalitis with cellulitis (most common)
3. Omphalitis with systemic infection
4. Omphalitis with necrotizing soft tissue infection

Some mild discharge of the umbilicus may be normal. Signs of cellulitis include erythema that extends to the abdominal wall and spreads rapidly over time (Figure 23.3). Crepitus and bullae are late findings of a necrotizing infection. Signs of systemic infection, including irritability, fever, lethargy, and poor feeding, are concerning for sepsis.

Differential Diagnosis

Other diagnoses to consider include periumbilical skin irritation, patent urachus (tract between bladder and umbilical cord; result in drainage), umbilical granuloma (soft, pink, velvety texture; bleed easily and serosanguinous discharge), vitellointestinal duct remnants (feculent discharge), and necrotizing enterocolitis.

Diagnostic Confirmation

The diagnosis of omphalitis is based on physical examination findings. If mild discharge or erythema is present, often observation with reassessment helps differentiate between local irritation and omphalitis. Immediate intervention is required with systemic or rapid progression.

Treatment

Treatment is based on the causative organism: aminoglycoside for gram-negative

(A)

(B)

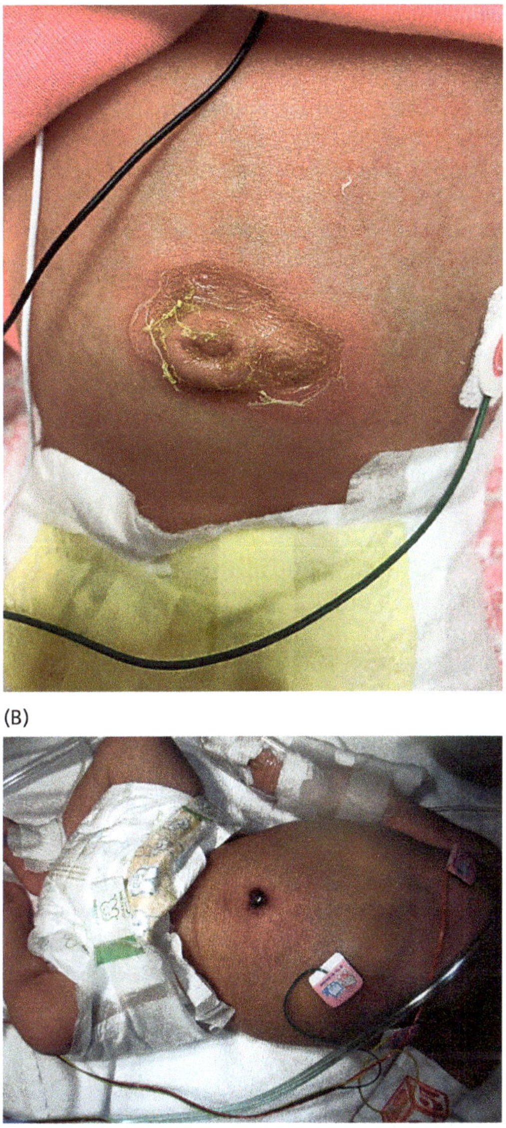

FIGURE 23.3 (A) Neonatal omphalitis. (B) Omphalitis in a patient who died a few days after admission.

Source: (A) Keya Manshadi. (B) Photo courtesy of Nobuaki Inoue.

coverage, such as gentamycin at 5 mg/kg intravenously (IV) daily; a broad-spectrum penicillin such as ampicillin 50 mg/kg IV q6h for gram-positive coverage, with addition of methicillin-resistant *Staphylococcus aureus* (MRSA) bactericidal vancomycin 15–20 mg/kg IV daily if needed; and anaerobic coverage with clindamycin 20–40 mg/kg daily in q6–8h divided doses or metronidazole 1.5 mg/kg IV q12h if concerned about maternal history of chorioamnionitis. Treatment is typically for a minimum of 10 days.

Clinical Algorithm

A detailed history should be obtained, including both birth history (labor length, location, and maternal risk factors) and recent history. A physical examination should be performed, with special focus on vital signs, systemic symptoms, poor feeding, skin discolorations, and irritability. If system symptoms are found, sepsis evaluation of the neonate should also be performed, which includes blood cultures, urine analysis and culture, lumbar puncture, C-reactive protein (CRP), wound culture, and complete blood count. Areas of erythema should be marked on first evaluation to monitor for progression. Early surgical consultation should be obtained if infection is progressive, extensively involves the abdominal wall, or there are signs of necrotizing soft tissue infection. Further imaging, such as computed tomography (CT), magnetic resonance imaging (MRI), and/or ultrasound, to determine the extent of infection should also be considered.

Disposition

All patients with any form of omphalitis should be admitted to the hospital for IV antibiotics and close monitoring. Intensive care unit (ICU) level of care is required for close monitoring.

Patients with mild erythema of the umbilical stump can be observed and reassessed in the emergency department if local irritation from the diaper or pants is suspected. Local irritation will quickly resolve if the stimulus is removed. Omphalitis will remain and/or progress.

Complications

Soft tissue necrotizing infections are the most common major complications (mortality rates of 60–85%), In addition, systemic infections may cause significant morbidity and mortality due to access of pathogens to the intra-abdominal cavity and bloodstream. These include thrombophlebitis of the portal and umbilical veins, peritonitis, intra-abdominal abscess infection, and bowel ischemia. If infection is rapidly progressing, antibiotics should be broadened, and surgical consultation should be obtained.

Key Points

- Omphalitis is umbilical inflammation with surrounding erythema including the abdominal wall.
- Omphalitis is a serious diagnosis of neonates that has significant morbidity and mortality.
- All cases of omphalitis require admission for IV antibiotics, monitoring, and possible surgical intervention if necrotizing fasciitis develops.

Pitfalls

- Omphalitis may appear as a benign/superficial cellulitis; it is not.
- Omphalitis can rapidly progress on a spectrum of severity; close monitoring and prompt diagnosis can decrease mortality and morbidity.

STAPHYLOCOCCAL SCALDED SKIN SYNDROME

Background

Staphylococcal scalded skin syndrome (SSSS) is an exotoxin-mediated superficial skin blistering disease caused by *S. aureus*. The disease more frequently occurs in neonates and children younger than age 5 years. Younger children and neonates are more susceptible to SSSS because of both a lack of protective antibodies against staphylococcal toxins (secondary to limited life exposure) and the decreased ability of their kidneys to excrete the exotoxin. Adults who contract the disease have a much higher infection burden and almost always have concomitant severe disease such as immunodeficiency, renal dysfunction, or serious illness.

Staphylococcus aureus is a common pathogen found in 35% of the population, often in the nares. *Staphylococcus aureus* can produce various toxins, but approximately 5% of the organisms contain particularly virulent exotoxin-producing strains. These exotoxins target the stratum granulosum in the epidermis. Cleavage induces bulla formation and eventual sheet-like desquamation. It can take approximately 24–48 hours for the exotoxin to bind to antibodies and/or to be renally cleared. Erythema and pain significantly decrease 2 or 3 days after initiation of treatment. Neonates have prolonged clearance of the toxin and a longer disease course.

Staphylococcal infections are easily transmitted, and the source is often impetigo or wound infections. The incubation period to development of clinical SSSS varies from 1 to 10 days after the initial infection.

Classic Clinical Presentation

The presentation often starts with a prodrome of irritability, fever, and malaise. Progressive cutaneous erythema and desquamation (mimicking a burn) then occur. Erythema and pain begin predominantly in the skin folds and then generalize. The initial *S. aureus* infection is often in the head and neck [often upper respiratory infection (URI), pharyngitis, and conjunctivitis], but in neonates it can also occur in the groin folds and umbilicus. Table 23.2 presents the timeline of skin changes. The flaccid bullae can spread from gentle palpation to neighboring skin as the skin separates from the upper epidermis. Gentle stroking of seemingly normal skin may desquamate (Nikolsky sign). Bullae may also extend to seemingly normal adjacent skin with gentle pressure (Asboe–Hansen sign). Even gentle friction on the skin can induce sheet-like desquamation, revealing underlying moist, erythematous skin.

TABLE 23.2 TIMELINE OF SKIN CHANGES IN STAPHYLOCOCCAL SCALED SKIN SYNDROME

Initial	<24 Hours	24–48 Hours	Days 3–5	>10 Days
Tender patches, faint and erythematous	Patches start to coalesce into confluent scarlatiniform erythema (sandpaper in texture)	Flaccid bullae appear in the erythematous areas; when ruptured, the underlining skin is red and moist, giving the term scalded	Fissuring begins; the open lesions start to dry out	Skin starts to heal

Fissuring commonly occurs around the mouth and in friction zones (groin). The crusting and fissuring around the mouth, nose, and eyes are frequently described as having the appearance of dried oatmeal. Mucosal membranes are typically spared.

Differential Diagnosis

Staphylococcal scaled skin syndrome can be mistaken for many other blistering diseases. The cleavage plane in SSSS is more superficial than in most other blistering conditions. Table 23.3 summarizes key differences between major blistering diseases. Differences vary with regard to the presence of *S. aureus* in bullae, the presence or absence of Nikolsky sign, mucosal involvement, and clinical history. The differential includes burns, child abuse, TEN, SJS, erythema multiforme, bullous pemphigoid, pemphigoid vulgaris, pemphigus foliaceus, toxic shock syndrome, KD, bullous impetigo, scarlet fever, drug rash with eosinophilia and systemic signs, and coxsackie infection.

Diagnostic Confirmation

Diagnosis is typically made by clinical history and skin findings in an at-risk patient population. Biopsy may help differentiate in atypical or unclear cases. Culture swabs may be obtained from involved areas, including groin, umbilicus, throat, nose, and skin lesions. However, it is important to note that skin findings are toxin mediated and the bullae do not contain *S. aureus*. Blood cultures can also be obtained but are less likely to be positive in children (because the disease is caused by the exotoxin).

Treatment

The treatment of SSSS begins with eradication of the underlying/causative infection. Initiate IV antibiotics with a penicillinase-resistant synthetic penicillin such as nafcillin, oxacillin, or flucloxacillin. First line is flucloxacillin at 50–100 mg/kg/day divided into four doses. Clindamycin can be used as adjunct due to its ability to inhibit exotoxin production. Vancomycin should be used if MRSA is

TABLE 23.3 SUMMARY OF KEY DIFFERENCES BETWEEN STAPHYLOCOCCAL SCALED SKIN SYNDROME AND DIFFERENTIAL DIAGNOSES OF MAJOR BLISTERING DISORDERS

Disease	Background	Clinical Features	Nikolsky Sign	Mucosal Membrane Involvement
SSSS	Neonates, children <5 years, and immunocompromised	Erythema, coalescing into bullae; when ruptured reveals scalded red skin	Positive	None
Pemphigus vulgaris	Middle-aged to older populations	Mucosal and skin flaccid bullae	Positive	Yes
Pemphigus foliaceus	Common in children	Clinically similar to SSSS; differentiated by biopsy	Positive	None
TEN/SJS	Drug reaction TEN >30%, SJS <10% of body	Progressive red rash with blistering and desquamation	Positive	Yes
Bullous impetigo	Neonatal	Localized areas of flaccid bullae; the bullae contain infection (*Staphylococcus aureus*, can be cultured) and will have crust when ruptured	Negative	Yes
Bullous pemphigoid	Older population; AI diseases against hemidesmosomal proteins	Tense blisters	Negative	Sometimes

SJS, Stevens–Johnson syndrome; SSSS, staphylococcal scaled skin syndrome; TSS, toxic epidermal necrolysis.

suspected. Cefuroxime or clarithromycin can be used with penicillin allergy.

Severe/refractory cases may benefit from experimental treatment with fresh frozen plasma or IVIG therapy. Both are theorized to help neutralize circulating toxin.

Supportive measures include IV fluids, maintenance fluids, monitoring for electrolyte abnormalities, and skin care. Topical emollients, saline-soaked gauze, and topical antibiotic ointments are discouraged because they lead to antibiotic resistance. Iodine and silver-containing dressings should also be avoided to prevent systemic absorption. Nonsteroidal anti-inflammatory drugs for analgesia should be avoided to avoid exacerbating any underlying renal insufficiency. Acetaminophen and opiates may be used as needed. Physical therapy should be done to encourage early range of motion.

Disposition

Most patients require hospitalization for IV antibiotics, fluids, and skin care. Patients with extensive involvement may particularly benefit from admission to a burn unit.

Complications

Most patients completely recover in 2 or 3 weeks without scarring. Complications include secondary infections (cellulitis, pneumonia, and sepsis) and complications due to fluid resuscitation (hyponatremia) and skin loss (hypovolemia, dehydration, and hypothermia). Extensive skin involvement and comorbidities correlate with a higher rate of complications and a higher mortality rate. The current mortality for children is 4%.

Key Points

- SSSS is a toxin-mediated condition caused by *S. aureus* infection.
- SSSS occurs in children younger than age 5 years; neonates are particularly at risk.
- SSSS begins with a prodrome of malaise, fever, and irritability.
- Skin manifestations include tender, widespread scarlatiniform erythema with flaccid bullae. Bullae are easy to spread and are Nikolsky sign positive. Rupture of bullae reveals red hot scalded skin. Skin heels in 10–14 days.
- There is no mucosal membrane involvement.
- Treatment is IV antibiotics for 7–10 days with penicillinase-resistant synthetic penicillin, addition of MRSA coverage if clinically indicated, hydration, and skin care.

Pitfall

- Failure to admit and administer antibiotics early

STEVENS–JOHNSON SYNDROME AND TOXIC EPIDERMAL NECROLYSIS

Background

Stevens-Johnson syndrome and TEN are severe mucocutaneous reactions characterized by extensive epidermal necrosis and detachment. Most cases are febrile. SJS/TEN are both triggered by recent medication exposure/re-exposure and, less commonly, infection. Most cases (90%) have mucous membrane involvement. They are classified based on body surface involvement [total body surface area (TBSA)]. SJS involves <10% TBSA, and TEN involves >30% TBSA. Cases that involve 10–30% TBSA are called SJS/TEN overlap. SJS is more common than TEN, and mortality roughly correlates with involved TBSA.

The most common inciting medications are antiepileptics and antibiotics (particularly sulfa), but many medication classes may induce SJS/TEN. Symptoms typically develop within the first 8 weeks of medication initiation (and within days of medication re-exposure). Less commonly, infection triggers the reaction. *Mycoplasma* is the most common associated infection. HIV increases the risk of SJS/TEN 100 fold.

Significant skin necrosis occurs secondary to direct keratinocyte cell death. Skin necrosis may be partial to full thickness.

Classic Clinical Presentation

Drug exposure is often 1–4 weeks prior to onset of symptoms (average, 14 days). The acute phase occurs over 8–12 days. An initial prodrome of fever (usually >39°C), flu-like symptoms, malaise, myalgias, conjunctivitis, dysuria, and pain with swallowing commonly occurs. These symptoms can precede lesions by

1–3 days. Pain is often widespread, in all areas of mucocutaneous involvement.

Any mucosal surface may be involved. Pharyngeal mucosa is affected in nearly all patients, and most patients describe odynophagia. Approximately 80% of patients have ocular involvement ranging from dry eye to corneal ulceration and panophthalmitis. Photophobia and pruritus are common. Urethritis develops in up to two-thirds of patients and presents as dysuria or with urinary retention. Genital erosions may occur. Less commonly, mucosal lesions of the bronchial, tracheal, esophageal, and intestines can occur.

Skin lesions are painful and start as ill-defined, erythematous, coalescing macules that can have purpuric centers. Lesions start on the trunk and face and spread symmetrically. The anterior face and trunk are more predominantly involved, with relative distal extremity sparing. Lesions often spare the palms, soles, and scalp. Lesions progress to vesicles and bullae and start to slough. Applying lateral gentle pressure causes more sloughing (Nikolsky sign), and applying direct pressure to the bullae can cause extension to unaffected skin (Asboe–Hansen sign). Epidermal sloughing may generalize, leaving large areas of raw, painful, denuded skin. See Table 23.4 for a detailed list of locations and clinical manifestations. Re-epithelialization begins after 1 week and can take 2–4 weeks for healing. Delayed skin and nail peeling may occur.

Atypical Presentation

The vast majority of cases have some skin involvement. Rarely, skin findings may be absent, with only mucosal and intraorgan involvement.

Differential Diagnosis

Like many of the blistering diseases, SJS/TEN have a wide differential diagnosis. Key differences are the presence of fever, Nikolsky sign, Asboe–Hansen sign, mucosal involvement, and histological findings. (See Table 23.7 for distinguishing lesion characteristics.) Additional diagnoses include erythema multiforme, acute graft versus host disease, drug-induced linear immunoglobin A (IgA) bullous dermatitis, phototoxic eruptions, acute generalized exanthematous pustulosis, generalized bullous fixed drug eruptions, erythroderma and erythematous drug eruptions, and paraneoplastic pemphigus. See Table 23.5 for comparisons.

Diagnostic Confirmation

There are no firm diagnostic criteria. Histologically, SJS/TEN can look similar to other diseases. Inclusion of the following clinical features would make the diagnosis of SJS/TEN likely:

- Recent drug exposure followed by febrile illness
- Prodrome with fever, flu-like symptoms
- New drug exposure in the preceding 1–4 weeks or a recent re-exposure

TABLE 23.4 SUMMARY OF CUTANEOUS AND MUCOSAL INVOLVEMENT OF STEVENS-JOHNSON SYNDROME/TOXIC EPIDERMAL NECROLYSIS

Location	Clinical Manifestations
Ocular	Conjunctivitis, corneal scaring/xerosis, sandy sensation, photophobia, vision loss
Ears, nose, and throat	Auditory canal stenosis, hypopharyngeal stenosis, dental growth abnormalities, gingival and labial lesions, stomatitis and mucositis (which impairs oral intake)
Cutaneous	Macular rash, vesicular and bullous rash, epidermal separation, dyspigmentation, hair and nail thinning, oncyholysis, eruptive melanocytic nevi
Respiratory	Bronchiectasis, chronic obliterative bronchitis, bronchiolitis obliterans
Gastrointestinal tract/liver	Small bowel obstruction, intestinal ulcers, chronic cholestasis, ischemic hepatitis, esophageal stricture and webs
Urogenital	Vaginal stenosis, fusion of labia minora/majora, hematocolpos, hydrocolpos, vulvar and vaginal adenosis
Renal	Glomerulonephritis

TABLE 23.5 DIFFERENTIAL DIAGNOSIS OF STEVENS–JOHNSON SYNDROME/TOXIC EPIDERMAL NECROLYSIS

Disease	Mucosal Involvement	Fever	Skin Manifestations	Onset	Features
SJS/TEN	Yes	Yes	Dusky red skin maculose/ patches that progress to vesicles/bullae and skin sloughing; Nikolsky positive	Acute	Drug induced; mycoplasma induced
SSSS	Yes	Yes	Erythematous rash; coalesces; tender; forms bullae that when ruptured reveal scalded skin; Nikolsky positive	Acute	Children <5 years; immunocompromised adults; staph infection not always found; blisters sterile
Erythema multiforme	Yes	Sometimes	<10% of body surface; raised, targetoid lesions symmetrically found on distal extremities	Acute	Often in setting of HSV, mycoplasma pneumonia
Erythroderma and erythematous drug eruptions	No	Sometimes	Maculopapular erythema; generalized and symmetrical	Acute	Common drug reaction
Acute generalized exanthematous pustulosis	No	Yes	Superficial pustules	Acute	Reaction to a β-lactam antibiotic
Paraneoplastic pemphigus	Yes	No	Flaccid bullae	Gradual	Can be one of the first presentations of malignancy; often in non-Hodgkin lymphoma
Acute graft vs. host disease	Rare	Yes	Bullae; erosion and morbilliform rash	Acute	Can mimic TEN
Drug-induced linear IgA bullous dermatosis	Rare	No	Subepidermal bullae; tense; Nikolsky negative	Acute	Autoimmune disease

HSV, herpes simplex virus; IgA, immunoglobulin A; SJS, Stevens–Johnson syndrome; SSSS, staphylococcal scaled skin syndrome; TEN, toxic epidermal necrolysis.

  - To determine if the drug is likely the culprit, an algorithm of drug causality for epidermal necrolysis (ALDEN) was developed. Each possible drug is assigned a score based on parameters such as drug presence, drug notoriety, previous history of exposure same drug.
- Painful, rapidly progressing rash
  - Initially erythematous macules/ patches that progressed to vesicle and bullae
  - Bullae Nikolsky sign positive and may have Asboe–Hansen sign
  - Sloughing of dermis
- Mucosal lesions

Treatment

Determination and withdrawal of the culprit drug should be done immediately. Determine ALDEN scores for all potential drugs. Supportive care includes wound care (surgical debridement and silver-impregnated antimicrobial dressings); nutritional support (nasogastric feeding may be required); fluidized air beds to help with dependent areas of skin involvement; pain control with anxiolytics, opioids, and non-opioid analgesics; fluid resuscitation to maintain adequate urinary output; and maintaining room temperature at 30–32°C to decrease caloric expenditures due to skin loss. Rigorous care to prevent infection should be implemented.

Eye care can be guided based on ocular score involvement—from none to very severe (ocular surface epithelial defects and pseudomembrane formation). Artificial tear and lubrication are initial treatments. Topical corticosteroids may also be used, and broad-spectrum antibiotic eye drops can be applied four times a day if patients have some mild ocular involvement. For higher grades, an amniotic membrane transplantation may be required.

There are no established treatments beyond supportive care and removal of inciting medication. Adjunctive therapies for SJS/TEN are controversial, with conflicting data. Systemic corticosteroids and IVIG have been used with mixed results. Cyclosporine and TNF inhibitors may halt disease progression.

Disposition

All patients with suspected SJS/TEN should be admitted to the hospital. If the patient meets TEN criteria (>30% BSA), has severe mucous membrane involvement, or has significant comorbidity, the patient should be admitted to the ICU. All patients with TEN require burn unit level of care. Prompt evaluation by ophthalmology is advised to examine ocular manifestations and start treatment; evaluation by gynecology is advised to examine vaginal lesions and initiate possible interventions (creams and vaginal molds) to prevent vulvovaginal sequelae.

Complications

Mortality of TEN is as high as 25–34% in the general population; it is lower in pediatric populations. In a recent study performed in the United States, mortality for children was 0% for SJS, 4% for SJS/TEN, and 16% for TEN. The leading cause of death is sepsis. Complications of SJS/TEN are numerous due to the multiorgan nature of the disease. The most common complications are ocular, which develop in 50-90% of patients. These involve dry eyes, vision loss, trichiasis, keratitis, corneal scarring, photophobia, and, less commonly, blindness. Patients may develop ocular complications years after the acute SJS/TEN event. Cutaneous sequelae include hyper- and hypopigmentation, scarring, chronic nail changes, and skin lesions with concomitant infections. Renal complications of glomerulonephritis can lead to chronic kidney disease. Vaginal dryness, urinary retention, dyspareunia, and vaginal adenosis commonly occur in females. Pulmonary complications include bronchiectasis and obstructive changes. Long-term psychiatric complications are also frequently described.

Key Points

- SJS/TEN are severe mucocutaneous reactions.
- The involved TBSA varies (SJS <10%, <10–30% is SJS/TEN overlap and >30% TEN)
- Mucous membrane involvement (pharynx, oral mucosa, ocular, and genitourinary) occurs in 90% of patients.
- Cutaneous changes are dusky red skin macules/patches that progress to vesicles and bullae that slough. Nikolsky sign and Asboe-Hansen sign may help differentiate bullous lesions.
- Stop the inciting medication as soon as possible.
- Supportive care with IV fluids, wound care and pain control, ophthalmological evaluation, and gynecological evaluation (for females) are important.
- TEN, severe involvement, or significant comorbidities require intensive care. Burn unit care should occur with TBSA involvement >30%.

Pitfall

- Failure to thoroughly evaluate mucosa in a patient with a skin rash may result in a missed diagnosis.

MENINGOCOCCEMIA

Background

Neisseria meningiditis is the leading cause of bacterial meningitis in children and young adults and has a significant mortality rate (10–20%). It is responsible for epidemic meningitis and progressive shock.

Classic Clinical Presentation

Meningococcal disease can present with meningitis, shock, or a combined presentation. The disease often begins with mild upper respiratory symptoms and sore throat, followed by a sudden onset of fever, headache, painful myalgias, and nausea/vomiting. Common initial specific symptoms include leg pain, cold hands/feet, and skin mottling/pallor.

Disease progression is notoriously rapid. Younger children progress more rapidly than adolescents; infants may progress over a few hours, and adolescents typically presents <24 hours after symptom onset.

The associated rash is most commonly nonblanching, 1- or 2-mm petechiae, and half of patients have a rash on presentation. The trunk and lower extremities are most commonly involved, but the rash may be present anywhere on the body, including the mucous membranes. Areas of dependence often develop the rash first (e.g., under a blood pressure cuff or pant elastic and buttock/legs). The rash frequently coalesces to purpuric/ecchymotic lesions (Figure 23.4).

Skin lesions in fulminant meningococcal septicemia are frequently extensive, hemorrhagic in appearance, with central necrosis.

Atypical Clinical Presentation

Up to 20% of children with meningococcemia do not develop a rash. In addition, the rash may mimic a viral exanthem and be transiently macular or papular. The rash may also be located on the head, palms, soles, and mucous membranes.

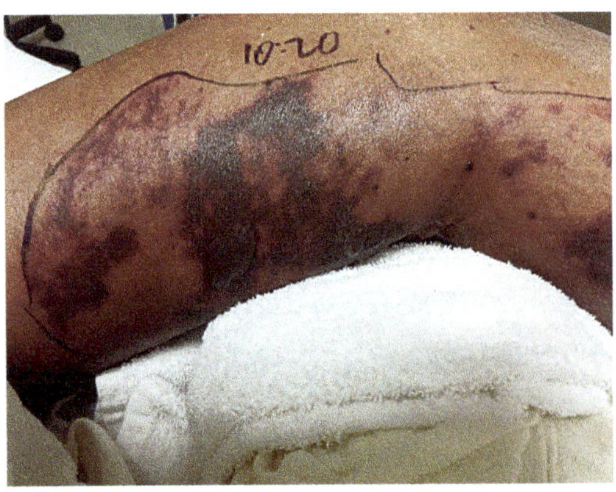

FIGURE 23.4 Purpura fulminans in a patient with meningococcemia.

Source: Photo courtesy of Garrett Sterling,

Patients with bacteremia may present with many different symptoms of bacterial seeding, including abdominal pain.

Differential Diagnosis

Many other etiologies of meningitis as well as systemic bacterial and viral infections may mimic meningococcal disease. The key distinguishing characteristic of meningococcus is its rapid progression. The most common mistaken diagnosis is viral syndrome, particularly because meningococcus frequently initially presents with URI symptoms and pharyngitis.

Diagnostic Confirmation

The initial diagnosis is suspected clinically. Blood and cerebrospinal fluid cultures and gram stain should be obtained in suspected cases.

Treatment

Early antibiotic administration [IV ceftriaxone or cefotaxime (100 mg/kg)] is essential to stop bacterial proliferation. In most cases, waiting to give antibiotics until after a lumbar puncture unnecessarily delays definitive treatment and may result in increased morbidity and mortality. Concomitant septic shock should be aggressively managed (see Chapter 12 on pediatric sepsis).

Disposition

All cases of suspected meningococcemia should be admitted to a monitored setting with droplet precautions.

Because meningococcus may initially present with URI symptoms, it is important to reassess any patient who develops a rash during the visit and give return precautions.

Complications

Meningococcal infections have significant morbidity and mortality rates. Untreated, the mortality rate is up to 90%. Concurrent complications include septic shock, disseminated intravascular coagulation, purpura fulminans, Waterhouse–Friderichsen syndrome, acute respiratory distress syndrome, myocarditis, septic/reactive arthritis, and limb necrosis. Long-term survivor sequelae include seizures, sensorineural hearing loss, focal neurological deficits (including cranial nerve dysfunctions), vasculitis, and intellectual disability.

Key Points

- Meningococcus is a rapidly progressive infection that infects otherwise healthy children (particularly infants and adolescents).
- Initial symptoms may be subtle and mimic a viral infection.
- Early recognition and prompt antibiotic administration are essential.

Pitfalls

- Failure to consider the possibility of meningococcal disease in a patient with fever and a rash
- Failure to reassess a patient diagnosed with a URI who suddenly develops a rash
- Failure to give return instructions to patients

NECROTIZING FASCIITIS

Background

Necrotizing soft tissue infections have significant associated morbidity and mortality. Prompt recognition and intervention are required. Necrotizing fasciitis is a subset of the broader category of necrotizing soft tissue infections.

Risk factors for necrotizing fasciitis include neonates, diabetes, cirrhosis, multiple comorbidities, and conditions or medications inducing immunocompromised states. Polymicrobial infections are more common in adults, but a single pathogen (e.g., group A *Streptococcus* or MRSA) and truncal involvement are more common in children.

Classic Clinical Presentation

Patients typically present with localized swelling, pain, and erythema of the affected area (Figure 23.5). Rapid progression is a hallmark of the disease. Pain is classically out of proportion to the clinical appearance and may frequently be present beyond the area of erythema. With disease progression, the area may become anesthetic due to the destruction of the associated cutaneous nerves. Later findings include bullae, crepitus, and necrosis. Associated fever is common, but it occurs in only half of all patients at initial presentation. Systemic symptoms such as myalgias, anorexia, nausea/vomiting, and diarrhea may also be present.

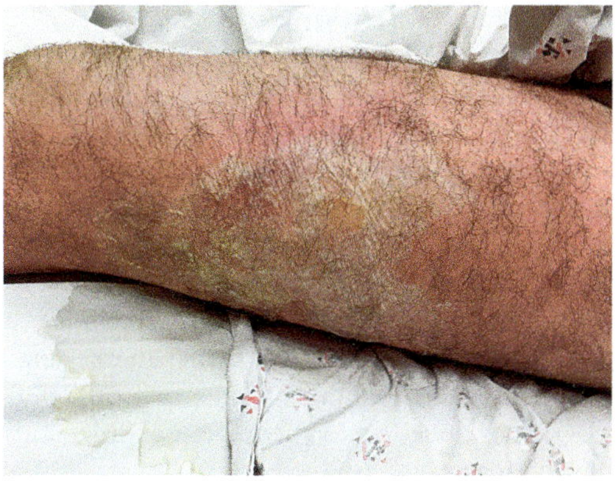

FIGURE 23.5 Necrotizing fasciitis involving the thigh with rapidly expanding erythema, extensive bullae formation, and "dishwater" drainage from the affected area.

Source: Photo courtesy of Emily Rose.

Atypical Clinical Presentation

Necrotizing infections may occur with a more gradual spread of disease. Necrotizing MRSA infections occur more commonly in children and often are associated with a relatively slower progression of disease.

Diagnostic Confirmation

The diagnosis is primarily made clinically based initially on history and physical examination. Laboratory evaluation and diagnostic testing may assist in equivocal cases. Definitive diagnosis is made upon surgical exploration.

Laboratory values demonstrating inflammatory states are nondiagnostic but can be suggestive of leukocytosis, hyponatremia, hyperglycemia, anemia, and elevated creatinine and erythrocyte sedimentation rate/CRP.

Plain films may demonstrate gas along fascial planes. This finding is not sensitive but is specific for a necrotizing infection. CT has a higher sensitivity for the presence of gas. MRI has even greater sensitivity, but the lack of availability and time to completion render it less useful in the evaluation of an emergent necrotizing infection. Point-of-care ultrasound is also commonly used and can visualize subcutaneous tissue thickening, abnormal fluid collections, and subcutaneous air. If the diagnosis remains equivocal after labs/imaging, a bedside incision of the area may be made to evaluate for necrotic tissue and/or fluid (often described as "dirty dishwater" in character; see Figure 23.4).

Treatment

Definitive treatment for necrotizing fasciitis is surgical debridement. Important adjunctive therapy includes aggressive fluid resuscitation and broad-spectrum antibiotics. Clindamycin is recommended in all necrotizing infections for its potential toxin-suppression effects. Triple therapy is recommended while awaiting operative intervention. This includes a β-lactamase inhibitor or carbapenem (e.g., piperacillin-tazobactam or meropenem) plus MRSA coverage (e.g., vancomycin or linezolid) plus clindamycin.

Vasopressor agents may be required during resuscitation, but their use should not delay operative intervention. A patient with a necrotizing infection will not stabilize until definitive operative debridement occurs.

Disposition

All patients with suspected necrotizing infections should have emergent operative debridement. Only equivocal/unclear cases should be admitted to a medical unit.

Complications

Without appropriate treatment, there is a nearly 100% mortality rate with necrotizing fasciitis. There is an overall 17–30% mortality rate, which increases to up to 45% if the trunk is involved.

Aggressive life-saving operative debridement may be required, resulting in significant disfigurement and morbidity. Complete limb amputation is sometimes required.

Key Points

- Necrotizing fasciitis should be considered in any musculoskeletal complaint with pain out of proportion to clinical examination.
- Definitive therapy is operative debridement.
- IV fluids and triple antibiotic therapy are adjunctive therapy only.
- Rapid progression is common.

Pitfalls

- Failure to consider the diagnosis of necrotizing fasciitis in a patient with minimal skin findings but significant discomfort.
- Failure to advocate for the patient and insist on emergent operative intervention.
- Do not be overly reassured by the effectiveness of IV fluids and antibiotic administration in the management of necrotizing fasciitis. The treatment is surgical intervention.

TICK-BORNE ILLNESSES: ROCKY MOUNTAIN SPOTTED FEVER AND LYME DISEASE

Background

The majority of tick-borne illnesses occur from April to October, but they can occur year-round. Patients are frequently not aware of a preceding tick bite. RMSF and Lyme disease are some of the most clinically important diseases (due to both frequency and severity of sequelae) spread by a tick bite. Although reported in all regions of the continental United States, RMSF occurs most commonly in the southeastern and south-central United States, and Lyme disease is most commonly seen in northeastern and upper Midwestern states as well as the Pacific Northwest.

RMSF (caused by *Rickettsia rickettsia*) directly infects vascular endothelial cells and causes a systemic vasculitis. Symptoms typically appear 3–12 days after the initial tick bite.

Lyme disease is more complex and can involve the dermatologic, neurologic, and cardiovascular system.

Classic Clinical Presentation

Rocky Mountain spotted fever classically begins with fever and then a rash that begins on the wrists and ankles and then spreads up the extremities to include the torso. The rash may be initially macular and become petechial over time. The rash most commonly appears between the third and fifth days of illness. Although a rash on the palms and soles is characteristic of RMSF, it typically occurs later in the disease course.

Associated symptoms include fever, headache, myalgias, and malaise. Nausea with or without vomiting frequently occurs, and children may also have abdominal pain (which is sometimes severe). Hyponatremia is common. RMFS is a clinical mimic of bacterial meningitis, particularly meningococcemia. Systemic vascular injury can result in clinical syndromes such as interstitial pneumonitis, myocarditis, and encephalitis.

Lyme disease classically presents in three stages: early localized, early disseminated, and

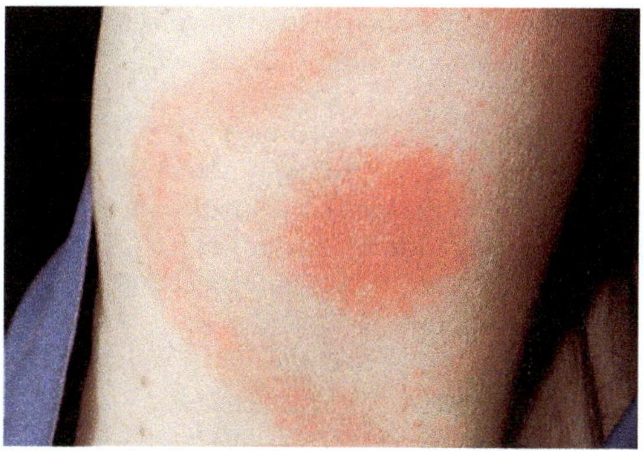

FIGURE 23.6 Erythema migrans.

Source: From Centers of Disease Control and Prevention (https://www.cdc.gov/lyme/signs_symptoms/rashes.html).

late disease. Early localized disease presents with erythema migrans, a solitary erythematous targetoid lesion at the site of a tick bite (typically within 1 or 2 weeks after the bite; Figure 23.6). Untreated, this rash expands to an erythematous lesion with or without central clearing that is 5–70 cm in diameter.

The early disseminated stage occurs weeks to months after the bite if Lyme disease is untreated after initial presentation. Symptoms include disseminated erythema migrans lesions and neurologic and cardiac sequelae. Neurologic symptoms vary and may be mild or severe, ranging from peripheral neuropathy/palsies (bilateral cranial nerve VII palsy is almost always caused by Lyme disease) to meningoencephalitis. Cardiac sequelae are most commonly atrioventricular (AV) block and sometimes myopericarditis. The AV node blockade is typically self-limited (lasting days) but may require intervention if symptomatic. Late disease presents as arthritis (and rarely with subtle neurologic symptoms) and occurs months to years after initial infection. Lyme arthritis occurs most commonly in one or several large joints, particularly in the knee.

Atypical Clinical Presentation

Rocky Mountain spotted fever may present initially without a rash, or the rash may be localized to one body area. The rash may be confluent with areas of skin necrosis in severe disease. The disease may also present with predominantly gastrointestinal symptoms, including abdominal pain, nausea, vomiting, and diarrhea. Headache may be absent.

Disseminated erythema migrans, arthritis, or neurological symptoms may less commonly be the initial presentation of Lyme disease.

Although tick bites more commonly occur in less populated areas, they may be acquired even in inner-city parks in endemic areas.

Differential Diagnosis

Bacterial meningitis is the most important clinical mimic of RMSF. Other conditions that present similarly include viral syndromes, scarlet fever, and KD.

The cutaneous findings of the initial erythema migrans lesion of Lyme disease may mimic nummular eczema, tinea corporis, cellulitis, and erythema multiforme.

Diagnostic Confirmation

Rocky Mountain spotted fever is a clinical diagnosis. No rapid confirmatory tests are available, and treatment should be initiated as soon as possible to decrease morbidity and mortality rates. Serologic testing may not be positive early in the disease because it requires 7–10 days to develop serum antibodies. Hyponatremia and thrombocytopenia may be helpful diagnostic clues but are less common early in the disease course.

Similarly, serological diagnostic testing is not useful in Lyme disease for localized disease because it is only positive in the minority of patients early in the disease course. Up to 90% of patients with early disseminated infections will have positive serology.

Treatment

Doxycycline is the most effective treatment for RMSF and should be used in nearly all cases in both adults and children. A 5- to 7-day course is typically curative. The mortality rate without treatment has been historically as high as 30%.

The treatment of early Lyme disease includes oral amoxicillin, doxycycline, or cefuroxime. Doxycycline has the best penetration into the cerebrospinal fluid and most effectively treats potential co-infecting organisms. Treatment is typically given for 10–21 days. Severe cases require IV antibiotics, and late disease requires treatment up to 1 month. A Jarisch–Herxheimer reaction may occur in the first 24 hours of treatment. Symptomatic AV nodal blockade may require a temporary pacemaker (typically only for several days). Most patients have resolution of symptoms within 3 weeks after treatment initiation.

Disposition

Mild disease with RMSF may be treated on an outpatient basis. Severe symptoms require hospitalization. Due to the significant associated mortality rate and potential complications, most patients diagnosed with RMSF should be admitted and monitored for complications. Early antibiotic administration is important to reduce morbidity and mortality.

Most patients with Lyme disease may be treated on an outpatient basis. Patients who require IV antibiotics or those with severe complications (e.g., meningoencephalitis or AV nodal blockade) may require admission.

Complications

Complications of RMSF include death, meningoencephalitis, cerebral edema, acute renal failure, cardiopulmonary complications, shock, seizures, and potential long-term sequelae such as focal neurologic deficits.

Key Points

- The life-threatening tick-borne illnesses of RMSF and Lyme disease are both diagnosed clinically.
- The most effective treatment for tick-borne illnesses is doxycycline.

Pitfalls

- Failure to consider the diagnosis of a tick-borne infection in an ill patient
- Failure to consider the diagnosis of RMSF in a patient without a rash

Further Reading

Kawasaki Disease

McCrindle BW, Rowley AH, Newburger JW, et al. Diagnosis, treatment, and long-term management of Kawasaki disease: A scientific statement for health professionals from the American Heart Association. *Circulation*. 2017;135:e927.

Omphalitis

Sinha A, Sazawal S, Pradhan A, Ramji S, Opiyo N. Chlorhexidine skin or cord care for prevention of mortality and infections in neonates. *Cochrane Database Syst Rev*. 2015;2015(3):CD007835.

Stewart, D, Benitz, W. Umbilical cord care in the newborn infant. *Pediatrics*. 2016;138(3):e1.

Staphylococcal Scaled Skin Syndrome

Leung AKC, Barankin B, Leong KF. Staphylococcal-scalded skin syndrome: Evaluation, diagnosis, and management. *World J Pediatr*. 2018;14(2):116–120.

Malburg L, Pacheco, GS. Staphylococcal scalded skin syndrome. In Rose E, ed. *Life-Threatening Rashes: An Illustrated Practical Guide*. Cham, Switzerland: Springer; 2018:127–140.

Mishra AK, Yadav P, Mishra AA. Systemic review on staphylococcal scalded skin syndrome (SSSS): A rare and critical disease of neonates. *Open Microbiol J*. 2016;10(1):150–159.

Staiman A, Hsu DY, Silverberg JI. Epidemiology of staphylococcal scalded skin syndrome in U.S. children. *Br J Dermatol*. 2018;178(3):704–708.

Stevens–Johnson Syndrome and Toxic Epidermal Necrolysis

Alerhand S, Cassella C, Koyfman A. Stevens–Johnson syndrome and toxic epidermal necrolysis in the pediatric population: A review. *Pediatr Emerg Care*. 2016;32(7):472–476

Hsu DY, Brieva J, Silverberg NB, Paller AS, Silverberg JI. Pediatric Stevens–Johnson syndrome and toxic epidermal necrolysis in the United States. *J Am Acad Dermatol*. 2017;76(5):811–817.e814.

Huq, F, Omer, T, Behar, S. Stevens–Johnson syndrome and toxic epidermal necrolysis. In Rose E, ed. *Life-Threatening Rashes: An Illustrated Practical Guide*. Cham, Switzerland: Springer; 2018:37–54.

24

Skin and Soft Tissue Infections

NICHOLAS M. OROZCO AND JESSICA LANGE OSTERMAN

INTRODUCTION

Skin and soft tissue infections (SSTIs) are a common presenting complaint to acute care centers. SSTIs include folliculitis, furuncle, carbuncle, impetigo, ecthyma, erysipelas, cellulitis, and abscess. These infections are caused by methicillin-resistant and methicillin-susceptible *Staphylococcus aureus* (MRSA and MSSA, respectively) and streptococcus species. Importantly, the type of SSTI often correlates with the bacterial species, which in turn guides management and antibiotic choice. Other important considerations in managing pediatric patients with an SSTI include pain control, diagnosis of abscess, decision to sedate or not for abscess drainage, disposition, and follow-up.

BACKGROUND

Folliculitis is a superficial bacterial infection of the hair follicle within the epidermis (Figure 24.1). When purulent material develops around the follicle extending into the dermis creating a small abscess, it is known as a *furuncle* (Figure 24.2). Coalescence of multiple furuncles with opening of follicles to the surface and purulent drainage is known as a *carbuncle* (Figure 24.3). These infections are typically caused by MSSA or MRSA.

Impetigo is a contagious superficial skin infection caused by streptococcus, staphylococcus, or both species (Figure 24.4). Lesions progress from papules to vesicles, pustules, and finally crusts. *Bullous impetigo* occurs with infection of staphylococcus that produces exfoliative (epidermolytic) toxin A—a toxin that causes loss of cell adhesion in the superficial epidermis by targeting the protein desmoglein (Figure 24.5). These lesions typically begin as vesicles and enlarge to flaccid bullae. *Ecthyma* is impetigo that involves the epidermis

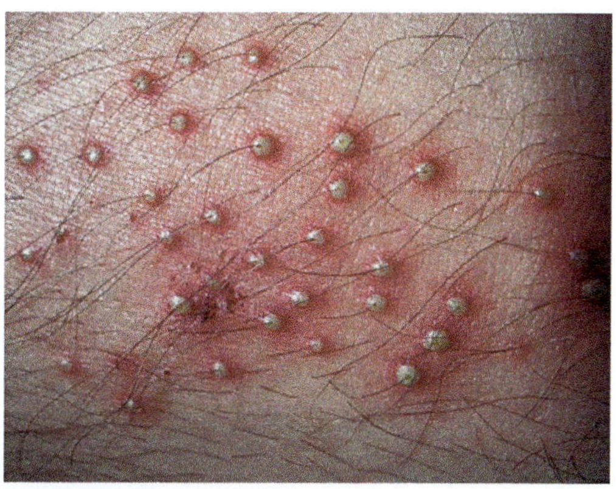

FIGURE 24.1 Folliculitis—pustules within the hair follicles.

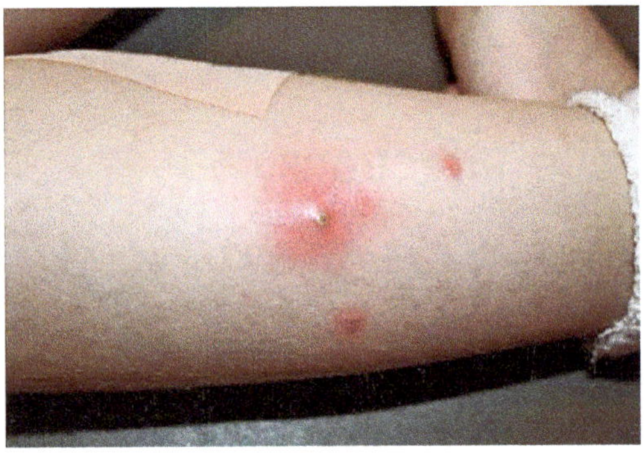

FIGURE 24.2 Furuncle—purulent material extending into dermis, creating a "boil" or small abscess.

extending deep into the dermis, forming an ulcer with yellow crusting and violaceous borders (Figure 24.6).

Erysipelas entails a distinct streptococcal infection of the uppermost layers of the subcutaneous tissues and superficial lymphatics (Figure 24.7). Characteristic of erysipelas is a well-demarcated margin of infected skin that is raised compared to uninfected skin. Often, there is edema that causes the skin to appear as an orange peel or "peau d'orange." *Cellulitis* represents infection of the deep dermis and subcutaneous fat tissue typically caused by streptococcus or staphylococcus (Figure 24.8). An *abscess* is a collection of pus within the dermis and deeper subcutaneous tissue caused by MSSA or MRSA (Figure 24.9).

CLINICAL PRESENTATION

Folliculitis presents with follicular pustules and papules with an erythematous base. Pruritus is the most common symptom, although patients

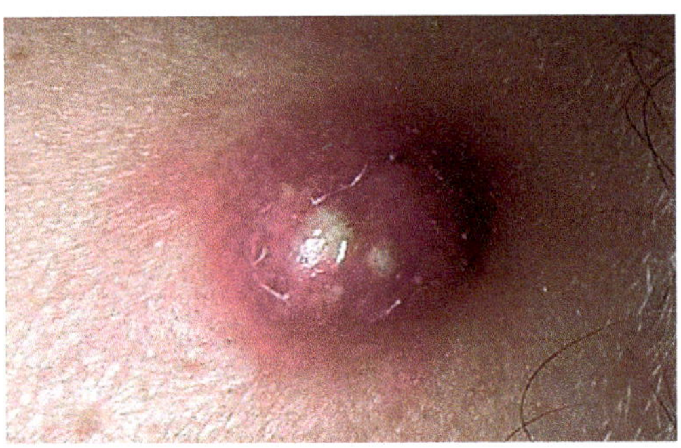

FIGURE 24.3 Carbuncle—coalescence of multiple furuncles.

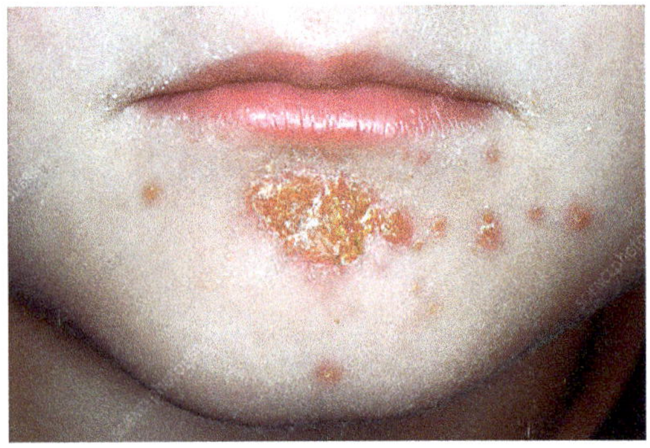

FIGURE 24.4 Impetigo—honey-crusted lesions on the face.

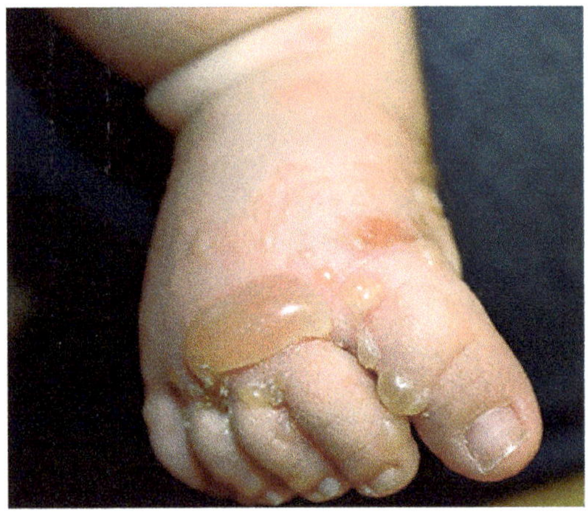

FIGURE 24.5 Bullous impetigo—fluid-filled bullae caused by exfoliative toxin produced by *Staphylococcus aureus*.

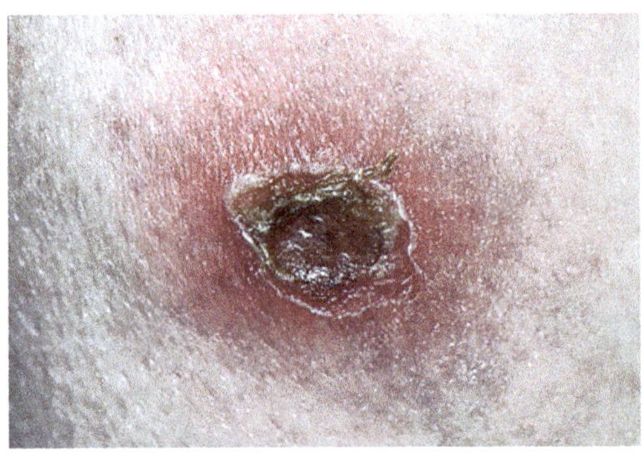

FIGURE 24.6 Ecthyma—"punched out" ulcer that extends deep into the subcutaneous tissue with darkened crusting.

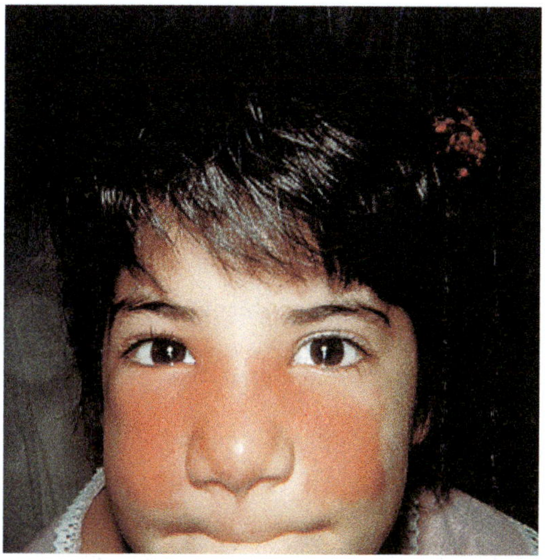

FIGURE 24.7 Erysipelas—well-demarcated margins of raised erythema with "butterfly" appearance over cheeks and nasal bridge.

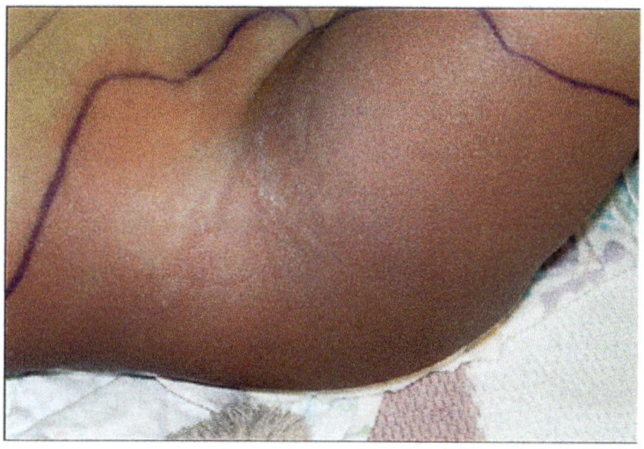

FIGURE 24.8 Cellulitis—erythema to thigh and buttock with outlined borders to demarcate area of infection.

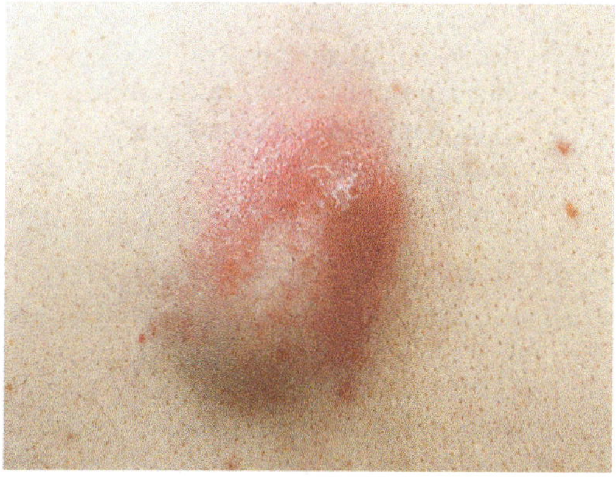

FIGURE 24.9 Cutaneous abscess—indurated with area of fluctuance indicative of pus that has extended into subcutaneous tissue.

may also experience pain. Although folliculitis can occur in any area of the body with hair follicles, certain body distributions correspond to different etiologies. It is most common on the face and scalp, upper trunk, buttocks, and legs; however, MRSA folliculitis is more likely to occur on the chest, flank, scrotum, and umbilical area. Another common type of folliculitis is "hot tub folliculitis" caused by *Pseudomonas aeruginosa*. This occurs after spending time in a contaminated hot tub or heated pool usually 8–48 hours after exposure. Distribution is typically along the trunk and buttocks area where the bathing suit was worn. Other types of folliculitis exist, including fungal and viral folliculitis, and should be considered when treatment has failed.

Impetigo is most commonly seen between the ages of 2 and 5 years. The lesions begin as small vesicles that grow quickly to vesiculopustular lesions which then rupture, releasing purulent discharge. This then gives rise to the characteristic adherent yellow or honey-crusted lesion. The lesions are often painless without erythema or warmth and typically asymptomatic, although there can be pruritus, which helps spread the infection. They occur most often on traumatized skin (e.g., scratch or abrasion) and exposed body surfaces such as the face (nose and mouth) or extremities, with the palms and soles unaffected. Impetigo tends to occur more frequently during warmer temperatures with increased humidity. It is highly contagious and spread among family members and especially preschool children; poor hygiene is a risk factor.

As mentioned previously, bullous impetigo is an infection with *S. aureus*, most commonly seen in newborns, infants, and children aged 2–5 years. Typical findings of bullous impetigo include vesicles that enlarge to flaccid bullae, which are serous initially and then become pus-filled. There can be a single lesion or few or multiple lesions scattered over different areas. The bullae are typically oval or round without surrounding erythema. One of the pathognomonic findings of bullous impetigo is the scaly rim after the bulla has ruptured; Nikolsky sign is absent (see Chapter 23 on dermatologic emergencies). In addition, unlike impetigo, lesions of bullous impetigo occur in covered areas, including the trunk, perineum, buttocks, and extremities, and do not have a seasonal predilection (e.g., warm or cold environments). Bullous impetigo lesions typically heal without scarring.

Ecthyma lesions begin similarly to impetigo but penetrate the entire thickness of the epidermis into dermis. They begin as vesicles that rupture and then appear as discrete, punched-out ulcers covered with dark crusts. They can sometimes appear as cigarette burns and are a child abuse mimic. These lesions are most common on the legs, seen in children of all ages, and are more frequent during summer. Frequently, there is preceding minor skin trauma such as an abrasion, scratch, or insect bite. In distinction to impetigo, ecthyma lesions tend to cause scarring.

Erysipelas involves a fiery red or salmon-color infection of the uppermost layers of the subcutaneous tissue and, importantly, the cutaneous lymphatic system. It is often hot, tender, and indurated, with sharp demarcated borders distinguishing it from uninfected skin. It is commonly described as having an orange peel appearance. It is frequently seen in infants and young children after a predisposing lesion such as an abrasion, laceration, or some other break in the skin. Risk factors for erysipelas include diabetes mellitus, malnutrition, lymphedema, and local lymphatic dysfunction (e.g., venous stasis). The infection is typically abrupt in onset, with constitutional symptoms such as fever, chills, malaise, and headache. The most common sites are the face and extremities. On the face, there may be a butterfly appearance involving both cheeks and the nasal bridge. Sometimes the edema from the infection can cause the formation of vesicles and tense bullae to form that rupture and crust over. Given that the infection creates issues with lymphatic drainage, a single infection often leads to recurrence as lymphatic vessels become obstructed, causing lymphedema. Associated fever is common.

Unlike erysipelas, cellulitis involves the dermis and subcutaneous tissues and contains poorly demarcated margins. Left untreated, cellulitis can develop into an abscess in which purulent material accumulates and tracks into the dermis and deeper subcutaneous tissue, requiring drainage; however, an abscess without surrounding cellulitis may also develop. Cutaneous abscesses are painful and tender, fluctuant, red nodules often with surrounding erythema. Differentiating between abscess and cellulitis can be challenging when there is heavy induration, making the decision for incision and drainage difficult.

DIFFERENTIAL DIAGNOSIS

- Folliculitis
  - Acne vulgaris
  - Rosacea
  - Perioral dermatitis
  - Drug-induced folliculitis
  - Keratosis pilaris
  - Hidradenitis suppurativa
  - Scabies
- Impetigo, bullous impetigo, and ecthyma
  - Herpes simplex virus
  - Varicella
  - Tinea corporis
  - Localized acute pustular psoriasis
  - Bullous arthropod bite
  - Poison ivy
  - Autoimmune blistering disease (e.g., pemphigoid, pemphigus, linear immunoglobulin A disease, epidermolysis bullosa)
  - Child abuse (burn injury)
  - Ecthyma gangrenosum
- Erysipelas and cellulitis
  - Butterfly rash of systemic lupus erythematous
  - Deep vein thrombosis or thrombophlebitis
  - Contact dermatitis
  - Necrotizing soft tissue infection
- Furuncle, carbuncle, and abscess
  - Vascular malformation
  - Kerion
  - Myiasis
  - Herpetic whitlow
  - Hidradenitis suppurativa
  - Sexually transmitted infection (e.g., lymphogranuloma venereum)
  - Sporotrichosis
  - Cat scratch disease

DIAGNOSTIC CONFIRMATION

Diagnosis is primarily dependent on history and physical examination findings, as discussed previously. However, the physical examination does have limitations, and there is diagnostic variability among clinicians. Although needle aspiration may facilitate diagnosis, it can lead to multiple attempts/needle sticks and false negatives if not aspirating from an area of purulence.

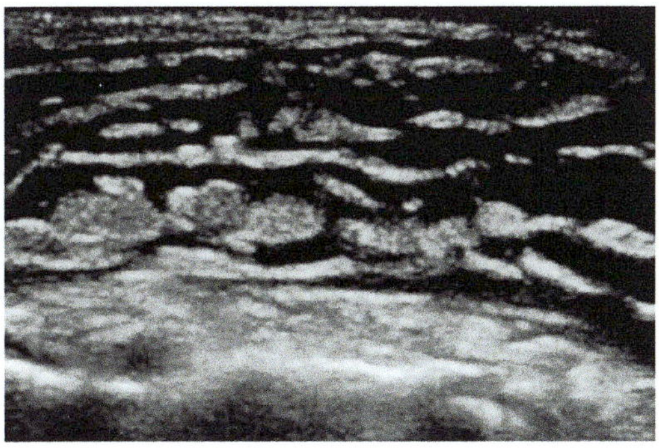

FIGURE 24.10 Cobblestoning—pattern created by edema on ultrasound; seen in cellulitis without a definitive pocket of fluid to suggest abscess formation.

Ultrasound (US) increases both sensitivity and specificity in diagnosing superficial abscesses when done by physicians with point-of-care US. This is particularly useful in children for both diagnosis in equivocal cases and avoiding unnecessary invasive procedures. Cellulitis will demonstrate tissue edema on US termed "cobblestoning" without a hypoechoic fluid collection (Figure 24.10), whereas an abscess will have a hypoechoic fluid-filled pocket (Figure 24.11).

TREATMENT

Nonpurulent Skin and Soft Tissue Infections

Folliculitis and impetigo are superficial localized SSTIs. Topical antibiotics can be used if there is no evidence of systemic infection. This includes mupirocin or retapamulin ointment applied twice daily for 5 days or until all lesions have cleared.

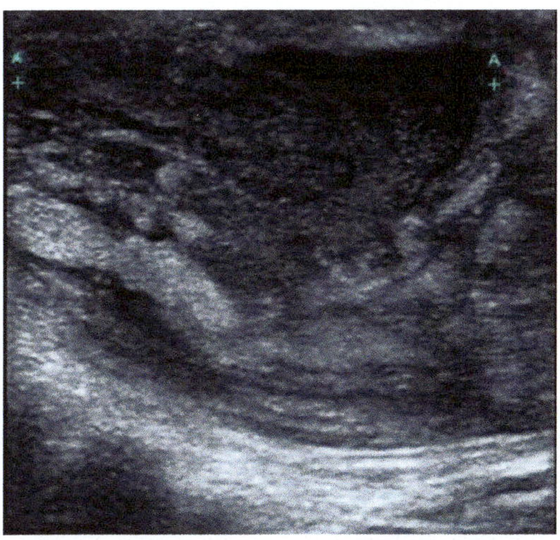

FIGURE 24.11 Abscess as seen on ultrasound image with definitive pocket of fluid and debris.

For patients with multiple lesions in different areas of the body or in households with multiple outbreaks and in patients with ecthyma, oral antibiotic therapy is recommended. Oral therapy should cover MSSA or streptococcus and includes dicloxacillin or cephalexin for a 7-day course. In patients with suspected or confirmed MRSA infection, doxycycline, clindamycin, or sulfamethoxazole–trimethroprim (SMX-TMP) is recommended.

For cellulitis and erysipelas in hemodynamically stable patients without risk factors for MRSA, coverage for streptococcus and MSSA is recommended with oral antibiotic therapy. This includes first-generation or second-generation cephalosporins (e.g., cephalexin and cefuroxime) or dicloxacillin. Patients with suspected or confirmed MRSA infection require coverage for streptococcus and MRSA. This includes monotherapy with clindamycin or combination therapy with a β-lactam antibiotic (e.g., amoxicillin or cephalexin) plus SMX-TMP or doxycycline. The preferred treatment is clindamycin for these infections unless there is a prevalence of clindamycin-resistant MRSA >15%. The recommended treatment duration is 5–7 days, although this may be extended if infection does not resolve.

Children with systemic signs and symptoms should have more of a diagnostic workup, including laboratory studies and initiation of parenteral therapy. These signs and symptoms include the following:

- Fever >38.4°C
- Tachycardia
- Hypotension
- Rapid progression of erythema
- Signs of necrotizing soft tissue infection or ischemic limb, such as crepitance, bullae, pain out of proportion to examination, decreased pulses, or other evidence of ischemia
- Children with underlying medical problems that are likely to have poor response to therapy or complications (e.g., immunodeficiency, malignancy, diabetes mellitus, and sickle cell disease)
- Inability to tolerate oral medication
- Children with SSTI close to an implanted device

Purulent Skin and Soft Tissue Infections

The mainstay of treatment for purulent SSTIs is incision and drainage (I&D). This includes cutaneous abscesses, large furuncles, and carbuncles if there is large enough of a purulent collection to drain. To effectively treat purulent SSTIs, I&D, probing, and deloculation of the wound must be done. Needle aspiration both alone or with the guidance of US is not effective to cure the abscess. Thus, US should be used for diagnosis alone and not needle aspiration because this can lead to unsuccessful treatment.

In pediatric patients, I&D is one of the most painful procedures undergone in the emergency department. Topical anesthetic should be given when performing an abscess I&D. This may include lidocaine/tetracaine patch or cream, subcutaneous lidocaine, or, preferably, a combination of the two (see Chapter 48 on pain management and procedural sedation). Oral agents and/or intranasal fentanyl may also be useful adjunctive therapy. Additional procedural sedation agents (most commonly ketamine) may be required to facilitate drainage, particularly in young children.

Once the abscess has been drained, simply covering the wound with a dry dressing has been shown to be most effective in pediatric patients. Packing abscess cavities is no longer recommended because it increases pain and does not improve outcomes. After I&D, systemic antibiotics have not been shown to increase cure rates, even in those with MRSA infections. However, systemic antibiotics should be given to patients with signs and symptoms of systemic infection and those with severely impaired host defenses.

DISPOSITION

Most SSTIs can be managed on an outpatient basis, although occasionally infections with systemic signs may require observation or hospital admission. Pediatric patients with impetigo or folliculitis can return to school 24 hours after beginning treatment, with draining lesions covered. Crusted lesions can be gently washed, and handwashing is important to reduce the spread of infection.

Hospitalization is recommended for patients with systemic signs and symptoms, with hemodynamic instability, or with significant risk factors for complications. Factors to be considered for observation include the following:

- Neonates (≤28 days of age)
- Children aged 29 days–11 months with SSTI ≥3 cm (1.2 in.) in diameter (including surrounding erythema or cellulitis) or aged 12 months–4 years with SSTI ≥4 cm (1.6 in.) in diameter
- Children younger than age 5 years with abscesses on the face or perineum
- Children of any age with multiple sites of nonsuperficial infections (e.g., infections other than impetigo, ecthyma, and folliculitis) or any systemic signs or symptoms

For borderline cases, the first one to two antibiotic doses can be given in the emergency department observation unit if available.

COMPLICATIONS

Rare complications from untreated SSTIs include more severe infections such as sepsis, septic arthritis, osteomyelitis, pyomyositis, and necrotizing soft tissue infections (see Chapter 37 on orthopedic emergencies and Chapter 23 on dermatologic emergencies).

KEY POINTS

- SSTIs include nonpurulent (folliculitis, impetigo, ecthyma, erysipelas, and cellulitis) and purulent infections (furuncle, carbuncle, and cutaneous abscess) typically caused by streptococcus, MSSA, or MRSA.
- Folliculitis and impetigo represent infections localized to the epidermis and are typically treated with topical antibiotics such as mupirocin.
- Ecthyma represents an ulcerating infection extending deeper into the dermis.
- In patients with ecthyma or multiple sites of impetigo or folliculitis, oral antibiotic treatment with a cephalosporin is recommended.
- Erysipelas and cellulitis represent deeper subcutaneous infections and require oral antibiotic therapy typically with a cephalosporin.
- When MRSA is suspected, the preferred oral antibiotic is clindamycin.

- Purulent infections extend into the dermis and require I&D.
- Ultrasound can be used to decipher equivocal cases of abscess versus cellulitis and improves sensitivity and specificity.
- Adequate pain control with topical anesthetic, analgesia, and sometimes sedation is necessary for I&D.
- After I&D of abscesses, packing and oral antibiotics have not been shown to increase cure rate.
- Consider observation and hospitalization for patients with systemic signs and symptoms or with risk factors for treatment failure (e.g., multiple infection sites, facial and perineal infections, neonates, and immunocompromised).
- Rare complications include sepsis, septic arthritis, osteomyelitis, pyomyositis, and necrotizing soft tissue infections.

PITFALLS

Failure to recognize and perform an I&D on an abscess can result in prolonged, worsening infection or some of the complications noted previously. Multiple attempts at treatment without a definitive I&D may lead to antibiotic resistance in patients solely treated with antimicrobial therapy. US guidance can help decipher a purulent SSTI versus a nonpurulent SSTI.

Abscess mimics should not undergo I&D in the emergency department. These include vascular malformation, kerion, herpetic whitlow, hidradenitis suppurativa, sexually transmitted infections, cat scratch disease, and sporotrichosis. US can help decipher these mimics (e.g., blood flow in a vascular malformation).

Last, several types of abscesses require surgical drainage because of the high rates of complications. These include abscesses of the perirectum and rectum, anterior and lateral neck, hand, areas adjacent to vital nerves and vessels (e.g., facial nerve and carotid or femoral artery), breast, and the central triangle of the face formed by the corners of the mouth and nasal bridge because they pose a risk of intracranial extension via the cavernous sinus.

Further Reading

Duong M, Markwell S, Peter J, Barenkamp S. Randomized, controlled trial of antibiotics in the management of community-acquired skin abscesses in the pediatric patient. *Ann Emerg Med.* 2010;55:401–407.

Fenster DB, Renny MH, Ng C, et al. Scratching the surface: A review of skin and soft tissue infections in children. *Curr Opin Pediatr.* 2015;27:303–307.

Gorowitz RJ. A review of community-associated methicillin-resistant *Staphylococcus aureus* skin and soft tissue infections. *J Pediatr Infect Dis.* 2008;27:1.

Stevens DL, Bisno AL, Chambers HF, et al. Practice guidelines for the diagnosis and management of skin and soft tissue infections: 2014 update by the Infectious Diseases Society of America. *Clin Infect Dis.* 2014;59(2):e10–e52.

Talan DA, Mower WR, Krishnadasan A, et al. Trimethoprim–sulfamethoxazole versus placebo for uncomplicated skin abscess. *N Engl J Med.* 2016;374:823.

25

Pediatric Burns

NEAL MOEHRLE AND JESSICA LANGE OSTERMAN

THERMAL BURNS

Pathophysiology of Burns

Understanding the pathophysiology of burns provides insight into the primary goals of burn management in the emergency department. The primary functions of the skin are to prevent free water loss, to prevent the entry of microorganisms, and to regulate body temperature. Disruption of this protective barrier leads to significant fluid losses and hypovolemia, increased risk of secondary bacterial infections, and hypothermia. Over the course of the first 24 hours after a thermal burn, the release of inflammatory cytokines leads to increased capillary permeability, resulting in tissue edema and additional fluid losses. In large burns, myocardial depression can occur, resulting in burn shock. The pathophysiology of burns is fundamentally similar in adults and pediatrics; however, because children typically have thinner skin than adults, burns tend to penetrate more deeply in children and cause more tissue damage.

Burn Classification

Burn management and ultimately patient disposition are dependent on the type of burn involved. Burns are described by two classification systems. One method takes into account only the depth of an individual burn and the types of tissues involved. The other, put forth by the American Burn Association, takes a more global approach and considers the depth, total body surface area (TBSA), location, and other associated injuries in order to guide disposition.

Classically, burns have been described as first, second, third, and even fourth degree, but the terminology has shifted to include the burn depth as superficial, partial thickness, and full thickness:

1. Superficial burns are analogous to sunburns; only the epidermis is involved, which will be erythematous, warm, blanching, dry, and painful (Figure 25.1). No bullous lesions are present, but after 7–10 days, the epidermis sloughs off without scar formation.
2. Partial-thickness burns occur when the burn extends deeper into the dermis, and the resulting lesions are erythematous, wet appearing, and painful (Figure 25.2). Partial-thickness

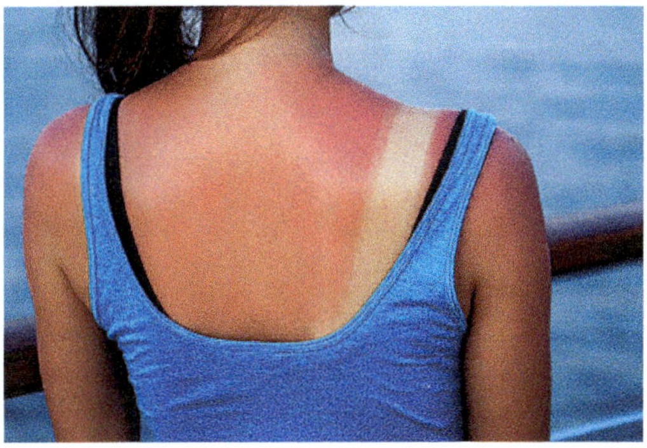

FIGURE 25.1 Superficial burn.

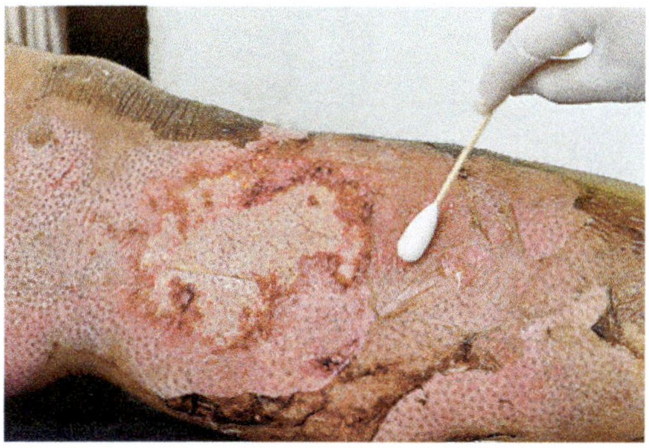

FIGURE 25.3 Deep partial-thickness burn.

burns can be further subdivided into superficial and deep components, both of which involve bullae formation. Superficial partial-thickness burns involve only the papillary layer of the dermis, whereas deep partial-thickness burns extend into the reticular layer as well. The two can be differentiated by the degree of erythema and pain. Capillaries and sensory nerve fibers are often damaged in deeper burns; as a result, deep partial-thickness burns tend to be paler, nonblanching, and less painful than their superficial counterparts (Figure 25.3).

3. Full-thickness burns occur when burns extend past the dermis into the subcutaneous tissue. These burns have a dry, leathery, and waxy appearance, and they are insensate (Figure 25.4). Muscle, tendon, and bone may be exposed, creating a fourth-degree burn. Deep partial-thickness and full-thickness burns will ultimately result in scar formation and typically require surgical management and skin grafting because the regenerative tissues are damaged by the initial insult.

Accurately identifying the type of burn is imperative to guiding management and also in counseling the patient on cosmetic outcome and determining the need for surgical consultation.

Estimation of Total Body Surface Area

Once burns are adequately classified, the emergency provider must be able to adequately estimate the surface area of skin involved because this plays directly into the resuscitation of the patient. Only partial- and full-thickness burns are included in this calculation. Several techniques are available to help guide providers in this estimation. In the palm method, the size of the patient's palm (including fingers) is

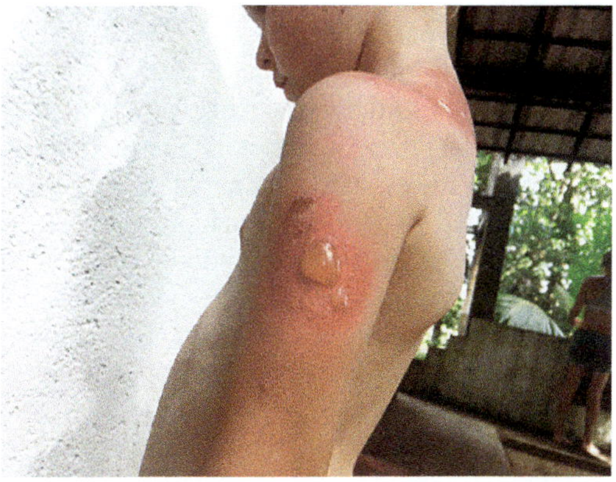

FIGURE 25.2 Superficial partial-thickness burn.

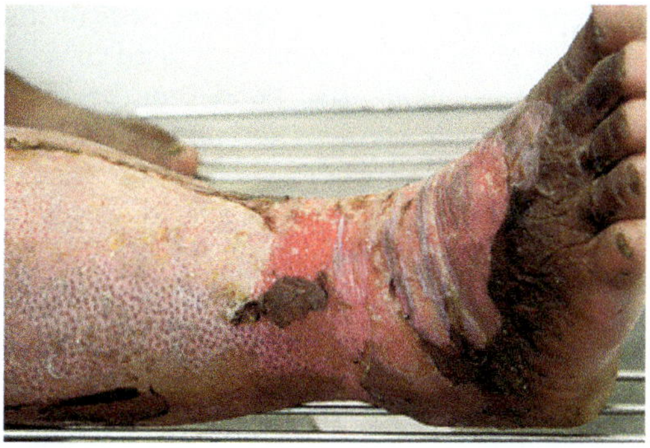

FIGURE 25.4 Full-thickness burn.

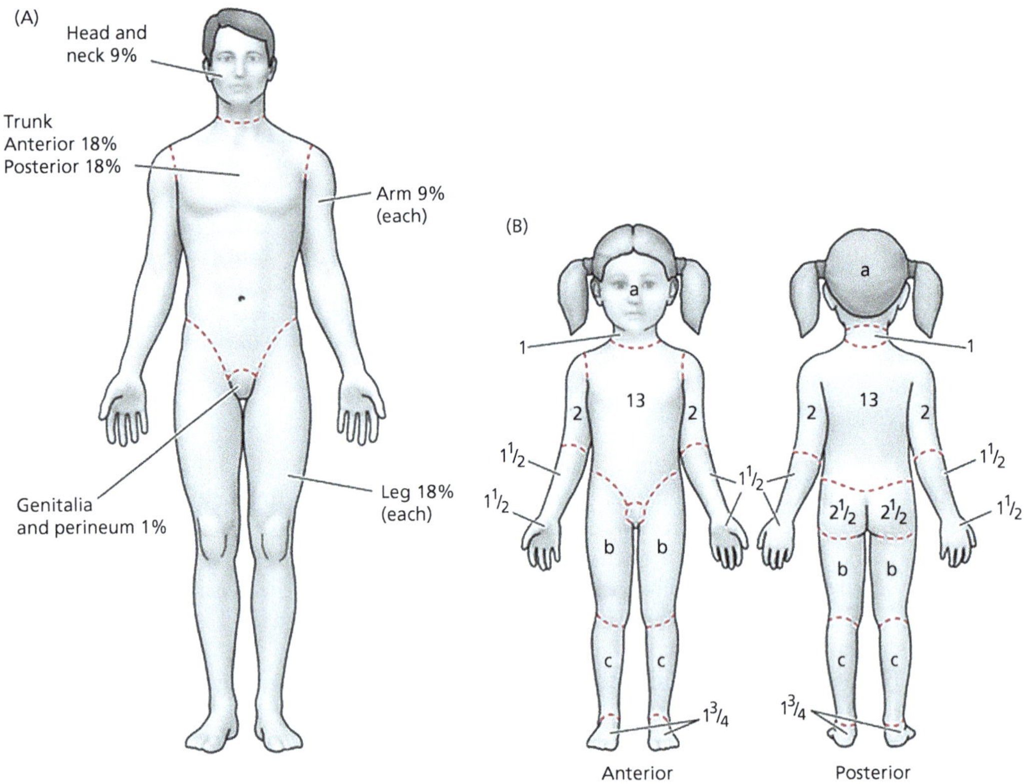

Relative percentage of body surface area (% BSA) affected by growth

	Age				
Body Part	0 yr	1 yr	5 yr	10 yr	15 yr
a = ½ of head	9½	8½	6½	5½	4½
b = ½ of 1 thigh	2¾	3¼	4	4¼	4½
c = ½ of 1 lower leg	2½	2½	2¾	3	3¼

FIGURE 25.5 Lund–Browder chart.

approximately 1% of TBSA, which may be more helpful for irregularly shaped burns or those with patchy involvement and is the basis for the "rule of nines" that is commonly used in adult burn resuscitation. The Lund–Browder chart more accurately accounts for proportional differences in body parts as children age (Figure 25.5). Head size decreases and lower extremity size increases with age, and it is important for emergency providers to take this into consideration when making this calculation.

Initial Management

Emergency department management of burns involves a full traumatic assessment including airway, breathing, and circulation; fluid resuscitation; initiation of wound care; and, importantly, pain control.

Fluid Resuscitation

With interruption of the skin barrier, significant fluid losses can result, which are often compounded by the third spacing that occurs as a result of increased capillary permeability. Maintaining intravascular volume is not only important to account for these losses but also essential to prevent hypoperfusion to potentially salvageable tissues. A modified version of the Parkland formula can be used by emergency providers to calculate the volume of fluid necessary for resuscitating pediatric burn patients:

Total volume in the first 24 hours = 3 mL/kg × %TBSA + weight-based maintenance fluids (in children <30 kg)

Half of this volume is given over the first 8 hours, with the second half given over the subsequent 16 hours. Typically, lactated Ringer's is the fluid of choice because normal saline can cause a normal anion gap metabolic acidosis when used in large quantities. In children <20 kg, 5% dextrose-containing fluids are used for maintenance because baseline smaller glycogen stores increase their risk for hypoglycemia.

The modified Parkland formula should be used as an initial estimation of fluid management, but the rate and volume should be adjusted based on the patient's fluid status. A Foley catheter should be placed to accurately track urine output, with a goal of 1–2 mL/kg/hr in children <30 kg and 0.5–1 mL/kg/hr in children >30 kg. In addition, other signs of perfusion (skin perfusion, lactate, serum bicarbonate, etc.) should also be used as data points to evaluate for adequate resuscitation.

Wound Management

Although burn wounds are generally cared for in a specialized burn unit, emergency providers must have a basic understanding of the principles of wound management. If transport to the referring burn center is delayed, wound care should begin in the emergency department to minimize risk of infection, fluid loss, and hypothermia. Pain medications, typically intravenous opioids, should be given prior to wound care because this process can be extremely painful for patients. An initial dose of morphine 0.05–0.1 mg/kg intravenously (IV) or hydromorphone 0.05 mg/kg IV can be given, and re-dosing may be required as needed.

Once pain is adequately controlled, the wounds should be cleansed with mild soap and water. Ruptured bullae should be debrided with saline-soaked gauze or sterile forceps to decrease rates of infection. Whether unruptured bullae should be debrided remains more controversial because there is no clear evidence regarding whether leaving blisters intact is advantageous for wound healing or infection prevention. Many providers, however, choose to debride large unruptured blisters as well as those that cross major joints.

After cleaning and debriding, all nonsuperficial burns should be covered with a topical antibiotic. Numerous options exist for this purpose, with silver sulfadiazine, bacitracin, and triple antibiotic ointment being the most frequently used topical formulations. Silver sulfadiazine 1% cream, applied twice daily, has been shown to decrease bacterial colonization of burn wounds, but its benefit in preventing bacterial infection is uncertain. It is contraindicated in infants younger than age 2 months and in patients with allergies to sulfonamides. Other side effects include transient leukopenia and oculotoxicity, and it should be avoided on facial burns because it temporarily causes skin discoloration. In burns with smaller surface area or on more sensitive areas, bacitracin and triple antibiotic ointment are superior alternatives. When used in large quantities, however, these medications can be absorbed and cause systemic nephrotoxicity. The wounds should then be covered with a nonadherent dressing prior to transfer.

In circumferential burns, emergency providers should be familiar with the steps of performing an escharotomy. This procedure is ideally performed by an experienced burn surgeon, but if transfer to a burn receiving center is delayed or if long transport times are expected, the procedure should be performed in the emergency department prior to transfer. An escharotomy is often not indicated on initial evaluation. However, as compartments become more edematous with aggressive fluid resuscitation, the procedure may be necessary because the consequences can be life- or limb-threatening. Circumferential chest burns can prevent full chest excursion and impair ventilation, which can be avoided by making incisions in the bilateral anterior axillary lines and a transverse incision connecting the two across the lower chest. Children may require thoracic escharotomy even if the burn is not completely circumferential, and escharotomy should be performed if ventilation becomes impaired in a child with significant thoracic burns. In circumferential extremity burns, an escharotomy may be indicated for elevated compartment pressures, reduced distal pulses, delayed capillary refill, or oxygen saturation <90% on a pulse oximeter placed on the distal digits. Incisions are typically made laterally (with hands supinated in anatomical position) with a depth only to the subcutaneous tissue/fat, with special precaution not to violate the underlying fascia. The decision to perform an escharotomy prior to transfer should be made in conjunction with the consulting burn specialist.

Prior to transfer, tetanus prophylaxis should be given if clinically indicated. A booster vaccine should be given to those children whose tetanus has not been updated within 5 years, and the immune globulin should be given to all un-/underimmunized children (see Chapter 26 on wound care for more detailed recommendations on tetanus prophylaxis).

Inhalational Injury

In the clinical approach to a burn patient, all emergency providers must consider whether or not a patient may have an inhalational injury. Inhalational injury typically occurs in the setting of enclosed fires, as the combustion of organic materials releases toxins that can cause airway damage down to the terminal bronchioles. Upper airway injury occurs early in the course of inhalational injury, as the direct effect of the heat can cause ulceration and edema, which is exacerbated by fluid resuscitation over the first day. Injury in the tracheobronchial tree leads to bronchoconstriction, especially in children with reactive airway disease, as well as edema within the smaller airways. Airway inflammation leads to exudate formation and obstruction, causing atelectasis and fluid accumulation within alveoli, ultimately leading to ventilation–perfusion mismatch and hypoxemia. Impaired mucociliary clearance, combined with dysfunction of alveolar leukocytes, increases risk for developing pneumonia.

The presence of inhalational injury is difficult to predict and may not correlate well with physical examination findings. Assessment for intubation should occur early in the primary survey, and it should be performed if the patient has significant altered mental status; respiratory distress such as stridor, retractions, grunting, and tachypnea; full-thickness burns on the face or mouth; and circumferential neck burns. More subtle signs of possible inhalational injury include singed facial hairs or carbonaceous sputum or soot in the posterior oropharynx. If the patient requires transfer to a burn center, emergency physicians should consider intubating the patient prior to transfer if there is concern for possible inhalational injury because progressive edema will increase the likelihood of a difficult airway.

Baseline chest radiographs should be obtained on all patients with respiratory complaints or an abnormal pulmonary examination. Imaging is often normal early in the course of inhalational injury, and any parenchymal disease may indicate more severe injury and worse prognosis.

Not only does smoke inhalation cause direct damage to the entire respiratory tract but also inhaled gases pose more systemically toxic effects. Carbon monoxide, for example, is a colorless, odorless gas that binds to hemoglobin with >200 times affinity than oxygen and impairs oxygen delivery to tissues. The end result of this is tissue hypoxia, end organ ischemia, and multisystem organ failure. Carboxyhemoglobin levels can be obtained by either a venous or arterial blood gas. All patients with suspected inhalational injury should be placed immediately on oxygen high-flow non-rebreather to displace inhaled carbon monoxide until the carboxyhemoglobin level is <5%. Similar to carbon monoxide poisoning, inhaled cyanide gas also leads to diffuse ischemia, via a slightly different mechanism. Cyanide uncouples the electron transport chain in mitochondria, causing all cells to shift to anaerobic metabolism for energy production. The end result is a severe lactic acidosis, which is the main laboratory finding in cyanide toxicity. Although there is no specific test to easily diagnose cyanide poisoning in the emergency department, consider empiric treatment in burn patients who have significantly elevated lactate and are in cardiac arrest or altered. Treatment is hydroxycobalamin 70 mg/kg IV in a single dose and should be empirically given in patients with smoke inhalation, altered mental status, hypotension, or if the lactate is >10 mmol/L.

All patients with signs of inhalational injury should be admitted to a monitored setting, even if not intubated. Although clinical judgment should be used to determine individual need for admission, patients who have a reported syncopal event, an elevated carboxyhemoglobin level, a metabolic acidosis, or pulmonary symptoms are considered high risk and should be admitted. Patients who remain asymptomatic and with normal vital signs after 4–6 hours of observation in the emergency department can be discharged home.

Disposition

The American Burn Association uses the depth of the burn and estimation of the TBSA to help providers determine need for hospital admission or transfer to a burn center. With the exception of children younger than age 10 years, children with superficial or partial thickness <10% TBSA are eligible for outpatient management. Other factors to consider when determining if a child can be discharged are the presence of comorbidities, willingness of parents to properly tend to wound care, adequate pain control, and reliable follow-up with a pediatrician in 24–48 hours for a re-evaluation. Prior to discharge, parents should be educated on the signs and symptoms of infection and should be taught how to properly care for a burn wound. Criteria for transfer to a burn center include the following:

- Burns in children younger than age 10 years
- Partial-thickness burns >10% TBSA
- Full-thickness burns of any size
- Burns of the face, hands, feet, genitals, perineum, and joints
- Electrical and chemical burns
- Inhalational injury
- Burns in children with preexisting conditions that could complicate management, prolong recovery, or affect mortality
- Burns in children in a hospital without personnel or equipment to care for children
- Burns in patients who will require social, emotional, or rehabilitative interventions
- Burns in patients who also have concomitant trauma in which the burn poses the greatest risk of morbidity and mortality

ELECTRICAL INJURIES

Electric shock injuries are not uncommon reasons for pediatric visits to the emergency department each year. In the pediatric population, electrical injuries occur among two age groups: toddlers and adolescents. Children younger than age 6 years are more likely to suffer household injuries from lower voltage power outlets or electrical cords, whereas teenagers generally suffer injuries related to higher voltage power lines. Fortunately, lightning-related accidents are extremely rare, but when they occur, they often result in death or disability. Emergency providers should be equipped to handle both low- and high-voltage electrical injuries.

Pathophysiology

Understanding the pathophysiology of electrical burns requires a brief discussion of the physics behind electrical energy and its impact on various tissues. The degree of injury depends on the amount of current [in amperes (A)] traveling through the body, which is proportional to the voltage of the energy source and inversely proportional to the resistance of the tissue through which it travels. Tissues with high fluid and electrolyte content—such as nerves, muscles, blood vessels, and moist skin—have low resistance and thus generate more current, whereas tissues such as bone and fat have higher resistances. Approximately 4–10 mA is required to generate pain, and 50–100 mA is enough to induce ventricular fibrillation. Electric shocks cause damage not only directly via current but also through heat generation and the thermal burns they produce. Electrical shocks with longer durations of contact and over larger surface areas tend to generate more heat and subsequently result in more severe burns. The type of current, whether alternating or direct, also has clinical implications. Alternating current (AC) is often found in households and refers to currents that alternate directions cyclically, which can cause muscular tetany that results in prolonged exposure to the electrical source. Direct current (DC), often in power lines and batteries, has unidirectional current and is more likely to result in a patient being thrown from the source, increasing the risk for other traumatic injuries but reducing prolonged exposure to the electrical shock.

Electrical burns can be classified as either low- or high-voltage electrical injuries. Low-voltage injuries are those that occur from sources with <1,000 V, including home outlets, whose voltage ranges from 120 to 240 V. High-voltage injuries are defined as those that occur from >1,000 V, with lightning strikes being approximately 10 million volts. In classic electrical injuries, the patient becomes part of the circuit, with entrance and exit wounds indicating where the electrical current entered and left the body. Despite these skin findings, it is very difficult to predict the true path of the electrical current and, in turn, the extent of internal damage and tissue necrosis; even wounds that appear minor may have catastrophic internal injuries. A less common type of electrical injury is a flash burn, in which an electrical arc generates a significant wave of energy and heat, causing varying degrees of burns on the skin. However, because the current in arc burns does not penetrate the skin, there are usually no associated internal injuries.

Clinical Findings

Cardiovascular

The most immediate life-threatening injuries associated with electrical burns are cardiac dysrhythmias, which occur in approximately 15% of electrical injuries. Of those that lead to sudden cardiac arrest, low-voltage AC injuries tend to be associated with ventricular fibrillation, whereas high-voltage DC injuries are more likely to induce asystole. Less fatal arrhythmias include atrial tachyarrhythmias, atrioventricular nodal block, and QT prolongation. Not all causes of cardiac arrest after an electrical injury are due to a cardiac etiology; electrical current can cause tetanic contractions of the diaphragm, leading to hypoxemia and respiratory arrest. Cardiopulmonary injury should be considered in all electrical injuries in which the path of the current crosses the thorax, whether from one hand to the other or from head to toe.

Neurologic

Electrical injuries have variable effects on the nervous system, especially on peripheral nerves, causing paresthesias, paralysis, and peripheral neuropathies. Symptoms can be transient or permanent, as well as immediate or delayed. The central nervous system can also be affected, leading to various upper and lower motor neuron presentations.

Musculoskeletal

In electrical injuries, muscles undergo repetitive contractions that, if forceful and large enough, can cause fracture of the underlying bones. A significant amount of heat is generated in the soft tissues, which results in coagulative necrosis of the muscle and third spacing of fluid into extremity compartments, increasing the risk for compartment syndrome and rhabdomyolysis. In addition, in the extremities, electrical currents can cause arterial thrombosis or aneurysm formation.

Skin

Skin findings in electrical injuries range from superficial to partial-thickness and full-thickness thermal burns. Not surprisingly, more severe burns result from higher voltage electrical injuries and longer durations of contact with the electrical source. The severity of the burn does not necessarily correlate with internal injuries because even the most minor surface burns can be associated with significant tissue necrosis.

Initial Evaluation and Management

Similar to the management of thermal burns, patients with electrical burns may have a wide array of injuries and initial evaluation should include both a traumatic and a medical assessment, beginning with airway, breathing, and circulation. For patients presenting in cardiac arrest, the Pediatric Advanced Life Support (PALS) algorithm should be followed. Once deemed stable enough after the primary survey, a careful history of the event and physical examination can help providers determine the need for advanced imaging for possible traumatic injuries. Patients who are thrown from the electrical source may have experienced head or neck trauma, and their cervical spine should be immobilized until underlying injuries can be ruled out. Extremities should be evaluated for tense compartments, bony deformities, diminished peripheral pulses, and electrical burns.

Standard protocols have often included a screening electrocardiogram (ECG) in all pediatric patients. Although this recommendation is still valid for victims of high-voltage injuries, emerging evidence suggests that ECGs may not be necessary for patients with low-voltage injuries, especially in the absence of symptoms of high-risk features (history of syncope, seizures, tetany, prolonged exposure, moist skin, and prior cardiac history). Providers should use their clinical judgment to determine if a screening ECG is clinically warranted.

In more significant injuries, a basic metabolic panel, creatine kinase, and a urinalysis should be obtained to evaluate for rhabdomyolysis, acute kidney injury, and hyperkalemia. These laboratory studies, in addition to the degree of myoglobinuria, should be trended to determine response to treatment. Intravenous fluid resuscitation should be started to maintain renal perfusion and dilute renal tubular concentrations of myoglobin to minimize kidney damage. The rate of fluid administration should be titrated to a urine output of 1.5–2 mL/kg/hr. Over time, the tissue necrosis and third spacing of fluid may lead to compartment syndrome, at which point a surgical fasciotomy or amputation of the extremity may be required.

Superficial burns should be managed as thermal burns, which were discussed previously. Among toddlers, one of the common patterns of injuries is an oral burn after biting an electrical cord, which often damages the labial commissure. Although typically only superficial injuries, these oral burns may have functional and aesthetic consequences. Injury to the labial artery is a feared complication and often presents as delayed hemorrhage when the eschar sloughs off approximately 1 week after the initial insult. These patients should be referred to an oral or plastic surgeon for definitive and cosmetic repair.

Disposition

Children who suffered from a low-voltage electrical injury who are asymptomatic and have no evidence of arrhythmia on cardiac monitoring can be safely discharged home. Even in the presence of mild symptoms, patients can be safely discharged home with outpatient follow-up if their laboratory studies and ECG are normal. Conversely, all high-voltage electrical injuries should be admitted for a period of monitoring on telemetry, regardless of symptoms. Other indications for admission are high-risk features including an abnormal ECG or arrhythmia, loss of consciousness, prior cardiac history, tetany, seizures, or wet skin. Patients with extensive burns should be transferred to a burn center for further care.

KEY POINTS

- Identifying the depth of burn—first, second, or third degree—can help guide burn management.
- Estimating the TBSA burned is essential in guiding fluid resuscitation and volume management. Physicians can use the Palm method in children or the Lund–Browder chart to estimate the area involved.
- In children, fluid resuscitation should follow the modified Parkland formula: total volume in the first 24 hours = 3 mL/kg × %TBSA + weight-based maintenance fluids. Half of this volume is given over the first 8 hours, and the second half is given over the subsequent 16 hours.
- Lactated Ringer's is the fluid of choice for resuscitation in burn patients.
- Wound management should be initiated in the emergency room if a burn unit is not immediately available.
- Pain control, usually with opioid medications, should be a management priority.
- Emergency physicians should have a low threshold to intubate patients for airway protection, especially if the patients were in an enclosed-space fire, have signs of inhalational injury, or require transport to another facility.
- Patients should be evaluated for carbon monoxide poisoning and cyanide toxicity.
- High-voltage electrical injuries can cause significant internal necrosis and tissue damage even if there is little evidence of injury to the skin.
- Electrical injuries carry a higher risk of rhabdomyolysis, which should be evaluated especially in patients with higher voltage injuries.

PITFALLS

The most significant pitfalls in the management of pediatric burn patients are the failure to secure an airway early in a patient who is at high risk for inhalational injury, inadequate fluid resuscitation during the first 24 hours after a burn injury, and inadequate pain and temperature control. These should be early priorities for any emergency physician to ensure adequate outcomes.

Emergency physicians should also be aware of the indications for transfer to a burn center and facilitate early transfer to a higher level of care if burn specialists are not in-house. Patients at risk for inhalational injury should often be intubated prior to transport because significant airway-compromising edema can develop rapidly.

Another pitfall is the inability to recognize the risk of significant tissue necrosis and internal organ injury in the setting of high-voltage electrical injuries that have very few or no superficial skin findings. Emergency physicians must maintain a high index of suspicion and thoroughly evaluate these patients with advanced imaging in the proper setting.

Further Reading

Arbuthnot MK, Garcia AV. Early resuscitation and management of severe pediatric burns. *Semin Pediatr Surg*. 2019;28(1):73–78.

Glatstein MM, Ayalon I, Miller E, Scolnik D. Pediatric electrical burn injuries: Experience of a large tertiary care hospital and a review of electrical injury. *Pediatr Emerg Care*. 2013;29(6):737–740.

Kang S. *Fitzpatrick's Dermatology*. 9th ed. New York: McGraw-Hill; 2019.

Krishnamoorthy V, Ramaiah R, Bhananker SM. Pediatric burn injuries. *Int J Crit Illness Injury Sci*. 2012;2(3):128–134.

26

Wound Care

SHWETA R. IYER AND EE TEIN TAY

INTRODUCTION

Pediatric injuries, including wounds, are among the top reasons for children's visits to the emergency department (ED). There are many different ways to repair wounds, which vary based on the wound properties and age and cooperation of the patient. This chapter discusses how to approach pediatric wounds and determine further care and management.

HISTORY AND PHYSICAL EXAMINATION

The history should include the mechanism of injury, when the wound occurred, and vaccination status. Consideration of potential infectious exposure such as a bite, a crush injury involving bone, a weapon-related injury, an injury with risk of retained foreign body in tissue, and time since injury should be elicited. These details will direct imaging and wound exploration.

Physical evaluation should determine the type, contour, length, depth, and approximation of the wound edges. Analgesia may be required for full evaluation. A careful neurovascular examination should be undertaken, including assessing pulses and circulation, sensation, strength, and movement of the affected body part. Bleeding should also be controlled by direct pressure, and a tourniquet should be applied if necessary.

If there is concern for contamination, the wound should be probed for foreign body removal, and imaging should be obtained. The wound should be appropriately cleaned and irrigated, and any devitalized tissue should be debrided prior to repair.

ANALGESIA

It is important to consider anxiolytics and pain control for pediatric patients who are not able to sit still for a physical examination due to anxiety, pain, and/or fear. See Chapter 48 for further discussion on analgesia and sedation in children. The topical combination of lidocaine, tetracaine, and epinephrine (LET) in a gel form can be applied for pain relief prior to repair and should be liberally used in children. Lidocaine can be additionally injected immediately prior to the procedure for further analgesia. Ibuprofen or acetaminophen may provide additional pain relief but should be given 20–30 minutes prior to the procedure. Table 26.1 presents anesthetic and pain medication options.

Children are anxious about wound repair. Several options exist to calm the pediatric patient during the procedural repair, including

TABLE 26.1 PAIN CONTROL OPTIONS

Medications	Route	Indication
LET (lidocaine, epinephrine, tetracaine)	Topical	Superficial gel; can be applied for 30 minutes prior to repair
Lidocaine ± epinephrine	Injectable	Can be injected a few minutes before repair at the wound site
Versed, fentanyl, ketamine	Intranasal, IV, or IM	Noninvasive method (intranasal) has a good absorption rate and is preferred; however, these medications can be given as injectables if needed.
Opioids	IV or IM	Morphine most common

IM, intramuscular; IV, intravenous.

achieving appropriate analgesia, providing anxiolytics during the procedure, and utilizing distraction techniques. Parental involvement can occur both in holding and distraction. Papooses may be available in some hospitals in order to keep a child still during repair, but if unavailable, wrapping the child tightly in a bed sheet will accomplish the same goal. If none of these are viable options, procedural sedation may be required. Ketamine is favored by most practitioners due to its low side effect profile and quick onset. See Chapter 48 on pain management and procedural sedation.

PREPARATION

Prior to repair, bleeding should be controlled with direct pressure, and wounds must be copiously irrigated with sterile water, tap water, or normal saline to reduce post-repair infection. Typically, 50–100 mL of liquid per 1 cm of laceration length is recommended, given via a pressurized method such as a syringe. Dirty wounds may require additional debridement and more extensive irrigation. LET and/or additional analgesia should be applied prior to wound cleaning. A careful exploration of the wound should be undertaken to ensure the wound is clean and any foreign bodies are removed prior to repair.

If a foreign body is suspected and not visible, imaging should be obtained prior to repair. X-rays should be performed in patients who have point tenderness over a joint/extremity or have difficulty moving an extremity to evaluate for fracture. In addition, any patient with an open fracture should receive prompt neurovascular evaluation, be immobilized for comfort, and receive appropriate analgesia and antibiotics.

DIAGNOSTIC IMAGING

Imaging of affected extremities/body parts should be performed with associated trauma or crush injury. Patients with suspected foreign bodies also warrant imaging to evaluate for the type of foreign body and depth of penetration. Many objects and some types of glass may not be radiopaque on X-rays. In these cases, soft tissue ultrasounds may be helpful in locating the foreign body. Computed tomography scan may be indicated in cases of significant blunt or penetrating injuries suspected of interrupting blood vessels or damaging internal organs.

CONSULTS

Neurovascular deficits, tendon injury, and open fractures typically require emergent surgical consultation (see Table 26.2 for specific recommendations). Large tissue defects, cosmetically delicate locations, and some complicated lacerations may require plastic surgery consultation for initial or delayed repair, debridement, or skin grafting.

TABLE 26.2 EMERGENT VERSUS URGENT INJURIES

Emergent	Urgent/Possible Consultant Referral
Open wounds/fractures	Extensor tendon injuries
Flexor tendon injuries	Large wounds
Nerve injury (e.g., neurovascular deficits)	Cosmetic wounds (e.g., facial wounds)
Joint injury	Genital wounds
Blood vessel injury (e.g., arterial tear)	Wounds with debrided tissue

TABLE 26.3 WOUND CLOSURE OPTIONS

Type	Indication
Sutures	Deep, gaping, or jagged-edged wounds; wounds on areas of tension; wounds requiring multiple layers of closure
Staples	Scalp wounds, thick skin on extremities/trunk, surgical wounds
Tissue adhesives	Small (<5 cm) well-approximated wounds; quick application, no follow-up needed
Surgical adhesive strips	Small superficial wounds or to secure thin, absorbable sutures
Hair apposition technique	Scalp wounds; few complications; can be used for nonbleeding wounds with hair of at least 3 cm length

WOUND REPAIR OPTIONS

Many methods of wound repair are available and are detailed in Table 26.3. Ideally, the least invasive method with acceptable cosmetic outcome should be chosen in children.

The type of repair depends on the location of the laceration, the appearance of wound edges, and the wound depth. More complicated laceration repairs usually require suturing. Special suturing techniques may be warranted for wounds under high tension, wound flaps, or large wounds with edges that may not approximate well without subcutaneous sutures. Tissue adhesives are preferred for simple, linear lacerations (usually <5 cm) not overlying hair that are easily approximated into a straight line. This is favored by most providers because it is less invasive, quick, and usually does not require procedural sedation.

For scalp lacerations, staples are preferred due to ease of application and good cosmetic outcome. The hair apposition method may also be used, which involves taking hair on both sides of a scalp laceration and apposing (i.e., interlocking) it with a twist. Tissue adhesives are used to further secure the apposed hair and close the wound. There is no need for follow-up because the hair will unravel in approximately 7 days. The technique has been shown to be equal to suturing and stapling for scalp lacerations, with fewer complications.

SUTURE TYPES AND INDICATIONS

The type of suture used for wound repair depends on the type of laceration and indication (Table 26.4).

TABLE 26.4 COMMON SUTURE MATERIALS AND INDICATIONS

Suture Type	Brand Name	Absorption (Days)	Indications/Notes
		Absorbable	
Chromic catgut	Chromic Gut	21	For tongue, oral mucosa, nail bed lacerations
Plain catgut	Plain Gut	10–14	Good tensile strength
Fast absorbing surgical gut	Fast Absorbing Plain Gut	5–7	Less tensile strength; used for epidermal sutures and facial lacerations
Polyglactin 910	Vicryl	60–90	Buried sutures for tongue, oral mucosa, deep lacerations, nail bed lacerations
Polyglactin 910	Vicryl Rapide	10–14	For simple lacerations on extremities/trunk
Poliglecaprone 25	Monocryl	90–120	Good tensile strength; for subcuticular closure and deep facial lacerations
		Nonabsorbable	
Nylon	Ethilon	—	Nylon sutures with high tensile strength
Polypropylene	Prolene	—	Blue dyed suture, more difficult to tie but cause less scarring than nylon
Silk	PERMA-HAND Silk	—	Low tensile strength; mostly used for securing central lines and chest tubes

TABLE 26.5 SUTURING TECHNIQUES

Method	Indication
Simple interrupted	Deep or multilayer wounds
Running/subcuticular	Long, low-tension wounds with straight, even edges; surgical wounds
Vertical mattress	Eversion of skin edges
Horizontal mattress	Gaping, high-tension wounds or fragile skin
Corner	Closure of a flap wound or edge of skin

In pediatrics, it is common to choose absorbable sutures to bypass removal of sutures at a later date. Absorbable sutures have similar cosmetic outcomes as nonabsorbable sutures in pediatric patients with no increase in adverse effects. However, in certain circumstances, nonabsorbable sutures may still be required, such as for high-tension regions, wounds over joints, and deep wounds. Only fast-absorbing gut should be used on the face because other absorbable sutures will remain too long and cause increased scarring. To stabilize sutures and prevent removal by children, one option includes applying a layer of Dermabond or Steri-Strips over the absorbable sutures.

SUTURING METHODS

Various options exist for suturing techniques, as detailed in Table 26.5. A deep layer of absorbable sutures may need to be placed to better approximate wound edges in gaping wounds, which allows for better cosmesis and superficial closure.

TETANUS

Tetanus is a rare but important complication of wounds. *Clostridium tetani* typically enters the body through a contaminated wound and flourishes in anaerobic conditions. Tetanus should be updated and immunoglobulin administered if insufficient immunity as indicated in Table 26.6.

Children receive the DTaP (diphtheria, tetanus, pertussis) vaccine at ages 2, 4, 6, and 15–18 months as part of regular pediatric care. The Tdap (tetanus, diphtheria, pertussis) vaccine is provided to teens at age 11 or 12 years, and Td (tetanus, diphtheria) boosters are recommended every 10 years as adults.

ANTIBIOTICS

Routine antibiotics are not indicated for most wounds. Box 26.1 details the indications for which antibiotics should be prescribed. Prophylactic antibiotics are not indicated for simple, superficial human bites or uncomplicated dog bites in the head and neck region.

SPECIAL CONSIDERATIONS

Animal Bites

Animal bites are common in children, with dog bites being the most frequent followed by cat bites. Various factors increase the risk of infection from animal bites, including bites to the extremities, puncture wounds, traumatic or crush injuries, and cat bites. Patients with underlying illnesses, immunosuppression, and delayed presentation are at higher risk of developing infections. Common bacteria found in most animal flora include *Pasteurella, Capnocytophaga, Bartonella,* and various anaerobes. The median time to infection from a dog bite is 24 hours, whereas a cat bite can present with infection in as early as 12 hours due to the wound typically being a deep puncture wound.

Imaging is usually not necessary for animal bites unless underlying injury is suspected. Wound care management for animal bites is the same as general wound care management.

TABLE 26.6 TETANUS CHART

Patient's Vaccine Status	Clean Wound	Dirty Wound
Vaccine <3 doses or unknown	Vaccine	Vaccine and immunoglobulin
Vaccine >3 doses (immunized)	Vaccine if last dose ≥10 years ago	Vaccine if last dose ≥5 years ago

> **BOX 26.1**
> **INDICATIONS FOR ANTIBIOTIC TREATMENT FROM BITES**
>
> Patients who are immunocompromised or at high risk for infections
> Extremity bites (hands and feet)
> Cat bites
> Deep human bites
> Bites near joint spaces
> Deep wounds
> Crush injury
> Open fractures
> Concern for cellulitis or other infection

Proper wound irrigation and removal of any foreign bodies decrease risk of local infection. Wound closure for certain animal bite wounds is not recommended; these wounds should heal by secondary intention due to risk of infection from suturing (Box 26.2):

Animal bite wounds are typically treated with amoxicillin–clavulanate if indicated (i.e., cat bites, extremity bites, and deep bites).

Rabies prophylaxis is not necessary in a bite from a healthy animal, with a known owner, and when the animal can be observed for 2 weeks. Bats, raccoons, and skunks have a higher potential to be rabid, and prophylaxis includes a regimen of human rabies immunoglobulin and human rabies diploid cell vaccine on days 0, 3, 7, and 14. The vaccine is given intramuscularly, whereas the immunoglobulin is given around the wound site and the rest of the dose intramuscularly at another body location.

> **BOX 26.2**
> **INDICATIONS FOR SECONDARY INTENTION HEALING FROM BITES**
>
> Crush injuries
> Puncture wounds
> Hand and foot wounds[a]
> Cat bites
> Human bites[a]
> Wounds in the immunosuppressed
> Wounds that appear infected
> Wounds that are >12 hours old[a]
>
> [a]Without large cosmetic defect.

Nail Bed Lacerations

Nail injuries can vary in type and have significant aesthetic and functional morbidity. Subungual hematomas are among the most common types of nail injuries, and they typically do not necessitate removal unless significant underlying damage is noted. A subungual hematoma indicates an underlying nail bed laceration, but its presence does not always require nail removal and repair. If the nail and its margins are intact, good outcomes occur even if a significant percentage of the nail is involved. If the nail is intact and there is discomfort associated with a subungual hematoma, nail trephination should be performed.

If trephination is to be attempted, the nail should be cleaned, but alcohol should be avoided due to flammability with an electrocautery device. If a trephinator is not available, other items, including a scalpel or an 18-gauge needle, can be used to puncture the nail and release pressure from the hematoma. Nail trephination typically has a good outcome with relief of symptoms.

Indications for nail removal include significant nail damage, if the nail margins are not intact, or significant tissue disruption. If the nail is to be removed, typically a hemostat is used to spread and free the nail from the bed of the finger or toe with care not to further damage the underlying matrix. After the nail is removed, absorbable sutures (5.0 or 6.0 chromic gut or similar) can be used to repair the open wound and nail bed. Glue has been used to repair the nail bed with similar functional and cosmetic outcomes as sutures. Topical adhesives may be better tolerated in children but require a dry surface prior to application.

DISPOSITION

Following repair of simple lacerations, most patients can be discharged with appropriate follow-up for suture or staple removal, depending on the type of suture material used and the location of the wound. Suture/staple removal and wound checks to evaluate for appropriate wound closure can usually be performed in a primary care physician's office. Patients should be told to avoid direct water pressure over the wound and to keep the area dry for 24–48 hours to avoid reopening or wound contamination. Wounds should remain clean and covered for the initial healing process. Moist (not wet) covered wounds heal best, and topical antibiotic cream may be utilized to promote healing. Patients should always be told to return for fevers, drainage from the wound, increasing pain, or erythema to the laceration site. If a patient has a wound with an increased concern for infection (i.e., a contaminated wound, a bite wound, etc. as described in Table 26.6) upon discharge, wound check should be arranged in 2 or 3 days post repair to ensure that the wound is healing optimally.

Outpatient consultation follow-up may be required for retained foreign body, significant burn injuries (see Chapter 25), or large tissue defects. Operative wash-out and hospital admission are typically indicated for open fractures.

SUTURE AND STAPLE REMOVAL

See Table 26.7 for recommended timing of suture removal. Absorbable sutures should be removed if still present by date of recommended removal.

COMPLICATIONS

It is important that discharged patients return for any concern of infection because this may necessitate suture removal and/or antibiotic treatment. Post-repair infection rates are quite low in children due to their generally healthy status; infection rates have been reported in the literature to be 1–5% for uncomplicated wounds.

TABLE 26.7 TIMING OF SUTURE REMOVAL

Body Part	Time to Removal (Days)
Face	3–5
Neck	3–4
Scalp	7–10
Trunk, upper extremities	7
Lower extremities	8–10
Laceration over joint or high-mobility location; regions of high tension	10–14

Abscess formation may occur and require intervention and possible incision and drainage.

Puncture wounds, especially over the foot and hand, can lead to risk of infection. This risk is increased in patients with comorbidities such as diabetes because they can develop osteomyelitis. In addition, infection risk is increased in patients who have deep penetration of the wound, foreign bodies, or wound contamination. Patients who wear shoes and have plantar puncture wounds are at risk of pseudomonal infection, which can lead to osteomyelitis.

Necrotizing fasciitis is a rare but severe complication of contaminated wounds. Risk is increased with underlying immunosuppressive disease.

Occasionally, topical adhesives do not approximate and close the wound appropriately. Patients may return with complaints of open wound and lack of healing. Typically, these patients should receive sutures due to failure of topical adhesive treatment. In addition, if the incorrect suture material and/or suture size is used for a wound (i.e., using absorbable, small-sized sutures over areas of high tension such as a knuckle), the wound may not close and heal, and the patient will need appropriate suture closure of the wound.

SCAR PREVENTION/ TREATMENT

Certain wounds have greater potential for scarring, such as wounds that are oriented perpendicularly to the normal draping of the skin. Wounds heal best if kept moist during the initial phases of healing, and tension over the wound should be minimized to avoid scarring. Avoidance of sun exposure and use of sunscreen are important adjuncts to limit hyperpigmentation and scarring. In addition, many topical treatments, such as Mederma and silicone gel, have been thought to help in collagen organization and reduction of hypertrophic scarring, but large randomized trials have not been performed.

KEY POINTS

- A history and physical examination are paramount to proper wound management.
- Various options exist for analgesia and anxiolysis, including child-friendly techniques and topical, oral, intranasal, and injectable medications.

- Appropriate imaging and consults should be obtained prior to repair, when relevant.
- Many options exist for wound repair, including nonsuture techniques that may be favorable in children when appropriate (hair apposition technique, tissue adhesives, etc.).
- Absorbable sutures are preferred in children when sutures are indicated.
- Tetanus and antibiotics should be given when indicated, depending on the nature of the wound.
- Appropriate discharge instructions are key to wound repair because complications can infrequently occur and necessitate immediate emergency management.

PITFALLS

- Failure to copious irrigate and debride wounds prior to closure
- Failure to explore wounds for retained foreign body
- Failure to recognize that many foreign bodies are radiolucent
- Failure to further secure absorbable sutures in a toddler
- Failure to give adequate wound care and return instructions

Further Reading

Aziz H, Rhee P, Pandit V, Tang A, Gries L, Joseph B. The current concepts in management of animal (dog, cat, snake, scorpion) and human bite wounds. *J Trauma Acute Care Surg.* 2015;78(3):641–648. doi:10.1097/TA.0000000000000531

Clark TA, Reingold A, Sawyer M, et al. Prevention of pertussis, tetanus, and diphtheria with vaccines in the United States: Recommendations of the Advisory Committee on Immunization Practices (ACIP). *MMWR Recomm Rep.* 2018;67(2):1–44. doi:10.15585/mmwr.rr6702a1

Harman S, Zemek R, Duncan MJ, Ying Y, Petrcich W. Efficacy of pain control with topical lidocaine–epinephrine–tetracaine during laceration repair with tissue adhesive in children: A randomized controlled trial. *CMAJ.* 2013;185(13):E629–E634. doi:10.1503/cmaj.130269

U.S. Department of Health & Human Services. Tetanus: Protect your family with vaccines. https://www.cdc.gov/tetanus/index.html. Accessed March 13, 2019.

Xu B, Xu B, Wang L, et al. Absorbable versus non-absorbable sutures for skin closure: A meta-analysis of randomized controlled trials. *Ann Plast Surg.* 2016;76(5):598–606. doi:10.1097/SAP.0000000000000418

27

Renal Emergencies in Children

LIZA KEARL AND MAUREEN MCCOLLOUGH

INTRODUCTION

Renal emergencies in children range from more common conditions such as acute kidney injury due to simple gastroenteritis to less common but more serious conditions such as hemolytic uremic syndrome. Treatment for renal emergencies may range from intravenous rehydration for a simple kidney injury to the need for emergent peritoneal or hemodialysis for a child with hemolytic uremic syndrome. Some renal emergencies, such as acute glomerulonephritis, may present with more obvious signs, such as gross hematuria or tea-colored urine. Others, such as nephrotic syndrome, may present with more nonspecific signs, such as periorbital edema or weight gain, which can delay the ultimate diagnosis. Emergency department providers must be aware of the presenting signs and symptoms of renal emergencies in children as they care for this vulnerable population.

ACUTE KIDNEY INJURY

Background

Acute kidney injury (AKI) can result from simple dehydration that is easily resolved to more serious causes such as sepsis or trauma. Previously known as acute renal failure, AKI results from impaired glomerular filtration rate (GFR), and this in turn can affect blood pressure, fluid management, acid–base balance, and removal of nitrogenous waste. The most commonly used laboratory test to make the diagnosis of AKI is a rise in the serum creatinine over the baseline. Early impairment of GFR may not yet show a rise in creatinine because there has not been adequate time for the accumulation of nitrogenous waste.

AKI is often classified into three categories: prerenal, renal or intrarenal, and postrenal. Prerenal causes involve decreased renal perfusion; examples include volume depletion (e.g., severe vomiting and diarrhea, burns, or hemorrhage), shock (e.g., anaphylaxis or sepsis), and congestive heart failure. Compromise to vascular flow, such as obstruction of the renal artery or thrombosis of the renal vein, can also result in AKI.

Renal or intrarenal causes involve damage directly to the nephrons. Glomerular insults include post-streptococcal glomerulonephritis (PSGN), systemic lupus erythematosus (SLE) nephritis, hemolytic uremic syndrome, and sepsis causing hypoperfusion of the parenchyma. Tubular insults can be caused by hemoglobin–myoglobin from a crush injury, burn, hemolytic crisis, or heavy metal poisoning. AKI has also been reported from use of nonsteroidal anti-inflammatory drugs in dehydrated children. In hospitalized children, nephrotoxic medications such as furosemide, aminoglycosides, vancomycin, piperacillin–tazobactam, antiviral medications, and angiotensin-converting enzyme inhibitors have been associated with AKI. Intravenous contrast does not appear to be associated with AKI in severely injured pediatric trauma patients. Comorbid conditions such as congenital heart disease requiring surgery, stem cell transplants, liver transplants, nephrotic syndrome, or sickle cell disease also place patients at higher risk for AKI.

Postrenal injury involves obstruction in the urinary tract caused by infection, stones, tumor, or post-urethral valves. Obstruction of both kidneys is generally required to develop acute renal failure.

Classic Clinical Presentation

The clinical presentation will also vary depending on the ultimate cause of the AKI. AKI can present with signs and symptoms due to the decreased renal function, such as edema, decreased urine output, and macro- or microscopic hematuria. AKI may present as simply as a parent or caretaker noticing a significant decrease in urine output due to volume loss such as vomiting or diarrhea. A history of bloody diarrhea 3–7 days before oliguria may suggest hemolytic uremic syndrome. Pharyngitis or impetigo a few weeks prior to the onset of hematuria or peripheral edema suggests poststreptococcal glomerulonephritis (PSGN). A nonblanching vasculitic rash with lower extremity joint swelling may indicate Henoch–Schönlein purpura (HSP). Edema may indicate nephrotic syndrome or glomerulonephritis; hypertension may also indicate glomerulonephritis. Evidence of volume overload or respiratory distress may indicate heart failure. A palpable kidney may indicate renal vein thrombosis or polycystic kidney disease.

AKI can result in life-threatening difficulties such as hyperkalemia, hypocalcemia, hyponatremia, metabolic acidosis, pulmonary edema, hypertensive encephalopathy, seizures from encephalopathy, or septic shock from renal obstruction or pyelonephritis.

Severe AKI in critically ill children is associated with increased mortality. The combination of decreased urine output and elevated creatinine also has also been reported to have worse outcomes.

Atypical Clinical Presentation

Acute kidney injury may be found secondarily during the workup for other presenting conditions such as sepsis, heart failure, or HSP vasculitis.

Differential Diagnosis

Box 27.1 presents potential etiologies of AKI.

Diagnostic Confirmation

Urinalysis may be normal in patients with an AKI; hematuria and/or proteinuria may be a sign of an intrinsic AKI such as glomerular

BOX 27.1

ETIOLOGIES OF ACUTE KIDNEY INJURY IN CHILDREN

Prerenal

Decreased intravascular volume or dehydration
Burns or hemorrhage
Third spacing
Sepsis
Decreased cardiac output
Cardiac shock
Decreased renal artery blood flow

Intrarenal

Glomerular disease
Post-streptococcal and other glomerulonephritis
Pyelonephritis
Systemic causes
Hemolytic–uremic syndrome
Henoch–Schönlein purpura or other vasculitides
Systemic lupus erythematosus
Sepsis or other causes of prolonged decreased perfusion
Toxins
Heavy metal poisonings, such as lead and gold
Myoglobin or hemoglobin deposits
Antibiotics such as aminoglycosides
Anticonvulsants such as phenytoin
Radiocontrast dyes

Postrenal

Obstructive lesions
Nephrolithiasis or tumor
Post-urethral valves
Intra-abdominal tumor obstructing urinary flow
Infection
Renal vein thrombosis

disease or tubular necrosis. Elevated blood urea nitrogen (BUN) and creatinine are diagnostic for renal involvement. Other diagnostic tests will depend on the clinical presentation.

AKI is generally defined as rise in the creatinine over the baseline. Normal creatines vary by age:

- Newborn: 0.3–1 mg/dL (27–88 μmol/L)
- Infant: 0.2–0.4 mg/dL (18–35 μmol/L)
- Child: 0.3–0.7 mg/dL (27–62 μmol/L)
- Adolescent: 0.5–1 mg/dL (44–88 μmol/L)

Because of the wide range of creatine by age group, subsequent measurements of the creatine every 12–24 hours showing an increase may be required.

Moderate to severe dehydration can result in a decrease in urine output, resulting in BUN typically rising more than creatinine. Classically, BUN >20 is indicative of a prerenal cause. After hydration and improved intravascular volume, urine output should improve and the elevated BUN and creatinine concentrations should resolve.

Fractional excretion of sodium (FENa) is often used to differentiate a prerenal cause from an intrinsic cause of the AKI. Smartphone calculator "apps" are often used to calculate the following formula:

$$\text{FENa, percent} = \frac{\text{UNa} \times \text{SCr}}{\text{SNa} \times \text{UCr}} \times 100$$

U = Urine
S = Serum

FENa is a measurement of the renal handling of sodium. FENa <1% suggests a prerenal cause with sodium reabsorption due to decreased perfusion. FENa >2% suggests acute tubular necrosis (ATN). FENa between 1% and 2% is nondiagnostic. In preterm and term infants, FENa <2% is often used to indicate prerenal cause; FENa >2.5% indicates ATN. Previous fluid administration or diuretic therapy may limit the usefulness of the FENa score.

The urinalysis may be normal or may show evidence of infection. Red cell casts can indicate glomerulonephritis. Brown granular casts or epithelial cell casts can be a sign of ATN. White blood cells casts or pyuria may be seen with urinary tract infections, tubular or interstitial disease, or sometimes acute glomerulonephritis. Elevated specific gravity >1.020 often indicates a prerenal cause. Loss of the kidneys' concentrating ability is often an early sign of ATN with a specific gravity <1.010. Prerenal causes will generally have urine osmolality >500 mOsmol/kg; ATN generally has urine osmolality <350 mOsmol/kg. Microangiopathic hemolytic anemia and thrombocytopenia with an AKI are diagnostic of hemolytic uremic syndrome; anti-streptococcal antibody testing (ASO titer) can be diagnostic for PSGN.

Ultrasonography is often used to evaluate obstructive causes of renal failure. Ultrasonography may also reveal small kidneys due to congenital hypoplasia or parenchymal loss as evidence of chronic kidney disease. A noncontrast computed tomography urography can also identify an obstructive cause and avoids the use of nephrotoxic radiocontrast material. A voiding cystourethrography can show extrinsic pressure on the bladder by posterior urethral valves.

Treatment

If the AKI is thought to be due to a prerenal cause such as dehydration or blood loss, then rehydration using crystalloid in boluses of 20 mL/kg over 30 minutes is warranted; bolus may be repeated twice as needed. Significant delays in rehydrating the patient can result in ATN. If there is no urinary response after two or three boluses and no improvement in renal function and the patient is now considered euvolemic with no evidence of obstruction, then bladder catheterization or bladder scanning for urinary volume by ultrasound is recommended to confirm anuria. Ultrasound can also confirm the hydration status by evaluation of the inferior vena cava. Ongoing losses in the emergency department, such as vomiting and diarrhea, should be accounted for.

Diuretics should be considered in any patient who has had no response to two or three crystalloid boluses or in any patient who is considered volume overloaded or with evidence of heart failure or pulmonary edema. A diuretic such as furosemide, 1 mg/kg per dose every 2–6 hours intravenously, may be tried. If there is no response within 2 hours of the initial dose, furosemide should not be continued due to the risk of ototoxicity and renal toxicity from furosemide. Bumetanide, 0.015–0.1 mg/kg per dose every 6–24 hours intravenously, may be tried if furosemide yields no success. Mannitol, 0.75 mg/kg per dose every 6 hours intravenously, may also be tried but is contraindicated if there is evidence of obstruction.

Renal replacement therapy such as hemo- or peritoneal dialysis should be considered in critically ill children with an AKI and fluid overloads exceeding 10% with multiorgan failure; oliguric despite diuretic therapy; hyperkalemia >6.5 mEq/L unresponsive to traditional lowering therapies; uremia defined as a BUN >80–100 mg/dL; or potentially life-threatening conditions such as pulmonary edema, heart failure, or hypertension unresponsive to traditional pharmacological therapy. Nephrology consultation should be obtained.

If hypertension with encephalopathy develops as a result of the AKI, then a controlled 10–20% reduction of the blood pressure should be obtained using intravenous agents such as labetolol or nicardipine. See Chapter 19 on neurovascular emergencies.

Hyperkalemia from the AKI is often asymptomatic but can result in nausea, malaise, and muscle weakness. Hyperkalemia can cause cardiac arrhythmias, and potassium levels >6.5 mEq/L may cause peaked T waves or widened QRS complexes on electrocardiogram. Significant electrocardiogram changes such as loss of P waves or widened QRS complexes should be treated emergently. Calcium gluconate (10%) given intravenously helps stabilize the action potential of the cardiac cells, decreasing the risk of arrhythmias. Glucose (25% dextrose in water for children younger than age 3 years and 50% dextrose in water for children older than age 3 years) should be given along with regular insulin to help shift the potassium temporarily into the cells. Nebulized albuterol can also help shift potassium temporarily into the cells and can lower serum potassium by 1–1.5 mEq/L. Emergent dialysis may be required for severe cases or those associated with renal failure.

Metabolic acidosis can be the result of impaired renal excretion of acid and impaired reabsorption of bicarbonate. Acid production may be increased due to shock or sepsis. Patients may hyperventilate to correct the acidosis. Initial fluid boluses using normal saline alone may often correct the acidosis; lactated Ringer's solution is often recommended for ongoing replacement fluid therapy. Sodium bicarbonate remains controversial because of its adverse effects, and its use should be limited to life-threatening situations.

Hypocalcemia is often seen in AKI and is due to increased serum phosphate and decreased renal conversion of vitamin D to its active form. Rhabdomyolysis can also contribute to significant hypocalcemia. Metabolic acidosis can increase the portion of ionized calcium, the active form. Rapid correction of metabolic acidosis with bicarbonate can decrease the concentration of ionized calcium and precipitate hypocalcemia symptoms such as muscle weakness, tetany, seizures, and cardiac arrhythmias. Hyperphosphatemia can also contribute to hypocalcemia and can result from tissue breakdown such as in tumor lysis syndrome or rhabdomyolysis.

Seizures may result from hypertensive encephalopathy or metabolic changes such as hyponatremia. Intractable hyponatremic seizures may require the use of hypertonic saline (3% sodium chloride, 3–5 mL/kg). Each 1 mL/kg should increase the sodium by 1 mEq/L. Once the seizures have terminated, the sodium correction must occur more slowly to avoid central pontine myelinolysis. Correcting the sodium no faster than 10–12 mEq/L in the first 24 hours is recommended.

Normal saline (0.9%) is relatively hypertonic compared to serum and may be helpful in correcting the hyponatremia. Restricting the intake of water along with intravenous normal saline may be a temporary solution because hyponatremic patients may require dialysis.

Disposition

Disposition of the child will depend on a number of factors, including the degree of AKI based on the BUN and creatinine, the cause of the injury, and the treatment required. An AKI from dehydration due to vomiting and diarrhea resulting in a mild increase in BUN and creatinine can likely be treated with rehydration in the emergency department and discharge home with return precautions. Antiemetic medication such as ondansetron may be helpful in the rehydration process. Parents should be instructed to continue rehydration efforts at home using small aliquots, 5–20 cc at a time, of rehydration fluids such as Pedialyte with strict return precautions to return if the child is unable to keep down any oral fluids.

Key Points

- Causes of AKI range from benign gastroenteritis to more significant cause such as sepsis or vasculitis.
- Resolution of the injury will be primarily due to the ultimate cause of the AKI. AKI due to simple dehydration will be more readily resolved than AKI due to severe sepsis or other severe systemic disorders.

Pitfalls

- Failure to obtain laboratory testing including BUN, creatinine, and electrolytes in children with signs of significant dehydration such as ill appearance, altered mental status, hypotension, or significant decrease in urine output
- Failure to act quickly in correcting significant electrolyte disturbances such as hyperkalemia, especially when associated with changes on the electrocardiogram

HEMOLYTIC UREMIC SYNDROME

Background

Hemolytic uremic syndrome (HUS) is one of the most common causes of AKI in children, presenting with microangiopathic anemia, thrombocytopenia, and AKI. HUS typically occurs in children younger than age 5 years but may also rarely occur in adults.

The most common cause of HUS is infection, and Shiga toxin-producing *Escherichia coli* (STEC) serotype O157:H7 is responsible for >90% of cases. Transmission can occur from person-to-person contact, and can also occur through contaminated food, such as unpasteurized dairy or beef. Petting zoos have also been implicated. Acquired causes of HUS include infections (e.g., STEC, *Shigella* organisms, *Aeromonas*, and HIV), autoantibodies to complement factors, drugs (chemotherapy or transplant anti-rejection drugs), or rare idiopathic causes such as pregnancy or lupus. *Streptococcus pneumoniae* is thought to cause up to 5% of cases in children, most commonly due to complicated pneumonia. Urinary tract infection is also a known cause.

Damage to renal endothelial cells is the primary cause resulting in arteriolar and capillary microthrombi (thrombotic microangiopathy). Renal vascular injury is caused by either viral or bacterial agents or the toxins released. Microangiopathic hemolytic anemia then results from red blood cells (RBCs) damaged by injured narrowed blood vessels. Platelets, complement, and fibrin also deposit in the glomerular lumen. Thrombocytopenia, a decrease in GFR, and overt renal failure can result.

Classic Clinical Presentation

The classic presentation of HUS includes watery diarrhea, crampy abdominal pain, and, occasionally, fever. Within days, patients will experience increased abdominal pain, with 50–85% developing bloody stools. Sudden onset of hemolytic anemia, thrombocytopenia, and acute renal insufficiency, with possible progression to renal failure, will occur in up to 10% of cases. Morbidity and mortality are still high in cases of HUS, with up to 60% of diarrhea-associated HUS cases requiring dialysis and 12% developing end-stage renal disease or succumbing to the disease. Dehydration upon presentation appears to increase the risk of renal failure. Thrombotic microangiopathy is thought to cause extrarenal sequelae. Pancreatic insufficiency resulting in insulin-dependent diabetes mellitus has also been reported. Neurological sequelae tend to be the most common life-threatening extrarenal manifestation; seizures may develop in up to 40% of patients with HUS. Hypertension occurs in up to 50% of patients; encephalopathy may develop. Other manifestations include dilated cardiomyopathy, pulmonary hemorrhage, or bowel perforation and necrosis. HUS recurrences have been associated with a 30% mortality rate.

Atypical Clinical Presentation

Atypical forms of HUS usually refer to those due to a noninfectious cause and most likely a mutation of genes that code for proteins involved in the complement system. Atypical forms will usually present with fulminant hemolytic anemia, thrombocytopenia, and kidney failure. Atypical forms may have a trigger such as an upper respiratory infection or viral gastroenteritis that can make it difficult to distinguish from STEC–HUS. Other atypical forms can present with subclinical anemia, fluctuating thrombocytopenia, and delayed renal manifestations; symptoms may include nonspecific fatigue and anorexia delaying the diagnosis. Sequelae of atypical HUS include similar neurologic, cardiac, or pulmonary manifestations due to the thrombotic microangiopathy.

Differential Diagnosis

Differential diagnosis of HUS includes HSP, thrombocytopenic thrombotic purpura, ulcerative colitis, intussusception, and other causes of acquired hemolytic anemia. Dehydration caused by infectious diarrhea may lead to an increase in BUN and creatinine levels. A diagnosis of HUS can only be made with laboratory confirmation of microangiopathic anemia and thrombocytopenia.

Diagnostic Confirmation

A family member or close contact with concurrent history of HUS suggests an infectious disease source. A previous history of HUS or remote family history of HUS suggests a genetic or complement-mediated source. Exposure to a possible source such as undercooked beef or a petting zoo should be investigated by public health officials. Laboratory testing showing significantly higher leukocyte counts and C-reactive protein levels is more common in patients with toxin-producing *E. coli* O157:H7. The peripheral blood smear shows microangiopathic changes such as teardrop cells, helmet cells, microspherocytes, and burr cells. Additional laboratory testing may show a platelet count of <50,000/μL. Hemoglobin may be as low as 5 g/dL due to the rapid hemolysis.

Treatment

Supportive therapy and early peritoneal dialysis have resulted in a mortality rate of <5%. Early and adequate hydration using parenteral fluids should be the goal, monitoring for signs of volume overload. Hyperkalemia is commonly seen and should be managed with the classic treatment of sodium bicarbonate, calcium gluconate or chloride, dextrose and insulin, and sodium polystyrene sulfonate (Kayexalate). Dialysis may be required for patients with severe hyperkalemia, hyperphosphatemia, or severe metabolic acidosis.

Transfusion of packed RBCs (5 mL/kg over 4 hours) is generally recommended if the hemoglobin falls below 6 g/dL. Platelet transfusions are required only for life-threatening bleeding or before an invasive procedure. Hypertension is responsive to usual treatment of calcium channel blockers, labetalol, captopril, or nitroprusside in refractory cases.

Seizures will typically respond to benzodiazepines and phenytoin. For hyponatremic-induced seizures, treatment with 3% saline (3–5 mL/kg) is warranted. Pancreatic islet cell necrosis from HUS may result in hyperglycemia, ketonemia, and acidosis; all can be managed with insulin therapy.

Treatment with gastrointestinal antimotility agents may lead to toxic megacolon and is not recommended. Antibiotic treatment may increase risk of HUS in STEC enterocolitis and should not be used.

Atypical HUS due to compliment dysregulation has classically been treated with plasmapheresis, especially if there is neurologic involvement. Steroid and monoclonal antibody treatments are often used. Transplant is not always curative because atypical HUS can recur.

Disposition

All patients diagnosed with HUS require hospital admission. Consultation with a pediatric nephrologist should occur urgently. Early dialysis and supportive therapy can significantly improve renal function back to baseline in up to 90% of patients with acute renal failure.

Key Points

- Early recognition through the combination of bloody diarrhea, anemia with evidence of microangiopathic changes, and elevated creatinine can lead to earlier treatment.
- Treatment includes correction of volume status, blood pressure if significantly elevated, and anemia if hemoglobin is <6 g/dL.

Pitfalls

- Failure to recognize bloody diarrhea as a potential first sign of HUS.
- Laboratory testing for evidence of anemia or renal compromise is important.

NEPHROTIC SYNDROME

Background

Nephrotic syndrome is classically characterized by significant proteinuria, hypoalbuminemia, hyperlipidemia, and edema. Primary, or idiopathic, nephrotic syndrome usually occurs in children younger than age 5 years, is limited to the kidney, and has no identifiable systemic cause. Renal biopsy may be used to determine therapeutic plans and prognosis. Secondary nephrotic syndrome, usually occurring in older children, results from systemic illnesses such as PSGN. Other secondary causes include SLE, hepatitis B and C, and HIV. Congenital and infantile nephrotic syndromes occur in children younger than age 1 year and can be primary or secondary (usually due to infection) diseases; two-thirds of cases will have a poor outcome.

Primary nephrotic syndrome causes 90% of cases, with the vast majority due to minimal change disease, which is responsive to corticosteroid treatment.

Classic Clinical Presentation

The classical presentation of nephrotic syndrome begins with the onset of edema that may be insidious, starting with periorbital edema, typically worse in the morning, which may be mistaken for allergies. Edema of feet and legs is typically more noticeable at the end of the day. Pants and shoes may not fit as edema and weight increase. The child does not usually appear ill unless pulmonary edema or ascites is present. Other signs and symptoms may include headache; fatigue; or anorexia, nausea, and vomiting secondary to edema of the intestine. Anasarca may be present. Foamy urine may be a presenting complaint. Hypertension may be present, especially in cases due to glomerulonephritis; it is less likely in cases due to minimal change disease. Children with nephrotic syndrome, especially minimal change disease, despite having increased extracellular volume, can present with signs of hypovolemia such as tachycardia, peripheral vasoconstriction, and decreased urine output. Diuretics, ongoing volume loss such as diarrhea, or sepsis can worsen the child's condition.

Historical findings may include fever, joint pain or swelling, rash, mouth ulcers, hair loss, or malaise syndrome.

Differential Diagnosis

Edema and weight gain may also be a presenting complaint with glomerulonephritis and renal failure. Hypoproteinemia may be seen in gastrointestinal disorders such as cirrhosis, cystic fibrosis, and protein-losing enteritides.

Diagnostic Confirmation

Proteinuria in nephrotic syndrome can be defined as excretion of >50 mg/kg per 24 hours. This corresponds to 3+ or 4+ on the dipstick reading. Specific gravity may be elevated due to the proteinuria. Total protein:creatinine ratio on a spot urine >3 mg protein/mg creatinine is concerning for nephrotic syndrome. Microscopic hematuria also may be found on urinalysis along with proteinuria. Gross hematuria is more indicative of glomerulonephritis.

Other findings include decreased total serum protein, decreased serum albumin, hyperlipidemia, and hyponatremia. BUN and creatinine concentrations are usually normal, but an AKI can occur.

Treatment

Despite the edema, children with signs of hypovolemia or shock need to be resuscitated with crystalloid. Hypertension requires prompt recognition and treatment. Consultation with a pediatric nephrologist is key to the management of pediatric patients with nephrotic syndrome. In general, patients aged 1–10 years with no hypertension, no gross hematuria, no significant increase in serum creatinine, and with normal complement levels are assumed to have minimal change disease and can be treated with corticosteroids (and often not require a renal biopsy). Prednisone at 2 mg/kg/day taken orally, divided two or three times a day, is initiated for 6 weeks.

Complications of fluid overload and infection must also be identified and treated.

Disposition

Hospitalization may be required for newly diagnosed patients for an initial evaluation, treatment, and education of both the child and the parents. Acute complications including shock and respiratory distress require emergent stabilization and intensive care.

Complications

Nephrotic syndrome increases the risk of thromboembolic complications due to change in kidney permeability and loss of anticoagulant factors. Renal vein thrombosis, one of the most frequent thromboses, is characterized by flank pain, hematuria, and worsening renal function. Deep vein thrombosis and pulmonary embolus may also be complicating factors.

Concomitant corticosteroid use has many associated side effects, including irritability, behavioral changes, and insomnia, as well as increased susceptibility to infection.

Key Points

- Evidence of volume overload and edema are usually the first presenting signs of nephrotic syndrome in children.
- Large proteinuria and low serum protein and albumin are diagnostic features.

Pitfalls

- Failure to recognize subtle signs of edema, including periorbital edema, weight gain, and ill-fitting shoes
- Failure to pursu further diagnostic studies

ACUTE GLOMERULONEPHRITIS

Background

Glomerulonephritis (GN) is an inflammatory process that involves the nephrons of the kidney causing generally edema, hematuria, decreased renal function, and sometimes hypertension. The exact cause is not understood but involves an autoimmune response that results in glomerular inflammation and injury. Primary GN, such as PSGN or membranoproliferative GN, is intrinsic to the kidney; secondary GN, such as lupus nephritis, is due to some other systemic cause. PSGN is the most common cause of acute GN; children who do not have a clear presentation of a poststreptococcal cause will likely undergo a renal biopsy to identify the etiology.

PSGN is a sequelae of both streptococcal pharyngitis and, less frequently, streptococcal skin infections. Overall incidence of PSGN is declining, but it still remains an issue in developing countries. Antibiotic treatment of streptococcal pharyngitis dose not decrease the incidence of PSGN, but it does decrease the incidence of acute rheumatic fever. PSGN is believed to result from deposition of circulating immune complexes in the kidney that trigger complement activation and inflammation and resultant decreased glomerular filtration.

Classic Clinical Presentation

Although many cases of PSGN are asymptomatic, classic PSGN presents in children older than age 3 years with a history of a febrile pharyngitis 2 weeks prior or a skin infection up to 6 weeks prior to the onset of GN. PSGN can range from simple asymptomatic microscopic hematuria to more classic symptoms, including gross hematuria and flank pain, and less specific symptoms, such as lethargy and generalized edema. Urine may look smoky, tea-colored, or cola-colored. Blood pressure may range from mildly to severely elevated due to salt and fluid retention. In some cases, more serious clinical signs, such as pulmonary edema, cardiac arrhythmias, and hypertensive encephalopathy, may be present. Magnetic resonance imaging may show posterior reversible encephalopathy. AKI is a classic finding, and 2% have renal failure.

Atypical Clinical Presentation

Atypical presentation may be less urinary tract specific with more generalized weakness or lethargy as the main complaint. Gross hematuria may be absent. Some children may present with hypertensive encephalopathy or pulmonary edema but minimal urinary findings.

Diagnostic Confirmation

For the diagnosis of PSGN, key elements are hematuria, proteinuria, edema, oliguria, and hypertension along with documentation of a previous streptococcal infection through cultures or serological tests. The urinalysis in PSGN shows significant blood and protein with RBC casts in 60% of cases. Pyuria with granular or hyaline casts also may be found. Nephrotic ranges of proteinuria are not common. Variable decline in GFR may be manifested as a rise in creatinine. Acute renal failure requiring dialysis is not common.

The ASO titer is typically elevated in PSGN due to pharyngitis. The rise of the ASO titer may be blunted due to previous antimicrobial treatment of the streptococcal pharyngitis.

Treatment

If the acute streptococcal infection is still present when PSGN presents, then treatment with antibiotics such as penicillin, or erythromycin if allergic, is indicated. Management of PSGN is mostly supportive but can include restriction of fluid and salt intake and sometimes use of diuretics if there is evidence of volume overload. Initial furosemide dosing is 1 or 2 mg/kg per day in divided doses. Hypertensive encephalopathy should be treated immediately with intravenous blood pressure-lowering agents for better control. (See Chapter 19 on neurovascular emergencies.) Some children may require dialysis, depending on the level of renal dysfunction (BUN typically >90–100 mg/dL), life-threatening volume overload, or hyperkalemia refractory to medical management. Consultation with a pediatric nephrologist is recommended.

Disposition

A well-appearing child with normal blood pressure and mild symptoms may be managed as an outpatient with urgent follow-up, typically less than 1 week, with a pediatric nephrologist. Return precaution for worsening or new symptoms is vital. Any patient with significant hypertension, congestive heart failure, or uremia requires hospitalization for inpatient management and often consultation with a pediatric nephrologist.

Complications

Complications include volume overload, pulmonary edema, cardiac arrhythmias, hypertension, and renal failure. Recurrence of PSGN is rare.

Key Point

- Glomerulonephritis is most commonly caused by a previous streptococcal infection and can range from asymptomatic microscopic hematuria to full-blown nephritic syndrome with hematuria, proteinuria, edema, and hypertension.

Pitfalls

- Failure to recognize a new presentation of hypertension or volume overload in a child as a sign of glomerulonephritis.
- Evaluation of the urine for signs of hematuria and proteinuria is vital in this situation.

Further Reading

Hahn D, Hodson EM, Willis NS, Craig JC. Corticosteroid therapy for nephrotic syndrome in children. *Cochrane Database Syst Rev.* 2015;2015(3):CD001533.

Kaddourah A, Basu RK, Goldstein SL et al. Oliguria and acute kidney injury in critically ill children: Implication for diagnosis and outcomes. *Pediatr Crit Care Med.* 2019;20(4):332–339.

Metz DK, Kausman JY. Childhood nephrotic syndrome in the 21st century: What's new? *J Paediatr Child Health.* 2015;51(5):497–504.

Mody RK, Luna-Gierke RE, Jones TF, et al. Infections in pediatric postdiarrheal hemolytic uremic syndrome: Factors associated with identifying Shiga toxin-producing *Escherichia coli. Arch Pediatr Adolesc Med.* 2012;166(10):902–909.

Paul KM, Johnson J, Garwe T, et al. Computed tomography with intravenous contrast is not associated with development of acute kidney injury in severely injured pediatric patients. *Am Surg.* 2019;85(1):e1–e5.

Wang C, Greenbaum LA. Nephrotic syndrome. *Pediatr Clin North Am.* 2019;66:73–78.

28

Pediatric Hematologic Emergencies

JACQUELYN BASKIN AND JERANIL NUNEZ

INTRODUCTION

Children often present to the emergency department (ED) for evaluation of a variety of hematologic complaints, from pallor to bruising and bleeding. Some may require emergent evaluation and treatment, whereas others pose more of a diagnostic challenge. A detailed history and physical examination along with laboratory evaluation can aid in appropriate diagnosis and management of these patients. This chapter discusses pediatric anemia, bleeding disorders, and clotting disorders.

ANEMIA

Background

Anemia occurs when the concentration of hemoglobin (Hgb) or red blood cell (RBC) volume is below normal for age. This causes a decrease in the oxygen-carrying capacity of blood and, when significant enough, a decrease in oxygen delivery to tissues. In pediatric patients, the normal level of Hgb varies with age, with a mean nadir of 11.5 g/dL at 2–6 months of life. Newborns and adolescent males tend to have higher Hgb values, with an expected decrease seen in infants at approximately 2 months of age (physiologic anemia) from a reduction in erythropoietin production. Anemia is usually a sign of an underlying condition, either inherited or acquired, and appropriate evaluation should be undertaken to determine the etiology. Acquired forms of anemia can result from blood loss, destruction of RBCs, or decreased production of RBCs. The chronic anemia seen in patients with inherited forms of anemia is typically in a compensated state but can worsen in the face of an acute hemolytic or aplastic crisis. Severe anemia requires prompt evaluation because it can lead to hypoxia, congestive heart failure, and death.

Classic Clinical Presentation

Patients with mild anemia tend to appear well, whereas patients with severe anemia or significant underlying disease (sepsis, malignancy, hemolysis) appear ill. Clinical symptoms of moderate anemia include fatigue, exercise intolerance, and lightheadedness, whereas severe anemia can cause acute dizziness, shortness of breath, syncope, and signs of heart failure. Physical examination findings in the anemic patient can vary by etiology as well as acuity and severity of illness. Findings can include tachycardia, hypotension, pallor, jaundice, scleral icterus, petechiae, purpura, new murmur, hepatosplenomegaly, signs of congestive heart failure, or congenital physical abnormalities related to the underlying disorder.

Differential Diagnosis

Important details in the medical history that can aid in diagnosis are a history of prematurity (anemia of prematurity), prenatal infections (TORCH syndrome, cytomegalovirus), jaundice at birth (ABO/Rh incompatibility, sepsis, congenital hemolytic anemia), patient ethnicity and familial anemia (African or Mediterranean descent, sickle cell anemia), family history of splenectomy or cholecystectomy (inherited hemolytic disorders), recurrent jaundice [glucose-6-phosphate dehydrogenase (G6PD) deficiency, hemoglobinopathies], excessive milk intake or dietary restrictions (iron deficiency), pica (lead toxicity, iron deficiency), medications (sulfa drugs, anticonvulsants), acute or chronic blood loss (trauma, gastrointestinal bleed, hematuria, irregular menses), acute infections [Epstein–Barr virus (EBV), parvovirus, hemolytic uremic syndrome (HUS)], and chronic disease (renal, liver, rheumatologic, gastrointestinal).

Diagnostic Confirmation

A thorough medical history, family history, physical examination, and laboratory evaluation will help guide diagnostic confirmation. Initial laboratory values that should be obtained in anemic patients include a complete blood cell count (CBC) with RBC indices, reticulocyte count, and peripheral blood smear. Evaluation of the reticulocyte count and mean corpuscular volume help classify the anemia and aid in determining the next steps in diagnosis of the underlying etiology. Anemia with a low reticulocyte count suggests impaired production of RBCs, whereas a high reticulocyte count suggests blood loss or RBC destruction. Figure 28.1 presents an algorithm for evaluating patients with anemia.

Treatment

In the following sections, we discuss some of the more common causes of anemia in pediatric patients requiring emergent evaluation, as well as recommendations for diagnosis and treatment. Specific treatment and patient management recommendations will depend on the underlying etiology and severity of anemia.

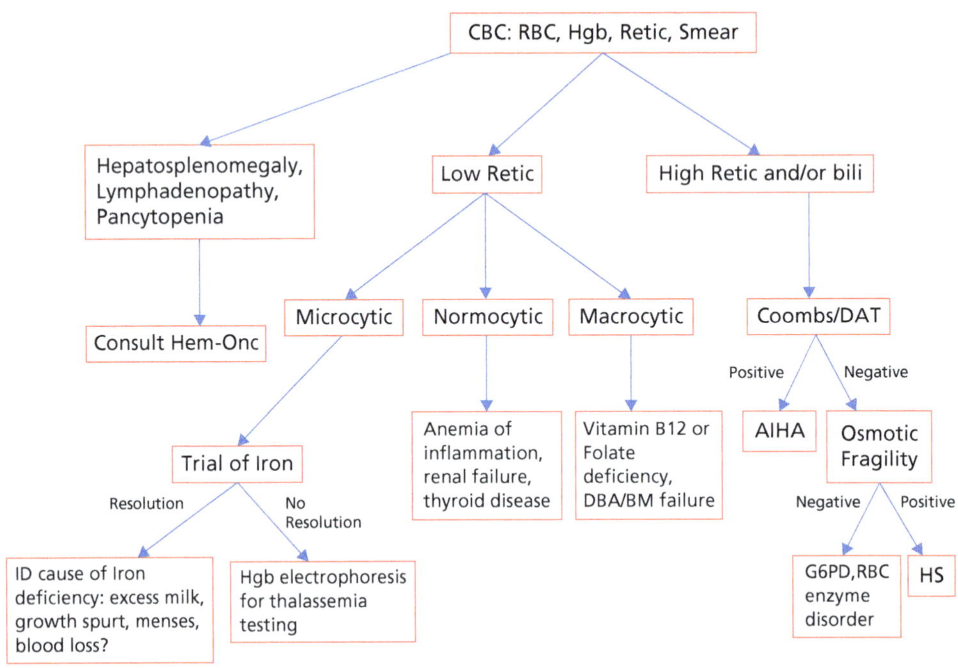

FIGURE 28.1 Clinical algorithm for evaluating patients with anemia. AIHA, autoimmune hemolytic anemia; CBC, complete blood count; DAT, direct antiglobulin test; G6PD, glucose-6-phosphate dehydrogenase; Hgb, hemoglobin; Hem-Onc, hematology–oncology; HS, hereditary spherocytosis; RBC, red blood cells; Retic, reticulocyte count. DBA: Diamond-Blackfan anemia, BM: bone marrow failure.

SICKLE CELL DISEASE

Sickle cell disease (SCD) is an inherited hemoglobinopathy most commonly seen in people of African descent. The disease is caused by a mutation in the hemoglobin gene, leading an unstable form of hemoglobin (Hgb S). RBCs carrying Hgb S become rigid and deformed (sickled) in the setting of hypoxia or acidosis. The sickled-shaped RBCs aggregate and occlude capillary beds, causing ischemic tissue injury, organ damage, and pain. This recurrent and progressively destructive process leads to acute and chronic complications in various organ systems. SCD has wide phenotypic variability with multiple genotypes, the most severe being HbSS. It is associated with significant morbidity and a shortened life span compared to that of the general population. Newborn screening for early detection of disease is offered in all states. Definitive diagnosis and further classification of SCD are made by Hgb electrophoresis. Acute complications of SCD frequently seen in children are discussed next, as are life-threatening conditions.

Complications

The most common complication of SCD is an acute episode of severe pain, or vaso-occlusive crisis (VOC). Precipitating factors include fever, infection, dehydration, cold exposure, and hypoxia. Children may begin to have painful crisis episodes as early as age 6 months, often presenting as dactylitis, or hand–foot syndrome. This is usually the first physical manifestation of SCD in an infant. Presentation before age 24 months predicts an increased risk for severe SCD with frequent complications. Infants with dactylitis will have bilateral painful swelling of the hands and feet due to infarction of the small metacarpal and metatarsal bones. Progression of disease leads to destructive bony changes that can later be seen on radiographs. VOCs in older children tend to follow adult patterns and occur most commonly in the extremities, chest, and back. Pain in other sites (head, chest, abdomen) may represent VOC episodes or other acute complications [stroke, acute chest syndrome (ACS), splenic sequestration] and disease entities (appendicitis, cholecystitis). Investigation for other possible etiologies of pain should be undertaken for patients presenting with atypical VOCs or when clinically indicated. Management of VOCs includes intravenous hydration and adequate analgesic therapy guided by patient report of pain severity.

Fever in patients with SCD should be considered a potential life-threatening emergency. Bacterial sepsis is a significant cause for morbidity and mortality in infants and very young children with SCD. Impaired splenic function from splenic infarction leads to an increased risk of severe bacterial infections by encapsulated organisms (*Streptococcus pneumoniae, Hemophilus influenzae, Nisseria, Mycoplasma pneumoniae*). Penicillin prophylaxis is therefore started early in infancy for all children with SCD. Infants as young as age 2 months can have splenic impairment with increased susceptibility for meningitis, bacteremia, and sepsis. Other life-threatening infections include acute chest syndrome and osteomyelitis (*Staphylococcus aureus, Salmonella*). In patients with bone pain and extremity swelling or erythema, osteomyelitis should be considered and managed accordingly. Children with SCD presenting with fever require emergent evaluation and prompt treatment with parenteral antibiotics that provide coverage against *Streptococcus pneumoniae* and gram-negative enteric organisms. Diagnostic tests should be sent according to presenting symptoms to identify the source of fever (blood and urine cultures, chest X-ray, etc.) along with CBC with differential and reticulocyte count. Rapid intravenous fluid resuscitation should be initiated promptly if sepsis is suspected. Tachycardia is the earliest sign of sepsis in pediatric patients. Criteria for admission for patients with fever and SCD include ill appearance, age younger than 1 year, white blood cell count <5/>30, temperature >39.5°C, the presence of other SCD complications (ACS, splenic sequestration), or if the patient is unable to return for follow-up care.

ACS is the second most common reason for hospital admissions in children and adults with SCD and the most common cause of death. The clinical picture of ACS resembles that of pneumonia (cough, shortness of breath, retractions, abnormal lung examination) with a new infiltrate on chest radiography. Children tend to have fever and single lobe involvement, whereas adults are more often afebrile with multilobe involvement. It occurs more frequently in people with asthma and with prior episodes of ACS. Although ACS most commonly results from infection, fat embolism, pulmonary infarction, atelectasis, and pulmonary edema can also lead to this complication. Patients with severe disease can develop respiratory failure or multiorgan system failure. Treatment includes broad-spectrum antibiotics, supplemental oxygen, intravenous hydration, analgesics, bronchodilators, PRBC transfusion, and, if severe, exchange blood transfusion.

Acute splenic sequestration, which can be life-threatening, mostly occurs in children aged 6 months to 4 years, although it may also be seen in older children or adolescents with hemoglobin SC, S-β-thalassemia(+), or those on hydroxyurea. Infants may present with acute, severe anemia and hypovolemic shock. Children will complain of left-sided abdominal pain and often have a recent or concurrent febrile illness. They can have signs of acute hemolysis with tachycardia and scleral icterus, as well as splenomegaly on examination. Large amounts of blood and platelets can rapidly become sequestered in the spleen, leading to hypovolemic shock and cardiovascular collapse. Examination of the abdomen should begin from the pelvis so as not to miss massive splenomegaly. Hemoglobin levels are usually reduced by at least 2 g/dL from baseline and frequently associated with thrombocytopenia. Early recognition of symptoms and rapid initiation of therapy with packed RBCs may be life-saving. Care should be taken not to overcorrect the anemia because this may lead to an elevated hematocrit, which is associated with complications from hyperviscosity. It is recommended to transfuse packed RBCs in small aliquots with frequent reassessment to determine response. Recurrence rate is high, and splenectomy may be recommended after critical or recurrent events.

Aplastic crisis is due to bone marrow suppression from infection, typically a viral infection, potentially parvovirus B19 or fifth disease. It can lead to a rapid, profound decrease in hemoglobin level in affected patients. Children will have worsening fatigue, increasing pallor, and shortness of breath with decreasing reticulocyte count in the face of worsening anemia. Tachycardia is typically prominent, with signs of heart failure in severe cases. Patients may have significantly low hemoglobin levels (3–6 g/dL) compared to their baseline, with minimal or no reticulocytes. Treatment is supportive care with packed red cell transfusions as needed to maintain adequate hemoglobin level until aplastic crisis has resolved.

Stroke (see Chapter 19 on neurovascular emergencies) is a devastating complication of sickle cell anemia with a peak incidence between ages 6 and 9 years. Without prevention, as many as 10% of children with HbSS will have acute strokes, and up to 30% will have silent cerebral infarcts. Transcranial Doppler screening along with regular blood transfusions and hydroxyurea therapy in high-risk patients decreases their risk. Most strokes in children are caused by ischemia or stenosis of the internal carotid or middle cerebral artery. Transient ischemic attacks may herald overt strokes but may not be initially detectible on neuroimaging. Children will show signs similar to acute strokes in adults: weakness, hemiplegia, ataxia, dysarthria, aphasia, visual disturbance, seizures, coma, or other focal neurologic deficits. Events may be precipitated by any complication that causes acute anemia (ACS, aplastic crisis, etc.). Brain computed tomography (CT), magnetic resonance imaging (MRI), and magnetic resonance angiography (MRA) should be obtained emergently and exchange transfusion initiated in consultation with hematology.

Several other acute complications of SCD that require emergent evaluation and management to preserve organ function include priapism and ocular emergencies such as hyphema, central retinal artery occlusion (CRAO), orbital compression syndrome, and orbital infections/infarctions. Delay in management of priapism, a painful erection lasting more than 4 hours, may lead to impotence. If symptoms do not resolve with vigorous hydration and analgesic therapy, urology should be consulted for possible penile aspiration, use of α-adrenergic agents (corpus irrigation or oral), or surgical intervention. Exchange transfusions have not been shown to be beneficial. CRAO is a rare complication seen mostly in children and young adults that presents with sudden unilateral or bilateral painless visual loss. Ocular emergencies in people with SCD can result in permanent visual loss and should be co-managed with an ophthalmologist and hematologist.

HEMOLYTIC ANEMIAS

Hemolysis of RBCs can be caused by acquired disease processes (immune-mediated, infectious, medications) or by an acute precipitant in people with certain inherited disorders (hemoglobinopathies, thalassemia, red cell membrane defects, or enzyme deficiencies). Destruction of RBCs may lead to significant anemia if the bone marrow is unable to compensate for the loss.

Autoimmune Hemolytic Anemia

Autoimmune hemolytic anemia (AIHA), in which the body forms antibodies against its own RBCs, can sometimes lead to severe anemia in children. AIHA can be due to a primary autoimmune disorder or secondary to an underlying systemic illness (infections, malignancy, inflammatory conditions, etc.). Patients usually present with a sudden onset of pallor, jaundice, and dark urine. They may be significantly ill with signs of congestive heart failure at presentation if the anemia is severe. Treatment is discussed later.

Glucose-6-Phosphate Dehydrogenase Deficiency

G6PD is the most common inherited RBC enzyme deficiency. G6PD allows RBCs to detoxify oxidants. In its absence, RBCs can become damaged by oxidant exposure, leading to rapid hemolysis. Oxidants (e.g., sulfa drugs and fava beans) and stress/infections can induce acute hemolysis in affected patients. A quantitative enzyme assay can confirm the diagnosis in suspected cases.

Hereditary Spherocytosis

Hereditary spherocytosis (HS) is an inherited RBC membrane disorder in which RBC membranes are abnormally shaped with increased fragility and deformability. Patients with HS have variable clinical presentations, with intermittent jaundice and episodes of acute hemolytic or aplastic crisis associated with viral infections, splenomegaly, and cholelithiasis.

Clinical Presentation and Differential Diagnosis

Important family history to obtain includes a history of anemia, autoimmune disease, splenectomy or cholecystectomy (inherited hemolytic disorders), recurrent jaundice (G6PD deficiency, hemoglobinopathies), and medication use (sulfa drugs). Patients with intravascular hemolysis may have back pain or dark urine. The presence of lymphadenopathy or splenomegaly suggests an underlying malignancy, systemic illness (systemic lupus erythematosus, infection), or an inherited disorder (sickle cell disease, spherocytosis). Liver disease, abetalipoproteinemia, vitamin E deficiency, Wilson disease, prosthetic valves, and disseminated intravascular coagulation (DIC) may also cause hemolytic anemia.

Diagnostic Confirmation

Laboratory values in hemolytic anemia will show anemia with elevated reticulocyte count, elevated indirect bilirubin, elevated lactate dehydrogenase (LDH), and decreased haptoglobin. Spherocytes or schistocytes on a peripheral blood smear and hemoglobinuria on urinalysis also indicate hemolysis. In autoimmune hemolytic anemia, the direct antiglobulin test (DAT) or Coombs test will be positive.

Treatment

Treatment depends on the underlying etiology and degree of anemia. Corticosteroids are the first line of therapy for warm, autoimmune hemolytic anemia, which is typically immunoglobulin G (IgG) mediated. For patients with severe symptomatic anemia (Hgb <6 to 7 g/dL with hypoxia or congestive heart failure), intravenous corticosteroids (methylprednisolone 0.5–1 mg/kg per dose every 6–8 hours) should be given until the hematocrit stabilizes. Blood transfusions can lead to worsening hemolysis and transfusion reactions from blood incompatibility due to the presence of nonspecific antibodies in the patient's serum and should be reserved for patients who are hemodynamically unstable. Blood transfusion should be initiated in small aliquots of 5 mL of ABO/Rh-compatible blood over 15 minutes, with frequent reassessments for signs of worsening hemolysis. Additional immunosuppressive medications, such as Rituximab or Cellcept, may be warranted in refractory cases. Patients with mild to moderate anemia can be started on oral prednisone 2 mg/kg/day. Corticosteroid therapy can be weaned slowly when the hematocrit has improved to a safe level. For patients found to have a cold autoimmune hemolytic anemia, which is typically IgM mediated and associated with viral infections (mycoplasma or EBV), the treatment consists of supportive care with packed RBC transfusions as needed. Admission for observation and treatment response is recommended for most patients in consultation with a hematologist.

IRON DEFICIENCY ANEMIA

Clinical Presentation

Iron deficiency anemia is the most common cause of anemia in children. Depleted iron stores, poor intake of iron-rich foods, and excessive cow's milk intake in toddlers [>20 oz (600 mL) daily] can lead to iron deficiency anemia. Adolescent girls with heavy menstrual flows are also at increased risk. Patients will have various degrees of clinical presentations depending on the degree of anemia, with pallor and fatigue seen more commonly. Hemoglobin levels as low as 4 or 5 g/dL can be well tolerated due to the chronicity of illness.

Diagnostic Confirmation

Initial diagnostic studies include a CBC with differential consistent with a microcytic anemia and high RBC distribution width and, if obtained, a low serum ferritin level. Further studies are not indicated in patients with mild anemia and a clinical history consistent with iron deficiency anemia. Iron deficiency anemia in older children is less common, and other causes for anemia should be considered depending on the clinical picture.

Treatment

Treatment consists of a trial of iron supplementation (ferrous sulfate 3–6 mg/kg of elemental iron, once daily) along with an increase in iron-rich foods and, when applicable, decreased milk intake. A repeat CBC should be obtained within 4 weeks to assess response to treatment. Children with severe symptomatic anemia may require admission for RBC transfusion and further diagnostic studies.

KEY POINTS

- For patients with SCD presenting with atypical VOCs from their baseline, consider other possible etiologies of pain.
- Fever in patients with SCD should be considered a potential life-threatening emergency and requires immediate evaluation and prompt treatment with parenteral antibiotics.
- In splenic sequestration, early recognition of symptoms and rapid initiation of therapy with packed RBCs may be life-saving.
- Blood transfusion therapy in patients with autoimmune hemolytic anemia should be initiated with care because it can lead to worsening hemolysis and transfusion reactions.
- In iron deficiency anemia, hemoglobin levels as low as 4 or 5 g/dL can be well tolerated due to the chronicity of illness.

PITFALLS

- Abnormalities in multiple blood cell lines indicate a bone marrow disease process. Bone marrow aspirate is indicated in these cases to evaluate for bone marrow failure or malignancy.
- For SCD patients presenting with signs concerning for a stroke, imaging (brain CT, MRI, MRA) should be obtained emergently and exchange transfusion initiated in consultation with hematology.

BLEEDING DISORDERS

Background

Hemostasis is achieved by complex interactions between platelets, coagulation factors, and the vascular endothelium. Defects in any of these components lead to increased bleeding. Injured endothelium secretes von Willebrand factor, which facilitates platelet activation and aggregation. The liver synthesizes procoagulant proenzymes involved in the coagulation cascade. It can sometimes be challenging to diagnose the underlying etiology of excessive bleeding or bruising in children. The type and location of bleeding, along with screening tests, can aid in differentiating between primary and secondary hemostatic disorders and help determine diagnosis. In this section, we discuss the more common hemostatic disorders and their management.

Classic Clinical Presentation

Defects in primary hemostasis typically indicate a problem with platelets, von Willebrand factors, and/or vasculature. Symptoms include increased bruising, petechiae, mucocutaneous bleeding (prolonged epistaxis/gingival bleeding), prolonged bleeding after surgery or dental extractions, and, less frequently, hematuria or gastrointestinal bleeding. Female patients may present with heavy menstrual bleeding.

Defects in secondary hemostasis typically indicate a defect with the coagulation cascade (e.g., hemophilia) and are associated with bleeding into soft tissues, muscle, or joints as well as delayed bleeding with lacerations or following surgery. Some patients may also present with mucocutaneous bleeding. Infants with prolonged bleeding after circumcision and patients with spontaneous intracranial hemorrhages or significant mucosal bleeding should also be evaluated for possible defects in their coagulation factors.

Differential Diagnosis

Details in the medical history that can aid in diagnosis are a history of recurrent epistaxis, heavy menstrual bleeding since menarche (von Willebrand disease, platelet dysfunction, thrombocytopenia), bleeding with circumcision (hemophilia A or B or other rare factor deficiencies, congenital thrombocytopenia, von Willebrand disease), intracranial hemorrhage in infancy (neonatal alloimmune thrombocytopenia, hemophilia A or B, congenital thrombocytopenia, factor XIII deficiency), associated anemia with neurologic changes [thrombotic thrombocytopenic purpura (TTP)], or isolated thrombocytopenia [idiopathic thrombocytopenia purpura (ITP)]. Hemophilia is an X-linked disorder that affects mostly males. Duration of symptoms may differentiate between congenital and acquired syndromes. Conditions that can result in secondary coagulopathies include renal disease (acquired platelet dysfunction), liver disease (acquired coagulopathy), vitamin K deficiency, medications (thrombocytopenia), ingestions (warfarin), and sepsis (DIC).

Neonatal Hemostasis

Although neonates have a balanced hemostatic system, many facets of the neonatal coagulation system are different from those of older children and adults. In neonates, platelets are thought to be hyporesponsive with impaired aggregation. Due to liver immaturity, all coagulation factors are low, except factor VIII, von Willebrand factor, and fibrinogen, leading to normally increased activated partial thromboplastin time (aPTT) and prothrombin time/international normalized ratio (PT/INR) levels in this population. Most of these factors will reach normal levels at approximately age 6 months. Increased levels and function of von Willebrand factor along with decreased production of both pro- and antithrombotic proteins create a balanced hemostatic system in neonates.

Diagnostic Confirmation

Initial screening tests for the child with bleeding of unknown etiology include a CBC with differential, peripheral blood smear, and coagulation studies (PT/INR and aPTT). A type and screen or crossmatch should be sent on any patient who may require a blood transfusion. Imaging studies in children with bleeding disorders who present to the ED with acute bleeding are dependent on the presenting complaint and acuity of illness:

- CBC: Assess for quantitative defects in platelets and hemoglobin level for severity of bleeding. Abnormalities in multiple cell lines are concerning for leukemia or bone marrow failure syndrome.
- Peripheral blood smear: Excludes platelet clumping and RBC microangiopathy.
- Isolated elevated PT/INR: Factor VII deficiency, vitamin K deficiency, or liver disease.
- Isolated elevated aPTT: Low levels of factors 8, 9, 11, or 12, heparin contamination, or lupus anticoagulant. An elevated aPTT may also be associated with severe von Willebrand disease (vWD). If the aPTT is elevated, send a 1:1 mixing study to determine if there is a factor deficiency (aPTT will normalize) or the presence of an inhibitor such as the lupus anticoagulant (aPTT would not completely correct).

Treatment

Treatment for patients with moderate to severe bleeding and abnormal coagulation studies in the ED depends on the underlying etiology and hemostatic defect. Hemoglobin levels should be obtained before and after initiation of treatment, and blood transfusions should be given if needed. Irrespective of underlying etiology, treatment for all cases of mild mucocutaneous bleeding discussed next begins with local measures, including pressure, topical therapy (topical thrombin/fibrin sealant), and antifibrinolytics if not otherwise contraindicated.

Patient disposition for all causes depends on location of bleed and severity of illness. In all cases, hematology should be consulted to help guide management.

HEMOPHILIA

Background

Hemophilia is an X-linked recessive bleeding disorder caused by deficiency of factor VIII (hemophilia A) or factor IX (hemophilia B). Hemophilia can also be caused by de novo mutations in patients with no family history of the disease. Severity of illness is determined by the level of clotting factor activity, with patients with <1% of normal clotting factory activity classified as severe.

Clinical Presentation

Patients can have variable clinical presentations depending on the severity of disease. Patients with mild disease generally do not have frequent bleeding episodes and usually present with bleeding after surgery or significant trauma. Patients with moderate disease can bleed with mild trauma, whereas patients with severe disease are more likely to have spontaneous bleeding events, with or without trauma, usually in joints and soft tissues. Patients with spontaneous joint bleeding or intracranial hemorrhage should have an evaluation for a bleeding disorder.

Diagnostic Confirmation

Patients with hemophilia will have prolonged PTT with a normal PT and normal platelet count on laboratory testing. Assays for levels of factor VIII and factor IX can be sent for confirmation of disease in the patient with unknown diagnosis. For ED patients with known hemophilia who present with bleeding episodes, empiric factor dosing for treatment is used without the need to check factor levels. Factor levels after treatment can help assess for the presence of an inhibitor.

Treatment

Treatment involves replacing the missing factor to optimize the coagulation system either as prophylaxis to prevent bleeding episodes or as needed in response to spontaneous bleeding or trauma. Patients with hemophilia who present to the ED with symptoms of bleeding should be evaluated emergently and factor given promptly for bleeds with significant morbidity or mortality prior to obtaining confirmatory imaging studies. Typical bleeding presentations in patient with hemophilia and their management are shown in Table 28.1.

Inhibitors to Replacement Factor

Patients with a family history of inhibitors or increased exposure to replacement factor early in life are at risk for developing inhibitors. Inhibitors are antibodies that block the function of the replacement factor given. The presence of inhibitors should be suspected in patients who are provided optimal factor replacement and are still not responding as anticipated based on factor levels or clinical improvement. Although testing exists to evaluate for the presence of inhibitors, bypassing agents, such as an activated prothrombin complex concentrate [i.e., FEIBA (50–100 U/kg q 12 hr) or Novo-7 (90 μg/kg q 2–3 hr)], can be given to critical patients or patients with known inhibitors. Novo-7 can be given for two or three doses, with re-evaluation for efficacy. Some patients may benefit from a loading dose of 270 μg/kg followed by 90 μg/kg dosing after 2–4 hours. FEIBA should not be used with antifibrinolytics or given to patients already on emicizumab (Hemlibra), which is a newly approved monoclonal antibody that is used as prophylaxis to prevent bleeding episodes in patients with hemophilia A with or without inhibitors.

VON WILLEBRAND DISEASE

Background

Von Willebrand disease can result in either a quantitative or a qualitative defect in the von Willebrand antigen, subsequently impacting its activity. There are three general types of vWD: Type 1 is a mild quantitative defect accounting for 75% of patients, the various type 2 subtypes are different qualitative defects impacting von Willebrand factor (vWF) interaction with platelets or factor VIII and account for 25% of patients, and type 3 is a severe quantitative defect leading to virtual absence of the protein and is rare (<1% of patients).

Clinical Presentation

The most common symptoms are epistaxis, gingival bleeding, and, in most females with vWD, heavy menstrual bleeding after

TABLE 28.1 HEMOPHILIA COMPLICATIONS AND MANAGEMENT RECOMMENDATIONS

Hemophilia	Bleeding Type	Symptoms	Imaging	Treatment[a]	Disposition/Recommendation
Life-threatening Emergent factor replacement *before* imaging	Intracranial hemorrhage	Infants: irritability, vomiting, bulging fontanelle, lethargy Older children: persistent headaches, altered mental status, seizures, focal neurologic changes	Brain CT Negative head CT does not always rule out an ICH	Factor replacement emergently to maintain levels at 80–100% × 7 days	ICU admission, neurosurgery/ hematology consultation Maintain airway Neuroprotective measures Seizure prophylaxis
	Spinal bleed	Trauma, back pain, peripheral neuropathy, recent lumbar puncture	CT/MRI spine	Factor replacement prior to lumbar punctures	
	Airway	Signs of upper airway obstruction (stridor, grunting, retractions)	CT scan if indicated	Factor should be initiated prior to confirmatory imaging	ICU admission, maintain patent airway
	Iliopsoas	Pain in lower abdomen, back, or groin; hip held in flexed position; pain on hip extension; paresthesia of the medial aspect of upper thigh	Can try US, but usually need CT scan/MRI	Factor replacement to 80–100% for first few days, then lower dose long term for healing	Admission, strict bed rest until symptoms improving
	Gastrointestinal	Hematemesis, hematochezia, and/or melena		Factor replacement Antifibrinolytics	Admission, serial hemoglobin levels
	Hip	Hip held in flexed position, pain on hip extension, limp	Hip US	Factor replacement, analgesics, RICE, joint immobilization	
	Retroperitoneal	Back pain	US or CT scan	Factor replacement	Admission, serial hemoglobin levels
	Multisystem trauma	Variable clinical presentation, suspect intra-abdominal bleed if bruising/ abdominal tenderness present or hypotension	Imaging as dictated by severity of illness	Factor replacement to a goal of 100%, direct pressure to bleeding area, joint immobilization, ± blood transfusions	ICU admission, maintain airway patent, serial hemoglobin levels

(continued)

TABLE 28.1 CONTINUED

Hemophilia	Bleeding Type	Symptoms	Imaging	Treatment[a]	Disposition/Recommendation
Less severe	Hemarthrosis	Joint pain, swelling, decreased range of motion or warmth/redness over joint; small children—refusal to bear weight or utilize the extremity, pain with passive movement	Routine imaging not needed Extremity trauma: X-rays	Factor replacement, analgesics, RICE, joint immobilization	Discharge home with ongoing factor replacement—duration dictated by hematologist Admission: pain management, unable to give at home
	Muscle bleed	Bruising, swelling, pain over site	Not indicated	Factor replacement for 2 or 3 days	Bleeding in forearm/calf: risk for compartment syndrome → requires admission and may require fasciotomy
	Mucocutaneous	Epistaxis, gingival bleeding, prolonged bleeding after dental procedures		Direct pressure, nasal packing/cautery, topical pro-coagulants, antifibrinolytic, factor replacement	Discharge if bleeding controlled Continue factor outpatient
	Hematuria	Painless or post-traumatic	Renal US	Bed rest, hydration Factor replacement if symptoms are not improving/increased pain/anemia	Antifibrinolytics contraindicated due to risk of urinary obstruction
	Lacerations	Prolonged bleeding		Direct pressure, factor prior to repair	

[a]Factor VIII replacement: factor level desired × weight (kg) × 0.5. Factor IX replacement: factor level desired × weight (kg).

CT, computed tomography; ICH, intracranial hemorrhage; ICU, intensive care unit; MRI, magnetic resonance imaging; RICE, rest, ice, compression, and elevation; US, ultrasound.

menarche. In type 2N and type 3, hemophilia type bleeds such as hemarthrosis can also be seen because these patients also have low levels of factor VIII. Although extremely rare, intracranial hemorrhage is possible.

Diagnostic Confirmation

If there is suspicion for vWD based on the patient's history, screening tests include vWF activity/ristocetin cofactor and antigen, factor VIII levels, and a blood type.

Treatment

Treatment depends on the severity and type of bleeding episode as well as the type of vWD present. Less severe episodes of mucocutaneous bleeding can be managed by local methods, including pressure for epistaxis and fibrin sealants, or the use of antifibrinolytics. Contraindications to antifibrinolytic use include the presence of hematuria, DIC, or increased thrombotic risk. For females with heavy menstrual bleeding, hormonal control with estrogen-containing medications can be used.

For type 1 vWD patients, if these measures are insufficient, desmopressin acetate (DDAVP) can be given either intranasally (one 150-μg puff per nostril in children >40 kg, one puff in one nostril for children <40 kg) or subcutaneously/intravenously (0.3 μg/kg). DDAVP facilitates the release of vWF from the endothelium, temporarily increasing circulating levels, which may improve hemostasis. Overuse of DDAVP can lead to fluid overload, hyponatremia, and potentially seizures, particularly in very young children (younger than age 3 years). Patients should not receive more than once-daily dosing because more frequent administration leads to increased side effects and decreased efficacy.

DDAVP may not be effective in a subset of patients with vWD (type 1 nonresponders and those with types 2 and 3). In these patients, the next step in treatment for uncontrolled bleeding episodes is vWF:factor VIII concentrate or recombinant vWF to replace the missing factors, with an initial dose of 40–60 IU/kg for major bleeding episodes. If these are not available, cryoprecipitate can be given because it contains both vWF and factor VIII protein.

FACTOR VII DEFICIENCY

Of the rare congenital bleeding disorders, factor VII deficiency is the most common and has variable presentations from minimal to life-threatening bleeding episodes. Factor VII level does not always correlate with bleeding risk. Factor VII deficiency is suspected in patients with an isolated elevated PT/INR level in whom liver disease and vitamin K deficiency have been ruled out, which can be done if there is no response to a trial of parenteral vitamin K. Initial treatment is based on significance of bleeding episode. Mucocutaneous bleeding can be managed as discussed previously. For patients with more severe bleeding episodes, factor VII replacement may be necessary. The most common form used is recombinant factor VIIa 15–30 μg/kg. Alternative therapies include direct factor VII concentrates, prothrombin complex concentrates such as Kcentra (25 U/kg), or fresh frozen plasma (FFP; 15–20 cc/kg).

FACTOR XI DEFICIENCY

Although rare, factor XI deficiency has been noted with increased frequency in certain populations, including those of Ashkenazi Jewish background. Factor XI deficiency would be suspected in those with an isolated, elevated PTT, frequently more than twice normal levels, and normal factor VIII, IX, and XII levels. Factor XI protein levels do not correlate with bleeding risk; rather, family and personal history may dictate chance of having bleeding episode. Mild mucocutaneous bleeding episodes can frequently be managed with topical treatment and/or antifibrinolytics, with hormonal control used for females with heavy menstrual bleeding. For patients with significant bleeding episodes, factor replacement should be considered. Although a recombinant factor XI exists, it is frequently unavailable; therefore, most patients are treated with FFP, approximately 20 mL/kg, for replacement therapy.

FACTOR XIII DEFICIENCY

Factor XIII is required for cross-linking fibrin and strengthening clots laid down for hemostasis. Deficiency of this protein leads to an unstable clot and delayed bleeding symptoms as well as poor wound healing. Patients may have prolonged or delayed bleeding from the umbilical stump or poor healing as well as risk for intracranial hemorrhage. On laboratory examination, the PT/PTT would be within normal limits, so if a bleeding disorder is suspected, a factor XIII level should be sent. In these cases, the factor XIII level correlates with bleeding risk. Prophylaxis is frequently instituted in patients with severe factor XIII deficiency or with prior symptomatic bleeding episodes, particularly because patients can be dosed every 3 or 4 weeks due to the long half-life of this protein. Options for replacement therapy include recombinant factor XIII (although only effective for those missing the A subunit), FFP at 15–20 mL/kg, or cryoprecipitate at 1 U/10 kg. Because this protein does have a long half-life, repeat dosing is not necessary in the acute setting.

AFIBRINOGENEMIA/ HYPOFIBRINOGENEMIA

Fibrinogen disorders can be due to either quantitative defects (low or absent levels of fibrinogen) or defective protein. For quantitative defects, fibrinogen levels correlate with risk of bleeding. Afibrinogenemia patients may have increased bleeding from the umbilical stump or skin, musculoskeletal bleeding, gastrointestinal/gastrourinary bleeding, or intracranial hemorrhage. Patients with hypofibrinogenemia may have variable degrees of bleeding symptoms. Screening coagulation studies (PT/PTT levels) will be elevated with decreased fibrinogen activity level. Mild episodes can be treated with local measures and antifibrinolytic therapy. More severe bleeding episodes can be treated with replacement therapy (recombinant fibrinogen concentrate, cryoprecipitate 1 U/ 5–10 kg, or FFP 10–15 mL/kg) with a goal of raising the fibrinogen level to 100–150 g/L of plasma.

PLATELET DISORDERS

Thrombocytopenia is defined as a platelet count <150,000/μL. Thrombocytopenia can be caused by decreased production or increased destruction of platelets.

IDIOPATHIC THROMBOCYTOPENIA PURPURA

Background

Idiopathic thrombocytopenia purpura is the most common cause of acute, isolated thrombocytopenia in children, with a peak incidence between ages 2 and 5 years. It is caused by antibodies directed against platelet membrane antigens leading to increased destruction of platelets primarily in the spleen. Although the etiology of primary ITP is unknown, a large percentage of patients have a prior viral illness within 1 month of the onset of ITP. Thrombocytopenia usually resolves within 6 months, with a small percentage of patients developing chronic ITP. Secondary causes of ITP include autoimmune disorders, immune deficiencies, collagen vascular disorders, and chronic infections.

Clinical Presentation

Most patients with ITP are healthy and well-appearing with signs of cutaneous or mucosal bleeding. The presence of other signs or symptoms (i.e., ill appearance, fever, weight loss, bone pain, hepatosplenomegaly, lymphadenopathy, chronic illness) or a family history of bleeding disorders warrant further evaluation for other disease processes. Most patients with acute ITP do not have serious bleeding despite having significantly low platelet counts (even <10,000/μL). Children with ITP will present with petechiae and/or increased bruising, with some patients also having prolonged epistaxis and/or bleeding gums and, less frequently, hematuria or gastrointestinal bleeding. Mucosal bleeding is more common in patients with platelet counts <20,000/μL. Severe bleeding occurs in <3% of patients. Intracranial hemorrhage is very rare (<1%) but should be suspected in any patient with a headache or an abnormal neurologic examination and thrombocytopenia.

Diagnostic Confirmation

Most patient have platelet counts significantly lower than 100,000/μL on presentation, with all other CBC cell indexes normal. Thrombocytopenia should be confirmed on peripheral blood smear because automated CBC counters can inaccurately report decreased platelet counts when platelets clump together. PT and PTT are usually normal and do not need to be routinely checked unless the patient presents with severe, excessive bleeding not predicted by the degree of thrombocytopenia. In these cases, coagulation studies should be sent as well as D-dimer, fibrinogen, and a screen for vWD. Blood type and a direct antiglobulin test (Coombs test) may also be checked. The direct antiglobulin test is negative in isolated ITP but may be positive in patients with Evan's syndrome, which is the combination of ITP and AIHA. In infants younger than age 1 year, ITP is less common, and additional testing for an immunologic disorder, including HIV, should be considered. HIV testing and antinuclear antibody screening should be also considered in older children with isolated thrombocytopenia. Bone marrow biopsy is reserved for patients with symptoms suggestive of another cause for thrombocytopenia, prior to the initiation of treatment with glucocorticoids, or if the patient fails to respond to treatment.

Treatment

Most patients will have resolution of symptoms within 3 months and do not require pharmacologic treatment. Initial management includes supportive care, avoidance of medications with antiplatelet activity (aspirin, nonsteroidal anti-inflammatory drugs, warfarin), and monitoring for bleeding. Participation in physical activity with risk of trauma is discouraged for all patients, and protective gear is recommended for all sports. Patients with significant bleeding or needing a surgical procedure require pharmacologic treatment and hospitalization. Treatment is also suggested for patients with an underlying bleeding disorder or those who need anticoagulation therapy. Treatment options include intravenous immunoglobulin (IVIG), glucocorticoids, and intravenous anti-D immune globulin (anti-D). Initiation of pharmacologic therapy is recommended in conjunction with hematology consultation. Platelet transfusions are mostly contraindicated with the exception of life-threatening hemorrhage or signs of an intracranial bleed. Patients with intracranial hemorrhages should also receive IVIG, methylprednisolone, and anti-D. Emergent splenectomy may be indicated in patients with active hemorrhage who do not respond to medical management.

DISSEMINATED INTRAVASCULAR COAGULATION

Background and Diagnostic Confirmation

Disseminated intravascular coagulation is a result of activation and dysregulation of the coagulation system with ongoing consumption of coagulation factors and impaired fibrinolysis. This leads to multiorgan failure from extensive deposition of fibrin with occlusion of small and medium-sized blood vessels (thrombosis) as well as depletion of coagulation factors (hemorrhage). DIC can result from sepsis, trauma, leukemia such as acute promyelocytic leukemia, certain vascular anomalies, along with other causative factors. Diagnostic studies include thrombocytopenia, low fibrinogen, elevated D-dimer from ongoing fibrinolysis, elevated PT/PTT, and schistocytes on peripheral blood smear. In cases in which factor levels are measured, one would see decreased factor V, factor VIII, protein C/S, and antithrombin III.

Treatment

Treatment consists of treating the underlying cause and monitoring response. Considering the potential for both bleeding and clotting complications, targeted treatment such as anticoagulation for vascular thrombus or prothrombin complex concentrate/activated factor VII for bleeding is usually reserved for life- or limb-threatening complications.

HEMOLYTIC UREMIC SYNDROME

Background and Diagnostic Confirmation

Hemolytic uremic syndrome is characterized by thrombocytopenia, microangiopathic hemolytic anemia, and renal dysfunction. At least 70% of cases are in children younger than age 5 years, and more than 90% of cases are associated with infection with *Escherichia coli* O157:H7. Symptoms include bloody diarrhea and renal insufficiency. Up to 50% of patients require dialysis, and 20% may have seizures or other neurologic changes. Diagnosis of typical cases of HUS includes CBC with peripheral blood smear in which one would see low platelets and red cells and likely schistocytes as evidence of microangiopathic hemolytic anemia, along with an elevated LDH level, low haptoglobin, and negative DAT.

Treatment

Treatment for these patients includes management of the renal dysfunction and platelet or packed RBC transfusions as needed for support. Approximately 10% of cases are not related to infection with *E. coli* and are considered atypical HUS. A defect in the complement cascade leads to vascular endothelial damage and platelet aggregation. This can be associated with post-transplant complications, autoimmune disorders, or various medications.

Additional testing includes assays for Shiga toxin and the ADAMTS13 metalloprotease, the results of both of which should be negative to differentiate these cases from typical HUS and TTP, respectively. These patients need more directed therapy to address the complement dysfunction along with hematology and nephrology consultations.

THROMBOTIC THROMBOCYTOPENIC PURPURA

Background and Diagnostic Confirmation

Thrombotic thrombocytopenic purpura is also a microangiopathic process that consists of microangiopathic hemolytic anemia, severe thrombocytopenia, and neurologic/renal dysfunction. Patients will present with neurologic complaints (headaches, seizures, or altered mental status). Renal dysfunction, if present, is usually mild. TTP is associated with decreased ADAMTS13 due to either congenital decreased production or antibody-mediated increased destruction. This leads to increased levels of ultra-large vWF, which results in microthrombi in the small arterial vessels. Patients have severe thrombocytopenia (platelet count <20,000/μL), mild/moderate anemia, elevated reticulocyte count, schistocytes on peripheral blood smear, increased LDH, and decreased haptoglobin. Coagulation studies (PT/PTT and fibrinogen) are typically normal.

Treatment

Definitive treatment is usually initiated as an inpatient and depends on the underlying etiology of TTP. Patients with antibody-mediated TTP are treated with plasma exchange as soon as the diagnosis is suspected to prevent ongoing vascular and organ damage. Some patients may also require other forms of immunosuppression, such as steroids or Rituximab. Patients already determined to have the congenital form should receive treatment with FFP, which provides the missing ADAMTS13 protein.

KEY POINTS

- Patients who should have an evaluation for a bleeding disorder include infants with prolonged bleeding after circumcision and patients with spontaneous intracranial hemorrhages or significant mucosal bleeding, spontaneous joint bleeding, prolonged heavy menses, or delayed bleeding after minor trauma.
- Patients with hemophilia and head trauma or signs of increased intracranial pressure should be given factor replacement emergently in the ED prior to obtaining confirmatory brain imaging.
- Treatment of most mild to moderate mucosal bleeds entails direct pressure, topical procoagulants, antifibrinolytic medication, and ice.
- Emergent splenectomy may be considered in patients with ITP with active hemorrhage who do not respond to medical management.
- DDAVP may not be effective in some patients with vWD, and severe bleeding episodes should be treated with a vWF:factor VIII concentrate or, if this is not available, cryoprecipitate.

PITFALLS

- Factor administration in patients with hemophilia who have bleeds with significant morbidity or mortality should never be delayed by imaging.
- Early recognition of an iliopsoas bleed in hemophilia patients is essential because they can lose a large amount of blood, leading to severe anemia or intra-abdominal compartment syndrome.
- A negative head CT does not always rule out an acute intracerebral hemorrhage, and patients with persistent symptoms should be admitted for monitoring and possibly further diagnostic testing.
- Platelet transfusions in patients with ITP are mostly contraindicated with the exception of life-threatening hemorrhage or signs of an intracranial bleed.
- In infants younger than age 1 year and adolescent patients with isolated thrombocytopenia, ITP is less common, and additional testing for an immunologic disorder, including HIV, should be considered. Other disease processes should also be considered in patients with thrombocytopenia and systemic symptoms or hepatosplenomegaly.

CLOTTING DISORDERS

Background and Diagnostic Confirmation

Diseases associated with increased probability of development of vascular thrombi include SCD, protein C/S deficiency, factor V Leiden, homocystinuria, nephrotic syndrome, systemic lupus erythematosus, and malignancy.

Treatment

Many factors impact the decision to initiate anticoagulation therapy in pediatric patients with a known thrombus. The goals of therapy are to decrease the risks of treatment complications, disease progression, recurrence, and development of post-thrombotic syndrome. A venous thromboembolism (VTE) that is an incidental finding and has been asymptomatic may not require anticoagulation and at times can be observed initially.

Initial therapy for most children is initiation of a heparin-based product, either unfractionated heparin (UFH) or a low-molecular-weight heparin (LMWH). Clinically unstable patients or those with increased bleeding risks are usually started on UFH, which has a shorter half-life. More stable patients with minimal bleeding risk can be started on LMWH (enoxparin 1 mg/kg every 12 hours or fondaparinux 0.1 mg/kg daily). Coagulation studies, CBC, and renal clearance labs (PT/PTT/INR and fibrinogen) should be checked prior to treatment. Admission for further management and education is recommended for all patients with a diagnosed thrombus.

Patients with life- or limb-threatening thromboembolism may require thrombolysis. Absolute contraindications to the use of thrombolytics include recent intracranial hemorrhage or stroke, known cerebrovascular abnormality, and malignant intracranial neoplasm. Relative contraindications include recent major surgery, uncontrolled hypertension, and recent significant bleeding episode. Tissue plasminogen activator (tPA) is most frequently given systemically (dose) and should be done in consultation with hematology. Catheter-directed tPA is reserved for severe extremity deep vein thrombosis (DVT) and requires both hematology and interventional radiology expertise for administration. Thrombectomy may be required for patients who are post cardiac surgery and have an intracardiac clot.

PULMONARY EMBOLUS

Risk factors for the development of a pulmonary embolus (PE) in children are similar to those for adults: prior/current central venous catheter, immobility, use of estrogen-containing oral contraception, recent surgery, malignancy, vascular malformations, nephrotic syndrome, and lupus. Approximately 50% of patients will also have a concurrent lower extremity DVT, and ultrasound (US) evaluation should be completed. Symptoms include shortness of breath, pleuritic chest pain, cough, dyspnea, and tachycardia. Initial changes on chest X-ray or echocardiogram could be suggestive of a PE; however, CT or MRA is needed for definitive diagnosis. Anticoagulation with either UFH or LMWH is first-line therapy. Hemodynamically unstable patients with cardiac compromise may require thrombolysis or thrombectomy if tPA is unsuccessful or contraindicated.

ARTERIAL THROMBOEMBOLISM

Indwelling catheters, cardiac catheterization procedures, as well as some uncorrected congenital cardiac lesions place children at risk for extremity arterial thromboemboli. On examination, the affected extremity may be cool, dusky, and pale with decreased pulses and prolonged capillary refill. Decreased or absent arterial blood flow on US with Doppler confirms the diagnosis. Indwelling catheters should be removed and a repeat US obtained to assess for improvement in blood flow. For patients with a symptomatic arterial clot, heparin products (UFH or LMWH) can be given until resolution of symptoms. For patients with more severe thrombus with significant life- or limb-threatening symptoms, consider emergent thrombolysis or thrombectomy.

ARTERIAL STROKE

An acute ischemic stroke is a rare event in pediatrics, with an incidence of approximately 2.4/100,000 per year and 25% of cases seen in neonates. These events are more common in patients with cardiac disease, particularly with shunt physiology or SCD. In neonates, various factors contribute to stroke risk that are not necessarily hematologic in nature, with some strokes having occurred in utero. Symptomatic neonates may present with lethargy, seizures, or coma, whereas older children may have acute focal neurologic changes.

The preferred imaging modality for diagnosis is brain MRI/MRA; however, this may not be feasible for young pediatric patients in the ED setting. Although a brain CT is easier to obtain in the ED, small lesions and acute events (<12–24 hours) may be missed. An electrocardiogram and echocardiogram should be obtained in all children with strokes to assess for a possible cardioembolic source, and neurology should be consulted.

Neuroprotective measures include fever reduction, seizure control, maintaining normoglycemia, and avoiding hypotensive episodes. There remains controversy regarding the use of antiplatelet versus anticoagulation therapy in pediatric patients. Anticoagulation therapy is recommended for patients with a cardioembolic source or arterial dissection. Contraindications to initiation of anticoagulation therapy include increased risk of hemorrhagic conversion, severe hypertension, or other risk for intracranial bleeding. Neurology and hematology can aid in ED management and disposition of patients.

KEY POINTS

- Initial therapy for acute, symptomatic VTE is anticoagulation with a heparin-based product. Patients who are clinically unstable, at risk for bleeding, or require surgical procedures should be given IV heparin.
- Patients with a PE should also be evaluated for extremity DVT.
- Duration of anticoagulation therapy for VTE is much longer than that needed for arterial clot.
- Venous or arterial thrombotic events that are life- or limb-threatening may require thrombolysis, if not otherwise contraindicated, or thrombectomy.

PITFALLS

- An incidental VTE found in asymptomatic patients may not require anticoagulation and can be observed for resolution.
- Renal function should be assessed prior to initiation of heparin-based anticoagulation because it is renally cleared.
- Arterial central venous catheters can cause vasospasm with clinical symptoms identical to those of an arterial clot. Re-imaging with Doppler US should be done after arterial catheter removal prior to initiation of therapy.
- Brain CT in evaluation of a stroke may miss small lesions or acute events (<12–24 hours).

Further Reading

Subramaniam S, Chao JH. Managing acute complications of sickle cell disease in pediatric patients. *Pediatr Emerg Med Pract*. 2016;13(11):1–28.

U.S. Department of Health and Human Services. *Evidence-Based Management of Sickle Cell Disease: Expert Panel Report, 2014*. Bethesda, MD: U.S. Department of Health and Human Services.

World Federation of Hemophilia. *Guidelines for the Management of Hemophilia*. 2nd ed. Montreal, Quebec, Canada: World Federation of Hemophilia; 2012. doi:10.1111/j.1365-2516.2012.02909.x.

Zapotocka E, Curtin JA, Blanchette VS. Managing hemophilia in children and adolescents. In: Blanchette VS, Brandão LR, Breakey VR, Revel-Vilk S, eds. *SickKids Handbook of Pediatric Thrombosis and Hemostatis*. 2nd ed. Basel, Switzerland: Karger; 2017:71–96.

29

Pediatric Oncologic Emergencies

ARA FESTEKJIAN

INTRODUCTION

Although relatively rare in children, patients with cancer often present with life-threatening conditions that require recognition and intervention. Oncologic emergencies may be due to the underlying oncologic process or result from the therapy initiated to treat the disease. Patients undergoing therapy for their cancer will have compromised immune systems and decreased function of vital organs from chemotherapeutic agent toxicity, sometimes resulting in diagnostic and therapeutic dilemmas and hastening their demise.

MEDIASTINAL MASS

Background

The mediastinum is the area in the chest cavity that separates the lungs from other vital organs, including the heart, aorta, esophagus, thymus, and trachea. Mediastinal tumors can originate in the anterior, middle, and posterior portions of the mediastinum.

Anterior mediastinal masses include germ cell tumors, leukemia, lymphoma (including Hodgkin's and non-Hodgkin's), thymomas, and thyroid masses. Middle mediastinal tumors include bronchogenic cysts, pericardial cysts, sarcoidosis, histiocytosis, and tracheal tumors. Posterior mediastinal tumors include neurogenic tumors originating from the sympathetic nerve chains such as neuroblastoma, sarcoma, and ganglioneuroblastoma.

Clinical Presentation

Most clinical presentations of mediastinal tumors result from their mass effect:

- Tracheal compression may lead to vocal cord paralysis, severe breathing problems, and acute airway compromise.
- Superior vena cava syndrome results from obstructed veins preventing normal venous return of blood and may cause facial swelling, orthopnea, and plethora. Superior vena cava syndrome and tracheal compression often occur jointly given their anatomic proximity.
- Esophageal compression may lead to severe dysphagia.
- Pediatric patients will commonly present with respiratory complaints, whereas adult patients will present with chest pain or be asymptomatic.

Special Consideration: Critical Mediastinal Mass Leading to Acute Airway Compromise

Concerning features of mediastinal masses for life-threatening emergencies include the following:

- Anterior mediastinal location
- Histological diagnosis of lymphoma
- Symptoms and signs of superior vena cava syndrome
- Radiological evidence of vessel compression or displacement
- Pleural and pericardial effusions, with the latter predisposing to pericardial tamponade

Classic Clinical Presentation

The typical presentation of a mediastinal mass involves a teenager who has recurrent and persistent cough or chest pain despite trial of common therapies. Diagnosis is typically made on screening chest radiograph. These patients are commonly initially misdiagnosed with upper respiratory infections due to the nonspecific nature of symptoms.

Atypical Clinical Presentation

Superior vena cava syndrome may uncommonly be the presenting syndrome. Varicose veins on the chest may serve as a clue. Horner's syndrome and periorbital ecchymosis may result from the mass effect of neuroblastoma in the posterior mediastinum. A small subset of children will have significant airway involvement at the time of presentation, and lying supine may precipitate complete airway collapse.

Diagnostic Confirmation

Mediastinal masses are diagnosed with imaging, and exact histopathology is needed to determine underlying etiology. There can be multiple radiographic findings, including widened mediastinum, pleural effusion, pericardial effusion, and airway collapse.

Treatment

Therapy for mediastinal masses depends on the underlying tissue diagnosis and can include surgical resection, radiation therapy, chemotherapy, and corticosteroids. Each diagnosis has its own predetermined regimen depending on histopathology, and children with airway involvement are treated by a multidisciplinary team aimed at minimizing consequences from procedures and anesthesia.

Potential complications (including death) may arise from anesthesia and lying supine for imaging. High-risk features include orthopnea, facial edema, and dyspnea at rest. Children with significant tracheal compression require intensive care monitoring and may have emergent radiation therapy even prior to tissue diagnosis.

Disposition

Patients with mediastinal masses should be hospitalized; intensive care unit admission is indicated with significant airway compression.

Complications

The most serious complication is complete airway obstruction leading to respiratory failure and cardiac arrest.

Key Points

- Anterior mediastinal masses may potentially completely obstruct the airway.
- Concomitant superior vena cava syndrome is more likely to have associated significant airway involvement.

Pitfalls

- Failure to anticipate airway compromise in mediastinal masses may have devastating consequences.
- Avoid sedating mechanisms and supine positioning.
- Failure to consider this rare diagnosis in common presentations such as recurrent wheezing and cough will further delay diagnosis.

CENTRAL NERVOUS SYSTEM ONCOLOGIC EMERGENCIES

Background

Brain tumors are the most common solid tumors in childhood. Brain tumors elevate intracranial pressure with a delayed diagnosis. Headache, particularly early morning headache, is the most common presenting complaint.

Classic Clinical Presentation

Headaches that are occipital in location, persistent or unremitting, associated with focal neurological symptoms or vomiting, and cause awakening at night have a higher likelihood of associated intracranial findings on radiographic studies. Focal weakness without headache may also be a presenting complaint for some brain tumors. When associated with increased intracranial pressure, headaches tend to be worse in the morning with vomiting and tend to improve during the day when the child is more upright. In the younger infant, findings may include increasing head circumference and persistently open cranial sutures. Patients may present for several visits with headache prior to diagnosis.

Atypical Clinical Presentation

Papilledema may be present with increased intracranial pressure and the initial clue to diagnosis. Torticollis in the infant may be an intracranial mass in the brainstem. Hydrocephalus with increased intracranial hypertension may also be an initial finding with delay in care or a missed diagnosis. Other presenting symptoms include ataxia, gait abnormalities, and seizures (generalized or focal).

Diagnostic Confirmation

Magnetic resonance imaging (MRI) is the preferred imaging modality in patients with concern for brain tumor. A computed tomography (CT) scan may be performed if MRI is unavailable.

Treatment

Definitive therapy (e.g., surgical resection, chemotherapy, and radiation) is determined by biopsy and tumor location. Emergent ventricular shunting may be required to treat intracranial hypertension prior to definitive therapy.

Disposition

Most children diagnosed with an intracranial mass are admitted for diagnostic and therapeutic intervention. Associated hydrocephalus requires intensive care-level monitoring.

Complications

Intracranial hypertension may result in brain herniation and death if not diagnosed and appropriately managed. Focal weaknesses may be permanent. Hydrocephalus may occur and require emergent ventriculoperitoneal shunt placement. Acute brain tumor hemorrhage may present with seizure, acute worsening pain, or new neurologic deficits. Metastatic lesions involving the spinal cord may have permanent devastating neurological sequelae.

Key Points

- Headache is the most common presentation of a brain tumor. Concerning features include occipital location; nighttime awakening/early morning worsening; and persistent, associated focal neurologic deficits.
- A thorough neurologic examination (including visual fields and assessment for papilledema) should be performed on every patient presenting with a headache, even if they appear well.
- Hydrocephalus may develop initially when first being diagnosed or subsequently as a result of recurrence of the mass, usually in the posterior fossa.

Pitfalls

- Posterior fossa masses may be missed on CT imaging alone.
- Lumbar punctures in patients suspected of having increased intracranial hypertension are contraindicated and may precipitate herniation if there is sufficiently increased intracranial pressure.

TUMOR LYSIS SYNDROME

Background

Tumor lysis syndrome (TLS) is an oncologic emergency resulting from tumor cell breakdown releasing potassium, phosphates, and nucleic acids, leading to hyperuricemia, symptomatic hypocalcemia, and secondary renal failure and cardiac dysrhythmias. TLS occurs in malignancies such as leukemia and lymphoma, due to rapid cell turnover and high tumor burden. TLS can manifest prior to the initiation of therapy or as a consequence of starting chemotherapy, particularly corticosteroids.

Classic Clinical Presentation

Tumor lysis syndrome is usually suspected in high-risk conditions prior to becoming symptomatic. If diagnosis is delayed or hyperuricemia is not suspected, symptoms can include fatigue; muscle cramps/twitching; vomiting; decreased urine output; edema; hematuria; and, in severe cases, seizures, cardiac dysrhythmias, and death due to multiorgan failure. Renal insufficiency and dehydration at the time of diagnosis increase the risk of developing TLS.

Atypical Clinical Presentation

Hyperkalemia leading to cardiac dysrhythmias and cardiovascular collapse may be a presentation of TLS.

Diagnostic Confirmation

Every new diagnosis of leukemia and lymphoma should be evaluated for TLS. Laboratory testing includes complete blood count, electrolytes (serum potassium, calcium, magnesium, phosphate, uric acid, and urea nitrogen), cardiac monitoring, and electrocardiograms to assess a widened QRS complex and peaked T waves in the setting of hyperkalemia and renal failure.

Treatment

Hydration with close monitoring of intake and output is critical to preventing TLS. Intravenous (IV) fluids without potassium and allopurinol (300 mg/m^2 PO, divided TID) are started prior to the initiation of cytolytic therapy. Urine alkalinization (urine pH goal of 6.5–7.5) aids in the excretion of uric acid. Those at higher risk can also be given rasburicase (urate oxidase) to help metabolize uric acid. This is contraindicated in glucose 6-phosphate deficiency, pregnancy, and lactation. Hyperkalemia (>6.0 mEq/L) that is asymptomatic may be treated with sodium polystyrene sulfonate (1 g/kg PO every 6 hours). Hyperkalemia that is symptomatic or >7.0 mEq/L is treated with the following:

- Glucose, dextrose 25 (2 mL/kg) IV with regular insulin (0.1 U/kg IV)
- Calcium gluconate 150 mg/kg IV

Dialysis or renal replacement therapy may be necessary for hyperkalemia and hyperphosphatemia not responding sufficiently to the therapies previously discussed.

Disposition

All patients with or at risk for developing TLS require inpatient hospitalization. Intensive care may be required for severe cases.

Complications

Renal failure, cardiac arrhythmias, and death can occur without appropriate monitoring and therapy.

Key Points

- High tumor burden and rapidly proliferating malignancies predispose to TLS.
- Hydration, urine alkalinization, allopurinol, and, at times, rasburicase and dialysis may be necessary to treat TLS.
- TLS can happen even prior to the start of initiating cytolytic therapy.

Pitfalls

- Rasburicase is contraindicated in glucose 6-phophate deficiency, pregnancy, and lactation.
- Failure to recognize TLS can lead to renal failure and fatal cardiac arrhythmias.
- Excessive urine alkalinization (urine pH >7.5) may lead to precipitation of calcium phosphate and xanthine crystals.

FEBRILE NEUTROPENIA AND SEPTIC SHOCK

Background

The combination of immunocompromise, neutropenia, and indwelling central venous catheters makes children susceptible to serious infections that are life-threatening if not recognized and treated promptly.

Classic Clinical Presentation

Fever in the possibly neutropenic patient is defined as a temperature >38.2°C (101°F) or two consecutive temperatures >38.0°C (100.4°F) taken orally in a 12-hour period. Rectal temperatures should never be performed in patients receiving chemotherapy. The absence of fever does not exclude infection, especially if a patient's chemotherapy regimen involves the use of steroids. Clinically significant neutropenia occurs when the absolute neutrophil count (ANC) is <500/μL. The febrile neutropenic patient may have varying areas that serve as a nidus for infection, including oral lesions, the perirectal area, and central venous access sites. These patients may also present in florid septic shock without an identified source.

Atypical Clinical Presentation

With significant immunocompromise, pneumonia may be present without chest radiography infiltrates. Typhlitis, or neutropenic enterocolitis, may present with right lower quadrant tenderness and diarrhea (due to transmural inflammation of the cecum). The ascending colon and ileum may be involved in severe cases. Necrotizing enterocolitis may develop and should be suspected with persistent abdominal pain. These patients require surgical consultation, broader antibiotic coverage, and are at risk for bowel perforation. Syncope and hypotension may be the presentation of shock or sequelae of some cancer treatments.

Diagnostic Confirmation

Laboratory testing includes a complete blood count [to evaluate for neutropenia and complications such as disseminated intravascular coagulation (DIC)], electrolytes, assessment of renal function with blood urea nitrogen/creatinine, and blood cultures obtained peripherally or from a dwelling central line.

Chest radiographs should be performed in suspected pneumonia, pulmonary edema, or hypoxia. Ultrasound or CT scans may be indicated with abdominal pain.

Treatment

Fever in the possibly neutropenic cancer patient is approached aggressively with specific treatment protocols and nationally accepted best practice algorithms. Rapid initial assessment and empiric broad-spectrum antibiotics covering gram-negative organisms (after obtaining blood cultures) should be administered expeditiously (within 30–60 minutes) after arrival to the emergency department. Monotherapy is typically sufficient, with the exact drug chosen varying based on institutional organism susceptibility patterns and including pseudomonal coverage. Cefepime, ceftazidime, piperacillin–tazobactam, and meropenem are commonly utilized. When treating sepsis, gram-positive coverage with vancomycin is added along with a second gram-negative covering antibiotic such as amikacin or gentamicin. Vancomycin should be given with toxic appearance, severe mucositis, and typhlitis. Metronidazole should be given with typhlitis and perirectal findings. Despite routine preventative treatment for *Pneumocystis jirovecii,* this diagnosis should be suspected with severe hypoxemia. Persistent abdominal pain should prompt imaging and surgical consultation for potential operative intervention for perforation.

Septic shock not responsive to volume resuscitation will also require inotropes and escalation of care. Corticosteroids may be required (i.e., for those receiving prednisone as part of their chemotherapy regimen or as treatment of graft-versus-host disease). Blood products including platelets, packed red blood cells, and fresh frozen plasma may also be required when treating septic shock, bleeding, or DIC. (See Chapter 12 on pediatric sepsis.)

Disposition

All patients with febrile neutropenia with an ANC <500/μL require hospitalization and possibly in the intensive care unit if septic shock or typhlitis is present.

Complications

The febrile neutropenic patient may have overwhelming septic shock and succumb to this disease. With typhlitis, they may have intestinal perforation requiring operating room intervention, which carries a high mortality. Cancer patients with DIC may have intracranial, pulmonary, or gastrointestinal bleeding. Severe pancreatitis may exist in conjunction with sepsis. Pericardial effusions resulting from radiation therapy or infections may lead to cardiac tamponade.

Key Points

- Any cancer patient receiving chemotherapy is at risk for overwhelming infection and requires prompt resuscitation.
- Adherence to nationally available guidelines for fever neutropenia and septic shock improves outcomes in febrile neutropenic patients.
- Frequent monitoring and re-examination are vital in caring for the febrile neutropenic cancer patient.

Pitfalls

- Failure to administer antibiotics, volume resuscitation, and inotropes in a timely manner can lead to greater harm to the neutropenic cancer patient.
- Earlier use of inotropes with concomitant lower total volume

resuscitation may be needed in patients receiving cardiotoxic chemotherapy agents.

SYNDROME OF INAPPROPRIATE ANTIDIURETIC HORMONE

Background

Excessive secretion of antidiuretic hormone (ADH) is known as syndrome of inappropriate antidiuretic hormone (SIADH). Excessive water resorption by the kidneys results in euvolemic hyponatremia, increasing the risk for hyponatremic seizures. SIADH is a common cause of hyponatremia in oncology, occurring in brain tumors, as a paraneoplastic syndrome, or induced by chemotherapy drugs. Vincristine is the cause of SIADH in the treatment of pediatric acute lymphoblastic leukemia (ALL). It causes neurotoxicity on the hypothalamic–pituitary axis, affecting the normal osmolality control of ADH secretion.

Classic Clinical Presentation

Occasionally, SIADH be asymptomatic and discovered on routine testing of electrolytes during treatment regimens. When present, its effects may be seen or anticipated approximately 4–7 days after receiving chemotherapy. Symptoms include nausea, vomiting, tremors, and cramping. These types of symptoms in a patient at risk should trigger one to perform blood and urine testing to determine if SIADH is present.

Atypical Clinical Presentation

More severe symptoms include irritability, altered mood, memory impairment, confusion, and hallucinations. In the worst cases, patients may have seizures and stupor or coma.

Diagnostic Confirmation

Persistent urinary excretion of sodium occurs despite the presence of hyponatremia and low intake of sodium. Additional brain imaging may be indicated to evaluate for intracranial hemorrhage or mass effects.

Treatment

The cornerstone of therapy for SIADH is fluid and water restriction. Vasopressin may be used to inhibit the action of ADH. Surgical removal should be performed in an ADH-secreting tumor. In active seizure or significant altered mental status, 3% sodium chloride should be administered until the patient clinically recovers, and then a slower correction is warranted.

Complications

Patients who present with neurologic impairment or have severe hyponatremia even in the absence of symptoms may go on to develop permanent neurologic impairment. Cerebral edema leading to cerebral herniation may occur when plasma osmolality decreases rapidly (faster than 10 mOsm/kg/hr).

Key Points

- Vincristine in the treatment for pediatric ALL is known to cause SIADH.
- Most common treatment for SIADH is fluid and water restriction.
- In severe cases, rapid but judicious treatment with 3% sodium chloride may be indicated.

Pitfalls

- Failure to anticipate and test for SIADH following administration of vincristine may worsen morbidity and mortality.
- SIADH may occur from multiple causes, and it is prudent to have a broad approach depending on the context of specific patient presentations.
- In asymptomatic patients particularly, rapid correction of serum sodium may lead to permanent impairment from central pontine myelinolysis.

SPINAL CORD COMPRESSION

Background

Spinal cord compression can result from malignant tissue invading the vertebrae (metastatic or direct spread) and causing pressure and collapse of the spinal cord. It can be one of the more devastating presentations for cancer. Vertebral venous plexus compression may also cause venous hemorrhage, cord edema, and ischemia resulting in tissue injury similar to a stroke. Spinal cord compression can occur at the time of diagnosis, with tumor progression, or with recurrence. Spinal cord compression, even if recognized promptly, may lead to permanent neurologic damage. The spine is a site for metastatic disease due to its rich blood supply and extensive lymphatic drainage. Many pediatric malignancies can lead to spinal cord compression, including leukemia, Wilms' tumor, sarcomas, neuroblastoma, lymphoma, and metastases of primary central nervous system tumors.

Classic Clinical Presentation

Spinal cord compression may present with neurologic symptoms stemming from the area of tissue compression, ischemia, or damage. Symptoms include progressive pain, sensory loss, motor weakness to paralysis, spinal deformity, and loss of sphincter control. The findings can develop insidiously (usually over 2 months), resulting in diagnostic delay.

Atypical Clinical Presentation

Spinal cord compression may be the initial presentation of malignancy given the insidious onset from pain to neurologic symptoms. Back pain in patients with prior malignancy should be thoroughly evaluated for potential spinal cord involvement. Thoracic spinal lesions may present with spasticity rather than weakness. In contrast to musculoskeletal back pain, back pain in spinal cord compression occurs higher in the spine and improves with activity.

Diagnostic Confirmation

Magnetic resonance imaging with gadolinium contrast enhancement is the modality of choice in diagnosing spinal cord compression.

Treatment

Emergent neurosurgical intervention is the most important therapy in acute spinal cord compression. The main goal in the treatment of spinal cord compression is preserving and, if diagnosed sufficiently early, reversing any neurologic manifestations, although full recovery after the onset of motor symptoms is rare. Adjunctive therapies include steroids, directed chemotherapy, and physical therapy aiming to preserve motor function. Radiation therapy either alone or in combination with other modalities is also utilized.

Complications

Neurologic consequences including paralysis and loss of sphincter control are devastating complications of spinal cord compression. Very rarely do patients have full recovery from spinal cord compression, and those with milder symptoms and earlier recognition and therapy have better outcomes.

Key Points

- Spinal cord compression can occur in many types of tumors either as primary or as metastatic spread.
- Spinal cord compression can have devastating consequences, including paralysis and loss of sphincter control.
- Magnetic resonance imaging with gadolinium contrast enhancement is the most sensitive method to diagnose spinal cord compression.

Pitfalls

- Failure to recognize that back pain in a patient with malignancy may be the first symptom of spinal cord compression may lead to delays in diagnosis.
- Failure to recognize differences in musculoskeletal from spinal cord compression back pain may lead to delays resulting in poorer outcomes.

Further Reading

Boussios S, Cooke D, Hayward C, et al. Metastatic spinal cord compression: Unraveling the diagnostic and therapeutic challenges. *Anticancer Res.* 2018;38:4987–4997.

Chen CH, Wu KH, Chao YH, Weng DF, Chang JS, Lin CH. Clinical manifestations of pediatric mediastinal tumors, a single center experience. *Medicine.* 2019;98(32):e16732.

30

Endocrine Emergencies

DAVIDA HEMMY, HENRIK GALUST, AND KATIE BAKES

INTRODUCTION

Endocrinology is the study of the system of glands that secrete hormones. Hormones are unique chemical structures that "communicate" with target cells, controlling growth regulation, metabolism, reproduction, and homeostasis. At the heart of the endocrine system is the hypothalamic–pituitary axis. A resplendent and nuanced feedback control center, this axis regulates the activity of the adrenal cortex, the thyroid gland, and the gonads through circulating hormones. Even endocrine glands outside the direct control of the hypothalamic–pituitary–adrenal (HPA) axis, such as the pancreas, are subject to regulation governed by the feedback of serum glucose and calcium levels. Despite the complexities of the endocrine system, clinical endocrinology can be approached simply by learning to recognize the signs and symptoms of hormone excesses and deficiencies (Box 30.1).

PITUITARY DISORDERS

Background

The pituitary gland sits within the sella turcica, at the base of the brain, and coordinates the function of other endocrine glands throughout the body, including the thyroid gland, the adrenals, and the gonads. The pituitary gland also connects to the hypothalamus and forms the hypothalamic–pituitary axis, which regulates growth, metabolism, temperature, sexual function, and stress response.

The pituitary gland is composed of two lobes: the anterior lobe, or adenohypophysis, and the posterior lobe, or neurohypophysis. The anterior pituitary is stimulated by hypothalamic-releasing hormones (e.g., growth hormone-releasing hormone, corticotropin-releasing hormone, thyrotropin-releasing hormone, and gonadotropin-releasing hormone) to release trophic hormones: adrenocorticotropic hormone (ACTH), growth hormone, thyrotropin [i.e., thyroid-stimulating hormone (TSH)], follicle-stimulating hormone (FSH), luteinizing hormone (LH), and prolactin. The posterior pituitary stores and releases oxytocin and vasopressin.

Like all endocrine pathology, pituitary pathology occurs from an excess or deficiency of its hormones. Central diabetes insipidus, for example, is due to inadequate vasopressin (antidiuretic hormone) production in the setting of posterior pituitary dysfunction. Patients with pituitary dysfunction may present with signs or symptoms of one or more hormone irregularities, and these findings are often quite subtle.

BOX 30.1
GENERAL SIGNS AND SYMPTOMS OF PEDIATRIC ENDOCRINE EMERGENCIES

- Central nervous system
  - Altered mental status
  - Apnea
  - Cheyne–Stokes respirations
  - Coma
  - Hyperreflexia
  - Hypotonia
  - Irritability
  - Lethargy
  - Seizures
  - Weakness
- Cardiovascular
  - Hypotension
  - Shock
  - Tachycardia
- Metabolic
  - Anorexia
  - Exercise intolerance
  - Failure to thrive
  - Kussmaul respiration
  - Nausea
  - Vomiting
  - Weight loss

CUSHING'S DISEASE

Background

Cushing's syndrome is a rare disorder that results from prolonged exposure to excess glucocorticoid hormone concentrations; approximately 10% of new cases occur in the pediatric population. Among pediatric cases, most (75–80%) are caused by Cushing's disease (CD)—that is, an ACTH-secreting pituitary adenoma. The median age of presentation of pediatric CD is 14.1 years, with an equal incidence of CD among males and females.

Classic Clinical Presentation

The key presenting features in children with CD are weight gain (98%), facial plethora (100%), virilization (44%), and growth failure (37%). The mean duration of symptoms prior to diagnosis in pediatric patients is 2.5 ± 1.7 years. If from a pituitary tumor that compresses the optic chiasm, patients may have cuts to their temporal visual fields.

Atypical Clinical Presentation

Although it is unusual, non-pituitary tumors (Cushing's syndrome) may be responsible for excess ACTH. Common locations for such tumors include the lungs, pancreas, and thyroid. However, even a case involving a neonatal sacrococcygeal teratoma has been reported. Although rare, inherited multiple endocrine neoplasia type 1 is a familial syndrome that can cause ACTH-producing tumors.

Differential Diagnosis

The differential diagnosis includes exogenous glucocorticoid use and hormone-secreting tumors of the brain, pituitary, and adrenals.

Diagnosis

The diagnosis of Cushing's syndrome first requires clinical suspicion. The diagnosis is subsequently confirmed by elevated salivary cortisol levels, 24-hour urinary free cortisol levels, or a positive dexamethasone suppression test. Figure 30.1 shows a simple algorithm for determining the etiology of Cushing's syndrome. Pituitary magnetic resonance imaging (MRI) is the imaging of choice for pituitary visualization and surgical planning.

Treatment

Trans-sphenoidal surgery is the first-line therapy for removal of a pituitary adenoma, with up to 98% of children in remission post-surgery. For those with persistent disease, pituitary radiotherapy is second-line therapy. Long-term medical therapy has not been well studied in children. However, in acutely ill patients, adrenal steroidogenesis inhibitors, such as ketoconazole and metyrapone, can be used to lower cortisol levels.

Disposition

Lasting remission is seen in younger children, in those with smaller tumors, and in those without cavernous sinus or dural invasion. In adults, recurrence has been seen up to 15 years post-surgery. Thus, lifelong follow-up with an endocrinologist is recommended for all children with CD.

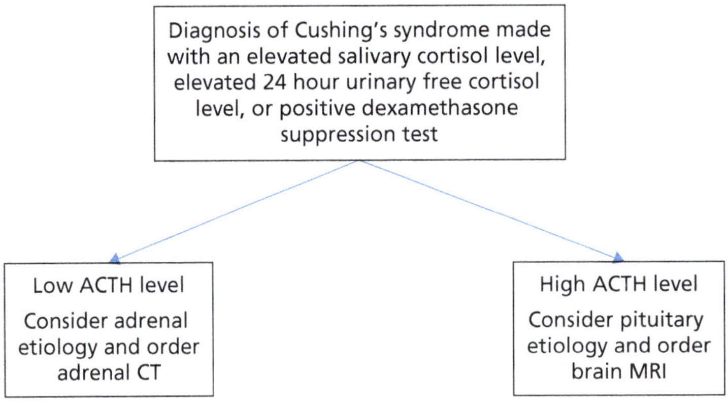

FIGURE 30.1 Diagnostic algorithm for Cushing' syndrome.

Complications

Prolonged exposure to elevated levels of glucocorticoids is associated with hypercoagulability, metabolic syndrome, growth impairment, osteopenia, obesity, and psychiatric sequelae. Reports have shown that hypertension persists in 16% of patients with CD and 21% of patients with ACTH-independent Cushing's syndrome.

Key Points

- Pediatric patients make up approximately 10% of patients diagnosed with Cushing's syndrome.
- Surgical resection of pituitary adenoma is first-line therapy.
- Despite a 98% post-surgical remission, close follow-up with an endocrinologist is important to mitigate consequences of prolonged exposure to elevated glucocorticoid levels and to ensure continued remission.

PITUITARY APOPLEXY

Background

The word *apoplexy* originates from Greek and means the sudden impairment of cerebral function. Pituitary apoplexy is most commonly the result of hemorrhage from an underlying adenoma; however, it can also be due to trauma or infarct. The sudden increase in sellar volume compresses surrounding structures, resulting in both endocrine and neurologic signs and symptoms. Pituitary apoplexy, or sudden complete pituitary dysfunction, is a medical emergency, and recognition of the condition and rapid hydrocortisone administration may be life-saving. In more than 50% of patients, clinical apoplexy will be the first indication of an underlying adenoma. However, up to 25% of hemorrhages due to pituitary adenomas occur without symptoms, referred to as "subclinical apoplexy." As stated previously, pituitary apoplexy is most commonly caused by hemorrhage, but it can also be due to infarction of the pituitary gland. When this occurs in women around childbirth due to hypotension secondary to peripartum hemorrhage, it is called Sheehan's syndrome.

Classic Clinical Presentation

Acute severe headache is the most common and earliest symptom of pituitary apoplexy. Patients may also exhibit nausea and vomiting. Third, fourth, fifth, and sixth cranial nerve palsies occur with cavernous sinus involvement. Clinically, this is seen in as many as 70% of patients. Fever, neck stiffness, photophobia, and decreased level of consciousness can also occur. Galactorrhea and amenorrhea are often present at the time of diagnosis. An MRI of the brain is the test of choice and can identify tumor and hemorrhage of the pituitary.

Atypical Clinical Presentation

Studies in children with traumatic brain injury (TBI) have demonstrated various endocrinopathies, the most common of which are growth hormone deficiency (6–48%) and ACTH deficiency (2–43%). Direct mechanical injury, hypoxic insult, edema, and compression from hemorrhage may all contribute to pituitary dysfunction after TBI. Autoimmunity is also thought to play a role in pituitary dysfunction after TBI. Clinical signs of anterior hypopituitarism or subclinical apoplexy are subtle and can be masked by the sequelae of TBI, making diagnosis difficult without clinical suspicion.

Differential Diagnosis

The differential diagnosis of pituitary apoplexy includes subarachnoid hemorrhage (SAH), cavernous sinus thrombosis, meningitis/encephalitis, and brainstem infarction or lesion.

Diagnosis

The diagnosis of pituitary apoplexy should be considered in any patient with severe headache if SAH and meningitis have been ruled out; the patient has neuro-ophthalmic signs; or the patient has a pre-existing pituitary tumor. However, 80% of patients will have no prior history of pituitary pathology.

Treatment

Surgical decompression and corticosteroid therapy are the mainstays of treatment for pituitary apoplexy caused by tumors. Subclinical apoplexy or anterior hypopituitarism has been less well studied. However, hormone levels should be closely followed and symptoms addressed when they present.

Disposition

Postoperative patients should be followed closely by specialists in neurosurgery and endocrinology. Patients with anterior hypopituitarism due to TBI are a more unique entity. Pediatricians and specialty consultants should consider symptom monitoring and routine screening for pituitary hormone dysfunction. Common symptoms by hormone deficiency include the following:

ACTH: fatigue, pallor, anorexia, weight loss

ADH: polyuria, polydipsia

TSH: neurodevelopmental delay, amenorrhea, delayed puberty, short stature

Growth hormone: fall from growth curve

LH and FSH: delayed or absent puberty

Key Points

- Pediatric patients with pituitary apoplexy or subclinical apoplexy tend to exhibit more indolent symptoms than the adult population and may have more favorable neurologic and endocrine outcomes.
- Research suggests that children may be less susceptible to infarction and more tolerant of hemorrhage compared to adults.

DISORDERS OF THE THYROID GLAND

The thyroid gland plays a critical role in neurocognitive development as well as in normal growth and development. Consequently, early identification and treatment of thyroid disease in young patients are critical for continued healthy growth and development. Thyroid function is so diverse, and its hormones act on such a wide variety of cells throughout the body, that its dysfunction can present in many forms. Table 30.1 lists the clinical manifestations of thyroid dysfunction by organ system.

HYPOTHYROIDISM

Background

Hypothyroidism is characterized by low or absent thyroid hormone levels, and it can be either congenital or acquired. Autoimmune thyroiditis (Hashimoto's disease) is the most common cause of acquired hypothyroidism. Although less common, congenital hypothyroidism is the second leading cause of endocrine emergencies in neonates after hypoglycemia. Testing for congenital hypothyroidism is part of all newborn screening programs in the United States, and it is performed in most developed nations. The most common cause of congenital hypothyroidism is thyroid dysgenesis. Central hypothyroidism (e.g., low TSH) is less common; associated with pituitary dysfunction; and patients often present with signs or symptoms of other endocrine abnormalities, such as microphallus, hypoglycemia, or jaundice. Table 30.2 lists the causes of hypothyroidism.

Classic Clinical Presentation

Signs and symptoms of hypothyroidism may be subtle in children. Fatigue, cold intolerance, constipation, and menstrual irregularities are the most common symptoms of hypothyroidism. Younger children may also

TABLE 30.1 CLINICAL MANIFESTATIONS OF THYROID DYSFUNCTION

Organ System	Hypothyroidism	Hyperthyroidism
Cardiovascular	Decreased cardiac output, bradycardia, pericardial effusion	Supraventricular tachycardia, atrial fibrillation, decreased peripheral resistance, increased cardiac output
Respiratory	Pleural effusion, obstructive sleep apnea	Decreased vital capacity
Gut	Weight gain, constipation, achlorhydria	Weight loss, diarrhea, nausea and vomiting, celiac disease
Genitourinary	Delayed puberty	Delayed puberty
Renal	Decreased renal blood flow, decreased glomerular filtration rate	Increased renal blood flow and glomerular filtration rate
Metabolism	Decreased appetite, cold intolerance, low body temperature, increased insulin sensitivity	Decreased glucose tolerance, increased appetites
Musculoskeletal	Poor growth and maturation of bone	Demineralization of bone, hypercalcemia, weakness
Neuro	Cretinism, depression	Tremor, hyperkinesia, emotional lability, nervousness
Skin	Myxedema, dry skin, brittle hair and nails	Onycholysis of nails

Source: Adapted from Nussey S, Whitehead S. *Endocrinology: An Integrated Approach.* Oxford, UK: BIOS Scientific; 2001.

present with either delayed or precocious puberty.

Atypical Clinical Presentation

Acquired hypothyroidism may occur with ingestion of amiodarone, expectorants, anticonvulsants, interferon-α, lithium, and medications used to treat hyperthyroid conditions

TABLE 30.2 CAUSES OF HYPOTHYROIDISM

Primary disorders	Common
	Hashimoto's thyroiditis
	Post-radioiodine therapy
	Post-thyroidectomy
	Uncommon
	Thyroiditis
	Anti-thyroid drugs
	Impaired T_4 synthesis
	Rare
	Thyroid hormone resistance
	Loss of function TSH receptor mutations
Secondary disorders	Hypopituitarism
	Impaired TSH synthesis
Tertiary disorders	Hypothalamic dysfunction due to tumors, radiotherapy, trauma

TSH, thyroid-stimulating hormone.

Case Example

A 5-year-old female without routine access to medical care presents to the emergency department with a complaint of cough, congestion, and fever for 5 days. She has had headache, vomiting, and altered mental status for the past day. Her parents report she was a term infant, with normal development and growth for the first 2 years of life. For the past 3 years, she has had little height growth and decreased exercise tolerance. Her current vital signs are notable for hypothermia, bradycardia, hypotension, and hypoxia. A chest X-ray reveals pneumonia. TSH is high, and free triiodothronine (T_3) and free thyroxine (T_4) levels are low.

This case represents myxedema coma, an extreme manifestation of hypothyroidism in patients who are undertreated, and is often precipitated by an infection such as pneumonia. Hashimoto's thyroiditis is one of the most common endocrine deficiencies encountered in pediatric patients. It is characterized by autoimmune destruction of the thyroid gland, and although not uncommon, it may be overlooked in pediatric patients until a concomitant illness unmasks severe symptoms. Pediatric patients with myxedema coma often present with altered mental status or coma, hypothermia, hypoventilation, bradycardia, hypotension, and hypoglycemia. Myxedema coma carries a 30–60% mortality risk.

Case Example

A preterm 28-week gestation neonate weighing 1,200 g is brought to the emergency department after home birth with respiratory distress and difficulty feeding. Newborn screening tests are performed at this time, which show a low total T_4 and normal TSH. Free T_4 is normal.

In premature infants, the findings described in this case are due either to hypothalamic–pituitary axis immaturity or to low thyroid-binding protein levels. They are most often seen in very premature (<30 weeks' gestation) or very low-birth-weight (<1,500 g) newborns. Although close follow-up is needed, total and free T_4 levels typically normalize in 6–10 weeks, with <10% of patients requiring prolonged treatment. However, if left untreated, congenital hypothyroidism can result in gastrointestinal, cardiac, musculoskeletal, and renal anomalies such as umbilical hernia, decreased cardiac contractility, mitral and tricuspid valve insufficiency due to chordae tendineae laxity, delayed bone maturation, hypotonia, and glomerulonephritis.

Diagnostic Confirmation

Diagnostic confirmation of hypothyroidism requires collection of serum TSH and free T_4 levels. In autoimmune thyroiditis, laboratory tests show anti-thyroid peroxidase antibodies, low concentrations of free T_4, and high concentrations of TSH. TSH levels are important in diagnosing hypothyroidism and in monitoring its treatment. T_4 directly represents the hormone production by the gland. Although it is the active form of the hormone, T_3 only indirectly represents gland function because 80% of T_3 production occurs extracellularly and requires the additional step of monodeiodination of T_4 to be formed. *Subclinical hypothyroidism* is the term used to describe a scenario in which TSH is elevated but free T_4 or T_3 levels are normal. Debate exists about whether subclinical hypothyroidism leads to adverse health outcomes in pediatric patients. As such, expectant management with periodic monitoring of thyroid function tests is appropriate.

Treatment

In infants with true congenital hypothyroidism, hormone replacement should be started immediately. The goal of therapy is to normalize thyroid hormone levels as quickly as possible because studies have demonstrated an inverse relationship between the age at normalization of hormone levels and intelligence quotients (IQ). Treatment of choice is intravenous (IV) levothyroxine at initial dosing of 80 μg/m²/day.

The treatment of acquired hypothyroidism is the same. Dose adjustments are made by monitoring serum TSH levels. In severe cases of hypothyroidism or in myxedema coma such as in those patients with impending respiratory failure, persistent hypotension or altered mental status, intensive care unit (ICU) admission, close monitoring, and hydrocortisone may also be required. Dosing for IV hydrocortisone is typically 2 mg/kg/day.

Disposition

A pediatric endocrinologist should be consulted for children with hypothyroid emergencies. In children with congenital hypothyroidism, hormone levels should be monitored every 2 weeks until they normalize and then every 1–3 months for the first year of life and every 2–4 months during the next 2 years. At age 3 years, children should be evaluated for continued hormone replacement needs. Children with Hashimoto's (autoimmune) thyroiditis will require lifelong hormone replacement and monitoring.

Complications

Delayed diagnosis of congenital hypothyroidism can have lasting impacts on neurocognitive development: hearing impairments, speech delays, decreased motor skills, and attention deficits. Chronic untreated hypothyroidism in older pediatric patients can result in potentially fatal myxedema coma during times of illness.

Key Points

- Congenital hypothyroidism requires immediate thyroid hormone replacement.
- Fatigue, cold intolerance, constipation, and menstrual irregularities are the most common symptoms of hypothyroidism. Younger children may also present with either delayed or precocious puberty.
- Goiter is the most common physical examination finding in hypothyroidism.
- Diagnosis is based on abnormal TSH and free T_3/T_4 levels.

Pitfalls

- Myxedema coma is extremely rare in children, but it is potentially lethal. Consider it in all children who present with altered mental status and hypothermia.
- Consider congenital hypothyroidism in a newborn or young infant who may not have had access to newborn screening tests and is presenting with any of the following symptoms: lethargy, prolonged jaundice, poor feeding, constipation, umbilical hernia, macroglossia, hypotonia, and mottled skin.

HYPERTHYROIDISM

Background

The most common causes of hyperthyroidism include Graves' disease (GD), toxic multinodular goiter, and toxic adenoma. GD is an autoimmune disorder in which the TSH receptor is stimulated by thyrotropin receptor antibodies, resulting in increased thyroid hormone production and release. The majority of cases of childhood thyrotoxicosis (i.e., excess thyroid hormone) are diagnosed during adolescence. Although GD is an autoimmune disorder, the condition may be precipitated or exacerbated by neck surgery, trauma, infection, parturition, medication noncompliance, or iodine ingestion. GD demonstrates the classic signs and symptoms of hyperthyroidism.

Classic Clinical Presentation

Case Example

A 16-year-old female presents to the emergency department for increased somnolence. She is complaining of shortness of breath. Her vital signs are significant for heart rate of 130 beats per minute (bpm) and temperature of 101.9°F. Review of systems indicates recent vomiting and diarrhea, cough, shortness of breath, palpitations, heat intolerance, and unintentional weight loss. Physical examination is notable for large goiter, lid lag, and exophthalmos.

Atypical Clinical Presentation

Case Example

A 2-year-old female presents to the emergency department after having ingested her mother's 30 tablets of levothyroxine. The child has a normal examination and is found to have elevated T_3 and T_4 serum levels. Poison control is contacted and recommends activated charcoal and admission for close observation. The child later develops fever with a heart rate of 200 bpm, lethargy, and tremulousness. Propranolol, IV fluids, and corticosteroids are initiated to manage thyroid storm.

Differential Diagnosis

The differential diagnosis includes infection/sepsis, malignancy, heat exhaustion/stroke, ingestions, and illicit drug use.

Diagnostic Confirmation

Serum TSH is the most sensitive and specific test for the evaluation of thyrotoxicosis. A normal TSH precludes the diagnosis of thyrotoxicosis. Low or undetectable levels of TSH and elevated levels of T_3 and free T_4 confirm the diagnosis of hyperthyroidism. When a patient presents with a uniformly enlarged thyroid, ophthalmopathy (exophthalmos, lid retraction, lid lag, proptosis, and ophthalmoplegia), and moderate to severe hyperthyroidism (low TSH), the patient most likely has GD. If the presentation is atypical, then measurement of thyrotropin receptor antibodies or radioactive iodine uptake is used to further determine the etiology of the disease.

Thyroid storm is diagnosed in patients with evidence of severe hyperthyroidism, a precipitating factor, and any of the following: hyperpyrexia, tachycardia, arrhythmias, heart failure, delirium, psychosis, coma, renal failure, hepatic failure, nausea, vomiting, or diarrhea. Precipitating factors include cessation of anti-thyroid medication, thyroidectomy, other surgeries in a patient with unrecognized thyrotoxicosis, and acute illness such as infection.

Treatment

For exogenous thyroid hormone overdoses, charcoal may be indicated for significant ingestions (>3 mg).

Treatment of thyroid storm includes the following:

Methimazole 0.8–1.2 mg/kg orally for one dose, then 0.6–0.8 mg/kg q8 hours to block new hormone synthesis

2–10 drops of Lugol's solution every 8 hours for 1 or 2 days to decrease additional thyroid hormone synthesis via iodine organification inhibition (Wolff–Chaikoff effect)

Propranolol: 0.015 mg/kg IV over 10 minutes, repeat up to three times as necessary to control adrenergic symptoms such as tachycardia and hypertension

For severe cardiovascular symptoms: IV methylprednisolone 1 mg/kg initial dose, then 0.25 mg/kg q6 hours to inhibit peripheral conversion of T_4 to T_3

Cooling blankets as needed

Long-term treatment of thyrotoxicosis is methimazole 0.5–0.7 mg/kg/day divided in two doses.

Disposition

Thyroid storm is a life-threatening emergency and carries a mortality rate of 10–30%. Causes of death include hyperthermia, arrhythmia, and multiorgan failure. Patients undergoing treatment for thyroid storm should be admitted for close neurologic and cardiopulmonary monitoring in the ICU setting. For newly diagnosed thyrotoxicosis, serum T_4 and T_3 should be checked 1–3 months after initiation of therapy. Serum TSH may remain suppressed for months after starting therapy. Once a patient becomes euthyroid, the dose of methimazole can be decreased by approximately 50%. Typically, medical therapy is continued for 1 or 2 years.

Approximately 30% of children with GD will go into remission, whereas the majority will require more treatment and may need long-term medical management. The majority of children with GD will also require either radioactive iodine ablation therapy (RAI) or surgery. RAI should be avoided in children younger than age 5 years due to increased lifetime risk of thyroid cancer. Thyroidectomy should be pursued in children younger than age 5 years for whom medical therapy has failed. The goal of both RAI and surgery is to render the patient hypothyroid. Total thyroidectomy has a 0% risk of recurrence, whereas subtotal thyroidectomy has an 8% risk of recurrence.

Key Points

- Thyroid storm is a clinical diagnosis and should be made in patients with severe thyrotoxicosis and evidence of systemic decompensation.
- Thyroid storm caries a high mortality rate and should be treated in the ICU setting for cardiovascular and mental status monitoring.
- More than 70% of children with thyrotoxicosis will require long-term management and definitive radiation or surgical interventions.
- Due to increased cancer risk, RAI should be avoided prior to age 5 years.

Complications and Pitfalls

- The U.S. Food and Drug Administration has issued a block box warning for propylthiouracil (which, like methimazole, is a thionamide that blocks thyroid hormone synthesis) in children because it carries up to a 1 in 2,000 risk of fulminant hepatic failure, which may be fatal or require liver transplantation.
- Because agranulocytosis is a reported side effect, methimazole should be stopped and white blood cell counts checked immediately in children who develop fever, arthralgia, pharyngitis, or malaise.

DIABETIC KETOACIDOSIS

Background

Diabetes mellitus (DM) is a complex endocrinological disorder marked by hyperglycemia in the setting of decreased insulin secretion, insulin resistance, or both (Box 30.2). The dysfunction between insulin and target tissues results in systemic abnormalities of carbohydrate, protein, and fat metabolism. Although the etiologies of DM can be multifocal, most cases are categorized as either type 1 or type 2. DM type 1 remains the most common form seen in children and is characterized by an absolute decrease in insulin production. Although pediatric incidence of DM type 2 is becoming increasingly common, it is still predominantly seen in older populations and occurs as a result of impaired insulin secretion and insulin resistance. Clinicians should suspect DM in children with the classic symptoms of polyuria, polydipsia, polyphagia, nocturia, enuresis, blurred vision, and unintentional weight loss.

Diabetic ketoacidosis (DKA), which has a known incidence of up to 25% in children with

BOX 30.2

DIAGNOSTIC CRITERIA FOR DIABETES MELLITUS

- Presence of classic symptoms of diabetes mellitus in addition to random plasma glucose concentration ≥200 mg/dL (11.1 mmol/L)
  Or
- 2-Hour oral glucose tolerance test ≥200 mg/dL (11.1 mmol/L)
  Or
- Fasting plasma glucose concentration ≥126 mg/dL (7 mmol/L)
  Or
- HbA1c >6.5%

type 1 DM, is marked by the triad of hyperglycemia, anion gap metabolic acidosis, and the presence of ketosis (Box 30.3 presents the diagnostic criteria for DKA). Risk factors for DKA in children include a history of DKA, insulin noncompliance, and concurrent illness (e.g., sepsis, gastroenteritis, and hyperthyroidism). Box 30.4 provides a more complete list of risk factors.

Classic Signs and Symptoms of Diabetic Ketoacidosis

- Clinical signs of dehydration (e.g., decreased urine output, dry oral mucosa, and decreased skin turgor)
- Tachycardia for age
- Hypotension for age
- Tachypnea for age
- Kussmaul respirations (deep and labored breathing pattern)
- Fruity odor (acetone) to breath
- Nausea and emesis
- Abdominal pain
- Change in mental status (drowsiness, confusion, and eventual loss of consciousness)

Atypical Clinical Presentation

Case Example

A 9-year-old female with no significant past medical history presents to the emergency department with her parents for reported headache during the past 24 hours in the setting of recent flu-like symptoms. Her parents also endorse associated weakness, fatigue, nonbloody or bilious emesis, confusion, recent bed wetting, and "not quite acting like her usual self." Her examination is notable for tachycardia, tachypnea with Kussmaul breathing, and mild fever. She is able to follow commands, but her Glasgow Coma Score is 14 due to mild confusion. Point-of-care glucose is 552 mg/dL, and venous blood gas shows a pH of 6.99, pCO_2 of 22 mmHg, and HCO_3 of 5 mmol/L. This is a

BOX 30.3

DIABETIC KETOACIDOSIS DIAGNOSTIC CRITERIA

Criteria for the diagnosis of diabetic ketoacidosis (DKA) must include all of the following:

Hyperglycemia: serum glucose concentrations ≥200 mg/dL (11 mmol/L)

Metabolic acidosis: serum pH <7.3 or serum bicarbonate concentration <15 mmol/L

Ketosis: presence of ketonuria and ketonemia (acetone, acetoacetic acid, and β-hydroxybutyric acid)

Severity of DKA is distinguished by degree of acidosis: mild, pH <7.3 or serum bicarbonate <15 mmol/L; moderate, pH <7.2 or serum bicarbonate <10 mmol/L; severe, pH <7.1 or serum bicarbonate <5 mmol/L

BOX 30.4
RISK FACTORS FOR PEDIATRIC DIABETIC KETOACIDOSIS

History of diabetic ketoacidosis
Insulin noncompliance
Concurrent illness (e.g., sepsis)
Insulin pump failure
Drug abuse (e.g., sympathomimetic abuse, ethanol abuse)
Glucocorticoid use
Pregnancy
Psychiatric illness
Limited medical access
Challenging family and social circumstances
Prepubertal and pubertal adolescent girls
Children with poor metabolic control (high HbA1c levels)

case of pediatric DKA presenting with findings concerning for early cerebral edema.

Specific Organ System Manifestations of Diabetic Ketoacidosis

Acute Kidney Injury

Acute kidney injury (AKI) is a well-described complication of DKA and may be seen in up to one-third of children admitted to the intensive care setting for DKA. AKI is associated with prolonged hospital length of stay, increased likelihood of requiring vasopressor therapy, possible need for mechanical ventilation, higher incidence of cerebral edema, and higher mortality outcomes.

Hypokalemia

Hypokalemia (serum K^+ <3.5 mEq/L) is seen in <5% of pediatric patients with DKA. Because potassium shifts from the intracellular to the extracellular space in the setting of insulin deficiency and acidosis, potassium values may appear normal, even with total body potassium deficits of up to 3–6 mEq/kg. Profound hypokalemia (serum K^+ <2.5 mEq/L) is associated with life-threatening cardiac dysthymias, particularly when insulin, which shifts serum potassium back to the intracellular space, is administered prior to potassium repletion. Thus, treatment with insulin should be delayed until serum potassium levels are 3.0 mEq/L or higher.

Respiratory Failure

The presence of metabolic acidosis stimulates respiratory counter mechanisms in an effort to partially offset CO_2 levels and correct acidemia. In general, for every 1 mEq/L drop in serum bicarbonate, reflexive tachypnea decreases 1.2 mmHg of measured arterial CO_2 concentration. Without timely intervention, however, compensatory tachypnea may devolve to eventual respiratory collapse as muscle fatigue sets in. Pulmonary edema may occur from both circulatory fluid overload and cytokine dysregulation (with risk of progression toward acute respiratory distress syndrome).

Cerebral Edema

Cerebral edema, although uncommon, accounts for up to 90% of all pediatric DKA deaths. In addition to high mortality rates, up to 25% of survivors experience some form of permanent neurological sequelae. Most pediatric patients with cerebral edema (66%) will demonstrate symptoms within the first 7 hours of treatment for DKA. The exact pathophysiology of cerebral edema is yet to be elucidated, but several mechanisms have been postulated. Potential pathophysiologic mechanisms include cerebral osmotic edema in the setting of excessive fluid replacement, idiopathic blood–brain barrier dysfunction with resultant vasogenic edema, and brain tissue ischemia and cytotoxic edema due to critical hypoperfusion. Factors shown to be associated with the development of cerebral edema in DKA are listed in Box 30.5. Diagnostic criteria for cerebral edema in pediatric DKA are presented in Table 30.3 (sensitivity, 92%; specificity, 96%).

Differential Diagnosis

The differential diagnosis of DKA includes other causes of anion gap metabolic acidosis, ketoacidosis, and metabolic encephalopathy (Box 30.6).

Treatment and Clinical Algorithm

Patients presenting with signs and symptoms of DKA require rapid evaluation to determine severity of illness and quickly initiate treatment. Initial examination should include a complete set of vital signs to determine the

BOX 30.5

FACTOR ASSOCIATED WITH CEREBRAL EDEMA IN DIABETIC KETOACIDOSIS

New-onset diabetic ketoacidosis
Age younger than 5 years
Severe metabolic acidosis (pH <7.1)
Severe hypocapnia ($PaCO_2$ <20 mmHg)
Hyponatremia
Elevated blood urea nitrogen levels
Overcorrection of dehydration with IV fluids
Insulin treatment within the first hour of fluid resuscitation
Treatment with bicarbonate

presence of shock; weight measurement to determine fluid and insulin dosing; and physical examination, including regular focused assessments of neurologic status. Diagnostic workup for suspected pediatric DKA includes the following:

- A point-of-care blood glucose >200 mg/dL confirmatory for hyperglycemia
- Serum electrolytes (including creatinine, blood urea nitrogen, calcium, magnesium, phosphorous, anion gap, and bicarbonate)
- Venous blood gas (venous pH and pCO_2)
- Complete blood count
- Ketones (serum β-hydroxybutyrate or urine ketones)
- Electrocardiogram to evaluate for morphologic changes observed in hypokalemia (U waves) and hyperkalemia (peaked T waves, P wave flattening with PR prolongation, QRS widening, or sine wave appearance)

The treatment of DKA includes IV fluids to correct dehydration, insulin administration to reverse ketosis and correct hyperglycemia, electrolyte repletion to correct for any deficiencies, continuous monitoring for complications of DKA, and identification and treatment of adverse outcomes. Figure 30.2 provides an overview of the management of pediatric DKA.

Fluid Repletion

Bedside clinical estimations of dehydration have been shown to be unreliable and inaccurate in pediatric patients presenting with DKA. However, clinicians can safely assume up to 5% total volume deficits in mild cases of DKA and up to 10% in more severe cases.

Initial volume expansion of 10–20 mL/kg of isotonic crystalloid solution [0.9% normal saline (NS) or Ringer's lactate] is recommended during the first 1 or 2 hours. An additional 10–20 mL/kg of isotonic crystalloid should be given for hemodynamic instability.

After completion of resuscitative fluids, the goal of rehydration is to correct the remaining fluid deficit during the following 24–48 hours with either IV 0.45% or 0.9% NS, Ringer's lactate, or Plasmalyte, depending on the patient's hydration status, serum osmolarity, and serum sodium concentration. A number of IV hydration protocols have been described, and they vary depending on institution preference. Importantly, the rate of fluid administration during this phase must take into account both the maintenance fluid rate and the additional calculated volume deficit. The rate of total fluid

TABLE 30.3 DIAGNOSIS OF CEREBRAL EDEMA IN DIABETIC KETOACIDOSIS (DKA)[a]

Diagnostic Criteria	Major Criteria	Minor Criteria
Abnormal motor or verbal response to pain Decorticate or decerebrate posture Cranial nerve palsy Abnormal neurological respiratory pattern	Altered mentation or fluctuation of consciousness Heart rate decelerations (>20 beats per minute) not improved with hydration or sleep Age-inappropriate incontinence	Vomiting Headache Lethargy or difficulty arousing from sleep Diastolic blood pressure >90 mmHg Age <5 years

[a]One diagnostic criterion *plus* two major criteria *or* one major and two minor criteria.

> **BOX 30.6**
> **DIFFERENTIAL DIAGNOSIS OF FINDINGS IN DIABETIC KETOACIDOSIS**
>
> Anion gap metabolic acidosis
> - Ketoacidosis
> - Lactic acidosis
> - Starvation ketosis
> - Ethanol ketosis
> - Salicylate toxicity
> - Acetaminophen toxicity
> - Methanol or ethyl glycol intoxication
> - Metformin toxicity
> - Iron toxicity
> - Uremia
>
> Metabolic encephalopathy
> - Hypoglycemia
> - Primary central nervous system disease
> - Hepatic failure
> - Renal failure
> - Sepsis
> - Seizure

administration should not exceed twice the maintenance rate (Box 30.7).

Insulin

Timely administration of insulin is critical for reversing hyperglycemia, optimizing cellular metabolism, limiting lipolysis, and inhibiting ketosis. However, to prevent cardiac arrhythmias from iatrogenic hypokalemia, insulin should only be given after the serum potassium is confirmed to be at least 3.0 mEq/L. Insulin should be administered intravenously and started at drip rates of 0.05–1 U/kg/hr. To prevent precipitating hypoglycemia during insulin therapy, 5% dextrose should be added to the IV crystalloid solution when plasma glucose concentrations are near 300 mg/dL (17 mmol/L). Fluids with up to 12.5% dextrose may be needed if serum glucose drops precipitously. Patients may transition to subcutaneous (SQ) insulin once DKA is resolved (Box 30.8) and they are able to adequately tolerate oral intake. SQ insulin should be given half an hour prior to discontinuing IV therapy (to prevent reflexive hyperglycemia), and be administered before a meal.

Electrolyte Repletion

As previously discussed, all children presenting with DKA suffer significant total body potassium deficits, even with normal serum laboratory values. In patients presenting with hyperkalemia, potassium repletion should be held until urinary output is confirmed. To prevent cardiac arrhythmias, patients with serum hypokalemia should be corrected to a potassium level of 3.0 mEq/L or higher prior to insulin therapy.

Serum sodium concentrations can vary significantly between patients with DKA. Pseudo-hyponatremia is commonly encountered because sodium values may be falsely low due to the osmotic effects of hyperglycemia. Importantly, patients whose serum sodium concentrations fail to normalize with treatment may be at higher risk for cerebral edema. Clinicians can correct for pseudo-hyponatremia with the following formula: Corrected plasma sodium = measured plasma sodium + (1.6 mEq/L × every 100 mg/dL serum glucose over normal).

As in serum potassium concentrations, pediatric patients with DKA suffer deficiencies in total body phosphate stores. Rarely, symptoms of profound hypophosphatemia may manifest as severe muscle weakness, rhabdomyolysis, or even cardiac dysrhythmias. Phosphate levels should be routinely monitored in concert with other measured electrolytes and replaced accordingly.

Disposition

Patients presenting with severe manifestations of DKA, hemodynamic instability, and risk for developing cerebral edema should be admitted to specialized pediatric intensive care units (PICUs) for close monitoring and treatment. Patients with moderate forms of DKA may alternatively be admitted to regular pediatric floors if the unit is capable of close observation, frequent laboratory draws, and administration of continuous IV insulin therapy. Children with very mild forms of DKA who demonstrate satisfactory recovery and resolution of DKA may be discharged if they have reliable guardians, close follow-up, an adequate supply of medications and equipment to check their blood glucose levels, and are able to promptly reaccess medical care if necessary.

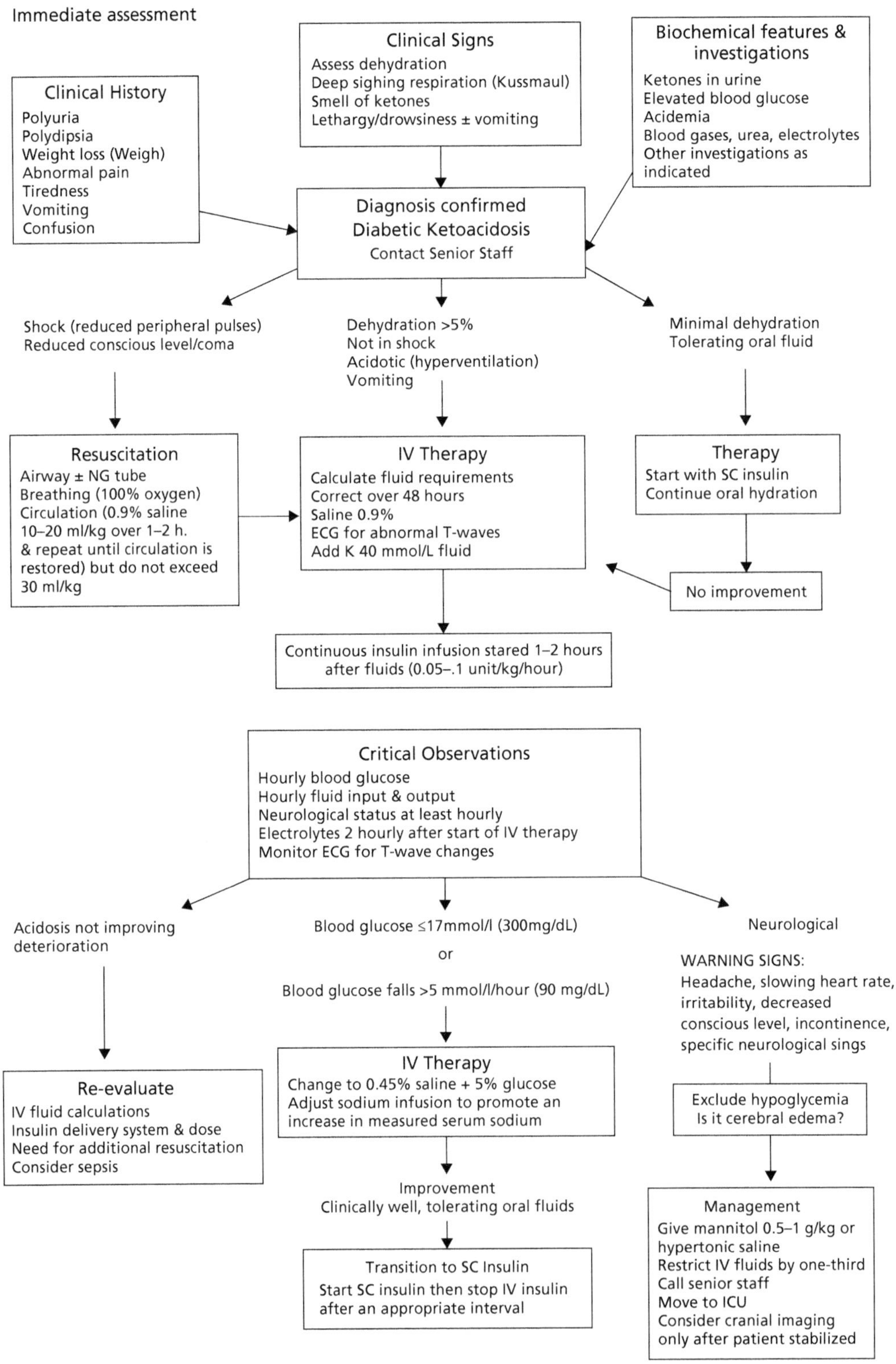

FIGURE 30.2 Treatment algorithm for pediatric DKA.

BOX 30.7

4-2-1 RULE FOR CALCULATING PEDIATRIC FLUID MAINTENANCE RATES

- 4 mL/kg/hr for the first 10 kg of body weight
  Plus
- 2 mL/kg/hr for the second 10 kg of body weight
  Plus
- 1 mL/kg/hr for each additional kilogram above 20 kg of body weight

Complications

The most frequently encountered complications of DKA during the course of therapy are iatrogenic hypoglycemia and hypokalemia. Frequent laboratory draws are necessary to closely trend electrolyte shifts and allow for timely intervention. Cerebral edema remains the most dreaded complication and may portend devastating outcomes. If clinicians suspect evolving cerebral edema based on clinical examination, initial steps include quickly reducing fluid administration by 33% and elevating head of the bed to reduce intracranial pressure. Next, hyperosmolar therapy should be initiated with either 3% hypertonic saline (5–10 mL/kg IV over 30 minutes) or mannitol (0.5–1 mg/kg IV over 20 minutes; may repeat within 30 minutes to 2 hours if no response).

BOX 30.8

CRITERIA FOR DIABETIC KETOACIDOSIS RESOLUTION

- Serum glucose <200 mg/dL (11 mmol/L)
  And
- pH >7.3 or serum bicarbonate >15 mEq/L
  And
- Closed anion gap or β-hydroxybutyrate <1 mmol/L (<10.4 mg/dL)

Key Points

- Diabetes mellitus commonly presents with increased thirst, increased urination, weight loss, and other nonspecific symptoms including commonly abdominal pain.
- Insulin noncompliance and infections can precipitate DKA.
- To avoid cardiac arrhythmias, in children with DKA and hypokalemia, insulin should be held until potassium is 3.0 mEq/L or higher.
- Goals of DKA treatment include fluid replacement, serum glucose correction, serum acid–base normalization, electrolyte replacement, and monitoring for cardiac arrhythmias and cerebral edema.
- Fluid composition or rates have not been associated with the occurrence of cerebral edema. However, once cerebral edema is recognized, current treatment includes a prompt 33% reduction in fluid administration and hyperosmolar therapy (3% hypertonic saline or mannitol).

ADRENAL INSUFFICIENCY

Background

Adrenal insufficiency (AI) is a life-threatening condition arising from either intrinsic adrenal gland failure or dysfunction along the HPA axis. Acute AI results from either absolute or relative reduction in serum corticosteroid concentrations, with or without concomitant adrenal androgens or mineralocorticoid deficiencies.

AI is classified as primary, secondary, or tertiary, depending on etiology. Primary AI occurs with destruction or dysfunction of the adrenal cortex, resulting most importantly in deficiencies of glucocorticoids such as cortisol and, of lesser consequence, deficiencies of mineralocorticoids or adrenal androgens. In pediatric populations, nearly three out of four cases of primary AI are due to congenital adrenal hyperplasia (CAH), most notably due to 21-hydroxylase deficiency.

Secondary AI occurs when ACTH production is impaired within the pituitary gland. Tertiary AI results from inadequate secretion of corticotropin-releasing hormone from the hypothalamus. Secondary and tertiary AI may collectively be classified under the umbrella term central AI. The most common cause of central AI is iatrogenic suppression of the HPA axis due to long-term glucocorticoid use.

Classic Clinical Presentation

Children and adolescents often present with vague and nonspecific symptoms, such as weakness, fatigue, abdominal pain, headache, weight loss, and salt craving. Classic signs include hypotension, vomiting, diarrhea, hyperkalemia, hyponatremia, hypoglycemia, and hyperpigmentation (only in primary AI) or vitiligo (indicating autoimmune pathology). Clinicians should consider AI secondary to CAH in infants who have additional findings of atypical genitalia (e.g., virilization in females), lethargy, and failure to thrive. Without timely intervention, patients can progress toward the most dreaded complications of AI, acute adrenal crisis and subsequent cardiopulmonary collapse. Adrenal crisis is often precipitated by acute events such as serious infections, stress, corticosteroid withdrawal, adrenal hemorrhages, or primary central nervous system insult. Adrenal crisis carries a pediatric mortality rate of up to 25%.

Atypical Clinical Presentation

Case Example

A 19-year-old female with a past medical history of type 1 diabetes presents to the emergency department with several weeks of fatigue with associated nausea, nonbloody emesis, and near syncopal episodes. On examination, she is found to be mildly hypotensive, hyperpigmented, and laboratory tests reveal mild hyponatremia and hyperkalemia. Both TSH and free T_4 levels are found to be low. Oral levothyroxine is initiated given a concern for new-onset hypothyroidism; however, soon after therapy, her clinical condition deteriorates, requiring urgent resuscitation and admission for intensive care.

This is a case of missed acute adrenal insufficiency in a patient presenting with symptoms ascribed to hypothyroidism. Both conditions may present with similar and nonspecific symptoms; however, clinicians should suspect adrenal insufficiency in light of additional findings, such as skin hyperpigmentation, hyponatremia, and hypokalemia. Unfortunately, patients with type 1 diabetes often have other autoimmune conditions, and as many as one in four with Addison's disease also have hypothyroidism. Of note, in patients with AI, initiating T_4 therapy before steroid replacement can precipitate an adrenal crisis.

Differential Diagnosis

The differential diagnosis for adrenal insufficiency includes causes of shock, electrolyte abnormalities, or other etiologies that can explain the symptoms that mimic AI. Importantly, these causes may also predispose AI patients to developing adrenal crises (Box 30.9).

Diagnosis

A definite diagnosis of AI is a multistep process that can be challenging in the emergency department due to the time requirements of testing. If clinicians are suspicious of acute adrenal crisis, particularly in patients with a known history of AI, we recommend initiating prompt empiric therapy with stress doses of corticosteroids prior to confirmatory results. (See Box 30.10 for steps to confirm and categorize AI.)

BOX 30.9

CAUSES AND MIMICS OF ADRENAL CRISIS

Sepsis from any cause of infection
Major trauma
Intracranial hemorrhage
Malignancy
Diabetic ketoacidosis
Appendicitis
Celiac disease
Thyroid dysfunction
Toxic ingestion
Anorexia
Hyperemesis gravidarum
Interstitial nephritis
Chronic kidney disease

Treatment

The treatment of children presenting with clinical manifestations of acute AI includes resuscitation from shock, administration of stress dose steroids, correction of electrolyte derangements, and treatment of any precipitating factors. Correction of dehydration and hypotension should begin with volume expansion, 0.9% NS at a dose of 20 mL/kg intravenously, repeated for persistent hypotension. Vasopressor therapy may be necessary in refractory states.

In patients highly suspected of having an adrenal crisis, stress dose hydrocortisone, adjusted for age, should be administered promptly without awaiting confirmatory testing: ages 0–3 years, 25 mg IV; ages 3–12 years, 50 mg IV; and ages 12 years or older, 100 mg IV—all given at presentation and repeated every 6 hours during the following 24 hours. Hypoglycemia should be corrected with 25% dextrose solution (D25W) at a dose of 2–4 mL/kg. Hyperkalemia may be present initially yet often improves with prompt management; additional correction may be necessary with glucose and insulin in more severe cases. During the resuscitation phase of treatment, steps should also be taken to address and treat potential precipitating factors, such as severe infection or trauma.

Management and prevention of AI are achieved through daily administration of oral hydrocortisone: 7 mg/m^2/day in children and 12 mg/m^2/day in infants. Other glucocorticoids, such as prednisolone or dexamethasone, may serve as alternatives. Hydrocortisone is preferred, however, because of its shorter half-life and lower potency—making it more amenable to titration in children. Of note, children with AI secondary to CAH may require double the usual glucocorticoid dosages. In addition, children with concomitant mineralocorticoid deficiencies require repletion therapy with oral fludrocortisone (dose of 0.05–0.2 mg daily).

BOX 30.10

ADRENAL INSUFFICIENCY TESTING

Step 1: Confirm diagnosis of adrenal insufficiency (AI). Measure early morning serum cortisol levels; diagnosis of AI is confirmed if <5 μmg/dL or <138 mmol/L.

Step 2: Determine primary versus central etiology of AI by measuring plasma ACTH levels.

A high level (>200 pg/mL or 200 pmol/L) confirms the diagnosis of primary AI.

A low ACTH level (<10 pg/mL or 2.2 pmol/L) supports the diagnosis of central AI.

If an ACTH level is indeterminate, perform an ACTH stimulation test. (Note that this test does not differentiate between primary or central AI but, rather, is confirmatory for the diagnosis of AI in the setting of equivocal findings.)

Step 3: In consultation with an endocrinology specialist, determine and treat the underlying cause.

Disposition

All children presenting with clinical evidence of adrenal crisis should be admitted to the PICU for ongoing resuscitation needs, frequent laboratory assessments, close observation, and continuous hemodynamic monitoring. Patients presenting with more chronic symptoms of AI may be discharged if they are able to demonstrate satisfactory symptom control, have remained hemodynamically stable during their stay, have timely follow-up available to them, and are able to immediately seek care when necessary. Patients should be educated on the prevention of adrenal crisis, the need for an increase in steroid dosing when they experience acute stressors, and that dosages will require titration depending on illness severity. In general, mild stressors (afebrile cases of viral upper respiratory infections) do not require dosage adjustments. More moderate episodes of stress (febrile illness with temperature >38°C) require doubling the daily dose until recovery. Severe stress episodes (temperature >39°C, gastroenteritis, and trauma) require triple doses. Upon discharge from the emergency department, patients should be given a prescription for an intramuscular hydrocortisone injection kit (50 g/m^2) to be used if they are unable to tolerate oral intake during illness. Patients should also be encouraged to wear medical alert identification (e.g., bracelets or necklaces) and carry emergency cards to inform medical personnel of their AI status in the event of a medical emergency.

Complications

Long-term glucocorticoid therapy is the mainstay in the treatment of AI but is associated with long-standing consequences in pediatric patients. In addition to the well-known Cushingoid effects of excessive exogenous steroid use (e.g., hypertension, immunosuppression, dyslipidemia, and skin atrophy), children are also prone to growth restrictions and short stature when exposed to supratherapeutic doses. Also, children are particularly sensitive to ophthalmologic complications of chronic steroid use, such as cataracts and glaucoma. It is imperative to stress the importance of frequent outpatient clinical surveillance and the need for vigilant monitoring of both under- and overdosing.

Key Points

- Among pediatric endocrinological emergencies, adrenal crisis has one of the highest rates of morbidity and mortality.
- Prompt recognition, resuscitation, and glucocorticoid replacement ("stress dose steroids") are paramount in preventing the catastrophic consequences of acute AI.

Further Reading

Thyroid Disorders

Azizi F, Amouzegar A. Management of thyrotoxicosis in children and adolescents: 35 years' experience in 304 patients. *J Pediatr Endocrinol Metab.* 2018;31(2):159–165.

Hanley P, Lord K, Bauer AJ. Thyroid disorders in children and adolescents: A review. *JAMA Pediatr.* 2016;170(10):1008–1019.

Kalplowitz PB. Neonatal thyroid disease: Testing and management. *Pediatr Clin North Am.* 2019;66:343–352.

Diabetic Ketoacidosis

Agrawal S, Baird GL, Quintos JB, et al. Pediatric diabetic ketoacidosis with hyperosmolarity: Clinical characteristics and outcomes. *Endocr Pract.* 2018;24(8):726–732.

Craig ME, Jefferies C, Dabelea D, et al. ISPAD clinical practice consensus guidelines 2014: Definition, epidemiology, and classification of diabetes in children and adolescents. *Pediatr Diabetes.* 2014;15(Suppl 20):4–17.

Gupta A, El-Wiher N. Therapeutic challenges in management of severe acidosis and profound hypokalemia in pediatric diabetic ketoacidosis. *Glob Pediatr Health.* 2019;6:2333794X19840364.

Kuppermann N, Ghetti S, Schunk JE, et al. Clinical trial of fluid infusion rates for pediatric diabetic ketoacidosis. *N Engl J Med.* 2018;378(24):2275–2287.

Parajuli B, Angurana SK, Baalaaji M, Williams V. Acute kidney injury in children with diabetic ketoacidosis: A real concern. *Pediatr Crit Care Med.* 2019;20(6):590–591.

Adrenal Insufficiency

Bornstein SR, Allolio B, Arlt W, et al. Diagnosis and treatment of primary adrenal insufficiency: An Endocrine Society clinical practice guideline. *J Clin Endocrinol Metab.* 2016;101(2):364–389.

31

Rheumatology

MEGHAN MALONEY AND C. ANTHONEY LIM

INTRODUCTION

Rheumatologic diagnoses are less common in the pediatric population compared to adults. There is some overlap in disease, such as systemic lupus erythematosus (SLE), which can begin in adolescence and continue into adulthood; some diagnoses are unique to pediatrics. As with adults, rheumatic disease in children can involve multiple organ systems and require care from various subspecialists. The presentation of rheumatic disease in children is often prolonged with insidious symptoms that can lead to delay in diagnosis. Serious life-threatening disease complications including organ failure can occur in children and adolescence with known rheumatic disease, but they may also be in the initial presentation in a patient who was previously undiagnosed. Although treatments for the diseases have improved, infection remains a leading cause of morbidity and mortality in this population.

JUVENILE IDIOPATHIC ARTHRITIS

Background

Juvenile idiopathic arthritis (JIA) is the most common pediatric rheumatologic diagnosis, comprising 10–20% of pediatric rheumatologic disease (although overall a rare disease). The diagnosis can be classified into four main subgroups depending on the number of joints affected and the presence of extra-articular symptoms. Oligoarticular disease involves fewer than five joints, whereas polyarticular disease involves five or more joints. Extra-articular symptoms can include systemic symptoms (systemic-onset JIA) or enthesitis-related JIA (inflammation of the insertion point of ligaments and tendons on bones). Although not comprising independent subgroups, JIA can also have associated psoriasis (psoriatic arthritis) and may be rheumatoid factor (RF) positive or negative.

Classic Clinical Presentation

Diagnostic features include chronic joint pain for 6 weeks or longer as well as immobility or morning stiffness for more than 30 minutes. Oligoarthritis is the most common type, comprising 50% of patients with JIA. In oligoarthritis, often medium to large joints are affected, and involvement can be asymmetric. Leg length discrepancy may occur due to increased blood flow and growth factor production in the affected leg. Polyarticular is the next most common type, accounting for approximately 35% of JIA patients. In this type, both large and small joints are affected, but it is usually symmetric. Systemic-onset JIA, otherwise known as Still's disease, comprises approximately 10–15% of diagnoses. These patients present with high fevers (39–40°C) occurring one or two times per day, usually with an associated salmon-colored macular rash coinciding with fever. These patients are often ill-appearing and at high risk for complications. Finally, the least common form, enthesitis-related JIA, typically occurs in males older than age 10 years. The large joints of the lower extremities are usually affected, and the enthesopathy often affects the tibial tuberosity or heel, but patients may also have sacroiliitis or lower back pain.

Atypical Clinical Presentation

A child presenting with persistent daily fevers and associated weight loss should trigger a workup for various systemic diseases including malignancy. These signs/symptoms are also associated with an atypical presentation of systemic-onset JIA. Another less typical presentation includes single joint involvement associated with fever. Although suggestive of infection, this may also be early onset systemic JIA.

Differential Diagnosis

For children presenting with symptoms concerning for JIA, a broad differential must be considered. Orthopedic conditions often present similarly. Hip pain in a school-age child may be Legg–Calve–Perthe syndrome or slipped capital femoral epiphysis in an overweight adolescent. Knee pain in school-age children may be due to Osgood–Schlatter disease or chondromalacia patellae. If the patient reports a recent prodromal illness, consider reactive arthritis, which can occur with rheumatic fever, streptococcal illness, Henloch–Schönlein purpura, or an upper respiratory infection (transient synovitis). These typically last at most 4–6 weeks and may improve with nonsteroidal anti-inflammatory drugs (NSAIDs). Joint infection must be considered when there is fever associated with joint pain or effusion, particularly if there is a single joint affected or the patient is toxic appearing. Symptoms may be due to bacterial pathogens, tick-borne illness, or direct viral infections. Neoplasm or malignancy including bone tumors, hematologic cancers such as leukemia and lymphoma, rhabdomyosarcomas, and neuroblastomas may also present with arthritis. These should be suspected if the patient has systemic symptoms as well as inflammatory markers that are elevated out of proportion to the arthritis. Finally, pain syndromes from overuse, growth pain, or complex regional pain syndrome in addition to other rheumatologic diseases such as SLE or dermatomyositis may also present with joint pain.

Diagnostic Confirmation

The diagnosis of JIA is one of exclusion. To meet criteria, the patient must have had continuous pain in at least one joint for 6 weeks or more. There is no confirmatory laboratory testing, but based on clinical suspicion for alternative diagnoses, these must be ruled out. In patients with fever, a joint aspiration is typically recommended to rule out infectious and reactive etiologies. These patients typically present with elevated inflammatory markers and leukocytosis. However, patients with JIA may also have elevated inflammatory markers, especially in polyarticular or systemic-onset disease. If a joint aspiration is performed, septic arthritis is more common if the joint effluent demonstrates leukocytosis of >50,000 white blood cells/μL. A gram stain and culture should be sent. Consider Lyme enzyme-linked immunosorbent assay (ELISA) with confirmatory Western blot if there are risk factors for Lyme disease. If malignancy is suspected, consider imaging for local neoplastic infiltration or sending a lactate dehydrogenase (LDH) and blood smear for blood cancers. If concern remains high, a bone marrow biopsy may be indicated. An antinuclear antibody (ANA) may not be helpful in distinguishing JIA from other joint disease because there is a high rate of false-positive results. Furthermore, rheumatoid factor (RF) is only positive in 5–10% of patients with JIA and is of little diagnostic assistance. If advanced imaging is required, magnetic resonance imaging (MRI) with gadolinium can confirm synovitis and may show early joint damage.

Treatment

Treatment of JIA consists of NSAIDs, disease-modifying agents, and corticosteroids. Most patients are initiated on NSAID therapy with ibuprofen, naproxen, or meloxicam. Typically, improvement occurs within 1 month, but it may take up to 12 weeks. If patients continue to have symptoms despite NSAID therapy, disease-modifying antirheumatic drugs (DMARDs) or biologics may be employed, with methotrexate most commonly prescribed, although newer biologics including rituximab may be gaining some favor. Other options may include antipyrimidines such as leflunomide; tumor necrosis factor-α (TNF-α) inhibitors such as etanercept, infliximab, or adalimimub that must be given parenterally; or corticosteroids given either orally or as joint injections for patients with severe or systemic disease.

Disposition

Most patients presenting with uncomplicated JIA may be discharged home. They will need close follow-up with rheumatology and ophthalmology due to the risk of associated uveitis. Admission may be considered depending on concern for complications that will need more aggressive management. Transfer to a tertiary care center should be considered for ill children because they may require consultation with multiple specialists.

Complications

Additional organ systems may be affected in patients with JIA, resulting in a broad range of complications.

The most common complication of JIA is uveitis, affecting up to 30% of patients with oligoarticular disease. Although uveitis typically presents with eye pain, erythema, or vision changes, patients with JIA may have very mild symptoms. However, uveitis can lead to blindness if undiagnosed and untreated. Routine slit-lamp examination every 3–6 months is recommended depending on disease type for the first 4 years after onset of joint symptoms. Examinations continue annually thereafter if the patient has not developed any evidence of disease. Initial treatment for uveitis is with topical steroids.

Cardiac complications may also occur with JIA, including pericardial effusion or tamponade. Pericarditis is most commonly associated with older children with systemic-onset JIA. Consideration of autoimmune conditions should occur in patients with a pericardial effusion because they account for up to 30% of cases. Pleuritis and restrictive lung disease are rare but serious potential complications.

Direct musculoskeletal complications, including subluxations, deformities, and ankylosis, are possible. Care should be taken in the airway management of patients with JIA. The cervical spine may be affected in prolonged, severe disease, resulting in an increased risk of atlantoaxial subluxation or cervical stenosis. In addition, there can be micrognathia if the temporomandibular joint is affected.

Hematologic and infectious complications are common in patients with JIA, especially if undergoing immunomodulatory treatment with corticosteroids or TNF-α blockers. Septic arthritis may occur as a complication of the disease and may be overlooked as an exacerbation. While undergoing treatment, fever may be absent, so infection should be suspected if there is a monoarticular or pauciarticular flare, especially if there is overlying erythema or other local signs of infection. Viral illnesses including parvovirus B19 may also be problematic in this population and can cause severe persistent anemia, neutropenia, and thrombocytopenia associated with a typical slapped cheek or stocking-glove rash. Diagnosis by DNA polymerase chain reaction is preferred in patients with rheumatologic disease, and treatment is supportive with administration of blood products as needed and intravenous immunoglobulin (IVIG). Use of oral steroids and NSAIDs can also lead to gastrointestinal complications such as gastritis, which can be mitigated by the use of H2 blockers and proton pump inhibitors.

A rare but potentially lethal complication of systemic-onset JIA is macrophage activation syndrome (MAS), which presents with fever, pancytopenia, hepatosplenomegaly, lymphadenopathy, and liver dysfunction. It is frequently associated with Epstein–Barr virus (EBV) and has similarities to hemophagocytic lymphohistiocytosis. Providers should have a high suspicion in the setting of worsening cytopenias, particularly neutropenia and thrombocytopenia. Other laboratory abnormalities are associated, including elevated ferritin, elevated fasting triglycerides, low fibrinogen, and coagulopathy. Treatment includes pulse steroids with methylprednisolone, repletion of cytopenias with blood products as needed, and antimicrobial coverage. Adjunct treatments may include IVIG, cyclosporine, and anakinra (Kineret, an interleukin-1 receptor antagonist). This complication can also be seen, although even more rarely, with SLE and Kawasaki disease. The associated mortality rate is estimated to be 7–12%.

Key Points

- JIA may present with one to many involved joints, enthesitis, predominantly systemic symptoms, or a combination of symptoms.
- RF and ANA have little diagnostic value in JIA.
- Initial treatment is with NSAIDs.
- The most common complication is uveitis, but many organ systems may be affected.
- MAS is a potentially lethal complication that presents with fever, lymphadenopathy, hepatosplenomegaly, pancytopenia, and liver dysfunction.

Pitfalls

- JIA may be difficult to distinguish from septic arthritis without a joint fluid aspiration and culture. Septic arthritis may be a complication but can be mistaken for a flare.
- Consider JIA in patients with pericarditis for whom there is no other clear etiology.
- Treatment options including DMARDs, steroids, and NSAIDs are all associated with potential side effects, in particular increased risk of infection.

SYSTEMIC LUPUS ERYTHEMATOSUS

Background

Systemic lupus erythematosus is primarily a disease of adults but can present in adolescents and rarely in younger children. Symptoms are due to overactivation of the innate and adaptive immune systems with overproduction of specific autoantibodies. In adolescence, the disease is more common in females, who overall comprise 90% of the affected population. Presentation in childhood occurs equally in males and females but is exceedingly rare. Several ethnic groups are more commonly affected, including people of African, Asian, and Hispanic descent.

Classic Clinical Presentation

The typical presentation occurs in an adolescent female between ages 9 and 15 years. Symptoms vary depending on which organs are affected by immune complex deposition, but common symptoms include fever, photosensitive rash (discoid or malar), fatigue, oral ulcers, arthritis, chest pain or pleurisy, Reynaud's phenomenon, and alopecia; 75% will have mucocutaneous involvement. Renal complications may be the initial presentation in children. Laboratory abnormalities include a positive ANA; cytopenias; elevated inflammatory markers; elevated liver enzymes; and urinary abnormalities including hematuria, proteinuria, or the presence of cellular casts.

Atypical Clinical Presentation

Systemic lupus erythematosus can present with disease complications. It is less commonly seen in males and in young children.

Differential Diagnosis

The differential diagnosis for SLE is broad, given the many systems that can be affected over time. There is significant overlap with all of the other rheumatologic diseases that can present in children, including systemic-onset JIA, mixed connective tissue disease, and vasculitides. Symptoms may overlap with infectious causes as well, including acute rheumatic fever and viral illnesses such as EBV, parvovirus B19, and HIV. Malignancies, especially blood cancers, may also present with similar symptoms such as fever and fatigue, and they should be considered. Organ-specific diseases may also be confused with SLE because it can cause disturbances in nearly every organ system in the body.

Diagnostic Confirmation

Systemic lupus erythematosus is associated with a positive ANA, an essential component of diagnosis. However, this is nonspecific and can be seen with other autoimmune disorders, medications, malignancy, and in 25% of healthy children. As such, there are two sets of criteria to make a diagnosis of SLE, which are the same for adult and pediatric patients. The American College of Rheumatology (ACR) has created the ACR criteria, which is 96% sensitive and specific (Box 31.1).

The second set of criteria has been put forth by the Systemic Lupus International Collaborating Clinics. It includes at least one clinical finding and one immunological criterion from a similar list as that of the ACR

BOX 31.1 ACR CRITERIA FOR SYSTEMIC LUPUS ERYTHEMATOSUS

Patient Must Have Four or More of the Following Clinical and Immunological Findings

1. Malar rash (photosensitive)
2. Discoid rash: an annular, scaly rash typically involving the scalp, face, and/or extremities
3. Photosensitivity: increased rash or symptoms after sun exposure
4. Mucus membrane ulcers: painless, on the hard palate and/or nasal septum
5. Arthritis: non-erosive arthritis of large and small joints, typically symmetric
6. Serositis: pericarditis and or pleuritis
7. Renal dysfunction: proteinuria (>0.5 g/day) and/or the presence of cellular casts in the urine
8. Neurologic abnormalities: seizures, psychosis
9. Blood cell count abnormalities
   a. Leukopenia (<4,000 WBC/mm^3)
   b. Lymphopenia (<1,500 lymphocytes/mm^3)
   c. Coombs positive anemia with reticulocytosis
   d. Thrombocytopenia (<100,000 platelets/mm^3)
10. ANA$^+$
11. Presence of other autoantibodies: anti-dsDNA, anti Smith, anti-cardiolipin Abs, lupus anticoagulant, false-positive RPR

ACR, American College of Rheumatology; ANA, antinuclear antibody; RPR, rapid plasma reagin; WBC, white blood cells.
Sources: Adapted from Tan EM, Cohen AS, Fries JF, Masi AT, McShane DJ, Rothfeld NF, et al. The 1982 revised criteria for the classification of systemic lupus erythematosus. *Arthritis Rheum.* 1982;25:1271–1277; and Hochberg MC. Updating the American College of Rheumatology revised criteria for the classification of systemic lupus erythematosus. *Arthritis Rheum.* 1997;40:1725.

criteria or a biopsy-proven lupus nephritis in combination with a positive ANA or anti-dsDNA.

Treatment

In a patient presenting with suspected new-onset uncomplicated SLE, symptomatic treatment can be given until a definitive diagnosis is made and the disease is more specifically classified. This may include NSAIDs for joint pains or pleuritis, topical corticosteroids for rash, and antihypertensive medications. Definitive care should be arranged with a rheumatologist, who may prescribe more specific therapies. Systemic corticosteroids are the mainstay of treatment, with a side effect profile including Cushing's syndrome, adrenal suppression, aseptic necrosis (most commonly of the femoral head), osteoporosis, and risk of infection. In children, growth can also be affected. Those with more severe disease are treated with pulse methylprednisolone (30 mg/kg/dose to a maximum of 1 g daily for 3 days) or high-dose prednisone (typically 2 mg/kg/day), which may be adjusted based on clinical and laboratory parameters of disease. Other medications that may be utilized for treatment of SLE include hydroxychloroquine, an antimalarial with anti-inflammatory and immune stabilizing properties; steroid-sparing agents such as mycophenolate mofetil, azathioprine, or cyclophosphamide; and DMARDs such as belimumab or rituximab. Of note, these DMARDs are not U.S. Food and Drug Administration approved for pediatric use, but they may be employed nonetheless. Adjunct treatments may include acetylsalicylic acid 81 mg daily for patients with antiphospholipid Abs due to the increased risk of thrombosis and antimicrobials if there are any signs of infection.

Clinical Algorithm

Although there is no specific clinical algorithm, there are additional labs recommended as part of the evaluation, in addition to those that comprise the diagnostic criteria. A complete blood count (CBC) can assess for various cytopenias. A complete metabolic panel (CMP) can be used to detect renal dysfunction, electrolyte disturbances that can occur with renal disease, and hypoalbuminemia which can be seen with proteinuria. Inflammatory markers including erythrocyte sedimentation rate (ESR) and C-reactive protein (CRP) may be helpful because ESR is often elevated in SLE, but CRP is usually normal and an elevation may prompt a broader differential or point to an infectious etiology. Complement levels including both C3 and C4 can be low due to formation of immune complexes. A urinalysis including microscopy should be completed to evaluate for hematuria, proteinuria, and the presence of cellular casts, as early renal disease may be clinically silent. A complete ANA profile as noted in the diagnostic criteria, including anti-dsDNA, anti-Smith, anti-ribonucleic proteins (anti-Ro, anti-La), and Sjögren's specific Ab A and B, should be obtained. These can help characterize the disease. Finally, it is recommended to send anticardiolipin Ab and lupus anticoagulant to assess for the risk of thrombosis.

Disposition

The disposition of patients with SLE is similar to that for JIA. New-onset or suspected new-onset patients with uncomplicated SLE, along with those with stable known disease, may be discharged home with outpatient follow-up. Follow-up with rheumatology and potentially other specialists, most commonly nephrology, should be arranged depending on the organ systems involved. The decision to admit these patients should be based on the presence of complications that require immediate treatment or close monitoring. If admission is required for significant complications, management should be discussed ideally with the patient's own rheumatologist, and providers should consider transfer to the patient's home institution for multidisciplinary management.

Complications

Because SLE is a disease that can affect nearly any organ system, so can the complications. The disease may be insidious in the pediatric population, and undiagnosed patients may present initially with a significant disease complication.

Infection is the leading cause of morbidity and mortality due to immune dysfunction associated with disease and with risk further increased by the use of immunomodulatory treatments. Although respiratory and urinary infections are the most common, bacteremia and subsequently sepsis has the highest rate of mortality. There are no specific guidelines for the approach to fever in a pediatric patient with SLE, but a low threshold should be maintained to perform an infectious workup including blood and urine cultures, throat culture, and echocardiogram for septic emboli or vegetations. Empiric antibiotics may need to be initiated during workup. Additional markers for infection may be useful, including CRP or procalcitonin level. Patients are at risk for common infections as well as more rare or opportunistic organisms. All patients should be screened for tuberculosis prior to starting treatment because the use of anti-TNF therapy can lead to reactivation of disease. In addition, patients who are receiving immunosuppressant therapy should not receive live vaccines. Viral infections may also occur, and EBV has been implicated in MAS in SLE patients as well as those with systemic-onset JIA. Confirmed or suspected influenza should be treated with antiviral medication. Opportunistic infections including fungal infections from *Aspergillosis, Cryptococcus, Pneumocystis* pneumonia (PCP), or endemic mycoses can occur; PCP in particular is associated with a high mortality.

Thrombosis is the most common hematologic complication and is associated with antiphospholipid syndrome. Catastrophic antiphospholipid syndrome occurs when there are disseminated microvascular thrombi that lead to multiorgan failure. This entity is often triggered by infection, but it can also develop after trauma, surgery, with concurrent neoplasia, use of oral contraceptives pills, or warfarin withdrawal. It can mimic disseminated intravascular coagulation or overwhelming infection with shock and organ failure. Treatment consists of parenteral anticoagulation and high-dose glucocorticoids, with IVIG and plasmapheresis as second-line treatments. Due to the increased risk of thrombotic events, patients with positive antiphospholipid antibodies or positive anticardiolipin antibodies are typically anticoagulated with a goal international normalized ratio of 2 to 3. More localized thrombosis may also lead to deep vein thrombosis or pulmonary embolism. Dural sinus venous thrombosis can also occur, as can cerebral strokes, either from antiphospholipid disease (large vessel) or SLE-related arteritis (small vessel). Patients with SLE can also develop bleeding diatheses, cytopenias, or thrombotic thrombocytopenic purpura.

Cardiac complications may occur, with pericarditis being the most common and affecting approximately 25% of patients. Myocarditis and endocarditis can also occur. Libman–Sachs endocarditis may lead to valve destruction and the need for replacement, or lesions may embolize or become infected. Coronary disease may be caused by a combination of premature atherosclerosis and, less commonly, coronary arteritis. Effusions leading to tamponade are relatively rare.

SLE can have several neurological complications. Posterior reversible encephalopathy syndrome occurs when the cerebral circulation is unable to autoregulate in response to acute changes in blood pressure. It typically affects the posterior circulation, but it can also affect other watershed zones of the brain. Both the cortical and subcortical tissues may be affected. Lupus cerebritis is another complication that may present with altered mental status, psychosis, seizure, coma, or focal neurological deficits. Although rare, SLE can also be a cause for transverse myelitis due to central nervous system (CNS) vasculitis or arterial thrombosis. This presents with lower extremity neuropathies and is often associated with bladder dysfunction. Meningitis, both aseptic and infectious, may occur. Therefore, if meningeal involvement is suspected, a lumbar puncture should be performed to differentiate between the two.

Pulmonary complications commonly include pleuritis associated with effusion, which can occur in 50–80% of patients. Pulmonary embolism can be seen especially in patients at increased risk of thrombosis. In addition, patients may suffer from pulmonary artery hypertension, which is associated with a poor prognosis, and/or acute lupus pneumonitis, which is rare but leads to loss of pulmonary function.

Finally, a rare but highly lethal complication affecting the pulmonary system is pulmonary artery hemorrhage, which can present with dyspnea, fever, and a new infiltrate on chest X-ray. There is limited specific information regarding this complication in pediatrics, but approximately 50% of adults with this complication present with hemoptysis. Consider this diagnosis especially in patients with new or worsening anemia and glomerulonephritis. Bronchoscopy can provide confirmation with visualization of hemosiderin-laden macrophages, and treatment is with pulse dose methylprednisolone.

There are two important gastrointestinal complications. SLE enteritis is a mesenteric vasculitis leading to bowel ischemia that can be diagnosed via computed tomography scan. Pancreatitis can also occur, either related to primary disease or as a complication of medical management.

The kidneys are very often affected in children with SLE, with up to 80% of patients experiencing lupus nephritis. Initial presentation with renal disease is common in pediatrics, and renal complications occur frequently, including acute renal failure, hypertensive crisis, and renal vein thrombosis. The latter will typically present with acute flank pain, macroscopic hematuria, and worsening renal function.

There are obstetric and neonatal complications of disease that should also be considered. Neonatal heart block can occur in infants of mothers with SLE, and it is possible even if the mother has undiagnosed disease. It is often detected on prenatal evaluation between 16 and 30 weeks of gestation, but there is risk for its development until delivery. Heart block resulting in fetal bradycardia may lead to hydrops fetalis, pericardial effusion in the developing fetus, or congestive heart failure in the newborn. If diagnosed prenatally, the mother is treated with glucocorticosteroids, and postnatal treatment can involve β-agonist treatment or cardiac pacing of the infant.

Key Points

- SLE is a multisystem inflammatory disease that can involve the skin, joints, serosa, bone marrow and blood, kidneys, and CNS.
- Diagnosis requires a minimum of four clinical and laboratory features, but patients can present with a large range of symptoms.
- There is a broad spectrum of complications from both disease and complications of medical management, with infection and thrombosis being among the most common.

Pitfalls

- Initial symptoms may be vague and nonspecific, and they may mimic other diseases.
- Presentation may be due to the presence of complications.

GRANULOMATOSIS WITH POLYANGIITIS

Background

Granulomatosis with polyangiitis (GPA), formerly Wegener's granulomatosis, is a chronic anti-neutrophil cytoplasmic antibodies (ANCA)-associated necrotizing vasculitis due to the production of autoantibodies against myeloperoxidase or proteinase-3. This disease affects predominantly the small vessels. It is primarily an adult disease, with rare onset in childhood; however, it is the most frequent ANCA-associated vasculitis in the pediatric age group. Even among pediatrics, onset is typically in the second decade, and unlike in adults, there is a slight female predominance. It is important to have a high suspicion for this disease because the mortality is very high if untreated—approximately 90% within 1 year.

Classic Clinical Presentation

The classic clinical presentation is similar in pediatrics to that in adults, with a triad of upper and lower airway inflammation associated with renal disease. Pulmonary symptoms are due to granulomatous inflammation, and renal disease is typically due to glomerulonephritis. Renal biopsy, if performed, shows a pauci-immune crescentic necrotizing glomerulonephritis, and serum studies can confirm the presence of ANCA antibodies. The most common clinical symptoms are ear, nose, and throat (ENT) complaints, including nasal discharge, epistaxis, crusting, ulcerations, acute otitis media (AOM), and hearing loss. In addition, pediatric patients are more likely to also have subglottic stenosis, which occurs in 20% of this population at the time of presentation. These patients may have hoarseness, stridor, and barking cough. Vague constitutional symptoms including malaise, fatigue, and weight loss are also common, as are respiratory complaints of cough, wheezing, hemoptysis, or dyspnea. Fixed lung infiltrates may be noted on chest X-ray. Renal findings may include hypertension or edema, and protein or blood may be seen on urinalysis. Mucus and skin findings occur in more than half of patients and can include mucosal ulcers, palpable purpura, petechial rash, livedo, and subcutaneous nodules. There is no specific atypical presentation for this disease in pediatrics.

Differential Diagnosis

This diagnosis may be difficult in children due to the overlap of symptoms with common viral or bacterial infections seen frequently in this age group. Symptoms may mimic recurrent viral upper respiratory infection, recurrent pneumonia, sinusitis, and AOM. In addition, the skin findings of petechiae and palpable purpura may be difficult to distinguish from those seen with Henoch–Schönlein purpura, a typically self-resolving vasculitis also seen in pediatrics.

Diagnostic Confirmation

New criteria for childhood GPA have been established and validated by several European groups, including the European League Against Rheumatism, Paediatric Rheumatology International Trials Organization, and Paediatric Rheumatology European Society (EULAR/PRINTO/PRES). To make the diagnosis, the patient must have three of the six criteria listed in Box 31.2.

Treatment

There are no specific pediatric guideline for treatment of GPA; the treatment modalities are extrapolated from adult data and based on expert consensus. Induction treatment usually includes corticosteroids and cyclophosphamide (2 mg/kg/day) to induce remission. Methotrexate may be used in mild disease instead of cyclophosphamide, but some studies show that it may be slightly less effective. Mycophenolate mofetil may also replace cyclophosphamide in less severe cases, but it may be associated with increased risk of relapse. Rituximab is also increasingly being used as part of initial treatment. Once remission is achieved, lower doses of steroids and azathioprine or other disease-modifying agents (rituximab, methotrexate, leflunomide, or mycophenolate mofetil) are typically continued for at least 2 years. In relapsing disease, IVIG can be helpful, and plasmapheresis may also be employed for relapse as well as for rapidly progressive glomerulonephritis or diffuse alveolar hemorrhage. During infection, high-dose steroids are given in combination with antimicrobials.

Disposition

It is unlikely that a new diagnosis of GPA is made during an emergency department visit because the criteria may require biopsies or

BOX 31.2

EULAR/PRINTO/PRES CRITERIA FOR DIAGNOSIS OF CHILDHOOD GRANULOMATOSIS WITH POLYANGIITIS

Patient Must Have Three of the Six Following Criteria

1. Histopathology showing granulomatous inflammation within the wall of an artery or perivascular/extravascular areas
2. Upper airway symptoms
   a. Chronic purulent or bloody nasal discharge/epistaxis, crusting, granulomata
   b. Perforation of the nasal septum
   c. Saddle nose deformity
   d. Chronic/recurrent sinus inflammation
3. Laryngo-tracheo-bronchial involvement, often stenosis
4. Pulmonary symptoms or imaging (CXR/CT) showing nodules/cavities/fixed infiltrates
5. Renal symptoms
   a. Proteinuria (>0.3 g/24 hr) or urine albumin:creatinine ratio >30 mmol/mg on a morning sample
   b. Hematuria (>5 RBC/HPF) or red cell casts, ≥2+ hematuria on dipstick
   c. Necrotizing pauci-immune glomerulonephritis
6. ANCA positive: immunofluorescence or ELISA

ANCA, anti-neutrophil cytoplasmic antibodies; CT, computed tomography; CXR, chest X-ray; ELISA, enzyme-linked immunosorbent assay; EULAR/PRINTO/PRES, European League Against Rheumatism, Paediatric Rheumatology International Trials Organization, and Paediatric Rheumatology European Society; HPF, high power field; RBC, red blood cells.
Source: Adapted from Ozen S, Pistorio A, Iusan SM, Bakkaloglu A, Herlin T, Brik R, et al.; Paediatric Rheumatology International Trials Organisation. EULAR/PRINTO/PRES criteria for Henoch–Schönlein purpura, childhood polyarteritis nodosa, childhood Wegener granulomatosis and childhood Takayasu arteritis: Ankara 2008. Part II: Final classification criteria. *Ann Rheum Dis.* 2010;69:798–806.

blood work that have some delay to result. If a new case is suspected but the patient is otherwise stable, they can likely be discharged with outpatient rheumatology/ENT/renal follow-up. Expeditious follow-up should be ensured, however, given the risk of mortality with untreated disease. If the child is presenting with a complication of illness or more severe symptoms, they may need admission for treatment such as parenteral steroids. This is best done in a children's hospital with a range of subspecialists who can be consulted to help with management.

Complications

With treatment, GPA has a low mortality in pediatrics, reported from 0% to 10%. However, there is increased risk for relapse compared to adult patients. One of the more severe complications is pulmonary renal syndrome, which consists of diffuse alveolar hemorrhage associated with rapidly progressing glomerulonephritis. It should be suspected if there is acute anemia associated with a new infiltrate on chest X-ray. This complication has a high mortality and requires prompt treatment with antimicrobials, immunosuppressive therapies, and high-dose corticosteroids; plasmapheresis may also be used. Rapidly progressive glomerulonephritis alone can occur as well and may require more intensive treatment. Subglottic stenosis is common; it requires immediate ENT evaluation with laryngoscopy, and tracheostomy may be required in severe cases. Surprisingly, this finding is not related to overall severity of disease and is often corticosteroid resistant. Other complications of disease include osteoporosis and avascular necrosis, as well as infertility.

Key Points

- GPA is a rare but life-threatening disease in childhood.
- The disease primarily affects the upper airway, lower airway, and kidneys.
- Serious complications involve the lungs and kidneys, but many organ systems may be impacted.
- Treatment is with immunosuppression.

Pitfalls

- Failure to consider the diagnosis and make appropriate referrals due to significant mortality rate.

- ENT symptoms overlap with many common pediatric disorders, so one needs to maintain a high suspicion.

DERMATOMYOSITIS

Background

Dermatomyositis (DM) is a small vessel vasculitis affecting primarily the skin and muscles. The exact pathogenesis is unknown, but it is thought that both genetic and environmental factors trigger disease. The incidence and prevalence in pediatrics are not well known, but they are thought to be similar to those of SLE. The age group most commonly affected is school-age children, and it is rare in younger patients. There are three disease courses that can occur: monophasic with resolutions; relapsing with variable outcome; and severe ulcerative disease, which has the highest morbidity and mortality.

Classic Clinical Presentation

The classic presentation for DM is a characteristic rash associated with proximal muscle weakness and elevated muscle enzymes. However, the onset of weakness is usually insidious and may be reported as increased fatigue with activities. Later in the course, proximal muscle weakness may interfere with performance of daily tasks such as difficulty combing hair (upper extremity), getting up from a chair (lower extremities), loss of head control (neck), and even difficulty swallowing (pharyngeal). Weakness is typically symmetric. The rash of DM has several well-described features. Patients may have a heliotrope rash, which is violaceous discoloration of the upper eyelids and is specific to DM. They may also have Gottron's papules, which are smooth, flat, nontender papules over the extensor surface of the metacarpophalangeal or proximal interphalangeal joints of the fingers. Occasionally, patients may have a malar rash, an eczematous rash over the extensor joints, or gingival erythema.

Atypical Clinical Presentation

Although skin and muscle symptoms are typical, other systems may be involved as part of the presenting picture, most commonly gastrointestinal (GI) and respiratory complaints.

Differential Diagnosis

Dermatomyositis must be distinguished from other forms of myositis, such as acute infectious myositis. One example is myositis due to influenza infection. Influenza typically has a more acute onset; is often painful; and affects a different distribution of muscles, with the calves most commonly being affected. There is also overlap with other rheumatologic diseases, including SLE, which may present with similar symptoms, and mixed connective tissue disease, an uncommon diagnosis used to describe patients with features of multiple rheumatologic conditions.

Diagnostic Confirmation

The set of criteria used to diagnose DM remains that developed by Bohan and Peter in 1975. It includes five features as outlines in Box 31.3.

Muscle biopsy may not be necessary for diagnosis any longer, if the patient meets the other criteria. However, it remains a helpful tool for establishing prognosis. MRI is often done prior to biopsy to identify areas of muscle injury and establish a location for the biopsy. Typically, the pelvis and thighs are imaged for this purpose. Other laboratory tests may

BOX 31.3

BOHAN AND PETER CRITERIA FOR THE DIAGNOSIS OF DERMATOMYOSITIS

1. Characteristic skin findings
2. Elevated muscle enzymes: CK (variable), AST, LDH, aldolase
3. Proximal muscle weakness on manual examination
4. EMG showing muscle wasting; now can use MRI findings of muscle wasting instead of EMG
5. Muscle biopsy showing characteristic inflammation and muscle cell injury

AST, aspartate transaminase; CK, creatine kinase; EMG, electromyography; LDH, lactate dehydrogenase; MRI, magnetic resonance imaging.

Source: Adapted from Bohan A, Peter JB. Polymyositis and dermatomyositis (first of two parts). *N Engl J Med.* 1975;292:344–347.

also be performed to rule out other diagnosis because creatine kinase is not always elevated in DM and aspartate transaminase, LDH, and aldolase are nonspecific. With DM, CBC and CMP may show nonspecific changes; inflammatory markers may be normal or elevated. Unlike in adults, myositis autoantibodies are not particularly helpful because they are often negative in this population. ANA may be checked to evaluate for other rheumatic disease because it is not produced in DM and, if positive, may point to an alternative diagnosis.

Treatment

As with most rheumatologic diseases reviewed, corticosteroids are the mainstay of treatment. Severe disease is often treated with pulse methylprednisolone. However, methotrexate given at a low dose weekly is becoming increasingly popular as a first-line therapy to reduce steroid use. Hydroxychloroquine is used to control dermatologic manifestations and may also permit reduced steroid use. Alternative immunomodulatory therapies have also been used for pediatric patients, although there are fewer studies in this population. Such drugs include cyclosporine, tacrolimus, azathioprine, and mycophenolate mofetil. Acute, severe symptoms can be treated with IVIG, and rituximab or cyclophosphamide are also being used in severe cases.

Disposition

Dermatomyositis is unlikely to be diagnosed in the emergency room given that diagnostic criteria include an electromyogram/MRI and possible muscle biopsy. However, most patients with suspected new or stable DM without complications can be discharged with outpatient follow-up with rheumatology. Patients with airway involvement or respiratory involvement may need admission for stabilization, whether or not diagnosis is firmly established. These admissions are also best for a children's hospital with available subspecialists who can manage complicated disease or potentially confirm diagnosis.

Complications

The main concerning complications from DM are respiratory and GI. Chest wall weakness can lead to respiratory distress, and patients may require respiratory support. They can also suffer from esophageal dysmotility, which puts them at risk of aspiration and pneumonia. Other GI complications include superficial ulcerations or more severe transmural perforation, which can occur anywhere along the GI tract. Rarely, patients may experience GI hemorrhage, volvulus, infarction, peritonitis, or pneumatosis intestinalis. The presence of GI complications is a poor prognostic indicator, and GI perforations are the leading cause of mortality in these patients. Any GI vasculitis should be treated with pulse dose methylprednisolone.

Key Points

- DM has an insidious onset of symptoms.
- DM is characterized by proximal muscle weakness and specific skin findings, including heliotrope rash and Gottron's papules.
- Important complications include compromised airway, respiratory distress, and GI perforations.

Pitfalls

- Symptoms may be mistaken for infectious myositis or other rheumatologic disease.
- Official diagnosis may require advanced testing not available in every emergency room.

Further Reading

Akikusa J. Rheumatologic emergencies in newborns, children, and adolescents. *Pediatr Clin North Am.* 2012;59:285–299.

Jariwala M, Laxer R. Primary vasculitis in childhood: GPA and MPA in childhood. *Front. Pediatr.* 2018;6:226.

Reyhan I, Gottlieb BS, Goldberg BR. Common presentations of pediatric rheumatologic diseases: A generalist's guide. *Curr Opin Pediatr.* 2013;25(3):388–396.

Shulman A, Punaro M. Critical care of the pediatric patient with rheumatic disease. *Curr Opin Pediatr.* 2011;23:263–268.

Vehe R, Riskalla M. Collagen vascular diseases: SLE, dermatomyositis, scleroderma, and MCTD. *Pediatr. Rev.* 2018;39(10):501–515.

32

Pediatric Head Injury

Evaluation and Management Across the Spectrum

JAMES L. HOMME

INTRODUCTION

Traumatic brain injury (TBI) is a common complaint and reason for presentation to an acute care provider. Although the vast majority of pediatric TBI is classified as minor head injury, it is important to remember that blunt head trauma (BHT) remains the leading cause of trauma-related death and disability in children worldwide. Anyone who cares for children in an acute care setting must be knowledgeable in both the evaluation and the management of pediatric head injury across the spectrum to avoid unnecessary exposure to ionizing radiation in those at low risk for injury and increased morbidity and mortality in patients at high risk.

The Centers for Disease Control and Prevention maintains the most recent data on pediatric TBI-related injuries (https://www.cdc.gov/traumaticbraininjury/data/tbi-edhd.html) as well as current recommendations for evaluation and management of mild traumatic brain injury (mTBI) with an emphasis on concussion (https://www.cdc.gov/traumaticbraininjury/PediatricmTBIGuideline.html). Differentiation of concussion from other forms of TBI, often referred to as TBI on computed tomography (CT) (i.e., structural head injury), is a critical educational element for health care provider discussions with patients and caregivers seeking care for minor BHT. Falls account for the majority of injuries in children younger than age 13 years. Assault, sports-related injuries, and motor vehicle accidents constitute the top three causes in children aged 13–18 years.

For clinicians evaluating BHT, the specter of more severe structural brain injuries looms large even though the rates of TBI on CT are <10% in children with minor head trauma [Glasgow Coma Scale (GCS) score of 14 or 15] and only 0.1% require neurosurgical intervention. The temptation remains to "rule out" anything serious through utilization of CTs, and studies show that in the United States, clinicians opt for imaging in one-third to one-half of pediatric patients with minor head injury presenting to the emergency department (ED). CT utilization for minor head injury varies significantly between institutions and clinician type. Irrespective of injury severity, suburban and general academic EDs (without pediatric specialists), as well as general emergency medicine practitioners, consistently image at higher rates. Clinical decision rules (CDRs) have been developed to help decrease this variability.

CLINICAL DECISION RULES FOR PEDIATRIC MINOR HEAD TRAUMA

PECARN, CATCH, and CHALICE

Investigators in the United States [Pediatric Emergency Care Applied Research Network (PECARN)], Canada [Canadian Assessment of Tomography for Childhood Head Injury (CATCH)], and Europe [Children's Head Injury Algorithm for the Prediction of Important Clinical Events (CHALICE)] have independently prospectively derived clinical prediction rules for use in evaluation of pediatric patients with minor BHT. These decision rules and performance statistics are summarized in Table 32.1. Primary and secondary endpoints for the studies varied; however, the endpoints established in the PECARN study have emerged as the most frequently utilized and cited. The primary endpoint of PECARN was clinically important traumatic brain injury (ciTBI), defined by the composite endpoints of death from TBI, neurosurgical intervention for TBI, intubation for more than 24 hours for TBI, or hospitalization for more than two nights for TBI. Notably, there were no deaths reported in the study of 42,412 patients. PECARN also reports rates of TBI on CT for patients who underwent imaging.

CATCH and CHALICE both performed very well in their derivation studies citing high sensitivities, specificities, and negative predictive values (NPVs). PECARN combined derivation and validation into a single study, reporting sensitivity of 100% and an NPV of 100% for those younger than age 2 years and sensitivity of 96.8% and an NPV of 99.95% for those aged 2–18 years in the validation portion of the study.

A large prospective study comparing the three rules was performed across 10 different EDs in Australia and New Zealand. More than 20,000 children younger than age 18 years were enrolled, although due to different inclusion criteria, all patients were not evaluated by all three rules. PECARN had the highest sensitivity across rules, not missing any patients with ciTBI younger than age 2 years and only a single patient older than age 2 years. All three CDRs had similar NPVs (PECARN: both <2 and 2–18 years, 100%; CATCH, 99.4%; and CHALICE, 99.8%). CATCH and CHALICE had higher specificities (56% and 78%, respectively).

All three CDRs are highly sensitive, weighted toward not missing injuries, although PECARN seems to have a slight edge over CATCH and CHALICE. Specificity favors CATCH and CHALICE, although many clinicians and caregivers favor sensitivity of a rule over specificity in order to not miss important injuries. How, then, should one choose which rule to utilize?

Clinical decision rules are derived in an attempt to improve upon current standard practices in establishing or excluding certain diagnoses. Decision rules take the form of one-way or two-way rules. One-way rules are typically used as a "rule out" by identifying patients at very low risk for a condition who require no further investigation. They *are not* meant to imply that patients who do not meet all criteria of the rule are at high risk of having the condition—a common misunderstanding of how to employ the rule. Patients who cannot be "ruled out" by the one-way CDR often require additional information for further risk stratification. Two-way rules are designed to *direct action* toward confirmation or exclusion of the condition in question depending on if criteria of the rule are met. Patients meeting all criteria of the rule can forgo testing, whereas those who do not meet all criteria undergo additional testing.

Clinicians could utilize these minor head injury CDRs as one-way injury exclusion rules—and for this application PECARN seems superior. However, both PECARN and CATCH stratify patients into varying risk categories based on the presence of certain "higher risk" variables. In these instances, imaging is suggested—making the rules into "two-way" rules.

Numerous studies have shown that if clinicians were to image all patients who did not meet all of the rule criteria required to be classified as very low risk, imaging rates would increase after adoption of the CDR—nullifying any value of the rule. Therefore, in practice, these CDRs are most appropriately applied in a "stepwise" manner—initially as a one-way rule to determine if the patients can be deemed at very low risk and not requiring neuroimaging. If these conditions are not met, then clinicians should further risk stratify patients into higher or lower risk groups based on the presence of high-risk variables or a combination of lower risk variables. Due to the magnitude of the

TABLE 32.1 CLINICAL DECISION RULE VARIABLES AND VALIDATION STATISTICS

Predictor Variable	PECARN <2 (*N* = 10,718)	PECARN ≥2 (*N* = 31,695)	CATCH (*N* = 3,866)	CHALICE (*N* = 22,772)
Mechanism of injury	Severe mechanism of injury (MVC with patient ejection, death of another passenger, or rollover; pedestrian or bicyclist without helmet struck by motorized vehicle; falls >0.9 m; or head struck by high-impact object)	Severe mechanism of injury (MVC with patient ejection, death of another passenger, or rollover; pedestrian/bicyclist without helmet struck by motorized vehicle; falls >1.5 m; or head struck by high-impact object)	Dangerous mechanism of injury (e.g., MVC; fall from elevation ≥3 ft. (≥91 cm) or ≥5 stairs; or fall from bicycle with no helmet)	High-speed RTA as pedestrian, cyclist, or occupant (defined as accident with speed >40 mph or 64 km/hr); fall >3 m in height; or high-speed injury from projectile or object
History	LOC for ≥5 seconds Not acting normally per parent report	Any LOC History of vomiting Severe headache	History of worsening headache	Witnessed loss of consciousness for >5 minutes Three or more discrete episodes of vomiting after head injury Amnesia (antegrade or retrograde; >5 minutes) Suspicion of non-accidental injury (any suspicion by the examining doctor) Seizure in patient with no history of epilepsy
Examination	GCS score <15 Other signs of altered mental status (agitation, somnolence, repetitive questioning, slow response to verbal communication) Palpable or unclear skull fracture Occipital, parietal, or temporal scalp hematoma	GCS score <15 Other signs of altered mental status (agitation, somnolence, repetitive questioning, slow response to verbal communication) Clinical signs of basilar skull fracture (e.g., hemotympanum, "raccoon" eyes, otorrhea or rhinorrhea of CSF, Battle's sign)	GCS score <15 at 2 hours after injury[a] Irritability on examination[a] Any sign of basal skull fracture (e.g., hemotympanum, "raccoon" eyes, otorrhea or rhinorrhea of CSF, Battle's sign) Suspected open or depressed skull fracture[a] Large, boggy scalp hematoma	GCS score <14, or <15 if aged <1 year Abnormal drowsiness (in excess of that expected by examining doctor) Positive focal neurology (motor, sensory, coordination, or reflex abnormality) Signs of basal skull fracture (hemotympanum, "raccoon" eyes, otorrhea or rhinorrhea of CSF, Battle's sign, facial crepitus, severe facial injury) Suspicion of penetrating or depressed skull injury, or tense fontanelle Presence of bruise, swelling, or laceration >5 cm if aged <1 year
Statistics[b]				
Sensitivity, % (95% CI)	100.0 (90.7–100.0)	99.0 (94.4–100.0)	88.7 (82.2–93.4)	92.3 (89.2–94.7)
Specificity, % (95% CI)	53.8 (52.3–55.4)	45.8 (44.9–46.8)	56.4 (55.0–57.8)	78.1 (77.5–78.7)
PPV, % (95% CI)	2.0 (1.4–2.8)	1.6 (1.3–1.9)	5.6 (4.7–6.7)	7.9 (7.2–8.7)
NPV, % (95% CI)	100.0 (99.8–100.0)	100.0 (99.9–100.0)	99.4 (99.1–99.7)	99.8 (99.7–99.9)

[a]High-risk predictors for CATCH (need for neurological intervention).
[b] Data from Babl FE, et al. Accuracy of PECARN, CATCH, and CHALICE head injury decision rules in children: A prospective cohort study. *Lancet.* 2017;389:2393–2402.
CATCH, Canadian Assessment of Tomography for Childhood Head Injury; CHALICE, Children's Head Injury Algorithm for the Prediction of Important Clinical Events; CI, confidence interval; CSF, cerebrospinal fluid; GCS, Glasgow Coma Scale; LOC, loss of consciousness; MVC, motor vehicle crash; NPV, negative predictive value; PECARN, Pediatric Emergency Care Applied Research Network; PPV, positive predictive value; RTA, road traffic accident.

sample size of the derivation and validation cohorts and the information they provide for risk stratification, PECARN has distinguished itself as the clear frontrunner in CDRs for minor head injury.

RISK STRATIFICATION IN MINOR BLUNT HEAD TRAUMA

PECARN rule patients without any risk factors have a very low risk for ciTBI (<2 years, 0.02%; 2–18 years, <0.05%), and therefore imaging is generally not recommended. Those with certain high-risk factors, such as GCS score <14 or other signs of altered mental status, signs of a palpable skull fracture, or signs of a basilar skull fracture are at higher risk of ciTBI (<2 years, 4.4%; 2–18 years, 4.3%), and imaging is considered appropriate for the majority of these patients. For the patients that fall into the intermediate risk category (~30%), rates of ciTBI are collectively 0.9%. Although sufficiently high for some clinicians or caregivers to warrant CT scanning, many others believe that the potential risks of ionizing radiation on the developing brain, cost of the testing, or discovery of incidental findings may outweigh the small risk of missing an injury. In reality, the intermediate risk group is an amalgam of patient groups with significant variability in *actual* rates of ciTBI. Through a series of preplanned secondary analyses of the PECARN parent data, each variable was further examined in isolation or in combination with one other variable to determine their predictive values. In addition, investigators also expanded the definition of an isolated variable to exclude other factors that have been associated with TBI in other studies. For each study, the variable in question was excluded from the following list to form the extensive definition: no history of loss of consciousness (LOC), acting normally per parent/guardian, pediatric GCS score of 15, no signs of altered consciousness (sleepiness, agitation), no palpable skull fracture, no scalp hematoma or other signs of traumatic scalp findings, no signs of basilar skull fracture, no neurologic deficits (motor or sensory abnormalities), no vomiting after head trauma, no seizure after head trauma, no headache, and no amnesia. Data from all these studies are summarized in Figure 32.1 in the form of a risk matrix that can be utilized to determine predicted rates of ciTBI. Intersection of row and column provides risk estimate with 95% confidence intervals for the variable(s) of concerns. These data "refine" the rule for intermediate risk patients—further stratifying them within the heterogeneous 0.9% ciTBI group. Additional data are also included in Figure 32.1 on patients with a combination of intermediate-risk and high-risk variables (final two columns).

For patients with isolated extensive definition of severe mechanism of injury, rates of ciTBI range between 0.1% and 0.3% depending on age group. Similar low rates of ciTBI are present in isolated extensive vomiting (0.2%), isolated non-frontal scalp hematoma (0.4%), and isolated LOC (0.2%). Patients with isolated extensive "not acting normally per parent" and "severe headache" had no cases of ciTBI. Review of each study results in the similar conclusion that ciTBI is rare in the setting of an isolated PECARN "intermediate" risk variable. In addition, some patients with non-isolated findings are also at sufficiently low risk of ciTBI that neuroimaging may not be indicated.

VALUE OF OBSERVATION IN MINOR BLUNT HEAD TRAUMA

In head injury, signs and symptoms may evolve over time—sometimes worsening and sometimes resolving. The most feared manifestation of this phenomena is observed in the patient with an expanding epidural hematoma who presents with the classic "lucid interval" followed by rapid deterioration. Much more commonly encountered in minor BHT is the patient suffering a concussive head injury who is initially confused, amnestic to events, very nauseated, dizzy, and complaining of a severe headache that gradually improves with rest, often quite dramatically over the first several hours post injury. Clinicians should therefore incorporate the timing of the assessment into their calculus when deciding on need for neuroimaging. Studies performed by Nigrovic and colleagues demonstrated decreasing head CT rates among patients who were observed prior to imaging. Clinical symptoms improved for the majority of observed patients. More than 75% of patients with abnormal mental status returned to normal, 78% of vomiting children older than age 2 years had cessation of vomiting, 66% of children older than age 2 years with severe headache improved, and 100% of children younger

< 2 Years Old-Rates of ciTBI

Intermediate Risk Variables	Isolated – Extensive definition	Isolated – PECARN rule based definition	Severe mechanism of injury	Nonfrontal scalp hematoma	Loss of consciousness +5 sec	Not acting normally per parent	High Risk Variables: Palpable or unclear fracture	GCS <15 or Altered Mental Status
Severe mechanism of injury	**0.1%** (1/756) (0–0.7CI)	**0.3%** (4/1327) (0.1–0.8CI)		**3.5%** (9/257) (2–7CI)	**3.5%** (2/57) (0.4–12 CI)	**0.6%** (1/156) (0–4CI)	**0%** (0/21) (0–16CI)	**3%** (3/103) (0.6–8CI)
Nonfrontal scalp hematoma	**0.4%** (12/2998) (0.2–0.7CI)	**0.5%** (4/820) (0.1–1.2CI)	**3.0%** (7/233) (1.2–6.1CI)		**0%** (0/16) (0–20.6CI)	**1.7%** (1/59) (0–9.1CI)	**1.4%** (1/72) (0–7.5CI)	**2.2%** (1/45) (0.1–11.8CI)
Loss of consciousness +5sec	**0.2%*** (1/576) (0–1.0CI)	**0.6%** (1/157) (0–3.5CI)	**3.5%** (2/57) (0.4–12 CI)	**0%** (0/16) (0–20.6CI)		**0%** (0/20) (0–16.8CI)	Data Not Available	**0%** (0/16) (0–20.6CI)
Not acting normally per parent	**0%** (0/188) (0–1.9CI)	**0.2%** (1/411) (0–1.3CI)	**0.7%** (1/143) (0–3.8CI)	**1.7%** (1/59) (0–9.1CI)	**0%** (0/20) (0–16.8 CI)		**0%** (0/10) (0–30.8CI)	**0.8%** (4/494) (0.2–3.0CI)
Vomiting	**0.2%*** (2/815) (0–0.9CI)	**0%** (0/567) (0–0.6CI)	**0.6%** (1/181) (0–3.0CI)	**0%** (0/76) (0–4.7CI)	**5.6%** (1/18) (0.1–27.3CI)	**0.6%** (1/158) (0–3.5CI)	**0%** (0/5) (0–52.2CI)	**0%** (0/35) (0–10CI)

*Aggregate data for all patients <18 years

2–18 Years Old-Rates of ciTBI

Intermediate Risk Variables	Isolated – Extensive definition	Isolated – PECARN rule based definition	Severe mechanism of injury	Loss of consciousness	Vomiting	Severe headache	High Risk Variables: Signs of basilar skull fracture	GCS <15 or Altered Mental Status
Severe mechanism of injury	**0.3%** (2/730) (0–1.0CI)	**0.6%** (12/1975) (0.3–1CI)		**2.3%** (14/601) (1–4 CI)	**4.5%** (5/110) (1–10 CI)	**0%** (0/27) (0–12.8 CI)	**0%** (0/12) (0–26CI)	**3.8%** (10/261) (2–7CI)
Loss of consciousness	**0.2%*** (1/576) (0–1.0CI)	**0.5%** (12/2623) (0.2–0.8CI)	**2.3%** (14/601) (1–4 CI)		**0.9%** (3/321) (0.2–2.7CI)	**0%** (0/121) (0–3.0CI)	**10%** (2/20) (1.2–31.7CI)	**1.9%** (13/695) (1.0–3.2CI)
Vomiting	**0.2%*** (2/815) (0–0.9CI)	**0.7%** (10/1501) (0.3–1.2CI)	**4.5%** (5/110) (1–10 CI)	**0.9%** (3/321) (0.2–2.7CI)		**1.4%** (1/69) (0–7.8CI)	**18.8%** (3/16) (4–45.6CI)	**1.8%** (9/487) (0.8–3.5CI)
Severe headache	**0%** (0/2462) (0–0.1CI)	**1.4%** (3/209) (0.3–4.1 CI)	**0%** (0/27) (0–12.8 CI)	**0%** (0/121) (0–3.0 CI)	**1.4%** (1/69) (0–7.8 CI)		**0%** (0/3) (0–70.8 CI)	**2.7%** (2/74) (0.3–9.4 CI)

*Aggregate data for all patients <18 years

FIGURE 32.1 Risk estimates of clinically important traumatic brain injury (ciTBI) in children younger than age 2 years and those aged 2–18 years with minor blunt head trauma based on one or two PECARN variables. GSC, Glasgow Coma Scale.

than age 2 years initially described as not acting normally returned to baseline. Observation is more common in patients presenting early to the ED after injury and in patients with intermediate risk for ciTBI (60% observed), and it has resulted in a significant decrease in overall imaging rate (5% in observed versus 34% in non-observed). Remarkably, each hour of observation resulted in an average reduction of 70% in CT utilization. Although observation did increase ED length of stay, the median duration was 2.5 hours, a difference of only 1.0 hour longer than that of those not observed. Optimal length of ED observation remains elusive; however, a large retrospective study of children younger than age 14 years with minor BHT demonstrated that only 5% of patients were diagnosed with intracranial hemorrhage more than 6 hours post injury. The necessary ED observation length is likely to be much shorter than 6 hours, and it is reasonable to consider active observation at home with appropriate caregiver instruction.

DELAYED PRESENTATION FOR BLUNT HEAD TRAUMA

Observation prior to imaging has been shown to decrease rates of imaging without increasing rates of missed injuries. Can this fact be extrapolated to patients who present in a delayed manner? PECARN excluded patients who presented more than 24 hours after injury and therefore the CDR is not validated for evaluation of patients presenting after this time. Few data exist to direct clinicians. Borland et al. provide some information through a planned secondary analysis of a study evaluating performance of minor BHT CDRs across 10 EDs in Australia and New Zealand. In their cohort of nearly 20,000 patients, 5% (981 patients) presented more than 24 hours after BHT. Patients younger than age 2 years made up 28% of patients with low-impact (<1 m) falls, constituting the most common mechanism of injury. The CT rate for patients with delayed presentation was 21.7% compared to 8.6% for those presenting before 24 hours. Clinically important TBI occurred in 8 (0.8%) of these patients, with 2 patients requiring neurosurgical intervention for hematoma evacuation. There were no deaths or intubation for longer than 24 hours due to BHT. The TBI on CT rate was 3.8% for delayed versus 1.2% for early presentation, with the factors of suspicion for depressed skull fracture and presence of nonfrontal scalp hematoma most closely association with a positive CT.

SHARED DECISION-MAKING

Patients with minor head injury are unique with individualized risk factors. In addition, they are often accompanied by caregivers with distinct values and preferences. Therefore, it stands to reason that individualization of care is not only reasonable but also optimal, especially when more than one rationale option may exist. The decision to actively observe a patient versus CT scanning should be made jointly between provider and caregiver through the process of shared decision-making. Decision aids (DAs) are tools that are designed to assist this process, having been shown to increase patient knowledge and engagement in decision-making as well as improve accuracy of risk perception. Shared decision-making, with or without the assistance of DAs, occurs when patients/caregivers are provided with evidence regarding the condition of concern (in an accessible format) while clinicians learn about patient/caregiver values and preferences. Equipped with this knowledge, together they determine the course of action. DAs for pediatric minor BHT were developed at the Mayo Clinic and prospectively studied in a multicenter trial. Utilization of the DAs resulted in increased caregiver knowledge, decreased decisional conflict, and increased involvement in decision-making regarding utilization of imaging versus observation compared to the usual care group. These DAs are available for download from the Mayo Clinic Shared Decision Making National Resource Center (https://shareddecisions.mayoclinic.org/decision-aid-information/head-ct-choice-decision-aid). In practice, patient/caregiver dyads are provided with the specific DA based on PECARN-based risk estimates for ciTBI. The DA is utilized in the discussion of imaging versus observation. DAs are not utilized for patients at very low risk for ciTBI. For this group of patients, clinicians make a specific recommendation (imaging is not indicated) rather than participate in shared decision-making.

Integration of evidence-based recommendations into imaging practices along with caregiver engagement in decision-making should be part of any individual or institutional practice for evaluation of minor BHT. Figure 32.2 provides an example of a protocol for minor head trauma that integrates these concepts.

APPLICATION OF PECARN TO SELECT PATIENT POPULATIONS

Sports-Related Traumatic Brain Injury

Sports-related BHT is common and increasing in incidence. As clinicians, we need to understand whether sports-related BHT is somehow different from non-sports-related BHT and therefore warrants a different approach. In addition, it is critical to clearly articulate the difference to patients/caregivers between concussions and other forms of

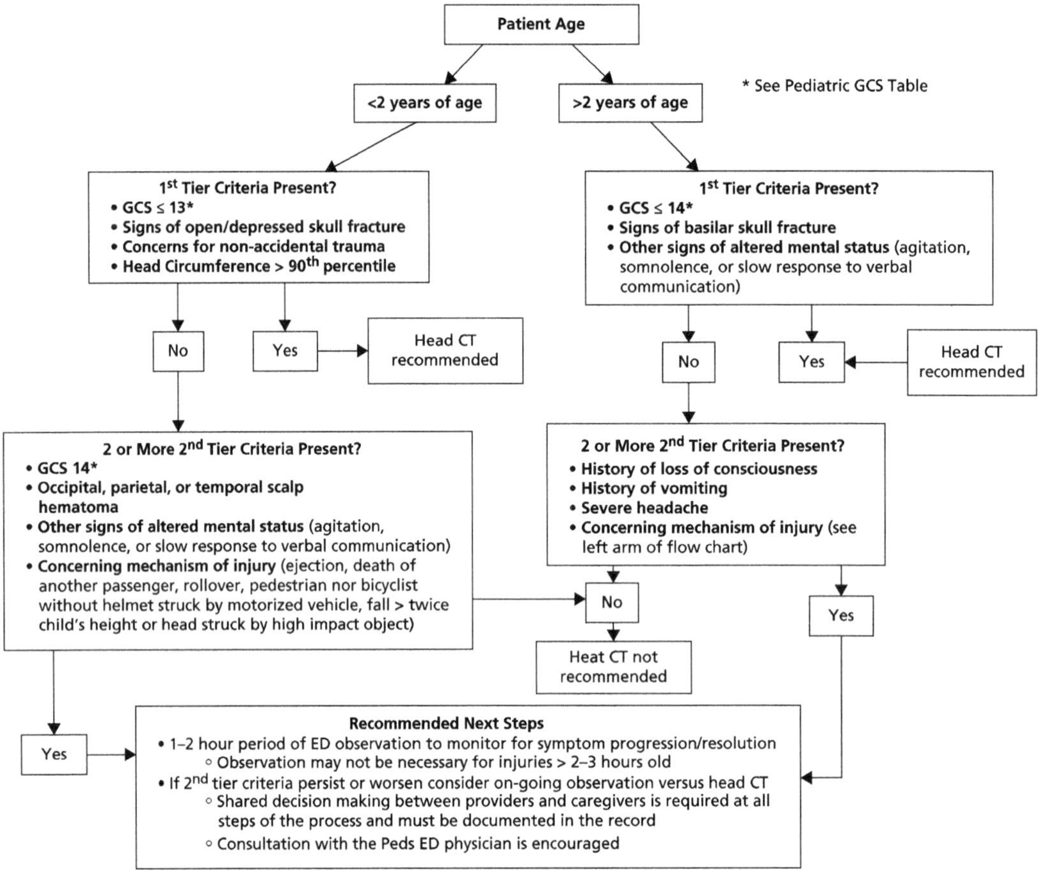

FIGURE 32.2 Example protocol for evaluation of pediatric minor blunt head trauma. CT, computed tomography; GSC, Glasgow Coma Scale.

Source: Adapted from the Mayo Clinic (Rochester, MN).

structural TBI. Concussions are diagnosed clinically because standard neuroimaging studies can be completely normal in symptomatic patients.

Glass et. al report data from a prospective study of more than 23,000 patients aged 5–18 years with sports-related BHT. The vast majority of sports-related BHT is minor, with 98% of patients exhibiting a GCS score >14 and >90% with a GCS of 15. Compared to the non-sports-related cohort, sports-related injury patients underwent scanning at higher rates (53% vs. 41%) but had lower rates of TBI on CT (4% vs. 7%) and no difference in rates of ciTBI. When queried as to the rationale for imaging, providers cited mechanism of injury, LOC, presence of headache, and parental preference as primary drivers. Participation in equestrian, snow, and wheeled sports (e.g., skateboarding, roller-blading, and riding scooters) carried the highest risk of TBI on CT. Based on these data, it is reasonable to conclude that children presenting with sports-related BHT should be evaluated in a similar manner as any other child with BHT.

Bleeding Disorders

Patients with either congenital or acquired bleeding disorders are often considered at higher risk of TBI on CT after minor blunt head trauma. PECARN investigators analyzed patients in their cohort with bleeding disorders and outcomes based on CDR variables. Of the 230 patients in the study, 56 had hemophilia, with 60% of these patients characterized as severe (factor level <1%). Other forms of disorders included von Willebrand disease (19.6%), thrombocytopenia (14.8%), anticoagulation therapy (6.5%), functional platelet disorder (2.6%), and other (0.4%). Imaging rates were very high (81%), with only 2 patients with intracranial hemorrhage (ICH; 1.1%)—both of whom were symptomatic and neither required neurosurgical intervention. Delayed presentation of bleeding is a possibility because patients were not enrolled more than 24 hours after injury; however, none of the enrolled patients returned with delayed ICH. The PECARN investigators concluded that "although patients with congenital or acquired bleeding disorders are at risk for ICH, the low rate of ICH suggests that they may not routinely require cranial CT imaging after minor blunt head trauma in the absence of signs or symptoms of ICH." Patients discharged without imaging require clear counseling on worrisome signs and symptoms that indicate the need for re-evaluation.

POST-TRAUMATIC SEIZURES

Post-traumatic seizures (PTS) occur in 0.6–4% of all cases of pediatric head trauma, with the largest prospective series reporting a rate of 1.3%. Overall TBI on CT rates after PTS are 15.5%, with an inverse relationship between GCS and CT findings (GCS 15 = 6.0%, GCS 14 = 38.8%, and GCS 3–13 = 46.4%). Increased seizure duration and delayed onset of seizure from time of injury correlate with higher TBI on CT rates. Overall recurrence risk for PTS is 3.7%, but it is only 0.3% in patients with a GCS score of 15. There is a low-risk group of patients with PTS, in whom seizure occurred at the time of injury and lasted <1 minute. The rate of TBI on CT in this low-risk group was 3.9%, with no patients requiring neurosurgical intervention—suggesting that these patients can likely be discharged safely from the ED, some even without imaging. For all other patients with PTS, strong consideration should be given to neuroimaging due to their high rates of TBI on CT. Negative CT scans in these patients facilitate discharge from the ED because recurrence risk for seizure is low and they do not require neurosurgical intervention.

ABUSIVE HEAD TRAUMA

Abusive head trauma (AHT) is the leading cause of death from traumatic injury in infants. It has been estimated that AHT occurs in approximately 1 in 3,000 infants. Victims of AHT are at twice the risk of death compared to those with accidental head injury. Even minor AHT injuries herald potentially more serious injury in the future. Although clinicians may be tempted to utilize the PECARN rule to determine need for neuroimaging in patients with suspected AHT, this temptation should be avoided. The PECARN rule was derived based on the assumption that clinical information obtained at the time of the initial ED encounter is accurate. Details surrounding the events leading to AHT are often misrepresented or unknown. In addition, the focus of the PECARN rule is identification of patients at risk for specifically defined ciTBI, not the primary goal of evaluation of AHT, which focuses on injury detection. TBI on CT in an accidental setting may not be deemed clinically important, whereas in AHT all findings are clinically relevant, including isolated skull fractures, which PECARN did not include in its definition of a TBI on CT. Finally, the aim of the PECARN CDR is to reduce unnecessary CT utilization in low-risk patients. Infants and young children who are victims of abuse are at high risk of morbidity and mortality even in the absence of any neurologic or physical examination findings. In these cases, injury identification outweighs any theoretical risks of radiation exposure from neuroimaging. The American Academy of Pediatrics and the American College of Radiology both recommend a head CT for all infants and children younger than age 2 years with any history or physical examination findings concerning for abuse.

Up to one-third of children ultimately diagnosed with AHT will have been evaluated previously by a physician for symptoms potentially compatible with brain injury. Identification of these at-risk patients is problematic due to nonspecific presentations. The Pittsburgh Infant Brain Injury Score (PIBIS) was derived and validated for clinical use to guide in the evaluation of infants with nonspecific signs or symptoms who should undergo cranial imaging for evaluation of possible AHT. The PIBIS CDR is a 5-point scale: abnormality on dermatologic examination (2 points), age 3 months or older (1 point), head circumference >85 percentile (1 point), and serum hemoglobin <11.2 g/dL (1 point). When applied to afebrile, well-appearing infants aged 30–364 days presenting without a history of trauma and a symptom associated with risk of AHT (Table 32.2), utilization of a score of 2 as the threshold for

TABLE 32.2 INCLUSION CRITERIA FOR PITTSBURGH INFANT BRAIN INJURY SCORE

Inclusion Criteria (All Four Must Be Met)	Seeking Medical Evaluation for One of the Following Symptoms
1. 30–364 days of age	1. ALTE/BRUE/apnea
2. Well-appearing	2. Vomiting (>4 episodes) without diarrhea
3. Temperature <38.3°C	3. Seizures or seizure-like activity
4. No history of trauma	4. Soft tissue swelling of the scalp
	5. Bruising
	6. Other nonspecific symptoms, such as lethargy, fussiness, or poor feeding

ALTE, apparent life-threatening event; BRUE, brief, resolved, unexplained event.

imaging produced a sensitivity and specificity for abnormal neuroimaging of 93% and 53%, respectively.

GUIDE TO DISPOSITION AFTER CT SCANNING

Normal Cranial CT Scan

When imaging is indicated, a clinician still must determine what to do with the information obtained. More than 90% of imaged children with minor BHT will have a normal scan. Holmes et al. reported outcomes for patients with negative cranial CT from a large prospective multicenter trial. In their cohort of more than 12,500 patients with an initial GCS of 15 and a normal ED CT scan, 83% were discharged and 17% were hospitalized. For the nearly 1,000 patients with an initial GCS of 14 and a normal ED CT scan, 61% were discharged and 39% were admitted. Two percent of discharged patients had repeat imaging, with the rate of new findings only 0.04% (GCS 15) and 0.2% (GCS 14). No discharged patients with a normal initial ED CT scan required neurosurgical intervention. Hospitalization resulted in a threefold increase in repeat imaging (6%), with the rate of new findings 0.5% (GCS 15) and 1% (GCS 14). No admitted patients with a normal initial ED CT scan required neurosurgical intervention, resulting in an NPV of a normal ED CT scan for neurosurgical intervention for patients with an initial GCS of 14 or 15 of 100%. These data support adoption of a standard practice of discharge for patients with a GCS of 14 or 15 and negative ED CT scan unless there are alternate reasons beyond concern for neurologic deterioration prompting inpatient observation or treatment.

Isolated Linear Skull Fractures

Isolated non-depressed linear skull fractures are some of the most common injuries detected in patients imaged for BHT. Retrospective review studies published in the neurosurgical, pediatric surgical, and emergency medicine literature suggest that neurologically normal patients with isolated accidental skull fractures do not require transfer for evaluation or admission for observation. PECARN investigators added prospective data to bolster these findings by reviewing 350 patients with isolated linear skull fractures—63% of whom were younger than age 2 years and 57% admitted to the hospital. Admission was associated with high rates (21%) of repeat imaging, with only 2.5% of studies revealing any new findings. No patients required neurosurgical intervention. Of the 149 discharged patients, 13.4% underwent repeat imaging with no new traumatic findings. Based on all these studies, clinicians can feel comfortable that neurologically normal patients with isolated linear skull fractures after BHT do not require inpatient observation and likely do not require follow-up imaging. Caregivers should be advised to watch for the development of a growing scalp mass at the site of the fracture, which can be a sign of a leptomeningeal cyst (i.e., growing skull fracture). These are seen in approximately 1% of all skull fractures. If this condition is suspected, repeat CT scan is indicated.

Isolated Cerebral Contusions

Isolated cerebral contusions also pose a disposition conundrum for clinicians. Do these patients need to be observed in an intensive care unit (ICU) setting for neurologic deterioration? Prospective outcome data from

PECARN provide some guidance. Patients with an initial GCS of 14 or 15 and isolated cerebral contusions on ED CT scan (54 total patients) had no adverse outcomes, including death, neurosurgical intervention, or intubation for >24 hours for TBI. In this study, isolated cerebral contusions tended to be small and occur in patients with normal mental status. The authors concluded that patients with a GCS of 14 or 15 after minor blunt head trauma and small isolated cerebral contusions do not generally require ICU admission or prolonged hospitalization.

Isolated Pneumocephalus

Patients with isolated pneumocephalus, as defined by not having any other findings of TBI on CT except for non-depressed skull fracture or basilar skull fracture (BSF), were reviewed from a large data set for adverse outcomes, including death, neurosurgical intervention, or intubation for >24 hours for TBI. In nearly 15,000 pediatric patients with BHT who underwent imaging, pneumocephalus was observed in 1% (148 patients). Isolated pneumocephalus occurred in 36.5%, with a strong association with BSF (77.8%). Fifteen percent of cases had only linear skull fracture, and 7.4% had no associated fracture. The most common location for the pneumocephalus was the temporal region. Eighty-three percent of these children were hospitalized, and there were no reported adverse events specifically due to the pneumocephalus. The authors concluded that the management of these children seems most appropriately aimed at other injuries sustained.

SEVERE TRAUMATIC BRAIN INJURY

Presentations for minor head injury provide the educational opportunities for acute care providers to stress the importance of primary prevention through use of seat belts, helmets, as well as safety regarding motorized vehicles and falls. When patients present with TBI in the moderate (GCS 9–12) or severe (GCS 3–8) range, little controversy regarding imaging and management exists. Guidelines have been published for the optimal care of these patients, with the primary goal of decreasing secondary brain injury from hypoxia and hypotension, which lead to worsened outcomes. Neurosurgical interventions for space-occupying lesions or brain swelling causing severe increased intracranial pressure (ICP) unable to be managed through other modalities are also key elements of care. Decisions regarding surgical therapies are typically collaborative involving neurosurgical services, with the rare exception of life-saving skull trephination for expanding epidural hematoma leading to brainstem herniation. The remainder of this chapter focuses on the medical interventions for severe TBI.

Identification of severe TBI and early intervention are critical to optimize outcomes. GCS is used to classify injury severity as minor (13–15), moderate (9–12), and severe (3–8). Evidence suggests that the motor score component is most predictive of overall mortality, as other nontraumatic transient factors may have greater influence on the verbal and eye components of the score. Recognition of deterioration is also important and requires frequent patient reassessment, especially in the comatose intubated patient. The following should be routinely evaluated and documented for trends: pupillary dilatation, responsiveness, and symmetry; hypertension, bradycardia, and spontaneous respiratory pattern (which can be signs of intracranial hypertension); and motor responsiveness. Herniation may occur at various levels, with clues provided by physical examination findings. Transtentorial herniation is accompanied by pupillary dilatation and bradycardia. Foramen magnum herniation is signaled by downbeat nystagmus and Cushing's triad of bradycardia, bradypnea, and hypertension. If unilateral or bilateral weakness is detected, without a structural correlate on imaging, this suggests subfalcine herniation. An understanding of the variations of decorticate and decerebrate motor responses can also help localize the level of brain dysfunction. Adjuncts such as ICP monitoring, brain tissue partial pressure oxygen monitoring ($PbrO_2$), advanced neuroimaging, and electroencephalography (EEG) are also utilized in the care of patients. Although many of these modalities may not be available in the acute care setting, recognition of their need guides decision-making regarding urgency, route, and destination for patients requiring transfer.

After injury identification and attention to acute stabilization and management issues, the goals of care focus on three primary areas: maintenance of physiologic normalcy, avoidance of cerebral ischemia, and treatment of intracranial hypertension. Guidelines outline key elements of initial or "baseline care." These include (1) neutral head positioning and elevation of the head of the bed, (2) maintenance of the appropriate level of analgesia and sedation, (3) controlled mechanical ventilation, (4) ensuring appropriate intravascular volume status and glucose monitoring, (5) maintenance of minimum hemoglobin level, (6) normothermic core temperature and prevention of fever, (7) treatment of coagulopathy, and (8) consideration of antiepileptic therapy and use of continuous EEG for seizure treatment or detection. Table 32.3 summarized these baseline elements of care.

CRITICAL CONCEPTS IN MANAGEMENT OF SEVERE TRAUMATIC BRAIN INJURY

Cerebral Perfusion Pressure

The cranial compartment is a closed space, so any increase in volume of one of the main contents (brain, spinal fluid, and blood) must result in a decrease in one of the other contents. Cerebral perfusion pressure (CPP) is the difference between the mean arterial pressure (MAP) and intracranial pressure (CPP = MAP – ICP). In normal physiology, cerebral autoregulation maintains CPP at a fairly constant level. In the injured brain, an increasing ICP leads to a lowering of the CPP, which results in a compensatory rise in systemic blood pressure and cerebral vasculature dilatation. These physiologic changes further increase ICP, producing a vicious cycle ultimately leading to hypoperfusion and ischemia in the absence of intervention. Minimum age-adjusted acceptable values for CPP in the setting of severe TBI are 40–50 mmHg, with the lower levels tolerated in infants and higher values in adolescents. Many interventions to maintain CPP can be employed, with first-tier actions focused on intravascular volume and second-tier use of vasopressors. However, a strategy directed at CPP alone is inadequate because herniation can occur due to increased ICP even in the setting of adequate CPP.

Intracranial Pressure Management

Intracranial pressure is measured directly through placement of a transducer within the cranial vault, ideally with the additional capability of drainage of cerebrospinal fluid (CSF) to aid in lowering ICP if necessary. Knowledge of ICP in the acute care setting is often limited to inference based on clinical signs and symptoms. However, this does not preclude attempts at management. Strategies to lower ICP include elevation of the head of the bead to 30°, temporary hyperventilation to a goal $PaCO_2$ of 35 mmHg, sedation, neuromuscular blockade, and use of hyperosmolar therapy such as hypertonic saline or mannitol. A recommended starting point for hyperosmolar therapy with 3% NaCl is a 10 cc/kg bolus given over 30 minutes followed by 0.1 cc/kg/hr infusion. Rates and volumes of administration may be titrated based on clinical situation. Use of 23% NaCl is also an option, but it should be administered through a central line, typically in 10-mL aliquots based on weight. If there are contraindications to hypertonic saline utilization or it is unavailable, mannitol can be given through a peripheral intravenous catheter at a dose of 0.5–1 g/kg/dose. Careful consideration of the impact of all therapies aimed to lower ICP or CPP must be taken into account because some types of sedation may decrease cardiac output and mannitol can cause a fluid diuresis, lowering intravascular volume. When ICP can be directly measured, a level >20 mmHg for more than 5 minutes or >25 mmHg at any time should be rapidly addressed. Signs of impending herniation also warrant aggressive measures to lower ICP.

Care of severe TBI begins immediately upon recognition, and while following general strategies, it must be tailored to the individual patient needs in order to optimize outcomes. Acute care clinicians have the ability to positively influence these outcomes by understanding and adhering to key management principles.

KEY POINTS

- Discussion of risks for TBI after BHT must clearly differentiate between concussive head injury and other forms of structural brain injury.
- CDRs such as the PECARN head injury rule are not designed to determine if a patient has sustained a concussion.
- Minor head injury is far more common than severe TBI, with <10% of imaging studies showing any findings and <1% requiring neurosurgical intervention.

TABLE 32.3 ESSENTIAL ELEMENTS OF "BASELINE CARE" IN SEVERE TRAUMATIC BRAIN INJURY

Element of Care	Rationale and Recommendations
Neutral head position Elevation of head of bed	Venous obstruction can increase ICP. Neutral (midline) head position and elevation of the head of bed 30° improves venous drainage.
Appropriate analgesia and sedation	Sympathetic response to pain from injury or interventions can increase ICP. Lidocaine has not been demonstrated to blunt sympathetic response and is not recommended. Most regiments include combination therapy with benzodiazepines and opiates. Ketamine can be utilized as a single agent for analgesic, dissociative sedation, maintenance of CPP, and as a neuroprotective agent through NMDA receptor antagonism.
Controlled mechanical ventilation	Hypoxia worsens neuronal injury. Hypocarbia may produce excessive vasoconstriction. Target saturation between 92% and 99% or PaO_2 90–100 mmHg. Target $PaCO_2$ between 35 and 40 mmHg.
Intravascular volume and glucose management	Hypotension increases ischemic damage. Osmolar shifts can worsen cerebral edema. TBI increases cerebral metabolic demand. Euvolemia with a target CVP of 4–10 mmHg and neutral fluid balance is ideal. Hypotonic fluids should be avoided. Target serum Na^+ should be >140 mEq/L. Maintain normoglycemia (<180 mg/dL) with consideration of insulin therapy for consecutive high blood sugar measurements. Dextrose-containing isotonic fluids may be needed to prevent hypoglycemia.
Maintain minimum hemoglobin level	Blood oxygen carrying capacity decreases with decreasing hemoglobin levels. A minimum target hemoglobin >7.0 mg/dL should be maintained. Higher levels may be indicated.
Maintain normothermia and prevent fever	Hyperthermia after TBI increases morbidity and mortality. Studies of therapeutic hypothermia in children had worse outcomes than normothermia. Targeted temperature management should aim for a core body temperature between 35.5° and 37.0°C. Antipyretics and other measures may be required to prevent temperatures >38.0°C.
Treat coagulopathy	Traumatic intracranial bleeding and intraoperative or postoperative bleeding may be worsened by coagulopathy. No definite recommendations exist for optimal coagulation parameters, and overcorrection of the INR with FFP may worsen coagulopathy. Correction should be targeted toward active bleeding and not specific laboratory parameters.
Prevent and/or treat seizures	PTS increase cerebral metabolic demand. PTS are more common in the young (<2 years) and in patients with a lower GCS (<8). Levetiracetam (20–40 mg/kg) prophylaxis or treatment of PTS is easier to administer than fos-phenytoin (20 mg/kg), but both are considered acceptable. Continuous EEG monitoring should be considered throughout management, especially in the setting of neuromuscular blockade.

CPP, cerebral perfusion pressure; CVP, central venous pressure; EEG, electroencephalography; FFP, fresh frozen plasma; GCS, Glasgow Coma Scale; ICP, intracranial pressure; INR, international normalized ratio; PTS, post-traumatic seizures; TBI, traumatic brain injury.

- ciTBI is defined by death, neurosurgical intervention, intubation for >24 hours for TBI, or hospitalization for >48 for TBI.
- The PECARN head injury decision rule classifies patients into very low risk, intermediate risk, or high risk for ciTBI.
- Observation of patients with minor BHT results in decreased imaging rates without increased risk of missed ciTBI.
- Patients presenting for initial evaluation of minor BHT >24 hours after injury often have less severe mechanisms of injury, with the factors of suspicion for depressed skull fracture and non-frontal hematoma most closely associated with TBI on CT.
- The decision to image patients not classified as very low risk by PECARN should utilize risk stratification based on combinations of risk factors and shared decision-making with caregivers.
- Utilization of DAs increases caregiver knowledge and engagement in decision-making regarding imaging or observation in minor BHT.
- Delayed or prolonged post-traumatic seizures increase risk for TBI on CT.
- Patients with no TBI on CT can be safely discharged unless alternative indications for admission exist.

PITFALLS

- Clinicians should not overestimate the risk of ciTBI based on factors such as mechanism of injury, isolated vomiting, or loss of consciousness with have classically resulted in high imaging rates.
- CDRs are meant to help guide, not dictate, clinical decision-making.
- Shared decision-making does not occur for patients at very low risk of ciTBI—where a clear recommendation (no imaging necessary) exists.
- Clinicians should avoid the temptation to apply the PECARN CDR to children with suspected non-accidental trauma.
- Certain accidental injuries detectable on CT are not classified as clinically important by PECARN—most notably non-displaced skull fractures.
- Neurologic deterioration can occur at any time, and therefore careful reassessment, especially in intubated and paralyzed patients, is critical.
- Clinicians must modulate environmental conditions to maintain normothermia.
- Hyperosmolar therapy with mannitol can detrimentally lower cerebral perfusion pressure by decreasing intravascular volume through diuresis.

Further Reading

Babl FE, et al. Accuracy of PECARN, CATCH, and CHALICE head injury decision rules in children: A prospective cohort study. *Lancet.* 2017;389:2393–2402.

Berger RP, et al. Validation of the Pittsburgh Infant Brain Injury Score for Abusive Head Trauma. *Pediatrics.* 2016;138(1):e20153756.

Borland M, et al. Delayed presentations to emergency departments of children with head injury: A PREDICT study. *Ann Emerg Med.* 2019;74(1):1–10.

Hamilton M, Mrazik M, Johnson DW. Incidence of delayed intracranial hemorrhage in children after uncomplicated minor head injuries. *Pediatrics.* 2010;126(1):e33–e39.

Holmes JF, et al. Do children with blunt head trauma and normal cranial computed tomography scan results require hospitalization for neurologic observation? *Ann Emerg Med.* 2011;58(4):315–322.

Homme JL. Pediatric minor head injury 2.0: Moving from injury exclusion to risk stratification. *Emerg Med Clin North Am.* 2018;36:287–304.

Kochanek PM, et al. Management of pediatric severe traumatic brain injury: 2019 consensus and guidelines-based algorithm for first and second tier therapies. *Pediatr Crit Care Med.* 2019;20:269–279.

Kuppermann N, et al. Identification of children at very low risk of clinically-important brain injuries after head trauma: A prospective cohort study. *Lancet.* 2009;374(9696):1160–1170.

Leetch AN, Wilson B. Pediatric major head injury: Not a minor problem. *Emerg Med Clin North Am.* 2018;36:459–472.

Osmond MH, et al. CATCH: A clinical decision rule for the use of computed tomography in children with minor head injury. *CMAJ.* 2010;182(4):341–348.

33

Spinal Trauma

EMILY MACNEILL

INTRODUCTION

Spinal trauma can lead to lifelong morbidity and even death. Although the incidence of injury is low (cervical spine injuries occur in 1% of all major pediatric trauma victims), the serious consequences of a diagnosis make the evaluation of the pediatric spine a high-stakes endeavor. Numerous challenges then add to the complexity of this evaluation. The pediatric spine changes drastically during the first two decades of life, leading to injury patterns not seen as frequently as those in adults. Second, clinicians may assess nonverbal and/or uncommunicative patients (by virtue of age, fear, or concomitant head injury). Children also engage in activities for which no guideline exist. (What "rule" does a clinician follow for the gymnast who sustained an axial load after a fall from the balance beam?) Finally, the current costly imaging modalities confer real yet poorly defined risks for patients, adding to the complexity of evaluating injured pediatric patients.

This chapter discusses the injury patterns most frequently seen in children and attempts to delineate the appropriate evaluation for children with suspected spinal trauma, focusing on answering two questions: Who needs to receive imaging for potential injury and what imaging will have sufficient sensitivity while causing minimal harm? Harm, in this context, refers to cost, radiation exposure, and the risks of sedation required for young children to get definitive imaging [e.g., magnetic resonance imaging (MRI)]. The majority of this chapter attends to cervical trauma because most spinal injuries in children occur in this region. As with all pediatric trauma pathology, prospective, randomized data are scarce. The recommendations in this chapter arise from (1) large retrospective reviews, (2) regression modeling for imaging criteria, (3) small single-center trials, and (4) expert opinion. Clinicians will have to gain comfort with ambiguity; no perfect algorithm exists that will identify every injury. Timely, deliberate, and shared decision-making with families is crucial to performing this evaluation well.

COMPARISON/CONTRAST WITH ADULT ANATOMY AND PHYSIOLOGY

Different body proportions, bony development, and weak musculature lead to unique injury patterns in the pediatric population. Young children have disproportionately large, heavy heads, in addition to weak neck muscles. Combined, these lead to a higher fulcrum of injury in the cervical spine the younger the patient. As the child grows, the fulcrum moves from C2–C3 in infancy to C3–C4 at the age of 5 years, C4–C5 by age 10 years, and C5–C6 in adulthood. This results in a pattern of injury from the occiput to C2 in young children, almost never seen in adults, with high degrees of instability and high morbidity and mortality.

The rigidity of the spinal column of an adult means that the application of sufficient stress will lead to fracture of the bony elements. In the child, however, the growing and incompletely ossified spine allows for enough motion to cause spinal cord injury without causing damage to the column itself. Facet joints, which have a 60–70° angulation in adults, have only a 30° angulation in children. This, along with shallow occipital condyles, allows for significant anterior–posterior motion. Undeveloped uncinate processes cause an increase in rotation and lateral motion along the column. Ligaments in the pediatric spine have much more laxity, further increasing mobility. Thus, the spinal column has flexibility in all plains of motion, up to the point of subluxation, without damage to the integrity of the structure. The cord that this column protects does not tolerate this degree of movement. Although the pediatric spinal column can stretch along its axis 2 in. without sustaining injury, damage occurs to the spinal cord after less than one-fourth of an inch of stretch. This phenomenon explains spinal cord injury without radiographic abnormality (SCIWORA).

CERVICAL SPINE INJURY

Background

Adults have a higher likelihood of cervical spine injury after polytrauma (5–10%) than do children (1% or 2%). Of all pediatric spinal injuries, cervical spine trauma constitutes the majority of injury patterns with severe consequences: a 40% mortality rate and a 61% prevalence of permanent neurologic damage. In large database studies, cervical spine injuries most commonly arise from motor vehicle collisions (MVCs), followed by falls and sports. The mechanisms will change as the child grows and engages in higher risk activities with a spine that becomes increasingly rigid.

Classical Clinical Presentation

Children with cervical spine injury present to the emergency department (ED) in four ways. Following high-velocity mechanisms of trauma, children in most areas of the United States receive rapid transportation to EDs with "spinal precautions." Ideally, this immobilization would include an appropriately sized backboard (contoured for small children to allow space for the relatively large occiput) with an age-appropriate collar. Not all emergency medical services agencies have this equipment, and younger children especially may present from an MVC with makeshift methods to hold the spine in line. Once in the ED, the clinician needs to determine if the child requires that immobilization technique (which may include application of a rigid collar if the original technique utilized alternate methods). In the next two presentations, which occur with lower velocity trauma (MVCs, sports injury, or falls), children arrive by private vehicle with isolated neck pain and/or neurologic symptoms. The clinician needs to decide what imaging to pursue, if any, and if the child requires the placement of an immobilization device. The fourth presentation is specific to infants with altered mental status for whom non-accidental trauma is a concern. Shaken babies can sustain ligamentous injuries to their spine, with few clinical clues; clinicians must ensure stabilization of the cervical spine during the assessment and resuscitation of these patients.

Differential Diagnosis

In a child with neck pain after trauma, the differential includes less serious diagnoses such as muscular strain. Although muscular injuries and isolated transverse process fractures can lead to a need for follow-up and outpatient therapy, the focus of this chapter is injuries that damage the structural integrity of the spinal column or the spinal cord. Cervical spinal column injuries are classified into one of two categories: axial (from occiput to C2) and subaxial (from C3 to C7 and sometimes T1).

Axial Injuries

Axial injuries lead to substantial morbidity and mortality—the highest for all cervical spine injuries. Once considered almost universally fatal, improvements in prehospital and pediatric trauma have led to more children with axial injuries presenting to EDs and surviving (some even without neurologic damage). This section discusses some of the notable pathologies and their causes. Note, however, that injury patterns occur more randomly than a chapter can delineate, and damage can occur at any bony and/or ligamentous structure.

Craniocervical Dislocation

The etiology of craniocervical dislocation includes atlanto-axial dislocation and atlanto-occipital dislocation—injuries that portend a high morbidity and mortality. The majority of patients who survive transport to the ED present with irreversible primary spinal cord damage with quadriplegia, quadriparesis, and potentially apnea and spinal shock. Concomitant injury to the brain commonly occurs, and the associated altered mental status makes spinal evaluation even more challenging. In the largest review of these injuries in 27 patients over 12 years at a level 1 pediatric trauma center (again demonstrating the rarity of this process), 10 died (37% mortality), 10 survived with significant neurologic symptoms, and 7 survived intact. These patients had a median age of 5 years with a maximum age of 9 years, reiterating that this is an injury pattern seen in younger children. These injuries do not result from low-mechanism events: MVCs made up the majority, one-third resulted from pedestrians being struck, and non-accidental trauma occurred in 1 patient. A large percentage of these patients had concomitant injuries; patients with craniocervical dislocation will require extensive radiologic evaluation and treatment at a trauma center.

Atlanto-Axial Rotatory Subluxation

This injury pattern, in which the lateral masses of C1 sublux relative to C2, constitutes a substantial proportion of spinal column trauma. Unlike other pathologies referenced herein, lower force mechanisms produce the majority of injuries (approximately one-third are secondary to simple mechanical falls), and they have good outcomes. Approximately 20% of patients will have a delayed presentation (after 24 hours) because their symptoms are attributed to "muscle strain." Atlanto-axial rotatory subluxation, also known as traumatic torticollis, occurs most commonly in young children with ligamentous laxity who present with the head tilted to one side and rotated to the opposite side. Children with traumatic torticollis who present directly from a higher velocity mechanism require close evaluation for other injuries and spinal cord damage.

Jefferson Fracture

A direct axial load can lead to a burst fracture of C1; diving into shallow water, unrestrained rollover MVC, etc. can cause this type of fracture. Because young children rarely experience these mechanisms, they rarely sustain this injury pattern. It increases in incidence in older school-age children and adolescents. Although this injury leads to high levels of instability because of ligamentous damage, the bony fragments tend to spread outward movement and do not cause spinal cord injury initially.

Hangman's Fracture

This eponym describes traumatic spondylolisthesis of C2 on C3 with sparing of the odontoid from a hyperextension force along the pars interarticularis, the weakest part of the spine at this juncture. Although a common axial cervical spine in adults, it is rare in children.

Odontoid Fracture

Significant mechanisms, such as high-velocity MVCs, can lead to odontoid fractures, although they occur only rarely in children. These fractures have favorable outcomes; if isolated, spinal cord damage rarely happens. Common causes of morbidity in adult patients are avascular necrosis of the odontoid fragment and malunion, which do not happen in children secondary to a high degree of vascularization in the distal portion of the bone.

Subaxial Fracture

The incidence of subaxial fractures increases with age as the fulcrum of injury moves inferiorly. By adolescence, the injury pattern mirrors that of adults.

Diagnostic Confirmation

As discussed previously, providers must answer two questions when confronted with patients who have potential cervical spine injuries: Who needs imaging and what imaging should be obtained? Answering these two questions has a higher degree of complexity for children than for adults. The adult literature demonstrates excellent sensitivity for numerous decision rules, which have been validated and prospectively studied, to guide in the decision of who to image. Regarding imaging, computed tomography (CT) has superior sensitivity and specificity. For children, answering this question carries more complexity. To collect sufficient positive outcomes with a rare process such as cervical spine injuries in children to enable building retrospective rules would be nearly impossible. These would then require prospective study and validation. In addition, the "pediatric" population as it pertains to cervical spine injuries includes three disparate groups of patients: a nonverbal "infant–toddler" group with an immature spine (younger than age 3 years), a verbal "school-age" group with an immature spine (aged 3–8 years), and an older child "adolescent" group with a mature cervical spine (older than age 8 years). Partitioning into these three segments also helps clinicians consider the risk of radiation from CT imaging, which disproportionately affects younger children.

Who Needs Imaging?

Three main clearance guidelines exist and have relevance to children: the National Emergency X-radiography Utilization Study (NEXUS), the Canadian C-Spine Rule (CCR), and the Pediatric Emergency Care Applied Research Network (PECARN). Appropriate use of these guidelines to reliably rule out cervical spine injury requires understanding their characteristics. Table 33.1 presents the various criteria for these rules.

The NEXUS study prospectively observed 34,069 patients in 21 centers that varied in their trauma accreditation, volume, and location. Attributes of this rule that have made it impactful include its simplicity and ease of use and its high degree of sensitivity (a crucial aspect of a clearance rule). For adults, it can safely rule out injury, and it substantially decreases the need for imaging studies. Of this large cohort, however, only 3,701 patients were younger than age 19 years, and fewer than 1,000 were younger than age 8 years. Forty-four

TABLE 33.1 COMPARISON OF RULES FOR IMAGING: NATIONAL EMERGENCY X-RADIOGRAPHY UTILIZATION STUDY, THE CANADIAN C-SPINE RULE, AND THE PEDIATRIC EMERGENCY CARE APPLIED RESEARCH NETWORK

	NEXUS	CCR	PECARN
Rules	No posterior midline tenderness No evidence of intoxication Normal level of alertness No focal neurologic deficit No painful distracting injuries	No high-risk factors[a] Simple rear-end MVC[b] or sitting in the emergency department or ambulatory or delayed onset of pain or absence of cervical spine Able to rotate 45° left and right	Altered mental status Focal neurologic findings Neck pain Torticollis Substantial torso injury[c] Conditions predisposing to cervical spine injury[d] Diving High-risk mechanism[e]
No. of pediatric patients	3,701	None	540 patients with injury and 2,774 controls
Sensitivity	0.57 (0.18–0.9) 0.98 (0.91–1.0) 1.00 (0.88–1.00)	0.86 (0.42–1.00)	0.98 (96–99)
Specificity	0.35 (0.25–0.45) 0.54 (0.45–0.62) 0.20 (0.18–0.21)	0.15 (0.08–0.23)	0.26 (0.23-0.29)

[a]High-risk factors: age >65 years, fall from >3 feet or five stairs, axial load (diving), MVC high-speed (>100 km/hr) or rollover or ejection, collision with motorized vehicle, and bicycle collision.
[b]Does not include being pushed into oncoming traffic, being hit by a large vehicle such as a truck or a bus, being struck by a vehicle at a high rate of speed, or if there is a rollover.
[c]This includes injuries from the clavicles down to the pelvis, spinal injuries, and solid organ and bony injuries.
[d]Numerous conditions can predispose children to cervical spine injury in the setting of trauma. Congenital abnormalities that affect the musculoskeletal system (Down syndrome, achondrodysplasia, Ehlers–Danlos syndrome, Marfan syndrome, osteogenesis imperfecta, etc.) and acquired abnormalities (juvenile rheumatoid arthritis, rickets, etc.) as well as previous history of cervical spine injury/surgery are all risk factors for injury after trauma.
[e]Diving, fall >10 feet, hanging, pedestrian/bicyclist/rider hit by car, MVC with head-on collision/rollover/ejection, death in the crash, speed >55 mph, motorized vehicle that is not a car, axial load, and clotheslining.
CCR, Canadian C-Spine Rule; MVC, motor vehicle collision; NEXUS, National Emergency X-radiography Utilization Study; PECARN, Pediatric Emergency Care Applied Research Network.

patients (1%) had cervical spine injury, and none of the injured patients were younger than age 2 years, making this rule difficult to apply in this population. NEXUS does not account for the mechanism, and its success depends on the ability of the patient to communicate. Can it then be used for a 2-year-old in a rollover motor vehicle accident? Although the literature demonstrates that numerous institutions utilize this rule in pediatric patients, case reports exist of young children with clinically significant spinal injuries despite screening negative by NEXUS.

The CCR has greater sensitivity and specificity than NEXUS in adults, and it does take mechanism into account, which makes it more appealing for use with younger children. However, the youngest patient in the original series was aged 16 years. One study, published in 2009, applied the CCR to a pediatric population and compared its sensitivity and specificity directly against those of NEXUS. Although the original paper showed that it performed well in comparison, and may in fact be superior, a Cochrane review elicited different results from the data for which there was no explanation. Again, although many institutions utilize CCR, the literature lacks strong evidence to support it.

In an effort to address the previously mentioned issues, PECARN performed a large retrospective case–control study to search for factors associated with cervical spine injury. Note that this study demonstrates a model and not a "rule" that has been prospectively and externally validated. As a guideline, this model, with eight separate elements, has some advantages. Data from a large number of injured pediatric patients from multiple centers and age- and mechanism-matched controls underwent multiple logistic regression modeling. A total of 540 of children had cervical spine injuries, and more than 2,500 children served as age and mechanism controls. Mechanism of injury (as in CCR but missing in NEXUS) emerged as a risk factor; this finding is supported by the existence of pediatric populations that have a higher risk of injury after trauma (children with trisomy 21, Ehlers–Danlos syndrome, etc.). This first study demonstrates a strong sensitivity and, yet again, external validation, and further study is needed. Again, Table 33.1 presents the elements of the PECARN, NEXUS, and CCR rules.

The PECARN model makes intuitive sense, especially for younger children, with its combination of examination findings, mechanism, and understanding of pediatric-specific pathologies. NEXUS has advantages with adolescents, who have adult anatomy and physics and the ability to communicate. Clearance of the cervical collar can occur with a thorough physical examination regardless of mechanism; this can help reduce radiation exposure. With younger children, the mechanism may need to have more impact on decision-making. Regardless of the methodology chosen, no perfect rule will ensure 100% sensitivity with minimal risk of radiation exposure. Having a guideline, developed locally with the input of multiple disciplines, appropriate for the resources of a specific ED, enables emergency medical practitioners to better make decisions with the added comfort of having the support of local specialties.

Imaging

Radiation Risk

Pediatric imaging decisions necessitate a discussion of the difficult assessment of radiation exposure risk, specifically from CT scans. Given the rarity of malignancies in young adulthood, studies require long periods of follow-up and large numbers of patients. Radiology technology improves rapidly, and the data from patients imaged in the machines from 10–15 years ago may not apply to patients imaged in the scanners of today. Clearly, radiation exposure is a risk for cancer, and the thyroid gland has the greatest sensitivity to radiation. Higher doses of exposure and younger age at the time of exposure lead to increased risk, but with regard to the exact numerical risk, the data lack clarity. In 2012, a study published in *Lancet* examined more than 170,000 patients and found that, in the 10 years following a head CT, one excess case of leukemia and one excess case of brain cancer occurred per 10,000 head CTs. In the ear, nose, and throat literature, a systematic review of 16 studies examining head and/or neck CT showed a borderline increase in all cancers after neck CT, with a significantly increased risk of thyroid cancers in an almost 10-year follow-up (incidence rate ratio = 1.78; 95% confidence interval, 1.24–2.58). When talking to families about CT scans for cervical spine injury, keep the range of these numbers in mind. The risk is present but small. Clinicians should limit CT radiation whenever possible, but for patients involved in high-mechanism traumas, the risk will not outweigh the benefit of identifying an injury to the spine.

The vast majority of children in the United States receive emergency care in non-academic, non-pediatric EDs, in which the literature has demonstrated a trend toward increased imaging after trauma. Numerous factors play a role in this difference, including the following: potential lack of comfort/confidence in the care of children, a need for rapid disposition, a lack of feasible specialist follow-up, and a decreased ability to "admit for observation" for pediatric trauma patients. Many factors play a role in each of these issues, many of which lie outside the realm of emergency providers. Also noted in the literature is a reduced administration of radiation per CT scan in academic centers and level I and II trauma centers in comparison to community hospitals. ED providers should engage directly with their radiology departments to ensure that the lowest possible radiation doses are delivered to pediatric patients.

Plain Film

Ideally, plain films could sensitively screen children for pediatric cervical spine injury (they impart less radiation, efficiently and at low cost), but numerous factors make this a challenge. First, the higher fulcrum of injury in younger children leads to injuries in areas more difficult to evaluate by plain radiography. Second, numerous normal variants in the pediatric cervical spine can be misconstrued as injury (e.g., pseudo-subluxation of C2 on C3 and C3 on C4, large prevertebral spaces, C1 lateral mass displacement "pseudo-Jeffersonian fracture," and an absence of lordosis). Not all EDs have pediatric radiologists who are comfortable ruling out injuries using this modality. Normal radiographs will not rule out ligamentous injury, and SCIWORA (discussed later) can occur in the pediatric spine. However, numerous publications continue to advocate that the combination of careful clinical examination and plain radiographs provides a judicious and safe way to evaluate young children for cervical spine injury. In a review of 32 of the 44 pediatric patients in NEXUS who had plain radiographs, all patients would have been identified as having an injury (the extent of injuries was not appropriately identified), and sensitivity throughout the literature ranges from 80% to 95%.

Odontoid views and flexion–extension radiographs, two other options broached in the pediatric literature, appear to have limited utility. The current evidence shows that the odontoid view adds little to the evaluation and can prove challenging in younger patients who cannot reliably hold the positions necessary to obtain it. Protocols that include plain radiographs should allow for two-view imaging (anteroposterior and lateral) for those aged 5 years or younger, with the possibility of three-view imaging (adding the odontoid) for older children. Flexion–extension radiographs do not have the sensitivity and specificity to merit utilization for routine pediatric trauma patients. Some clinical scenarios may warrant and some consultants may request these images. It is important to permit only active flexion and extension; children with persistent pain should never have their neck moved by another person in order to obtain ideal images.

Computerized Tomography

The data are clear for adult trauma patients that CT imaging is superior to plain films for the clearance of the cervical spine. For this reason, it seems reasonable to apply these same data to adolescent patients, for whom the physics mirror that of adults. For younger children, however, because the risk of radiation increases and the chance of injury decreases, this strategy confers excessive risk. There is currently not sufficient evidence to support a protocol of CT screening of all pediatric trauma patients who fail clinical clearance. Because significant barriers exist to following the large numbers of patients required to examine the benefits and risks of CT versus plain radiographs, one particularly interesting study created a hypothetical decision tree analysis using current available data for each decision point (including sensitivity of different studies, malignancy risk, and risk of missed injury). When the risk of malignancy was weighed against the risk of injury, performing CT first was not found to be the best approach. Instead, clinical clearance and screening radiographs provided the optimal risk:benefit ratio.

The data may support a protocol with a "focused CT" approach. This includes getting CT imaging of the occiput through C3 and plain radiographs for the remainder of the cervical spine. The majority of injuries in young children happen in the axial portion of the cervical spine, an area challenging to evaluate with plain radiographs. Visualization of these complex three-dimensional structures with CT allows for clinical clearance in higher risk patients. Limiting CT to this region also allows for the shielding of the thyroid (the most radiosensitive organ in the body). Thus, some institutions have algorithms for scanning down to C3 when scanning the head in pediatric trauma patients and obtaining plain radiographs for the subaxial cervical spine evaluation.

Magnetic Resonance Imaging

Utilization of MRI in the ED has increased during the past decade. The advantages of MRI in the evaluation of pediatric cervical spine injury are clear: zero radiation exposure and improved imaging of the soft tissue allowing for diagnosis of ligamentous injuries. This technology, however, has its own unique challenges and has not demonstrated superiority in the screening for injuries. First, MRI costs a great deal more than CT imaging or plain radiographs. Second, young children require sedation, a challenge for patients with cervical collars and with real associated risk. Finally, the incredible sensitivity of MRI for soft tissue abnormalities will likely demonstrate mild injuries that lack management guidelines. Practitioners may then unnecessarily immobilize patients and subject them to the burden of increased consultations and follow-up.

Although currently not useful as a screening tool, indications do exist for MRI of the pediatric cervical spine in the trauma setting. Clearly, any child with neurologic symptoms will need an MRI. Intubated children will need an MRI to rule out ligamentous injury to allow for easier clinical care in the intensive care unit (ICU); obviously, this imaging lies outside the initial ED encounter. Infant non-accidental trauma victims may represent a distinct population with regard to cervical spine injury, for which the literature demonstrates MRI of the spinal column as a diagnostic tool may help diagnose abuse through the identification of ligamentous injuries. Again, although this currently lies outside the purview of most EDs, it may be an important consideration when deciding disposition.

Clinical Algorithm

Many pediatric and trauma institutions have published and shared their pediatric cervical spine algorithms. Figure 33.1 is an example of a clearance guideline developed by a multidisciplinary team of emergency medicine, pediatric emergency medicine, neurosurgery, trauma, and pediatric radiology. This clearance guideline allows for differing decision-making based on age, for some practitioner preferences (e.g., the option to use either NEXUS or CCR for older children), and permits some shared decision-making with families. The guideline contains two separate algorithms that serve the three group of patients: school-age children and adolescents (ages 3–18 years; Figure 33.1a) and nonverbal infants/toddlers (younger than age 3 years; Figure 33.1b).

Regarding clearance of 3- to 18-year-olds (Figure 33.1a), recall that although the decisions for these age groups are similar, the spine at the beginning age of this range is vastly different than that at the end. When utilizing this algorithm for 9- to 18-year-olds, the spine resembles that of adults. This group can also communicate symptoms clearly, assuming the absence of traumatic brain injury, an underlying issue, or intoxication. Obtunded patients should receive CT imaging of the neck and brain. Although not in the purview of the ED, the guideline also recommends MRI for obtunded and intubated patients within the first 48 hours of care. This will potentially decrease ICU stays and cost of patient care because clearance of the cervical collar allows for easier and improved care of the intubated patient. For patients who do not require head imaging, the next step is clinical clearance, if possible. As per the previous discussion, both NEXUS and CCR apply to older children with reasonable sensitivity. Thus, for those aged 9 years or older, clinicians can use either NEXUS or CCR; with this algorithm, clinicians have some leeway to use the rule they believe is most appropriate. Due to the lack of current data regarding CCR, this algorithm recommends use of NEXUS for younger patients (ages 3–9 years).

If the child screens positive with neurologic findings, they will require MRI and consultation with neurosurgery or orthopedics. If the patient screens positive without neurologic findings, clinicians can pursue imaging with either CT or X-ray utilizing the PECARN

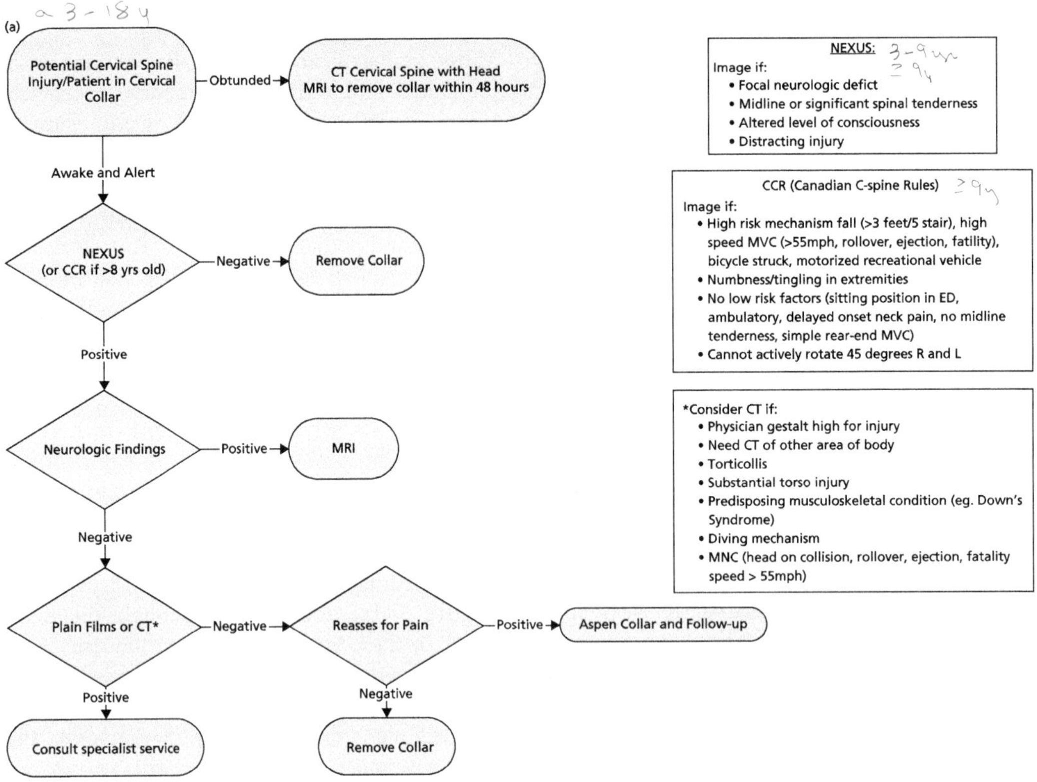

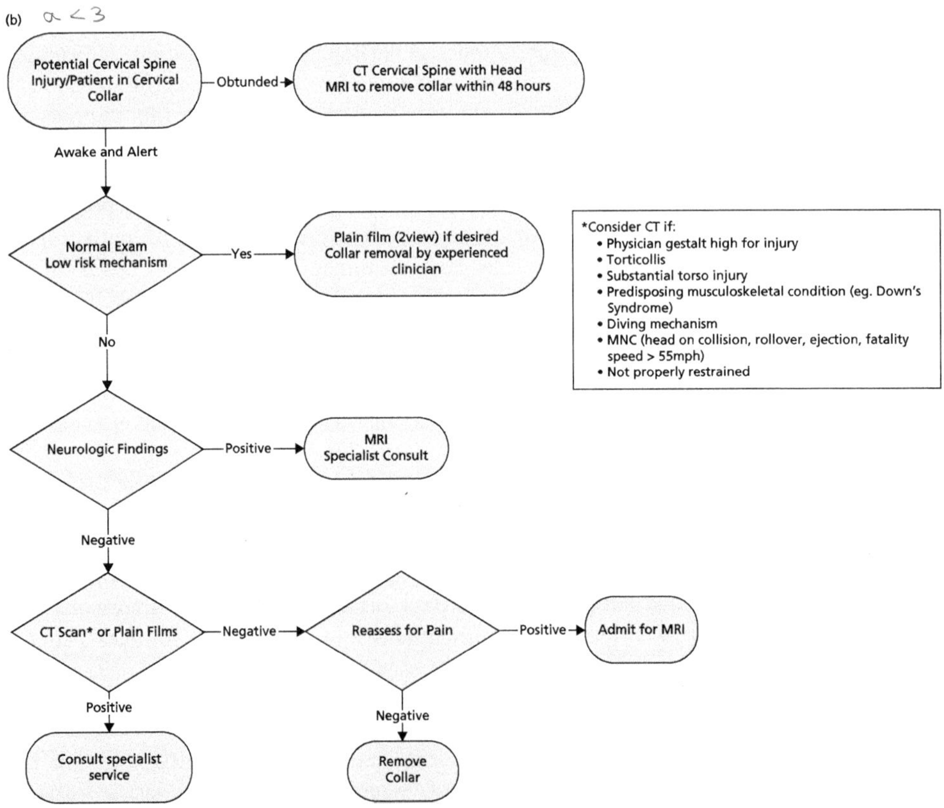

FIGURE 33.1 Cervical spinal clearance algorithms.

factors associated with injury as a guide for decision-making. If the patient has pain and sustained a concerning mechanism, the algorithm recommends CT. Young children with persistent pain despite mild mechanism would warrant plain films to mitigate radiation exposure. Patients who have persistent pain with negative imaging continue their immobilization with an Aspen collar and follow up as an outpatient in a subspecialty clinic (if available) in 3–7 days.

For the verbal child who has a pediatric spine (ages 3–8 years), the same algorithm (Figure 33.1a) can be used with two significant considerations. The algorithm no longer recommends use of the CCR to perform a clinical clearance because this age group was not represented in the initial data state and sufficient support does not yet exist in the literature for the application of this rule in younger patients. For patients who screen positively, the algorithm advises either CT or plain film. Clinician gestalt and comfort, family preference, associated injuries, and mechanism of injury (and other factors as noted by the PECARN study) all play a role in this decision. The remainder of the algorithm remains the same.

The population of children younger than age 3 years includes individuals who may not have the capacity to communicate pain or injury with accuracy. The literature supports using clinical examination for infants and toddlers; regardless of age, infants and toddlers will indicate pain with movement or pressure if they have a clinically significant injury. Because this population has the lowest risk of cervical spine injury from trauma of any age group and the highest risk of complication from the testing, clinicians must gain comfort with trusting their clinical examination. Restraint plays into this portion of the algorithm because rear-facing car seats provide excellent protection from cervical spine injury. Improperly restrained or forward-facing infants/toddlers require more conservative management. Again, altered or obtunded patients require CT of the cervical spine and the head. Awake, alert patients who are negative by screening (using NEXUS or PECARN) can have the collar removed by an experienced physician; if considered necessary, plain films can assist in the evaluation. If the screening is positive, the clinician can use plain films or CT for clearance, with a suggestion of CT in the setting of high-risk features (again derived from the PECARN algorithm).

Persistent Symptoms

Persistent neurologic symptoms after negative CT imaging will require urgent MRI and consultation with a spine specialist. EDs with these resources readily available can accomplish this on the initial encounter. More commonly, however, providers will encounter patients without neurologic symptoms but with persistent pain despite negative imaging. These patients can present a challenge to the emergency medicine provider. A combination of a conservative approach with the use of a pretest probability is likely the best methodology. Consider, for example, an adolescent with persistent neck pain after a low-mechanism MVC and negative plain films. If the pain is truly midline and the clinician is uncomfortable clearing the collar, the adolescent can either undergo a CT scan or have placement of a hard cervical collar and follow-up with a specialist in 7–10 days. Providers must engage in shared decision-making in this scenario. For patients with sports-related injuries, with less predictable mechanisms and screening rules less applicable, a conservative approach would be to obtain CT images and place in a collar if the patient has continued pain and follow-up with specialist.

A retrospective study in Boston demonstrates that a judicious use of imaging with utilization of outpatient follow-up safely decreases imaging. This study examined nearly 300 patients discharged from a level 1 pediatric trauma center in a hard collar. The vast majority of these patients received plain radiographs only; 20.8% had CT and 8.3% had an MRI. At follow-up (median 10 days), the specialist clinic provider cleared the collar on the first visit. Only 25 (13.2%) additional patients received MRI. This cohort had only six injuries identified, and none had instability or required surgical intervention. This study supports plain radiographs and good clinical decision-making. For discharged patients with low suspicion but persistent pain, a protective collar and good follow-up can replace a CT scan In the entire cohort of 289 patients, 64 (33%) had neck CT, 264 (91.4%) had plain radiographs, and 49 had MRI (21.5%). Compared to adult populations in which close to100% of trauma patients with neck pain get a CT scan, this appears to limit radiation in a cost-effective way to manage patients with persistent symptoms. Children may not require CT on primary evaluation when clinical suspicion is low.

Treatment

The ED provider has a limited role in the definitive management of cervical spine injuries, and consulting a specialist will ensure appropriate disposition and treatment. The mainstays of ED treatment are stabilization, immobilization, alleviation of pain, and consultation. Children victims of polytrauma have a higher likelihood of sustaining multilevel injuries in comparison to adults, and providers must ensure a thorough examination of the entire spinal column is performed once they have identified an injury.

Key Points

- Clinical clearance guidelines are available for children and should be utilized when evaluating a pediatric patient after trauma.
- Plain films, although imperfect, do have a good degree of sensitivity and can be used for clearance of lower risk and younger patients.
- CT scanning of the neck should be considered if the patient receives head imaging.

Pitfalls

- Using CT imaging as the only diagnostic tool for neck injury: Radiographs are safe and fairly reliable, especially in the setting of a lower mechanism injury.
- Avoidance of CT altogether to mitigate radiation exposure: There is a definitive use for CT in the evaluation of the pediatric cervical spine. As long as it is done with careful consideration for the likelihood of injury and radiation and in discussion with the family, clinicians should utilize CT imaging for high-mechanism traumas and sports-related traumas.
- Assuming that the cervical spine of an infant cannot be cleared clinically: If a toddler is appropriately restrained in a car seat and the vehicle is traveling at a moderate rate of speed when an MVC occurs, the risk of cervical spine injury is exceedingly low. Clinicians can use their judgment and a thorough physical examination to determine if any imaging is needed to clear a collar.
- Minimizing the risk of cervical spine injury in athletes: Unlike MVCs, the direct force to the cervical spine during athletic activities is difficult to assess. Careful consideration should be given to the athlete with neurologic symptoms or persistent pain. This does not mean that MRI is necessary in the acute setting for persistent pain. Patients can be sent home in a hard cervical collar and have follow-up arranged with a spine specialist.

THORACOLUMBAR INJURY

Background

While cervical spine trauma in pediatric patients is rare, thoracolumbar (TL) injuries are even more uncommon: <1% of all spinal trauma cases are pediatric injuries to this region. These injuries arise from high-velocity mechanisms and, as with cervical trauma, the most common etiologies are appropriate to the activities and restraints of the age. Young children protected from high-risk endeavors and who usually travel with appropriate restraints sustain few injuries of the TL region. Injuries in this age group stem from being struck as a pedestrian or from falls at great height. Children in regular seat belt restraint (school age and older) have an increased incidence of lumbar injuries due to MVCs compared to the younger group. With adolescence and an increase in high-risk activities, injuries are most commonly associated with MVCs and sports.

As with the cervical spine, the early development of the TL spine allows for greater flexibility of the elements of the spinal column. SCIWORA, described later in this chapter, can occur in this region as well. Some distinctions from the cervical spine warrant consideration. The rib cage and sternum immobilize and protect the thoracic spine from injury, especially from lateral forces. Compression fractures comprise the majority of injuries seen from T2 to T8. At the transition point between the neck and thorax (T1), more complex injuries may occur. T11 and T12, at the base of the thorax, lack circumferential ribs, and the transition point between the immobile thoracic and the mobile lumbar vertebra sustains the most injury. The majority of thoracic injuries from acceleration/deceleration will be found in this lower zone from T9 to L2 as a result of flexion forces. The lordotic and more mobile lower lumbar sustains injury from an axial load.

When evaluating the TL spine, consider the spinal column in three segments: anterior (the anterior half of the vertebral body and anterior longitudinal ligament), middle (posterior half of the vertebral body and posterior longitudinal ligament), and posterior (remainder of the posterior bony ring alternating with ligamentous complexes). Disruption of two or more segments is required to cause instability.

Classic Clinical Presentation

Much like with the cervical spine, clinicians will find it easier to assess the spine of the awake and alert, communicative patient. The evaluation will not differ from that of an adult, with careful palpation along each vertebral body and a careful neurologic examination. Obviously, younger children present a larger challenge. An important question to ask verbal pediatric trauma patients is whether they experienced "breath arrest" or a sensation of being unable to breath for a few seconds after the injury. In combination with thoracic tenderness, this has a high degree of sensitivity and a fair degree of specificity for thoracic spine injury.

Differential Diagnosis

Compression Fractures

Compression fractures, the most common subtype of fracture in the TL spine, occur most frequently at the TL junction. They often occur as a result of MVCs or sports-related trauma, and they do not always develop from axial loads. The kyphotic thoracic spine hyperflexes forward, compressing the anterior portion of the vertebral body. Less than 30% compression yields a good outcome, but compression greater than 50% has a higher association with injury to the posterior elements of the spinal column. The involvement of these two areas of the spinal column causes spinal instability, warranting an MRI for these greater compression injuries. High-velocity mechanisms (e.g., MVCs) produce a higher likelihood of abdominal injuries and multilevel spinal injuries.

Burst Fractures

Higher velocity trauma can give rise to burst fractures, most commonly in the lumbar spine. Axial loading to this region drives the nucleus pulposus of the intervertebral disc into the vertebral body, causing fracture of the anterior and middle columns of the spinal column. Fracture fragments push into the spinal canal (retropulsion), and urgent decompression may be necessary. Without retropulsion, neurologic abnormality, or signs of instability, these fractures may be managed conservatively with thoracolumbosacral orthosis bracing.

Apophyseal Ring Injury

The ring apophysis is the region of the vertebral body that attaches to the annulus fibrosis of the intervertebral disc. It is cartilaginous in children and thus a "weak" point where disc protrusion can occur. Whereas adults can sustain traumatic disc herniations, children will experience apophyseal ring fractures. Patients present with intractable back and radicular leg pain and have positive, yet often subtle, CT imaging.

Chance Fracture

This unique injury pattern arises from MVCs in which children, restrained in a lap belt, experience a rapid deceleration event in which a seat belt compresses the abdominal viscera against the lumbar spinal column, which then hyperflexes over the fulcrum of the belt. In addition to abdominal injury (often bowel), children will sustain damage to the posterior and middle elements of the spinal column, most commonly at the level of L2 and L3. The hyperflexion damages the spinal cord in approximately 40% of these cases and leads to instability, especially in a state of flexion.

Diagnostic Confirmation

No clearance guidelines exist for clearing the thoracic or lumbar spines. Expert opinion suggests that careful physical examination and plain films should be the first step in evaluation. Although the sensitivity of plain films is not perfect, it is important to weigh the benefits of CT imaging with the inherent risk of radiation. If there are abnormalities of the plain films or they do not appear to match the examination, CT images can be pursued. Even with CT, due to malleability of the spinal column, subtle abnormalities may indicate more serious injury. As with the cervical spine, neurologic findings or symptoms warrant CT scans.

Disposition

Any definitive injury to the pediatric spine requires specialist consultation. Injuries from high-mechanism traumas, even if minor from a spinal standpoint, suggest that the body has sustained massive forces and warrants observation to monitor for other injuries. Compression fractures, sustained from lower mechanisms such as falls or sports injuries, often receive conservative bracing and may do well managed as an outpatient with close follow-up. Damage to the end plate even in mild injuries can lead to chronic deformity and require close observation. Compression fractures of more than 50% of the vertebral height necessitate further imaging with MRI to ensure integrity of the posterior elements of the spinal column. MRI is likewise indicated for any neurologic signs/symptoms, burst fractures with retropulsed fragments, and all apophyseal ring injuries (which will necessitate surgical management).

Key Points

- TL spinal injuries are rare in pediatric patients. The vast majority are compression fractures and occur near the transition of the relatively immobile thoracic spine to the more mobile lumbar spine.
- It is imperative to mitigate radiation exposure, and CT should be used sparingly.
- Many injuries require only bracing and close follow-up in the outpatient setting, although high-velocity mechanism trauma victims, even with mild spinal damage, likely warrant observation.

SPINAL CORD INJURY WITHOUT RADIOGRAPHIC ABNORMALITY

Background

The tremendous mobility, in all planes, of the pediatric spine allows for the rare occurrence of SCIWORA in children (and very rarely in adults). The spinal column can sublux out of place temporarily, cause spinal cord injury, and then reduce spontaneously without any disruption to the structural elements. It was first described in 1977 before routine utilization of MRI, which begs the question, If an MRI is positive, does the patient truly have SCIWORA? The consensus in the literature is "yes" because MRI is not used as a screening examination for trauma and many institutions do not have ready availability of MRI for pediatric patients. "Real SCIWORA" refers to patients with negative MRI findings as well to those who mostly have good outcomes. For the purposes of this chapter, SCIWORA refers to negative imaging on CT scan and plain film.

Classic Clinical Presentation

The mechanism of injury for SCIWORA changes with age. For younger children (ages 0–10 years), motor vehicle accidents predominate. After the age of 10 years, sports injuries are the most common mechanism, and for adults, the cause is most frequently falls. By definition, patients will present with signs or symptoms of spinal cord injury and may or may not have spinal pain. SCIWORA can occur at any level of the spinal cord, but cervical injuries predominate. This pathology does not usually occur in isolation; the vast majority of children (especially younger children) have concomitant injuries, most often in the head.

Differential Diagnosis

Recall that SCIWORA occurs uncommonly within an already small population. For the cervical spine, of the 1% or 2% of pediatric trauma victims who have cervical spine injuries of any kind, SCIWORA represents only 13–19% of that group. Thus, fracture should remain highest on the differential diagnosis for patients with neck pain and/or neurologic findings or symptoms. The relative distribution of SCIWORA injuries in the spine mirrors that of fracture/dislocation; the cervical spine comprises the majority of the cases, with upper cervical spinal cord injuries most common in younger children.

Diagnostic Confirmation

All children with neurologic symptoms after trauma require imaging to the point of MRI. It is important to note that initial MRI may be negative. There are numerous cases of SCIWORA patients showing evidence of spinal cord edema and injury 3–5 days post injury, after initial studies were completely negative. Thus, a negative MRI does not rule out SCIWORA if symptoms are legitimate and persistent. Follow-up MRIs in these patients correlate well with symptoms, with a higher degree of edema associated with a higher degree of symptomatology.

Treatment

The treatment for SCIWORA is conservative and relies on immobilization and potentially steroids. Patients with cervical SCIWORA, if discharged, will require a hard collar, and thoracolumbar bracing will be necessary for injury to the lower spine.

Key Points

- SCIWORA is more commonly found in younger children and has a high association with other injuries.
- Although treatment is mostly conservative and supportive, observation is warranted for close monitoring for other injuries.

Further Reading

Hannon M, Mannix R, Dorney K, et al. Pediatric cervical spine injury evaluation after trauma: A clinical decision analysis. *Ann Emerg Med.* 2015;65:239–247.

Hazbaun R, Muñoz A, Krafft PR, et al. Craniocervical dissociation in pediatric patients: Pearls and pitfalls in diagnosis and management. *Pediatr Emerg Care.* 2019;epub ahead of print.

Leonard JR, Jaffe DM, Kupperman N, et al. Cervical spine injury patterns in children. *Pediatrics.* 2014;133:e1179–e1188.

Leonard JR, Kupperman N, Olsen C, et al. Factors associated with cervical spine injury after blunt trauma. *Annal Emerg Med.* 2011;58:145–155.

Pearce MS, Salotti JA, Little MP, et al. Radiation exposure from CT scans in childhood and subsequent risk of leukaemia and brain tumors: A retrospective cohort study. *Lancet.* 2012;380:499–505.

Srinivasan V, Jea A. Pediatric thoracolumbar spine trauma. *Neurosurg Clin North Am.* 2017;28:103–114.

34

Pediatric Facial Trauma

CHRISTOPHER S. AMATO

STATISTICS AND ETIOLOGY

The vast majority of pediatric facial trauma is blunt in nature. The most common cause varies by age, with falls the most common cause of injury in younger childhood and blunt trauma or motor vehicle injury the most common causes of injury in older children.

Motor vehicle injury and penetrating injury have a higher incidence of multiple facial fractures and increased morbidity. Nasal bone fracture is the most common facial bone fracture. Sports-related injury has a higher incidence of midface and upper midface fracture. Assault is noted to result in isolated mandible fracture. A seasonal variation, with peak incidence in warmer months, is found and related to increased outdoor activities.

PATHOPHYSIOLOGY

Due to their compact size and physiology, when children suffer corporeal trauma, it is more likely to affect multiple systems than a single system. Children are also more prone to secondary injury due to a higher surface area-to-body ratio, increased metabolic demands, and a critical airway that responds vigorously with edema. This pattern does not seem to hold sway with facial trauma. The smaller area of the midface of a child younger than age 5 years results in decreased facial fracture because the larger skull takes the brunt of the injury. This changes as children age, with downward and forward facial growth. Facial fracture, however, is still limited due to a thicker layer of underlying adipose with more elastic immaturity of their skeleton. Further protection is afforded by the lack of aeration of their sinuses and the stabilizing effect of the dental buds. In general, orthopedic injury will require less surgical intervention due to growth potential and higher vascular function. Pediatric facial fracture patterns are similar to those of adults but occur less commonly and may be clinically more difficult to diagnose compared to those of adults. Therefore, the evaluation of facial trauma should be performed using a stepwise approach ending with the evaluation of any lacerations. Although cosmesis is key to patient outcome, a strong suspicion of underlying bony abnormality must be maintained. It is easy to assume there is injury when there is gross overlying edema, ecchymosis, and/or bleeding; however, even when these are lacking, a thorough examination with the assumption that there is an abnormality to be found, as opposed to "all looks well so it should be well," is preferred. Close examination searching for any asymmetry as well as any motor dysfunction should be performed in all trauma patients.

The amount of force required to fracture a facial bone is classified into two categories: high impact (>50 times gravity) and low impact (<50 times gravity). Based on simple physics, injury will be related to mass, velocity, and location of impact. For example, 200 times gravity is required to cause a fracture of the supraorbital rim, whereas only 30 times gravity is required to break the nasal bones. Consider the facial bones similar to crumple zones in a car. They are, in a sense, present to absorb and deflect trauma forces away from the brain. The mandible illustrates this in that it is considered to be one of the strongest bones in the body, but the condyles are often fractured due to absorption of traumatic force aimed toward the brain. A mandibular fracture at the condyle, a thinner and more vascular component, is more common in pediatrics than in adults and is the most common facial fracture associated with hospital admission.

Up to 60% of patients presenting with severe facial trauma have concomitant multisystem trauma with possible airway issues. Up to 20–50% have traumatic brain injury, 1–4% with associated cervical spine injury, and up to 3% may have eye injury leading to blindness. Facial fracture may be seen in up to 2% of non-accidental trauma with typical involvement of the head, face, mouth, and neck. Higher risk groups are newborns, infants, and preschool children. Reporting of any suspected child abuse is a legal obligation.

AIRWAY/BREATHING ISSUES

The pediatric airway is extremely reactive to any inflammation or trauma leading to rapid edema, which could lead to an inability to ventilate the patient. Airway maneuvers, including chin lift or jaw thrust, should be performed with cervical stabilization. Suctioning is often needed to better visualize the glottic opening when performing advanced airway stabilization. Due to the potential for airway compromise, care should be taken with a rapid sequence approach because the airway may be so edematous as to preclude intubation, and no attempt should be made at a nasotracheal intubation with facial trauma due to potential for inappropriate tube placement.

CIRCULATION

Bleeding control is best obtained using direct pressure, or in the case of nasal bleeding, packing or tamponade may be utilized to control hemorrhage. Use of tranexamic acid (TXA) is becoming more common based on a growing literature regarding its use in trauma patients. An adult study that utilized TXA in maxillofacial trauma patients requiring surgical repair showed an overall decreased blood loss in patients receiving TXA compared to placebo. In this instance, hypotension was induced to further diminish bleeding. In pediatric patients, hypotension is an extremely late sign because children can maintain their blood pressure with up to a 33% loss of blood volume. As with any trauma patient, early and aggressive fluid resuscitation, including use of whole blood 10 mL/kg, should be strongly considered in the pediatric patient presenting with hypotension. The addition of either continuous infusion or press-dosed vasopressors also should be considered in the pediatric patient.

HISTORY

Use of the following questions to the awake and orient the patient may help elucidate specific injuries:

- Pain with eye movement?
- Sensation of paresthesia on a specific area?
- Ability to open mouth or pain with opening?
- Sensation of asymmetry of dentition/bite?

EXAMINATION

Facial stability and symmetry are some of the first factors a clinician should examine, but overlying edema and poor cooperation may make this difficult.

Boney examination for tenderness, crepitus, or step-off should be performed. An intraoral approach to the zygoma may diminish misinterpretation of overlying soft tissue versus bone injury.

Ophthalmic examination should include pupil reactivity and shape, extraocular muscular movement, and examination of periorbital rims, and a visual acuity test should be performed in those capable of such. Evaluation of all structures of the eye, including fluorescein testing for corneal injury, examination of the anterior chamber for hyphema, and examination of the posterior chamber for retinal injury, should be performed.

Ear examination should include palpation of the pinna as well as evaluation of the tympanic membrane for possible hemotympanum. Nasal examination should include evaluation for septal hematoma and any active epistaxis.

Dental examination with digital examination of each tooth searching for luxation or other signs of trauma should be performed, as should "tongue blade" testing for mandibular stability.

RADIOGRAPHY

Plain radiography is less sensitive in pediatric patients because of suture lines, poor sinus evolution, and obscured landmarks due to developing skeletal maturity. Computerized tomography (CT) has the highest resolution and capability for evaluation of facial fractures, but it exposures immature patients to ionizing radiation. (Pediatric patients have more radiosensitive tissues, more time for propagation of a mutation in themselves or in genetic material for progeny, and more time to accumulate further radiation.) Therefore, it should be used judiciously by the practitioner. Currently, CT is considered the gold standard for evaluating the traumatic patient.

SPECIFIC INJURIES

Frontal Bone/Sinus Fracture

Typically, this type of fracture is due to direct blunt trauma and is associated with intracranial injury with possible dural tear or orbital injury. A head CT should be obtained to evaluate for a frontal sinus fracture, naso-ethmoid fracture, as well as an intracranial bleed or injury. Radiographs may include the following:

Waters view: X-ray is beamed at the orbitomeatal line (the line passing through the lateral canthus and external auditory canal) and views the sinuses (maxillary, frontal, and sphenoid), ethmoidal cells, and possibly the odontoid.

Caldwell view: The X-ray is performed with the patient's face on the plate and the beam is sent at a 15° to 20° angle from the posterior aspect to the plate for best evaluation of anterior wall fractures.

Lateral view: This is a non-angulated view of the lateral skill with which to view the entire skull.

Non-displaced or isolated anterior wall fractures may be treated in an outpatient setting after consultation with neurosurgery. Any depressed skull fracture or those with associated posterior wall injury are likely to need neurosurgical or ear–nose–throat (ENT) consultation with potential admission for intravenous antibiotics. Sequelae for intracranial injuries include dural tear, epidural empyema, orbital roof fracture, mucopyocoele, cerebrospinal fluid (CSF) leak, and even development of meningitis.

Naso-Ethmoid-Orbital Fracture

This type of fracture may impact the lacrimal ducts and is associated with dural tear. A high suspicion should be held if there is trauma over the nose (flattening of the nasal bridge or saddle deformity, widened nasal bridge, CSF rhinorrhea, tenderness with or without crepitus of nasal bones, tenderness or injury of the medial orbit especially if there is movement of the medial canthus, or pain with eye movement). X-ray evaluation is not deemed sensitive enough, so a CT with coronal images of the medial orbits should be obtained.

Nasal Bone

The most common facial bone fracture is classified into three types: depressed, laterally displaced, and non-displaced. Examination searching for deformity of the nasal bridge, facial hypoesthesia, epistaxis, or bony mobility with crepitus is helpful for diagnosis. Some ENT or plastic surgeons may advise delayed treatment for the minimally displaced nasal fracture because overlying edema may prohibit improved cosmesis initially. Emergent consultation is utilized in grossly deformed nasal bones that require emergent reduction. A non-displaced fracture or simple edema of the overlying tissues does not require consultation and may be followed by the primary physician alone.

Orbital Blowout

This type of injury has a strong association with direct blow to the periorbital frame, specifically the inferior orbital rim. Clinical signs include soft tissue swelling, tenderness, and ecchymosis. Enophthalmos (sunken eye) is pathognomonic for this injury, as is impaired ocular movement. Radiographs may show air–fluid levels in the sinus and even orbital emphysema, but CT evaluation is indicated for this type of injury to better evaluate for extent of bony injury as well as evidence of entrapment.

If there is associated orbital injury, then emergent consultation with ophthalmology is warranted. If there is no associated orbital injury, a blowout fracture may be cared for on an outpatient basis with ENT or oral and maxillofacial surgery (OMFS) consultation. Common instructions include use of nasal decongestant, consideration of prophylactic antibiotics, as well as avoidance of strenuous activity and specific avoidance of blowing of nose or Valsalva maneuvers.

Zygoma

This bone has two components: the arch and the body. Arch fractures are most common, whereas tripod fractures can have serious implications:

Arch fracture: A fracture can occur in the middle or lateral to either end of the arch. Clinical examination will be notable for complaints of pain with opening of the mouth, hypoesthesia of the infraorbital nerve, or even a palpable bony step-off.

Tripod fracture: This is a fracture through the zygomatic arch, zygomatico-frontal suture, and the infraorbital rim and floor. Globe injury may be associated with this type of fracture.

A CT with coronal three-dimensional reconstruction is most illustrative as opposed to facial radiographs including Waters, submental, and Caldwell views. Disposition will depend on the extent of injury, eye involvement, reliability of follow-up, as well as pain control. Typical treatment will involve nasal decongestants, application of ice, pain control, and consideration of antibiotic prophylaxis. If there is displacement of the tripod fracture, surgical intervention may be warranted earlier.

Maxillary (Le Fort) Fracture

The treatment of these types of fractures should include airway management; elevating the head of the bed to approximately 40 degrees; consultation of OMFS, ENT, or a trauma surgeon; and likely admission with prophylactic antibiotics.

Le Fort I

Le Fort I is a horizontal fracture of the maxilla at the level of the nasal fossa. The nasal bridge will remain stable while there is motion of the maxilla. The fracture will involve the nasal aperture, the inferior maxilla, and the lateral wall of the maxilla.

Clinically, it is associated with facial ecchymosis and edema, with findings of malocclusion of the teeth.

Le Fort II

Le Fort II is a triangular fracture of the maxilla, the nasal bones, and the medial aspect of the orbital rim.

Clinically, it is associated with nasal flattening, epistaxis or CSF rhinorrhea, and increased distance between the medial canthi.

Le Fort III

Le Fort III is a fracture of the maxilla involving the nasal bones, the ethmoid bone, and zygoma, extending into the base of the skull.

Clinically, it is associated with "dish face" deformity; epistaxis and CSF rhinorrhea; and motion of the maxilla, nasal bones, and zygoma; It can be associated with severe airway compromise.

Mandible Fracture

Mandible fracture is the third most common facial fracture and has a high association with assaults and falls onto the submental area. Multiple fractures can be seen in more than half of the injured. Cervical spine injury can occur in up to 5% of patients, so cervical spine immobilization should be maintained. Classic clinical findings are malocclusion of teeth, dental separation with bleeding, trismus, as well as a positive tongue blade test. If the fracture is non-displaced, treatment will include analgesia and soft diet. Antibiotics should be considered in all cases. Case discussion of non-displaced or displaced fractures should occur with OMFS or dentistry.

CONCLUSION

Although rare in pediatrics, facial trauma with resultant fracture requires a thorough examination, a strong suspicion because many fractures may be missed, as well as consideration of the type of imaging and ultimately case discussion with either ENT or OMFS.

35

Pediatric Neck Trauma

KIM NEWTON

INTRODUCTION

Pediatric neck injuries are rare. Familiarity with an institution-specific algorithm is imperative for expedited diagnosis, stabilization, and treatment. Any hemodynamically unstable patient with hard signs of neck injury should be taken to the operating room (OR) immediately. Assurance of airway stability in all other pediatric patients with neck injury should take first priority. Bedside tests, including the extended focused assessment with sonography for trauma examination and plain films of the neck and chest, are readily available and can provide helpful information. High-resolution computed tomography with angiogram (CTA) has been shown to be the superior imaging study when evaluating the neck for vascular or aerodigestive injury. Additional diagnostic modalities are based on clinical suspicion, signs and symptoms, injury location, and CT results. Signs and symptoms of aerodigestive and vascular injury are categorized as hard or soft signs of injury (Table 35.1). Hard signs imply likely viscerovascular injury a with great potential for decompensation. Soft signs of injury in a hemodynamically stable patient are also concerning and should prompt an aggressive evaluation for injuries that require therapeutic intervention.

Neck trauma can be classified into three major categories: penetrating, blunt, and strangulation/near hanging, with the latter being subsets of blunt injury. Injury types can be thought of structurally, with the main categories being vascular, laryngotracheal, and esophageal. Trauma is the leading cause of morbidity and mortality in children. Fortunately, pediatric neck trauma is a rare entity, leading to a relative paucity of research in this age group. Because of this lack of information, much of the diagnostic and therapeutic principles are extrapolated from more commonly published adult neck trauma literature. The incidence of blunt pediatric neck trauma is much more common than that of penetrating injuries (approximately 80% vs. 20%).

Blunt neck trauma in the pediatric group is most commonly caused by motor vehicle crashes, but it can also be caused by sports injuries, clothesline trauma, assaults, and near hanging or strangulation.

Penetrating neck injury in the older child includes such mechanisms as stab wounds, debris from glass or shrapnel, gunshot wounds, and explosion debris from flammable materials. Younger children more often sustain penetrating neck injuries (PNIs) during play when they fall on a sharp object.

TABLE 35.1 HARD AND SOFT SIGNS OF NECK INJURY

Soft Signs of Injury	Hard Signs of Injury
Dysphagia	Severe active hemorrhage
Odynophagia	Airway compromise
Hoarseness	Respiratory distress
Subcutaneous or deep gas	Expanding or pulsatile hematoma
Stable hematoma	Massive subcutaneous emphysema
Focal neurologic deficits	Pulse deficit
Hematemesis/hemoptysis	Shock (fluid nonresponsive)
Oropharyngeal blood	Decreased/absent radial pulse
Dyspnea	New stroke-like symptom
	Vascular bruit/thrill

ANATOMY

Neck trauma should be thought of categorically as injury to any of the following:

- Airway (larynx and trachea)
- Digestive track (pharynx and esophagus)
- Vascular
- Neurological (cervical spine)
- Miscellaneous (salivary, thyroid, parotid glands, muscle, etc.)

The neck is unique because of the large number of structures confined in tight, fascial compartments. This translates to limited tolerance for bleeding or swelling, which can rapidly lead to airway distortion, compression, or obstruction. In addition, because the extremes of the neck are contiguous with the upper thorax and the base of the skull, traumatic injuries to the neck can also be associated with injury to these adjacent regions. For example, a stab wound to the base of the neck might also injure mediastinal structures.

Violation of the platysma muscle is considered a potential marker of visceral–vascular injury and defines penetrating neck trauma. The platysma muscle is sandwiched between the superficial fascia and the deep cervical fascia. These fascial divisions lead to compartmentalized regions of the neck. Airway distortion in the setting of excessive bleeding or swelling is a real concern when treating neck trauma. Conversely, these tight, localized spaces can limit bleeding via a tamponade effect. Likewise, the spread of deep space infections can also be contained within a defined space. The superficial fascia is located between the skin and platysma. Immediately deep to the platysma is the deep cervical fascia, which is composed of three distinct layers: the investing layer, the pretracheal layer, and the prevertebral layer. The investing fascial layer surrounds the entire neck just deep to the platysma. As it courses 360° around the neck, it splits to fully encompass both the sternocleidomastoid and trapezius muscles. The pretracheal fascia is deep to the investing layer and surrounds the esophagus, trachea, thyroid gland, and infrahyoid muscles. It attaches to the hyoid and thyroid cartridges and courses deep to the sternum to attach to the anterior pericardium. The prevertebral fascia surrounds the cervical spine and prevertebral muscles, extending caudally to the thorax. The pretracheal layer carries great clinical significance because of its anatomical relationship with the mediastinum. Mediastinitis is the feared complication from a missed aerodigestive injury because of this continuity.

The neck is divided into three regions or zones, with each carrying anatomic, diagnostic, and therapeutic implications. For many decades, zone nomenclature has been the most popular way of describing the location of penetrating neck wounds. Zone 1 (base of neck) begins at the clavicles and sternal notch and continues cranially to the cricoid cartilage. Zone 2 (mid-neck) begins proximally at the cricoid cartilage and extends superiorly to the angle of the mandible. Zone 3 (upper neck) includes the structures between the mandibular angle and base of the skull. Table 35.2 describes the contents contained in each zone.

TABLE 35.2 ANATOMICAL CONTENTS OF ZONES 1–3

Zone 1	Zone 2	Zone 3
From clavicles/sternal notch to the cricoid cartilage	From cricoid cartilage to the angle of the mandible	From mandibular angle to base of the skull
Apices of lungs	Carotid artery and branches	Cranial nerves IX–XII
Esophagus	Esophagus	Distal internal carotid artery
Major vessels of upper mediastinum	Jugular veins (internal and external)	Distal jugular vein
Proximal common carotid artery	Larynx	Pharynx
Spinal cord	Pharynx	Salivary and parotid glands
Subclavian artery	Recurrent laryngeal nerve	Spinal cord
Trachea	Spinal cord	Vertebral artery
Thyroid gland	Trachea	
Thoracic duct	Vagus nerve	
Vertebral artery	Vertebral artery	
Vagus nerve		
Aortic arch		
Jugular veins		

HISTORICAL PERSPECTIVE

Historically, in an attempt to avoid missing injuries while preventing unnecessary operations, many surgeons have relied on a selective, zone-based approach to decide on diagnostic testing and who would benefit from operative intervention. Currently, with the advent of high-resolution multidetector CT, wound trajectory and proximity wounds can be viewed in great detail. It is evident that many penetrating wounds that involve only one zone via skin inspection actually traverse two or more zones based on CT images. From this discovery came the recent concept of a "no-zone" approach for PNIs. As CTA has become a staple in screening neck injuries, less reliance on zones to dictate therapeutic treatment is expected, although zone nomenclature and selective algorithms are still in use today.

VASCULAR TRAUMA

Overview

Vascular injury to the neck can present dramatically in the setting of active exsanguination. However, these injuries have the potential to be insidious, with delayed symptom onset. Having a high index of suspicion, knowing the mechanisms of injury most associated with these lesions, and being confident in which patients will benefit from imaging or ancillary tests will afford the best outcome. In contrast to penetrating injuries, which typically involve the common carotid artery, blunt carotid trauma involves the internal carotid artery in 90% of cases. Bleeding from these vessels can result in exsanguination, hematoma expansion, airway distortion or compromise, and a variety of neurological sequelae including stroke symptoms. Injury types include puncture wounds, partial or complete vessel transection, intraluminal occlusion, pseudoaneurysm, and dissection. The feared and potentially delayed complication from blunt vascular injuries is stroke resulting from cerebral ischemia. Neurologic symptoms are often seen at the time of injury, but it is not uncommon for a delayed presentation of days to weeks. In the setting of neck trauma and new evidence of anterior or posterior circulation insufficiency, if the screening CT head is negative, a vascular source should be pursued.

Penetrating Vascular Injury

Pediatric penetrating neck trauma occurs rarely, with an incidence of 0.28%. These injuries are easiest to categorize in terms of stab or puncture wounds (glass, knives, bites, etc.) versus missiles or projectiles (firearms and other high-velocity mechanisms). This distinction is important because the tissue injury from stab or puncture wounds is directly related to and immediately within the path of the sharp object. The tissue destruction seen from high-velocity mechanisms results in both local injury from the projectile and remote tissue injury related to the cavitation effect from the transfer of kinetic energy.

Clinical Features

Penetrating injury to the great vessels of the neck comprises 10% of all vascular injuries, with the carotid artery being injured 17% of the time. Penetrating vascular wounds of the neck carry mortality rates as high as 50% and exsanguination is the leading cause of immediate death. Soft or hard signs of vascular injury are defined below. In general, any unstable patient with PNI and hard signs is taken expediently to the OR. Those with soft signs of vascular injury who are hemodynamically stable follow a more conservative algorithm. These hard and soft signs are specifically for vascular injury and differ from the more general terms noted in Table 35.1:

- Hard signs of vascular injury
  - Severe, pulsatile bleeding
  - Rapidly expanding hematoma
  - Fluid nonresponsive shock
  - Massive hematemesis or hemoptysis
  - Focal neurological deficit
- Soft signs of vascular injury
  - Minor hematemesis or hemoptysis
  - Stable hematoma
  - Slow vascular ooze

Diagnostic Confirmation

The diagnosis and management of PNI continues to advance, with all initial recommendations based on adult studies. Patients in extremis and essentially all with hard signs of injury fare best in the OR. Those with soft signs of injury are more controversial, and their management strategies continue to evolve. Today, despite the introduction of selective management protocols for pediatric patients, the pediatric literature on this topic remains less robust because of the lower incidence of PNI in children.

In the stable patient with soft signs of injury, a chest X-ray and bedside ultrasound are often performed as the initial screening studies. These modalities are fast and easily available, and they allow for quick assessment of adequate lung sliding, pleural or pericardial effusion, and the presence and location of metallic foreign bodies or free air in the soft tissues of the neck. In addition to these bedside tests, CTA has emerged as the first-line diagnostic test, replacing catheter angiography as the initial study of choice for excluding vascular injury. With newer generation equipment, these images are able to assess the trajectory and its proximity to adjacent structures noninvasively. Based on CTA results, the need for further diagnostic intervention such as endoscopy, esophagoscopy, or surgery can be determined. Because of the detailed information now afforded by CTA, less reliance on zone-based selective management protocols is evolving. CTA for penetrating trauma has a sensitivity of 100% and specificity of 97.5%; thus, it is highly sensitive, specific, and accurate for PNIs.

Duplex ultrasound has been successfully used for PNI in patients with soft signs of injury. It has a sensitivity of 91% and a specificity close to 100%, with a positive predictive value of 100% and a negative predictive value of 99%. Although use of ultrasound is advantageous in children because of the lack of radiation exposure, it has disadvantages, including technical difficulty imaging distal arteries (vertebral and internal carotid), operator dependency, and lack of 24/7 availability at some centers. It also requires patient cooperation, which may not be possible in younger patients.

Magnetic resonance angiography (MRA) has been evaluated in children in the setting of PNI. Like ultrasound, it has no radiation exposure, making it an attractive option. Because of the long scan time, difficulty monitoring patients, possibility of metallic foreign bodies, and need for sedation in many patients, it is not a first-line option.

Clinical Algorithm

PNI with no signs or symptoms of injury: Patients with PNI who exhibit no signs of vascular injury after meticulous physical examination should either be monitored for a change in their condition via serial physical examinations or undergo CTA with further management based on those results. The type of selective algorithm used is institution specific.

PNI with soft signs of injury: Most pediatric patients with soft signs of vascular injury should undergo CTA. Further management is based on those results and determined in consultation with the trauma team or surgeon.

PNI with hard signs of injury: Unstable patients or those with hard signs of vascular injury should be definitively treated in the OR with few exceptions.

Treatment

Definitive treatment is rarely provided in the emergency department unless the asymptomatic patient presents with PNI and no CTA evidence of proximity wounds. In that case, appropriate wound care (wash out and possible wound closure) may be all that is indicated after discussion with a trauma surgeon. This type of presentation is uncommon because almost all children with PNI will be minimally observed under the supervision of a trauma surgeon. When there are hard signs of injury, definitive treatment is essentially always provided in the OR with rare exception. In those with soft signs of vascular injury, ancillary studies used to determine if aerodigestive or vascular injury is present are often indicated. There are varied treatment options and much debate regarding penetrating arterial injuries of the neck. Some surgeons prefer carotid artery ligation, whereas others elect to accomplish reconstructive surgery. There are many variables to be considered by the surgeon when making these decisions, including overall neurological appearance, the presence of other injuries, injury location, patient age, and hemodynamic stability.

Key Points

- Many algorithms exist for the management of PNI. Most are based on adult studies.
- CTA is the initial imaging modality of choice in all patients who remain stable with soft signs of vascular injury.
- Management protocols are varied and often institution specific.

Pitfalls

- Delays in diagnosis or false reassurance that no vascular injury exists due to lack of adequate imaging can lead to catastrophic airway decompensation.
- Sending the patient for remote imaging and/or ancillary tests without assurance of stable airway or when hemodynamically unstable.

Blunt Vascular Injury

The incidence of blunt cerebrovascular injury (BCVI) has been reported to be as low as 0.03% in the pediatric trauma registry compared to 1% or 2% in the adult population. More recently, the incidence of pediatric BCVI has been cited at 0.3–0.9%. Despite the low incidence of BCVI in children, mortality rates range from 25% to 50%, including those who eventually manifest stroke sequelae. BCVI is well studied in the adult population. Risk factors, diagnostic algorithms, and protocols are established. Unfortunately, there are few large, prospective studies in the pediatric literature to establish similar guidelines. Because of this, adult foundational studies are often used to diagnose and manage young patients.

Clinical Features

Hard signs of vascular injury such as copious external bleeding and/or rapidly expanding hematoma often seen with PNI are reliable indicators of vascular insult. When these signs are absent, the diagnosis of pediatric vascular injury requires a high index of clinical suspicion and careful clinical examination, including the affected and contralateral extremity, skin color, capillary refill, and pulse examination. Pediatric patients have an increased propensity to undergo vasospasm unrelated to vascular injury. This can result in diminished or absent pulses. Coupling a detailed physical examination with a hospital-specific screening protocol, such as the modified Denver criteria or Utah Score, will help guide the physician to the best initial approach for these patients.

Many cases of BCVI present without overt signs or symptoms, which means the injury can be overlooked or missed altogether, especially in the setting of multitrauma. Screening criteria have been established in an attempt to avoid missing these potentially devastating injuries. Further complicating the issue, not all patients who have sustained injury to their carotid or vertebral arteries will have immediate neurological sequelae, whereas others may never manifest symptoms. The onset of delayed stroke symptoms can remain clinically occult for days or even weeks following vascular insult.

Normal anatomic variation, commonly seen in the general population, might explain why some vascular injuries remain clinically silent while others result in profound cerebral ischemia. The circle of Willis provides collateral flow for both anterior and posterior circulation. Without collateral circulation, a significant unilateral vascular insult would predictably result in neurological sequelae. In the patient with hypoplastic or absent anterior or posterior communicating arteries, these unilateral insults can result in stroke symptoms due to the lack of collateral circulation from the contralateral vessels. In the older population, in which significant coronary artery disease can be seen in cerebral arteries (i.e., distal to the Circle of Willis), even with an intact circle of Willis and thus good collateral circulation, these patients are still at greater risk of developing stroke symptoms following BCVI. This may in part explain why younger patients, with patent distal vasculature, seem to have a lower incidence of BCVI injuries compared to adults with variable amounts of atherosclerotic disease. It is possible that some of these asymptomatic children actually did sustain BCVI but never manifested ischemic symptoms because of patent vessels and good collateral circulation. In these instances, it is also possible that the children were never imaged, which would also explain the lower incidence of injury compared to that of adults.

Carotid and vertebral artery injuries differ with regard to mechanisms, clinical presentations, and onset of neurological sequelae. One of the criticisms of the widely used screening criteria for BCVI is that many diagnostic algorithms and treatment protocols consider both anterior and posterior circulation as one entity rather than considering each separately.

Injury mechanisms leading to BCVI are well delineated, with a common characteristic of stretching, shearing, or impingement of the great vessels. The most commonly reported mechanisms are high energy with rapid deceleration; extreme neck movement (flexion or extension) with contralateral rotation; blunt force trauma to the head, neck, face, and upper torso; and intraoral trauma. Each of these mechanisms has the potential to cause injury to carotid or vertebral vessels, leading to intimal tearing, platelet aggregation, and thrombus formation. Vessel wall damage can also lead to dissection. Pseudoaneurysm is another potential result of BCVI.

Symptoms seen in the setting of blunt vascular insult are highly variable and depend on the location of the injury and the patency of distal vasculature.

Anterior Circulation

When the carotid artery is involved, it can lead to cerebral ischemia and contralateral sensorimotor deficits in the setting of a large, central vessel occlusion. In other instances, an isolated Horner's syndrome might be the only manifestation of a potential vascular violation because the sympathetic chain courses next to the external carotid artery in the neck. If Horner's syndrome is noted (partial ptosis, miosis, and lack of sweating on the ipsilateral side of injury), then one should aggressively search for a vascular insult.

Posterior Circulation

Detecting injury to the vertebral arteries presents a similar challenge because many present asymptomatically. These injuries have a very high association with upper cervical spine fractures, but they are also seen following repetitive motion (swimming) or chiropractor neck manipulation. These latter injuries can be seen in combination with underlying ligamentous laxity or collagen vascular diseases. Presentation can vary from no symptoms to transient neurological complaints and acute stroke symptoms in the basilar artery territory. Unilateral traumatic vertebral artery injury is estimated to manifest symptoms in only 20% of patients because of extensive collateral supply within the posterior circulation. Delayed presentation of neurological sequelae is relatively common, but case reports have documented extreme delays as late as 3–6 months after the traumatic insult. Symptoms related to traumatic vertebral artery injury result from diminished blood flow to the cerebellum, brainstem, and visual cortex. Symptoms include dizziness, vertigo, diminished coordination, disequilibrium, ataxia, nausea and/or vomiting, neck or head pain, altered sensorium, speech (dysarthria) and visual deficits (double vision and nystagmus), lower cranial nerve palsies, and medial or lateral medullary syndrome.

Diagnostic Confirmation

Stroke is one of the most feared outcomes of BCVI, with a reported overall incidence of 10–13%. Approximately 50% of patients who develop neurologic sequelae will have stroke symptoms upon arrival to the emergency department. Among asymptomatic patients with BCVI, aggressive screening and timely treatment have been shown to decrease the incidence of stroke to <1%. Screening protocols have been published to aid in the determination of which patients should be imaged. These have been accepted in adults, but due to the smaller number of similar injuries in the younger population, validation is ongoing. The physician must consider radiation exposure versus missing the injury when deciding on the best diagnostic course of action to take, particularly with younger patients.

High-impact chest trauma (especially in association with clavicle fractures) or severe head injury (with either basilar skull fracture or intracranial hemorrhage) should increase one's suspicion for BCVI in the pediatric population. The controversial finding of a cervical seat belt sign has also been debated as a potential marker of BCVI in children. This latter finding, without other high-risk features, has not been independently shown to increase the risk of vascular injury in children. Despite recent skepticism regarding use of this sign in isolation, the cervical seat belt sign remains within the Memphis criteria, Boston criteria, and Denver criteria, as well as many institutional screening protocols.

Because so much controversy exists regarding which injury mechanisms are high-risk markers associated with BCVI, screening protocols have been established, including the Denver and modified Denver criteria, the Memphis and modified Memphis criteria, the Utah criteria, the Boston criteria, and the McGovern Screening Score. These tools serve to increase the physician's index of suspicion for BCVI in the asymptomatic patient by proposing conditions more highly associated with the injury. Using a liberal pediatric screening strategy should predictably increase BCVI detection rates, but concerns regarding the oncogenic effects of ionizing radiation can limit widespread applicability in young patients.

In 2009 and 2010, the Western Trauma Association (WTA) and the Eastern Association for the Surgery of Trauma (EAST) published guidelines, without providing strong scientific evidence, supporting the use of the modified Denver criteria to screen for BCVI in all ages (Table 35.3). During the next few years, multiple studies found that use of the modified Denver criteria alone missed approximately 20% of these injuries. These findings led to the expanded Denver criteria, which contains new inclusion criteria (mandibular fractures, complex skull fractures, traumatic brain injury with thoracic injuries, scalp degloving, and thoracic vascular injuries) in addition to previously described screening criteria. To date, the modified Denver criteria appears to be the

TABLE 35.3 MODIFIED DENVER SCREENING CRITERIA FOR BLUNT CEREBROVASCULAR INJURY: CLINICAL ALGORITHM

Signs/Symptoms of BCVI	Risk Factors for BCVI
Arterial hemorrhage from neck/nose/mouth	High-energy transfer mechanism with
Cervical bruit in patients <50 years	Le Fort II or III
Expanding cervical hematoma	Mandible fracture
Focal neurological deficit	Complex skull fracture/basilar skull fracture/occipital condyle fracture
Neurological exam incongruous with head CT findings	Severe TBI with GCS<6
Stroke on secondary CT scan	Cervical spine fracture, subluxation or ligamentous injury at any level
	Near hanging with anoxic brain injury
	Seat belt abrasion with significant swelling, pain, or altered mental status
	TBI with thoracic injury
	Scalp degloving
	Thoracic vascular injury
	Blunt cardiac rupture
	Upper rib fracture

BCVI, blunt cerebrovascular injury; CT, computed tomography; GCS, Glasgow Coma Scale; TBI, traumatic brain injury.

TABLE 35.4 UTAH SCORE FOR PREDICTING PROBABILITY OF BLUNT CEREBROVASCULAR INJURY IN THE PEDIATRIC POPULATION

Variable	Score
GCS ≤8	1
Focal neurologic deficit	2
Carotid canal fracture	2
Petrous temporal bone fracture	3
Cerebral infarct on CT	3
Total	11

CT, computed tomography; GCS, Glasgow Coma Scale.

most studied and is endorsed by both WTA and EAST.

Because BCVI incidence is much lower in children, there is a paucity of recommendations and validated studies to draw from. EAST supports the use of the modified Denver criteria in the pediatric population. One study found more than two-thirds of pediatric patients presenting with strokes resulting from BCVI did not meet vascular screening criteria based on accepted adult protocols. Studies such as this underscore the need for improved screening criteria tailored to this age group in an attempt to balance diagnostic accuracy with radiation risk.

The Utah Score (Table 35.4) is a scoring protocol that was initially based on a retrospective study examining BCVI in pediatric patients. The Utah Score was compared to the modified Denver criteria in children, and it was found that the Utah Score detected more vascular injuries than did the modified Denver criteria. A Utah Score ≤2 implies a low risk of BCVI (<7.9% risk based on initial study and <2.7% risk based on validation study), whereas a Utah Score ≥3 puts the patient at higher risk of BCVI (39.3% risk based on initial results and 18.1% risk based on validation study). It was also proposed in the study that a delayed MRA be used in place of a CTA with a Utah Score <2. Further investigation and validation are required to support the use of delayed MRA in lieu of CTA.

Imaging

CTA: With improved technology such as 16-section or higher CT scanners, CTA is considered the screening modality of choice for BCVI, with a sensitivity and specificity that approach 100%. CTA has many advantages over other diagnostic options. It is readily available, rapid, noninvasive, sensitive even for smaller vessels, maintains its sensitivity and specificity in children, and gives simultaneous information of surrounding structures. Timely CTA-based screening was shown to reduce the time to diagnosis 12-fold, giving the physician more time to decide on treatment options in an attempt to reduce neurological sequelae produced by vascular trauma. More timely diagnosis in turn was found to reduce injury-related stroke rate 4-fold, underscoring why a desired characteristic of imaging should be immediate access and rapid completion time.

Digital subtraction angiography: Digital subtraction angiography (DSA) is still touted to be the gold standard for detecting vascular injury, yet its use today pales in comparison to that of CTA. DSA in an invasive procedure with a complication rate of 1–3%, including a 0.5% risk of stroke. DSA is not readily available at many centers; takes considerably more time to perform; and requires transport to the angio suite, which may not be optimal for the semi-stable patient.

MRA: Despite limited, unvalidated recommendations for the use of delayed MRA in low-risk pediatric patients with suspected BCVI, the use of MRA acutely to detect BCVI is not widely accepted. Limitations making MRA unsuitable include long scan times; safety challenges related to patient monitoring; poor characterization of acute intravascular hematomas; possible contraindications when metallic foreign bodies are present; and lack of ubiquitous, 24/7 access.

Duplex ultrasound: Duplex ultrasound is an attractive option in that it is often a bedside test and is not invasive. The disadvantage is that it suffers from poor sensitivity (86% for carotid injuries and 38.5% for combined carotid and vertebral injuries). In addition, many of the distal carotid as well vertebral lesions are technically inaccessible. Ultrasound is highly operator dependent and carries an increased chance of missing dissection. Other technical limits include assessing vertebral vessels that may be obscured by bone, stiff necks or cervical collars making optimal positioning difficult, and artifacts from central venous catheters or metallic foreign bodies. EAST has not supported the use of ultrasound to diagnose these injuries.

Treatment

Among asymptomatic patients with BCVI undergoing aggressive screening and early treatment, the incidence of stroke has been shown to decrease from roughly 13% to <1%.

The optimum management strategy for BCVI has not been universally accepted due to a paucity of controlled trials in both adults and children. However, depending on the location and grade of injury, EAST and WTA support one of four options: observation only, surgical repair, endovascular management, or antithrombotic therapy. When active treatment is indicated, antithrombotic is often the chosen modality. Several options are available, including unfractionated heparin, low-molecular-weight heparin, and antiplatelet agents (aspirin vs. clopidogrel). Because of a paucity of BCVI in children, further studies are needed to elucidate which of these options is most ideal.

Key Points

- Various screening criteria help predict high-risk patients for BCVI.
- Isolated seat belt sign has not been proven to be a high-risk feature, despite its inclusion in some screening protocols.
- Many BCVIs are not diagnosed until after the onset of neurological sequelae.
- Neurological morbidity (stroke syndromes and focal deficits) as well as overall increased mortality rates increase significantly following a delay in the diagnosis.
- CTA is the study of choice in pediatric patients when BCVI is suspected.
- High-risk mechanisms include basilar, mid-face, or cervical fractures; Glasgow Coma Scale <8; and hanging attempt with anoxic brain injury.

Pitfalls

- Overlooking the possibility of BCVI in a multitraumatized patient can lead to a missed diagnosis. The risk is higher when the patient is altered or unable to cooperate with the examination.
- Attributing neurological sequelae resulting from BCVI to severe traumatic brain injury without a thorough inspection of the neck vasculature can result in a missed diagnosis.
- Failure to consult surgery during the window following BCVI while still asymptomatic can result in a delay in treatment, which in turn can result in a poorer outcome and increased mortality.

ESOPHAGEAL TRAUMA

Overview

Esophageal injury in the pediatric age group is uncommon, with the cervical esophagus more commonly injured than the thoracic region. Penetrating trauma occurs more often than blunt injury. Signs and symptoms that can be seen with esophageal injury are often nonspecific, making clinical diagnosis difficult without supporting diagnostic tests. Early diagnosis reduces both short- and long-term morbidity and mortality. Because of the paucity of these injuries in children, much of the recommendations are based on adult studies and algorithms. The overall mortality associated with esophageal perforation can approach 20%, and delay in treatment of more than 24 hours after perforation can result in a doubling of mortality.

Clinical Features

Signs and symptoms for both blunt and penetrating cervical esophageal injuries are nonspecific and often lacking, which can delay clinical suspicion and therefore definitive diagnosis and treatment. Some of the more commonly reported findings associated with esophageal perforations include dysphagia, dysphonia, hematemesis, drooling, neck or upper chest pain, neck crepitus, and saliva exiting the wound. Gas is often seen on plain films or CT scan of the neck. Less often, blood in oral or oral/nasal gastric tube secretions has been reported. Fever and tachycardia are considered late findings and, when seen, can present as a spectrum beginning as an inflammatory reaction from oral content spillage and later resulting in overt sepsis resulting from mediastinitis. Sepsis is most commonly seen following perforation of the thoracic or abdominal esophagus as opposed to the cervical esophagus. Anatomically, esophageal injuries in the cervical esophagus can spread to the mediastinum because of the pretracheal fascia originating in the neck and inserting in the mid-chest. This anatomical continuity provides a pathway for saliva or gastric contents leaking from esophageal wounds to reach the chest and result in mediastinitis.

Diagnostic Confirmation

The 24-hour mark seems to be a turning point after which increased morbidity and mortality are expected when esophageal injuries remain undetected. Because they can be innocuous or completely asymptomatic initially, a high index of suspicion for esophageal violation is required and, if considered, diagnostic testing should be aggressively pursued.

High-resolution contrast CTA of the neck is the initial imaging modality of choice in both penetrating and blunt neck trauma victims presenting with nonspecific symptoms. Because not all esophageal injuries will be detectable using CT scan, institution-specific algorithms should be relied on for stable patients. These should be considered as the next step when clinically indicated. Clinical indication for further investigation is based on CT proximity/trajectory or the presence of paraesophageal air or fluid on CT scan. Likewise, CT can safely eliminate the need for further imaging in appropriate settings in which no proximity lesions are noted and clinical suspicion is eliminated. It is important to remember that esophageal injury or perforation may not be seen on CT scan. When mechanism or presentation suggests this as a possible diagnosis, further evaluation is warranted.

WTA recommends flexible esophagoscopy as a first-line confirmation test, with appreciation that it has limited application as a sole diagnostic study. Although numbers vary, one study found a sensitivity of 100% and a specificity of 92.4% with a negative predictive value of 100% and a positive predictive value of 33% using this technique. In addition, compared to other techniques, flexible esophagoscopy better detects proximal injuries (hypopharynx and cervical esophagus).

If endoscopy is inconclusive, esophagography using fluoroscopy is indicated. A water-soluble, rapidly resorbing contrast solution (e.g., gastrografin) is initially used to minimize the risk of mediastinal fibrosis. It is important to recognize that approximately one in five injuries will be missed with water-soluble contrast, but these can be subsequently detected via thin barium esophagography. The other potential disadvantage is that contrast esophagography requires a stable and cooperative patient.

Helical CT esophagography may be a viable alternative. In adults, one study found CT esophagography to have a sensitivity and specificity of 95% and 91%, respectively, for cervical esophageal injuries.

Treatment

Traumatic esophageal perforation can be life-threatening. The type of treatment will vary depending on time from injury, type/size/location of the perforation, patient stability, other associated conditions, and physician judgment. Unstable patients with traumatic neck injury should be taken to the OR for immediate exploration.

Stable patients with cervical esophageal injuries should remain NPO. Many will require a nasogastric tube, which is best placed under direct visualization via endoscopy. Broad-spectrum antibiotics covering both anaerobes and aerobes can be initiated in the emergency department when esophageal injury is suspected, confirmed, or if there is any suggestion of sepsis.

Key Points

- Esophageal injuries can be very insidious; they require a high index of suspicion.
- CT scan can miss the injury, especially in children. When negative or inconclusive, endoscopy should be considered.

Pitfalls

- Sole reliance on CT scan can lead to missed injuries.
- Patients should be treated aggressively when diagnosis is likely but not confirmed. Broad-spectrum antibiotics should be considered early.

LARYNGOTRACHEAL INJURIES

Overview

The incidence of laryngotracheal (LT) trauma in children is rare, with blunt trauma the most common mechanism. Mortality rates in children are reported at 8.7%. A large number of blunt cases result from multisystem trauma. These cases often present with other distracting injuries, which can lead to a delay in diagnosis by masking a stable LT injury. LT injuries can result from any type of high- or low-velocity, penetrating trauma (bullets, knives, glass, bites, etc.) or blunt trauma (motorized vehicles, clothesline wounds, strangulation or near-hanging, sports accidents, bicycles, etc.). Currently, no algorithm has been uniquely established for children.

Pediatric airways differ from those of adults, leading to differences in incidence, injury patterns, and management algorithms. Children have shorter necks, with their larynx as high as C2 early in life. The larynx descends during the mid-teens years until it reaches the adult position of C6–C7. In young patients with a more cephalad larynx, the mandible affords protection, which explains why there are fewer LT injuries in this age group. The pediatric airway diameter is smaller than that of an adult; thus, minor injury leading to mucosal edema can threaten a child's airway more readily. Thyroid cartilage ossification begins after the teen years. Prior, the airway is much more flexible due to the increased cartilaginous flexibility, leading to fewer fractures. As the cartilaginous structures ossify and lose elasticity, they become more prone to fractures.

Clinical Features of Blunt Laryngotracheal Injury

Blunt LT trauma in children is an uncommon occurrence, with the potential for immediate or insidious airway compromise. Mechanisms include clothesline injuries, sports injuries, strangulation or near-hanging, motorized vehicle accidents, bicycle accidents, falls, and objects striking the neck directly. Signs and symptoms are nonspecific and not unique to the larynx because laryngeal injuries can be seen simultaneously with esophageal injury. Patients can present with voice changes (aphonia, dysphonia, and hoarseness), odynophagia, dysphagia, stridor, acute respiratory distress, anterior neck swelling or pain, and crepitus in soft tissues or over laryngeal cartilages.

In one study, neck pain, hoarseness, and dyspnea were the most common signs of injury in children with LT trauma. The presence of subcutaneous gas, which may be evident on a bedside X-ray or palpable clinically, is highly associated with LT injury. This should be taken seriously because one review reported that it was present in up to 84.8% of cases.

Diagnostic Confirmation of Blunt Laryngotracheal Injury

Airway stabilization must be ensured as the first priority; however, a number of patients are stable and can tolerate diagnostic evaluation without a preceding artificial airway. Conversely, a patient can appear stable with a life-threatening airway injury until enough soft tissue swelling ensues and leads to critical airway obstruction. This is why serial examination is crucial despite a stable clinical appearance.

If available, flexible fiberoptic laryngoscopy is a noninvasive approach to view the airway in the stable patient. CT scan remains the imaging modality of choice in the adult population at many institutions, and it is often used as a first-line approach in children with blunt neck trauma. The utility of CT scan has been examined in the pediatric population, and one review found a false-negative rate of 29.5%. This is believed to be related to skeletal immaturity and lack of ossification in young patients, making cartilaginous structures less well visualized by CT scan.

Spiral CT scan with intravenous contrast and multiplanar reconstruction with 1-mm cuts improves the sensitivity for visualizing LT injuries, including the nonossified laryngeal and tracheal cartilaginous structures in children. Sensitivity has been reported to be between 85% and 100%. If air is present in the deep tissues of the neck or mediastinum, the sensitivity of CT scan is increased. CT is less reliable for visualizing non-displaced cartilaginous fractures, small lacerations, and small mucosal disruption, all of which are unlikely to require surgical repair. CT is good at detecting significant LT or hyoid fractures or dislocations, significant internal or external LT hematomas, airway diameter measurement and vocal cord integrity.

Patients with a clinically unstable airway and a suspected LT fracture require immediate operative intervention; further diagnostic studies may be performed in the OR with the possibility of open repair.

Treatment of Blunt Laryngotracheal Injury

Delays in diagnosing LT injuries can result in conditions that negatively impact outcome, including pneumothorax, pneumomediastinum, and mediastinitis. In addition, diagnostic delays can lead to long-term sequelae such as dysphonia, dysphagia, and tracheal stenosis. Timely diagnosis and treatment offer the best chance at normal swallowing, speaking, and breathing. Differing treatment strategies have been proposed in the literature; the details of which are beyond the scope of this discussion. Some offer aggressive open surgical repair, whereas others support conservative management. Indications for surgical intervention or endoscopic repair are primarily based on direct visualization of the airway and/or CT scan results. Indications include cricotracheal or laryngotracheal disruption, cricoarytenoid dislocation, vocal fold paralysis, vocal fold avulsion, laryngeal cartilage fractures, degloving of the cartilage, and lacerations of the free edge of the vocal folds or anterior commissure.

Key Points for Blunt Laryngotracheal Injury

- Children lack mineralization of their airway cartilage and have higher airway positioning than do adults. This can lead to differences in injury patterns.
- Airway stabilization should always take top priority.
- CT scan can miss this injury in children; when clinically suspected, endoscopy should be considered.

Pitfalls for Blunt Laryngotracheal Injury

- Assuming a stable airway and not performing serial examinations can lead to airway catastrophe.
- Delayed diagnosis can lead to suboptimal outcomes for speech and breathing.

Clinical Features of Penetrating Laryngotracheal Injury

Penetrating laryngotracheal injuries can present in a number of ways. Patients may complain of shortness of breath, difficulty or painful swallowing, voice changes, or pain over the anterior neck. Physical findings can include bruising or tenderness over the anterior neck, aphonia, deviation of the LT complex, subcutaneous gas overlying the larynx, hoarseness, and hemoptysis. Bubbling from the wound implying an air leak is highly concerning for violation of the airway. Stridor, often resulting from airway impingement, can suggest the level of involvement. Inspiratory stridor implies supraglottic narrowing, whereas expiratory stridor typically points to a subglottic location. If biphasic inspiratory and expiratory stridor is heard, this suggests the obstruction is at the level of the glottis.

Diagnostic Confirmation of Penetrating Laryngotracheal Injury

Penetrating neck trauma allows for easier risk stratification when searching for LT injury and the potential for airway compromise than does concern for LT injury in the setting of blunt neck trauma. Detailed history and thorough physical examination alone will provide most of the information a physician needs to decide on the best management pathway. Unfortunately, there is no absolute consensus that all clinically significant LT lesions will manifest in the first hours post injury.

In the stable patient not requiring emergent surgical intervention or immediate airway stabilization, chest and neck X-rays are rapid bedside tests that can identify pneumothorax, pneumomediastinum, gas in the neck, or deviation of the airway. All of these findings are suggestive but not specific for an airway injury in the correct clinical scenario. Multiple modalities are available to confirm penetrating injury to the larynx or trachea. Diagnostic considerations include rigid or flexible laryngeal scopes or CT scan.

In the stable patient with PNI, the initial study of choice is CT scan. High-resolution helical CT is useful for detecting the trajectory of the penetrating object and its proximity to vital structures. When CT reveals deep emphysema in the tissue of the neck, it is highly suggestive of aerodigestive injury. A recent retrospective study suggested that when deep emphysema is absent, this virtually eliminates the possibility of an aerodigestive injury. This finding has not been validated in children.

Flexible nasolaryngoscopy (FN) is a bedside procedure that requires some level of patient cooperation, which can be difficult to achieve in the frightened child. FN can evaluate the endolarynx and assess for mucosal disruption. One disadvantage is that this equipment is not always readily available and requires an operator familiar with the technique. In addition to being a valuable adjunct to direct airway visualization, bedside FN can also be used to assist with intubation when indicated. Rigid laryngoscopy is another option for airway visualization of the distal larynx, but it requires general anesthesia.

Treatment of Penetrating Laryngotracheal Injury

The feared, either immediate or potentially delayed complication of LT injury is airway compromise. There is no "one-size-fits-all" algorithm for airway stabilization, with options including orotracheal intubation, intubation over fiberoptic scope, various intubating adjuncts, percutaneous transtracheal jet insufflation, retrograde tracheal intubation, cricothyrotomy, and tracheostomy. Most agree that direct visualization with a flexible nasopharyngeal scope is a safe first step, but that option is not always immediately available. In addition, excessive bleeding can impede the view, making this technique difficult or impossible. Many studies support gentle orotracheal intubation by an experienced intubator as a safe first approach. Using a tube one size smaller than anticipated to adjust for the potential of airway edema is prudent.

Many smaller injuries, such as mucosal tears, can be managed nonoperatively with antibiotics. Steroids should be considered in consultation with the surgeon. Higher grade injuries or unstable patients will require surgical intervention.

Key Points for Penetrating Laryngotracheal Injury

- Reliance on CT scan for wound trajectory is helpful when assessing proximity lesions.
- Endoscopy (rigid or flexible) is indicated if CT scan is nonconclusive in a high-risk patient.

Pitfalls for Penetrating Laryngotracheal Injury

- Assuming a stable airway and not performing serial examinations can lead to airway catastrophe.
- Delayed diagnosis can lead to suboptimal outcomes for speech and breathing.

36

Pediatric Thoraco-Abdominal Trauma

CHRISTOPHER S. AMATO

INTRODUCTION

Injury is the leading cause of death in the pediatric population. Thoraco-abdominal trauma is associated with a high morbidity and mortality. Abdominal trauma occurs in 25% of children with major trauma and is responsible for 9% of all trauma deaths. Because it can delay care, lack of recognition of intra-abdominal injury increases morbidity and mortality. Thoracic trauma comprises only 4–6% of pediatric trauma but is related to 14% of pediatric trauma-related deaths and is the second most common cause of mortality in pediatric trauma.

Comparison with Adult Physiology

In children, multiorgan injury is the rule rather than the exception. The pediatric patient is more compact, with little anterior musculature and subcutaneous adipose to protect the larger solid organs. The spleen and liver are the most common organs injured, with concomitant genitourinary injury found in up to 10% of cases. The bladder is intra-abdominal, whereas the kidneys are relatively larger and more inferior and, are therefore, at higher risk of injury in children. Identification of the injured tissue is more complicated in children because their tissue is more pliable and "rubbery," which may diminish outward signs of injury. History, more so than physical examination, should point the clinician toward blunt abdominal trauma. This can be augmented by repeated examination to identify any developing intra-abdominal injuries. Bowel perforation, as seen in lap belt injuries, is a key example of the additive value of repeat examination. An elastic rib cage causes further issues with thoracic trauma because the pliable nature of ribs allows for transmission of the kinetic energy with little visualized signs of injury. The force will therefore be directed inward toward the organs. They have a more mobile mediastinum, which can affect preload but will lead to decreased likelihood of aortic injury.

Vital signs are crucial to determine stability, but the pediatric patient has great compensatory mechanisms. In children, cardiac output, dependent on preload and rate, is maintained through tachycardia because they cannot affect stroke volume as adults can. An age-appropriate blood pressure can be maintained even after 25–33% loss of blood volume. Children consume oxygen at more than two times the adult rate but have a diminished functional residual capacity and so will desaturate quickly.

The developmental stage of the patient, any developmental delay, or any chronic disorders can make the clinician's job more difficult due to lack of ability to communicate. The examination is further inconvenienced with the physiologic response of fear and anxiety. Young children may be at higher risk due to their lack of motor coordination inhibiting their ability to protect themselves, whereas adolescents may engage in high-risk behaviors that can place them in harm's way.

CLASSIC CLINICAL PRESENTATION

Chest Trauma

- Vital sign abnormality, especially tachycardia or hypoxia, without other explanation
- Shortness of breath, persistent difficulty breathing, or pleuritic chest pain
- Abnormal breath sounds
- The presence of subcutaneous emphysema
- Jugular venous distension may connote a pericardial effusion. However, this is not a frequent finding in children and likely not found if the patient is hypovolemic with tamponade.

Abdominal Trauma

- Ecchymoses, abrasions, and patterned marks (handlebar or tire marking)
- Seat belt sign in restrained passengers from motor vehicle collisions
- Abdominal tenderness or distension, and fullness of a specific quadrant
- Absent bowel sounds
- Referred pain: to the back indicating pancreas injury or to the left shoulder (Kehr's) indicating splenic injury
- Peritoneal irritation: rigidity, rebound, and guarding
- Penetrating wounds through peritoneum: surgical consultation and operative exploration and repair
- A foreign body that has penetrated the abdomen should be left in place until definitive management can be performed.

Seat Belt Signs

Motor vehicle collisions are the most common mechanism of trauma and cause of blunt abdominal injury. Restraint systems for children are crucial for their well-being, but there is a three-fold increased risk for intra-abdominal trauma if they are incorrectly restrained. A seat belt sign is an area of erythema, ecchymosis, and/or abrasion across the abdominal wall resulting from seat belt restraints and compression of organs toward the spine. The presence of a seat belt sign, even without other clinical findings, should strongly prompt the clinician to consider adding radiographic imaging. The presence of this finding has a 25% sensitivity and 85% specificity for intra-abdominal injury, which can range from organ laceration to a hollow viscus or mesenteric injury. Seat belt syndrome is a term used to convey intra-abdominal pathology with a seat belt sign.

Blunt and Penetrating Thoraco-Abdominal Trauma

Non-accidental trauma should be considered in each case. Most rib fractures are related to abuse, but other organic causes, such as osteogenesis imperfecta and rickets, should remain in the differential. The mechanism involved in non-accidental trauma may lead to higher likelihood of intrathoracic injury. Mortality is directly correlated with each fractured rib (e.g., 1.79% without rib fracture and 5.81% with a single rib fracture), much like adult mortality is dramatically increased with more than six fractured ribs.

IMAGING

Focused Assessment with Sonography in Trauma Examination

Although a focused assessment with sonography in trauma (FAST) examination has become part of the primary survey of the traumatized patient, it does not bear out the same sensitivity and specificity in children. A variety of sensitivity and specificity ranges are reported for the Adult trauma patient in the literature, with some studies noting 94% for both while pediatric FAST has sensitivities from 66–68%. Because approximately 200 mL of fluid is required for a FAST examination to be "positive," many young children can have significant intra-abdominal bleeding that is not visualized on examination. In addition, pelvic free fluid may be normally seen in non-injured prepubescent males and females and does not necessarily represent acute injury.

Abdominal Computed Tomography

Computed tomography (CT) should be utilized cautiously because there are risks related to exposure to ionizing radiation. There are increasing data indicating that the "pan-scan" approach to the pediatric patient does not yield improved care compared with a customized approach. CT should be considered when the following are present:

- Concerns of intra-abdominal injury with positive seat belt sign
- High risk for intra-abdominal injury as determined by algorithm
- Laboratory findings of aspartate aminotransferase >200 IU/L or alanine aminotransferase >125 IU/L, and gross hematuria or microscopic hematuria with ≥50 red blood cells (RBCs) per high-power field in otherwise asymptomatic patients
- Falling hematocrit or hematocrit <30% without clear source of loss
- Increased fluid or blood requirements without source of loss
- Inability to perform adequate or serial abdominal examination (i.e., uncooperative children, altered mentation, or prior direct peritoneal lavage)
- Positive FAST examination in a hemodynamically stable patient

Contrast

Patients with blunt trauma should receive only intravenous (IV) contrast, rather than both IV and oral contrast. Studies have shown minimal difference in sensitivity and specificity with both oral and IV contrast. This has also borne out at trauma centers, where findings are similarly detected with IV contrast only. Oral contrast has been shown to delay CT as well as have more potential side effects.

TREATMENT OF PNEUMO-/HEMOTHORAX

Acute treatment of a tension pneumothorax is needle decompression using a large-bore needle placed in the second or third intercostal space in the mid-clavicular line. The needle is inserted above the rib so as to avoid vasculature. Placement in the fifth intercostal space in the mid-axillary line is also acceptable. If the patient is stable, asymptomatic, and there is a small pneumothorax, observation or even just aspiration may suffice. Aspiration may not need to be followed by a chest tube, whereas a definitive chest tube must be placed immediately after needle decompression for a tension pneumothorax. The size of the tube will vary with the size of the child and the underlying medical issue. Smaller pigtail catheters may be used in lieu of larger, more uncomfortable chest tubes, and these may provide drainage of air or fluid as needed. If there is a hemothorax, then a larger sized tube may be preferred, although tubes as small as 7 or 8 Fr can successfully drain a hemothorax if regularly flushed and declotted with thrombolytics as needed. The classic pediatric chest tube size is four time the endotracheal tube size (uncuffed formula = age/4 +4), with a minimal size of 36 Fr. However, much smaller tubes are used successfully in adults with hemothorax (28–30 Fr). Immediate drainage of >20 mL/kg is an indication for operative care with thoracotomy.

APPROACH TO RESUSCITATION OF HEMORRHAGIC SHOCK

As with any child who is showing signs of shock, a 20 mL/kg bolus of isotonic crystalloid, normal saline or Ringer's lactate, should be rapidly infused using a push–pull method as opposed to gravity or a regular pump, and it may be repeated up to three times (within 30–60 minutes) for patients without normalization of vital signs or clinical findings. Blood transfusion may be required in those who are not improving or in patients who are clearly having ongoing blood loss. For every 1 mL of blood loss, 3 mL of isotonic crystalloid is required for those in hemorrhagic shock. Blood is typically transfused in 10 mL/kg boluses. Studies have not shown improved outcome with use of colloid rather than crystalloid fluids. Vasopressors should not be considered in the hemorrhagic shock patient because the underlying issue is the loss of blood and the pressor may increase hypoxia.

Massive transfusion protocols (MTPs), with the goal of a 1:1:1 ratio for transfusion of fresh frozen plasma, packed RBCs, and platelets, have not been shown to be effective in improving outcome in children. MTPs have been found to improve the delivery time of blood products to the emergency department or trauma bay; however, overall mortality and morbidity have not shown consistent improvement.

Tranexamic acid (TXA) has become the standard of care in adult trauma patients with significantly reduced mortality when infused within 3 hours of injury, but there are only limited data on its use in children. It may decrease mortality in the severely traumatized child and has also been shown to decrease neurologic injury in those receiving significant transfusions, but again, there are limited data. Current suggested dosing is a loading dose of 15 mg/kg TXA (maximum 1g) over 10 minutes followed by 2 mg/kg per hour over 8 hours. There is expert opinion that the trauma resuscitation be guided by viscoelastic hemostatic assay to identify candidates with thrombolysis (elevated LY30) who may receive maximum benefit from TXA infusion.

EVIDENCE-BASED ALGORITHMS

PECARN Chest Trauma

1. Low systolic blood pressure
2. Elevated age-adjusted respiratory rate
3. Abnormal thoracic examination
4. Abnormal auscultation of lung fields
5. Femur fracture
6. Glasgow Coma Scale (GCS) score <15

This rule has a positive predictive value of 12%, a negative predictive value of 99%, and a sensitivity of 98% and specificity of 37% for thoracic injury.

It is important to weight the risks and benefits of any test that exposes the patient to ionizing radiation. A recent review found that there is a higher risk of cancer development than finding a thoracic aortic injury on chest CT in blunt trauma pediatric patients. The rule presented here is better adapted to help the clinician rule out the likelihood of intrathoracic injury than rule it in based on the negative predictive value.

Abdominal Trauma

1. No abdominal wall trauma or seat belt sign
2. GCS >13
3. No abdominal wall tenderness
4. No chest wall/thoracic tenderness
5. No complaints of abdominal pain
6. No decreased bowel sounds
7. No vomiting

This rule has a negative predictive value of 99.9% [95% confidence interval (CI): 99.7–100%], sensitivity of 97% (95% CI: 94–99%), and specificity of 42.5% (95% CI: 41.6–43.3%).

TREATMENT

The vast majority of pediatric trauma patients (~90%), even those with organ laceration (grades I–V), are observed without surgical intervention. Surgical exploration is typically performed in grade V laceration, although even with this degree of injury, patients may be cared for non-operatively as long as they remain stable. Surgery is also typical in children who are not hemodynamically stable or the clinical course is not consistent with the expected course (monitoring of vital signs, hemoglobin, and urinary output). Transfusion can occur in patients with liver or spleen lacerations. The approach to non-operative management has been systematically changed by the American Pediatric Surgical Association, which has devised an evidence-based approach that emphasizes clinical stability instead of degree of organ laceration.

Penetrating injuries are less common but often require operative management.

DETERMINANTS OF DISPOSITION

The pediatric trauma patient with an organ laceration is admitted for serial hemoglobin determination as well as possible repeat radiography. A liver injury has higher mortality due to hemorrhage, whereas bowel injury may not be seen on initial imaging and instead requires serial examination with possible repeat imaging. Emergency laparotomy is only utilized in patients with free intraperitoneal air, persistent hemodynamic instability despite aggressive resuscitation (i.e., transfusion >50% of total blood volume), gunshot or penetrating traumas, and evisceration of intraperitoneal contents. An intravenous pyelogram is typically performed in the operating room in stable patients noted to have gross hematuria or >20 RBCs in the aforementioned unstable patient. Bowel injury and perforation are also considerations.

DISPOSITION

If the blunt traumatized patient is stable and there are no findings on preliminary imaging, especially abdominal CT, discharge home is possible as long as the patient does not have continued abdominal pain, inability to tolerate fluids, and findings of seat belt sign; there are no concerns for non-accidental trauma and no other injuries; and close follow-up can be ensured.

Transfer to a designated pediatric trauma center (a center verified by the American College of Surgeons have significantly higher survival rates than do unverified centers) should occur in the following cases:

- Multisystem injury
- Persistently unstable or low trauma score despite resuscitative efforts
- Neurovascular injury/acute cord injury
- Requirement for subspecialty care

Caretakers should be comfortable with discharge home, and outpatient follow-up should be established. Signs or symptoms for the child to return to the emergency department include the following:

- Vomiting (bilious, blood)
- Increasing abdominal pain
- Difficulty urinating
- Poor oral intake/urine or stool output
- Fever/chills
- Difficulty breathing
- Difficulty swallowing

KEY POINTS

- Unintentional injuries are the leading cause of mortality in children.
- Children have excellent compensatory mechanisms and may have normal blood pressure despite significant hemorrhage/ serious underlying injury.
- Blunt trauma is far more common than penetrating trauma.
  - Liver and spleen are the most common organs injured.
  - Non-operative management is the treatment in 95% of cases.
- Penetrating injuries are less common but often require operative management.
- Multiorgan injury is common in children.
- Utilize algorithms/clinical decision rules to balance sensitivity of diagnosis with minimization of radiation in children.
- Optimize pediatric analgesia.
- Severely injured children have better outcomes when managed at a pediatric trauma center.

PITFALLS

- Non-accidental trauma must be considered in all children.
- If a rib fracture is present, this is an indication of significant impact and trauma.
- Mortality increases with each rib fracture found.

Further Reading

Arbra CA, Vogel AM, Plumblee L, et al. External validation of a five-variable clinical prediction rule for identifying children at very low risk for intra-abdominal injury after blunt abdominal trauma. *J Trauma Acute Care Surg.* 2018;85(1):71–77.

Arbuthnot M, Onwubiko C, Osborne M, Mooney DP. Does the incidence of thoracic aortic injury warrant the routine use of chest computed tomography in children? *J Trauma Acute Care Surg.* 2019;86(1):97–100.

Darling SE, Done SL, Friedman SD, Feldman KW. Frequency of intrathoracic injuries in children younger than 3 years with rib fractures. *Pediatr Radiol.* 2014;44(10):1230–1236.

Holmes JF, Lillis K, Monroe D, et al.; Pediatric Emergency Care Applied Research Network (PECARN). Identifying children at very low risk of clinically important blunt abdominal injuries. *Ann Emerg Med.* 2013;62(2):107–116.

Holmes JF, Sokolove PE, Brant WE, Kuppermann N. A clinical decision rule for identifying children with thoracic injuries after blunt torso trauma. *Ann Emerg Med.* 2002;39(5):492–499.

Lynch T, Kilgar J, Al Shibli A. Pediatric Abdominal Trauma. *Current Pediatric Rev.* 2018;14(1):59–63. doi:10.2174/1573396313666170815100547.

Rosenberg G, Bryant AK, Davis KA, Schuster KM. No breakpoint for mortality in pediatric rib fractures. *J Trauma Acute Care Surg.* 2016;80(3):427–432.

37

Pediatric Orthopedic Emergencies

JANET SEMPLE-HESS

INTRODUCTION

- Skeletal growth is dynamic in children; thus, children have several unique patterns of fracture and injury that differ from those of adults.
- The relative strength of the periosteum and ligaments in children, in contrast to the weakest area of the bone, the growth plate, accounts for the following unique fractures:
  - Buckle fractures (torus fracture)
  - Plastic deformities or bowing fracture
  - Greenstick fracture
  - Physeal (growth plate) fractures
- When evaluating a child's fracture radiologically, it is helpful to describe all physeal injuries using the Salter–Harris classification of physeal fractures:
  - I. Fracture within growth plate (physis)—may not be visible on radiograph or physis may be widened
  - II. "Above"—through physis and above (metaphysis)
  - III. "Below"—through physis and epiphysis
  - IV. "Above and below"—through physis, metaphysis, and epiphysis
  - V. "Crush"—compression fracture of physis
- Once the physes are closed (late adolescence), adult patterns of fracture are seen. Management should reflect this.
- Some pediatric fractures (e.g., type I supracondylar humeral fractures and tibial toddler's fractures) may not be evident in initial radiographs, and repeat radiographs in 7–10 days may be necessary to see new periosteal bone formation.
- For most pediatric fractures, because of the robust remodeling and callus formation, greater angulation and displacement may be acceptable, and non-union rarely occurs, except when noted in some unique fractures.
- Certain fracture patterns are suggestive of non-accidental trauma (NAT) or child abuse and warrant Child Protective Services evaluation. Particular attention should be paid to fractures in children younger than age 2 years, especially when there is unwitnessed trauma or the history of trauma does not fit the injury pattern seen, the child is non-ambulatory, or there was a delay in seeking care. Examples include (but are not limited to) the following:
  - Multiple fractures, in different stages of healing
  - Rib fractures

- Skull fractures in children younger than age 2 years
- Vertebral fractures
- Fracture patterns such as corner fractures or bucket handle fractures (metaphyseal), (pulling or twisting injury)
- Lower extremity (tibia, femur) fractures in non-ambulatory children

- Up to 50% of all fractures in infants (aged <1 year) are non-accidental. The most common fracture pattern in abusive injuries is a noncharacteristic long bone diaphyseal fracture. The diagnosis of inflicted injury should always be considered in the care of an injured child.
- Many pediatric fractures can be splinted with prompt follow-up with orthopedics in 1 or 2 days. In some institutes, reduction by emergency medicine physicians with casting is appropriate if immediate orthopedic consultation is not available.

PEDIATRIC UPPER EXTREMITY INJURIES AND FRACTURES

Clavicle Fractures

Introduction

- Clavicle fractures are fairly common in children, and they are the most common birth fracture seen in newborns. Unlike in adults and due to the rapid remodeling present in children, these fractures heal rapidly.

Classical clinical presentation

- A young toddler or school-age child, with fall on outstretch arm, either ground level or from a height

Atypical presentation

- A neonate, typically 1–4 weeks, presenting with a bump over clavicle or decreased movement of one arm. The mother may or may not remember any birth trauma.
- A child may come in days later, either complaining of using arm less after a fall or developing a bump (callus) over clavicle after a fall.

Differential diagnosis

- Shoulder dislocation (rare in younger children; more likely in the adolescent especially an athlete)
- Proximal humerus fracture (again, less common in younger children)
- Bony tumor (benign, malignant)—uncommon in this location

Diagnostic confirmation

- Anteroposterior (AP) view of clavicle; sometimes helpful to get bilateral view because some fractures are subtle

Treatment

- Most clavicle fractures encountered in children need no intervention, even if angulated.
- Simple sling, usually for 1 or 2 weeks, and nonsteroidal anti-inflammatory drugs (NSAIDs) for pain. Figure-of-eight immobilizations are associated with increased pain and may also delay healing.
- Most simple clavicle fractures do not need orthopedic follow-up.
- Advise families that acute fractures will start to heal in 1 or 2 weeks and the appearance of a "bump" (callus) may be noticed at the fracture site.
- Clavicle fractures requiring operative reduction and repair are unusual in children, and they usually involve high-impact sports (the adolescent football player) or high impact such as in motor vehicle accidents (MVAs).
- Tenting of the skin or open clavicle fractures, brachial plexus palsy or suspected underlying vascular injury, or medial sternoclavicular fracture with sternoclavicular dislocation are all indications for orthopedic consultation.
- Acromioclavicular ligament disruption is unusual in young children with lateral clavicular fractures.

Disposition

- The majority of patients with clavicle fractures can be discharged home.

Complications

- Non-union of a clavicle fractures is rare, and follow-up films are not necessary.
- In high-energy injuries, vascular or brachial plexus injury can occur.

Key point

- Clavicle fractures are a not uncommon birth injury in neonates and very common in childhood, most of which are uncomplicated and heal well with little intervention.

Pitfalls

- Not palpating over the clavicle when examining a child for arm injury or for complaints of not moving the arm
- Not getting bilateral views to detect subtle clavicle fractures

Proximal Humeral Fractures

Introduction

- These are fairly uncommon, usually caused by direct blow or fall on proximal arm. They are three or four times more common in boys.
- 80% of humeral growth in children occurs at proximal humeral physis; for that reason, children are able to remodel fractures in this area well, and malunion is unlikely.
- The epiphysis has three areas of ossification: humeral head (present at birth), greater tuberosity (at 3 years), and lesser tuberosity (at 5 years). Proximal humeral physis remains open until age 16–19 years. For this reason, radiographs may be difficult to interpret and may be misread.

Classical presentation

- Acute pain, not moving arm, minimal swelling after direct blow to shoulder/arm

Atypical presentation

- None or trivial injury (consider NAT in a young child)
- Unicameral bone cyst (consider pathologic fracture), neonate not moving arm (birth trauma)

Differential diagnosis

- Contusion, infection, tumor (malignancy)

Diagnostic confirmation

- Plain radiographs AP, lateral. Confirm that shoulder is not dislocated (rare) with axillary or Velpeau view.

Treatment

- Based on age and expected remodeling with growth. Prior to adolescence, most proximal humeral fractures are nonsurgical, sling or hanging arm casts, or coaptation splint for 3 or 4 weeks. No consensus exists for degree of angulation accepted, but the following guidelines are proposed (Pediatric Orthopaedic Society of North America):
  - <10 years old: any degree of angulation
  - 10–12 years old: up to 60–75° of angulation
  - >12 years old: up to 45° of angulation or two-thirds displacement
- Sling and swath, coaptation splint, hanging casts

Disposition

- Patient may be immobilized in the emergency department (ED) with splint and sling.
- Attention to pain control (non-opioid).
- Follow-up with orthopedics within 1 week.

Complications

- Radial nerve palsy (5%)—either primary or secondary due to manipulation of fracture.
- Vascular injury is uncommon.
- Malunion is uncommon.

Key points

- The majority of proximal humeral fractures are non-operative.
- Vascular injury is uncommon.

Pitfalls

- Not assessing for possible NAT (child abuse) in a child younger than age 2 years
- Not recognizing a pathological humeral fracture due to bone cyst or malignancy

Radial Head Subluxation ("Nursemaid's Elbow")

Background

- A common injury seen in toddlers (aged 1–4 years) with little or no trauma history, often but not always associated with a "pulled arm"

- Caused by a slipping of annular ligament into the radiohumeral joint, the radial head being relatively smooth at this age

Classical clinical presentation (50%)

- Child may present to the ED with a history of parent pulling child by arm (e.g., crossing the street or swinging a child by the arms); often parent does not remember the event. Child holds arm at side in partial flexion at elbow; full flexion and supination is painful.
- Elbow *is never swollen* with radial head subluxation (RHS).
- Pain is poorly localized to wrist, arm, or elbow.

Atypical clinical presentation (50%)

- History of fall or injury (usually very minor) or a very young child rolling over in bed and getting arm trapped underneath. Clinically examination is same as that for classic presentation.
- Child may hold wrist and parents may be concerned for wrist injury, but pain is clearly located at elbow when flexion is attempted.

Differential diagnosis

- Septic joint or osteomyelitis—swelling of the elbow, low-grade fever, elbow pain does not subside after attempted reduction
- Supracondylar humeral fracture—usually more significant trauma, with elbow swelling and/or point tenderness at elbow [typically supracondylar humeral fracture (SCH) type I]
- NAT (child abuse)—abnormal bruising or marks, fracture of elbow in a young child especially younger than age 2 year, with no explanation of trauma, such as a fall reported

Diagnostic confirmation

- Most RHS can be reduced without imaging; if imaging is ordered prior to seeing the patient, they may be reduced solely by positioning of the arm during imaging. So, unless there is some atypical feature on examination, such as swelling of elbow or deformity, or presentation in a child aged 5 years or older, imaging prior to attempted reduction is *not* warranted.
- Imagining will be normal in RHS.
- Reduction may be performed by either of two methods: supination/flexion method (more classically taught) or hyperpronation method. Warn parents that with either method of reduction child will often cry for a few minutes.
- The hyperpronation technique performs superiorly to supination/flexion (Number Needed to Treat [NNT] = 5).
  - If one method fails, it may either be repeated or the alternate method may be tried.
  - If a" click" is felt at radial head, this usually indicates success.
  - Usually children are still crying immediately after successful reduction, so explain to family that you will return to re-examine child in 10 minutes. Usually child will be moving arm by that time if reduction is successful.

Hyperpronation technique (Figure 37.1)

- With one hand at elbow, supporting fingers/thumb placed over radial head, with other hand at wrist, hyperpronate approximately 10–20°; click at radial head may be felt.

Supination/flexion technique (Figure 37.2)

- Support elbow with one hand, placing fingers/thumb over radial head, with the other head at distal forearm/wrist, apply gentle traction and fully supinate and flex child's arm in one simultaneous swift motion. Again, a click may be felt under finger at radial head, but it is not necessary for success.

Failed reduction

- If child does not begin to move arm after 10–20 minutes,

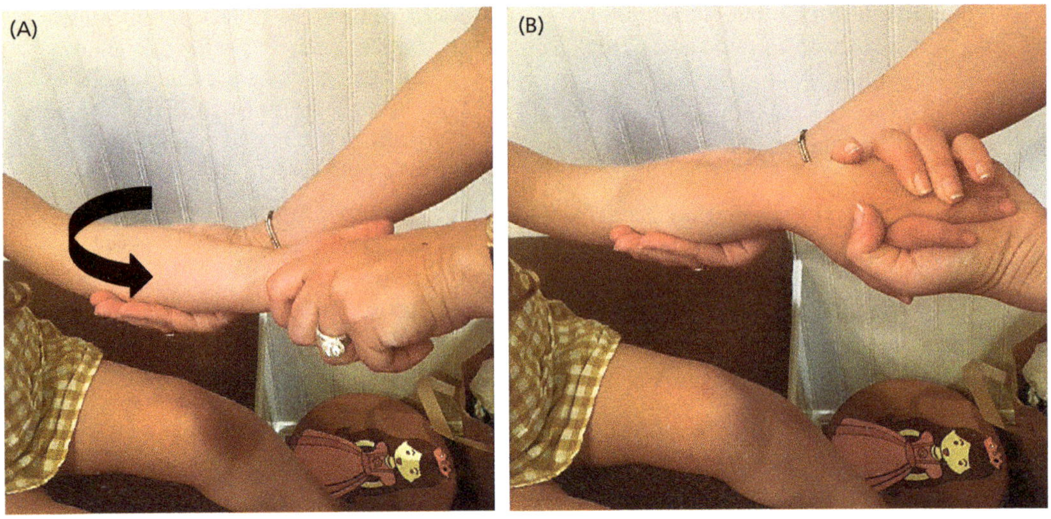

FIGURE 37.1 Radial head subluxation supination–flexion method. The thumb is placed over the radial head (A), and with the other provider's hand on the wrist, the arm is supinated and then immediately flexed (B).

radiographs of elbow, forearm, and wrist are indicated to evaluate to subtle fracture.

- If radiographs are negative for fracture, including no posterior fat pad, which may indicate at subtle type I SCH fracture, then discharging patient with splint and ibuprofen are warranted with close follow-up in 1 or 2 days with primary care physician. In the majority of these cases, the elbow is still "sore" or the child is still reluctant to move, but will begin moving normally again in 1 or 2 days.

Disposition

- The majority of children can be discharged with parental education regarding future prevention of RHS, as a small percentage of these children

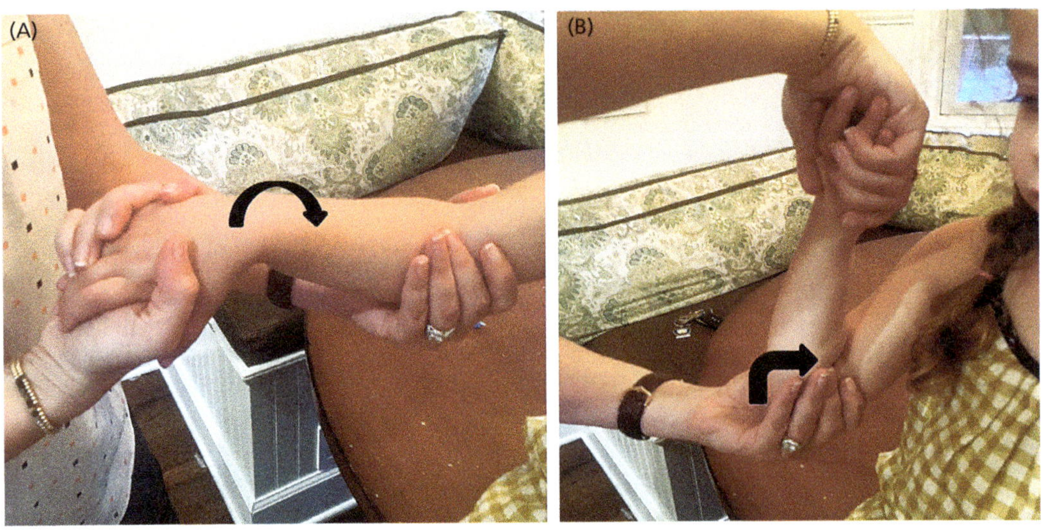

FIGURE 37.2 Radial head subluxation hyperpronation method. From the resting position, the arm is hyperpronated in one movement (A), and having a thumb or fingers over the radial head with the opposite hand allows one to feel the annular ligament slide into place (B).

will have recurrent RHS. NSAIDs as needed for pain, but most children leave the ED pain free.

- For the small number of children who are "failed reductions" and are sent home in splint, close follow-up within 1 or 2 days to ensure that a subtle fracture or possible septic elbow is not the case. Note that a few of these children have elbow soreness after reduction and so may not move the elbow well for 1 day.

Complications

- Complications arise when the initial diagnosis is incorrect.

Key points

- RHS is a relatively focused problem, occurring in toddlers aged 1–4 years classically, but not always with a history of arm being pulled.
- Be careful not to miss a subtle fracture of infection in child not moving arm. (RHS are not swollen!)
- No imaging is needed in advance of reduction of the subluxation.

Pitfall

- Diagnosis of RHS is very unusual in children older than age 4 or 5 years, and other diagnoses should be entertained first.

Elbow Fractures

Pediatric elbow fractures are particularly difficult to interpret, primarily because of several ossification sites that appear about the elbow starting at approximately age 1 or 2 years, until the elbow on radiograph appears as in adult films at age 16 years (Figure 37.3). For that reason, the mnemonic CRITOE (or CRITOL) is often used to remind clinicians, who may be confused by the appearance (childhood) and ultimate fusion (adolescence) of the ossification sites on radiographs. CRITOE stands for capitellum, radial head, *internal* (medial) epicondyle, trochlear, olecranon, *external or l*ateral epicondyle. Table 37.1 provides the ages of appearance and fusion of these ossification sites. Note that all ages are approximate, and females usually ossify/fuse 6–12 months sooner than males.

Because of the six ossification sites, and because certain fractures, such as supracondylar humeral fractures, are seen predominantly in children rather than adults and may have long-term complications related to future bone growth, it is important that clinicians familiarize themselves with these unique types of elbow fractures and potential pitfalls in diagnosis and treatment.

Supracondylar Humeral Fractures

Background

- The most common fracture of the pediatric elbow—90–95% are extension type [falls on outstretch hand (FOOSH)]—full extension of elbow into olecranon fossa, which is relatively thin in children and causes the distal humerus to displace posteriorly.
- Flexion type is uncommon (5–10%), where distal humeral fragment is anteriorly displaced.
- Peak incidence at ages 5–7 years; more common males (?).
- Many SCH fractures need surgical repair and may have associated

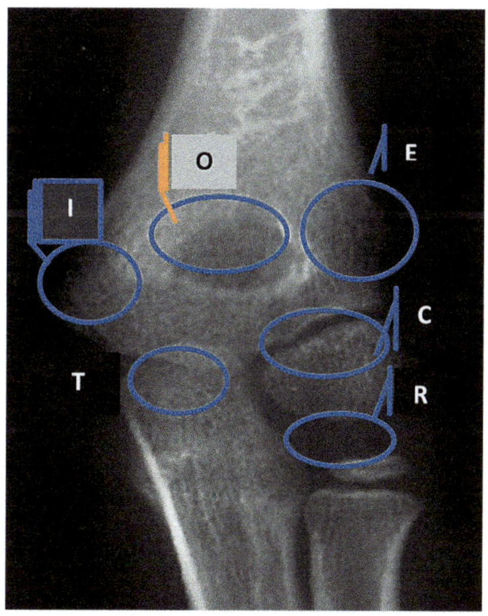

FIGURE 37.3 Radiograph with labeled ossification sites of the pediatric elbow. C-R-I-T-O-E. C = capitellum, R = Radial head, I = Internal (medial) epicondyle, T = Trochlear, O = Olecranon, E = External (lateral) epicondyle.

TABLE 37.1 OSSIFICATION SITES OF THE PEDIATRIC ELBOW (CRITOE)

Ossification Center	Age (Years) Ossification Appears (Radiographically)[a]	Age (Years) of Ossification Site Fusion (Radiographically)[a]
Capitellum	2	12–14
Radius	4	14–16
Internal (medial) epicondyle	6	16–18
Trochlea	8	12–14
Olecranon	10	15–17
External (lateral) Condyle	12	12–14

[a]Plus or minus 1 year (ossification sites and fusion may occur earlier in females than in males).
CRITOE, C = capitellum, R = radial head, I = internal (medial) epicondyle, T = trochlear, O = olecranon, E = external (lateral) epicondyle.
Source: Hahn S, Lee YH, Lee SH, Suh J-S. Easy way out—quick interpretation of musculoskeletal radiographs: The lower extremity. *J Korean Soc Radiol.* 2017;77(5):263–285. https://doi.org/10.3348/jksr.2017.77.5.263 (accessed August 20, 2019).

neurovascular injuries; Gartland classification is important to the decision to surgically treat.

Classic presentation

- For flexion type, full or outstretched arm, in full extension, from ground level or height (monkey bars). Olecranon forcibly extends into the thin olecranon fossae of distal humerus, causing a transverse fracture that may or may not extend to involve medial or lateral condyles.
- Elbow will be swollen (swelling may be more subtle in toddlers), tender, usually unable to fully flex to 90°, and held in some degree of extension (pain on supination and pronation).
- Neurovascular exam is key in this injury—brachial artery impingement, along with median nerve (anterior interosseous branch) with weak "ok" sign. Radial nerve injury (wrist extensor "thumbs up") may also occur.

Atypical clinical presentation

- Flexion type injury (5–10%) with anterior displacement (ulna nerve injury may occur).
- In young children (younger than age 2 years) with supracondylar fracture, potential for NAT should be considered.

Differential diagnosis

- Medial or lateral epicondyle fracture, radial head/neck, or olecranon fracture
- Septic elbow (low-grade fever, no history of significant injury)
- RHS (nursemaid's elbow)—arm held in extension, pain on flexion, but not swollen

Diagnostic confirmation

- AP, true lateral, and possibly oblique views
- Because these are very painful injuries and may require surgery, pain management [intravenously (IV) or PO], immobilization in splint, especially with suspicions of severe fracture, and keep NPO prior to radiographs.
- Anterior humeral line—radiographic line drawn down the anterior margin of the humerus—normally intersects the middle third of the capitellum. If it does not, this is suggestive of a fracture.
- Based on radiographic findings—extension-type supracondylar fractures can be described by Gartland classification system:
  - Type I—non-displaced fracture with evidence of elbow effusion (posterior fat pad sign, Figure 37.4), anterior humeral line transects middle one-third of capitellum. *Note*: Fracture line may not always be obvious on initial films, particularly if inadequate oblique views.
  - Type II—displaced fracture with intact posterior periosteum

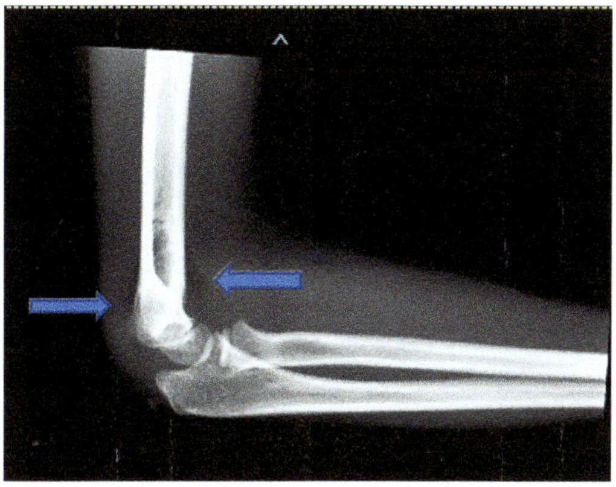

FIGURE 37.4 Pediatric elbow x-ray demonstrating the presence of fat pads (arrows). The thinner arrow on the left is the posterior fat pad and the arrow on the right is the abnormally large anterior (sail) fat pad.

anterior humeral line passing through interior one-third of capitellum or completely anterior to capitellum.

- Type III—displaced distal humerus fracture with disruption of anterior and posterior periosteum—may be displaced posteromedial (ulnar), posterolateral (radial nerve), or anterolateral. *These are at highest risk for neurovascular injury.*

Treatment

- Stabilize suspected supracondylar fracture in position of comfort—*do not attempt to position arm into 90° flexion.*
- Confirm NPO status and administer pain medication (orally, IV, or intranasally).
- Establish complete neurovascular examination—if radial pulse absent, or if hand cold/poorly perfused, confirm presence/absence of pulse with Doppler.
- Children with SCH fracture and absent pulse need emergent pediatric orthopedic consult; they may require partial closed reduction in ED to restore distal circulation if need transport to a facility with pediatric orthopedics.
- Assess for compartment syndrome (rare in SCH fractures, but can occur). Volkmann's contracture is rare but can occur.
- Suspected SCH fractures should be splinted in position of comfort (at the degree of flexion child is holding arm, usually 20–30° of flexion) before sending to radiology.
- Treatment is dictated by Gartland classification:
  - Type I fracture—long posterior splint with elbow at 90° of flexion, forearm neutral position. Consider splinting any swollen elbow with posterior fat pad but no obvious fracture line seen on radiograph.
  - Follow up with orthopedist within 1 week for observation or definitive casting.
  - Type II fracture—orthopedic consultation for operative closed reduction with percutaneous pin fixation.
  - Type III—urgent/emergent orthopedic consultation, careful consideration for neurovascular injury.
  - If concern for diminished perfusion or absent pulse, emergent orthopedic consultation; may require partial closed reduction in ED to restore circulation prior to operating room (OR).
  - Most type III if uncomplicated are closed reduced in OR with percutaneous pinning.

Disposition

- Gartland type I (or occult type I with join effusion but no obvious fracture) may be splinted and referred to orthopedics to be seen within 7 days.
- Gartland types II and III—require closed (rarely open) reduction with percutaneous pinning. If not available in your facility, transfer to a center with pediatric orthopedics. Occasionally, milder type II may be initially casted with close follow-up by orthopedist.

- For splinted or casted type I SCH fractures being discharged from ED, return precautions apply as in all fractures—numbness excessive or pain not controlled with NSAIDs, or pallor/cool distal extremities.

Complications

- Vascular injury, usually involving the brachial artery in up to 20% of SCH fractures, is most commonly seen in type II and III fractures, especially in those in which the proximal fragment is displaced posterolaterally. Pulses not improving after closed reduction and percutaneous pinning may need open vascular exploration; brachial artery may be trapped within the fracture site.

Nerve injury

- Seen in up to 20% in SCH fractures, especially in type III. Most nerve palsies are neuropraxias and therefore will resolve spontaneously; motor function usually recovers by 3 months and sensory changes by 6 months.
- Median nerve (anterior interosseous nerve branch)—in posterolateral distal fragment displacement
- Radial nerve—with posteromedial displacement
- Ulnar nerve—in flexion-type supracondylar fractures, so less common

Key points

- SCH fractures are the most common fractures in the pediatric elbow. If not diagnosed and treated appropriated, they may result in long-term deformity/disability.
- Gartland classification (types I–III) will determine orthopedic management.
- Vascular and nerve injury are potential complications, especially in type III fracture.

Pitfalls

- Misinterpretations of radiographs
- Failure to consult orthopedics urgently for type II and III supracondylar fractures
- Failure to evaluate radius pulse and nerve function distally when evaluating these fractures

Lateral Humeral Condyle Fractures

Background

- Lateral condyle fracture is the second most common fracture in the pediatric elbow, typically occurring in patients older than age 6 years.
- This fracture is at a higher risk of non-union, malunion, and avascular necrosis (AVN) compared with other pediatric elbow fractures.
- Salter–Harris IV fracture patterns of the lateral condyle are the most common.

Classic clinical presentation

- Avulsion fracture of the lateral condyle with the lateral collateral ligament intact, which results from the pull of the extensor muscles, or a fall onto outstretched hand with slight elbow flexion and adduction, which causes impaction of the radial head into the lateral condyle.
- Lateral elbow pain and swelling, which may be subtle if fracture is minimally displaced
- Examination lacks any obvious deformity as seen with supracondylar fractures, and swelling/tenderness is usually limited to the lateral side.
- Fractures originate proximally at the posterior aspect of the distal humerus metaphysis and extend distally and anteriorly across the physis and epiphysis into the elbow joint, or fractures may extend medially into the trochlear groove, making the elbow unstable and prone to posteromedial elbow dislocation.

Differential diagnosis

- Supracondylar fracture

Diagnostic confirmation

- AP, lateral, and oblique views of elbow—classification of the fracture depends on the amount of displacement of the lateral condyle (<2, 2–4, or >4 mm) and the integrity of the articular surface.

- Internal oblique views most valuable in demonstrating amount of fracture displacement because fracture is posterolateral.
- Optional views—contralateral elbow may be needed for comparison when ossification is not yet complete.
- Advanced imaging [computed tomography (CT), magnetic resonance imaging (MRI), and arthrogram] rarely needed in emergent setting.

Treatment

- Urgent consultation with a pediatric orthopedist is needed. If a pediatric orthopedist is not available in your institution, the patient should be splinted and transferred.
- Treatment is determined by the degree of articular displacement and may be operative or non-operative.
- Non-operative—long arm casting for 4–6 weeks indicated only if <2 mm displacements in all view with weekly follow-up with orthopedist to ensure healing.
- Operative—closed reduction percutaneous pins (CRPP) + 3–6 weeks in above elbow cast for fractures with 2–4 mm of displacement and have intact articular cartilage; open reduction (to align joint surface) and fixation + 3–6 weeks in above elbow cast if > 4 mm of displacement.
- Attention to pain control in ED (NSAIDs, opioids) and NPO status since operative repair may be indicated

Disposition

- Because these fractures require expert consultation with a pediatric orthopedist to determine treatment (operative vs. non-operative), these patients should receive urgent orthopedic consultation or transfer to a center that is able to provide this consultation.

Complications

- Delayed union—fracture may not heal with 6 weeks of immobilization, especially if fracture was not recognized and immobilized soon after initial injury.
- Non-union—lateral condyle fractures have higher rate of non-union compared with other elbow fractures. Nonsurgical management initially may be a contributor to this.
- Lateral condyle physeal arrest especially in severely deformed fracture, resulting in varus or valgus deformity
- Lateral overgrowth/prominence (spurring)—incidence up to 50% regardless of treatment; higher incidence in more severe fractures
- Ulna nerve palsy—due to stretching of nerve as fracture heals
- AVN—a late complication, occurs 1–3 years after fracture

Key point

- Due to a number of significant complications that can occur with these fractures, all lateral condyle fractures (suspected or confirmed) require urgent orthopedic consultation.

Pitfalls

- Failure to recognize this potential injury given the mechanism, and not obtain films, or misinterpret radiographs
- Failure to obtain orthopedic consultation

Medial Humeral Condyle Fracture

Background

- Accounting for up to 20% of all pediatric and adolescent elbow fractures; 75% are seen in boys aged 9–14 years, especially those involved in athletics
- Treatment controversial but usually non-operative

- May be associated elbow dislocation in 50–60% of cases, which may spontaneously reduce

Classic clinical presentation

- Excessive valgus stress with contraction causes medial epicondyle to avulse anteriorly.
- Pain over medial epicondyle after a fall or other injury with valgus stress; may not have impressive swelling.
- With more generalized swelling, this may indicate that elbow may have dislocated.

Differential diagnosis

- Chronic pain related to stress injuries, such as Little League elbow
- Elbow dislocation
- Supracondylar humeral fracture

Diagnostic confirmation

- AP and lateral radiographs of elbow; internal oblique view to evaluate displacement; distal humeral axial view may also be helpful to see displacement

Treatment

- After obtaining radiographs and controlling pain, ensuring NPO status, urgent orthopedic consultation is advised because treatment may be operative or non-operative.
- Non-operative long arm casting is indicated if <5 mm displacement; however, the amount of true displacement is difficult to determine and could result in non-union.
- Operative with open reduction internal fixation (ORIF) if fracture is displaced with entrapment of medial condyle fragment in joint space, or if involving articular surface, or with open fractures; operative management may also be considered if >2- to 5-mm displacement (controversial), >2 to 5 mm in valgus stress in athletes, or associated elbow dislocation or ulnar nerve dysfunction.

Disposition

- Discharge with outpatient orthopedic follow-up or admission/transfer depends on the decision for operative versus non-operative treatment.

Complications

- Non-union is the major complication long term; there are lower odds of non-union with operative management.
- Nerve injury—ulnar nerve injury reportedly 10%
- Missed incarceration of medial condyle fragment into elbow joint

Key points

- Medial condyle elbow fractures are not uncommon, seen in up to 20% of all pediatric and adolescent elbow fractures.
- Treatment is controversial but is usually non-operative unless the medial epicondyle is incarcerated in the joint or significantly displaced.

Pitfall

- Failure to recognize this injury and fracture and obtain orthopedic consultation when needed

Midshaft Forearm (Radius/Ulna) Fractures

Background

- These common pediatric fracture are also the most common of pediatric open fractures and the most common to be refractured in children.
- Unlike in adults, some degree of angulation may be acceptable, and many are close reduced.
- Galeazzi and Monteggia are seen less frequently in children (3% are Galeazzi); peak incidence occurs at ages 9–13 years in females and ages 4–10 years in males.

Classical clinical presentation

- In most incidences, FOOSH may be associated with multiple trauma if fall from a significant height.

- Tenderness over mid shaft, swelling and obvious deformity of arm if angulated; look for any puncture wounds (indicating open fracture). Limited range of motion (ROM).

Atypical clinical presentation

- History of a direct blow to the forearm
- Concern for NAT, particularly if the fracture is seen in children younger than age 2 years

Differential diagnosis

- Osteomyelitis (no immediate history of trauma is obtained)
- Bony mass or tumor (unusual in forearm)

Diagnostic confirmation

- AP and lateral radiographs are sufficient to identify this fracture.
- Elbow views may be needed if concern for dislocation.
- On radiograph, fracture may be described/classified as greenstick complex, comminuted, or plastic deformity ("bowing," usually of ulna with fracture of radius), and degree if angulation in lateral and AP view should be measured.
- If ulna bowing is suspected, may need comparison views of unaffected arm.

Treatment

- Attention to pain (NSAIDs); consider fentanyl intranasally (IN)/IV or morphine IV if severe fracture suspected.
- Temporary immobilization with sling or splint until radiographs can be done.
- Inspect forearm for any open wounds, especially associated with deformity of arm, and assess neurovascular status (median, radial, ulna nerve; radial pulse).
- Inspect elbow because 5% of pediatric forearm fractures are associated with supracondylar humeral fractures.
- Absent or weak pulse—although uncommon, some children may need emergent partial closed reduction to restore distal circulation, if orthopedic care is not readily available.
- Complete and greenstick fractures—because of the greater remodeling potential in children, a certain degree of angulation and malrotation is acceptable, so these children may be splinted and have outpatient orthopedic follow-up.
    - For children aged 0–10 years: <15% angulation, <45° malrotation
    - For children aged >10 years: <10% angulation, <30° malrotation
- Radius/ulna fracture with bayonet apposition
    - For children aged ≥10 years, no degree of bayoneting is acceptable.
    - For children aged ≤10 years, some small degree of bayoneting is acceptable (<1 cm shortening).
    - Plastic deformation: <20° is usually acceptable and will remodel; >20° needs closed reduction and casting.
- Special cases—Galeazzi and Monteggia fractures need orthopedic consult.

Disposition

- Most children who have undergone closed reduction and casting may be discharged from the ED; if splinted because angulation is within acceptable range, they can be similarly discharged. All should have close orthopedic follow-up within 5–7 days.
- Patients with open fractures or those needing operative repair should be admitted with urgent pediatric orthopedic consult or transferred if pediatric orthopedic care is not available at the institution.
- Pain control at home is with NSAIDs; rarely do children require opioid medications unless difficult reduction or multiple attempts at reduction.
- Discharge care with attention to the potential for compartment syndrome—usually not from the injury itself, but may be the result of a difficult reduction.

Complications

- Compartment syndrome—at-risk fractures include those due to high-energy trauma, or multiple attempts at closed reduction
- Malunion
- Refracture rate is 5–10%, especially in greenstick
- Loss of supination/pronation—a potential complication with ulna bowing fractures
- Galeazzi—ulnar physeal arrest, ulna nerve injury, radial nerve palsy, mal/nonunion of radius (due to ulnar subluxation)
- Monteggia—commonly due to missed radial head dislocation on radiographs during original injury; posterior interosseous nerve and ulnar nerve neuropraxia

Key points

- Midshaft radius/ulna fractures are common pediatric fractures, usually from FOOSH.
- Some may be splinted and obtain orthopedic consult outpatient, depending on the degree of angulation and malrotation. Many of those requiring urgent orthopedic consult can be treated with closed reduction and casting because children's bones have excellent remodeling potential.
- Galeazzi and Monteggia patterns are less common in children, and recognizing ulna bowing with radial fractures is important because it may affect future function.

Pitfalls

- Failure to recognize ulna bowing with isolated radius fracture, or Galeazzi/Monteggia fractures
- Failure to recognize an open fracture
- Failure to provide adequate pain control, or sedation for closed reductions

Distal Radial Fractures

Background

- Distal radius fractures are very common in childhood, accounting for up to 35% of pediatric fractures.
- Most of these fractures involve the metaphysis or physis of radius.
- Because of the robust remodeling that occurs to children's bones, many of these injuries can be treated non-operatively, with very select exceptions.

Classical clinical presentation

- Most distal radius fractures are obvious on presentation.
- Usually the mechanism is a FOOSH, usually from the child's height.
- Swelling, sometimes deformity and significant pain, limited ROM, especially to supination/pronation and flexion.
- Associated injuries (other fractures to same arm) are not seen unless more significant trauma is involved.

Atypical presentation

- Direct blow to the arm
- Any child younger than age 2 years with radius/ulna fracture (careful history to rule out NAT or bone disease such as osteogenesis imperfecta)
- Insignificant fall with later presentation (torus or buckle fracture)

Differential diagnosis

- Wrist sprain (unusual in children and not associated with swelling)

Diagnostic confirmation

- All suspected distal radius/ulna fractures should have true AP and lateral radiographs. Consider complete forearm and elbow views, especially if isolated ulnar fracture (look for radial head dislocation—Monteggia fracture).
- Advanced imaging is not necessary.
- The degree of angulation should be measured on radiographs because this will determine treatment.

Treatment

- Initial evaluation and treatment should include inspection for any open wounds (open fracture), especially if significant deformity, and assessment of radial, ulna, and median nerves (the most commonly injured), although neurovascular injuries are uncommon with these fractures.

- Attention to pain control, based on initial degree of injury suspected, NSAIDs orally, or fentanyl intranasal; fentanyl or morphine IV.
- In general, the majority of angulated metaphyseal radius/ulna fractures can be treated with splinting with or without closed reduction by ED physician or orthopedist if available.
- The degree of angulation tolerated and not requiring reduction in the ED, splinting:
  - For children aged <10 years: <15–20° of angulation on lateral view, 10–15° on AP view
  - For children aged >10 years: <15° of angulation on lateral view, 0° of angulation on AP view
- Closed reduction with conscious sedation with or without hematoma block is recommended for the following:
  - For children aged <10 years: >20° angulation on view, 10° angulation on view
  - For children aged >10 years: >15° angulation on lateral, >0° angulation on AP
  - After closed fracture reduction, remains casted for 4–6 weeks, although many will have a subsequent loss of reduction, so close orthopedic follow-up within 1 or 2 weeks is advised.
  - A small number of these fractures that are initially closed reduced and casted may ultimately need surgical management with percutaneous pins if the reduction is unstable.
  - Ulnar styloid fracture can occur in conjunction with distal radial fracture, and its treatment is determined by care of radial fracture *except* if ulnar styloid is fractured at base and is displaced (disruption of triangular fibrocartilage complex)—this may need surgical care.
  - Galeazzi fracture—although uncommon in children, may require surgical fixation of distal radioulnar joint, or alternatively closed reduction/casted by an orthopedist.
- Non-displaced metaphyseal (torus or buckle distal radius fractures)
  - Can be splinted with re-evaluation by an orthopedist in 5–7 days
- Physeal fracture of radius
  - Salter–Harris II fracture, non-displaced—volar splint and outpatient orthopedic follow-up
  - Salter–Harris II fracture, displaced—splint and follow-up within 1 week
  - Salter–Harris III and IV distal radius fractures—urgent orthopedic consultation because they may involve the joint (III, IV) and usually need operative repair
  - Salter–Harris V fracture (crush of growth plate)—difficult to detect on X-rays (but may be suspected based on history and physical examination); if suspected, prompt orthopedic follow-up is recommended (high risk of growth arrest)

Disposition

- Most patients with distal radius fractures involving metaphysis, either splinted without reduction or reduced and/casted, may be discharged home with elevation and pain control instructions (NSAIDs are usually sufficient).
- Metaphyseal fractures with significant angulation (>20° if <10 years old, >15° if >10 years old) that have been close reduced may have significant swelling and pain, so elevation, return precautions for swelling, compartment syndrome instructions, and prompt orthopedic follow-up within 7 days are needed.

- Operative fractures need hospital admission.
- Limited activity for up to 12 weeks to allow healing.

Complications

- The most common complication is loss of reduction (if reduced) and malunion, although remodeling occurs over 2 years.
- Long-term neurological issues are rare; short-term neuropraxias (especially median nerve) can occur.
- Displaced physeal fractures may lead to growth arrest (5%).
- Refracture of a distal radius fracture if not fully healed can occur.

Key points

- Because children have a robust ability to remodel, distal radial fractures in general are treated with casting or closed reduction and casting, with angulation in AP view up to 15–20° being acceptable for healing.
- Appropriate sedation and pain control for closed reduction and casting are necessary.
- Most distal radial fractures heal well with few complications.

LOWER EXTREMITY INJURIES AND FRACTURES

Pelvis

Introduction

- Most pelvis fractures are caused by high-energy accidents, as in adults, so suspicion for these injuries should accompany any workup for abdominal or lower extremity trauma.
- In children, because of the high proportion of cartilage, the pelvis is more deformable than in adults, so a higher energy is needed to produce pelvic fractures.
- The majority of pelvic fractures in children are to the pubic rami (53%) and iliac wing (29%). Acetabular fractures and hip dislocation are rarer in children. Unstable pelvis ring fractures are also uncommon (5%).
- The presence of a pelvic fracture in a child with no physical findings to the pelvis on examination and negative AP pelvis radiograph is <1%.
- Radiographic diagnosis and management in general are similar to those for adults.
- Most pelvic fractures in children require conservative treatment with bed rest, unless there is a displacement, unstable, or open fracture. Growth arrest is uncommon in pediatric pelvic fractures.
- Unique to pediatrics and associated with low-energy injuries are avulsion fractures of the pelvis.

Avulsion Fractures of the Pelvis

Background

- A unique fracture seen exclusively in adolescents, usually aged 13–15 year, it is an avulsion of one of the secondary ossification centers (apophyses), from the associated muscle group insertion, almost exclusively during athletic activities. See Figure 37.5.
- Knowledge of this type of fracture may eliminate extensive workups for the source of pain.

Classical clinical presentation

- Forced contraction against resistance of a particular muscle/tendon group while jumping, kicking, running, or sudden change in direction such as in soccer, football, track, or gymnastics.
- Most commonly involved
  - Anterior inferior iliac spine (AIIS) (rectus femoris)
  - Anterior superior iliac spine (ASIS) (sartorius)
  - Ischial tuberosity (hamstrings)
- Less commonly involved
  - Public symphysis (rectus abdominis)
  - Iliac crest (tensor fascia lata)
  - Pubic ramus (abductor muscle)

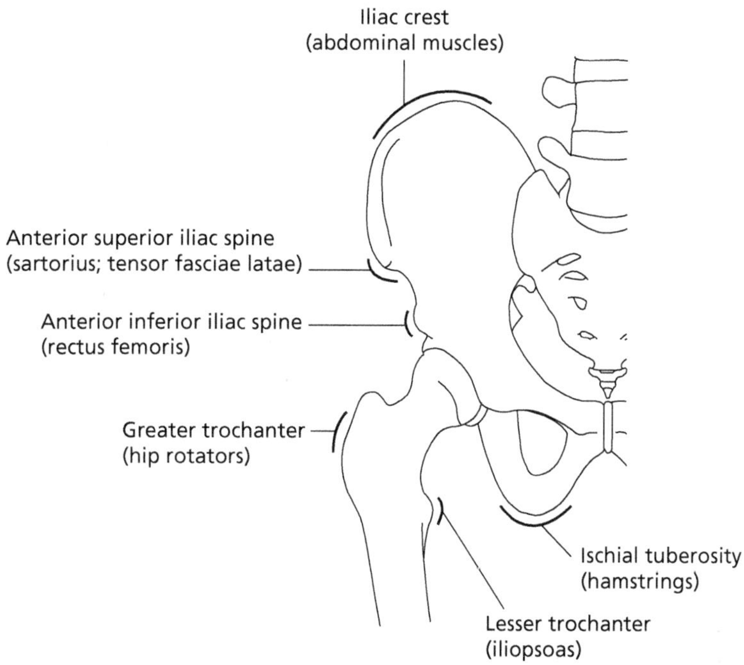

FIGURE 37.5 Muscle insertion locations in the pelvis prone to avulsion injuries.

- Patients report sudden "pop" or pain, localized, during sports activity.
- Pain is localized to one of the areas as noted previously—AIIS, ASIS, ischial tuberosity, etc.

Atypical presentation

- Pain noticed after strenuous activity as noted previously

Differential diagnosis

- Muscle strain/pull
- Apophysitis—more chronic, subacute
- Pathological fracture

Diagnostic confirmation

- AP pelvis for most suspected avulsion fractures; frog-leg hip view if AIIS avulsion is suspected.
- Radiographs for public symphysis avulsion fractures may be negative.
- If initial radiographs are negative, MRI is recommended if clinically suspected, but not emergently needed.

Treatment

- For most avulsion fractures, rest and non-weight-bearing, NSAIDs, and ice for 1 week, followed by physical therapy and partial weight-bearing. Return to full exercise and sports in 6-8 weeks.
- Most may follow up with orthopedics as outpatients to help with recovery and return to sports.
- Occasionally, for significantly displaced avulsion fractures, operative repair may be considered so orthopedic follow-up is more in such cases important.

Disposition

- All patients can be discharged home with rest, non-weight-bearing, NSAIDs, and outpatient orthopedic follow-up.
- Rarely, usually in the case of severely displaced fractures with considerable pain, is urgent orthopedic evaluation for operative repair needed.

Key points

- Avulsion fractures of the pelvis (ASIS, AIIS, pubic symphysis, ischial tuberosity their associated muscle groups) are very specific fractures seen in adolescent athletes, whose secondary ossification centers are not yet closed.

- Most are diagnosed with plain radiographs, and initial treatment is rest, non-weight-bearing, and NSAIDs.

Pitfalls

- Missing key historical points leading to suspicion of pelvic avulsion fracture and not ordering appropriate imaging
- Sending a patient with suspected pelvis avulsion fracture home to return to full athletic activity, thus aggravating the injury and possible prolonging recovery

Femur

Slipped Capital Femoral Epiphysis

Background

- A potentially devastating orthopedic issue of young adolescents, it is a common cause of hip pain not associated or minimally associated with injury.
- Prompt diagnosis, imagining, and orthopedic evaluation are essential.
- A misnomer, slipped capital femoral epiphysis (SCFE) is a proximal femoral metaphysis displacement anterolaterally in relation to the epiphysis in children, primarily young adolescents, with open physis.
- Males aged 9–16 years and females aged 8–15 years are at highest risk (60% in males); ethnicity (African American), and obesity also at increased risk.
- Traditionally classified as acute (sudden onset of symptoms for <3 weeks) or acute on chronic (pain for > 3 weeks with sudden exacerbation or injury), or chronic (symptoms for > 3 weeks).
- Approximately 5–15% are classified as "unstable SCFE." In patients with unstable SCFE, the epiphysis displaces acutely, and patients are unable to bear weight and will present for emergent care with extreme pain; these children have a higher incidence of complications.

Classical presentation

- A pre- or young adolescent, often obese, with complaints of hip, thigh, or knee pain (often families think that the knee is the problem) or limp, for days, weeks, could become acutely worse.
- Examination reveals groin pain with limited internal rotation of hip, and usually an antalgic gait.
- "Obligate external rotation"—affected leg as flexed at knee points out.

Atypical presentation

- Younger age
- Endocrine disorders—hypothyroidism, especially in younger children with SCFE (may be first presentation of hypothyroidism), growth hormone deficiency, and pituitary disease

Differential diagnosis

- Because of the chronicity of most cases, it is rarely confused with other orthopedic problems, but it is often ignored or minimized early on when a child presents with a limp (Table 37.2).
- Legg–Calve–Perthes (LCP) disease
  - Children are usually younger (5–9 years), often male and thin, and limp is less painful.
- Septic hip
  - Less likely again because of the chronicity at presentation; should be considered in any acute presentation.
- Bony tumor
  - Osteosarcoma peak age of 14 years
  - Ewing's sarcoma peak age of 12 years, so both should be considered when evaluating child with limp
  - Non-ossifying fibroma, benign bony tumors, such as aneurysmal bone cyst, unicameral bone cyst or exostosis

TABLE 37.2 ACUTE AGE-RELATED CAUSES OF LIMP

Toddlers (Age <3 Years)	Children (Ages 3–13 Years)	Adolescents (Ages 12–18 Years)
Toddler's fracture	Legg–Calve–Perthes disease (hip)	SCFE (may occur in rare cases as early as 8 years)
Other fracture (non-accident trauma to be considered)	Osgood–Schlatter disease	Osgood–Schlatter disease
Septic arthritis (usually hip)	Osteochondrosis (other-knee, calcaneal)	Overuse syndromes
Transient synovitis	Transient synovitis (less common in this age group)	Malignant tumors (osteosarcoma, Ewing's sarcoma)
Reactive arthritis	Reactive arthritis	Benign bony tumors
Osteomyelitis	Osteomyelitis	Myositis (viral, rheumatologic)
Malignancy-related bone pain (ALL, neuroblastoma)	JIA	JIA
Foreign body (knee, foot)	Myositis (viral) Benign bony tumor ALL (leukemia)	ALL (leukemia)

ALL, acute lymphoblastic leukemia; JIA, juvenile idiopathic arthritis; SCFE, slipped capital femoral epiphysis.

Diagnostic confirmation

- AP, lateral radiographs of both hips, as well as frog-leg views (except in potential unstable slips). See Figure 37.6.
- Subtle widening or irregularity of physis on symptomatic side may be an indication of "pre-slip" or early slip and warrants further investigation (MRI).

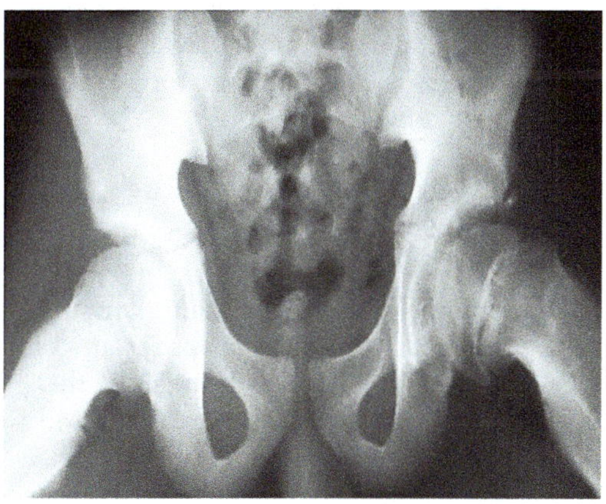

FIGURE 37.6 Left slipped capital femoral epiphysis. This image is a hip radiograph demonstrating a "slipped" femoral head on the left hip. A line drawn along the femoral head (Klein's line) does not intersect with the femoral head.

- Lateral radiographs are generally more sensitive than the AP images, particularly in the earliest phases of slipping.
- Because 33% of SCFEs are bilateral, both hips should be viewed.
- "Klein's line"—a line drawn along the superior border of the femoral neck should in a normal hip transect at least part of the femoral epiphysis. This measurement is classically used, although it will miss subtle slips.
- Modified Klein's line—the amount of the epiphysis that is lateral to the Klein line is compared between the two hips on the AP image, with a 2-mm side-to-side difference highly suspicious of SCFE.
- Southwick slip angle—measured on frog-leg view, it is a line drawn perpendicular to connect two points at anterior and posterior tips of epiphysis, with a third line down axis of femur; angle is between perpendicular line and line down shaft of femur. Used to classify degree of slip.

- Radiological classification of SCFE
  - Grade I: displacement of epiphysis <30% the width of femoral neck
  - Grade II: displacement of epiphysis 30–60% the width of femoral neck
  - Grade III: displacement >60% the width of femoral neck
- MRI is indicated if pre-slip suspected (strong history of symptoms) or to evaluate opposite side of SCFE patient to look for pre-slip.

Treatment

- Child should be made non-weight-bearing (given crutches or bed rest recommended, depending on severity of slip).
- Orthopedic consultation and urgent surgery are recommended depending on the center; some are admitted for surgery (concern that child may continue to weight-bear and potentially worsen slip) versus discharged home with absolute non-weight-bearing (crutches or wheelchair) with urgent follow-up appointment orthopedic.
- Treatment is surgical—most often this involves percutaneous single screw fixation (fluoroscopy-guided) through the center of the epiphysis; for unstable SCFEs, expert pediatric orthopedic decision is advised.
- Prophylactic fixation of uninvolved hip is controversial; one-third of patients develop SCFE on unaffected, usually within 18 months from first diagnosis.
- Many children with endocrine disorders and unilateral SCFE will develop bilateral disease, so prophylactic pinning should be considered in this group.

Disposition

- If child is not admitted to surgery, ensuring the ability for follow-up with an orthopedist is critical. Also critical is the family's understanding of the importance of timely surgery, non-weight-bearing, and return to the ED if there is a sudden worsening of pain.

Complications

- SCFE, even with timely diagnosis, may develop avascular necrosis. Although uncommon after repair of stable slips, in unstable SCFEs the incidence can be as high as 50%.
- Chondrolysis is less common (2%), and further slippage despite fixation can occur, although this is also uncommon.
- Femoral–acetabular impingement (bone spurs).

Key points

- SCFE should be suspected in any pre-adolescent/adolescent with any of the following—limps, knee or thigh pain, or hip/groin pain, regardless of length of time of these symptoms or absence of injury.
- Obesity (>95 percentile of weight for age) is a key risk factor.
- Timely diagnosis, imaging, and orthopedic evaluation are essential.

Pitfalls

- Missing an SCFE on radiographs or being reassured that there is not a subtle SCFE (pre-slip) that may need further imaging (MRI)
- Sending family home to arrange orthopedic follow-up and allowing child to weight-bear until further orthopedic evaluation

Legg–Calve–Perthes or Perthes Disease

Introduction

- Originally described more than 100 years ago, LCP disease is an idiopathic avascular necrosis of the femoral epiphysis, most common in the 5- to 9-year-old age group. To date, no one theory has explained its etiology.

Classical presentation

- More common in males than in females (4:1) and unlike SCFE, LCP disease is not associated with obesity.

Children present with limp and intermittent pain of either hip or knee, usually chronic (weeks/months).

- On examination, children usually have mild painful limp and decreases ROM of hip compared to the opposite side, especially internal rotation.

Atypical presentation

- Children as young as 18 months or as old as 18 years
- Painless or very painful limp, depending on stage of disease

Differential diagnosis

- Avascular necrosis of hip due to hemoglobinopathies, such as sickle cell (usually seen in slightly older children) or chronic steroid therapy
- Limp due to bony tumor (benign or malignant)
- Hypothyroidism
- Transient synovitis (early disease)

Diagnostic confirmation

- In the ED, AP and lateral pelvis radiographs.
- Early LCP disease will show increased density of the femoral head on radiograph.
- Severity of femoral head collapse is classified as group A (mildest) through group C (most severe).

Treatment

- No emergent orthopedic consult is needed. Follow-up is as outpatient with orthopedics.
- Immediate treatment is supportive care—NSAIDs for pain, limited physical activity, and physical therapy referral.
- Age of onset is the most important factor in prognosis.
- 50% of patients may develop degenerative arthritis in late adulthood.
- Younger children (younger than age 6 years) rarely need treatment. Older children (older than 8 years) with more severe disease may need surgery.

Disposition

- See treatment. If other more serious orthopedic issues have been ruled out (septic arthritis, malignancy), then children with LCP disease can be safely discharged home with outpatient orthopedic follow-up.

Key points

- LCP disease presents as mild limp with occasional pain, mostly in children aged 5–9 years, especially boys.
- No emergent orthopedic assessment is needed, but timely outpatient follow-up with orthopedics must be ensured.

Pitfall

- Not considering pelvic films in a child with a mild limp

Femur Fractures

Background

- Because of the relative strength of pediatric femurs, femoral head, neck, and distal femur fractures are uncommon and usually the result of high-energy forces, such as from MVAs or falls from a significant height.
- Most pediatric femur fractures are diaphyseal (shaft), and most heal and remodel rapidly, due in part to a rich blood supply.
- Treatment is age-dependent.

Classical presentation

- History and mechanism of injury are age-dependent.
  - Falls in infants and toddlers, rotary force (spiral fractures)
  - Special attention to young children, especially those younger than age 1 year, who are not ambulating, or who have a poor history, as NAT is of high concern
  - For older children and adolescents, falls, especially from heights, sports-related, or MVA auto vs. pedestrians
  - Younger children may present with just crying and not moving leg, with or without thigh swelling and localized tenderness.

- Older children/adolescents with high-energy injuries have thigh swelling and localized pain and may have associated other injuries or fractures as well.

Atypical presentation

- Fussy, crying infant (concern for NAT)
- Children with underlying conditions leading to osteopenia (cerebral palsy, spina bifida, osteogenesis imperfecta) may sustain femoral fractures with minimal movement or minor injury.

Differential diagnosis

- Bony tumor, benign (unicameral cyst) or malignant (osteosarcoma, Ewing's sarcoma), especially in older children/ adolescents
- Infection—osteomyelitis, pyomyositis, necrotizing fasciitis
- Pathology related to joint above or below femur (hip, knee)

Diagnostic confirmation

- AP and lateral radiographs of entire femur, including hip and knee joint
- Advanced imaging not necessary

Treatment

- For most femur fractures, pain control and stabilization are initial priorities.
- For the otherwise hemodynamically and neurologically stable child, IV/ IN opioids (fentanyl, morphine) or NSAIDs for milder pain.
- Splinting (avoid traction splints).
- Inpatient traction is generally less used in pediatrics.
- If concern for NAT (consider in children younger than age 2 years and especially those younger than age 1 year)—obtain skeletal survey and consult Child Protective Services. Consider transferring to a pediatric academic center with pediatric child abuse specialist/team.
- Urgent orthopedic consultation in ED. Definitive care from orthopedics depends on age, mechanism, and severity of fracture.
  - For infants, Pavlik harness may be used.
  - Older infants and toddlers—hip spica cast (this may be done in the OR).
  - School-age children, early adolescent—closed reduction and flexible intramedullary rod fixation.
  - Adolescents (closed physes)—treated as adults: rigid intramedullary nails.
  - External fixation is not commonly used, especially in children younger than age 12 years; usually used with comminuted fractures.

Disposition

- If candidate for hip spica cast, these are usually placed in OR. Similarly, any operative femur fracture requires admission.
- Dependent on Child Protective Services evaluation, a child younger than age 2 years with a fracture suspicious for NAT may be placed on hospital hold.
- Infants placed in Pavlik harness may be discharged home if pain is well controlled and there are no concerns for NAT.

Complications

- Immediate—neurovascular injury associated with fracture
- Postoperative—handware infection
- Long term—leg length discrepancy, which is usually minimal and may resolve later in growth; similarly, malunion or non-union are uncommon

Key points

- Diaphyseal femur fractures are the most common seen in children and heal rapidly, with few complications.
- Splinting, pain control, and orthopedic evaluation in the ED are priorities.
- Treatment of diaphyseal femur fractures is age-dependent.

Pitfalls

- Not evaluating for NAT in young children with femoral fractures
- Leaving a child in emergency medical services-placed traction device

- Not examining for any concomitant injuries and assessing neurovascular status

Injuries to the Pediatric Knee—Overview

- Acute traumatic knee pain in children, like adults, is usually ligamentous injury, with distal femur and proximal tibial injuries being less likely.
- Anterior cruciate ligament injuries in pediatrics have increased in frequency and severity.
- Ottawa knee rules (OKR) have been validated in children. In one study, OKR were 100% sensitive, with 43% specificity.
- More subacute, nontraumatic knee pain, especially in the presence of low-grade fever, should bring to consideration the possibility of septic arthritis, osteomyelitis, infectious patella bursitis, rheumatologic disease, or Lyme disease (in the appropriate geographic setting).
- See the section titled Overuse Injuries for a full discussion of subacute or acute-on-chronic knee pain, such as Osgood–Schlatter disease.
- Other causes of anterior knee pain, nonemergent, include synovial plicae of the knee, osteochondritis dissecans, and patellofemoral syndrome.

Patella Fractures (Sleeve Fractures)

Background

- Patella fractures in general are uncommon in children; patella sleeve fractures are uncommon as well but seen more in the pediatric population (1% of all children's fractures).
- Bipartite patella, seen in 20% of children, is a developmental variant that may be mistaken for patella fracture and is bilateral in 50% of children.

Classic presentation

- Usually seen in children aged 8–12 years, more commonly inferior (superior rare).
- Unlike typical patella fractures, this is an indirect injury caused by powerful contraction of the quadriceps muscle while the knee is flexed, usually the inferior pole.
- Knee has soft tissue swelling and is diffusely tender; there may be hemarthrosis, high-riding patella, and difficulty with extension of the knee.
- Because the patella is not fully ossified at this age, the cartilage separates and a "sleeve" is avulsed from the main part of the patella and ossified nucleus.

Differential diagnosis

- Sinding-Larsen-Johansson syndrome (for inferior pole injuries; *see Overuse Syndromes*)
- Bipartite patella

Diagnostic confirmation

- Lateral knee radiographs will show a small bony fragment that is separated from the inferior patellar pole. Significant patella baja or alta should raise suspicion of this fracture.
- Consider MRI or ultrasound (US) if diagnosis suspected but not clear on radiographs.

Treatment

- Non-operative—cast for 4–6 weeks in non-displaced fractures with intact extensor mechanism; however, most require ORIF
- Operative—open reduction and internal fixation: indications are >2- or 3-mm displacement or >2- or 3-mm articular step-off or disrupted extensor mechanism

Disposition

- Because the majority of these fractures require operative treatment, orthopedic consultation and possible admission for operative repair

Complications

- Malunion, non-union, difficulty with extension

Key point

- Patella sleeve fractures should be suspected in children without fully ossified patellae (ages 8–12 years) who have significant knee swelling and a radiograph suspicious for inferior pole avulsion. Most require operative repair.

Tibial Toddler's Fracture

Background

- As the name implies, this is a subtle, easily missed fracture primarily seen in toddlers; it is usually seen after a low-energy fall and is non-displaced.

Classical presentation

- Child/parent will have reported injury, usually rotational injury on a fixed foot. Whereas in older children this injury to the tibia may be sports-related, in toddlers it is usually due to a very minor fall.
- Child has pain localized to tibial shaft, usually without swelling or deformation, and refusal to bear weight or limping.

Atypical presentation

- Limping or refusal to bear weight with no reported injury, may present late (days later) due to milder symptoms.
- Findings on examination may be difficult to elicit.

Differential diagnoses

- NAT—tibial fracture seen in non-ambulating children (younger than age 1 year) or in the presence of multiple fractures with no high-energy incidence
- Osteomyelitis

Diagnostic confirmation

- AP on lateral radiograph; add oblique view if suspected fracture but not seen on AP/lateral.
- These fractures appear on radiographs as thin, hairline fractures, non-displaced, and can be missed even by radiologists or mistaken for a nutrient vessel.
- Older toddler's fractures (7–10 days after injury) may display callus or periosteal elevation as part of healing.

Treatment

- Splinting of toddler's fracture and making patient non-weight-bearing is appropriate ED management.
- Orthopedics follow-up is needed; follow-up can be arranged within 1 week.
- Most toddlers' fractures heal completely without complication.

Disposition

- All toddlers' fractures can be discharged home.
- The exception would be if the diagnosis or mechanism of injury is in question and NAT is still high in differential.

Complications

- Because toddler's fracture is non-displaced and its mechanism is low-energy falls, compartment syndrome risk is minimal, unlike for other more high-energy tibial fractures. There is very minimal risk of non-healing.

Key points

- Toddler's fractures should always be considered in children aged 1–3 years who are not bearing weight or are limping, with little or no significant trauma.
- NAT should be considered if the child with a toddler's fracture is non-ambulating (younger than age 1 year), concern for mechanism, or in the presence of other fractures.

Distal Tibial Fractures-Tillaux and Triplanar

Two distinct pediatric tibial fractures involving the distal tibial physis, both Tillaux and triplanar, can be difficult to assess and possibly missed on plain radiographs. Therefore, a high index of suspicion in adolescents is advised.

Tillaux Fractures

Background

- Tillaux fracture is usually seen in those aged 12–14 years and is considered a Salter–Harris type III fracture in which a portion of the lateral tibial physis is avulsed by the anterior tibiofibular ligament by an eversion injury (closure of the distal tibial physis proceeds from medial to lateral).

Classical presentation

- Children aged 12–14 years with eversion-type injury; swelling; tenderness over the medial, lateral malleolus;

and unable to bear weight or limited weight bearing

Atypical presentation

- Either younger or older than ages 12–14 years, perhaps due to accelerated or delayed growth plate closure

Differential diagnosis

- Osteomyelitis, septic joint, bony mass, or tumor (no distinct injury reported)
- Sprain
- Hemarthrosis
- Tibial fracture (other)

Diagnostic confirmation

- AP and lateral radiographs may fail to demonstrate a Tillaux fracture, especially if minimally displaced. A slight widening of lateral tibial physis is all that may be seen.
- If suspicious for Tillaux, get oblique, mortise views or CT to see fracture. CT is also helpful in determining more precisely the number of millimeters of displacement.

Treatment

- Closed reduction and casting for 3 or 4 weeks if <2 mm displacement; ORIF if >2mm displacement or CRPP

Disposition

- Patients with closed reduced fractures may be discharged home with pain control and return precautions for casting concerns—swelling, poor perfusion, or excessive pain.

Complications

- Early arthritis
- Because physeal closure has started, growth arrest is a rare complication
- May have associated fibular fracture

Key point

- Tillaux fractures should be suspected in children aged 12–14 years whose physis may be only partially closed, associated with an eversion-type injury and slight widening of lateral tibial physis. Have a low level of suspicion to obtain oblique, mortise views or CT to better evaluate this fracture.

Pitfalls

- Missing a Tillaux fracture on plain radiographs
- Not obtaining orthopedic consultation for Tillaux fractures

Triplane Tibial Fracture

Background

- Seen in children aged 10–17 years; fracture is a complex Salter–Harris IV occurring during physeal closure
- Seen at younger age than Tillaux fracture
- There are three types of triplane fractures
  - Two-part, three-part, and four-part fractures
- 50% of these have concomitant distal fibular fracture

Classical presentation

- Occurs during supination—external rotation (similar to Tillaux) or adduction injury
- Ankle pain, swelling, unable to bear weight

Atypical presentation

- Younger/older age (reported range 10–18 years)
- Minimal swelling

Differential diagnosis

- Tillaux fracture
- Salter–Harris II fracture

Diagnostic confirmation

- On AP/lateral radiographs, triplane may be mistaken for either a Salter–Harris III (AP view) or a Salter–Harris II (lateral view).
- Mortise view—best to assess degree of displacement.
- CT scan is usually required to better assess fracture pattern and articular involvement.
- If closed reduction is planned, CT should be done after to assess quality of reduction.

Treatment

- Prompt orthopedic consultation
- Closed reduction and casting if <2mm displacement, especially for

two fragment fractures; casting for 4–6 weeks
- CRPP or ORIF
  - >2mm displacement, especially in three and four-fragment fractures, then casting for 4–6 weeks

Disposition
- Depends on need for non-operative versus operative management
- If discharged from ED, careful return instructions for swelling, pallor of distal extremity, and excessive pain

Complications
- Growth arrests—can be seen in up to 20%, increased risk of residual fracture displacement after reduction
- Arthritis

Key points
- Triplane fractures are complex Salter–Harris type IV fractures seen in adolescents that may be missed on initial plain radiographs.
- CT is often needed to assess degree of displacement, type (two-, three-, or four-fragment), and articular surface involvement.
- Timely orthopedic assessment is needed because many triplane fractures are operative.

Pitfalls
- Missing a triplane fracture on plain radiographs
- Not obtaining orthopedic consultation for triplane fractures

PEDIATRIC BACK PAIN

See Table 37.3 for an extensive list of causes of back pain in children.
- Back pain in school-age children, specifically lower back pain, usually has

TABLE 37.3 CHILDHOOD CAUSES OF BACK PAIN

Etiology	Typical Age at Presentation
Structural	
Musculoskeletal	Late childhood/adolescent
Spondylolisthesis/spondylolysis	Early/late adolescence
Scheuermann's kyphosis	Early adolescence
Apophyseal ring fracture	Late adolescence
Infectious	
Osteomyelitis/discitis	Biphasic: toddlers(discitis) and adolescents
Epidural abscess	Any age—less common in children
Nonspinal infections (referred pain)	Spans childhood/adolescence
Pyelonephritis, pneumonia, PID, viral myalgias	Late childhood/adolescence
Potts' disease (tuberculous vertebral osteomyelitis)	Age range 4–15 years
Inflammatory	
Ankylosing spondylitis	Late adolescence
IBD-associated arthritis	Late childhood/adolescence
Neoplastic	
Leukemia/lymphoma	Spans all ages
Sarcoma, Ewing's	Peak 15–19 years
Sarcoma, osteogenic	Peak 13–16 years
Osteoid osteoma	Adolescence
Other: referred back pain	
Renal mass (Wilm's tumor, neuroblastoma)	Toddler/early childhood
UPJ obstruction (hydronephrosis)	Infant/early childhood
Pancreatitis	Childhood/adolescence
Cholecystitis	Adolescence

IBD, inflammatory bowel disease; PID, pelvic inflammatory disease; UPJ, ureteropelvic junction.

a nonspecific cause, such as mechanical (muscle strain), deconditioning, or obesity.

- However, there are red flag symptoms that should alert the clinician to a more serious pathology:
  - Any nontraumatic back pain in a child younger than age 8 years, fever (including low-grade), nighttime pain, weight loss, limp, other joint pain, any pain that is progressive or constant, morning stiffness, as well as any neurologic findings on examination
- In a 2015 study of 261 children aged 4–18 years, with symptoms of constant or night pain, radicular pain, or abnormal neurologic examination, MRI showed pathologic findings in more than one-third of patients.
- Unless severe, scoliosis is usually not by itself a cause of back pain in children.
- In adolescents involved in sports, spondylolisthesis and spondylolysis may be a cause of back pain (see the section titled "Overuse Syndromes"). Tumors such as Ewing's sarcoma and osteogenic sarcoma may present in this age group as back pain.
- Children at risk for compression fractures or other pathology such as any oncologic history, steroid-dependent illnesses, hemophilias, or chronic renal disease should have further investigation of back pain.
- Lumbar disc prolapse is very uncommon in adolescence and even rarer in children younger than age 9 years. Less than 10% of lower back pain in children is due to prolapsed disc.

BONY INFECTIONS

Osteomyelitis

Introduction

- Because children's bones have greater vascularity, osteomyelitis (OM) is most often hematogenous, although traumatic injury can be a factor in its development.
- Incidence is 4–5/100,000 per year in developed countries; males are at twice the risk as females.
- Lower extremity OM is more common than upper extremity OM, seen more often in proximal rather than distal bones; may also be seen in pelvis, skull, or spine in children.
- The most common bacterial sources are *Staphylococcus aureus* [methicillin-susceptible *Staph. aureus* (MSSA) and methicillin-resistant *Staph. aureus* (MRSA)], followed by *Streptococcus pyogenes* and *Strep. pneumoniae. Kingella kingae* is also a significant pathogen, more common in children younger than age 4 years.
- Younger than age 2 months—consider *Strep. agalactiae*, gram-negative organisms (*Escherichia coli*).
- Rare pathogens—fungal, mycobacterium, or *Bartonella henselae*

Classic presentation

- Because OM is more common in lower extremities, it most commonly presents as limp; with spinal OM back pain (back pain is an uncommon chief complaint in young children and should alert the clinician), initially may have low-grade fevers (99° or 100°F).
- Low-grade fevers (with MRSA high fevers seen)

Atypical presentation

- Because upper extremity OM is less common, a child not moving arm may be attributed to other causes before the clinician suspects OM.
- OM of spine presents as point tenderness at a focal spinal level. Because the disc space in children is vascularized until age 7 years, bacterial discitis is another consideration for focal back pain.
- Any non-ambulatory child younger than age 12 months having pain and not moving an extremity.

Differential diagnosis

- Leukemia (all ages) and neuroblastoma (primarily ages 1–6 years) may present as back pain, or bony pain/limp, either unilateral or bilateral and in addition may have fever

- Ewing's sarcoma or osteosarcoma may similarly present with focal long bony pain (user not febrile) or pelvic pain (less commonly focal back pain).
- Septic arthritis: It may be difficult in some cases to distinguish septic arthritis from OM, but evaluation is similar and some children may have both.

Diagnostic confirmation

- Complete blood count (CBC) with differential, C-reactive protein (CRP), erythrocyte sedimentation rate (ESR), and procalcitonin. Of all these, CRP is initially greatest value diagnostically and most easily available test. Initially, white blood cell (WBC) count may be normal but with left shift on differential.
- Plain films are less useful early in course of disease (first 1 or 2 weeks), periosteal elevation is an early sign, but radiographs may be helpful in ruling out Ewing's or osteosarcoma.
- Blood culture (may not always be positive).
- Scintigraphy (bone scan) with technetium is sensitive, but MRI is the best imaging method in most centers (may require anesthesia in young children); CT is a second choice if MRI is not available.
- If diagnosed confirmed/highly suspicious based on clinical symptoms/ examination, labs and imaging then confirmatory bone biopsy for culture should be performed.

Treatment

- If diagnosis is highly suspicious or confirmed in the ED, empiric treatment with clindamycin (covers *Staph. aureus*, the most common pathogen) or first-generation cephalosporins.
- Consider adding β-lactams for *K. kingae* and *Strep. pyogenes/ pneumoniae.*
- In unvaccinated children younger than age 4 years: consider coverage for *Haemophilus influenzae* type B—second- or third-generation cephalosporin
- Salmonella: sickle cell patients—third-generation cephalosporin, such as ceftriaxone or cefotaxime
- In neonates—oxacillin plus gentamicin

Disposition

- All children with OM suspected/confirmed should be admitted, orthopedic/ID consult, and empiric antibiotics started.
- For more equivocal cases, consider other diagnoses and admission versus close outpatient follow-up (24 hours).

Complications

- Sepsis, septic shock
- Subperiosteal abscess
- Pathologic fracture
- Bone growth, failure and limb length discrepancy—any (particularly if involved growth plate)

Key point

- Suspect OM in any child with long bone pain not suspected of having a fracture.

Pitfalls

- Believing that all children with acute OM are febrile (may not be, particularly very early in course)
- Relying only on insensitive CBC and plain films to diagnose OM
- Not consulting infectious disease specialist and orthopedist

Septic Arthritis

Background

- Like OM, septic arthritis is usually spread hematogenously and is more common in boys (2:1) and has an incidence of 5/100,000.
- It usually affects large joints of lower extremities, hip, knee, and ankle.
- *Staph. aureus* (MSSA and MRSA) is the most common bacteria isolated; *K. kingae* is increasingly identified in children younger than age 4 years.

- In neonates younger than age 2 months, *Strep. agalactiae* and gram-negative (*E. coli*) are most common.

Classical clinical presentation

- An acutely swollen erythematous, painful joint with limited ROM and fever, limping for younger children, refusal to bear weight, or pain on hip movement

Atypical clinical presentation

- Absent or low-grade fever, especially early in course
- History of trauma, which is then followed days later by worsening pain and fever
- Swollen erythematous joint without trauma in a sexually active adolescent (gonococcal)
- Neonates (can be late in presenting): fussiness, painful extremity, and fever

Differential diagnosis

- Transient synovitis (usually hip)—primarily younger children (ages 3–8 years)
- Juvenile idiopathic arthritis
- Osteomyelitis
- SCFE—in older children/adolescents with hip pain
- Hemarthrosis (previously undiagnosed hemophilia, or significant trauma)

Diagnostic confirmation

- Initial labs should include CBC with differential, CRP, ESR, procalcitonin if available, and blood cultures, especially if febrile.
- Kocher criteria (1999) for septic arthritis of hip may help distinguish from transient (toxic) synovitis. However, these criteria are not sufficiently sensitive and may miss subtle cases. Four criteria as follows:
  - Temperature >101.3°F (38.5°C)
  - WBC >12,000/µL
  - ESR >40 mm/hr
  - Inability to ambulate
  - One point for each criterion met: score of 3 or 4 has 93% or 94% sensitivity for septic arthritis of hip
- CRP >2 mg/dL is a strong independent predictor of septic arthritis.
- US of affected joint, especially hip because there is no reliable examination (redness, swelling), other than pain on ROM of hip. US of unaffected side of hip for comparison.
- A synovial fluid WBC >50 × 10^9/L with >75% polymorphonucleocytes is highly suggestive of septic arthritis.

Treatment

- Intravenous antibiotics and admission; consider transfer to pediatric center for orthopedics and infectious disease consultation if not available at your institution. Most orthopedists recommend antibiotics be started after joint aspiration so cultures may be obtained, but these should not be delayed if the child is septic or the time to aspiration/surgery is delayed.
- *Surgical drainage/aspiration—emergent.* This is a true orthopedic emergency. Surgical drainage of joint reduces risk of complications such as avascular necrosis of bone and permeant cartilage damage.
- Empiric treatment with oxacillin, cephazolin, or vancomycin if pen-allergic. In neonates—oxacillin plus gentamicin.

Complications

- Sepsis
- Joint destruction and ensuing arthritis

Key point

- Septic arthritis is a medical/surgical emergency, and it should be in the differential of any neonate/child who is not moving an extremity, has painful extremity not obviously due to fracture, or has red swollen joint.

Pitfalls

- Relying on plain radiographs and a CBC alone to rule out a diagnosis of septic arthritis
- Not obtaining emergent orthopedic consultation or not transferring

care to a center that has orthopedics and infectious disease consultants available

TRANSIENT SYNOVITIS

Background

- Transient synovitis is a benign, self-limiting inflammation of the synovium of the hip joint. It is the most common cause of hip pain in children. More serious causes of acute hip pain should be considered and evaluated for because transient synovitis is a diagnosis of exclusion.
- Importantly, children are well-appearing and not febrile with transient synovitis, and recent trauma is not present.
- Age range for transient synovitis is 3–8 years, with a mean of 4.7 years. It is not seen in adolescents.
- No real etiology has been identified, although there is evidence that as many as 40% may have historically had antecedent viral infection, usually upper respiratory.

Classical presentation

- Acute or subacute onset of groin or thigh pain without explanation. Usually, parents will notice child has a painful limp but will not automatically associate this pain as coming from the hip joint.
- Pain is unilateral (affecting only one hip joint). No fever (even low-grade temperature) is present.

Atypical presentation

- Thigh or knee pain
- Bilateral hip pain (reported in 1–4%)

Differential diagnosis

- Septic arthritis (most common among potential differentials)
- Unwitnessed trauma
- SCFE (usually in children older than age 8 years)
- Malignancy (leukemia, bony malignancy)
- Lyme arthritis
- Pyogenic sacroiliitis (usually febrile)
- Juvenile rheumatoid arthritis
- Transient synovitis is a diagnosis of exclusion.

Diagnostic confirmation

- CBC may be slightly elevated.
- CRP and ESR—more helpful in guiding clinical decision-making; CRP is usually < 2 mg/dL, ESR <20 mm/hr.
- Radiographs—AP/frog-leg views will be normal in transient synovitis.
- Ultrasound hips—in many cases, there is absence of hip effusion in transient synovitis, although some cases do have small effusions, thus making it difficult to rely on US alone.
- MRI—a newer modality for differentiating transient synovitis from septic arthritis; should be used when other diagnostic tests have not so far confirmed.
- Hip aspiration of effusion—usually difficult in children because of the need for sedation; nonetheless, if differentiating between septic arthritis and transient synovitis, it should be performed if significant effusion is present on US. A WBC $>50 \times 10^9$/L in the synovial fluid or a positive gram stain would confirm a diagnosis of septic arthritis, so absence of these two results may lead to a diagnosis of transient synovitis.
- Note that not all diagnostic tests need to be performed. Experienced clinicians may only obtain labs and/or US.

Treatment

- Transient synovitis is a benign, self-limiting disease. Supportive care (rest, limiting activity, non-weight-bearing if painful) is recommended.
- Most providers prescribe an NSAID for pain.
- Many cases of transient synovitis improve within 1 or 2 days; most are better by 1 or 2 weeks.

Disposition

- If the diagnosis of transient synovitis is certain, and other significant pathologies have been ruled out, then patients may be discharged home. Rarely do they need to be admitted for pain control.

- Good return precautions (return if fever, worsening pain) and follow-up with medical provider in 1 or 2 days are advised.

Complications

- None if diagnosis is correctly made, considering other potential diagnoses.
- 4% of children can have recurrence of transient synovitis, usually within the first few months after initial case.

Key point

- When diagnosed appropriately, and with consideration of more serious etiologies of acute hip pain in childhood, transient synovitis.

Pitfall

- Failing to work-up potential other causes of hip pain in a child aged 3–8 years.

OVERUSE INJURIES: OSTEOCHONDRITIS, APOPHYSITIS, AND EPIPHYSITIS

Background

- Seen primarily in active growing children and adolescents, these injuries are described as a disruption of the endochondral tissue or an osteochondrosis. (See Table 37.4 for a complete list.)
- These are non-emergent conditions, but children may appear in the ED for acute-on-chronic pain.
- The most common and well-known of these is Osgood–Schlatter disease.

Classic clinical presentation

- Pain during or after physical activity, usually sports, that has been ongoing, perhaps worsening for weeks to months
- Very specific point tenderness, such as over the tibial tubercle

TABLE 37.4 OVERUSE INJURIES: OSTEOCHONDROSIS

Osteochondrosis	Type	Location of Pain	Age Typically Affected (Sex if Applicable)	Sport/Activity
Panner's disease	Epiphysis	Elbow (capitellum)	6–10 years	Gymnastics, tennis
Osteochondrosis dissecans of capitellum		Elbow (capitellum)	>13 years (male)	Pitching, throwing
Little League elbow	Apophysis	Medial epicondyle	8–15 years	Pitching
Gymnast's wrist	Epiphysis	Distal radial physis	Adolescents	Gymnastics, tennis
Konig's disease		Femoral condyle (usually medial)	10–13 years (male)	
Osgood–Schlatter disease	Apophysis	Tibial tubercle	12–15 years (male); 8–12 years (female)	Basketball, track
Sinding–Larsen–Johansson syndrome	Apophysis	Inferior pole of patella	10–14 years (male)	Running, track (jumpers), weight lifting
Sever's disease (osteochondrosis of calcaneus)	Apophysis	Calcaneal at insertion of Achilles (calcaneal squeeze test)	8–13 years	Cleated sports, gymnastics
Osteochondrosis dissecans of talus		Medial foot	>10 years	Court sports (volleyball, basketball)

(Osgood–Schlatter disease) or calcaneus near Achilles insertion (Sever's disease)

Atypical presentation

- Sudden worsening of pain that has been chronic for weeks to months

Differential diagnosis

- Bony tumor or cyst (usually diaphyseal pain)

Diagnostic confirmation

- Although radiographs are not necessary in general to make this diagnosis, it may be helpful in ruling out other etiologies if the pain is more sudden in onset or there is an acute change.
- Occasionally, comparison views of unaffected extremity are helpful in interpreting the affected side.
- Radiographic findings are based on the location of osteochondrosis (see Table 37.4).
- MRI as outpatient if conservative therapy (temporary cessation of sports, rest) is not improving symptoms.

Treatment

- Curative treatment involves stopping the particular physical activity/sport for 4–6 weeks, on average, and in some severe cases permanently.
- Occasionally, surgery may be needed if there is articular surface injury and rest over time has not improved pain.
- Rest, in some cases crutches and non-weight-bearing, ice, and NSAIDs.

Disposition

- All of these children may be discharged home with outpatient follow-up with their primary care physician, sports medicine, or orthopedist, depending on severity of symptoms as well as competitive level of child.

Key point

- Overuse injuries such as Osgood–Schlatter, Little League elbow, and Sever's disease are seen in growing children and involve an inflammation or osteochondrosis at the junction of the tendon/ligament to bone. Treatment is primarily rest and temporary removal from sports.

Pitfall

- Overimaging—radiographs may be confusing to interpret because the diagnosis is clinical

Back Pain and Overuse Injuries: Spondylolysis and Spondylothesis

Background

- Spondylolysis is a stress fracture of the pars interarticularis of the vertebral arch, either uni- or bilateral, in the lower lumbar vertebra (L4 and L5 most commonly involved) and is a common cause of lower back pain in adolescent athletes.
- Spondylothesis occurs when an adolescent with spondylothesis (lower back pain) has an anterior slippage of the more cephalad vertebra over the more caudal vertebrae. This usually occurs 1 or 2 months after initial back pain from spondylothesis and is more common in younger athletes (younger than age 16 years).
- Both spondylolysis and spondylothesis are seen in athletes with repetitive spinal loads, either acute or due to overuse. Such activities involved more often are gymnasts, wrestlers, weight lifters, and high divers.

Typical clinical presentation

- Lower lumbar pain and focal tenderness are usually at L4/L5 in adolescents, but they can be as high as L1. Presentation also includes lumbar lordosis, pain with lumbar extension, and tight hamstrings.
- Most often, neurologic examination is entirely normal. Rarely, the L4/L5 nerve root may be involved in high-grade spondylothesis.
- The "stork test" may be positive but is nonspecific for spondylolysis.

Atypical presentation

- Children as young as age 7 years have been found to have spondylolysis radiographically, but usually this finding is not associated with pain in this age group. In young children, a further cause of back pain should be sought because most back pain in young children is pathologic.
- Pars interarticularis fractures can be due to trauma or congenital.

Differential diagnosis

- Scheuermann's (juvenile) kyphosis
- Sacroileitis or sacroiliac instability due to lumbar injury
- Osteomyelitis
- Osteoid osteoma (benign tumor)
- Malignancy (osteosarcoma, Ewing's sarcoma, neuroblastoma, leukemia)
- Scoliosis

Diagnostic confirmation

- AP and lateral radiographs are the first studies to be considered if spondylothesis is suspected. Radiographs will demonstrate up to 84% of fractures. Oblique views are not needed because "Scotty dog" sign, although classically taught, may not be as sensitive for fracture as originally thought.
- For patients who have not improved after a period of rest from athletics (few weeks), advance imaging such as MRI or single-photon emission computerized tomography (SPECT) bone scan can be pursued as outpatient. ED advanced imaging should only be considered if there are new neurological findings to suggest severe slip (spondylothesis).
- Slippage, when present on radiographs, is defined as the percentage of cephalad vertebra that is anteriorly displaced over the caudal vertebra, graded as I–V:
  - Grade I: ≤25%
  - Grade II: 26–50%
  - Grade III: 51–75%
  - Grade IV: 76–100%
  - Grade V: >100%

Treatment

- Rest from all athletic activities, especially those that incite pain, for a period of a few weeks to 2 months is appropriate for the majority of spondylolysis cases. Bracing (Boston Overlap Brace) is controversial with regard to clinical effectiveness.
- Patients with pain that has not improved with rest and physical therapy and low-impact cardiovascular exercise should be referred to a spinal surgeon. This includes pain not improving with rest in grade I spondylothesis or progression to grades II or higher.
- Immediate spinal surgeon consultation and MRI are needed for any patient with motor defect or cauda equina syndrome.

Disposition

- Most adolescents with suspected spondylolysis just diagnosed can be sent home with rest from sports and follow-up with sports medicine or orthopedist.
- Adolescents with more pain that is not improving should be sent home with urgent MRI and spinal surgeon referral.
- Adolescents with any neurologic findings should get emergent MRI and spinal surgeon consult.

Key points

- Spondylolysis is primarily an overuse injury, a fracture of the pars interarticularis, usually in the lumbar region and most commonly seen in adolescent athletes. Spondylothesis can occur when there is slippage of one vertebra over another. Slippage is graded I–V, with V being the worst.
- Lumbar back pain, either acute or subacute, and during activity, is the primary symptom, although there may be weakness in the L4/L5 distribution and uncommonly cauda equina syndrome,

and therefore patients should receive a complete neurologic examination.

- Plain radiographs identify most (84%) cases of spondylolysis/spondylothesis, and most patients who do not have any neurologic findings can be discharged home with athletic rest and outpatient follow-up, including outpatient MRI/SPECT if pain is not resolving.

Pitfalls

- Failing to develop a substantial differential diagnosis in children with back pain and to consider other diagnoses besides spondylolysis, especially in younger adolescents and non-athletes
- Failing to consult spinal surgeon with any patient having neurologic deficits with spondylothesis

38

Pediatric Otolaryngology Emergency Management

RYAN H. BELCHER AND PATRICK MUNSON

INTRODUCTION

Pediatric otolaryngology emergency department (ED) visits encompass a wide variety of symptoms and diagnoses. The symptoms within ear, nose, and throat are commonly encountered with significant complications if not treated or assessed appropriately. This chapter discusses many of these commonly encountered issues, including ear emergencies, neck masses/enlargement, nasal/sinus symptoms, and airway emergency management.

EAR

Otitis Media

In the United States, acute otitis media is the most commonly diagnosed pediatric illness.

Classic Clinical Presentation

There are two important distinctions of otitis media: otitis media with effusion (OME) and acute otitis media (AOM). OME is the presence of fluid in the middle ear without signs or symptoms of acute ear infection. Approximately 90% of children have OME before school age and develop four episodes of OME on average every year, with most of these episodes resolving within 3 months. Thus, it is not uncommon to see OME on routine otologic examination in any pediatric patient who presents to the ED. In contrast, AOM is considered to be "infectious" and presents with rapid onset of signs and symptoms, most often with ear pain and a bulging eardrum due to inflammation in the middle ear.

Atypical Clinical Presentation

In pediatric patients who have previously had tympanostomy ear tubes placed or a ruptured/perforated tympanic membrane (TM), AOM often presents with otorrhea, mostly purulent with foul odor in character. This does not occur if the TM is intact. Tympanostomy tube otorrhea is the most common sequela after the placement of ear tubes. OME can also present with distinct redness of the TM but without acute signs and symptoms from the patient; this should still be considered OME and not a criterion for prescribing antibiotics.

Differential Diagnosis

AOM

OME

Mastoiditis

Otitis externa

Temporal bone trauma

Dental pain

Temporomandibular joint pain
Pharyngitis
Tonsillitis

Diagnostic Confirmation

Physical examination and clinical history are the gold standard for diagnosis of otitis media, whether OME or AOM. Both OME and AOM will present with fluid in the middle ear. In OME, the TM is often cloudy with immobility on pneumatic otoscopy, with an air fluid level or bubble visible in the middle ear. Tympanometry or acoustic reflectometry can also confirm middle ear effusion, but these are often not available in the ED setting. In addition to the physical examination findings, AOM diagnosis requires acute onset of middle ear inflammation symptoms.

Treatment

Acute otitis media may resolve without treatment, and watch-and-wait therapy may be initiated (Table 38.1). Treatment with analgesics is indicated for discomfort (acetaminophen 15 mg/kg or ibuprofen 10 mg/kg). Topical lidocaine preparations may provide some additional pain relief but should not be used with perforated TM.

AOM is caused most often by typical nasopharyngeal pathogens *Streptococcus pneumoniae, Haemophilus influenzae,* and *Moraxella catarrhalis.* The first-line antibiotic therapy (if the TM is intact) is oral high-dose amoxicillin (90 mg/kg/day BID; maximum 3 g/day) for 10 days for children younger than age 2 years and 5–7 days for children older than age 2 years. Amoxicillin–clavulanate (Augmentin) should be given if the patient has concomitant purulent conjunctivitis (non-typeable *H. influenzae* is nearly 100% resistant to amoxicillin alone), if the patient has been treated with antibiotics in the past 30 days, or in children with persistent symptoms despite amoxicillin therapy. Alternatives for penicillin allergic patients include the following:

- Cephalosporins
  - Cefdinir 14 mg/kg/day in one or two doses (maximum 600 mg/day)
  - Cefpodoxime 10 mg/kg/day BID (maximum 400 mg/day)
  - Cefuroxime 30 mg/kg/day BID (maximum 1 g/day)
  - Ceftriaxone 50 mg/kg (maximum 1 g) intramuscularly once per day for one to three doses
- Lincosamides
  - Clindamycin 20–30 mg/kg/day TID (maximum 1.8 g/day)

If tympanostomy tubes are present in the setting of uncomplicated AOM with otorrhea, topical antibiotic therapy only, without oral antibiotics, is a strong recommendation in the consensus guidelines from the American Academy of Otolaryngology—Head and Neck Surgery (AAO-HNS). Several studies have investigated the merits of combination therapy of topical antibiotics with and without concurrent oral antibiotics, but no advantage has been identified with this combination therapy. Most common topical antibiotic therapies contain a fluoroquinolone (ofloxacin or ciprofloxacin–dexamethasone). Several studies have shown that addition of a corticosteroid to the topical antibiotic drops can reduce inflammation and days to cessation of ear drainage.

It is not recommended by the AAO-HNS guidelines to treat OME with antihistamines and/or decongestants because studies have shown them to be ineffective. Antimicrobials

TABLE 38.1 TREATMENT OF OTITIS MEDIA

Treatment with Antibiotics	Watch-and-Wait Therapy Acceptable
<6 months	Non-severe unilateral OM, 6--23 months
Bilateral OM if <24 months	OM in ≥24 months
Moderate–severe otalgia	
Otalgia >48 hours	
Temperature ≥39°C	

OM, otitis media.

and corticosteroids also do not have long-term efficacy and are not recommended for routine management. Although antimicrobial therapy, with or without steroids, has not been found to have long-term effectiveness in resolution of OME, therapy can be considered in some cases for short-term benefit if the parent or caregiver expresses a strong aversion to impending surgery.

Disposition

Uncomplicated AOM can be followed up with the patient's pediatrician, typically within 72 hours. If the patient is having recurrent episodes of AOM that are impacting quality of life, then follow-up with a pediatric otolaryngologist should be considered. Concerns for hearing, speech, and language development should also prompt follow-up.

Complications

Facial nerve paresis/paralysis

Hearing loss

Meningitis

Empyema

Cholesteatoma

Dizziness

Tympanic membrane perforation

Key Points

- Most cases of acute otitis media resolve spontaneously.
- Discomfort with AOM may be treated with oral analgesics.
- Observation and watch-and-wait therapy are reasonable in non-severe cases (see Table 38.1).
- If tympanostomy tubes are in place or TM perforation is visualized, use topical antibiotic drops; oral systemic antibiotics are not necessary.

Otitis Externa

Classic Clinical Presentation

Acute otitis externa (AOE) is diffuse inflammation of the external ear canal that can also affect the TM and/or the pinna. The vast majority of AOE in the United States is bacterial in etiology. The symptoms are of rapid onset (within 48 hours), with otalgia, fullness of the ear, otorrhea, cellulitis, and edema of the external auditory canal (EAC) as some of the more common presentations.

Atypical Clinical Presentation

Fungal AOE is extremely rare but can present in chronic otitis externa or after treatment of AOE with antibiotics. On otologic examination, one can often see white debris with hyphae or moist white deposits with black debris spotted throughout.

If the infection spreads outside of the EAC into the surrounding soft tissue and into the temporal bone causing osteomyelitis, it would be considered malignant otitis externa. Diabetic patients are at an increased risk of this developing, and the EAC examination may have granulation or polyp tissue.

Differential Diagnosis

Atopic dermatitis

Seborrheic dermatitis

AOM

OME

Furunculosis

Malignant otitis externa

Mastoiditis

Temporal bone trauma

Conditions with referred pain to the ear

Diagnostic Confirmation

Clinical history and physical examination including otoscopy are the mainstays of diagnostic confirmation of this disease. Culturing of the EAC can help tailor antibiotic selection. Imaging studies are not recommending in uncomplicated AOE, but if malignant otitis externa is suspected, then a computed tomography (CT) scan with and without contrast may be warranted. If intracranial complications are suspected, magnetic resonance imaging (MRI) of the brain should also be considered.

Treatment

Bacterial infection is the cause for 98% of AOE in the United States, so an antibiotic should be first-line therapy for uncomplicated AOE. Topical antibiotic drops should be first-line therapy for AOE unless there is extension outside of the EAC or other host factors that would indicate a need for systemic therapy. The most common pathogens are *Pseudomonas aeruginosa* and *Staphylococcus aureus*, so therapy should be targeted toward those pathogens as treatment with penicillins, macrolides, or cephalosporins have been shown to increase disease persistence with cephalosporins, causing increased recurrence of disease. Duration of therapy is typically 7–10 days to prevent relapse of infection or symptoms. If the ear canal is obstructed, performing aural toilet and/or placing an ear wick for several days is also recommended.

Acute pain should not be underappreciated nor inadequately treated in this disease process. The pain can be intense and severe due to the high sensitivity of the periosteum of the underlying bone that is in close proximity of the ear canal skin. Acetaminophen or a non-steroidal anti-inflammatory drug can help for mild to moderate pain, and a short course of opioids can be used at the discretion of the physician should the pain be significant.

Disposition

Patients should be reassessed by their pediatrician or otolaryngologist 48–72 hours after initiation of treatment to ensure symptoms are improving and the disease process has not spread beyond the ear canal. If malignant otitis externa is diagnosed, the patient may require inpatient admission with the administration of intravenous (IV) antibiotics to address the osteomyelitis.

Complications

Malignant otitis externa

Otomycosis

Facial nerve paresis/paralysis

Temporomandibular joint pain

Temporal headaches

Dysphagia

Key Points

- Uncomplicated AOE should be treated with topical antibiotics directed at the most common pathogens.
- If infection has spread to surrounding soft tissue, adding an oral antibiotic should be considered.
- Malignant otitis externa is an extension of infection into soft tissues and into surrounding bone, causing osteomyelitis. Cultures and appropriate imaging are warranted.

Mastoiditis

Classic Clinical Presentation

Any patient with AOM will almost assuredly have opacification of the mastoid air cells on imaging and essentially have mastoiditis, although the symptoms with AOM will be more prominent and the mastoiditis is not considered a separate entity. It is important to distinguish whether the patient has acute mastoiditis (AM) and whether it is coalescent. AM is the most common severe complication associated with AOM, and these patients usually present with a recent history of AOM, bulging TM, otalgia, fever, mastoid tenderness, ear swelling, and sometimes protrusion of the pinna.

Coalescent mastoiditis, which is a radiological diagnosis, describes the destruction of the bony septae in the mastoid, and mucoperiosteal disease extends to involve the bone. Extension of disease outside of the mastoid is more likely to occur when this happens, due to infection spreading to the bone and the accumulation of purulence inside the mastoid.

Atypical Clinical Presentation

Acute mastoiditis can still occur in the setting of tympanostomy tubes, despite the middle ear having a drainage pathway out into the ear canal. Infected fluid and purulence can be trapped in the mastoid with blockage of the antrum and thus mastoiditis can develop.

This disease can also present with no middle ear fluid and normal TM visualized on otoscopy. Less commonly, more extensive disease can have subperiosteal abscesses postauricularly, facial nerve paresis/paralysis, or intracranial extension of infection.

Differential Diagnosis

AOM

AOE

Temporal bone trauma

Adenopathy

Parotitis

Stroke

Sepsis

Diagnostic Confirmation

Confirmation of diagnosis is attained by clinical history and physical examination. Imaging, particularly CT scan or MRI, should be reserved for patients in whom intracranial extension or complications are expected, such as a subperiosteal abscess.

Treatment

The most common causes of AM are similar to the causes of AOM. *Streptococcus pneumoniae*, *H. influenzae*, and *Strep. pyogenes* are found most often in cultures in children with AM. Cultures from the site of infection help guide the antibiotics to be tailored to the particular organism.

Antibiotic choice and surgical intervention largely depend on the stage of the infection and the presence of complications. If simple AM in the setting of AOM is the diagnosis, then oral antibiotics are the initial treatment. If symptoms such as pain and persistent fevers do not improve over 48 hours or complications arise, antibiotic escalation should occur and imaging should be obtained.

If coalescent mastoiditis, particularly infection that has bony involvement, subperiosteal abscess, or extension of infection beyond the mastoid, is suspected and confirmed on radiographic imaging, then IV antibiotics should be given and otolaryngology consulted for potential surgical intervention. These patients can also be managed with tympanostomy tube placement, with or without mastoidectomy. Once tympanostomy tube is placed, topical antibiotic ear drops can be added to the antibiotic regimen to treat the infection. Neurosurgery consultation is also recommended with intracranial extension of infection.

Disposition

Simple AM: Follow-up with pediatrician or pediatric otolaryngologist in 48–72 hours to ensure improvement with antibiotic treatment

Coalescent AM: Admitted to hospital for IV antibiotic management and possible surgical interventions

Complications

Facial nerve paresis/paralysis

Subperiosteal abscess

Hearing loss

Labyrinthitis

Lemierre syndrome

Meningitis

Sigmoid sinus thrombosis

Empyema

Brain abscess

Seizures

Temporomandibular joint pain

Temporal headaches

Key Points

- Incidental finding of opacification or fluid in the mastoid is very common in the setting of AOM.
- Coalescent mastoiditis is a radiographic diagnosis and a more serious condition.
- Imaging (CT or MRI) should be reserved for patients in whom coalescent mastoiditis or extension of infection outside of the mastoid is suspected.
- Coalescent mastoiditis and extension of disease outside of mastoid most likely warrant IV antibiotics and consideration of surgical intervention by an otolaryngologist or neurosurgeon depending on the extension of disease.

NECK MASSES

Introduction

The vast majority of neck masses in the pediatric population are either congenital or inflammatory in nature. Although possible, it is rare for a pediatric neck mass to be malignant, with only 5% of all pediatric malignancies occurring in the head and neck. With the wide differential for pediatric neck masses, the history and a detailed physical exam are helpful in narrowing the possibilities. Particularly on the physical examination, delineating the location of the neck mass can further narrow the possible type of neck mass (Table 38.2). This section focuses on the most common presenting neck masses—cervical reactive lymphadenopathy, suppurative lymphadenitis/neck abscesses, branchial cleft cysts, thyroglossal duct cysts, and dermoid cysts—and other less common congenital neck masses.

Inflammatory Neck Masses: Reactive Lymphadenopathy/Abscess/ Congenital Neck Mass

Classic Clinical Presentation

Cervical lymphadenopathy is common, and even healthy children have been estimated to have palpable lymphadenopathy 38–45% of the time. Acute lymphadenopathy is defined as being present for less than 3 weeks and is most

TABLE 38.2 PEDIATRIC NECK MASS DIFFERENTIAL DIAGNOSIS BASED ON LOCATION OF OCCURRENCE

Type/Location	Anterocervical	Midline	Posterocervical
Inflammatory	Lymphadenitis Abscess Hematoma Sialadenitis Atypical mycobacterium	Lymphadenitis thyroiditis Infected dermoid/TGDC	Lymphadenitis
Congenital	Branchial cleft anomaly Hemangioma Vascular malformation Fibromatosis colli Torticollis	Thyroglossal duct cyst Dermoid cyst Thymic cyst Ectopic thyroid Vascular malformation Lymphocele	Hemangioma Vascular malformation Lymphatic malformation
Neoplastic (malignant and benign)	Lymphoma Carotid body tumor Sarcoma/fibrosarcoma Schwannoma Metastatic (nasopharyngeal carcinoma, neuroblastoma)	Thyroid mass Parathyroid Teratoma	Lipoma Sarcoma/fibrosarcoma Lymphoma

TGDC, thyroglossal duct cyst.

commonly found following or during a bacterial or viral (e.g., upper respiratory) infection. Enlarged lymph nodes are generally considered to be >1 cm, although deeper lymph nodes often need to be larger to feel with palpation. The lymph nodes are often mobile, small, bilateral, and without overlying skin changes. These patients can present with or without fever or tenderness on palpation.

Pediatric suppurative lymphadenitis can evolve from reactive cervical lymphadenopathy or can present independent from having prior lymphadenopathy. Suppurative lymphadenitis presents with fever in younger children, frequently with overlying skin changes and palpable fluctuance. These patients frequently have elevated inflammatory markers and may have previously failed a course of oral antibiotics.

Congenital neck masses are present at birth, but often they are subclinical and are not diagnosed until later in life. These masses can present similar to nonreactive lymphadenopathy or can be infected with fluctuance similar to suppurative lymphadenitis. If surrounding lymph nodes become infected and a conglomeration of suppurative lymphadenitis occurs, it can make the diagnosis of congenital neck mass difficult. Thyroglossal duct cysts (TGDCs) are the most common congenital pediatric neck mass, followed by branchial cleft anomalies and dermoid cysts. The location of these masses helps narrow the differential diagnosis. TGDCs and dermoid cysts occur most commonly in the midline of the neck, and branchial cleft anomalies (types 2–4) are more lateral in the neck, directly medial to the sternocleidomastoid.

Atypical Clinical Presentation

Supraclavicular lymph nodes, nodes firm and nontender or fixed to the skin or underlying structures, occurrence in patients older than age 8 years, associated lymphadenopathy in other areas outside of the neck (axilla, groin, etc.), and hepatosplenomegaly are all signs and symptoms worrisome for malignancy. Weight loss, persistent night sweats, fatigue, and fevers should also raise concern for malignancy or a chronic inflammatory condition.

A gradually enlarging lymph node in the submandibular or upper anterior cervical region with a violaceous skin discoloration (Figure 38.1) that persists despite antibiotics is most likely an atypical mycobacterial infection (*Mycobacterium avium-intracellulare* or *Mycobacterium scrofulaceum*). A subset of these

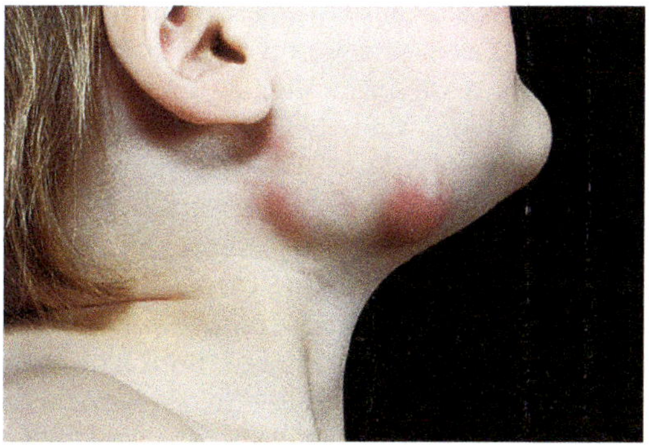

FIGURE 38.1 Atypical mycobacterium presentation. Note the mass' location in the submandibular region with focal erythema/violaceous hue and no diffuse swelling.
Source: Courtesy of Patrick Munson. Reproduced with permission.

patients may go on to develop a draining fistula tract. Surgical excision or medical management may be appropriate therapy, and the decision is often made in consultation with otolaryngology and infectious disease specialists.

Differential Diagnosis

- Reactive lymphadenopathy
- Suppurative lymphadenitis
- Peritonsillar abscess
- Viral causes (upper respiratory infection, mononucleosis via Epstein–Barr virus, measles, etc.)
- Bacterial causes (streptococcal infection, staphylococcal infection, atypical mycobacterium, lymphoma, cat scratch disease, anaerobic bacterial infections following dental procedures or in setting of poor dentition)
- Toxoplasmosis
- Malignancy
- Congenital neck mass

Diagnostic Confirmation

The diagnosis is most commonly confirmed by a targeted history and physical examination with careful consideration and inquiry of alternative etiologies and possible exposures. Patients should be asked about any recent dental procedures (anaerobic bacterial infection), contact with animals/pets (e.g., toxoplasmosis or cat scratch disease), immune status (measles, mumps, HIV, etc.), chronicity, weight loss, night sweats (e.g., malignancy), or recent illnesses. If suspicion of diagnosis is reactive lymphadenopathy, laboratory tests and imaging are not typically required. A complete blood count and inflammatory markers such as C-reactive protein and erythrocyte sedimentation rate may help evaluate treatment response.

Ultrasound (US) is the first-line imaging modality for evaluating pediatric neck masses, particularly lateral or central neck masses. US has both high sensitivity and high specificity in evaluation of purulent masses and does not expose a child to ionizing radiation. If US is not available, if there is concern for deep neck space involvement, or if there are worrisome features of neck mass (adherent to surrounding structures or supraclavicular lymph node enlargement), then a CT scan of the neck may be indicated. A CT scan gives more anatomical information compared to US, and this information can help determine the extent of infection and help guide surgical management.

Treatment

The majority of reactive lymphadenopathy in the pediatric population is benign and self-limiting, so clinical observation is appropriate in these patients with close follow-up with their pediatricians. If the lymphadenopathy or neck mass is of suspected bacterial etiology (overlying warmth or erythema), then treatment with antibiotics is indicated. *Staphylococcus aureus* is the most common bacteria involved with acute bacterial lymphadenitis in children aged 1–years, followed by β-hemolytic streptococcus infections, so antibiotic coverage should be targeted to these suspected pathogens (e.g., cephalosporins or clindamycin).

If the neck infection has persisted or enlarged despite a course of oral antibiotic treatment or if there is fluctuance on examination, then IV antibiotics with or without surgical intervention should be considered. Purulent lymphadenopathy >2 cm on imaging does not tend to improve with IV antibiotics alone and often requires surgical incision and drainage.

Newly diagnosed congenital neck masses that do not require immediate surgical drainage, unless secondary abscess formation has occurred, should have close follow-up with otolaryngology. These neck masses do not dissipate on their own and often require surgical excision to avoid recurrent infection.

Complications

Draining fistula

Neck immobility

Persistent infection despite antibiotic treatment (e.g., methicillin- or clindamycin-resistant *Staph. aureus*)

Airway compromise via mass effect

Mediastinitis

Key Points

- Clinical history and physical examination are essential in determining diagnosis. Particularly the location of the neck mass on physical examination can help narrow the differential diagnosis.
- *Staphylococcus aureus* is the most common bacteria involved with suppurative lymphadenitis, followed by β-hemolytic streptococcus.
- US is the first-line imaging modality for lateral and midline neck masses. CT scan of the neck should be considered with deep neck space involvement or worrisome features of the neck mass.

Pitfall

- Misdiagnosis of the neck mass (e.g., treating an atypical mycobacterial infection with antibiotics directed for suppurative lymphadenitis or not considering malignancy)

NASAL

Epistaxis

Background

Epistaxis is a common presentation and occurs in >50% of children older than age 5 years. It is most commonly spontaneous and self-limited, whereas severe epistaxis occurs more often in adults and elderly patients. A large database study of more than18,000 pediatric epistaxis ED encounters showed that 97% were routine, or uncomplicated, encounters. Seasonal changes, indoor heating (which can create relatively dry air), and direct irritation/trauma can damage the thin-walled blood vessels anteriorly in Kesselbach's plexus and trigger bleeding episodes.

Classic Clinical Presentation

Pediatric cases of epistaxis are rarely severe and often arise from digital trauma or rhinitis involving the anterior septum. Simple anterior epistaxis often lasts minutes and is self-resolving, although patients may have used digital pressure or self-packing to stop the bleeding. The bleeding can less commonly traverse posteriorly and drain down into the oropharynx and be swallowed. Both nares may be involved, and laterality may alternate in presentation.

Atypical Clinical Presentation

Recurrent epistaxis lasting longer than 20–30 minutes despite interventions, easy bruising, and a family history of hematologic disorders are all abnormal in presentation and should prompt a more thorough evaluation. Underlying coagulation disorders have been found to be present in as many as 4.5% of pediatric patients presenting with epistaxis to the ED. Other atypical presentations include facial pain, facial numbness, and/or fixed nasal obstruction.

Differential Diagnosis

Posterior nasal bleed

Coagulopathy (e.g., von Willebrand)

Thrombocytopenia

Medication induced (e.g., direct irritation from nasal sprays such as fluticasone)

Allergic rhinitis

Chronic sinusitis

Upper respiratory infection

Trauma

Non-accidental trauma (especially if younger than age 2 years)

Nasal cavity/nasopharyngeal tumor

Post-surgical from sinus endoscopy surgery

Adenoidectomy

Septoplasty

Diagnostic Confirmation

A thorough clinical history should be obtained that includes asking about the frequency, duration, severity, and laterality of the bleeding episodes as well as nasal spray use, facial pain, nasal obstruction, recent surgeries, easy bruising, and family history of hematologic disorders. Anterior rhinoscopy should be performed with physical examination, paying close attention to the anterior septum. The anterior septum can vary in its appearance depending on whether there has been recent or active bleeding. It can appear with hypervascularity in Kesselbach's plexus, which is often the inciting site of bleeding. If recently bleeding, this area may have crusting or dried blood that if manipulated can induce re-bleeding.

Laboratory testing, particularly checking hemoglobin, hematocrit, platelets, and prothrombin time/partial thromboplastin time, is indicated if bleeding has been prolonged, the patient is showing systemic signs of anemia, or there is concern for underlying disorder causing the epistaxis (von Willebrand, nasopharyngeal tumor, etc.). Imaging is not indicated in these patients unless there is high concern for a nasal tumor causing nasal obstruction and/or epistaxis.

Treatment

Conservative management and nasal hygiene comprise the first-line therapy for pediatric patients with simple anterior epistaxis. If not actively bleeding, counseling the family and patient on nasal mucosa hygiene can help prevent further episodes. Methods of nasal hygiene include avoiding picking nose or causing trauma to the septum, normal saline sprays or rinses at least once a day, placing a humidifier in the patient's room to help keep moisture in the air, and placing a small amount of Vaseline at the nasal sill and on the nasal septum prior to going to sleep. If the patient uses a nasal spray such as fluticasone, it is also common that improper positioning with the applicator pointed directly at the septum can cause nasal septal irritation and epistaxis. Discussing proper positioning of the nasal spray so that it is pointed into the nasal cavity and not directly at the nasal septum may also be helpful. Patients may need to discontinue nasal steroid spray until epistaxis improves.

If actively bleeding, treatment can include two to four sprays of oxymetazoline in the nasal cavity with digital pressure of the cartilaginous and soft tissue portion of the nose for 15–20 minutes or less if resolving. Packing the nose for anterior simple bleeds should be avoided if possible. In a controlled setting, silver nitrate cautery to the anterior septum on the side that has the hypervascularity or active bleeding can also help control the bleeding if not responding to conservative management. It is important to avoid cauterizing both sides of the anterior nasal mucosa so as to not cause a septal perforation.

Should the epistaxis be severe and not respond to treatments, the ED provider should be prepared to pack the nose or consult the otolaryngology team if the patient is stable. Expandable nonabsorbable packing such as Merocel or Rhino Rocket is helpful but can also be damaging to surrounding nasal mucosa, which can be problematic in a patient with thrombocytopenia or coagulopathy. There have been reports of toxic shock syndrome occurring with nasal packing, so there should be a strong consideration of placing the patient on prophylactic antibiotics if nonabsorbable packing is placed. In pediatric patients with an underlying coagulopathy or thrombocytopenia, absorbable packing (e.g., Floseal, thrombin-soaked gelfoam, and Surgicel) should be considered, if available.

Disposition

Patients with simple anterior epistaxis that is not recurrent can be discharged from the ED with education on nasal hygiene. If the epistaxis is a recurrent problem or requires cauterization, then patients should follow up with their pediatrician or pediatric otolaryngologist to discuss this further in the clinic setting.

Rarely do pediatric patients need to be admitted to the hospital for management or for complications related to their epistaxis. Younger patients requiring nasal packing often need to be admitted to the inpatient unit for observation. Patients with thrombocytopenia or newly diagnosed coagulopathy should have a hematologic consult. For severe epistaxis that does not respond to conservative treatments in the ED, otolaryngology consult should be considered because the patient may require nasal endoscopy and control of the epistaxis in the operating room setting.

Complications

Although rare in the pediatric population, if patients have hereditary hemorrhagic telangiectasia and are treated with nasal cautery, this may make the bleeding worse and difficult to control.

Key Points

- More than 97% of cases of pediatric patients presenting to the ED with epistaxis are simple and uncomplicated.
- Anterior septum at Kesselbach's plexus is the most common site of epistaxis in the pediatric population. Trauma (picking nose) and sinusitis are the most common irritants causing the epistaxis to start.
- If nasal cavity packing is needed in severe epistaxis, consider using absorbable packing, if available, particularly in pediatric patients with thrombocytopenia or underlying coagulopathy.
- If nonabsorbable packing is used, recommend placing patient on prophylactic antibiotics to potentially prevent toxic shock syndrome from occurring.

SINUSITIS

Background

Pediatric sinusitis can often present differently than in adults and can be difficult to diagnose. The symptoms can mimic other etiologies, such as viral illness or allergies. The maxillary and ethmoid sinuses are present at birth, but the sphenoid and frontal sinuses are not fully developed until late in the teen years, which can contribute to the variability in presentation of symptoms.

Classic Clinical Presentation

Children can present with a myriad of symptoms when they have acute sinusitis, including daytime cough, rhinorrhea including thick yellow-green nasal discharge, postnasal drip, headache (usually in children aged 6 years or older), irritability, fatigue, facial pain, swelling around the eyes, nasal obstruction, and fever. Pediatric acute sinusitis is most commonly viral in etiology, but it is very important to delineate whether the etiology may be bacterial. If the generalized symptoms last longer than the usual 7–10 days, then a bacterial sinus infection may be the cause. Any child with high-grade fever and purulent nasal discharge for at least 3 consecutive days should be considered to have a bacterial sinus infection.

Pediatric chronic sinusitis is defined as lasting 90 days or longer with symptoms of purulent rhinorrhea, nasal obstruction, facial pressure/pain, or a cough with corresponding endoscopic and/or CT findings. It is often not necessarily a "long infection" but is usually caused by prolonged inflammation. Patients can present with complaints of recurrent infections or persistent constellation of sinusitis symptoms that have not resolved despite medical treatments during that 90-day span.

Atypical Clinical Presentation

Diagnosing acute sinusitis can be difficult, particularly in younger children who do not have fully developed sinuses and are unable to articulate their generalized symptoms. Because of the generalized symptoms, sinusitis may not be diagnosed early, and orbital complications can present (Table 38.3). These symptoms can range from eyelid edema and erythema to orbital cellulitis and even as severe as an orbital abscess or cavernous sinus thrombosis.

TABLE 38.3 CHANDLER CLASSIFICATION FOR ORBITAL COMPLICATION OF SINUSITIS

Chandler Class	Diagnosis	Clinical Symptoms
I	Preseptal cellulitis	Erythema and eyelid edema; normal vision
II	Orbital cellulitis	Diffuse inflammation of orbital contents, but no abscess
III	Subperiosteal abscess	Subperiosteal abscess of lamina papyracea; can have pain and restriction with extraocular eye movement
IV	Orbital abscess	Purulence within the orbit; proptosis; ophthalmoplegia with decreased visual acuity
V	Cavernous sinus thrombosis	Bilateral ocular symptoms; proptosis; decreased visual acuity; meningismus

Source: Chandler JR, Langenbrunner DJ, Stevens ER. The pathogenesis of orbital complications in acute sinusitis. *Laryngoscope.* 1970;80:1414–1428.

Differential Diagnosis

Unrecognized nasal foreign body
Acute sinusitis
Chronic sinusitis
Viral illness/common cold/upper respiratory infection
Vasomotor rhinitis
Allergies
Adenoid hypertrophy
Adenoiditis
Immune deficiency
Ciliary dyskinesia
Tumor or mass of the sinuses

Diagnostic Confirmation

A thorough history and physical examination can usually lead to the correct diagnosis. Important questions include duration of symptoms, fevers, nasal discharge, recurrent infections, changes with smell, allergies, and vision changes. Anterior rhinoscopy should evaluate for turbinate hypertrophy, consistency of rhinorrhea, or any other anatomic abnormalities. It is also important to evaluate any signs of orbital extension of infection, including orbital edema, erythema, or impaired orbit movement. Laboratory testing is usually not helpful in obtaining a diagnosis unless there is concern for an immunodeficiency or cystic fibrosis.

Rigid endoscopy performed by the otolaryngologist is a safe procedure that can be done at the bedside with proper equipment, although it is often not required in the acute infectious setting unless there are complications from the infection.

Imaging is not indicated for uncomplicated acute sinusitis. It is only indicated in the acute setting if there is a complication from the infection, such as orbital cellulitis. For pediatric chronic sinusitis, a non-contrast CT scan of the face, including axial, coronal, and sagittal views, is recommended for patients when medical management and/or adenoidectomy have failed to control symptoms. If a patient is presenting to the ED for chronic sinusitis, consider obtaining the CT scan in the outpatient setting unless there are complications related to the current infection. Due to radiation safety concerns, imaging should be limited, especially in children younger than age 6 years.

Treatment

If the etiology for acute sinusitis is presumed to be viral, then no antibiotics are indicated and patients should be symptomatically treated. Antibiotics are reserved for suspected bacterial sinus infections. The most common bacteria involved with pediatric sinusitis include *Strep. pneumoniae, H. influenzae,* and *M. catarrhalis,* among others. Amoxicillin is a commonly used first-line therapy for 10–14 days. If the infections have been recurrent, a nasal steroid spray may be used in addition to daily, topical nasal saline irrigations. If allergies are playing a major role in the development of recurrent sinusitis, then an antihistamine such as cetirizine or loratadine can be added.

The acute infection in chronic sinusitis should be treated in addition to outpatient "maximal medial therapy." Surgery may be performed should these measures fail.

Patients with complications related to their sinusitis, including orbital or neural extension, should have empiric IV antibiotics started with appropriate consultations to pediatric ophthalmology, otolaryngology, and/or neurosurgery. A short course of systemic steroids, nasal irrigations, with or without oxymetazoline for 3 days decreases nasal inflammation and symptoms.

Disposition

Acute and chronic sinusitis patients can be treated in the ED setting and discharged with appropriate follow-up with their pediatrician or otolaryngologist. Allergist referral may be appropriate if allergies are playing a major role in symptoms. Hospital admission for IV antibiotics and possible surgery may be indicated if complications are present.

Complications

Epistaxis
Anosmia
Orbital cellulitis
Orbital abscess or subperiosteal abscess
Cavernous sinus thrombosis
Intracranial extension of infection, including abscess
Meningitis

Key Points

- Most sinus symptoms in children are of viral etiology and should be treated symptomatically.

- Acute bacterial sinusitis is diagnosed if symptoms (nasal drainage, cough, fevers, etc.) persist more than 10 days, symptoms are worsening, or the patient has high-grade fever with purulent nasal discharge for 3 days.
- Amoxicillin with or without clavulanate is first-line therapy for treatment of uncomplicated acute bacterial sinusitis.
- Imaging (e.g., CT scans) should be reserved for patients with complications from their sinusitis or for those who have chronic sinusitis.

LARYNGOTRACHEAL OBSTRUCTION/STRIDOR MANAGEMENT

Background

Pediatric patients with acute or chronic laryngotracheal obstruction presenting with stridor are encountered often in the ED setting. These cases have likely increased in recent years as younger and more fragile premature neonates survive intensive care via advanced technology relying on surfactant and often endotracheal intubation and ventilator support. This has allowed their previous lethal airway lesions or pathology to become manageable as they mature and grow.

The most common cause for stridor in a neonate is laryngomalacia, with other etiologies also contributing, including laryngotracheobronchitis, congenital abnormalities of the larynx and trachea, infectious causes (e.g., croup), trauma [e.g., subglottic stenosis (SGS)], and tumors or masses, although these are more rare in the pediatric population than in adults. Some studies have also shown that >25% of patients presenting with stridor have multiple locations of airway obstruction.

Some etiologies of pediatric stridor have decreased during the past few decades. Although epiglottitis can still occur in pediatric patients, the incidence has been dramatically reduced with the widespread use of the *H. influenzae* B vaccine. The knowledge and awareness of acquired SGS due to oversized endotracheal tubes and overinflated balloons have also led to a decreased incidence of SGS and improved airway management of the intubated child. As the number of patients receiving the human papilloma virus vaccine increases, there are also expectations and hopes that the number of pediatric patients with respiratory papillomatosis (RRP), which has a predilection for the larynx with a dysphonic and stridulous presentation, will decrease.

Classic Clinical Presentation

As these patients present to the ED, it is important to remember that stridor is a symptom and not a diagnosis. Stridor occurs as a result of partial obstruction of the airway, which leads to turbulent airflow that can create a vibratory effect on tissues that are closely approximated. The phase of respiration (inspiration, expiration, or both) can often correlate to the particular anatomic site at that partial obstruction is occurring. Stridor is anatomically and audiologically different from stertor, although they can occur at the same time (e.g., adenotonsillar hypertrophy with laryngomalacia). Stertor is caused by dynamic pharyngeal or nasopharyngeal collapse with the reverberation of soft tissue structures at that level, which can sound like snoring. Differentiation and recognition of the two different noises are paramount for proper management of airway obstruction.

Location and severity of the airway obstruction will often determine the constellation of symptoms with which pediatric patients present. Patients with mild or moderate obstruction can present with stridor along with coughing, choking, and feeding difficulties. Croup or subglottic narrowing can lead to a more barky cough. More severe laryngotracheal obstruction can present with apnea, lethargy, cyanosis, failure to thrive, and pulmonary hypertension. All type of laryngotracheal obstruction can present with suprasternal and/or intercostal retractions.

Atypical Clinical Presentation

Pediatric patients can be rather resilient, and their bodies can compensate despite chronic obstruction of their laryngotracheal airway. A child resting comfortably with stridor may have a severe airway obstruction along with CO_2 retention and poor pulmonary reserve.

Differential Diagnosis

Laryngomalacia

SGS

Laryngeal stenosis

Tracheomalacia

- Unilateral or bilateral vocal fold immobility
- RRP
- Foreign body aspiration
- Infantile hemangioma
- Epiglottitis
- Laryngotracheitis
- Angioedema
- Tumor

Diagnostic Confirmation

Patients with laryngotracheal obstruction with or without stridor most often present to the ED as the initial point of evaluation. It is therefore imperative for the ED physician to accurately assess any impending respiratory compromise. Vital signs, respiratory rate and effort, and oxygenation are paramount in the initial evaluation. If these parameters and the patient are stable and there is not an impending need for intubation or emergency airway interventions, then a more thorough history and physical examination can be performed.

When obtaining the clinical history, emphasis on the onset of symptoms is key. Patients with acute onset of stridor are more likely to have an etiology of infection, foreign body aspiration, or inflammation. More chronic stridor that has been present since soon after birth is most often laryngomalacia. If the stridor slowly develops at ages 2–4 months, then the diagnosis of infantile hemangioma may be considered, particularly if facial hemangiomas in a "beard distribution" are also present. Other important aspects to consider are the perinatal history; prematurity, including history of intubation; previous surgeries; intensive care unit history; exacerbating factors; apneas; cyanotic changes; positioning; feeding and growth history; and gastroesophageal reflux. Physical examination focuses on respiratory symptoms that include rate of respiration, retractions, cyanotic changes, quality of noise with breathing (stridor vs. stertor), and pulmonary auscultation.

In stable patients, flexible nasolaryngoscopy has been shown to be a very safe procedure to perform at bedside to assist in visualizing the site or potential source of laryngotracheal obstruction. This often requires consultation with the otolaryngology team. If available, an audio/video cart employed during the examination has been shown to be particularly useful because multiple providers as well as the family members can observe/visualize the laryngotracheal pathology, which can provide more meaningful dialogue and understanding of the potential management of the patient (Figure 38.2).

Treatment/Disposition

The differential for laryngotracheal obstruction is wide, and it is beyond the scope of this chapter to discuss each individual treatment pathway. If the patient has impending airway compromise, implementing a difficulty airway pathway with escalating airway adjuvants as needed is essential. Emergent consultation may be required in difficult or complex cases. Otolaryngology may be particularly

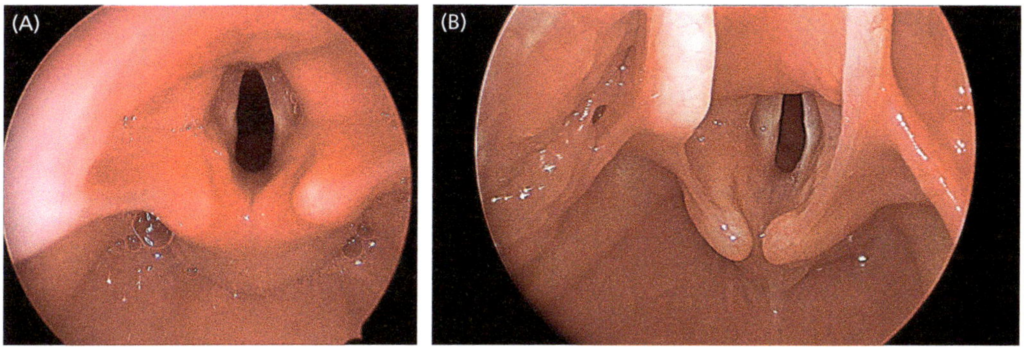

FIGURE 38.2 (A) Endoscopic picture of a normal pediatric larynx. No noted arytenoid edema, foreshortening of aryepiglottic folds, or partial obstruction of airway. (B) Endoscopic picture of a pediatric larynx with laryngomalacia. The aryepiglottic folds are foreshortened, leading to stridor with feeding.

Source: Courtesy of Patrick Munson. Reproduced with permission.

advantageous for the ability to visualize, diagnose, and potentially intervene at the site of airway obstruction with flexible nasolaryngoscopy prior to intubation.

Flexible nasolaryngoscopy can also aid in determining the treatment plan for a stridulous patient. If the cause is determined to be infectious (epiglottitis, bacterial tracheitis, etc.), then antibiotic therapy may be required. Inflammatory etiologies may be best managed with steroid treatment. In approximately 90% of patients, laryngomalacia can be conservatively managed, with surgical intervention usually reserved for those who have cyanotic spells, failure to thrive, and/or dysphagia.

Complications

Airway compromise
Respiratory failure
Failure to thrive
Pulmonary hypertension
Hypercapnia
Inability to intubate
Tracheostomy
Death

Key Points

- Stridor is a symptom and not a diagnosis. It is due to partial obstruction of the airway causing turbulent airflow.
- Knowing the anatomic and audiologic differences between stridor and stertor is helpful in making the correct diagnosis.
- When assessing a patient with laryngotracheal obstruction, it is important for the ED physician to accurately assess whether airway compromise is impending and if intubation is needed.
- Flexible nasolaryngoscopy is a safe procedure that can be performed at the bedside to help visualize the larynx and make the correct diagnosis and identify the location of laryngotracheal obstruction.

Further Reading

Otitis Externa

Rosenfeld RM, Schwartz SR, Cannon CR, et al. Clinical practice guideline: Acute otitis externa. *Otolaryngol Head Neck Surg.* 2014;150(1 Suppl):S1–S24.

Mastoiditis

King LM, Bartoces M, Hersh AL, Hicks LA, Fleming-Dutra KE. National incidence of pediatric mastoiditis in the United States, 2000–2012: Creating a baseline for public health surveillance. *Pediatr Infect Dis J.* 2019;38(1):e14–e16.

Laulajainen-Hongisto A, Saat R, Lempinen L, Aarnisalo AA, Jero J. Children hospitalized due to acute otitis media: How does this condition differ from acute mastoiditis? *Int J Pediatr Otorhinolaryngol.* 2015;79:1429–1435.

Marom T, Roth Y, Boaz M, et al. Acute mastoiditis in children: Necessity and timing of imaging. *Pediatr Infect Dis J.* 2016;35:30–34.

Inflammatory Neck Masses

Quinn NA, Olson JA, Meier JD, et al. Pediatric lateral neck infections: Computed tomography vs. ultrasound on initial evaluation. *Int J Pediatr Otorhinolaryngol.* 2018;109:149–153.

Quintanilla-Dieck L, Penn EB. Congenital neck masses. *Clin Perinatol.* 2018;45:769–785.

Rosenberg TL, Nolder AR. Pediatric cervical lymphadenopathy. *Otolaryngol Clin North Am.* 2014;47:721–731.

39

Ophthalmologic Emergencies

KATE KAUFMAN

COMPARISON WITH ADULT PHYSIOLOGY

The anatomy and size of the infant and child eye are surprisingly similar to those of the adult eye. In contrast to the 10-fold weight difference between an infant and a full-grown adult, there is only an approximately 1.8-mm difference between the corneal diameter of a neonate (10 mm) and that of an adult (11.8 mm). In addition, the orbit of an 18-month-old is approximately 75% the size of an adult orbit. Children, especially neonates, have a significantly less developed resistance to the systemic and central nervous system complications associated with ophthalmic infection and other ophthalmic findings.

PEDIATRIC EYE EXAMINATION TIPS

- Engage the child in a few minutes of play to gain trust
- Demonstrate the next step of the examination on an older sibling, a parent, or the child's doll
- When appropriate, touch equipment to the child's hand and then cheek to demonstrate it is not painful, then move on to the eye
- To test extraocular movements, have the child follow a moving toy or video; for an infant, have a parent move around and observe the eyes for tracking; "fix and follow" can roughly substitute for hand motion visual acuity, and "reacts to light" can roughly substitute for light perception
- To assess for abnormalities in neonates, dim the lights or block direct light to encourage opening of the eyes
- Saline can be dripped on a fluorescein strip directly into the eye or onto the medial canthus so it drains into the eye (child must be supine)
- Sometimes wide canthal folds can create the appearance of dysconjugate gaze; true dysconjugate gaze is unlikely if the corneal light reflex appears in the same spot on the cornea/iris in both eyes
- The eye may need to be pried open for full examination; a papoose and additional staff or parent are often required; sedation may be required in high-risk situations

CONJUNCTIVITIS

Conjunctivitis is by far the most common diagnosis for a pediatric eye-related emergency department (ED) visit and includes infectious, allergic, and chemical etiologies. Eye redness from bulbar conjunctival injection is the most defining feature of conjunctivitis. Other features include chemosis, inflammation of the palpebral conjunctiva, tearing, itching, foreign body sensation, and discharge. Mild blurriness is common; true vision changes suggest an alternative diagnosis. Most viral infections have associated upper respiratory infection symptoms. Bacterial conjunctivitis is relatively more common in children (especially under age 6 years-old), but usually self-resolves in 10–14 days without antibiotic drops. Clinical appearance is frequently indistinguishable between etiologies, and history may be more helpful for diagnosis (Table 39.1). Culture is only considered in resistant, recurrent, or severe cases. Test with fluorescein if there is concern for corneal involvement or a corneal abrasion. The American Academy of Pediatrics notes that conjunctivitis has transmission, duration, and disability similar to those of the common cold. Therefore, no recommendation is made for exclusion from school. However, many schools require 24 hours of antibiotic drops, or a doctor's note, before returning to class.

Differential Diagnosis

Adenovirus Pharyngoconjunctival Fever and Epidemic Keratoconjunctivitis

- Adenovirus is the most common cause of conjunctivitis when all age groups are considered; epidemics in day cares, schools, and universities
- Pharyngoconjunctival fever occurs in children; bilateral conjunctivitis, high fever 3–5 days, sore throat, malaise, headache, and tender preauricular lymphadenopathy
- Epidemic keratoconjunctivitis is most common in teens and adults less than 40 years old; severe injection (can include subconjunctival hemorrhage), chemosis, watery discharge, ipsilateral lymphadenopathy; progresses to bilateral in approximately 70% of cases; can cause pseudomembrane inside the lid (great diagnostic clue); lasts 7–21 days

TABLE 39.1 UTILITY OF CONJUNCTIVITIS SYMPTOMS FOR DETERMINING ETIOLOGY

Symptom	Significance
Lids stuck together in the morning	Factor most predictive of bacterial infection
Age <6 years	More likely bacterial (≥65%)
Copious purulent discharge	Suggests GC
Purulent discharge	Not helpful
Watery discharge	Slightly favors viral (including HSV) or allergic
Pseudomembrane on mucosal surface of lid	Adenovirus or GC
Purulent ear effusion	Conjunctivitis–otitis syndrome; nontypeable *H. influenzae*
Corneal lesion	HSV (ulcer, dendritic lesion) or GC (perforation)
Pain	HSV, enterovirus hemorrhagic conjunctivitis, corneal abrasion, uveitis
Preauricular lymphadenopathy	Suggests viral (but also includes GC and chlamydia)
Unilateral	May suggest viral (note adenovirus pharyngoconjunctival fever is bilateral) HSV and chlamydia commonly unilateral Allergic should not be unilateral
Bilateral	Not helpful
URI symptoms	Not helpful
Itching	Not helpful
Gradual onset, waxes and wanes, recurrent	Suggests allergic
Exposure to eye drops, pool, smoke, etc.	Chemical conjunctivitis

GC, gonococcus, HSV, herpes simplex virus, URI, upper respiratory infection.

Enterovirus/Coxsackie Hemorrhagic Conjunctivitis

- Pain; conjunctival petechiae that coalesce; highly contagious; self-limited (~7 days); complications rare

Herpes Simplex Virus (HSV) and Herpes Zoster Conjunctivitis and Keratitis

- Often unilateral; painful; surrounding skin may have vesicles or "punch lesions" but usually is normal
- Dendritic lesions with fluorescein examination confirm the diagnosis; full staining pattern may not be present
- Hutchinson's sign: preceding vesicle on the tip or side of nose (zoster affecting trigeminal nerve)
- Consider HSV when there is a failure to resolve with usual antibiotic treatment for conjunctivitis

Chlamydia Inclusion Conjunctivitis

- Spread by secretions and poor hand hygiene; children susceptible
- Question teens about sexual history, new partners, and concomitant urethritis or vaginitis
- Characterized by prominent follicles on the superior palpebral conjunctiva; may find a rough/bumpy appearance under the lid and failure to respond to routine ophthalmic antibiotics

Gonococcal Conjunctivitis

- Severe copious purulent discharge; hyperacute onset; ask about sexually transmitted infection history and urethritis/vaginitis
- Consider abuse, but an infected parent can inoculate a child through poor hand hygiene
- Neonatal cases decreasing due to maternal screening; cases in young men increasing due to epidemic

Conjunctivitis–Otitis Syndrome (Nontypeable *Haemophilus influenzae*)

- Classically, unilateral conjunctivitis with ipsilateral otitis media (but either feature can be bilateral)
- Commonly affects multiple children in a household (mimicking a viral pattern)
- *Haemophilus influenzae* type b vaccine is *not* protective

Perinaud Oculoglandular Syndrome

- Follicular conjunctivitis; impressive ipsilateral preauricular and submandibular lymphadenopathy; often fever and malaise
- *Bartonella* (cat scratch disease) is the most common cause; exposure to kittens imparts greatest risk
- Tularemia (rabbits and rural areas, higher fever, sicker patient); sporotrichosis (rose thorns or organic plant matter)
- Other causes are less common, including tuberculosis, syphilis, Epstein–Barr virus, leukemia, and lymphoma

Uveitis

- Deeper injection with ciliary flush/perilimbal involvement; painful; often miosis (see the section titled "Uveitis"; Figure 39.1)

Dacryostenosis (Obstructed Lacrimal sac/Nasolacrimal Duct)

- Epiphora (leakage of tears onto the face); the normal tear drainage is blocked by stenosis
- Light crusting or mild mucous discharge at the medial canthus
- Conjunctiva should be clear
- Skin over the lacrimal sac should be normal; erythema suggests dacryocystitis (infected lacrimal sac)

Atopic Keratoconjunctivitis

- History of atopic dermatitis and/or asthma; both eyes affected

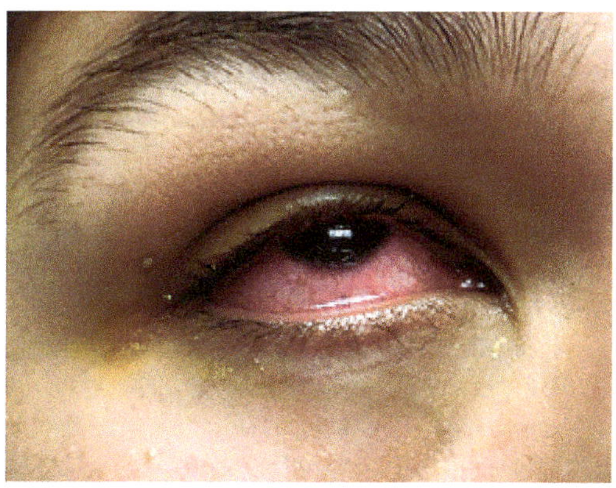

FIGURE 39.1 Uveitis with ciliary flush/perilimbal involvement.

- Year-round (nonseasonal) eye irritation and inflammation of bulbar and palpebral conjunctiva
- When severe, it can involve the cornea; fluorescein uptake

Kawasaki Disease

- Bilateral; perilimbal sparing; high fever >5 days; irritable or ill-appearing (see Chapter 24)

Treatment

See Table 39.2 which outlines treatment options for uncomplicated conjunctivits. A 7-day course is recommended for all of the regimens listed.

The Treatments for selected special cases of conjunctivitis are discussed below.

Chlamydia-Inclusion Conjunctivitis

- Oral azithromycin, one dose of 20 mg/kg (maximum 1 g)
- *Or* doxycycline 100 mg BID for 10 days (>8 years-old and 45 kg)
- For infants, use oral erythromycin 50 mg/kg/day divided QID for 14 days
- Add topical erythromycin ointment for 7 days

Gonococcal Conjunctivitis

- Ceftriaxone 50 mg/kg (maximum 1 g) given intramuscularly (IM) or intravenously (IV)
- Also cover for chlamydia with oral azithromycin or erythromycin

TABLE 39.2 COMMONLY PRESCRIBED TREATMENTS FOR UNCOMPLICATED CONJUNCTIVITIS[a]

Medication	Dosing	Comments
First-line Antibiotics		
Polymyxin B/trimethoprim (10,000 U/1 mg) per 1 mL solution	2 gtt QID	Common first-line agent
Erythromycin 0.5% ointment	½-in. ribbon BID–QID	Soothing effect for pain; greasy—blocks vision
Antibiotics for Contact Lens Users		
Ciprofloxacin 0.3% Ofloxacin 0.3%	2 gtt QID	Treat pseudomonas; first line for contact lens users; unnecessary in most uncomplicated cases
Moxifloxacin 0.5% Besifloxacin 0.6%	1 gtt TID	
Gentamicin 0.3%	½ in. or 2 gtt QID	Causes chemical irritation
Ocular Lubricants (all available over the counter)		
Purified water	1–2 gtt as needed	Helps with itching
Sodium chloride 0.9%	1–2 gtt as needed	
Sodium chloride 0.35% + hyetellose 0.44% (Natural Tears)	1–2 gtt as needed	
Mineral oil 42.5% + white petrolatum 57.3% (Lacri Lube)	¼ in. q3–4 hours as needed	Relieves dryness
Sodium carboxymethyl cellulose 0.25% drops	1–2 gtt as needed	Use thick gel form for overnight use
Sodium carboxymethyl cellulose 1% gel (Thera Tears)	¼ in. as needed	
Antihistamines		
Ketotifen 0.025% (= keto fumarate 0.035%) (Bausch+Lomb Children's Alaway is identical to regular Alaway—parents can buy either, or Zaditor)	1 gtt BID as needed (≥3 years old)	May have rebound effect with prolonged use but do not worsen infection
Naphazoline 0.027% + pheniramine 0.315% (Opcon-A, Visine-A, Naphcon-A)	1–2 gtt q6 hours as needed (≥6 years old)	More immediate rebound effect can occur

[a]Treat for 7 days.

Conjunctivitis–otitis Syndrome

- Treat with Augmentin; resistant to amoxicillin alone
- No additional antibiotic eye drops are needed

Key Points

- Approximately 60% of pediatric conjunctivitis includes bacterial involvement.
- Viral or bacterial conjunctivitis should self-resolve in 7–14 days.
- Treat with the least aggressive antibiotic and adjust management as needed.

Pitfalls

- Do not forget to consider gonococcus (GC) and chlamydia, especially in teens.
- Failure to recognize and treat uveitis can result in permanent eye damage.
- Signs of systemic illness can easily be missed.

NEONATAL CONJUNCTIVITIS (OPHTHALMIA NEONATORUM)

Neonatal conjunctivitis occurs within the first 30 days of life. It is predominantly contracted during birth from maternal vaginal flora; thus, sexually transmitted infections are a common cause. Other causes include chemical conjunctivitis and *Staphylococcus aureus.*

Most neonates will present to the emergency room with 1 or 2 days of eye redness and discharge without other symptoms. One or both eyes can be affected, and lid swelling may be present. The neonate may look well or ill-appearing. The most serious complications are sepsis and meningitis.

Differential Diagnosis

Chemical Conjunctivitis

- Day 1 of life
- Due to antibiotic prophylaxis, and less common now that erythromycin is used instead of silver nitrate
- Clear tearing due to irritation; can include mild lid swelling
- Scant or no discharge, absence of other symptoms, generally improves instead of worsening

Neisseria gonorrhea

- Days 2–5 of life
- Less than 1% of neonatal conjunctivitis in the developed world
- Severe copious mucopurulent discharge is suggestive of GC; watery discharge suggests against GC
- Systemic illness is more common

Chlamydia trachomatis

- Days 5–7 of life
- Most common, up to 40% of neonatal conjunctivitis; often a well-appearing infant
- Chlamydia conjunctivitis not only overlaps with the time frame of GC onset but also can be purulent and look identical to GC
- Milder case with lighter crusty discharge does suggest chlamydia

Herpes Virus

- Days 4–28 of life
- Mother may report a history of genital herpes or cold sores
- Watery discharge, injected eye; may appear ill or well
- Skin findings such as vesicles or "punch lesions" help confirm the diagnosis (but are frequently absent)
- Flourescein uptake may demonstrate dendritic lesions on the cornea (actually visualizing these lesions is difficult and probably impractical in a neonate, but lacey or patchy uptake is suspicious)
- Seizure or neurologic finding is also very suggestive of a herpetic infection

Staphylococcus aureus, Streptococcus pneumoniae, nontypable *H. influenzae*

- No specific timing; increasingly prevalent or increasingly recognized
- Purulent discharge; risk of bacteremia

Blocked Lacrimal Duct (Dacryocystocele)

- Tearing without conjunctival injection
- No fever or other symptoms
- A pink or bluish papule/cyst may be seen at medial canthus
- No treatment necessary; ophthalmologist probing or surgical repair if not self-resolved

Dacryocystitis

- Infection of the nasolacrimal gland, most common in neonates
- Erythema and edema/fullness/firmness in the space between medial canthus and nose

- High risk of complications including meningitis; (see section titled "Periorbital Cellulitis, Orbital Cellulitis, and Dacryocystitis")

Treatment

Treatment should be initiated immediately (Table 39.3), and laboratory confirmation may not be obtained in many cases. If possible, a Gram stain and culture of the discharge should be sent. A negative Gram stain does not rule out GC. Admitted infants should also have blood cultures, and a febrile or ill-appearing neonate requires a lumbar puncture. Testing for HIV and syphilis should also be performed.

Disposition

Chemical Conjunctivitis

- Rarely seen by providers outside of the newborn nursery
- Use great caution in deciding that an infectious cause is not suspected
- Can discharge home; advise recheck in 8–12 hours

Chlamydia Conjunctivitis

- May discharge home if the conjunctivitis is mild, the infant has no fever, the infant is feeding well, the infant seems otherwise normal to both the mother and the provider, and the caregiver is reliable
- Admit if the above criteria cannot be confirmed
- Follow up with pediatrician in 1 day
- Ophthalmologist if not resolved in 1 week

GC/HSV/Staph/Dacryocystitis/ Unclear Cause

- Admit or transfer to a facility with pediatric specialty care; involve ophthalmology

TABLE 39.3 TREATMENT FOR NEONATAL CONJUNCTIVITIS

Etiology	Day of Life	Topical	Systemic
Chemical	1	None or lubricant	n/a
GC	2–5	Saline lavage q2h Erythromycin ointment	Ceftriaxone 25–50 mg/kg ×1 dose IM/IV (maximum 125 mg)[a] *Or* Cefotaxime 100 mg/kg ×1 dose IM/IV
Chlamydia	5–14	Erythromycin ointment	Erythromycin 50 mg/kg/day PO divided QID ×14 days No. 1 CDC recommendation, No. 2 WHO[b] *Or* Azithromycin 20 mg/kg daily ×3 days IV/PO No. 1 WHO recommendation, No. 2 CDC[b]
Staph infection		Erythromycin ointment *or* Flouroquinolone	Cefotaxime 50–100 mg/kg IM/IV *Add* clindamycin or vancomycin if MRSA suspected
HSV	4–28	Gancyclovir *or* Trifluridine/vidarabine	Acyclovir 20 mg/kg IV
Septic		Erythromycin ointment	Ampicillin 50–100 mg/kg IV + Cefotaxime 50–100 mg/kg IV *Add* acyclovir if vesicles, seizure, neuro Consider cefotaxime + vancomycin for skin or soft tissue

[a]Ceftriaxone ×1 is a WHO and CDC recommendation. In many US pediatric centers, cefotaxime is preferred for infants younger than 44 weeks gestational age. By definition, essentially all cases of neonatal conjunctivitis are in patients younger than age 44 weeks.
[b]WHO cites a risk of pyloric stenosis when erythromycin is used in infants younger than age 6 weeks as the reason for recommending azithromycin. The CDC notes that both erythromycin and azithromycin have been linked to pyloric stenosis and recommends monitoring infants who have had either treatment.
CDC, Centers for Disease Control and Prevention; GC, gonococcus, HSV, herpes simplex virus; IM, intramuscularly; IV, intravenously; MRSA, methicillin-resistant Staphylococcus aureus; n/a, not applicable; WHO, World Health Organization.

Key Points

- Neonatal conjunctivitis is serious and requires systemic treatment; many cases should be admitted.
- Fever or ill appearance requires septic workup and lumbar puncture.
- Onset in the first 4 days makes GC more likely.
- Add acyclovir if conjunctivitis is accompanied by a neurologic finding.
- Well infants with suspected chlamydia can be treated as outpatients with close follow-up.

Pitfalls

- Even mild neonatal conjunctivitis should not be treated with topical medication only.
- Failure to treat associated sepsis or meningitis can result in neonatal death.

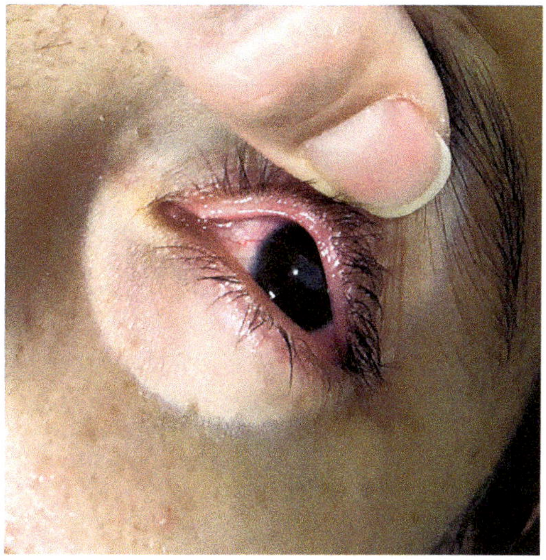

FIGURE 39.2 Corneal ulcer in a teen with suspected lupus.

KERATITIS AND CORNEAL ULCERS

Keratitis is an inflammation of the cornea. The greatest risk factor is contact lens-related infection, followed by trauma and, less commonly, immunocompromise. Children are at greater risk for long-term vision complications.

Keratitis shares many symptoms with conjunctivitis, including redness, itching, and foreign body sensation. Patients with keratitis almost always complain of some form of blurry vision, and they can also have significant pain and photophobia. A past medical history of diabetes, rheumatoid arthritis, transplant, steroid use, or other immunosuppression should raise the provider's suspicion that a red eye could be something more than simple conjunctivitis.

Examination reveals an injected eye and some sort of corneal irregularity. Corneal signs include stippling observed with fluorescein, white stippling visible with the naked eye or slit lamp, clouding/edema of the cornea, a white "immune ring" formed on the cornea by reactive infiltrates, and frank corneal ulcer. With progressive infection, a hypopyon may be visible on examination. Confirming a diagnosis of herpes, fungus, or acanthamoeba requires special culture and staining by an ophthalmologist. A corneal ulcer is due to erosion of the cornea. Infection is the most common cause. Other causes include allergic keratitis, trauma, thermal and chemical burns, and chronic irritation from entropion. Corneal ulcers (Figure 39.2) can arise during the course of conjunctivitis/keratitis or, in less common presentations, the only complaint is that the child or parent notices a white spot on the cornea.

Treatment

Aggressive and frequent topical treatment is required for any infection that involves the cornea. Severe cases will require specialized administration of antibiotics such as subconjunctival and intrastromal injection. Additional systemic treatment is sometimes required. Cycloplegics can be used for pain and to reduce scarring. Steroids are controversial because they may decrease inflammation but also have the potential to worsen infection. Admission may be required in severe cases. Urgent ophthalmology follow-up is required. Consider testing for HIV.

Bacterial Keratitis, Corneal Ulcer, and Initial Empiric Treatment

- Use a broad-coverage antibiotic; solutions penetrate better than ointments
- *Topical* fluoroquinolones can be used in children without concern
- See Table 39.4

HSV and Herpes Zoster Keratitis

- Initiate aggressive oral and topical antiviral regimen

TABLE 39.4 COMMONLY PRESCRIBED ANTIBIOTICS FOR KERATITIS OR CORNEAL ULCER

Antibiotic	Dosing	Comments
Besifloxacin 0.6% Gatifloxacin 0.5% Moxifloxacin 0.5%	Day 1 1 gtt q30–60 min 1 gtt q1h overnight Days 2 and 3 1 gtt q1h Day 4+ Per ophthalmologist	q15min loading *not* required More limited insurance coverage
Ciprofloxacin 0.3%	Day 1 2 gtt (½ inch) q15 min for 6h then q30 min while awake and q1h overnight Day 2 2 gtt (½ in.) q1h while awake Day 3+ 2 gtt (½ in.) q4h while awake	Considered less potent Better insurance coverage
Ofloxacin 0.3%	Days 1 and 2 1 gtt q30min while awake 1 gtt q4h overnight Day 3+ 1gtt q1h while awake	Considered less potent Usually covered by insurance
Levofloxacin 0.5%	Day 1 1 gtt q30min while awake 1gtt q2h overnight Days 2 and 3 1 gtt q1–2h while awake 1 gtt q4h overnight Day 4+ 1 gtt q2–4h while awake	
Cefazolin or vancomycin *plus* tobramycin or gentamicin	Load with 1–2 gtt q5–15min for 4 doses then q1h	Has been replaced by quinolones An alternative in certain settings
Ceftriaxone IV	50 mg/kg (maximum 1 g) IM or IV	If gonococcus suspected

IM, intramuscularly; IV, intravenously.

- Avoid steroids until after antivirals have been initiated and patient sees ophthalmology
- Check intraocular pressure (IOP) and consult ophthalmology if elevated
- Commonly prescribed antivirals for HSV and varicella zoster virus (VZV) are presented in Table 39.5.

Complications

Acute complications of keratitis and corneal ulcers are intraocular infection and corneal perforation. Long-term complications include scarring, astigmatism, and permanent vision loss. During the neuro-ophthalmologic development period from birth until 8 years-old, temporary vision loss from a corneal opacity can lead to amblyopia.

Key Points

- Keratitis and corneal ulcers are emergent conditions that require aggressive treatment.
- Treat immediately with broad-spectrum topical antibiotics.
- Emergent or urgent ophthalmology involvement is indicated.

TABLE 39.5 COMMONLY PRESCRIBED ANTIVIRALS FOR HSV AND VZV

Medication	Dosing	Duration
	Oral	
Acyclovir	20 mg/kg/dose PO QID If ≥40 kg, then 400 mg 5×/day If zoster present, then maximum 800 mg QID	7–14 days
Famciclovir	250 mg PO TID (not approved for children younger than age 12 years)	7–14 days
Valacyclovir	20 mg/kg/dose PO BID If >45 kg, then 1 g BID	5–14 days
	Topical	
Acyclovir 3% solution or ointment	½ in. 5–9×/day	Lacks data for children younger than age 2 years
Ganciclovir 0.15% gel	½ in. 5×/day	Lacks data for children younger than age 2 years
Trifluridine 1% (Viroptic)	Not preferred	Only approved for children older than age 6 years

HSV, herpes simplex virus; VZV, varicella zoster virus.

Pitfalls

- Missing early corneal abnormalities and settling on a diagnosis of conjunctivitis delays vision-preserving treatment.
- Discharging patients without ensuring they have access to antibiotic drops and explaining the complicated regimen will result in treatment failure.
- Failure to facilitate immediate or very prompt follow-up with an ophthalmologist also delays definitive care.

UVEITIS

Uveitis—the inflammation of the iris, ciliary body, and/or choroid—is less common in children but is still an important consideration when evaluating the red eye. Delayed diagnosis increases the risk of damage to the lens, retina, and optic nerve. Most cases are idiopathic, with traumatic iritis, HSV-1/2, and VZV also being common. The most common autoimmune cause in children is juvenile idiopathic arthritis.

Uveitis presents as injection of one eye or, less commonly, both eyes. Significant pain and lack of discharge are distinguishing features. Traumatic iritis typically appears a few days after the trauma. Examination includes ciliary flush (i.e., no perilimbal sparing; see Figure 39.1) and often miosis with lack of normal dilation when the lights are dimmed. Consensual photophobia is often present. A slit lamp examination can be used to detect cells (tiny, slightly white/gray, ghost-like leukocytes floating in the aqueous humor) or flare (smoky appearance of aqueous humor caused by protein/exudate). Leukocytes can settle and cause a hypopyon. Classic findings for HSV uveitis include dendritic lesions on fluorescein examination, increased IOP, and a layered collection of hypopyon and hyphema known as a "candy cane hypopyon." Complications of uveitis include scarring, glaucoma, cataract, and blindnesss. HSV can cause acute retinal necrosis, which is treated with IV acyclovir.

Treatment

Topical steroids constitute the principal treatment for uveitis, including that caused by HSV. See Table 39.6 for initial treatment guidelines. Nonsteroidal anti-inflammatory drugs can help relieve pain and inflammation. Arrange urgent follow-up with an ophthalmologist.

Key Points

- Uveitis is a serious condition that can lead to blindness.
- Children with autoimmune disease are at higher risk for uveitis.

TABLE 39.6 INITIAL TREATMENT FOR UVEITIS

Medication	Dosing	Comments
	Steroids	
Prednisolone acetate 1%	1 gtt ql–2h	Mainstay of treatment
Oral prednisolone 15mg/5mL	1 mg/kg PO Daily	Add if autoimmune disease present
	Cycloplegics	
Homatropine 5%	1 gtt BID-TID	Decrease photophobia and synechiae
Tropicamide 0.5%	1gtt q4–6h	
Cyclopentolate 1%	1gtt BID-TID	
	Antivirals	
Use oral antivirals	Various PO regimens	Add for suspected HSV; topical drops do *not* sufficiently penetrate the AC

Pitfalls

- Overlooking the key signs of ciliary flush, miosis, and consensual photophobia can lead the examiner to miss the diagnosis of uveitis.
- Do not discharge a patient with uveitis without starting steroid and cycloplegic therapy.

EYELID LESIONS

Hordeolum (Stye)

- Among the most common lid lesions presenting to a pediatric ED
- Caused by local infection of the gland of Zeiss (sebaceous gland of the eyelash hair follicle)
- Presents with a round erythematous mass on the eyelid margin
- Often painful
- May have discharge from the exit of the gland or from erosion of the overlying skin
- May cause conjunctival irritation if the lesion affects the mucosa or interrupts the lid margin
- Most common infectious etiology is staph (90–95%)

Treatment: erythromycin or mupirocin ointment and warm compresses applied to the eye for 10–15 minutes, three or four times a day

Chalazion

- Can be similar in presentation to the hordeolum but generally farther away from the lid margin
- Caused by obstruction or inflammation of a meibomian gland (exocrine gland that secretes an oily product to prevent evaporation of the tear film)
- More likely to have normal overlying skin (i.e., a bump on the lid but without erythema)
- Often painless unless infected or under pressure

Treatment: warm compresses, ophthalmology referral for resistant cases

Molluscum Contagiosum

- Caused by the poxvirus molluscum contagiosum; spread by touching or fomites, but with variable levels of transmission similar to that of warts
- One or more small skin-colored or pearly umbilicated lesions on the eyelid; may have a waxy discharge
- May or may not have lesions elsewhere on the body; 10–20 papules throughout body is not uncommon

Treatment: clears on its own in 12–18 months in most cases

Dermoid Cyst

- One of the most common orbital masses in children
- Appears under the brow or can present as a round mass protruding at the canthus of the eye
- Often appears in infancy as a tiny lump which later rapidly expands
- Round shape—can feel soft and rubbery or firm and immobile

Treatment: surgical resection while the cyst is still small, thus avoiding damage to nearby structures as the mass enlarges

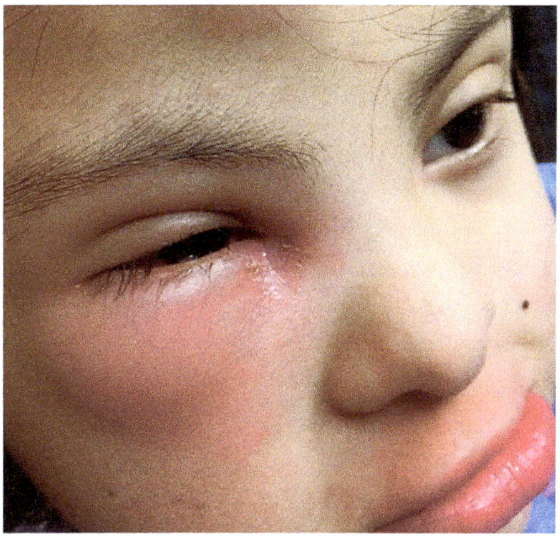

FIGURE 39.3 Periorbital cellulitis.

PERIORBITAL CELLULITIS, ORBITAL CELLULITIS, AND DACRYOCYSTITIS

Periorbital cellulitis (Figure 39.3), also known as preseptal cellulitis, can appear clinically similar to orbital cellulitis but only affects the tissues anterior to the orbital septum. Both conditions predominantly affect children and present as erythema and edema around the eye, with or without a preceding lesion or illness. Asymptomatic sinusitis is a common inciting factor. The more serious diagnosis of orbital cellulitis includes involvement posterior to the orbital septum and ranges from inflammatory changes to abscess, either periosteal or filling the orbital space. Current vaccination strategies and associated herd immunity have significantly decreased the incidence of orbital cellulitis. Table 39.7 summarizes the clinical differences between periorbital and orbital cellulitis. Definitive diagnosis is made by CT scan.

Dacryocystitis is an infection of the lacrimal sac that mimics periorbital cellulitis, and almost exclusively affects neonates. It is usually secondary to nasolacrimal duct obstruction and carries a high risk of complications.

Differential Diagnosis

Dacryocystitis

- Affects patients in the first 1 or 2 weeks of life (Figure 39.4)
- Erythema, edema, tenderness in the triangle between the nose and the medial portion of the lower lid
- Palpation of the area may express purulent drainage at the inferior lacrimal punctum
- History may include pre-exiting plethora (excessive tearing)

TABLE 39.7 CHARACTERISTICS OF PERIORBITAL AND ORBITAL CELLULITIS

Periorbital Cellulitis	Orbital Cellulitis
Usually well-appearing	Well-appearing or ill
No visual change	± visual change
Fever less common; vomiting rare	Fever and vomiting more common
Possible preceding superficial lid lesion, insect bite, trauma, maxillary tooth dental abscess	More commonly a deeper infection source such as sinusitis or trauma with fracture
88% have none of the signs of orbital cellulitis listed below	Any of the signs below suggests orbital cellulitis and dictates CT orbits or CT maxillofacial
Presence of any sign dictates CT for diagnosis	*All signs may be absent*; still maintain a high degree of suspicion in an ill child and obtain CT
Symptoms and Signs Significantly Associated with Orbital Cellulitis	
Proptosis	
Decreased visual acuity (or changes in color vision)	
Abnormal pupillary reflex	
Diplopia or ophthalmoplegia	
Pain with extraocular movements (with or without limitation in the movements)	
Chemosis	

CT, computed tomography.

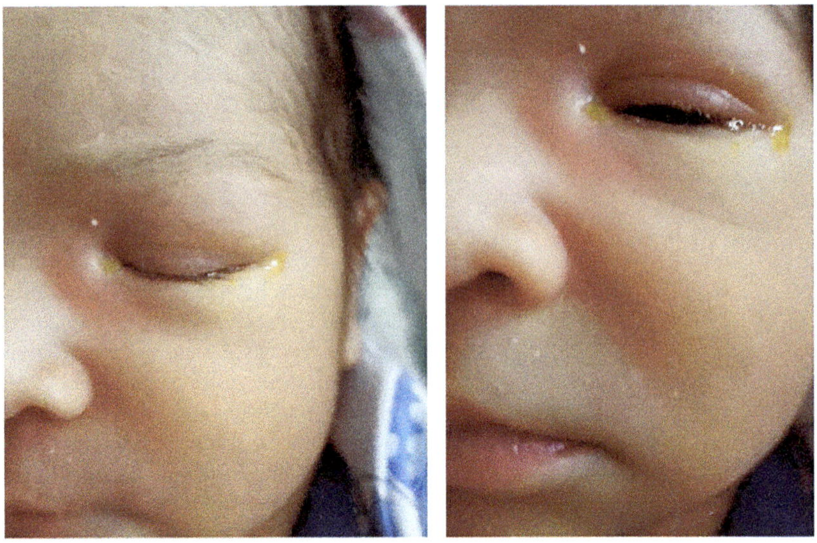

FIGURE 39.4 Dacryocystitis.

- May be febrile or septic; even mild-appearing cases carry a high risk of becoming febrile or septic

Treatment

In the post-*H. influenzae* era, *Staph. aureus* and *Streptococcus* species are the most common etiologies. Coverage must also include group A *Streptococcus* and, increasingly, methicillin-resistant *Staph. aureus* (MRSA). Specific treatment recommendations vary by institution and local susceptibilities.

Periorbital Cellulitis

- Trial of PO antibiotics if well-appearing, afebrile, age more than 1 year
- Clindamycin 10 mg/kg/dose (maximum 600 mg) PO TID for 7–10 days
- Alternative: amoxicillin–clavulanate 45 mg/kg/dose of amoxicillin component (maximum 1,000 mg) PO BID

Plus trimethoprim–sulfamethoxazole 4–6 mg/kg/dose of trimethoprim component (maximum 160 mg) PO BID

- Severe or worsening cases require admission and IV cephalosporin + vancomycin

Orbital Cellulitis

- Admit for IV antibiotics
- Ampicillin–sulbactam 50 mg/kg/dose of ampicillin component (maximum 2 g) IV q6h (age 1 year or older)
- Severe or suspect MRSA: add vancomycin 15 mg/kg/dose IV q6–8h
- Alternative (includes age younger than 1 year): ceftriaxone + vancomycin
- Consult ophthalmology; possible surgical drainage but many resolve with IV antibiotics alone; emergent decompression if IOP is elevated (see section titled "Orbital Compartment Syndrome")

Dacryocystitis

- Neonates are not yet vaccinated for *H. influenzae* or *Strep. pneumoniae*
- Neonates are at high risk for bacteremia and meningitis; initiate septic work-up
- Ampicillin 100 mg/kg/dose IV q8–12h (can reduce to 50 mg/kg/dose if lumbar puncture negative)

Plus gentamicin 5 mg/kg/dose IV q24h (adjust dose for preemies as per facility protocol)

- Alternative: cefotaxime or ceftazidime 50 mg/kg/dose IV q8h +

Plus vancomycin 15 mg/kg/dose IV q8–12h

- Alternative to vancomycin in a well-appearing infant: clindamycin 8 mg/kg/dose IV q8h
- Older children can be treated as periorbital cellulitis; consider atypical cause if not resolving
- Urgent ophthalmology consultation; probing to open nasolacrimal duct after antibiotics initiated

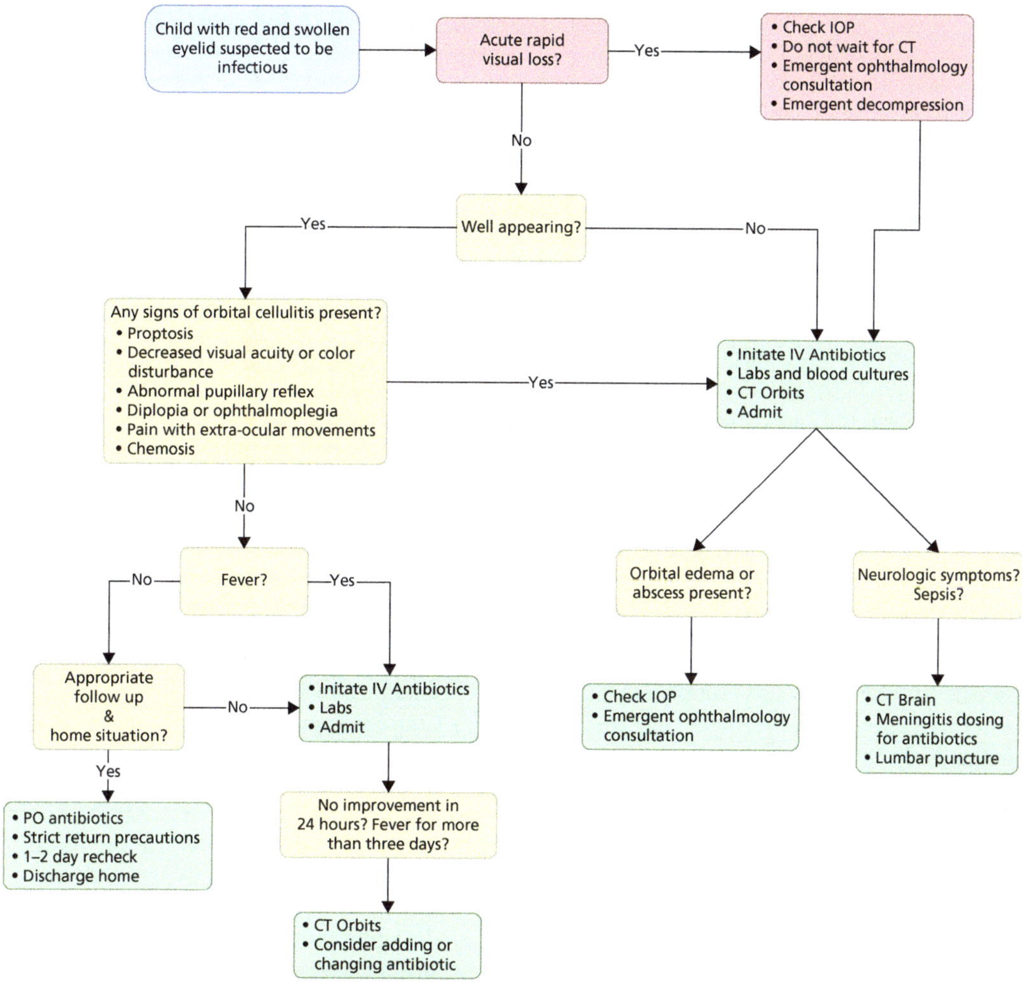

FIGURE 39.5 Clinical algorithm for a child with a red or swollen eyelid. APD, afferent pupillary defect; CT, computed tomography; IOP, intraocular pressure; IV, intravenous.

Clinical Algorithm

See Figure 39.5 for a clinical algorithm for a child with a red or swollen eyelid.

Complications

Complications of soft tissue infection around the eye include orbital abscess, orbital compartment syndrome with optic nerve and retinal ischemia, blindness, cavernous sinus thrombosis (rule out if there is bilateral eyelid edema), intracranial abscess, and sepsis.

Key Points

- Neonates with dacryocystitis, periorbital cellulitis, or orbital cellulitis should be admitted for broad-spectrum antibiotics and septic workup.
- Any sign of orbital cellulitis, most commonly pain with eye movements, warrants a CT scan and IV treatment for orbital cellulitis.
- Mild cases of periorbital cellulitis can be treated with PO antibiotics.

Pitfalls

- Failure to search for and recognize signs of orbital cellulitis can result in vision loss or progression to brain abscess.
- Do not miss a dental abscess that is causing periorbital cellulitis. Extraction may be required in order for treatment to be effective.

- Neonatal dacryocystitis is not a minor blocked tear duct or a localized periorbital cellulitis. Affected infants can quickly become septic.

CORNEAL ABRASIONS AND EYE FOREIGN BODIES

Symptoms include sudden onset of tearing and an irritated eye that often becomes red. A history of scratching the eye or being hit with a foreign object or a flying insect may be reported. Patients with corneal abrasion often have a foreign body sensation even when the offending object did not remain in the eye.

Some corneal abrasions can be seen with the naked eye, and all can be easily diagnosed with fluorescein staining and a cobalt blue light or Wood's lamp (Figure 39.6).

To evaluate for a foreign body, start by examining the eye with a light from several different angles. Retract the eyelids, and use a cotton swab to help evert the upper lid; inspect the fornices and subtarsal mucosa. Saline irrigation of the fornices may flush the foreign body into view. Slit lamp examination is indicated and allows detection of tiny corneal foreign bodies. If an embedded foreign body is found, use a fluorescein examination to evaluate for globe rupture (Seidel sign). A tiny brown rust ring visualized on the cornea with a slit lamp is a classic finding; it indicates the presence of a small metal foreign body embedded in the cornea at the center of the ring.

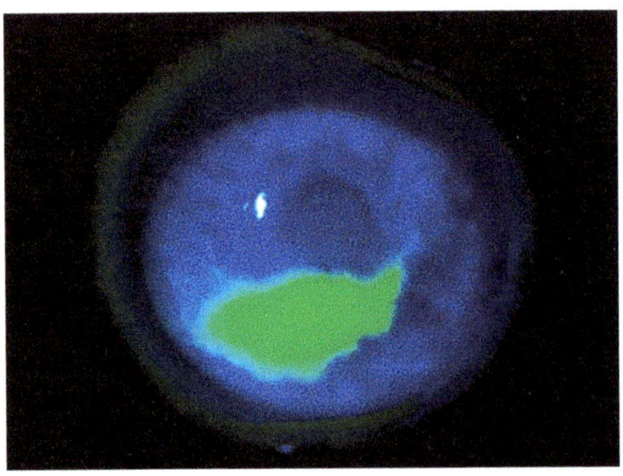

FIGURE 39.6 Fluorescein staining demonstrating a corneal abrasion.

Source: Roots J. Nonpenetrating eye injuries in children. *Clin Pediatr Emerg Med.* 2017;18(1):74–86. Reproduced with permission.

Treatment

Corneal Abrasion

- There is evidence that no treatment is necessary; good option especially if <1 mm
- Standard treatment consists of prophylactic antibiotics; ointment is soothing and may be preferred
- Always use antibiotics in contact lens users
- No benefit to patching the eye; randomized control study in children found increased discomfort and more trouble walking
- Studies also show cycloplegics have no benefit for pain or healing

Foreign Body

- Use anesthetic drops to increase tolerance of foreign body removal
- Loose foreign bodies can be flushed out with saline; retract the lids to inspect and irrigate the fornices
- Moisten a cotton swab so that the fibers will not stick to the eye; use the tip to retrieve the foreign body; press down gently on the foreign body and avoid dragging motions, especially across the cornea
- If a small child with a subtarsal foreign body is uncooperative, try having the parents pull the upper lid down over the lower lid and then releasing it; lower lashes may dislodge the foreign body
- If any corneal abrasion is present, it should be treated as discussed previously

Foreign Body in the Cornea

- Anesthetize the eye
- Use a 21-gauge needle to scoop out the foreign body; needle should be bevel out; the approach is parallel or "flat on" to the corneal surface—that is, angled in such a way that puncture into the globe will not likely occur
- If during removal the foreign body is deeper than expected or difficult, reapply fluorescein afterward to look for any sign of globe rupture

- The procedure is not different in a toddler and can be performed under ketamine sedation
- Discharge with antibiotic ointment; lubricating drops; ibuprofen

Key Points

- Most providers treat corneal abrasions with antibiotics.
- Many foreign bodies can be removed in the ED.

Pitfalls

- Kids are not great historians, so do not skip the fluorescein examination.
- Failure to recognize full-thickness penetration of a foreign body through the cornea, thereby an open globe, can lead to infection or vision loss.

SUBCONJUNCTIVAL HEMORRHAGE

Most presentations include a well-appearing patient with bright red blood in a localized area of one eye (see Figure 39.7). Bilateral cases can occur. The dramatic appearance of the blood leads to parental alarm. There may be a history of trauma, vomiting, or forceful coughing, or there may be no history at all. Small children cannot report a history of rubbing the eye or a minor trauma that occurred without the parent's knowledge.

Underlying abuse or comorbidities should be considered. Provide reassurance and education that resolution takes weeks but occurs without additional treatment.

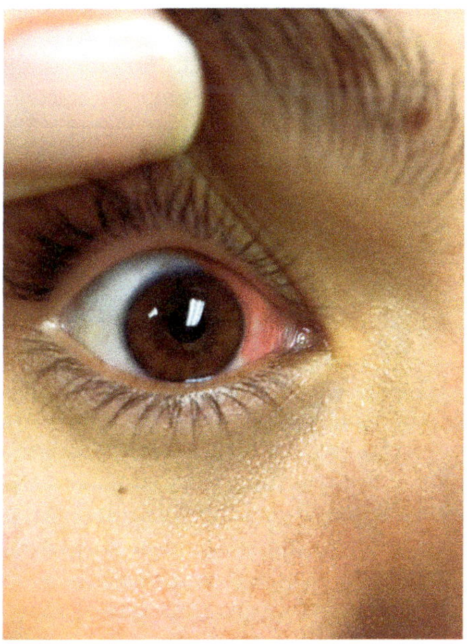

FIGURE 39.7 Subconjunctival hemorrhage.

TRAUMA

Selected Diagnoses

Eyebrow and Eyelid Lacerations

- The least concerning wounds involve the eyebrow or areas adjacent to the eyelids
- Wounds on the eyelid, but not involving the tarsal plate or the lid margin, require careful consideration
- Most concerning are the lacerations that disrupt the lid margin, penetrate the tarsal plate, or communicate with the mucosal surface of the eyelid
- If necessary, immobilize or sedate the child and manipulate the lids in order to see the full extent of a laceration, especially when it is hidden in the canthus
- In a deep upper lid laceration, look for ptosis, which could indicate levator muscle injury

Traumatic Hyphema

- Hemorrhage inside the globe; painful eye caused by blunt trauma (90% during play at home); the eye may or may not be injected
- A collection of blood is visible in the AC; usually appears as a small red crescent at the inferior rim of the cornea; with careful inspection, many small hyphemas can be seen without a slit lamp
- If blood level overlies the pupil, it can physically block vision; an "eight-ball" hyphema fills the entire AC
- Blood can clog the trabecular network and cause elevated IOP; nausea, if present, is a suggestive sign

Retinal Detachment

- Injury causing the retina to separate from the choroid and thus lose its blood supply
- Commonly presents as visual disturbance after a blow to the eye or

head; older children may be able to describe flashes of light, or a curtain or shadow over the visual field
- Outward examination is usually normal; fundus examination may detect a wavy or rippled and pale area
- Bedside ultrasound has excellent diagnostic sensitivity and specificity
- Due to young resilient tissues, retinal detachment is much less common in children

Ruptured Globe (Open Globe Injury)

- An injury that perforates the eyeball and creates an external exposure to the intraocular contents
- For pediatric cases of open globe, penetrating trauma is much more common than blunt trauma
- Obvious examination findings include deflated or sunken globe, imbedded foreign body, laceration of the cornea, peaked pupil, iridodialysis (separated space between a portion of the iris and the surrounding white rim of sclera), and uveal prolapse of iris extruded through the cornea (40–70% of cases)
- Full-thickness lid laceration should cause high suspicion for open globe
- Less obvious or less specific findings are hyphema (30%), afferent pupillary defect (20%), and hemorrhagic chemosis
- IOP <10 mmHg is highly suspicious; do not check pressure if there are other confirmatory signs
- Fluorescein may demonstrate Seidel's sign (aqueous humor exiting a wound in the globe creates a river-like clearing of the fluorescein stain)

Orbital Blowout Fracture

- Fracture of the bony orbit; usually the inferior wall
- Pain and swelling around the eye after blunt trauma; assault most common
- Evaluate carefully for signs and symptoms of extraocular muscle entrapment; untreated this leads to muscle ischemia and permanent limitation of eye movement
- Diplopia present in approximately 55% of pediatric cases; ocular movement restriction in approximately 55%
- Associated nausea predicts entrapment; enophthalmos is rare, and ecchymosis is less common in children
- CT is diagnostic

Retrobulbar Hematoma

- Bleeding in the confined orbital cavity behind the globe, which can put pressure on optic structures
- Visual disturbance (especially diplopia), blindness or proptosis after trauma to the eye; may be painful or painless
- Exam may show periorbital trauma or be fairly normal
- Afferent pupillary defect is a serious finding indicating ischemia of the optic nerve, and mandates emergent treatment
- Blood in the orbit is easily seen on CT, but clinical findings and elevated IOP are the most important diagnostic findings
- IOP ≥40 mmHg mandates emergent treatment

Orbital Foreign Body

- Patient may present with a visible foreign body in the eye, or may report a suspicious penetrating injury with a "missing" foreign object such as a BB or the end of a stick that broke off and can't be found (Figure 39.8)
- May have neurological symptoms if the object penetrated the orbit into the cranium
- CT is excellent for detecting metallic foreign bodies in the globe or orbit
- High clinical suspicion warrants ophthalmology involvement regardless of imaging results

Treatment

Eyebrow and Eyelid Lacerations

- Eyebrow lacerations can be repaired with tissue glue or sutures
- Lacerations on the lid that do not involve the lid margin, tarsal plate, or mucosal surface can be repaired in the ED; use 6-0 fast-absorbing gut and take care that a shallow approach is used so that the sutures do not violate deeper structures; sedation may be required
- Lacerations involving the tarsal plate, the mucosal surface, or the lid margin

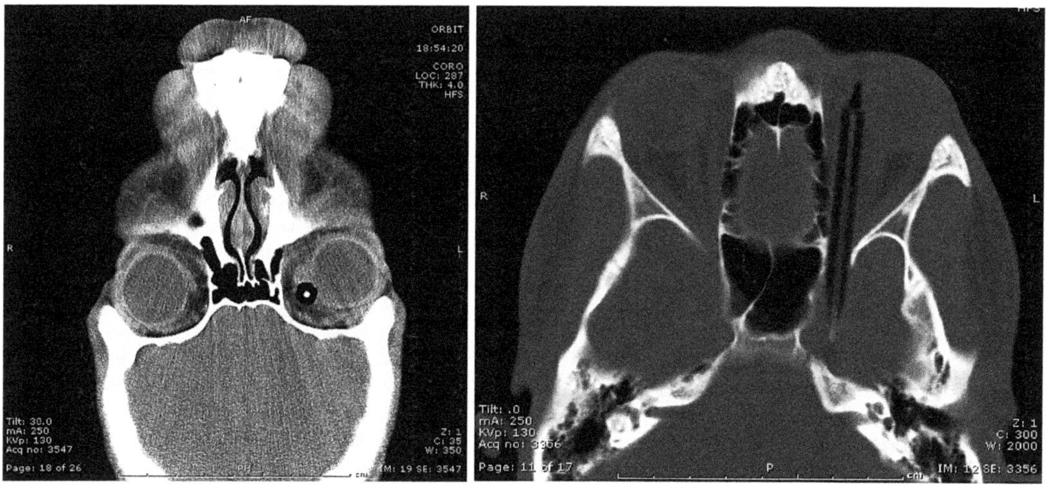

FIGURE 39.8 Foreign body (pencil) penetrating the globe and passing into the cranium. No foreign object was visible on examination, but the left pupil was blown.

require evaluation and repair by an ophthalmologist within a few hours

- Lid margin repair complications include overflow of tears due to structural damage, as well as eye irritation and corneal inflammation from lid scarring
- No prophylactic antibiotics are indicated

Hyphema

- Elevate head of bed to 30° or more; this allows blood to settle in the bottom of the AC and avoid obscuring the pupil
- Can worsen or recur; consult ophthalmology for possible inpatient monitoring
- Reverse coagulopathies; control nausea to avoid increased IOP from vomiting; pain control
- Treat increased IOP >21 mmHg with medication such as timolol 1% eye drops; consult ophthalmology; if medication is not effective, then surgical decompression is needed
- Do not use cycloplegics unless the IOP is controlled, because retraction of the iris toward the ciliary body can worsen obstruction of the trabecular meshwork
- After consultation with an ophthalmologist, cycloplegic medication such as cyclopentolate 1% may be part of management
- Patients with sickle cell disease have an increased complication rate, and acetazolamide use is contraindicated

Retinal Detachment

- Requires laser or surgical repair as soon as possible (particularly if the macula is not yet involved in the detachment); consult ophthalmology immediately
- Best result with surgical repair within 24–48 hours

Ruptured Globe (Open Globe Injury)

- Leave any projectile in place
- Elevate head of bed; bed rest with no bending, lifting, or Valsalva; NPO; antiemetic
- Immediate ophthalmology consultation
- Systemic antibiotics; cefazolin 50 mg/kg IV (maximum 1–2 g)
- If intraocular foreign body, give ceftazidime 30–50 mg/kg (maximum 1 g) + vancomycin 10 mg/kg (maximum 500 mg)

Orbital Blowout Fracture

- Surgical repair is required if there is evidence of entrapment
- Emergent decompression is required if there is evidence of orbital compartment syndrome
- NPO; pain control; antiemetics as needed

- Non-displaced fractures without entrapment or vision change do not require intervention
- Prophylactic antibiotics are commonly given (but there is little evidence to support this practice)

Retrobulbar Hematoma

- If no vision loss and no increased IOP, no treatment is needed but patient must be monitored
- Emergent decompression for increased IOP or deterioration of vision (see below)
- Decompression within 60–90 minutes from the onset of symptoms has the best outcome; if treated within 3 hours, approximately 80% of patients regain baseline vision, as opposed to 10% if treated after 3 hours
- Medical therapy (mannitol, acetazolamide, steroids) is *not* effective and should not be used

Orbital Foreign Body

- Ophthalmology consultation for surgical removal
- Neurosurgery consultation if the object enters the intracranial space
- Ceftriaxone 50 mg/kg IV (maximum 1–2 g)
- Address causes of elevated IOP if present

Orbital Compartment Syndrome

- Increased pressure inside the confines of the orbit, caused by retrobulbar hematoma or post-traumatic edema; leads to ischemia of nerve/muscle/ retina
- Requires emergent lateral canthotomy and cantholysis by ED provider (see section titled "Orbital Compartment Syndrome")

Fox Shield (Rigid Eye Shield)

- Convex metal disc with perforations used to protect an injured eye
- Use for hyphema, open globe, intraocular foreign body, possibly retinal detachment
- The idea is to protect from any pressure on the globe, so the edges should rest on the bones around the eye; do not put gauze or a soft patch underneath
- Use a paper cup or other improvised device if a shield is not available

Tetanus

- Tetanus status should be verified and/ or updated for all of the eye injuries discussed previously.

Clinical Algorithm

Figure 39.9 provides a clinical algorithm for the management of a child with orbital trauma.

Key Points

- Orbital compartment syndrome is the most urgent diagnosis in eye trauma.
- Globe rupture and retinal detachment are time-sensitive emergencies and require emergent ophthalmology consultation.
- Many cases of hyphema should be admitted and followed by ophthalmology.
- Most lid lacerations can be repaired by the emergency provider, but sedation may be needed.
- Lacerations involving the lid margins need to be repaired by an ophthalmologist.

Pitfalls

- An uncooperative child is at high risk for incomplete eye examination. Avoid letting this situation deter a proper evaluation of trauma.
- Examine carefully for subtle limitations in extraocular eye movements.
- A fear that the risks of lateral canthotomy are greater than the benefits can result in a missed opportunity to save a patient's vision.

CHEMICAL AND ENVIRONMENTAL EYE INJURIES

Chemical Injuries

Household chemicals cause almost all cases of pediatric chemical eye injury. Symptoms include pain, redness, and tearing of the eye. Lesions on the skin, such as blistering or eschar, suggest a serious exposure. A

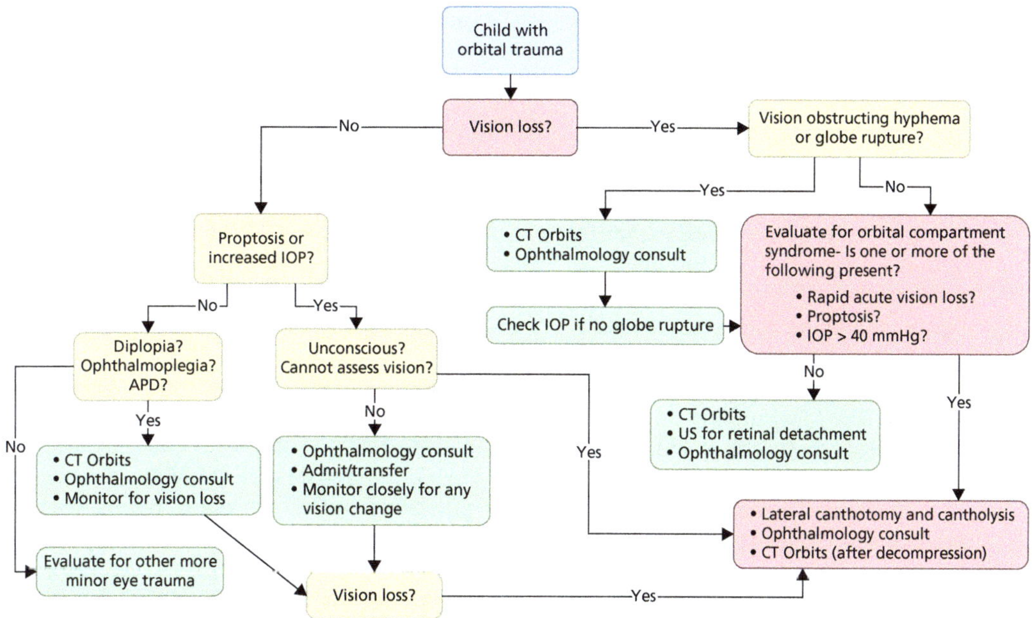

FIGURE 39.9 Clinical algorithm for the management of a child with orbital trauma. CT, computed tomography; IOP, intraocular pressure; US, ultrasound.

misty appearance of the cornea is a concerning sign; a clear cornea and minimal injection are reassuring. If the parents know the name of the product, poison control (1-800-222-1222 or http://www.poison.org) can help identify the chemical ingredients. However, acid and alkali burns appear similar on presentation, and emergency management is the same for both. Focus on initiating copious irrigation rather than determining the agent. Severe chemical burns are complicated by infection, scarring, corneal perforation, loss of tear control due to eyelid sagging, and potential blindness.

Acid Chemical Burns

- Generally considered less severe than alkaline burns
- Coagulative necrosis; acids denature proteins, causing their precipitation on the eye's surface, which lessens deeper penetration
- Hydrofluoric acid (rust remover) differs, and it penetrates the cornea (irrigate and then use calcium gluconate eye drops)
- pH paper reads acidic (below 6.5)
- Common acidic products: toilet bowl cleaner and hard water deposit remover, tile and mold cleaner, car battery

Alkali Chemical Burns

- More severe than acid burns
- Liquefactive necrosis; lipophilic and penetrate tissue more easily than acids; penetration of the cornea; "melting" effect of the eye tissues; may increase IOP
- pH paper reads alkaline (above 8.5)
- Common milder alkaline products: sodium hypochlorite (bleach), ammonia (Windex), laundry detergent, multisurface cleaners
- Sodium hydroxide: most common devastating agent; oven cleaner, drain cleaner, driveway cleaner, degreasers

Grading of a chemical burn depends on the appearance of the cornea and the presence and degree of limbal ischemia (white blanching of the tissue around the rim of the cornea). White (as opposed to red) appearance can be misinterpreted as reassuring, but a bright solid white area represents a loss of normal vasculature.

Treatment

Acid or Alkali Chemical Injuries

- Irrigate, irrigate, irrigate! Use saline or plain water; never delay—irrigation performed at the location where injury occurred leads to the best outcome
- Usually 1–5 L; may require 10–20 L in extreme cases; any corneal whitening probably warrants 12 hours of irrigation
- Flip lid and check fornices, especially for cement or powdered agents that may clump in recesses
- Standard size Morgan lens can be used for ages 6 months or older; give ibuprofen, anesthetic eye drops, and a pacifier; surprisingly, infants and toddlers will often fall asleep once irrigation is initiated
- If checking pH, have patient close the eyes for 5 minutes after ceasing irrigation and then test; acceptable pH 6.5–8.5
- Many eye drops (e.g., tropicamide) can alter pH for up to 40 minutes; ideally, test initial pH before eye drops; interpret subsequent pH tests with caution
- Once sufficient irrigation is finished, initiate ophthalmic antibiotics
- Consult ophthalmology

Thermal Burns

Mild burns from steam, vaporizers, fireplace embers, or glancing contact with a cigarette, can be treated as corneal abrasions. Serious burns warrant ophthalmology and burn specialist care.

Photokeratitis ("Snow Blindness")

Essentially a sunburn of the eye, photokeratitis commonly occurs from several hours spent on the snow (80% ultraviolet [UV] reflection) or water and sand (each ~25% UV reflection) without eye protection. Onset of symptoms typically begins a few hours after the exposure. Patients complain of red painful eyes with miosis and blurry vision. Punctate uptake in the cornea is seen with fluorescein. Treatment is supportive care and pain control.

Key Points

- Irrigate chemical burns immediately and copiously.
- Control pain.
- Whitening of cornea indicates a significant burn and should prompt consultation with ophthalmology.
- Photokeratitis is treated similarly to a corneal abrasion.

Pitfalls

- Avoid delayed irrigation or insufficient irrigation.
- Old, narrow-range, or light-exposed pH strips can be inaccurate.
- Do not discharge severe exposures. Admit or transfer to a specialist.

PAPILLEDEMA

Papilledema refers to optic nerve swelling caused by increased intracranial pressure. When the pressure increases, cerebrospinal fluid exerts that pressure along the length of the optic nerves. Therefore, it is almost exclusively bilateral. In common use, papilledema may refer to optic nerve swelling from any cause and be specified as unilateral or bilateral.

Patients complain of several days of headache accompanied by nausea or vomiting and often blurry vision. Blurry vision is usually vague, occurs with either or both eyes open, and may be transient. In advanced cases, the visual field may become smaller and more centralized. Visual acuity may still be 20/20 if central vision is preserved. Papilledema may be the only neurologic finding on examination. If a tumor is present, or as the pressure increases, other neurological findings may appear. Atypical cases can present with an isolated complaint of vision loss, altered colored perception, or pain.

Papilledema is diagnosed by visualizing a bulging optic disc on fundoscopic examination. Bedside ultrasound may facilitate diagnosis utilizing a 10.5 MHz or 13.6 MHz linear probe to measure the optic nerve sheath diameter (ONSD). An ONSD of >5 mm correlates with an intracranial pressure >20 mmHg, and it has a sensitivity of 88% and a specificity of 93%.

Differential Diagnosis

- Brain tumor
- Idiopathic intracranial hypertension (pseudotumor cerebri)

- Trauma with intracranial hemorrhage or diffuse axonal injury
- High-altitude cerebral edema
- Meningitis, notably from cryptococcal infection; also Lyme disease
- Hypoxia; anoxic brain injury
- Obstructive hydrocephalus
- Central venous sinus thrombosis
- Retrobulbar tumor
- Retrobulbar hematoma
- Optic neuritis; concerning for multiple sclerosis

Key Points

- The finding of papilledema indicates a serious condition is present and the cause must be investigated.
- Treatment depends on the underlying cause.

Pitfalls

- Examination of the fundus is often overlooked—a missed diagnostic opportunity.
- Early in the course of increased intracranial pressure, papilledema may not have developed yet.

ORBITAL COMPARTMENT SYNDROME

Orbital compart syndrome is an acute vision-threatening condition in which pressure within the confines of the bony orbit causes ischemia to the optic nerve and retina. Associated pain and proptosis are common. Trauma with retrobulbar hematoma is the most common cause of orbital compartment syndrome. Orbital cellulitis is also a notable cause among many other less common causes.

As in other types of compartment syndrome, the clock is ticking for ischemic time and permanent loss of function. Decompression should occur within 30–100 minutes. Patients with suspected or confirmed compartment syndrome should be admitted or transferred.

Signs of Orbital Compartment Syndrome

- Acute proptosis
- Elevated IOP 35–40 mmHg
- Rapid vision loss
- Ophthalmoplegia
- Fixed dilated pupil or a relative afferent pupillary defect

The emergency provider may need to perform a lateral canthotomy and cantholysis, particularly if an ophthalmologist is not immediately available.

Indications to Perform Emergency Lateral Canthotomy and Cantholysis

- Reasonable suspicion: trauma; significant cellulitis; severe eye pain or vomiting

Plus any *one* of the following

- Rapid vision loss
- IOP ≥40 mmHg (may use the presence of a very tense, firm globe upon palpation as a substitute finding)
- Proptosis

In an unresponsive patient, in a child too young to report visual loss, or in the case of uncertain vision function, the provider should rely on IOP or the presence of proptosis and should not delay the procedure. A patient with any of the previously mentioned criteria should not be transferred *before* decompression because vision loss could occur during transport.

Contraindication to Lateral Canthotomy and Cantholysis

- Ruptured globe

Lateral Canthotomy and Cantholysis Procedure

- Although seemingly invasive, lateral canthotomy and cantholysis are fairly easy to perform, heal well, and have low complication rates.
- Inject local lidocaine with epinephrine at the lateral canthus.
- Slide one jaw of a hemostat inside the lateral canthus, going from the eye toward the face.
- Clamp down the hemostat for approximately 90 seconds to decrease blood in the tissue; remove hemostat.
- Use iris scissors to cut a 1- or 2-cm opening, again sliding one side of the scissors under the skin at the lateral corner of the eye.

- Pull the skin down and find the Y-shaped canthal tendon; the two upper branches of the "Y" face toward the eye—one is the superior tendon and the other is the inferior tendon.
- Use the iris scissors to cut the inferior tendon.
- If the IOP does not decline to <40 mmHg within a few minutes, then cut the superior tendon.
- Cutting the lateral canthal common tendon (the base of the "Y") is less effective than cutting the inferior tendon alone.
- Again, this procedure is vision saving, can be performed with basic tools, and has few complications.

40

Oral and Dental Emergencies

THOMAS A. YAMAMOTO, NAM S. CHO, AND F. KYLE YIP

INTRODUCTION

Pediatric visits to the emergency department for oral- and dental-related complaints are common. Many are related to trauma. Nontraumatic emergency visits, mostly due to dental caries and associated infections, have increased over time and may account for 60–75% of oral- and dental-related visits to the emergency department. Explanations for this include increasing caries rate, poorer dental insurance coverage, and worsening access to primary dental care.

Few emergency departments have dental or oral and maxillofacial surgery consultants readily available for acute management. Furthermore, many conditions require specialized dental equipment, such as dental-specific radiography, for diagnosis and management. Fortunately, most dental- and oral-related conditions may be easily triaged in the acute setting and do not require immediate intervention. A fundamental understanding of the basic triage and management of dental- and oral-related conditions is worthwhile for today's emergency practitioner.

PEDIATRIC DENTOALVEOLAR ANATOMY AND PHYSIOLOGY

Pediatric Versus Adult Dentition

There are significant differences between pediatric and adult dental anatomy that impact clinical presentation and management. The following are clinical keys that may aid the emergency practitioner:

- Morphologic differences between pediatric (primary) and adult (permanent) dentition
  - Primary dentition has thin enamel, spindly roots, and large pulp chambers in comparison to permanent teeth (Figure 40.1).

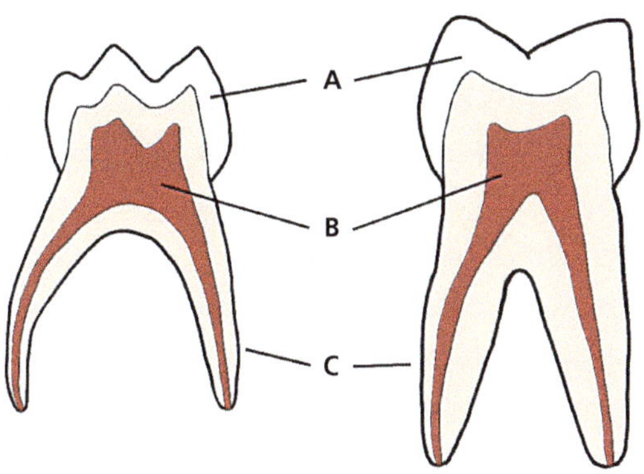

FIGURE 40.1 Pediatric and adult dentition have generally different characteristics. The hard, resilient enamel layer is thinner in primary teeth (A), the pulp chamber is larger and more susceptible to exposure (B), and the roots are thinner and more spindly (C).

As the permanent dentition begins to erupt, the roots of the primary dentition are resorbed.

Clinical pearl: Root resorption along with the bony plasticity of the pediatric maxillofacial skeleton contribute to a higher incidence of primary tooth luxation versus tooth crown fracture after trauma.

Pediatric dentition is composed of fewer teeth.

- Labeling dentition (Figure 40.2)
  - Pediatric dentition is termed ***primary*** teeth, which are labeled by consecutive letters (A–T; 20 total).
  - Adult dentition is termed ***permanent*** teeth, which are labeled by consecutive numbers (1–32; 32 total).
  - In the United States, labeling begins from the posterior of the right maxilla and proceeds around the arch to the posterior of the left maxilla (Primary A–J, Permanent 1–16), and it continues from the posterior of the left mandible around the arch to the posterior of the right mandible (primary K–T, permanent 17–32).

The dentition is referenced in quadrants. Each quadrant of the mouth is composed of the same set of teeth (Figure 40.3).

- Pediatric "primary"–five teeth per quadrant
  - Three anterior teeth: central incisor → lateral incisor → canine
  - Two posterior teeth: first molar → second molar (most posterior)
  - There are no premolar teeth in the primary dentition.
- Adult "permanent"—eight teeth per quadrant
  - Three anterior teeth: central incisor → lateral incisor → canine
  - Five posterior teeth: first premolar → second premolar → first molar → second molar → third molar (wisdom tooth)

Clinical pearl: Teeth can also be referred to by their quadrant and tooth type—for example, upper right central or lower left first molar.

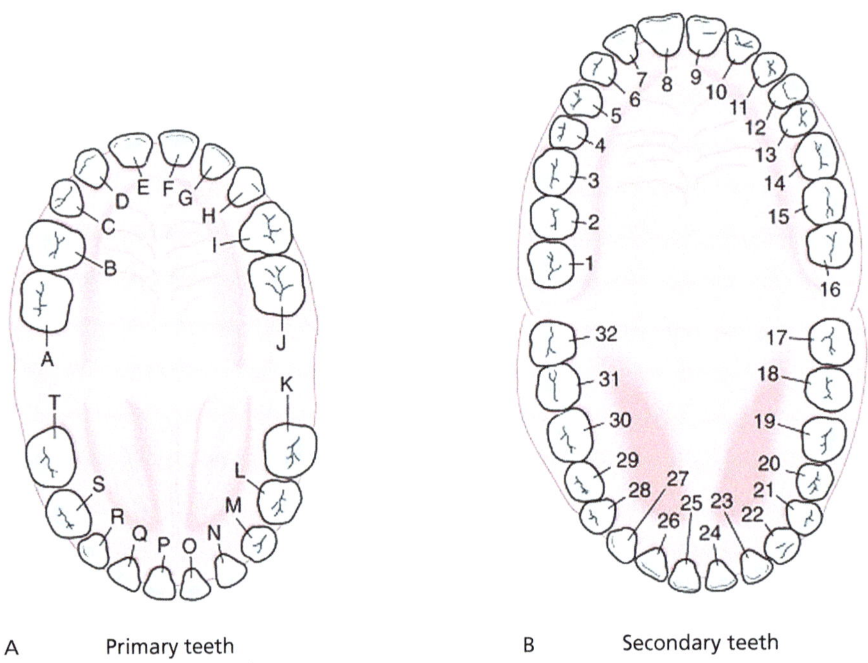

FIGURE 40.2 Numbering of both primary (pediatric) and secondary (permanent, adult) teeth begins from the maxillary right quadrant and terminates on the mandibular right quadrant. Primary dentition is labeled A–T (A), whereas secondary dentition is labeled 1–32 (B).

Source: Adapted from Martin B, et al. Oral disorders. In: Zitelli BJ, McIntire S, Nowalk AJ, eds. *Zitelli and Davis' Atlas of Pediatric Physical Diagnosis*. 7th ed. Philadelphia, PA: Elsevier; 2018:733–758.

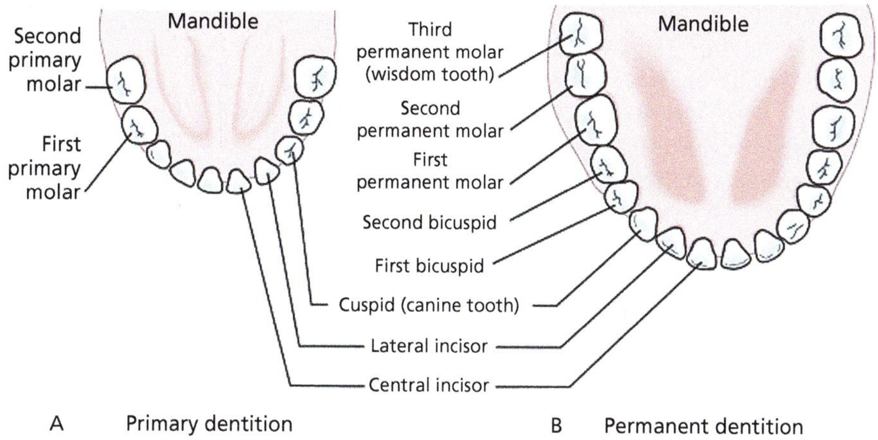

FIGURE 40.3 Each quadrant has the same set of teeth. (A) In the primary phase, there are five distinct teeth. (B) In the secondary phase, there are eight distinct teeth.

Source: Reprinted from: Martin B, et al. Oral disorders. In: Zitelli BJ, McIntire S, Nowalk AJ, eds. *Zitelli and Davis' Atlas of Pediatric Physical Diagnosis*. 7th ed. Philadelphia, PA: Elsevier; 2018:733–758.

Dental Eruption Patterns

The eruption pattern of human dentition has three broad phases (Figure 40.4):

- Primary dentition, ~6–24 months
  - Central incisors → lateral incisors → molars → canines
  - The mandibular incisors are usually first to erupt
- Mixed dentition, ~6–12 years
  - Presence of both primary and permanent dentition; begins with eruption of the first permanent tooth

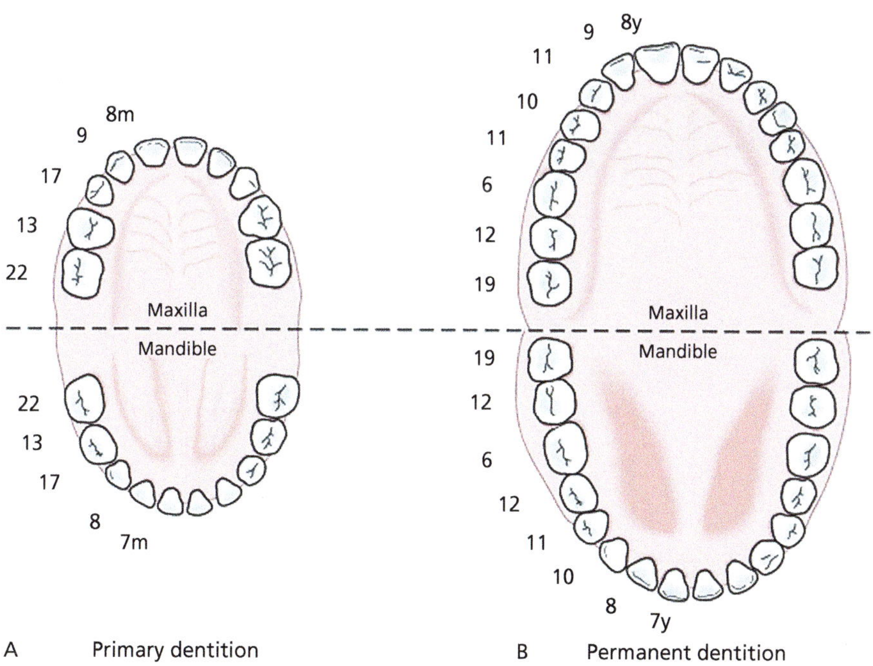

FIGURE 40.4 Eruption of teeth types follows a general pattern and timeline. (A) Primary teeth appear between 6 and 24 months. (B) Secondary teeth appear from 6 to 18 years. Note that teeth do not appear consecutively from front to back.

Source: Reprinted from Martin B, et al. Oral disorders. In: Zitelli BJ, McIntire S, Nowalk AJ, eds. *Zitelli and Davis' Atlas of Pediatric Physical Diagnosis*. 7th ed. Philadelphia, PA: Elsevier; 2018:733–758.

Completed by approximately 12 years of age when all primary dentition is lost

The first permanent teeth to appear are usually lower incisors with exfoliation of the associated primary tooth

First permanent molars begin to appear posterior to the primary dentition—*no associated exfoliating teeth*

The last primary teeth to exfoliate may be the primary molars or canines

Permanent (adult) dentition, ~12 years or older

Begins when last primary tooth is lost at approximately age 12 years

Continued eruption of permanent teeth occurs with permanent second molars (ages 12–14 years) and third molars (ages 16–20 years)

Clinical pearl: Understanding which dentition are age-appropriate will aid the emergency provider when evaluating dental trauma. Referring to a dentogram for labeling of dentition and general eruption ages will aid accuracy and diagnosis (Figure 40.5).

DENTOALVEOLAR TRAUMA—PRIMARY DENTITION

General Approach and Examination

Dentoalveolar trauma may present in isolation or in combination with other maxillofacial or head and neck injuries. Initial trauma surveys should be performed. The emergency provider should then begin by obtaining a thorough history of the injury. Common etiologies include falls and direct trauma from sports injuries. Child abuse or interpersonal violence are less common causes that should be considered, especially when the injury type is rare or inconsistent with the history. The dental history of any recently lost teeth prior to the injury will also aid with the examination of the existing dentition.

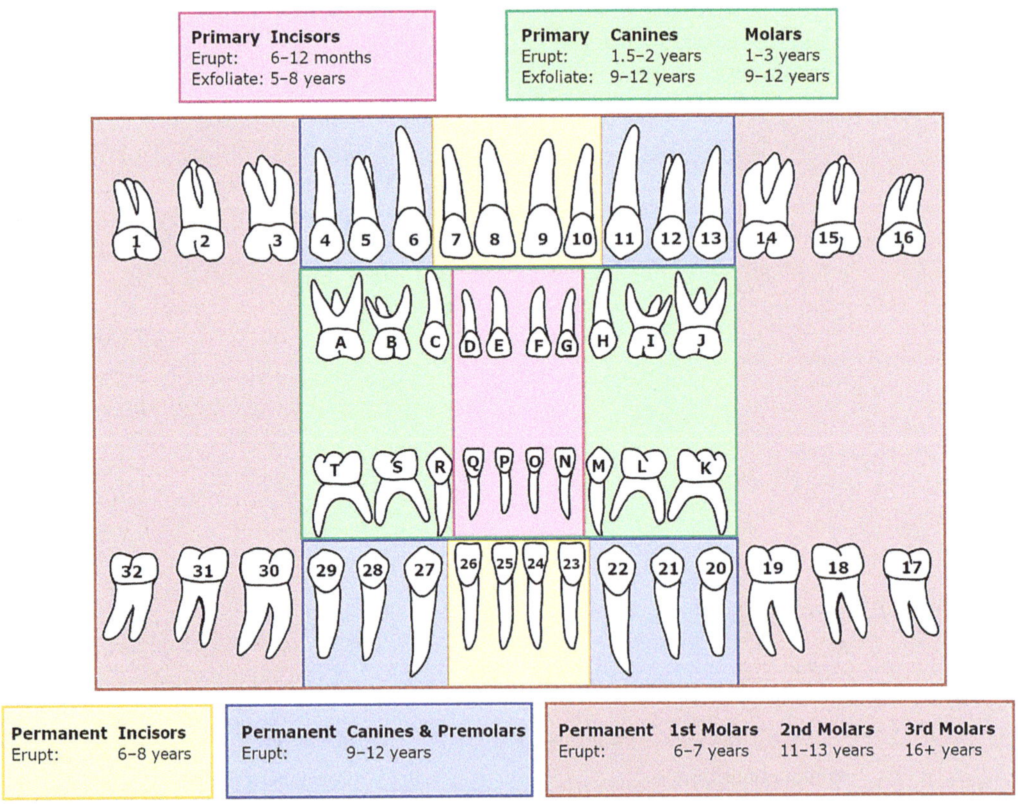

FIGURE 40.5 A dentogram summary of primary and secondary teeth is a useful reference to evaluate pediatric dentition. Children aged 5–12 years are typically in the "mixed" phase of dentition. This chart aids with labeling, and eruption and exfoliation ranges are listed for reference.

Clinical pearl: It is important to distinguish traumatized teeth from mobile primary teeth that are in the process of exfoliation from the underlying adult tooth.

The head and neck should be evaluated for traumatic stigmata, such as asymmetry, edema, contusions, or lacerations. Palpate the facial tissue for tenderness and crepitus, and evaluate the integrity of the underlying facial skeleton.

The oral examination begins with an extraoral evaluation focusing on the perioral tissue and lip vermillion. Blunt trauma in this area may lead to rapid edema. Tense or severe edema should be evaluated for expanding hematoma. Blunt external trauma may cause penetrating injury from the dentition, resulting in large mucosal injury.

A cursory temporomandibular joint (TMJ) examination may be performed by having the patient open maximally and measuring the inter-incisal distance between the anterior teeth. The normal range for adults is 45–50 mm. A 6-year-old child should be able to reach 40 mm. The mandible should open and close without deviation from the midline. Significant deviation or pain may indicate TMJ injury or mandible fracture.

The examination then proceeds intraorally with the aid of focused lighting. A systematic approach should be used to ensure that occult injuries are not missed. The lip vermillion and labial mucosa are inspected for laceration, followed by the buccal mucosa and vestibule of the maxilla and mandible. There are frenum attachments at the midline of the buccal maxillary and mandibular vestibules. The palate and pharynx are inspected, as well as the tongue dorsum and floor of mouth. Ecchymosis may be a sign of underlying fracture. The lingual frenum is inspected. Finally, the dentition should be inspected sequentially.

Clinical pearl: Children present as a challenging dental examination due to the mixed dentition of varying stages of development. The dentogram chart with accompanying eruption patterns should be referenced during the examination (see Figure 40.5).

Spacing between the teeth may be normal due to skeletal/alveolar growth, irregular eruption patterns, or exfoliated primary dentition with impending permanent (adult) dentition. Traumatic sequelae, on the other hand, may include tooth avulsion, complete crown fracture, or intrusion. The gingiva should be inspected for evidence of trauma such as bleeding, tissue void, and gingival laceration. Suspected tooth avulsion or crown fracture may warrant chest X-ray to rule out aspiration if the lost components are not accounted for by the patient.

Tooth Fractures

A tooth is composed of the crown and the root. The outer surface of the crown consists of enamel, which is a hard mineralized material that is generally resilient against traumatic force and decay and is insensitive. The inner surface consists of dentin, which is also mineralized but structurally softer than enamel and less resilient. The dentin color is yellow and darker in comparison to enamel. It may be sensitive to touch or temperature when exposed. The innermost aspect of the crown is the pulp, which is the neurovascular component of the tooth and continues apically into the root canal (Figure 40.6). It is responsible for the vitality of the tooth. The pulp may appear as pink blushing through the dentin layer or as overt bleeding from within the tooth crown (Figure 40.7). Exposure of the pulp necessitates repair that may also involve root canal therapy. Compromise of the pulp is responsible for tooth necrosis that may progress to dentoalveolar or odontogenic infections.

Tooth fractures are graded based on the degree of involvement of the previously discussed layers (Figure 40.8).

- Enamel/dentin fracture (Figure 40.8A–C)
  - Isolated enamel fracture is largely cosmetic. Dentin exposure may cause significant sensitivity and predispose the tooth to future decay. Fractures involving enamel and dentin do not require emergent treatment. If asymptomatic, dental consultation within 1 or 2 weeks should be encouraged. If symptomatic, consultation should be obtained within 72 hours to rule out other injuries to the tooth or surrounding tissues.
- Pulp exposure (Figures 40.7 and 40.8D, F)
  - Fractures involving the pulp should receive urgent evaluation and care from a dentist because pulp exposure may be very painful and contamination may

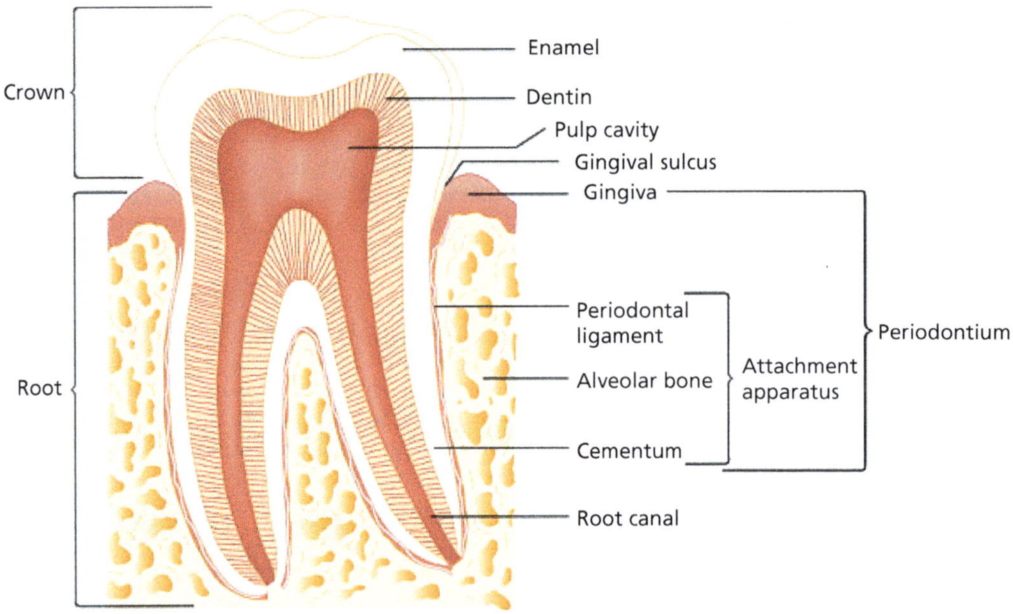

FIGURE 40.6 The dental apparatus consists of a tooth and its anatomic layers, the surrounding bone, and periodontal tissues.

Source: Reprinted from Pedigo RA, Amsterdam JT. Oral medicine. In: Ron M. Walls, Robert S. Hockberger, Marianne Gausche-Hill, eds. *Rosen's Emergency Medicine: Concepts and Clinical Practice*. 9th ed. Philadelphia, PA: Elsevier; 2018:771–789.

result in devitalization of the tooth and odontogenic infection.

If available, calcium hydroxide may be used for symptomatic relief of exposed pulp. If unavailable, the patient may be able to purchase temporary filling material at a drugstore to temporarily cover the sensitive dentin or pulp.

Dental consultation should be obtained within 72 hours.

Root fracture

Fractures that extend from the crown to the root surface have a poor prognosis and will likely need extraction (Figure 40.8E, F). Fractures of the root within the alveolus may require dental X-ray for diagnosis (Figure 40.8G). Retained roots from complete fracture of the crown will also need evaluation by a dentist (Figure 40.8H).

Dental consultation should be obtained within 72 hours.

Clinical pearl: All traumatized teeth require specific dental imaging by a dentist in order to evaluate any injury to the root structure or underlying, developing teeth.

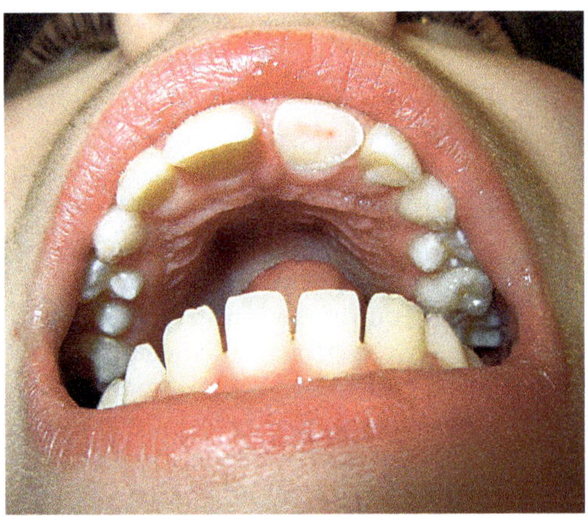

FIGURE 40.7 A fracture of the left central incisor, tooth No. 9, demonstrates the outer enamel layer, inner dentin layer, blushing of the pulp visible through dentin, and a pinpoint area of pulp exposure.

Source: Photograph by James Heilman, distributed under a CC BY-SA 3.0 license.

Tooth Displacement Injuries

Primary teeth have a higher likelihood of tooth displacement after trauma than do permanent teeth. Management may differ significantly depending on the type of displacement.

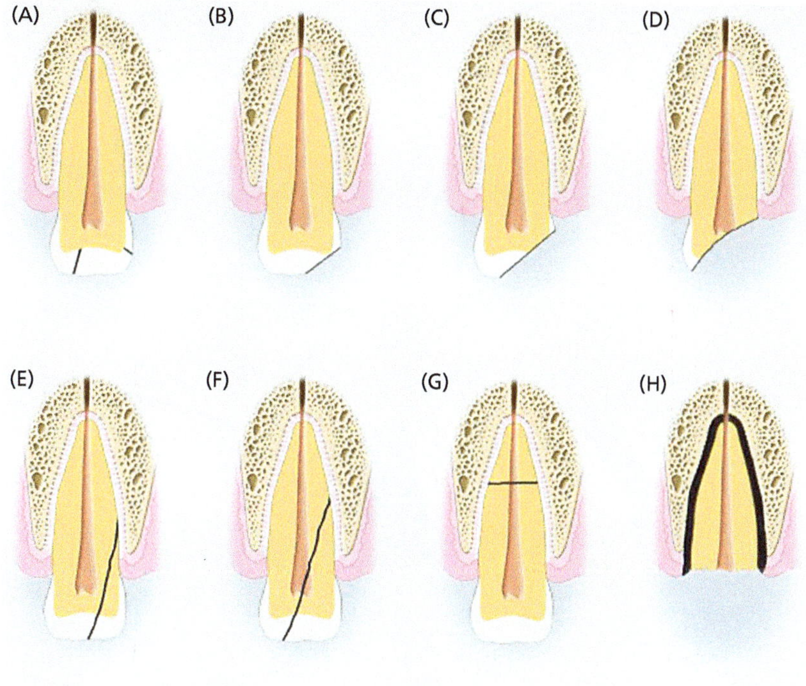

FIGURE 40.8 Tooth fracture injuries are characterized by the extent of involvement. The fracture may involve enamel only (A), enamel and dentin (B and C), pulp exposure (D), root surface (E and F), or isolated root fracture (G). The crown may be fully fractured, resulting in a retained root (H).

Source: Reprinted from Reynolds JS, et al. Diagnosis and management of dentoalveolar injuries. In: Fonseca RJ, Barber HD, Walker RV, Powers MP, Frost DE, eds. *Oral and Maxillofacial Trauma*. 4th ed. St. Louis, MO: Elsevier; 2013:248–292.

Furthermore, due to incomplete tooth development and the remaining regenerative capacity, the prognosis of permanent tooth displacement in children is often better than that in adults.

Displacement injuries are categorized into seven types (Figure 40.9):

- Concussion (Figure 40.9A): The tooth has sustained trauma but is otherwise stable and non-displaced.
  - Examination
    - Tooth appears non-displaced.
    - Tooth is nonmobile.
    - Tooth may be tender to percussion.
  - Management
    - Primary tooth: soft diet, follow-up with dentist within 48 hours
    - Permanent tooth: same
  - Prognosis
    - Primary tooth: good
    - Permanent tooth: good
  - Dental follow-up is necessary because sequelae, such as pulp necrosis, may develop in delayed fashion.
- Subluxation (Figure 40.9B): The tooth has sustained trauma and is unstable but non-displaced.
  - Examination
    - Tooth is non-displaced.
    - Tooth is mobile.
    - Tooth may be tender to manipulation.
    - There may be bleeding from the gingival sulcus.
  - Management
    - Primary tooth: soft diet, follow-up with dentist within 24 hours; may require splinting
    - Permanent tooth: same
  - Prognosis
    - Primary tooth: good
    - Permanent tooth: good

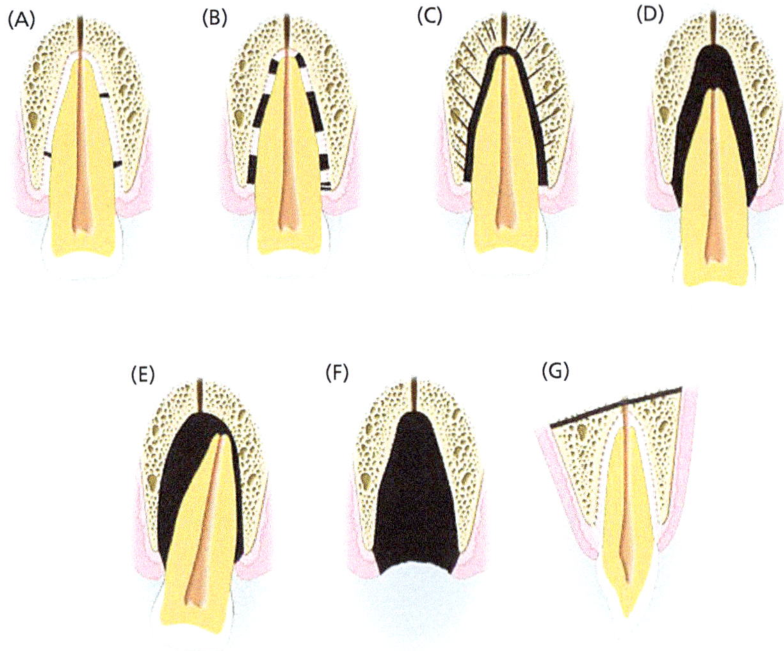

FIGURE 40.9 There are seven types of tooth displacement injury: concussion without displacement or mobility (A), subluxation without displacement but with mobility (B), intrusive luxation (C), extrusive luxation (D), lateral luxation (E), avulsion (F), and alveolar fracture (G).

Source: Reprinted from: Reynolds JS, et al. Diagnosis and management of dentoalveolar injuries. In: Fonseca RJ, Barber HD, Walker RV, Powers MP, Frost DE, eds. *Oral and Maxillofacial Trauma*. 4th edition. St. Louis, MO: Elsevier; 2013:248–292.

Follow-up is necessary because sequelae, such as pulp necrosis, may develop in delayed fashion. The alveolar bone may require imaging by the dentist to rule out alveolar fracture.

Intrusion (Figure 40.9C): The tooth has been displaced into the socket or alveolus.

Examination

The crown of the affected tooth is below the level of the adjacent occlusion. It may be driven beneath the gingiva, giving the appearance of an absent or avulsed tooth. It may be difficult to differentiate an intruded tooth from a partially erupted developing tooth. Referencing the eruption pattern of the tooth type (i.e., patient age) will aid diagnosis.

The affected tooth is typically nonmobile.

The tooth is usually nontender.

Percussion of the tooth with a small metal instrument may result in a metallic or tinny resonance compared to healthy teeth.

The surrounding gingiva may show evidence of trauma such as erythema or bleeding.

Management

Primary tooth: The intruded tooth is often extracted to prevent injury to the underlying tooth bud. It may be left to spontaneously erupt if there is no evidence of injury to the underlying tooth bud. A dentist will need to take X-rays to help with this determination.

Permanent tooth: The intruded tooth likely needs to be repositioned and splinted. Immature teeth may be observed for spontaneous eruption over 2–4 weeks. The tooth will likely need endodontic therapy (root canal).

Dental consultation should occur within 24–72 hours.

Prognosis

Primary tooth: poor

Permanent tooth: guarded-poor; the tooth may be salvageable but will require endodontic therapy and may be subject to resorption and ankylosis

Extrusion (Figure 40.9D): The tooth has been displaced out of the socket or alveolus but remains partially in the socket.

Examination

The crown of the tooth is hypererupted but remains in the socket.

The tooth is likely mobile.

The surrounding gingival sulcus may bleed, and gingiva may be tender.

Management

Primary tooth: The tooth should not be repositioned into its socket to avoid injuring the underlying tooth bud. The tooth should be referred to a dentist for evaluation and X-rays to determine if it can be repositioned. Extraction may be necessary.

Permanent tooth: The tooth should be repositioned and stabilized/splinted as soon as possible. The tooth can be repositioned in the emergency department and referred to a dentist for splinting and further management. Avoid chewing on the affected tooth.

Prognosis

Primary tooth: poor; the tooth will likely require extraction

Permanent tooth: good; the tooth may revascularize or require endodontic therapy (root canal) depending on the maturity of the root apex

Lateral luxation (Figure 40.9E): The tooth has been displaced laterally but is not significantly intruded or extruded.

Examination

The tooth is displaced in any axial direction, more often in the lingual/palatal direction than labial/buccal.

The tooth may or may not be mobile.

The tooth may be tender to manipulation.

There may be bleeding from the gingival sulcus, and there may be gingival laceration.

Management:

Primary tooth: The displaced tooth may be left in place if it is not prematurely contacting the opposing dentition on intercuspation. It may be extracted if it is suspected to be impinging on the underlying tooth bud. If the tooth is prematurely contacting the opposing dentition, the tooth will need to be repositioned or extracted.

Permanent tooth: The displaced tooth will need to be repositioned and splinted for a period of 2–4 weeks, depending on the condition of the alveolar housing. The tooth may need endodontic treatment (root canal).

Dental/oral and maxillofacial surgery consultation should be sought within 24 hours. If unavailable, basic management may be considered. For example, a tooth may be repositioned and the patient kept on a no-chew diet until consultation can be attained.

Prognosis

Primary tooth: variable; treatment goals are to prevent further injury to the developing permanent tooth

Permanent tooth: guarded; the tooth will likely need endodontic therapy (root canal) but is typically salvageable. There may be fracture of the tooth socket or alveolar housing.

Avulsion (Figure 40.9F): The tooth has completely displaced from the socket.

Examination

The tooth is absent and the socket is patent.

There may be bleeding from the socket.

Clinical pearl: A history of how long the tooth has been avulsed, how it has been stored, and how long it has been out of any liquid storage medium is critical. Successful replantation is inversely correlated with extraoral dry time, and necrosis is expected after 60 minutes. The goal is to maintain vitality of the periodontal ligament that envelopes the tooth root. The best storage medium is Hank's balanced salt solution (EMT Tooth Saver, Biochrom AG), followed by cold milk, and saliva or holding the tooth in the mouth. Water is a poor storage medium that lyses the cells of the periodontal ligament.

Management

Primary tooth: It is not recommended to replant primary teeth in order to avoid injuring the underlying permanent tooth. If replanting is necessary, primary teeth roots can be shortened by 2 or 3 mm to allow replanting and avoid injury to the underlying tooth bud.

Permanent tooth: The avulsed tooth can be replanted in the emergency department. Gently rinse the tooth with saline or water for 10 seconds and then replant into anatomic position. Inability to achieve some amount of stability on replantation is an aspiration risk, and it may indicate that there is interference within the socket or fracture of the socket housing. If stability is achieved, the tooth can be held in place by gently biting on gauze until a dental provider can splint the tooth. Urgent referral is indicated.

Prognosis

Primary tooth: poor; do not replant primary teeth in the emergency department

Permanent tooth: variable, depending on time to replantation and maturity of the tooth root apex. Endodontic therapy (root canal) is likely. Extended dry time prior to replantation has a poor long-term prognosis and will lead to tooth ankylosis and root resorption. When in doubt, replant a permanent tooth in the emergency department. Replanting the tooth regardless of long-term prognosis may have short-term benefits to esthetics, function, and maintenance of the surrounding bone and tissue while a long-term solution is prepared by the patient's dentist.

It may be difficult to differentiate an avulsed tooth from a fractured tooth that has retained the root in the alveolus. If the avulsed tooth is unavailable, chest X-ray is recommended to rule out aspiration. Dental X-rays should be taken to rule out retained fragments.

Alveolar fracture (Figure 40.9G): The alveolar housing around a tooth or set of teeth has been fractured and displaced from the basal bone, and the teeth themselves are fixed within the alveolar segment.

Examination

The traumatized dentition will be displaced in a segment, most commonly with two to four consecutive teeth.

The teeth are typically stable and nonmobile within the segment. The segment itself may be mobile, where the entire tooth–alveolus segment moves upon manipulation, or it may be relatively immobile.

There is typically bleeding and gingival laceration at the fracture margins.

Management

There is no difference in management whether primary or permanent dentition is involved. The segment will need to be reduced and stabilized with a bonded splint or Erich arch bars for 2–4 weeks. Complete reduction may be difficult due to interference from the tooth roots and comminution of the alveolar bone. Urgent consultation with an oral and maxillofacial surgeon or dentist competent in managing dentoalveolar trauma is indicated. The segment can be left alone en route to consultation, especially if it is not causing premature occlusion. Gauze packing may help with bleeding and separating the occlusion in the case of premature occlusal contact. Lacerations in the gingiva do not typically need primary repair.

Prognosis: good; the teeth may need vitality testing and endodontic therapy. The alveolus heals well with stabilization.

Note that primary teeth lost prematurely will need space maintenance in order to prevent migration of the adjacent teeth and disruption of the underlying permanent teeth's eruption. A pediatric dentist or orthodontist should evaluate the patient and determine if an appliance is necessary to maintain appropriate spacing.

Children in orthodontic treatment have dentition that is more mobile and vulnerable to luxation or avulsion injury. When repositioning teeth, existing braces may be used as a temporary splint until dental consultation is feasible.

Soft Tissue Injuries

Lacerations in the oral cavity heal rapidly with minimal sequelae. Scar formation is reduced in mucosa compared to skin and is particularly minimal in the keratinized surfaces of gingiva and palatal mucosa. Most lacerations do not require any intervention and may be left to heal by secondary intention, even if there is bone exposure. Repair may also be delayed and referred to a dentist or oral surgeon with instrumentation that facilitates repair within the oral cavity.

Immediate repair in the emergency department may be necessary if there is significant bleeding, discomfort, or if referral is not readily available within 24 hours. Note that resorbable sutures tend to break down more rapidly in the oral cavity due to the moist environment and salivary enzymes. Intermediate resorbing suture such as chromic gut or polyglycolic acid/polyglactin (Vicryl) is most commonly used and recommended.

Gingival Lacerations

Gingival lacerations often heal spontaneously and will remodel based on the underlying bone. When necessary, resorbable suture, such as 3-0 to 5-0 chromic gut, is preferred for any repair. Gingiva may be macerated and in poor condition to hold suture. In these cases, gauze pressure may be used to control hemostasis in lieu of repair with suture.

Tongue Lacerations

Lacerations to the tongue can be difficult to repair due to patient cooperation, mobility of the tongue, and the wet oral environment. Lacerations less than 1 or 2 cm do not typically require repair. Lacerations with significant bleeding, gaping, or those that bisect the anterior tongue are indicated for repair.

Local anesthesia may be administered via lingual nerve block unilaterally or bilaterally or via local infiltration. Local infiltration of anesthetic with epinephrine may decrease bleeding during repair. 3-0 or 4-0 resorbable suture such as chromic gut or Vicryl is appropriate. The tongue may be controlled by wrapping the uninjured portion with gauze and having an assistant secure the gauze between thumb and forefinger. Alternatively, a 3-0 silk or Vicryl suture may be passed through the center of the uninjured (and anesthetized) tongue and used for retraction.

The laceration should be repaired in interrupted fashion with thick bites through mucosa and muscle. This will minimize dehiscence of the wound as a result of constant tongue movement. The prognosis is good, and the patient may follow up with their dentist within 48 hours for evaluation. Ice may be used intraorally to aid with comfort and decrease edema.

Mucosal Lacerations

Mucosal lacerations heal well via secondary intention. Repair may be necessary as a result of uncontrolled bleeding or discomfort. Simple interrupted resorbable sutures, such as 3-0 or 4-0 chromic gut, with 3- to 5-mm bites of tissue are typically sufficient.

Lacerations to the frenula are uncommon. This may correlate with abuse in nonmobile children but may occur in an active child after trauma. Repair is not indicated.

Lip Lacerations

Lip lacerations should be repaired if significantly displaced or if involving the vermillion border. Realigning the vermillion border is critical for cosmesis and should be the first suture placed, preferentially with a finer suture such as 5–0 or 6–0 gut. The cutaneous portion may then be repaired as is typical for facial skin. The vermillion may be repaired with 4–0-or 5–0 gut. The wet mucosa may be left to heal by secondary intention or repaired with 4–0 or 5–0 gut.

NONTRAUMATIC DENTAL EMERGENCIES

Odontalgia, Caries, and Dentoalveolar Infections

Dental Decay/Caries

Caries, or dental decay, is a bacterially mediated disease process that results in tooth destruction. It is the direct result of acid-producing bacteria, such as *Streptococcus mutans*, in a carbohydrate-rich environment, and it is often associated with poor oral hygiene. The pediatric caries rate in the United States is rising and has resulted in a significant increase in related emergency department visits. Caries is particularly prevalent in low-income populations that are the least likely to have primary dental care. As the disease progresses to pain (i.e., toothache and odontalgia) or infection, patients then present to the emergency department as their primary form of treatment.

Caries begins in the hard enamel outer surface of a tooth (see Figure 40.6). This phase is largely asymptomatic, and progression is relatively slow. The enamel is eventually demineralized to expose the softer underlying dentin, which may also result in spontaneous pain and sensitivity. The tooth surface may show focal discoloration or cavitation. Progression through dentin may be rapid, and penetration into the pulp chamber results in pulpal necrosis and pain.

Dentoalveolar Infections

Once the enamel and dentin layers are compromised, an unimpeded path through the root canal system is available for bacterial colonization and spread into the alveolar bone around the tooth apex, resulting in periapical infection and abscess.

The path of least resistance is then followed through the alveolus and into the adjacent mucosal tissue. The patient may complain of spontaneous pain and severe toothache due to pressure from pus accumulation. If the abscess path is near the crest, the lesion may fistulize through the gingiva as a parulis and be visible as a small fluctuant mass or draining papule (Figure 40.10A). The patient may become asymptomatic at this point as the pressure is relieved. There are rarely any systemic signs of infection. If the lesion tracks below the mucosal attachment, however, infection may spread along anatomic tissue planes from the vestibule (Figure 40.11A) to facial spaces and deep neck spaces (Figure 40.11B, C).

Infection involving the fascial spaces of the head and neck is similar in presentation to that in adults. Maxillary spread of infection may progress via the canine space to periorbital or orbital compartments (Figure 40.11B). Infection in this area may involve the danger triangle of the face and result in intracranial spread and meningitis. Mandibular infection may involve the submental, sublingual, and submandibular spaces and may lead to airway distress via mass effect (Figure 40.11C). Infection may further progress to the lateral pharyngeal and retropharyngeal spaces and result in mediastinitis.

Examination

History

Systemic symptoms such as fever from odontogenic infections, even those involving deep facial spaces, are uncommon unless they become severe. Young children may have difficulty identifying the source of pain and may be uncooperative. They may be unwilling to eat or complain of pain with chewing. Older patients may report a history of toothache that is ongoing or has spontaneously resolved. Outright necrosis of a tooth may temporarily relieve pain as the tooth itself becomes insensate. Pain may return as surrounding inflammation and the accumulation of pus trigger sensation in the alveolar housing and adjacent soft tissue. Facial swelling may have appeared suddenly. Rapid progression may be indicative of more virulent pathogens. Trismus is indicative of masticator space involvement. Odynophagia is a concerning sign of lateral or retropharyngeal space involvement.

Head and Neck

The face and neck are inspected and palpated for appearance and symmetry. Cellulitis and

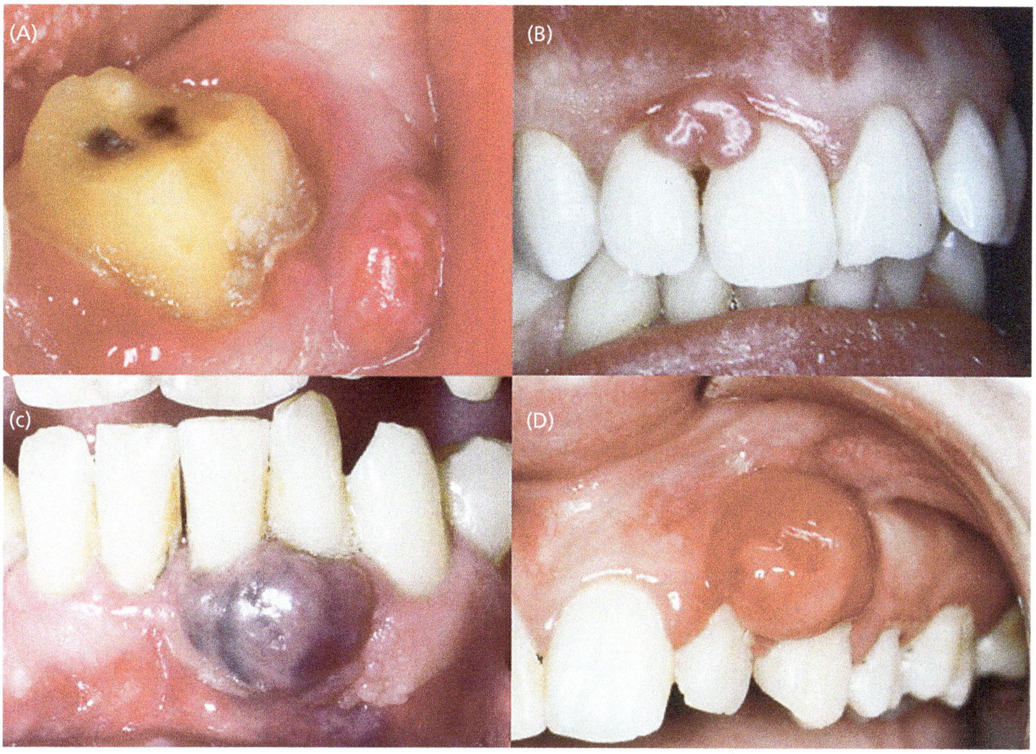

FIGURE 40.10 The "four P's" of gingival masses are difficult to distinguish clinically. Examples of parulis (A), pyogenic granuloma (B), peripheral giant cell granuloma (C), and peripheral ossifying fibroma (D) demonstrate their similar clinical appearance.

Source: B–D, reprinted from Neville B, et al. Soft tissue tumors. In: *Oral and Maxillofacial Pathology.* 4th ed. St. Louis, MO: Elsevier; 2016:473–532.

abscess may demonstrate swelling, induration, and overlying erythema of the involved space. Fluctuance may be observed in a chronic abscess (Figure 40.11).

- Canine or infraorbital space (Figure 40.11B)
  - Fullness over the ipsilateral malar region and may result in lip swelling, blunting of the nasolabial fold, and periorbital edema.
  - Periorbital and orbital cellulitis should be ruled out. Retrograde spread may cause cavernous sinus thrombosis.
  - The canine, primary molar, or permanent premolar are the most likely contributors.
- Buccal space (Figure 40.11C)
  - Fullness over the ipsilateral cheek, lateral and posterior to the canine space, and encompasses the maxilla and mandible.
  - Posterior teeth from either arch may be causative.
- Sublingual, submental, and submandibular spaces (Figure 40.11C)
  - These spaces are interconnected. The sublingual and submandibular spaces are paired, bilateral spaces, but they may interconnect across the midline via the submental space.
  - The sublingual space may show floor of mouth elevation.
  - Extraoral swelling and erythema may be present inferior and medial to the mandibular border in the submental and submandibular spaces.
  - Posterior teeth of the mandible are typically the causative agents.

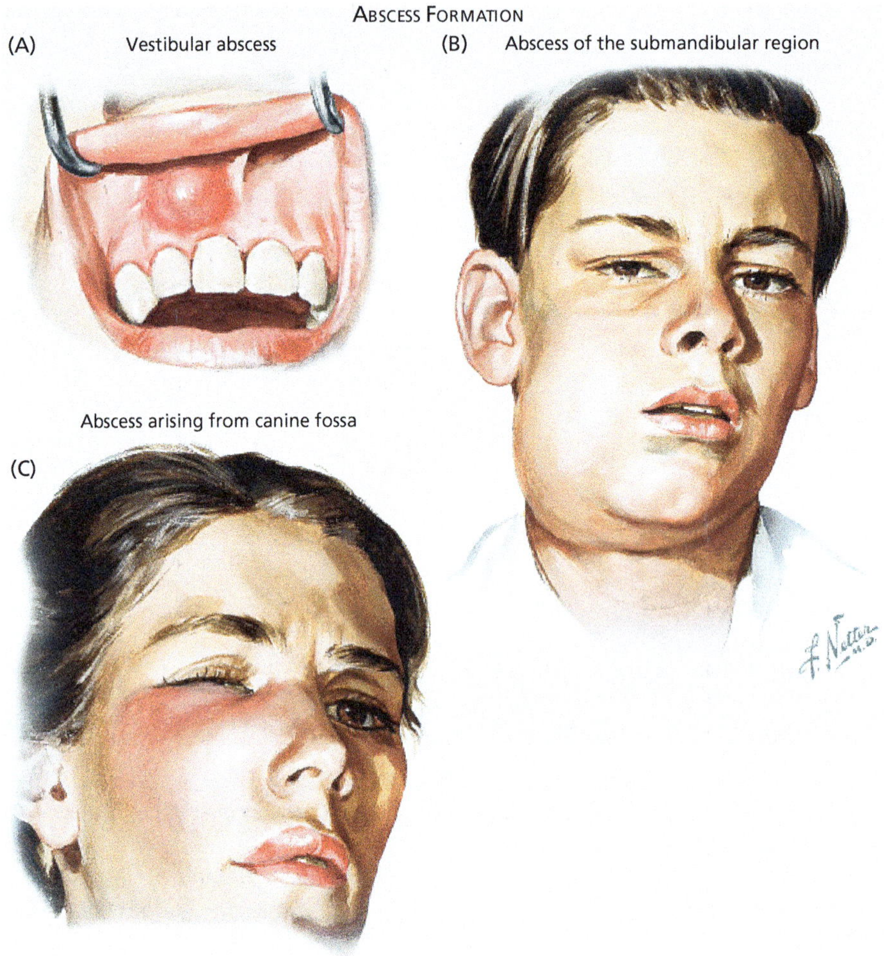

FIGURE 40.11 Odontogenic infections that spread through the local alveolus may spread to the adjacent vestibule (A) or deep fascial spaces such as the canine/infraorbital space (B) or buccal and submandibular space (C).

Source: Reprinted from Reynolds JC, et al. Mouth and pharynx. In: *The Netter Collection of Medical Illustrations: Digestive System Part I, Upper Digestive Tract*. 2nd ed. Philadelphia, PA: Elsevier; 2017.

Dentition

The suspected teeth are inspected for discoloration, cavitation, mobility, or tenderness to percussion. There may be adjacent erythema or edema of the gingiva or vestibular abscess (Figure 40.11A). A draining sinus tract or parulis may be present (Figure 40.10A).

Management

Source control (i.e., extraction or endodontic therapy)_is requisite for cure of any odontogenic infection. Antibiotics may provide temporary relief if source control is not immediately achievable. If infection does not appear to have advanced beyond the local alveolus or vestibule, however, tooth extraction is often sufficient without the need for any antibiotics in healthy individuals. Therefore, most odontogenic infections should be treated urgently by a dentist or oral surgeon in order to avoid unnecessary antibiotic use.

Severe infections, such as those extending beyond the local alveolus or whose progression has been rapid and aggressive, warrant intravenous antibiotics combined with urgent source control. Hospital admission is appropriate to monitor for disease progression and control.

Antibiotics

Odontogenic infections may be empirically treated with penicillin derivatives, which have excellent coverage of oral flora. Amoxicillin is the preferred oral variant because compliance is improved with its less frequent dosing interval compared to penicillin VK. For parenteral administration, intravenous penicillin G is appropriate. For penicillin-allergic patients, clindamycin is the first alternative for either oral or parenteral administration.

The preferred antibiotic for serious odontogenic infections is ampicillin plus sulbactam (Unasyn). This improves coverage against β-lactamase-resistant and anaerobic organisms. If penicillin allergic, clindamycin or moxifloxacin are suitable alternatives.

Clinical pearl: Tetracycline derivatives should be avoided in children with developing tooth buds because they will cause intrinsic staining.

Post-Extraction Complications

Bleeding

In healthy patients, typical bleeding after tooth extraction is easily managed with gauze and pressure. Prolonged bleeding may be due to poor compliance with post-extraction instructions. Small extraction spaces, such as those left after primary tooth extraction, may be difficult to apply direct pressure against. Patients may be biting on gauze with the adjacent dentition but not applying pressure directly against the extraction socket. It may be difficult for young patients to maintain continuous pressure on the extraction site. Pressure should be continuously maintained for 20–30 minutes. Many patients remove gauze packing too quickly to inspect the extraction socket, which allows for bleeding to restart without adequate coagulation. Saliva mixing with a small amount of blood may also be perceived as significant bleeding by the patient or parent.

Management

If concerned with post-extraction bleeding, the site should be gently rinsed of existing blood and clot with sterile irrigation. Exophytic clot, or "liver clot," may need to be removed to allow direct pressure onto the extraction site. If gauze and pressure fail to achieve hemostasis within 5–10 minutes, adjuncts may be considered. Hemostatic materials, such as gelatin sponge, oxidized cellulose, or microfibrillar collagen or collagen sponge, may be lightly condensed into the socket. Topical materials, including topical thrombin, aminocaproic acid, and tranexemic acid, may also assist with hemostasis. A figure-of-eight suture may help bring the tissue together and reduce the patency of the extraction socket, as well as hold in packing materials.

Failure to achieve hemostasis at this point may warrant evaluation for coagulopathy or bleeding disorders.

Pain

Pain is well managed by nonsteroidal anti-inflammatory drugs and acetaminophen, either alone or in combination, after extraction in pediatric populations. Persistent pain or pain refractory to oral analgesics may be indicative of abnormal postoperative healing. Two conditions may be considered: alveolar osteitis, known colloquially as dry socket, and postoperative infection.

Dry Socket

Alveolar osteitis, which is commonly referred to as dry socket, is a post-extraction condition that is relatively common and may cause severe discomfort to the patient. It is commonly expected to occur after 5–15% of posterior mandibular permanent tooth extractions and is particularly associated with third molar extractions. The pathogenesis is poorly understood but may involve early and abnormal fibrinolysis of the blood clot within the socket. There are few risk factors identified in adolescents, and it is rare before age 12 years.

Dry socket typically presents as severe pain associated with the extraction socket in delayed fashion, from 1 to 5 days after extraction. Patients may complain of radiating pain to the ear, low-grade fever, and halitosis or a foul taste or odor. These signs and symptoms often lead patients and parents to be concerned about post-extraction infection, which is rare but should be ruled out.

Clinical pearl: Alveolar osteitis/dry socket is diagnosed primarily by history and symptoms. Clinical signs are nonspecific and nondiagnostic, but they may support the diagnosis.

Examination

- The socket itself is typically patent and may or may not contain maturing clot or debris.
- The socket is not typically "empty."
- The surrounding tissue and gingiva may otherwise appear normal.

Mild swelling of the adjacent tissue or face may be present as a result of recent surgical extraction but is not necessarily related to alveolar osteitis.

Management

The condition is self-limiting and resolves within a few days.

Immediate relief is typically achieved only by direct socket dressing with a eugenol-based topical analgesic, which may require referral to the patient's dentist. This is typically administered with a small gelatin foam sponge or packable gauze, the latter of which requires later removal. If eugenol is unavailable, patients may be instructed to purchase clove oil, which contains eugenol, and apply it to the socket with packable gauze until they can be seen by their dentist.

Oral analgesics may provide brief relief but are otherwise poorly effective.

Antibiotics are not indicated and do not change the prognosis of alveolar osteitis.

Post-Extraction Infection

Postoperative infection is uncommon after extractions in pediatric populations. Extraction sockets are very tolerant of the oral environment and heal uneventfully without postoperative antibiotics. Initial pain, inflammation, and edema may be expected within 48 hours of extraction. Persistent pain may be indicative of a localized infection or aggressive, spreading infection where tooth extraction or pulp therapy was insufficient for control.

Examination

If erythema and exudate are localized to the socket, local postoperative infection may be considered.

Significant pain, erythema, or edema spreading into the adjacent vestibule or associated facial and neck spaces is concerning for worsening, uncontrolled infection and warrants further evaluation as mentioned previously.

Management

Localized postoperative infection

The site should be irrigated and referred back to the dentist for evaluation because this may be difficult to differentiate from alveolar osteitis. Local irrigation and debridement are typically sufficient, and antibiotics are not necessary unless there is concern for infection spreading beyond the local socket.

Persistent or spreading postoperative infection

Oral or intravenous antibiotics may be indicated, depending on whether the patient requires continued inpatient observation. Refer to the previous discussion on odontogenic infections.

Oral Lesions

Lesions within the oral cavity may appear suddenly and cause serious concern to children and parents. Fortunately, most oral lesions are benign and do not require urgent management. Immediate care may be indicated for lesions causing significant discomfort or, rarely, when there may be life-threatening sequelae.

A comprehensive review of possible lesions is beyond the scope of this chapter. The following is a review of common lesions and lesions that may warrant inpatient management.

Neonatal Lesions

White/nonpigmented lesions (Figure 40.12): occur commonly in the oral cavity, up to 50–85% of newborns, but may cause concern in the new parent and result in an emergency department visit

Appearance: solitary or clustered, white or yellow vesicles, may have smooth white surface appearance, 1–3 mm in size

Epstein pearls

Location: median palatal raphe

Bohn nodules

Location: hard and soft palate junction

Dental lamina cysts

Location: alveolar mucosa

Treatment: observation

Prognosis: self-resolving

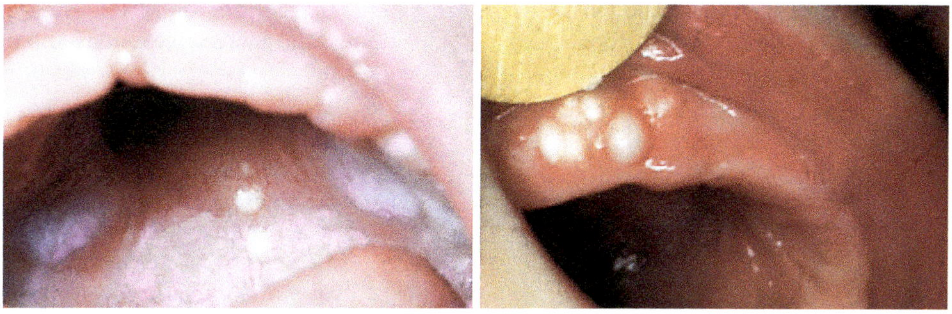

FIGURE 40.12 Small, white-yellow vesicular lesions in the newborn are generally classified based on location. Epstein pearls and Bohn nodules appear on the palate (left), whereas dental lamina cysts appear on the alveolus (right).

Source: Reprinted from Martin B, et al. Oral disorders. In: Zitelli BJ, McIntire S, Nowalk AJ, eds. *Zitelli and Davis' Atlas of Pediatric Physical Diagnosis*. 7th ed. Philadelphia, PA: Elsevier; 2018:733–758.

Melanotic neuroectodermal tumor of infancy: This is a rare neoplasm that occurs in the first year of life. Approximately 75% of these tumors occur in the oral cavity, with the vast majority in the maxilla over the mandible.

Appearance: They may appear as a rapidly expansile, pigmented blue or black lesion. The lesion is typically benign, although there is a 20% recurrence rate with enucleation, and some reported cases have demonstrated malignancy and metastasis.

Age: first year, may be present at birth

Treatment: surgical excision for biopsy and cure

Natal teeth: Newborns may be born with erupted teeth, termed natal teeth. They may be prematurely erupting primary teeth (normally expected after 6–8 months) or supernumerary teeth.

Age: birth

Treatment: likely extraction, depending on etiology. Referral to dentist is necessary to determine etiology.

Neonatal candidiasis: Approximately 5% of infants develop oral candidiasis (thrush). This is thought to be due to transfer of candida through the vaginal canal at birth and an undeveloped immune system.

Appearance: wipeable white film overlying an erythematous base

Age: birth through infancy

Treatment: Many cases may spontaneously resolve and may be observed. Otherwise, treatment is with antifungals and, in breastfeeding infants, may require concurrent treatment of the mother's breast.

Masses of the Oral Cavity

Eruption cyst/hematoma (Figure 40.13): An erupting tooth is surrounded by a sac-like covering known as the dental follicle. This allows the tooth to pass through the alveolar bone toward the gingival crest as it develops. The follicle

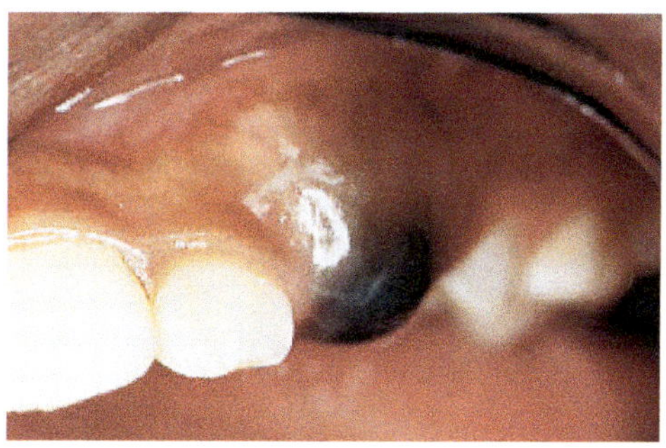

FIGURE 40.13 Erupting teeth and their associated eruption cyst may cause the overlying tissue to bulge and a small hematoma may form beneath, resulting in bluish discoloration.

Source: Reprinted from Martin B, et al. Oral disorders. In: Zitelli BJ, McIntire S, Nowalk AJ, eds. *Zitelli and Davis' Atlas of Pediatric Physical Diagnosis*. 7th ed. Philadelphia, PA: Elsevier; 2018:733–758.

may become fluid filled and fail to disperse prior to emergence through the gingiva. It is typically asymptomatic.

Appearance: cyst-like swelling that may be amber, blue, or red in color

Age: at the time of any erupting tooth

Treatment: This cyst may appear clinically concerning but typically self-erupts and spontaneously resolves.

Parulis (Figure 40.10A): A parulis is a soft tissue abscess typically associated with a periapical abscess that has penetrated through the bone.

Appearance: often reported as a bubble or "pimple" that bursts and leaves behind a 3- or 4-mm erythematous papule. A sinus tract from the lesion to the periapical abscess usually demonstrates purulent drainage.

Age: any age after tooth eruption

Treatment: Source control of the odontogenic infection is necessary, via either pulp therapy (pulpotomy/pulpectomy/root canal therapy) or extraction. Antibiotics are typically not necessary if dental treatment is prompt.

Pyogenic granuloma, peripheral giant cell granuloma, and peripheral ossifying fibroma: These lesions present as exophytic gingival lesions that are often grouped together because they are difficult to distinguish clinically (see Figure 40.10). Along with parulis, they are referred to as the "4 P's." They are thought to be reactive lesions and not true neoplasms.

Appearance: typically 5–20 mm but may grow rapidly in size and cause concern to patients and parents. Their surface appearance may be red to blue, smooth or ulcerated, sessile or pedunculated, and single or multilobulated. Pyogenic granulomas are very vascular in nature and may bleed easily.

Age: any age

Treatment: These lesions are non-emergent, and complete excision is typically utilized for both biopsy and cure. Identifying the source of irritation or trauma will decrease recurrence.

Clinical pearl: The adjacent teeth should be evaluated for caries and infection in order to rule out parulis.

Mucocele, ranula, and plunging ranula (Figure 40.14): Minor salivary glands may become obstructed and form localized, fluid-filled mucosal swellings termed mucoceles (Figure 40.14A). The equivalent lesion in the sublingual gland in the floor of the mouth is a ranula (Figure 40.14B). A plunging ranula occurs when there is extension through the mylohyoid into the neck and may result in significant extraoral swelling (Figure 40.14C). Obstruction of the gland is presumed to be due to trauma

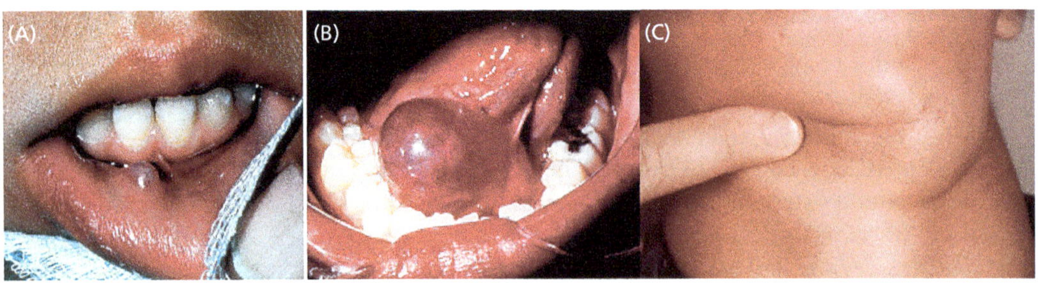

FIGURE 40.14 Mucous accumulation from obstructed salivary glands may form pseudocysts in the oral mucosa. (A) Mucoceles appear most typically in the lower lip. (B) They are termed ranulas if the sublingual gland is involved at the floor of the mouth. (C) A ranula becomes a plunging ranula when the underlying mylohyoid is disrupted, resulting in extraoral swelling.

Source: Reprinted from Wenig BM. Non-neoplastic diseases of salivary glands. In: *Atlas of Head and Neck Pathology*. 3rd ed. Philadelphia, PA: Elsevier; 2016:816–860.

resulting in injury of the gland's excretory duct. The patient will often provide a history of the lesion spontaneously rupturing and recurring.

- Appearance
  - There is translucent swelling with fluctuant core.
  - Minor salivary glands are found throughout the mouth, but most mucoceles occur in the lower lip.
  - Ranulas occur in the floor of the mouth and may have overlying erythema.
  - Plunging ranulas may demonstrate significant extraoral swelling.
- Age: any age
  - Most mucoceles and ranulas occur in the first three decades.
- Management: Excision of the lesion and the associated salivary gland(s) is necessary to prevent recurrence.

Ulcerative and Erosive Lesions

Ulcerative lesions that occur in the mouth of young patients are relatively common. Fortunately, the differential is finite and is generally self-limiting in mild to moderate cases. In severe cases, ulcerations may be very distressing and difficult to differentiate from erosive conditions associated with diseases of high morbidity.

Allergic Reaction

Ulcerations and erosions may occur from allergic reactions to virtually any material, natural or synthetic. Common allergens include foods or food ingredients such as cinnamon, or synthetic ingredients such as those found in toothpaste.

Aphthous Stomatitis

Aphthous ulcers are oral mucosal lesions caused by immune-mediated destruction of mucosa. Their cause is unclear, although several inciting factors have been identified, including local reaction to oral antigens (i.e., toothpaste ingredients) and systemic causes such as immuno- or nutritional deficiency or stress. When associated with fever, pharyngitis, and neck swelling, a diagnosis of PFAPA syndrome (periodic fever, aphthous stomatitis, pharyngitis, cervical adenitis) may be considered. Aphthous ulcerations have also been associated with several systemic diseases, such as Behçet syndrome.

- Presentation
  - Recurring aphthous ulcerations most commonly present as minor aphthous ulcers (80%), which are 3–10 mm in size and occur in low numbers (fewer than five at a time) and resolve within 1 or 2 weeks.
  - Larger ulcers (10–30 mm), termed major aphthous ulcers (10%), are also more severe in depth and may take several weeks to resolve.
  - Herpetiform aphthous ulcerations are the least common and present as very small, 1- to 3-mm lesions that are greater in number.
  - The pattern of ulcerations may resemble virally mediated ulcerations such as with primary herpetic gingivostomatitis.
- Management
  - The lesions may be observed or treated with topical corticosteroids.
  - Large lesions may take several weeks to resolve.
  - Referral to evaluate underlying causes is prudent to reduce the frequency or likelihood of recurrence and evaluate for the presence of related, occult systemic disease.

Virally Mediated Vesiculoulcerative Lesions

The following virally mediated lesions overlap in their presentation and may be difficult to distinguish. They may appear as few or abundant small vesicles that erupt over time into shallow ulcerations to confluent erosions. Location patterns and associated signs and symptoms may help distinguish the diagnoses; laboratory tests or cytology may be necessary for confirmation. Severe cases may resemble serious, erosive lesions discussed in the following section.

- Varicella (Figure 40.15A): Oral lesions may accompany varicella.
  - Presentation: typically few in number
  - Management: resolves without complication
- Acute herpetic gingivostomatitis (Figure 40.15B): The vast majority of people are exposed to herpes simplex virus 1 at a young age, but primary infection is

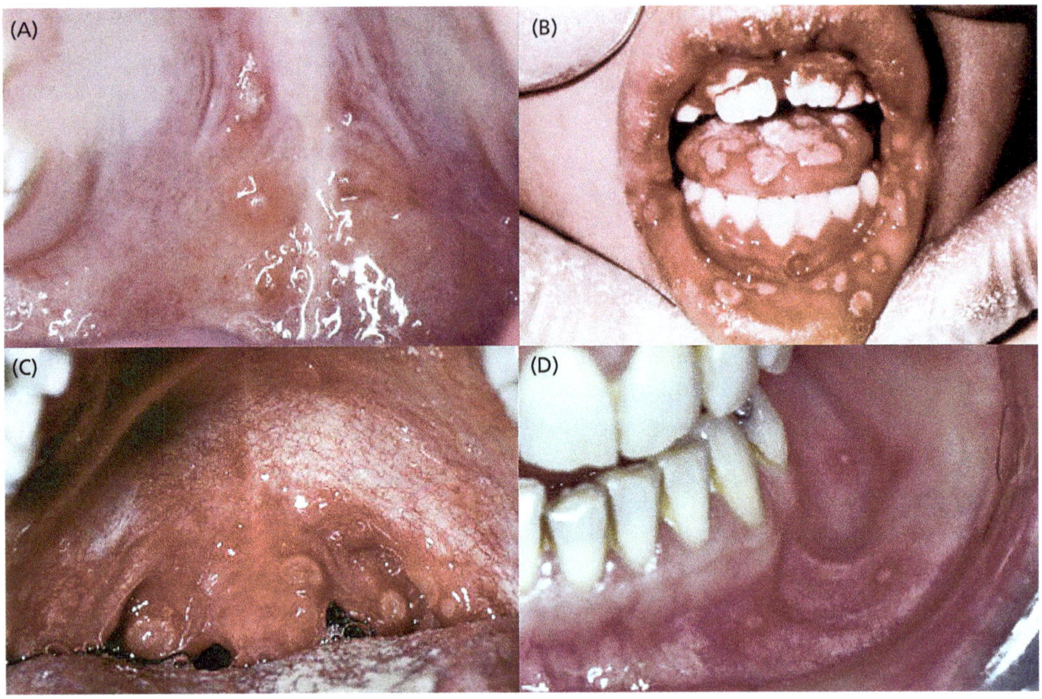

FIGURE 40.15 Viral lesions may cause oral ulcerations and erosions that are difficult to distinguish and may range in severity. (A) Varicella may have oral lesions to accompany skin lesions. (B) Primary herpes may cause severe acute herpetic gingivostomatitis. Herpangina is typically limited to the parapharyngeal tissue (C), whereas hand–foot–mouth lesions may be more broadly distributed (D).

Source: Reprinted from Neville B, et al. Soft tissue tumors. In: *Oral and Maxillofacial Pathology.* 4th ed. St. Louis, MO: Elsevier; 2016:473–532.

usually asymptomatic. The most common eruption pattern in those who are symptomatic is acute herpetic gingivostomatitis, usually between 6 months and 5 years.

Presentation

- The onset is sudden and may be accompanied by high fever, chills, lymphadenopathy, and loss of appetite.
- The oral lesions may be mild or severe.
- The lesions begin as numerous small vesicles that subsequently erupt and may coalesce to form large ulcerations and erosions.
- Any oral mucosa may be affected, including the vermillion of the lips.

Management

- Although the disease course is self-limiting, early treatment with antivirals (acyclovir suspension) has been shown to significantly reduce the time course of the outbreak.
- Mild cases resolve within 1 week, whereas severe cases may last more than 2 weeks.
- Symptomatic relief with antipyretics, analgesics, and oral rinse topical anesthetics may be helpful.
- Care should be taken with younger patients and excessive exposure to topical anesthetics, due to risk of methemoglobinemia.

Herpangina and hand, foot, and mouth disease (Figure 40.15C, D): Infection by enteroviruses, typically coxsackie virus but also echovirus and enterovirus, may result in oral eruption of vesicles, leading to ulcers. Naturally, patients typically complain of odynophagia and dysphagia, but they may also exhibit gastrointestinal symptoms such as vomiting, diarrhea, and anorexia. Patients may also have cough and fever. The symptoms overall are usually mild and resolve within 1 week.

Presentation

Herpangina lesions are limited to the peri-pharyngeal tissue; the soft palate and tonsillar pillars.

- Hand, foot, and mouth disease lesions are more distributed throughout the oral cavity. As the name describes, vesicular lesions are also commonly found on the hands and feet, particularly adjacent to the palms, soles, and on the ventral surfaces and sides of digits. Other symptoms are similar to herpangina.

Management

Supportive care

The disease course usually resolves in approximately 1 week.

Erosive and Erythematous Lesions

Necrotizing ulcerative gingivitis (NUG), trench mouth, and noma (Figure 40.16): NUG is an acute condition of the gingiva presenting as severe interdental inflammation. The condition is associated with physiologic stress, malnutrition, immunocompromise, or poor hygiene, and it is bacterially mediated. The condition may extend beyond the gingiva to the adjacent soft tissue (necrotizing ulcerative mucositis/stomatitis), and it may even extend to the skin of the face (noma/cancrum oris). It may occur at any age.

Appearance

Gingiva shows significant inflammation and surface erosion.

Severe recession of the affected tissue.

May bleed or show areas of necrosis and overlying pseudomembrane.

Management

NUG responds well to local debridement and infection control, which involves cleaning, scaling, and curettage of the teeth and gingiva, and frequent rinses with chlorhexidine or hydrogen peroxide.

Antibiotics such as penicillin or metronidazole may be used adjunctively.

For the emergency provider, prescription of an oral rinse and antibiotics with urgent referral to a dental provider are appropriate.

Erythema migrans (geographic tongue) (Figure 40.17): Erythema migrans is a benign condition that presents as erythematous patches on the dorsal surface of the tongue.

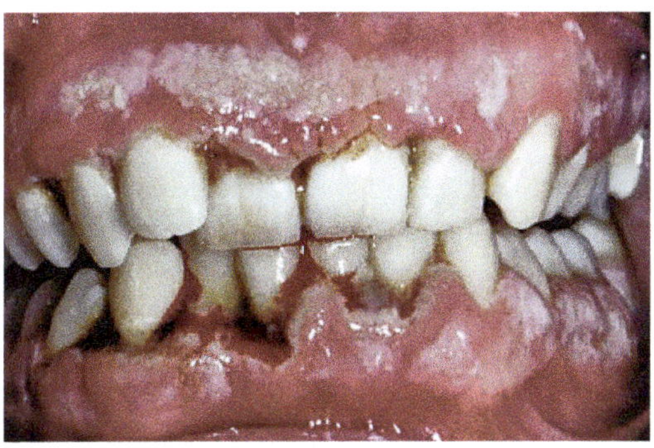

FIGURE 40.16 Necrotizing ulcerative gingivitis is characterized by severe gingival inflammation, erosion, bleeding, and recession.

Source: Reprinted from Neville B, et al. Soft tissue tumors. In: *Oral and Maxillofacial Pathology*. 4th ed. St. Louis, MO: Elsevier; 2016:473–532.

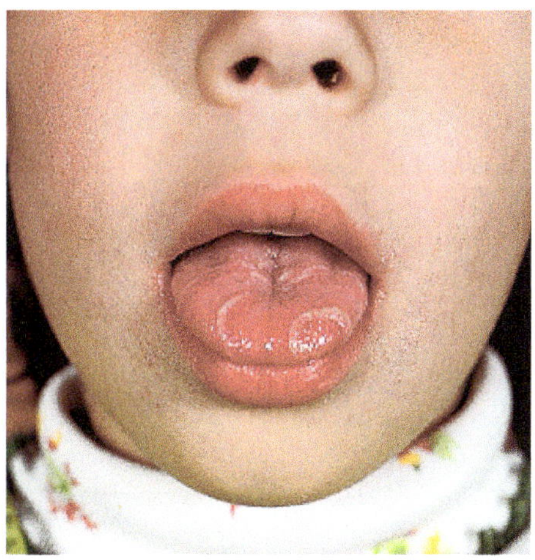

FIGURE 40.17 Erythema migrans, or "geographic tongue," typically shows smooth, red, and irregularly shaped lesions that may change shape and appearance over time (migration).

Source: Reprinted from Martin B, et al. Oral disorders. In: Zitelli BJ, McIntire S, Nowalk AJ, eds. *Zitelli and Davis' Atlas of Pediatric Physical Diagnosis*. 7th ed. Philadelphia, PA: Elsevier; 2018:733–758.

Appearance

Smooth, red, irregularly shaped lesions on the dorsal surface of the tongue.

The periphery may be encompassed by serpentine, white-yellow borders.

Lesions may uncommonly be found on other mucosal surfaces in the mouth, but they are usually also associated with tongue lesions.

The lesions frequently evolve and change location over time.

Erythematous candidiasis may appear similarly and should be ruled out.

Management

No treatment is typically necessary, although symptomatic treatment is occasionally indicated.

Candidiasis: *Candida albicans* is a component of normal oral flora, but overgrowth and opportunistic infections may occur with antibiotic use, corticosteroid use (topical or inhaled), immunosuppression, xerostomia, and prosthetic appliance use (i.e., orthodontic retainer).

Appearance

White film that wipes off, leaving an erythematous base (pseudomembranous candidiasis)

Erosive red, raw mucosal surface (erythematous candidiasis)

Management

Candidiasis is treated with antifungal medication. However, the differential diagnosis may be very broad, and the diagnosis should be confirmed and underlying causes evaluated prior to starting treatment.

41

Pediatric Gastrointestinal Emergencies

JOSHUA EASTER

Gastrointestinal (GI) problems are common among children. They present with unique signs and symptoms from adult gastrointestinal problems, and in younger children it can be particularly difficult to elicit reliable diagnostic information from the history and physical examination. Pediatric GI disease often requires surgical intervention, and delays in diagnosis may lead to significant morbidity and mortality.

The physical examination of the abdomen is paramount in children to differentiate benign and more serious causes of vomiting or abdominal pain. In order to facilitate the abdominal examination, it should be performed with the child relaxed. This is often accomplished with a young child in the caregiver's lap and with examination of the abdomen prior to other noxious physical examination maneuvers. Nonpainful areas of the abdomen should be examined first, with the examiner watching the child's face throughout the examination to determine if tenderness is present. Distracting children with nonmedical questions before and during the abdominal examination may facilitate assessment. In anxious children, it can be difficult to determine if they have tenderness because they tend to report pain with any palpation. The examiner may overcome this by palpating the areas of the abdomen with the stethoscope. Having the child jump on one foot or cough are alternate approaches to assess for peritoneal irritation in anxious children.

CONDITIONS MOST COMMONLY AFFECTING CHILDREN YOUNGER THAN AGE 3 MONTHS

Malrotation

Background

With malrotation, the cecum fails to rotate completely during fetal development, and Ladd bands of peritoneum attach the cecum to the right abdominal wall instead of its normal fixation to the retroperitoneum. The Ladd bands may compress the duodenum, leading to obstruction of the small intestine. In addition, the abnormal rotation and fixation of the cecum create a narrow stalk of mesentery that is prone to twisting/volvulus. This may impede blood flow to the bowel and cause necrosis.

Classic Clinical Presentation

Bilious emesis in a child younger than age 1 month is a surgical emergency until proven otherwise. Although parents often report green or yellow emesis, true bilious emesis is bright green or yellow; it is often helpful to show caregivers an image of bilious emesis to determine if the child's vomiting is bilious. Nearly half of neonates with bilious emesis have surgical pathology, and 15% have critical pathology that requires emergent treatment. The overall appearance of the child does not reliably distinguish patients with more benign causes of bilious emesis from those with sinister causes, and radiographic evaluation is always indicated.

The most common emergent cause of bilious emesis in a neonate is malrotation with midgut volvulus. This condition can rapidly lead to bowel necrosis, with children developing hematochezia and signs of peritonitis. Untreated, this progresses to septic shock and death. In contrast, malrotation without volvulus often presents with a more insidious onset of vomiting and abdominal pain. Children with malrotation but not volvulus may even be asymptomatic, with the malrotation detected while evaluating other conditions. Malrotation is more common in children with other congenital anomalies, such as diaphragmatic hernias, heart disease, abdominal wall defects, duodenal or biliary atresia, and Meckel's diverticulum.

Atypical Clinical Presentation

Many patients may be diagnosed in later childhood and even adulthood. Older patients tend to have more gradual onset of nonspecific symptoms such as abdominal pain and vomiting (including nonbilious emesis). Volvulus may also occur.

Diagnosis

All infants with bilious emesis require imaging. Malrotation may be identified on radiograph, ultrasound, or computed tomography (CT), but an upper GI series is the most accurate test. On plain radiographs, the presence of a double bubble sign with dilation of the stomach and proximal duodenum indicates small bowel obstruction, which increases the likelihood of malrotation. Radiographs are not sensitive, and their primary benefit is to identify pneumoperitoneum from perforation in an ill-appearing child with abdominal pain or vomiting. Regardless of the findings on plain radiography, all children with bilious emesis require further diagnostic evaluation.

A fluoroscopic upper GI series with contrast is the gold standard for diagnosing malrotation and volvulus. It will show a corkscrew duodenum with the ligament of Treitz, which is a suspensory muscle connecting the duodenum, jejunum, and mesentery, residing on the right side of the abdomen. With volvulus, the contrast often comes to a point that resembles a bird's beak. When reviewed by a pediatric radiologist, the upper GI series has a sensitivity of 96% and a specificity of 99% for malrotation. False positives may arise when the duodenum appears displaced due to other causes, such as improper technique when acquiring the images, gastric overdistension, or the presence of splenomegaly or abdominal tumors. The findings of malrotation and volvulus on an upper GI series can be subtle, and if there is any uncertainty, consultation with a pediatric radiologist or surgeon can aid in the diagnosis.

Although not as specific as upper GI for malrotation, ultrasound has reasonable sensitivity (87–100%) and should be considered if upper GI is not readily available. The most apparent sign of malrotation on ultrasound is the superior mesenteric vein residing to the left of the superior mesenteric artery. With volvulus, the twisting of the mesentery produces a characteristic whirlpool sign. Obstruction leads to dilatation of the proximal small bowel. Experienced emergency medicine ultrasonographers have successfully identified these findings at the bedside in the emergency department (ED). Ultrasound also has the advantage of being able to identify alternate causes of vomiting or pain in infants, such as pyloric stenosis or intussusception. However, patients with high clinical suspicion for malrotation require a subsequent upper GI series if the ultrasound is unrevealing. In addition, the specificity of ultrasound is lower than that of the upper GI series, and most patients with abnormal findings on ultrasound should undergo confirmatory testing with upper GI series prior to surgery.

CT can also identify malrotation when it displays the superior mesenteric vein to the left of the mesenteric artery. Other signs on CT include the proximal small intestine residing primarily in the right side of the abdomen and the third part of the duodenum residing outside its usual location between the mesenteric artery and aorta. Finally, as with ultrasound, the whirlpool sign from twisting of the mesentery suggests volvulus. CT is not the preferred imaging modality in infants due to radiation exposure and the need for the child to remain relatively still during image acquisition.

When there is a high clinical concern for malrotation with volvulus, and the child shows signs of sepsis, shock, or bowel ischemia, such as hematochezia or peritonitis, imaging should not be obtained. It delays definitive surgical treatment and increases morbidity and mortality. Acquisition of plain radiographs or bedside ultrasound may be performed while awaiting surgical consultation, but these tests should not delay definitive treatment.

Differential Diagnosis

Bilious emesis may arise from a number of emergent conditions in infants, including duodenal atresia, necrotizing enterocolitis (NEC), and intussusception (Table 41.1). Duodenal atresia is a congenital obstruction of the duodenum that may also be associated with malrotation. Infants with duodenal atresia develop bilious emesis and abdominal distension but may still pass meconium. Plain radiographs show the double bubble sign with air distending the stomach and proximal duodenum. Radiographs should be followed with an upper GI series to identify concomitant malrotation. Duodenal atresia requires surgical correction, although it is not a critically time-sensitive procedure like malrotation with volvulus. NEC, intussusception, and pyloric stenosis are discussed in more detail elsewhere in this chapter.

Treatment

Rapid recognition of volvulus and consultation with a surgeon are critical. Children should receive intravenous fluids, with boluses of fluid, if there are any signs of hemodynamic instability. Ill-appearing children or those with peritoneal signs should receive broad-spectrum intravenous antibiotics (e.g., ampicillin, gentamicin, and metronidazole) and emergent surgery. During the operation, necrotic portions of the bowel are excised. Areas of bowel with uncertain viability may be left in place and observed closely with subsequent surgical explorations. Laparoscopy for children without peritonitis or hemodynamic instability appears to be associated with less adverse events and more rapid recovery compared to open laparotomy.

Malrotation without volvulus is not a surgical emergency. With the Ladd procedure, a surgeon incises the Ladd bands, widens the mesentery, and ensures the bowel cannot rotate. The appendix is typically removed during the procedure because its atypical location may lead to delay in the diagnosis of appendicitis in the future. For asymptomatic children with malrotation without volvulus, the Ladd procedure can be performed electively after outpatient discussion of the risks and benefits of the procedure with a pediatric surgeon.

TABLE 41.1 EMERGENT CONDITIONS LEADING TO VOMITING IN INFANTS

	Condition				
	Malrotation with Volvulus	Pyloric Stenosis	NEC	Hirschsprung Disease	Intussusception
Age	<1 year	<3 months	<1 month	<1 year	<2 years
Presentation	Bilious emesis	Projectile emesis	Bilious emesis; abdominal distention	Bilious emesis; constipation; diarrhea if enterocolitis	Emesis may be bilious; colicky abdominal pain
Diagnosis	Upper GI	Ultrasound	X-ray	Contrast enema	Ultrasound
Secondary diagnostic tests	Ultrasound	Upper GI	Ultrasound	Biopsy	N/A
Treatment	Emergent surgery	Surgery	Antibiotics; surgery	Antibiotics and surgery if enterocolitis	Air or saline enema

GI, gastrointestinal; N/A, not applicable; NEC, necrotizing enterocolitis.

Complications

Delays in definitive surgical management of volvulus increase the risk of bowel necrosis, sepsis, and death. Children requiring transfer to another hospital for management are more likely to require bowel resection. Resection of bowel increases children's risk of short gut syndrome.

The vast majority of children with malrotation without volvulus heal without significant complications; although subsequent volvulus may arise in <10% of patients because surgical correction does not completely preclude future twisting of the mesentery.

Disposition

Children with volvulus require immediate surgery. Children with concern for malrotation (including neonates with bilious emesis) should undergo emergent upper GI series or ultrasound. If these are not available, these children should be transferred emergently to a hospital where they can be performed. Ill-appearing children should receive fluids and antibiotics prior to transfer. A neonate with bilious vomiting should ideally be evaluated by a pediatric surgeon given the limited utility of imaging (especially if interpreted by a non-pediatric radiologist) and the high risk of complications with delayed recognition of volvulus. Transfer to a center with a pediatric specialist should be considered prior to imaging in high-risk patients (even if initially well-appearing) to expedite evaluation.

Asymptomatic malrotation incidentally found does not require emergent surgery. However, outpatient surgery referral should occur due to future risk of volvulus.

Key Points and Pitfalls

- All neonates with bilious emesis should be assumed to have malrotation with volvulus until proven otherwise.
- Children may appear well with benign abdominal examinations but still have life-threatening volvulus.
- Emergent upper GI series and pediatric surgery consultation should be obtained if there is concern for volvulus, which may require transfer.
- Plain radiographs cannot rule out malrotation. Even an upper GI is not completely sensitive.
- Volvulus can occur in older children.

Pyloric Stenosis

Background

Pyloric stenosis arises with hypertrophy of the sphincter around the exit from the stomach into the duodenum. This enlargement limits the egress of food from the stomach. As the hypertrophy worsens, food can only exit the stomach through vomiting.

Risk factors include male, first born, prematurity, bottle-feeding, family history, maternal smoking, and maternal macrolide use.

Classic Clinical Presentation

Pyloric stenosis typically presents with projectile vomiting in an infant younger than age 3 months. In contrast to the more common gastroesophageal reflux and normal spitting up, the emesis of pyloric stenosis is forceful. Clarification and direct observation in the ED can help differentiate true projectile vomiting. Patients without projectile vomiting are unlikely to have pyloric stenosis; children born prematurely are an exception because they often do not have sufficient musculature to generate forceful vomiting. With pyloric stenosis, the emesis will typically arise within 30 minutes of feeding. Moreover, infants are typically hungry and feed voraciously. Bilious vomiting and hematemesis are uncommon but can rarely occur.

On physical examination, children are typically well-appearing early in the disease with a fairly benign abdominal examination. An olive-shaped mass on the right side of patients' epigastrum is best noted with significant abdominal musculature relaxation. The absence of a mass should not alter the level of concern for pyloric stenosis because it is sometimes difficult to appreciate.

Atypical Clinical Presentation

Infants presenting later in their disease course may appear ill and may have stopped gaining weight or even lost weight. They often have reduced vomiting because they no longer have the energy to attempt feeding. They may show signs of dehydration, with poor skin turgor and decreased urine output. Their weight declines. Severe alkalosis from protracted vomiting may lead to apnea. Hyperbilirubinemia and jaundice may occur.

There have been reports of children presenting with pyloric stenosis as young as age 1 week and as old as age 12 weeks. Vomiting beyond age 12 weeks should prompt evaluation for alternate etiologies.

Diagnosis

Laboratory evaluation is not required in the initial evaluation of a well-appearing child with vomiting. In children with pyloric stenosis, chemistries may reveal a hypochloremic, metabolic alkalosis due to vomiting of gastric acid. Children may also develop hypokalemia with persistent vomiting. However, nearly 90% of children do not have any electrolyte abnormalities. Notably, the presence of an acidosis should increase suspicion for an alternate etiology for vomiting. Other laboratory studies are not typically warranted unless additional clinical circumstances are present—for example, bilirubin should be measured if the infant is jaundiced.

Ultrasound is the gold standard for identifying pyloric stenosis. Signs of hypertrophy of the pylorus include pyloric length >15 mm, diameter >10 mm, and thickness of the muscle >3 mm. Other signs are the target sign in the transverse view (hypertrophied muscle outside of the pyloric mucosa) and failure to see stomach contents pass into the duodenum during the examination. When measured by an experienced ultrasonographer, including emergency physicians, these cutoffs have excellent diagnostic accuracy, with sensitivity and specificity approaching 100%. Feeding the child a small amount of sucrose before the ultrasound may improve accuracy by dilating the fundus. False negatives may arise with poor visualization of the pylorus or in small infants. The size of the normal pylorus may be proportional to the child's overall size, and therefore these cutoffs may be too large for small, premature infants. False positives arise with transient pylorospasm, which occurs in healthy infants.

An upper GI series can also visualize pyloric stenosis. It will show the string sign with contrast passing through an elongated pyloric canal or the beak sign with contrast gradually tapering as it reaches the pylorus. Unlike midgut volvulus, this beak sign is in the stomach with pyloric stenosis and not the duodenum. Upper GI series expose infants to radiation and should not be the first-line imaging modality for pyloric stenosis. It may be appropriate if alternate diagnoses are being considered (e.g., malrotation) or if ultrasound is not readily available.

Plain abdominal radiographs do not have sufficient sensitivity to rule out pyloric stenosis and should not be obtained unless there is concern for obstruction or pneumoperitoneum.

Differential Diagnosis

True forceful, projectile, and nonbilious emesis is rarely encountered with other conditions in infants (see Table 41.1). Forceful vomiting is typically bilious in intestinal obstruction or malrotation.

Treatment

Pyloromyotomy, a laparoscopic surgical incision of the pylorus, is the treatment.

Ill-appearing children require admission to the intensive care unit (ICU) and repletion of their intravascular volume (boluses of 20 cc/kg of isotonic fluids) and electrolytes (typically potassium chloride) prior to surgical repair.

Disposition

Pyloric stenosis is not a surgical emergency, and surgery is typically scheduled urgent next day. Children are at risk for dehydration with ongoing vomiting, but there is no inherent risk to the stomach or duodenum. Non-operative management with atropine to reduce muscle spasm and peristalsis may achieve resolution of pyloric stenosis within 2 weeks in up to 80% of children, but this practice is not standard of care in the United States.

Complications

The primary complication of pyloric stenosis is dehydration. This has become much less common because children present earlier in the course of their illnesses. The primary risks of pyloromyotomy are (1) incomplete incision of the pylorus leading to ongoing vomiting and (2) perforation of the stomach leading to pneumoperitoneum.

Key Points and Pitfalls

- Vomiting most frequently arises with gastroesophageal reflux or overfeeding in infants, but true projectile vomiting in an infant younger than age 2 months is typically pyloric stenosis.
- The presence of bilious emesis suggests potentially more ominous etiologies.
- Although children with pyloric stenosis can become severely dehydrated, most

children are well-appearing with normal physical examinations.
- Ultrasound is an excellent test for identifying pyloric stenosis, and most infants with projectile vomiting do not require other studies.

Umbilical Hernia

Background

All children have an opening at the umbilicus at birth for the umbilical cord. This tends to close within 1 week of birth. Failure to close leads to the formation of hernias, which arise in 20% of infants.

Classic Clinical Presentation

Most commonly, umbilical hernias will be encountered in the ED in the midst of examining a child for an unrelated concern. The hernia is usually apparent at birth but may increase in size. Umbilical hernias may be quite large, and crying may further increase their size. They are usually readily reduced when the child relaxes the abdominal muscles or when the child is sleeping. In contrast to inguinal hernias, <1% of unrepaired umbilical hernias incarcerate.

Diagnosis

Umbilical hernias that are readily reducible on examination do not require any diagnostic evaluation in the ED. Ultrasound can confirm the presence of bowel in umbilical masses that cannot be readily reduced in the ED.

Differential Diagnosis

Umbilical granulomas are pink, pedunculated lesions that are typically <1 cm. They may drain serous fluid. Weekly application of silver nitrate leads to their resolution.

Children can also develop hemangiomas, neurofibromas, lipomas, and skin malignancies at the umbilicus. These masses are initially small and cannot be reduced.

Hernias near the umbilicus that persist beyond age 5 years often are not umbilical but, rather, supraumbilical, indirect hernias. These are difficult to differentiate from umbilical hernias on physical examination. In contrast to umbilical hernias, they typically do not close spontaneously, and they require surgical repair.

Treatment

Unlike in adults, nearly all (>90%) umbilical hernias in children close spontaneously and do not require surgery. They typically resolve by age 1 year. Practice varies from repair only for symptomatic hernias to repair of all umbilical hernias that persist at age 5 years. Incarcerated or strangulated hernias require surgical repair.

Disposition

Patients with asymptomatic umbilical hernias identified in the ED should receive nonemergent outpatient referral to a surgeon to discuss the risks and benefits of elective repair. Children with signs of incarceration or strangulation are rare, but they require emergent surgical treatment.

Complications

After surgical repair, there is a 1% risk of infection and 1% or 2% risk of hernia recurrence.

Key Points and Pitfalls

- Umbilical hernias may be quite large, and their appearance may be distressing to parents. However, nearly all of them resolve spontaneously without intervention or complication.
- The ED evaluation of these hernias should focus on identifying incarceration and strangulation through the history and physical examination.

Necrotizing Enterocolitis

Background

Necrotizing enterocolitis is a life-threatening condition most commonly seen in the neonatal ICU but can less commonly present to the ED in term infants. NEC likely represents a spectrum of diseases, with inflammation, infection, and ischemia contributing to damage to the intestinal wall, most commonly the terminal ileum and colon. Nearly all (>95%) cases of NEC occur in children born before 32 weeks of gestation or with very low birth weight (<1,500 g).

Classic Clinical Presentation

Because NEC most commonly arises 1–3 weeks after birth in neonates born prematurely, it typically presents while children are in the neonatal ICU. Children who have previously been feeding without incident develop vomiting, which is often bilious. On examination, their abdomens become distended, and later in the disease they may also develop erythema and induration of the abdominal wall. Often, occult blood is present in the stool. The disease progresses rapidly over the course of hours. As the bowel necroses, infants develop peritonitis and hematochezia. Systemic inflammation may lead to shock with pallor, hypotension, temperature instability, and tachycardia or bradycardia. Bowel perforation may lead to peritoneal signs, with the abdomen developing a bluish hue.

Atypical Clinical Presentation

Necrotizing enterocolitis rarely may afflict infants born at term, particularly those with other congenital comorbidities or peripartum complications. The diagnosis should be considered in neonates with bilious emesis or abdominal distention in the first 1 or 2 weeks of life.

Diagnosis

The presence of air in the bowel wall or portal venous system on imaging (i.e., pneumatosis intestinalis) represents NEC until proven otherwise. Earlier in the disease, children may only have dilated bowel loops and thickened bowel walls. As the disease progresses, bowel perforation may lead to pneumoperitoneum.

Plain radiographs are the initial screening test for NEC. On radiographs, air appears as bubbles or linear railroad tracks within the bowel wall (Figure 41.1). It is most readily visualized in the right lower quadrant. The extent of the gas in the bowel wall does not correlate with disease severity. Gas in the portal venous system appears as a curvilinear radiolucency over the liver. False positives may arise from air in the stool. False negatives occur in 25% of cases and are more common early in the disease course when air is not yet visible in the bowel wall.

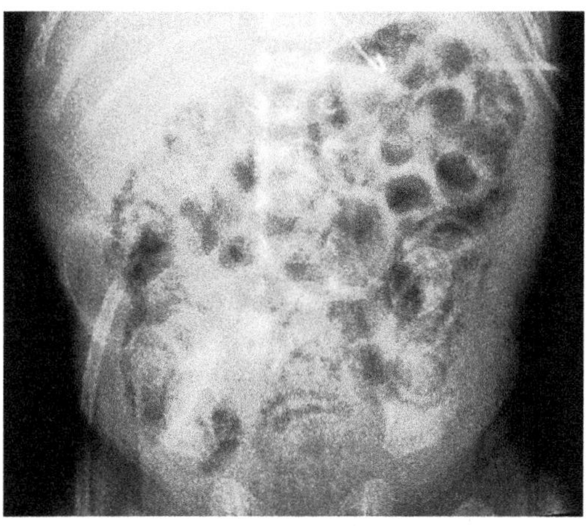

FIGURE 41.1 Plain film of necrotizing enterocolitis demonstrating air within bowel wall.

Ultrasound may allow detection of NEC earlier in the disease course compared to plain radiographs. It should be employed when plain radiographs are not diagnostic and there is clinical concern for NEC. With color Doppler, ultrasound also has excellent sensitivity for necrotic bowel and pneumoperitoneum.

CT is not typically required to diagnose NEC. Although it is highly sensitive and specific for NEC, it exposes neonates to significant radiation.

Children with pneumatosis or pneumoperitoneum should have laboratory studies obtained, including complete blood count, chemistries, coagulation panel, and blood culture. Approximately half of children will have bacteremia. Many develop metabolic acidosis, neutropenia, thrombocytopenia, and hyponatremia due to dehydration, disseminated intravascular coagulation, or sepsis.

Differential Diagnosis

Necrotizing enterocolitis should be considered as a potential etiology for any critically ill neonate because it may present with signs of sepsis, including multiorgan dysfunction, shock, or apnea. In particular, if hematochezia is present with these conditions, this suggests NEC. Both malrotation and NEC may present with bilious emesis (see Table 41.1). However, volvulus does not produce pneumatosis. There are alternate etiologies for pneumatosis in an infant, such as cow's milk protein allergy and food protein intolerance enterocolitis syndrome. These tend to arise later in childhood and should be considered only after ruling out NEC in a neonate with vomiting or abdominal distention.

Treatment

All infants with pneumatosis require surgical consultation, broad-spectrum intravenous antibiotics (e.g., ampicillin, gentamicin, and metronidazole), intravenous fluids (20 mL/kg of isotonic fluid, if there are any signs of volume depletion), and placement of a nasogastric tube. Exploratory laparotomy and resection of any necrotic bowel are necessary for children with pneumoperitoneum or evidence of bowel necrosis.

Disposition

All children with concern for NEC require emergent evaluation by a pediatric surgeon and admission to the ICU.

Complications

Necrotizing enterocolitis is associated with extremely high morbidity and mortality; nearly one-third of neonates with NEC die. Necrosis of the bowel wall may lead to short gut syndrome or the development of strictures and fistulas. The systemic inflammation of NEC may also adversely impact the brain, leading to microcephaly and developmental delay.

Key Points and Pitfalls

- Neonates may present with nonspecific symptoms; the presence of hematochezia or bilious emesis in a neonate younger than age 3 weeks, particularly if they were born prematurely, should prompt consideration of NEC.
- Because premature infants are now leaving the hospital earlier, NEC may be more frequently encountered in the ED.
- Plain radiographs may not show pneumatosis early in the course of NEC, and these patients may still develop bowel necrosis imminently. Therefore, any neonate with clinical concern for NEC should undergo close observation and surgical consultation, even if plain radiographs are unrevealing.

CONDITIONS MOST COMMONLY AFFECTING CHILDREN YOUNGER THAN AGE 2 YEAR

Hirschsprung Disease (Congenital Aganglionic Megacolon)

Background

The absence of ganglion cells in the distal large bowel results in loss of peristalsis and a functional large bowel obstruction. In <10% of cases, the disease extends beyond the colon into the small intestine. It is more common in children with trisomy 21 or other congenital anomalies.

Classic Clinical Presentation

Infants with Hirschsprung disease present with signs of obstruction, including feeding intolerance and bilious emesis. Almost all (90%) infants with Hirschsprung disease do not pass meconium within 24–48 hours of birth. On physical examination, infants with Hirschsprung disease will have abdominal distention. With rectal examination, they may have a large release of flatus or stool.

Atypical Clinical Presentation

Although classically Hirschsprung disease manifests as a bowel obstruction in a neonate, in approximately 10% of cases it presents beyond age 3 years with chronic constipation. Ongoing constipation that fails to improve with diet changes and laxatives should raise concern for Hirschsprung disease in older children.

One-third of children with Hirschsprung disease may also develop enterocolitis. Instead of constipation, these children have forceful diarrhea and vomiting with fever and abdominal distention. Unlike most cases of gastroenteritis, children with enterocolitis appear ill and may develop fulminant sepsis.

Failure to pass meconium within the first 48 hours of life, growth delays, or abdominal distention support the diagnosis of Hirschsprung disease in patients with atypical presentations.

Diagnosis

The gold standard for the diagnosis of Hirschsprung disease is rectal biopsy. However, in the ED, the primary diagnostic modality is ***plain radiography*** despite its poor diagnostic accuracy. It may demonstrate dilated loops of large and small bowel with a cone-shaped transition zone, but it is often normal. Notably, the combination of abnormal radiographs suggestive of obstruction and diarrhea in a neonate should raise concern for Hirschsprung disease and enterocolitis.

Treatment

Surgical repair removing the abnormal segment of bowel is the treatment of Hirschsprung disease. Ill-appearing children with potential Hirschsprung disease, including those with enterocolitis, should receive intravenous fluids, broad-spectrum antibiotics (e.g., piperacillin–tazobactam and metronidazole), nasogastric tube placement, and emergent surgical evaluation. Definitive treatment typically is delayed until the patient's condition stabilizes, although patients with enterocolitis may benefit from emergent surgery.

Complications

The most severe complication is sepsis in children with enterocolitis. Following surgery, children may develop renewed symptoms of constipation and obstruction. This arises as a result of mechanical obstruction from adhesions or failure to resect the entire aganglionic segment during surgery. Children may also develop encopresis due to hyperperistalsis or poor muscle function. These complications typically resolve spontaneously within a few years.

Key Points and Pitfalls

- The presence of diarrhea or fever in a neonate with an abdominal radiograph suggestive of bowel obstruction is concerning for Hirschsprung disease with enterocolitis. These children can deteriorate rapidly and require aggressive resuscitation, antibiotics, and surgical consultation.
- The presence of abdominal distention, vomiting, and constipation in a neonate, particularly in a child who did not pass meconium within 48 hours of life, should prompt further diagnostic workup.
- Well-appearing children with concern for Hirschsprung disease can be discharged safely with outpatient follow-up for rectal biopsy.

Meckel's Diverticulum

Background

Meckel's diverticulum is the most common congenital abnormality in the GI system. It is a remnant of an embryologic duct leading to an outpouching of bowel that contains all the layers of the small intestine and often contains heterotopic gastric, pancreatic, or colonic tissue. This excess tissue may lead to obstruction or diverticulitis. Heterotopic gastric tissue may release acid that damages the intestinal mucosa, leading to hemorrhage. Only a small minority of patients develop symptoms, but half of these cases present before age 10 years.

Classic Clinical Presentation

The most common presentation of Meckel's diverticulum is painless GI bleeding (bright red or melena). With prolonged bleeding, children may show signs of anemia with fatigue, lightheadedness, and pallor. With massive bleeding, children may have hemodynamic instability. Abdominal pain is uncommon, but mild cramping may occur.

Adults are more likely to present with obstruction; bleeding is typically melena when it less commonly occurs.

Atypical Clinical Presentation

In addition to bleeding, Meckel's diverticulum can cause intussusception, diverticulitis, and volvulus. The diverticulum may act as lead point for intussusception. These children present similarly to children with other causes of intussusception. However, after treatment with air enemas, children with diverticula may experience recurrent intussusception. The diverticula may also become inflamed, leading to diverticulitis, which is otherwise rare in children. As in adults, these children present with abdominal pain, vomiting, and fever, which often raises initial concern for appendicitis. Finally, the stalk attaching the diverticula to the bowel can act as a fulcrum for the bowel to twist around it, leading to volvulus. These children present with severe abdominal pain and vomiting.

Diagnosis

The appropriate diagnostic modality depends on the extent of bleeding. Meckel's diverticulum is not typically visible on plain radiographs, ultrasound, endoscopy, or colonoscopy. For children with mild to moderate bleeding (i.e., children with hemodynamic stability and only mild reductions in their hemoglobin), a Meckel's scan displays excellent sensitivity (90–97%) for detecting diverticula with ectopic gastric mucosa. A tracer, technetium-99m, with affinity for gastric mucosa is injected and then visualized on the scan. Rarely, false positives arise from inflammatory bowel disease and intussusception.

For patients with more severe bleeding, CT angiography has high diagnostic accuracy for active bleeding, with a sensitivity of 85% and a specificity of 92%. It does expose children to significant radiation and should be reserved for cases with concern for significant bleeding.

Finally, for patients with life-threatening bleeding, arteriography with interventional radiology has excellent diagnostic accuracy and also allows for treatment of alternate causes of life-threatening bleeding, such as arteriovenous malformations (AVMs).

Differential Diagnosis

A common alternate cause for red stool in young children is the ingestion of red substances, such as fruit punch or Cheetos. These result in stools that are hemoccult negative. Juvenile polyps may produce painless bleeding in young children. These can be identified and resected with colonoscopy. Most other causes of bleeding are associated with pain, including enteritis, colitis, inflammatory bowel disease, anal fissures, and ulcers. Other causes of painless bleeding encountered in adults, such as diverticulosis and malignancy, are rare in children.

Treatment

Children with significant bleeding require resuscitation with blood. This is followed by surgical resection of the diverticula. If the diverticula is particularly wide, removal of the surrounding bowel and anastomosis may be necessary.

Children with signs of obstruction or volvulus should receive nasogastric tube decompression followed by surgical resection of the diverticula.

Disposition

Patients with bleeding from Meckel's diverticula require admission to the hospital and to the ICU if there are signs of brisk bleeding or hemodynamic instability.

If a Meckel's scan is not readily available, observation may help determine the extent of the bleeding in children without initial signs of severe bleeding. Children with ongoing bleeding in the ED or signs of impending significant bleeding (tachycardia, anemia, etc.) should be transferred to a hospital with the ability to perform a Meckel's scan or CT angiography. Well-appearing children with minimal bleeding can be discharged with outpatient follow-up within 3 days.

When an asymptomatic diverticulum is visualized on CT, patients can be discharged with non-urgent outpatient follow-up with a pediatric gastroenterologist or surgeon. They should return to the ED if they develop bleeding, vomiting, or abdominal pain.

Key Points and Pitfalls

- Most gastrointestinal bleeding in children is benign, but bleeding from a Meckel's diverticulum can become severe, leading to shock.
- Conventional imaging is not sufficiently sensitive to rule out Meckel's diverticulum, and patients require a Meckel's nuclear scan or CT angiography.
- After a period of observation in the ED, well-appearing, hemodynamically stable children with a normal hemoglobin can be discharged for outpatient diagnostic evaluation.

Intussusception

Background

With intussusception, a proximal piece of intestine (typically the ileum) telescopes into a distal piece. Between 5% and 20% of cases in children have a pathological lead point that serves as a nidus for the intussusception, and these are more common in children older than age 5 years. Potential lead points include a Meckel's diverticulum, polyp, or tumor. Although the association of rotavirus vaccine with intussusception has received extensive publicity, the current vaccine is low risk (1 case per 20,000–100,000 vaccinations). Nearly one-third of children with intussusception experience a viral prodrome, such as gastroenteritis or an upper respiratory infection, which may produce hypertrophy of Peyer's patches in the bowel. These may then serve as nonpathological lead points for intussusception.

Classic Clinical Presentation

Most (80%) children present with intussusception before age 2 years. The incidence declines with age, although it can occur at any age, including adulthood. It is more common in males. The textbook triad of colicky abdominal pain with the knees drawn to the chest, an abdominal mass, and currant jelly stools is rarely encountered (25% of cases). The most common feature is severe, intermittent abdominal pain. Children may draw their legs up to their abdomen, curl into the fetal position, or cry inconsolably for 5–30 minutes at a time. Vomiting is initially nonbilious and nonbloody but may later contain bile (Table 41.1). In infants, vomiting may be the primary symptom. Currant jelly stools from the combination of mucus and blood are a late finding. Occult blood may be present.

Intussusception may be difficult to identify based on history and physical examination because patients often appear well between episodes of pain and vomiting. Moreover, most patients have normal abdominal examinations. Due to gaseous distention of the bowel, the classically described sausage-shaped mass in the right upper quadrant and flat right lower quadrant are rarely encountered in the ED.

Atypical Clinical Presentation

Children rarely develop bowel ischemia or perforation in the setting of intussusception. When present, these children appear ill and have peritoneal signs on examination.

Children may also present with lethargy, which may develop due to release of endogenous opioids. Like the other signs of intussusception, lethargy may be intermittent. This often leads to delays in diagnosis, as other emergent and common causes of lethargy are evaluated.

Small intestine to small intestine intussusception may cause similar symptoms to ileocolic intussusception or be asymptomatic and noted incidentally on imaging. Unlike ileocolic intussusception, most small intestine intussusceptions resolve spontaneously. If a long segment of bowel >3.5 cm is involved or the patient has ongoing significant symptoms, reduction may be warranted. Small bowel reductions require surgical intervention because enemas do not effectively reduce small bowel intussusception.

Diagnosis

Ultrasound is the preferred modality for identifying intussusception. It displays a target sign in the right abdomen, with intestine contained within intestine on cross section, or the pseudokidney sign in the longitudinal axis. Ultrasound has nearly perfect sensitivity and specificity when performed by an experienced ultrasonographer, including emergency physicians. It is readily performed at the bedside, inexpensive, and does not harbor any radiation. It also helps predict the likelihood of success with non-operative management. Identification of a pathologic lead point, free peritoneal fluid, the absence of blood flow with Doppler suggestive of bowel ischemia, or the presence of fluid trapped between the colon and telescoping small intestine are associated with failure of non-operative management.

CT also has excellent diagnostic accuracy for intussusception. However, its acquisition requires children to remain still, which is often difficult with the colicky pain of intussusception. In addition, it exposes children to harmful radiation.

Previously, air or contrast enema was employed for diagnostic purposes in children with high clinical suspicion for intussusception. An enema does not identify other potential etiologies for the patient's symptoms. It is invasive and exposes children to radiation. Therefore, ultrasound has supplanted enema for diagnostic purposes.

In patients with low pretest probability of disease, the presence of air in the terminal ileum or ascending colon on all views of a three-view abdominal radiograph reduces the likelihood of intussusception. However, for most children with concern for intussusception, plain radiographs do not demonstrate adequate diagnostic accuracy for routine use, with a sensitivity of approximately 50% and specificity of 20%. The identification of a soft tissue mass, dilated loops of bowel, or a target sign on radiographs increase the likelihood of intussusception.

Differential Diagnosis

Intussusception can be difficult to diagnose because severe, colicky abdominal pain coupled with vomiting in a young child can arise from multiple conditions. These include other critical illnesses, such as ovarian torsion, testicular torsion, strangulated hernia, or appendicitis, as well as more benign conditions such as constipation. Notably, the fluid surrounding a perforated appendix may look similar to an intussusception on ultrasound.

Rectal bleeding can occur in infants with Meckel's diverticulum, anal fissures, colitis, or food-induced allergic colitis. Unlike intussusception, these conditions do not yield currant jelly stools.

Treatment

Non-operative management is the first-line therapy for children, except those with peritonitis, hemodynamic instability, or sepsis. Air, saline, or water-soluble contrast enemas performed by a radiologist under fluoroscopic guidance are successful at reducing intussusception in approximately 75% of patients.

Compared to liquid enemas, air enemas have higher rates of success, require less radiation, are less expensive, and are safer if perforation occurs. Saline enemas allow reduction under ultrasound guidance, which is difficult with air enemas because air obscures images. Ultrasound-guided enemas reduce radiation exposure. Sedation is typically not required. Empiric antibiotics prior to reduction are sometimes given, but their benefit remains unproven.

Occasionally, enemas fail to reduce the intussusception. Failure occurs more frequently in infants younger than age 3 months, with symptoms longer than 2 days, and with a pathological lead point. However, enema should still be attempted prior to operative reduction in these patients because it may be successful and is safe. If there is a partial reduction of the intussusception and no pathologic lead point is apparent, a delayed repeat enema in 1 or 2 hours may provide complete reduction and obviate the need for surgical reduction in 50–80% of cases. Repeat enema is unlikely to provide benefit if the initial attempt did not provide any change in the intussusception.

Operative management is rarely necessary except with unsuccessful non-operative attempts at reduction, multiple recurrences, or signs of peritonitis or shock. These children should receive intravenous antibiotics prior to surgery. If no pathological lead point is visualized in the operating room, manual reduction under laparoscopic guidance is first line. If this fails or if a lead point is identified, children may require bowel resection and anastomosis. Surgical management has higher morbidity, mortality, and cost compared to enema therapy.

Interestingly, external manual compression of the abdomen with dynamic ultrasound visualization of the intussusception has been reported. This has many potential advantages but does not have sufficient evidence to supplant the current standard of care.

Disposition

Children undergoing successful non-operative reduction—that is, with radiographic confirmation of the reduction and resolution of their symptoms—can be discharged home. Routine admission after reduction does not reduce the risk of recurrence or perforation and therefore is not warranted. Patients should be instructed to return to the ED if they have renewed symptoms.

If ultrasound or enema are not available to diagnose intussusception, urgent transfer is necessary. If an enema is performed and leads to movement of the intussusception but not reduction, it can be repeated again prior to transferring the patient. Notably, if a patient becomes asymptomatic in transfer after an initial ultrasound showing intussusception, a repeat ultrasound should be obtained; occasionally, the intussusception will have resolved spontaneously.

If intussusception is identified incidentally while evaluating other etiologies, it can be evaluated further as an outpatient. Most of these asymptomatic intussusceptions resolve without intervention. Patients should return to the ED if they become symptomatic.

Complications

Less than 0.5% of children undergoing non-operative reduction sustain a perforation of their bowel requiring emergent surgical consultation and intravenous broad-spectrum antibiotics. Perforation appears to be more common in children younger than age 6 months, with prolonged symptoms, receiving sedation prior to reduction, and requiring higher pressures during reduction. Perforation rarely leads to tension pneumoperitoneum with air in the abdomen limiting ventilation and venous return. Children may develop a fever after their reduction. Typically, this is transient, reflecting inflammation and not sepsis or perforation.

Approximately 10% of children will experience recurrence of the intussusception. This is most common in the first 48 hours after the reduction but can occur at any point. Recurrence is more likely if there is a pathological lead point. Recurrent intussusceptions can continue to be managed non-operatively; surgical management becomes appropriate when there are multiple recurrences. Small studies suggest administration of dexamethasone around the time of reduction may reduce the risk of recurrence.

Key Points and Pitfalls

- The presence of colicky abdominal pain in a child younger than age 2 years should raise concern for intussusception.

- Many patients will not have vomiting or blood in their stool. Their abdominal examinations are often normal.
- Lethargy may be the sole presentation of intussusception or associated with vomiting.
- Ultrasound should be obtained on all patients with concern for intussusception. Plain radiography does not have sufficient sensitivity to rule out intussusception.
- Delayed repeat enema is often successful in children when the initial enema only accomplishes partial reduction of the intussusception.
- Well-appearing children with successful reduction of their intussusception do not require admission to the hospital.

CONDITIONS MOST COMMONLY AFFECTING CHILDREN OLDER THAN AGE 2 YEARS

Appendicitis

Background

As in adults, appendicitis in children arises when material in the bowel or an enlarged lymphoid follicle obstructs the lumen of the appendix. This allows bacteria to propagate and invade the wall of the appendix, leading to inflammation and peritonitis. If unchecked, eventually the appendix perforates.

Classic Clinical Presentation

Appendicitis can arise at any age but most commonly develops after age 9 years. The presenting signs and symptoms vary by age (Table 41.2). Children older than age 9 years present similarly to adults with abdominal pain that begins around the umbilicus and migrates to the right lower quadrant. Anorexia and vomiting commonly accompany the pain. Individual symptoms are poor predictors of appendicitis. In contradistinction, physical examination findings are better predictors of appendicitis, with rebound tenderness, guarding, Rovsing's sign, obturator sign, and psoas sign most suggestive of appendicitis.

Appendicitis is much less common in young children because the shape of the appendix early in life renders it less prone to obstruction. However, when appendicitis develops in young children, it is also more apt to perforate because the wall of the appendix is thinner in young children. Children younger than age 5 years with appendicitis have difficulty localizing their symptoms. Infants younger than age 2 years may present only with fever, irritability, or vomiting. Focal tenderness in the right lower quadrant is less common, arising in one-third of young children. Diarrhea is present in one-third of young children with appendicitis. As a result of these atypical presentations, substantial delays in diagnosis are common. Nearly all infants and half of children younger than age 5 years develop appendiceal perforation before diagnosis. These children present with abdominal distension and tenderness.

From age 5 years until adolescence, children have more typical presentations with abdominal pain, vomiting, and fever. However, these children continue to have difficulty localizing their pain. It may impact their gait and limit their willingness to hop on one foot or cough. Children usually have focal right lower quadrant tenderness on abdominal examination. Pain is greatest over McBurney's point,

TABLE 41.2 PRESENTATION OF APPENDICITIS BY AGE OF THE CHILD

	Age (Years)			
	<2	2–5	5–9	>9
Primary symptoms	Various; often perforated	Vomiting	Abdominal pain	Right lower quadrant pain
Associated symptoms	Irritability; fever; vomiting	Abdominal pain; fever	Vomiting; fever	Vomiting; fever; anorexia
Physical examination	Distention; diffuse tenderness	Tenderness on right or lower abdomen	Tender in right lower quadrant; + rebound	Tender in right lower quadrant; + rebound

two-thirds of the distance along an imaginary line from the umbilicus to the anterior superior iliac spine. The presence of rebound tenderness—that is, pain elicited when releasing the hand after applying 15 seconds of constant pressure—is the most useful sign, increasing the likelihood of appendicitis threefold. Psoas, Rovsing, and obturator signs increase the likelihood of appendicitis when present, but their absence does not reduce the likelihood of appendicitis substantially. Fever often arises after 1 or 2 days of symptoms, and the presence of fever increases the likelihood of appendicitis threefold. The absence of fever does not rule out appendicitis.

Atypical Clinical Presentation

Children with retrocecal or pelvic appendices present with atypical locations for their pain. Patients with retrocecal appendicitis may have tenderness on examination, but often the distended cecum mitigates pressure applied to the right lower quadrant. Occasionally, percussion of the right lateral or posterior abdomen may jostle the retrocecal appendix, eliciting pain. Similarly, pelvic appendicitis leads to pain inferior to the abdomen, and right lower quadrant tenderness is not often present. Notably, the other symptoms of appendicitis, such as nausea, anorexia, and fever, are not different in patients with atypical locations for their appendices.

Diagnosis

There are not any laboratory tests that display sufficient diagnostic accuracy to serve as isolated screening tests for appendicitis. Although they cannot rule in or rule out appendicitis, laboratory tests may help guide decision-making by increasing or decreasing the likelihood of appendicitis. At a white blood cell count threshold of 10,000/μL, the sensitivity for appendicitis is 90%, and it is 60% at a threshold of 15,000/μL. Leukocytosis is also not specific, with a specificity of 40% at a threshold of 10,000/μL and 84% at 15,000/μL. Studies report conflicting evidence on C-reactive protein, ranging from diagnostic accuracy comparable to the white blood cell count to slightly improved sensitivity. Regardless, laboratory testing should not be used in isolation to rule in or rule out appendicitis.

Various clinical prediction models, incorporating signs, symptoms, and laboratory values, exist, including MANTRELS, Pediatric Appendicitis Score, and pediatric appendicitis risk calculator. These models identify high-risk groups, which warrant imaging, and low-risk groups, which may not require any further workup. The models' diagnostic accuracies depend on the particular threshold employed. Studies comparing the different models are limited but suggest the MANTRELS score has the best diagnostic accuracy. This score is calculated by summing the following:

- Migration to the right lower quadrant (1 point)
- Anorexia (1 point)
- Nausea (1 point)
- Tenderness in the right lower quadrant (2 points)
- Rebound tenderness in the right lower quadrant (1 point)
- Elevated temperature (1 point)
- Leukocytosis (2 points)
- Shift of the white blood cell count to the left with >75% neutrophils (1 point)

A total score >6 increases a child's risk of appendicitis 4-fold, whereas a total score <7 decreases a child's risk of appendicitis 5-fold. A score <5 decreases the risk 20-fold; these patients likely do not require any further evaluation.

These prediction models have limitations. There is substantial interrater variability on the components of the rules. Validation studies also report variability in sensitivity and specificity, with most showing sensitivities and specificities of only 70–80%. Moreover, experienced clinicians' gestalt performs as well as the prediction models. Finally, with ultrasound supplanting CT as the first-line imaging modality for appendicitis, concerns regarding radiation exposure from acquisition of imaging have abated. This renders it less crucial to have a prediction model with high specificity. The primary role for the models is to augment clinical judgment by helping identify patients who require imaging and patients who can be safely discharged without imaging.

Ultrasound is the preferred initial imaging modality. It is inexpensive, radiation-free, and relatively easy to perform. It is recommended as first line by the American College of Emergency Physicians and the American

College of Radiology. Ultrasound results can be classified into three categories: positive, equivocal, and negative for appendicitis. A large, noncompressible tubular structure with wall thickness >2 mm or diameter >6 mm, appendicolith, or target sign constitute a positive study for appendicitis. The presence of large amounts of free fluid, phlegmon, or periappendiceal inflammation are highly suggestive of appendicitis. Inability to visualize the appendix is the most common equivocal ultrasound finding, whereas identification of a normal size and compressible appendix constitutes a negative study.

False positives and negatives are possible with ultrasound, and so results should be interpreted in the context of the clinician's level of suspicion for appendicitis. In a patient with a moderate or high clinical suspicion for appendicitis, which is nearly all patients undergoing imaging in the ED, an ultrasound showing the aforementioned positive signs increases the likelihood of appendicitis to a sufficient level that no further testing (e.g., CT) is required. In contrast, although a negative ultrasound reduces the risk of appendicitis, if the pretest probability of appendicitis is high, a negative ultrasound does not rule out appendicitis, and further testing or observation is required. If the pretest probability of appendicitis is moderate or low, then a negative ultrasound is typically sufficient to rule out appendicitis.

The frequency of equivocal or nondiagnostic ultrasounds varies greatly (25–60%) depending on the publication. Ultrasound is less likely to visualize the appendix in obese children or patients with significant abdominal tenderness. Prior evidence suggested an equivocal ultrasound was not helpful in ruling out appendicitis; however, recent studies suggest that when performed by an experienced ultrasonographer, nonvisualization of the appendix decreases the likelihood of appendicitis, with a negative predictive value of 85%. The next step in the evaluation of a child with an equivocal ultrasound depends on the level of concern for appendicitis. Clinician gestalt or the aforementioned prediction models can quantify risk. For example, among children with equivocal ultrasounds for appendicitis, 9% identified as low risk by the Pediatric Appendicitis Score had appendicitis, and 47% identified as high risk had appendicitis. This suggests that all children with high pretest probability of appendicitis, as determined by a prediction model or clinical gestalt, and an equivocal ultrasound, should undergo further evaluation. This may entail observation, repeat ultrasound in 12–24 hours, surgical consultation, CT, or magnetic resonance imaging (MRI). Children with low pretest probability of appendicitis and equivocal ultrasound are at low risk of appendicitis and should undergo observation in the ED or at home. If their signs and symptoms worsen—for example, new focal tenderness in the right lower quadrant develops—then further diagnostic evaluation is warranted.

Trained emergency physicians perform point-of-care ultrasound for appendicitis with sensitivity (85%) and specificity (90%) approaching the accuracy of radiologists. Although ultrasound is not as sensitive as CT for appendicitis, its widespread utilization has not resulted in increased frequency of perforation of the appendix or ED revisits.

Ultrasound is not as accurate for identifying perforated appendicitis. It has excellent specificity (93%) but only moderate sensitivity (44%) when performed by experienced ultrasonographers. Visualization of complex periappendiceal fluid on ultrasound increases the likelihood of perforated appendicitis 18-fold. Other findings suggestive of perforation are simple periappendiceal fluid, increased maximum diameter of the appendix, and an appendicolith.

CT demonstrates slightly improved sensitivity (94%) and specificity (95%) compared to ultrasound for appendicitis. However, it exposes children to harmful radiation. Intravenous contrast may improve detection of appendicitis, but oral or rectal contrast administration is unpleasant for the child and does not improve the diagnostic yield of CT. Notably, unlike ultrasound, if the appendix is not visualized on CT, the child is unlikely to have appendicitis. The sensitivity of CT for perforated appendicitis (60%) is higher than that of ultrasound but still limited. After decades of increased utilization, the frequency of CT acquisition for appendicitis has recently declined nearly 50%. CTs are utilized more routinely at general EDs compared to pediatric EDs. Typically, CT should be reserved for cases in which (1) ultrasound is not available, (2) ultrasound is equivocal and there is ongoing concern for appendicitis, or (3) there is concern for alternate etiologies for the patient's presentation.

MRI also has excellent sensitivity (96%) and specificity (96%) for appendicitis. It can be performed more rapidly without contrast, obviating the need for sedation. It does not subject children to any radiation exposure and, if readily available, results in similar ED lengths of stay as those for CT. As a result, when available, it is the preferred imaging modality for children with clinical concern for appendicitis and equivocal ultrasounds.

Differential Diagnosis

Mesenteric adenitis is the most common mimic of appendicitis. Subsequent to a viral infection, the lymph nodes in the mesentery swell. This produces abdominal pain, which often is maximal in the right lower quadrant. Ultrasound, CT, and MRI can differentiate mesenteric adenitis from appendicitis. Caution should be taken when swollen lymph nodes are identified in the right lower quadrant on ultrasound but the appendix is not visualized because this may arise with appendicitis. In females with lower abdominal pain, consideration of pregnancy, pelvic inflammatory disease, or ovarian pathology, including ovarian torsion, is warranted.

Treatment

Laparoscopic appendectomy is the primary treatment for appendicitis. Waiting up to 24 hours for surgery after the diagnosis of appendicitis does not adversely impact outcomes, including the frequency of perforation. Children should receive intravenous antibiotics, and there are multiple appropriate regimens, including ceftriaxone and metronidazole, cefepime, or gentamicin and clindamycin.

Non-operative management with antibiotics is an alternate therapeutic option. There is burgeoning evidence to support this approach, although the evidence in children is more limited compared to that in adults. The presence of an appendicolith is associated with lower frequency of success with non-operative management. This approach should not be employed in the ED without discussion of the risks with the family and the physician who will follow the child after they leave the ED.

The appropriate management of perforated appendicitis is less clear. Perforation is often uncertain because the sensitivity and specificity of ultrasound and CT for perforation are limited. If perforation is suspected, initial antibiotics followed by delayed appendectomy in 1 or 2 months are often employed. Whereas intravenous antibiotics are typically given for 24–48 hours, oral antibiotics are equivalent to intravenous antibiotics in efficacy. If present, an abscess may be drained by interventional radiology. Alternatively, early appendectomy can be performed. This approach may increase the risk of intraoperative complications but reduces the risk of readmission to the hospital. Ultimately, the decision about the appropriate management should be made in conjunction with the surgeon and the family.

Disposition

Patients with appendicitis require admission to the hospital. Patients with equivocal ultrasounds may benefit from inpatient observation if there is moderate or high clinical suspicion for appendicitis. If ultrasound is not readily available, transfer to a hospital for ultrasound may be appropriate after discussion with the family. In particular, if eventually the patient is going to require transfer for treatment of appendicitis, it may be beneficial to transfer them earlier in the workup for ultrasound rather than subject them to radiation from CT.

Complications

The primary complications after appendectomy are skin infections (2%) and formation of intra-abdominal abscesses (1%). Abscess formation occurs several days after surgery; therefore, imaging may not be needed to evaluate for this complication in the initial 2 or 3 days after the surgery.

Key Points and Pitfalls

- Administration of analgesics, including opioids, does not delay the diagnosis of appendicitis and may facilitate visualization of the appendix on ultrasound.
- Pyuria and bacteriuria are common with appendicitis; their presence increases the risk of appendicitis and should not preclude imaging.
- Plain radiography may identify an appendicolith, which is highly suggestive of appendicitis, but it is only present in 10% of children. Therefore, plain radiographs cannot rule out the diagnosis of appendicitis.

- An ultrasound that does not display the appendix does not rule out disease in a child with a moderate or high clinical suspicion for appendicitis.
- CT is rarely indicated as the first-line imaging modality for children with abdominal pain and concern for appendicitis.

Pancreatitis

Background

The release of pancreatic enzymes produces autodigestion of the pancreatic gland. Unlike adults, in whom alcohol and biliary tract disease are the most common etiologies of pancreatitis, in children it often stems from infections or trauma. Mumps, coxsackie virus, hepatitis, and *Streptococcus* all can cause pancreatitis. Trauma tends to arise following motor vehicle collisions or bicycle injuries, particularly handlebar injuries, which transmit force to the epigastrum. One-third of cases in children are idiopathic.

Classic Clinical Presentation

Although much less common in children, pancreatitis presents similarly in children and adults with recurrent episodes of vomiting and severe epigastric pain radiating to the back. Younger children may have difficulty localizing their pain. On physical examination, there is typically tenderness in the epigastrum or upper quadrants. Low-grade fever is often present. Signs of hemorrhagic pancreatitis, such as blue discoloration along the flank or umbilicus, are rare in children. The history should include assessment for potential etiologies, including medications, alcohol, marijuana, infections, and trauma.

Diagnosis

Lipase is elevated more than three times the upper limit of normal. Levels rise within hours of symptom onset and only normalize after 1 or 2 weeks. The extent of the lipase elevation is not correlated with the severity of illness. Lipase is more specific than amylase with comparable sensitivity. For the initial episode of pancreatitis, liver function tests and ultrasound should be obtained to evaluate for potential bile duct obstruction. Ultrasound can also identify pseudocysts. The presence of an associated ileus may limit image acquisition by ultrasound.

Prediction models, such as Ranson's criteria and the Modified Glasgow Coma Scale score, have low sensitivity for complications in children and should not be routinely employed to make treatment decisions.

Differential Diagnosis

The most common etiology of recurrent abdominal pain in children is functional pain. Unlike pancreatitis, vomiting is not usually present and laboratory studies are normal. Severe epigastric pain can also arise with esophagitis, gastritis, ulcers, obstruction, or choelilithiasis.

Treatment

Relief of symptoms and prevention of complications are the primary goals of therapy. Children should receive an initial bolus of 20 cc/kg of isotonic fluids followed by 1.5 times maintenance fluids. Intravenous opioids (e.g., 0.5 μg/kg of fentanyl) improve pain. Patients should take in nothing by mouth until their vomiting and pain have improved.

Disposition

Children with shock or signs of end organ damage require admission to the ICU. Children with a new diagnosis of pancreatitis typically benefit from admission to the hospital. Well-appearing children with recurrent pancreatitis who are tolerating liquids without substantial pain can attempt outpatient therapy. They should follow up with their pediatrician or gastroenterologist within 1 or 2 days and return to the ED if their symptoms escalate.

Complications

As in adults, recurrent pancreatitis can lead to pseudocysts, pancreatic insufficiency, and varices.

Key Point

- Pancreatitis is rare in children but presents similar to adults. Infections, trauma, and medications may be the cause.

Gallbladder Disease

Background

Cholelithiasis can occur at any age but is much more common in adolescents. The primary risk factors for gallstones in young children are cystic fibrosis, sickle cell anemia, and furosemide use. Risk factors in adolescents resemble those in adults, including obesity, oral contraceptive use, and pregnancy. Children rarely develop cholecystitis, and when present it usually is acalculous, with inflammation arising in the setting of an infection, such as Rocky Mountain spotted fever, *Salmonella* enteritis, *Shigella* enteritis, hepatitis, pneumonia, or scarlet fever. Cholangitis is even less common and tends to occur in children with prior instrumentation of their biliary tract.

Classic Clinical Presentation

Children with cholelithiasis present similarly to adults, with severe, colicky pain that often radiates to the right scapula and is brought on by eating and lasts for hours. They often have vomiting. With cholecystitis, a low-grade fever develops and the pain is constant in nature. On examination, they often have a Murphy's sign with arrest of inspiration when the examiner depresses the right subcostal region. With cholangitis, children have high fever and jaundice.

Diagnosis

As in adults, ultrasound should be the initial imaging modality. It is readily available, easy to perform, and highly accurate. The appearances of cholelithiasis and cholecystitis on ultrasound are similar to those for adults. With stones in the bile duct, ultrasound may show bile duct dilatation, but false negatives are common. Magnetic resonance cholangiopancreatography has excellent sensitivity and should be obtained if there is concern for a stone in the bile duct or for ascending cholangitis. Unlike CT, there is no radiation or need for contrast. Unlike in adults, nearly half of gallstones in children are radiopaque; nevertheless, plain radiographs should not be routinely obtained if ultrasound is available.

Transaminitis and hyperbilirubinemia may be present with a bile duct stone or cholangitis. The white blood cell count is nonspecific and is often elevated with cholelithiasis, cholecystitis, and cholangitis.

Differential Diagnosis

Right upper quadrant pain and vomiting may also arise with pancreatitis, hepatitis, or pneumonia.

Treatment

With a dearth of evidence specific to children, the treatment principles are the same in children as in adults for cholelithiasis, cholecystitis, and cholangitis. Children with symptomatic cholelithiasis often benefit from anti-inflammatories and opioids for refractory pain. If pain does not improve sufficiently, children may require urgent cholecystectomy. In contradistinction, if the child is well appearing and pain improves in the ED, elective cholecystectomy is appropriate. Children with asymptomatic gallstones do not require intervention. Children with acalculous cholecystitis require intravenous fluids and broad-spectrum antibiotics (e.g., piperacillin–tazobactam or ceftriaxone and metronidazole) as well as consultation with interventional radiology, surgery, or gastroenterology for percutaneous drainage. Children with calculous cholecystitis should also receive intravenous fluids and broad-spectrum antibiotics as well as consultation for laparoscopic cholecystectomy after they are stabilized. Acute cholangitis requires aggressive resuscitation with intravenous fluids and broad-spectrum antibiotics. As in adults, consultation with a gastroenterologist or interventional radiologist is needed for biliary drainage after the patient is stabilized.

Disposition

Well-appearing children with gallstones and pain or vomiting that has improved can be discharged with outpatient follow-up in 1 or 2 weeks with surgery or gastroenterology. Children with ongoing vomiting or pain require admission to the hospital. Children with cholecystitis and cholangitis require admission to the hospital and, if they are systemically ill, to the ICU.

Complications

As in adults, ascending cholangitis can be life-threatening, leading to fulminant sepsis.

CONDITIONS AFFECTING CHILDREN OF ALL AGES

Upper Gastrointestinal Bleeding

Background

Gastrointestinal bleeding is a less common cause for presentation to the ED in children compared to adults. Moreover, often the etiology is consumption of foods that mimic bleeding. Fruit juice, fruit punch, and beets often produce stools that appear red. Iron supplements, bismuth, blueberries, grapes, licorice, and spinach may produce stools that appear dark.

Moreover, when true GI bleeding is present in children, it is less likely to require emergent intervention compared to that in adults. Less than 5% of children presenting to a pediatric ED with GI bleeding required blood products or operative intervention.

Table 41.3 outlines the common and emergent causes of GI bleeding based on a child's age. The majority (80%) of GI bleeding in children is from the lower GI tract.

Classic Clinical Presentation

Children with upper GI bleeding often present with hematemesis and melena. Hematemesis may be bright red when fresh blood is vomited or dark (coffee grounds) from old blood. Blood turns dark as it passes through the digestive tract, leading to melanotic stools that are black and tarry. With brisk upper GI bleeding, the blood may not have had time to change appearance as it passed through the GI tract, leading to the passage of bright red blood from the rectum.

In the ED, the primary goal is to rule out emergent causes of bleeding. This can be accomplished by evaluating for signs of significant bleeding, such as tachycardia, hypotension, delayed capillary refill, a hemoglobin <8 g/dL, or decrease in hemoglobin of >2 g/dL. In addition, children with multiple episodes of hematemesis or melena in the ED are at risk for significant bleeding. Esophageal varices are the most common cause of severe upper GI bleeding in children. They arise from portal hypertension in the setting of liver disease or portal vein thrombosis. Children often have splenomegaly and may display other signs of liver disease, such as jaundice, easy bruising, or acholic stools. Children of all ages may also develop ulcers that bleed briskly. Whereas adolescents present similarly to adults, young children often do not localize the pain of a peptic ulcer to their epigastrum. As in adults, nonsteroidal anti-inflammatory drugs and steroids may induce peptic ulceration.

A myriad of causes can produce more benign upper GI bleeding in children. Because the causes vary by age, the presentation will often vary by age as well. In neonates, upper

TABLE 41.3 LOCATION, PRESENTATION, AND ETIOLOGY OF GASTROINTESTINAL BLEEDING

	Upper GI Bleeding		Lower GI Bleeding	
	Emergent	Non-Emergent	Emergent	Non-Emergent
Location	Esophagus; stomach; duodenum		Jejunum; ileum; colon; rectum	
		Presentation		
Vomiting	Hematemesis	Hematemesis	None	None
Stool	Melena; bright red	Melena	Bright red	Blood on outside of stool or toilet paper; constipation
Hemoglobin	Decreased or normal initially	Normal	Decreased or normal initially	Normal
		Etiology		
Neonate	Ulcer	Swallowed maternal blood; esophagitis	NEC; malrotation; coagulopathy; colitis	Anal fissure; Hirschsprung disease
Infant	Ulcer; AVM; coagulopathy	Gastritis; esophagitis	Intussusception; Meckel's diverticulum; HUS	Anal fissure; milk protein allergy
Toddler	Ulcer; AVM; caustic ingestion	Swallowed blood; gastritis; esophagitis; Mallory–Weiss tear	HUS	Anal fissure; HSP; colitis
>5 years	Ulcer; varices; AVM	Gastritis; esophagitis; Mallory–Weiss tear	IBD	Colitis

AVM, arteriovenous malformation; GI, gastrointestinal; HSP, Henoch–Schönlein purpura; HUS, hemolytic uremic syndrome; IBD, inflammatory bowel disease; NEC, necrotizing enterocolitis.

GI bleeding prompts concern but is typically benign. In breastfeeding infants, the most common cause is blood swallowed from the cracked nipples of the mother. Visualization of the mother's nipples after breastfeeding or pumping in the ED will show blood coming from the nipples. In infants, esophagitis often produces hematemesis or melena. These children typically have significant gastroesophageal reflux with increased fussiness and vomiting after feeding. Children with blood-streaked emesis after periods of prolonged nonbloody vomiting or retching likely have a Mallory–Weiss tear.

Atypical Clinical Presentation

Mimics of GI bleeding should also be identified. Hemoccult testing of stool or Gastroccult testing of emesis can help determine if blood is present. False positives may arise if the child has consumed red meat, broccoli, cauliflower, or cantaloupe. For emesis, Hemoccult testing is not as sensitive as Gastroccult testing. Blood can also arise from alternate sources, particularly from epistaxis.

Diagnosis

All children should have Hemoccult or Gastroccult testing to confirm the presence of blood. In the well-appearing child, if bleeding is minimal and resolves without intervention, no further testing is required. For all other children, a hemoglobin should be measured. Although a hemoglobin is a poor measure of acute hemorrhage, it can provide valuable clues to prior hemorrhage. Serial measurements can help assess for ongoing hemorrhage. If a clearly benign etiology for the bleeding cannot be identified based on the history and physical examination, additional laboratory testing may help. An elevated blood urea nitrogen suggests an upper GI bleed, but its absence does not rule out an upper GI source. Unlike in adults, there are no validated prediction models for upper GI bleeding in children.

For children with signs of significant hemorrhage or ongoing bleeding in the ED, type and crossmatch, chemistries, liver function tests, and coagulation panel should be acquired. Endoscopy can identify the source of bleeding and may also allow for treatment. For most children without severe hemorrhage, it is safe to delay endoscopy for 24–48 hours after presentation.

For children with life-threatening bleeding, CT angiography has high diagnostic accuracy for active bleeding, with a sensitivity of 85% and a specificity of 92%. It does expose children to significant radiation and should be reserved for cases with concern for significant bleeding. For patients with life-threatening bleeding, arteriography with interventional radiology has excellent diagnostic accuracy and also allows for treatment of alternate causes of life-threatening bleeding, such as AVMs.

Other specific diagnostic tests depend on the level of concern for particular diagnoses:

- The Apt–Downey test can confirm the diagnosis of swallowed maternal blood by differentiating maternal hemoglobin from fetal hemoglobin. Although simple to perform with sodium hydroxide and a centrifuge, this test is not always readily available.
- Ultrasound of the abdomen can identify portal hypertension.

Treatment

Given the infrequency of significant upper GI bleeding in children, there is a dearth of high-quality evidence to guide management. Most therapies are recommended based on their success in adults. Patients with hemodynamic instability require aggressive resuscitation with blood products and emergent consultation with a pediatric gastroenterologist and intensivist. Children with varices may benefit from intravenous octreotide, ceftriaxone, and a proton pump inhibitor while awaiting variceal ligation. Children with upper GI bleeding should receive acid-suppression therapy with a proton pump inhibitor. In adults, proton pump inhibitors reduce the risk of rebleeding and lengths of stay but do not appear to improve mortality.

Endoscopy is the mainstay of therapy for upper GI bleeds. For nonvariceal bleeding, endoscopy allows injection of hemostatic agents, cautery, and placement of clips or bands. For children with variceal bleeding, endoscopy should be performed within 12 hours. Banding is most effective at achieving hemostasis. Children with significant hemorrhage may require endotracheal intubation to minimize the risk of aspiration.

Disposition

Well-appearing children presenting with minimal bleeding and children in whom a benign etiology is evident based on their history and physical examination can be discharged without further diagnostic evaluation. For children who appear well but the etiology of their bleeding is not clear, a diagnostic evaluation (i.e., hemoglobin, electrolytes, liver function tests, and coagulation panel) and a 3- or 4-hour period of observation in the ED are appropriate. If these are normal, children can be discharged with outpatient follow-up with a gastroenterologist in 1 week and instructions to return if bleeding resumes. Children with significant bleeding or comorbidities that increase their risk of bleeding (e.g., liver disease or coagulopathy) require hospital admission. Although endoscopy does not have to be performed emergently, it is often warranted the next day. If pediatric endoscopy is not available, children require transfer to a hospital where it can be performed. Children with significant bleeding require admission to the ICU.

Key Points and Pitfalls

- Signs of significant bleeding include tachycardia, hypotension, delayed capillary refill, a hemoglobin <8 g/dL, or decrease in hemoglobin of >2 g/dL.
- Declines in blood pressure or hemoglobin are late findings, and their absence should not be used to rule out significant bleeding.
- Orthostatic vital signs have limited diagnostic accuracy and also should not be used to risk stratify bleeding.
- Well-appearing children with bleeding that has resolved do not require extensive evaluation.
- Children who present with splenomegaly or a history of liver disease should raise concern for bleeding from esophageal varices. Although rare, these patients may be critically ill, with a study reporting 19% die within 1 month of their hemorrhage.

Lower Gastrointestinal Bleeding

Background

Lower GI bleeding is much more common than upper GI bleeding in children, but the conditions share many of the same diagnostic and treatment principles. Similar to upper GI bleeding, the etiologies vary by age (see Table 41.3). Unlike in adults, most cases arise from relatively benign etiologies, although life-threatening bleeding can arise with Meckel's diverticulum, and bleeding can be the initial presenting symptom of other sinister diseases discussed in this chapter, such as NEC, malrotation, and intussusception.

Classic Clinical Presentation

In children with concern for lower GI bleeding, the character of the bleeding and stool as well as associated symptoms can aid in determining the likely etiology. The most common cause of lower GI bleeding in children younger than age 5 years is an anal fissure. Constipation with passage of large, hard stools or frequent stools with diarrhea lead to tears in the anus. Tears produce bright red bloody streaks on the surface of the stool, and the tears are visible on physical examination of the rectum. Children have pain with passage of stool.

As milk is introduced into the diet, children may develop a food protein-induced allergic colitis with hematochezia. There is substantial heterogeneity in the extent of the bleeding; children may have grossly bloody diarrhea or stools streaked with mucus but only containing occult blood. Most children appear well and continue to grow normally. Allergic colitis may occur with infant formula or while an infant is still breastfeeding from maternal consumption of cow's milk. Egg, soy, and corn may also induce colitis.

At any age, children may develop dysentery (bloody diarrhea) from infectious causes. Viruses are the most common etiology for diarrhea in children, but the presence of blood increases the likelihood of a bacterial or parasitic etiology. Children may develop associated fever and abdominal pain. The most common bacterial pathogens are *Shigella, Salmonella, Escherichia, Clostridium*, and *Campylobacter*.

Children with inflammatory bowel disease (IBD), particularly ulcerative colitis, may present with bloody diarrhea. Although IBD may occur at any age, it is most commonly encountered in early adolescence, and this diagnosis should be considered in adolescents with hematochezia. A family history of IBD, weight loss, recurrent abdominal pain, recurrent diarrhea, or perianal skin tags increase the likelihood of IBD. Although children can suffer the same extraintestinal manifestations as adults, most children do not have these upon initial diagnosis. As in adults, during acute exacerbations children may also have fever and abdominal pain.

Other etiologies of lower GI bleeding are discussed elsewhere in this chapter.

Atypical Clinical Presentation

The most likely etiology of significant ongoing hemorrhage in a young child is Meckels' diverticulum. Other less common sources of significant bleeding are juvenile polyps, duplication cysts, angiodysplasia, and AVMs. These can be diagnosed with nuclear imaging, angiography, or colonoscopy.

Diagnosis

All children with concern for GI bleeding should have Hemoccult testing of their stool to confirm the presence of blood. Similar to upper GI bleeding, children who are well-appearing with likely benign etiologies of their bleeding based on the history and physical examination do not require further diagnostic evaluation. Children with uncertain etiologies for their bleeding or concern for more significant bleeding should have their hemoglobin measured. Children with signs of significant bleeding should also have chemistries, coagulation panel, and type and crossmatch obtained.

Further testing depends on the suspected etiology of the bleeding. For infectious colitis, stool culture may identify the pathogen; polymerase chain reaction should be obtained if there is concern for *Clostridium difficile* infection. Blood cultures should be obtained in infants younger than age 2 months with bloody diarrhea or diarrhea and fever. Children with IBD typically have elevated white blood cell counts, erythrocyte sedimentation rates, and C-reactive protein levels.

Treatment

As in adults, treatment in critically ill patients focuses on resuscitation with blood products as well as identification and treatment of the underlying etiology. For anal fissures, stool softeners improve constipation and allow the fissure to heal, and sitz baths provide symptomatic relief. For food protein-induced allergic colitis, consider a food challenge, with elimination of the potential offending food from the child's diet to determine if symptoms resolve. Unlike adults, most well-appearing children with dysentery and concern for infectious colitis should not receive empiric antibiotics while awaiting stool culture results because antibiotics are associated with increased risk of hemolytic uremic syndrome in children infected with shiga toxin-producing *Escherichia coli*. For IBD, children more often present with severe exacerbations compared to adults. If they have profuse, grossly bloody diarrhea, severe abdominal pain, fever, or tachycardia, they should receive intravenous steroids and admission to the hospital. Children who appear ill also warrant empiric broad-spectrum antibiotics. In well-appearing children, initial therapy with 5-aminosalicylate (5-ASA), such as mesalamine or sulfasalazine, is as effective at achieving disease remission with less adverse effects compared to steroids. Disease refractory to 5-ASA agents may improve with oral steroids.

Disposition

Patients with signs of significant bleeding require admission to the ICU. Otherwise healthy and well-appearing children with anal fissures, food protein-induced allergic colitis, and infectious colitis can be discharged with outpatient follow-up with their pediatrician. Children with IBD may require admission if they have severe presentations (i.e., fever, profuse bloody diarrhea, dehydration, and inability to tolerate liquids). If their symptoms are mild, they can be discharged to outpatient follow-up with a pediatric gastroenterologist within 1 week. If the etiology of the bleeding is unclear and the patient appears well with a normal hemoglobin, a 2- to 4-hour period of observation in the ED will help determine if bleeding is significant and ongoing, meriting hospital admission.

Complications

Life-threatening lower GI bleeding is rare in children and most commonly arises with Meckel's diverticulum or AVMs.

Key Points and Pitfalls

- Many foods can produce red stools, and Hemoccult testing can differentiate this from hematochezia.
- Well-appearing, young children with bloody stools often have anal fissures that are visible on rectal examination or food-induced allergic colitis.

- Antibiotics increase the risk of hemolytic uremic syndrome and therefore should be avoided in children with suspected bacterial infectious colitis until the pathogen is identified on stool culture.

Constipation

Background

Functional constipation occurs when there is not an underlying anatomic or neurologic etiology. It tends to be self-perpetuating. Pain with defecation leads children to avoid stooling. As fecal material stays in the colon longer, not only does it get larger but also additional water is absorbed, making the stool harder. This renders the stool more painful with defecation. Eventually, the colon dilates, reducing the child's urge to have a bowel movement and exacerbating constipation. It most commonly arises when children transition to drinking cow's milk or a solid diet.

Classic Clinical Presentation

Children present with irregular and infrequent passage of painful, hard stools. Importantly, constipation should not be diagnosed solely based on the frequency of bowel movements because this may vary greatly between children. However, nearly all (95%) children aged 1–4 years have a bowel movement at least every other day; the mean is 1.2 bowel movements per day in children older than age 4 years. Similarly, crying with bowel movements in infants does not necessarily constitute constipation, if the resulting stool is soft. Rectal examination may detect anal fissures and reveals the amount and consistency of stool in the rectal vault.

Atypical Clinical Presentation

There are several red flags that should raise concern for alternate etiologies and warrant further testing. True constipation in infants younger than age 1 month is rare. Infants consuming formula may pass only one stool every 2 or 3 days. Infants who are breastfeeding may only have one bowel movement per week. It is crucial to question caregivers of infants with constipation about the timing of meconium passage; children who do not pass meconium within the first 48 hours of life or have an empty rectal vault on examination may have Hirschsprung disease. The presence of a pilonidal dimple or decreased lower extremity reflexes suggest a potential spinal cord problem, such as a meningomyelocele or tumor. Other potential concerning etiologies of constipation in infants include cystic fibrosis, hypothyroidism, and severe dehydration.

Diagnosis

Constipation is typically a clinical diagnosis. Testing is only required if there is concern for alternate etiologies. Numerous attempts at quantifying stool burden on abdominal radiographs have failed. Radiographs are not sensitive, and they also may be misleading; children diagnosed with constipation after radiography are more likely to have missed diagnoses compared to children who do not undergo radiography. Radiographs of children without any symptoms often demonstrate ample stool burden.

Treatment

In the United States, adjustments in diet can adequately relieve most constipation, which typically results from inadequate fiber intake and excess cow's milk. For infants and toddlers, addition of prune or white grape juice softens the stool. In older children, increased water intake and replacement of processed foods with foods high in fiber are helpful. Children should be encouraged to sit on the toilet for 5–10 minutes after meals to attempt to pass stool.

For toddlers, osmotic laxatives, such as polyethylene glycol (0.4–1.0 g/kg/day), are second-line treatments. These medications are relatively safe, and caregivers can adjust dosing until regular, soft stools are produced. Children should continue daily maintenance therapy for 1 month after symptoms resolve. For infants, glycerin suppositories may help expel stool in the rectum but should not be employed regularly because children may develop resistance to their effects.

Enemas should be reserved for rectal impaction. Soap suds and tap water enemas can lead to water intoxication in young children. Hypertonic phosphate enemas such as Fleet may produce profound hyperphosphatemia, hypernatremia, and hypocalcemia in infants and should be reserved for children older than age 2 years.

Disposition

Children with functional constipation can typically be managed as outpatients. Well-appearing children who do not improve with the aforementioned treatments should be referred to a pediatric gastroenterologist. Ill-appearing children with severe constipation refractory to therapies may require hospital admission.

Key Points and Pitfalls

- Most cases of constipation are benign and can be managed as outpatients with dietary changes.
- Onset before age 1 month, failure to pass meconium within 48 hours of birth, systemic symptoms such as fever or weight loss, and severe abdominal distension increase the risk of more concerning etiologies.
- Radiographs do not reliably distinguish constipation from more severe causes of abdominal pain.

Further Reading

Bachur RG, Callahan MJ, Monuteaux MC, Rangel SJ. Integration of ultrasound findings and a clinical score in the diagnostic evaluation of pediatric appendicitis. *J Pediatr.* 2015;166(5):1134–1139. doi:10.1016/j.jpeds.2015.01.034

Benabbas R, Hanna M, Shah J, Sinert R. Diagnostic accuracy of history, physical examination, laboratory tests, and point-of-care ultrasound for pediatric acute appendicitis in the emergency department: A systematic review and meta-analysis. *Acad Emerg Med.* 2017;24(5):523–551. doi:10.1111/acem.13181

Freedman SB, Thull-Freedman J, Manson D, et al. Pediatric abdominal radiograph use, constipation, and significant misdiagnoses. *J Pediatr.* 2014;164(1): 83–88.e2. doi:10.1016/j.jpeds.2013.08.074

Gluckman S, Karpelowsky J, Webster AC, McGee RG. Management for intussusception in children. *Cochrane Database Syst Rev.* 2017;2017(6):CD006476. doi:10.1002/14651858.CD006476.pub3

Polites SF, Lautz TB, Jenkins TM, Dasgupta R. Implications of transfer status on bowel loss in children undergoing emergency surgery for malrotation. *J Pediatr Surg.* 2019;54(9):1848–1853. doi:10.1016/j.jpedsurg.2019.01.061

42

Male Genitourinary Emergencies

DEBORAH R. LIU

INTRODUCTION

Pediatric male genitourinary complaints are common, with a few diagnoses being true emergencies. This chapter focuses on distinguishing between the varied non-emergent common diagnoses while highlighting the true emergencies that the clinician must consider in the differential diagnosis. Making this important distinction allows the emergency provider to either act immediately by performing organ-saving diagnostic testing and/or therapeutic procedures or to provide education and reassurance to the family. The easiest approach is to first distinguish if the patient has a disorder of the scrotum (e.g., testicular torsion, epididymitis-orchitis, torsion of the appendix testis, hydrocele, inguinal hernia, or a testicular tumor) versus a disorder of the penis (e.g., balanoposthitis, phimosis, paraphimosis, zipper injury, or tourniquet syndrome of the penis).

DISORDERS OF THE SCROTUM

Among the many pediatric disorders of the scrotum, it is most helpful to categorize these entities as either painful or painless. In younger infants and children who are unable to answer this question themselves, the best approach is to ask the caregiver if there has been any perceived pain, unusual crying, or inconsolability by history. Although the physical examination of the scrotum in a calm or distractible pediatric patient may readily identify tenderness, in infants and toddler-aged patients, it may be difficult to differentiate crying due to pain versus anxiety. The differential diagnosis of a painful scrotum includes testicular torsion, torsion of the appendix testis, epididymitis-orchitis, incarcerated inguinal hernia, traumatic rupture testis, traumatic hematocele, Henoch–Schönlein purpura, or cellulitis/abscess of the scrotum. If painless, common etiologies include hydrocele, nonincarcerated inguinal hernia, varicocele, spermatocele, testicular tumor, acute idiopathic scrotal edema, and nephrotic syndrome (scrotal edema associated with proteinuria, periorbital edema, extremity edema, or ascites). The remainder of this section focuses on the most common painful and painless scrotal complaints.

Testicular Torsion

Background

Testicular torsion is a true surgical emergency in which timely diagnosis and therapeutic intervention are critical to preserve the viability of the testis. Twisting of the spermatic cord results in diminished blood flow to the testicle. Testicular necrosis can occur without timely diagnosis and intervention. Testicular torsion has a bimodal age presentation, with one small peak in the immediate neonatal period and a much larger peak during puberty.

Classic Clinical Presentation

The most common clinical presentation of testicular torsion occurs in an adolescent (aged 12–18 years) who experiences a sudden onset of severe, unilateral testicular pain, usually accompanied by nausea and/or vomiting. The patient often walks with a wide-based gait to minimize the amount of contact the affected side of the scrotum has with the inner thigh. On physical examination, the affected testis is typically swollen, high-riding, and very tender to palpation. The torsed testis may have a horizontal lie, in contrast to the unaffected testicle's normal vertical lie. The scrotal skin may be erythematous and swollen as well, and with time, the scrotal skin in untreated testicular torsion becomes more edematous and indurated. The absence of the cremasteric reflex is usually seen with testicular torsion, although some males do not have a cremasteric reflex normally at baseline. In addition, the cremasteric reflex may be maintained in clinically confirmed testicular torsion.

Atypical Clinical Presentation

Although torsion most commonly occurs in adolescents, it can occur at any age. Many cases are spontaneous, but trauma or physical activity may be an inciting event. Perinatal torsion may also occur in utero. For those patients, it is controversial whether they should be taken immediately to the operating room because at the time of diagnosis, the testicle is usually already nonsalvageable and one must weigh the risks and benefits of general anesthesia in neonates. Intermittent testicular torsion and detorsion can occur, whereby the patient has a history of intermittent testicular pain followed by rapid spontaneous resolution of symptoms. The ultrasound may be negative. These patients are predisposed to acute complete testicular torsion.

Differential Diagnosis

Table 42.1 presents the causes of painful and painless scrotal swelling.

Diagnostic Confirmation

If the clinical diagnosis of testicular torsion is suspected, consultation with urology should occur immediately prior to diagnostic imaging in order to expedite surgical intervention and improve rate of testicular salvage. For less clear cases, the imaging modality of choice is ultrasound with color flow Doppler, which will show decreased or absent blood flow on the painful side with normal blood flow to the contralateral side. Because the testicular salvage rate decreases significantly after 6 hours of pain, it is imperative that the emergency provider does not delay obtaining a stat surgical consult while waiting for imaging in likely cases of testicular torsion. Currently, there is not enough evidence to recommend routine use of point-of-care ultrasound by emergency physicians to diagnose pediatric testicular torsion. Blood and urine testing are of limited diagnostic utility, although they may help identify alternate causes of pain, such as sexually transmitted infections causing epididymitis-orchitis in adolescents.

TABLE 42.1 CAUSES OF PAINFUL AND PAINLESS SCROTAL SWELLING IN CHILDREN

Painful Scrotal Swelling	Painless Scrotal Swelling
Testicular torsion	Hydrocele
Torsion of appendix testis	Incarcerated hernia (nonincarcerated)
Epididymo-orchitis	Varicocele
Inguinal hernia (incarcerated or strangulated)	Spermatocele
Traumatic ruptured testis	Testicular tumor
Traumatic hematocele	Nephrotic syndrome
Henoch–Schönlein purpura	Acute idiopathic scrotal edema
Cellulitis/abscess	Allergic reaction

Treatment

Emergent surgical exploration of suspected testicular torsion is critical to maximize the chance of maintaining viability of the testis. Surgical intervention should not be delayed for imaging, other testing, or for NPO status in highly suspicious cases. For patients who undergo surgical exploration with less than 6 hours of symptoms, the testicular salvage rate is approximately 90%. However, the salvage rate declines precipitously beyond 12 hours of symptoms and is near zero beyond 24–48 hours.

Manual detorsion may be a treatment option if surgical intervention is not immediately available. Before attempting manual detorsion, parental opioid analgesia, a dorsal penile block, procedural sedation, or a combination of these analgesic options should be administered. Because most cases of torsion twist medially, manual detorsion is performed by rotating the affected testis 180 degrees outward toward the thigh, which is often described as "opening a book." However, the spermatic cord may twist laterally and/or twist up to 360–720 degrees, so definitive surgical exploration with bilateral orchidopexy is still indicated to confirm complete detorsion.

Disposition

Patients with acute testicular torsion should undergo emergent surgical exploration and orchidopexy with likely admission following surgery. Patients with suspected intermittent testicular torsion who have a normal Doppler ultrasound in the emergency department (ED) and have complete resolution of pain can be discharged home with close outpatient urology follow-up and clear return precautions. The patient and caregivers should be aware of the testicular ischemia risk and counseled to return immediately to the ED if the testicular pain recurs.

Complications

The primary complication of acute testicular torsion is loss of the testicle due to inability to restore blood flow and tissue viability, leading to potential decreased fertility.

Key Points

- Testicular torsion most commonly occurs in adolescent males with sudden, severe, unilateral testicular pain.
- A torsed testis is high-riding, often with a horizontal lie and absent cremasteric reflex; overlying skin may be erythematous and edematous.
- Surgical exploration is the diagnostic method of choice in classic cases.
- Ultrasound may be performed in equivocal cases and should not delay operative intervention.
- Outcomes are best if detorsion occurs within 6 hours of symptom onset.

Pitfalls

- Failure to consider torsion in the setting of trauma
- Failure to recognize torsion in a patient with an intact cremasteric reflex or recognize that some patients without torsion may normally have an absent reflex
- Failure to recognize intermittent torsion–detorsion and provide adequate follow-up and return instructions

Torsion of Testicular Appendage

Background

Torsion of a testicular appendage is another common cause of acute scrotal pain in children. Two embryologic remnants, the appendix testis (attached to the superior portion of the testis) and the appendix epididymis (attached to the head of the epididymis), can each twist onto itself. This results in venous congestion of the testicular appendage, which ultimately leads to necrosis. Fortunately, these embryologic remnants have no physiologic function. Thus, although torsion of the testicular appendage causes pain, there are generally no long-term complications.

Classic Clinical Presentation

Torsion of the appendix testis or of the appendix epididymis classically presents in a male between ages 7 and 12 years who describes a somewhat insidious onset of mild to moderate testicular pain. There are usually no other systemic symptoms. As shown in Figure 42.1, torsion of the testicular appendage may show mild swelling and erythema of the hemiscrotum with point tenderness over the upper pole of the testis or epididymis. The testis should have a normal vertical lie. The clinician may see the "blue dot sign" over the scrotum, which represents the ischemic testicular appendage.

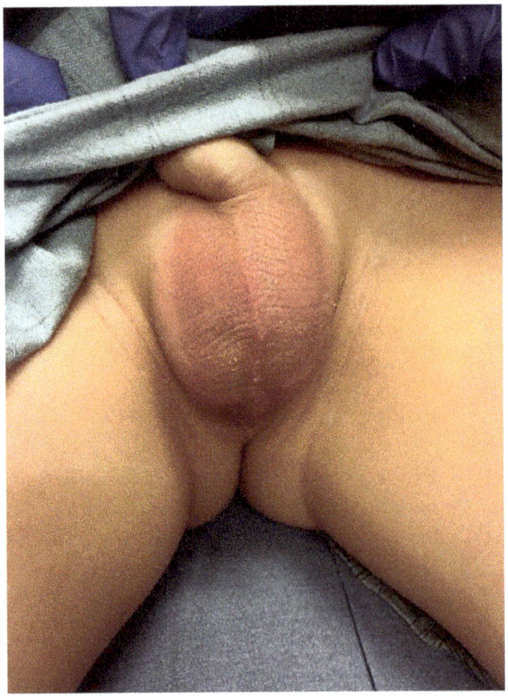

FIGURE 42.1 Seven-year-old patient with mild pain, erythema, and swelling of left hemiscrotum. Doppler ultrasound showed torsion of the left appendix testis.

Differential Diagnosis

See Table 42.1 for causes of painful and painless scrotal swelling.

Diagnostic Confirmation

Similar to other scrotal pathologies, ultrasound with color Doppler is the diagnostic imaging of choice for torsion of the testicular appendage. Ultrasound should visualize normal flow to both testes (thus excluding acute testicular torsion) and may show a small hyperechoic area adjacent to the testis, representing the infarcted testicular appendage. However, this is frequently not identified.

Treatment

Treatment for torsion of a testicular appendage is primarily supportive care. The patient should wear scrotal support (briefs style underwear instead of boxers), limit sports activities as tolerated, and use oral analgesics such as nonsteroidal anti-inflammatory agents.

Disposition

Patients with torsion of a testicular appendage do not require hospitalization and may be referred to a pediatric urologist as an outpatient. The patient and family should be counseled to return to the ED for significant worsening of the testicular pain.

Complications

Complications of torsion of a testicular appendage are highly unusual, but prolonged testicular pain and inflammation have been described.

Key Points

- Torsion of the testicular appendage typically occurs in boys aged 7–12 years.
- Pain is insidious and less severe than torsion.
- Mild erythema and scrotal swelling may be present with upper pole tenderness, sometimes with a "blue dot sign.
- Treatment is supportive care.

Pitfall

- Failure to recognize true testicular torsion in a younger patient or one with mild to moderate pain

Epididymo-orchitis

Background

Epididymitis (inflammation or infection of the epididymis) often presents in conjunction with orchitis (inflammation or infection of the testicle), whereby it is referred to as epididymo-orchitis. It is another relatively common cause of scrotal pain in the pediatric population. Although epididymo-orchitis can affect both prepubertal and postpubertal patients, the mean age of presentation is approximately 11 years, with most cases occurring between ages 10 and 14 years. In non-sexually active patients, the most common causes are adenovirus and enterovirus. A common cause of orchitis in a nonvaccinated patient is mumps (paramyxovirus). In sexually active patients, *Chlamydia trachomatis* and *Neisseria gonorrhoeae* are more common etiologies for epididymo-orchitis.

Classic Clinical Presentation

The typical presentation for epididymo-orchitis occurs in a preteen male who presents with an insidious onset of mild to moderate testicular pain, possibly with dysuria, urinary frequency, or a low-grade fever. Because many cases of epididymo-orchitis are associated with various viral infections or may present immediately following a viral infection, the patient may also endorse symptoms such as cough, congestion, or vomiting, although it is unusual for epididymo-orchitis itself to cause nausea or vomiting. This is in comparison to acute testicular torsion, which classically presents with sudden onset of severe testicular pain with nausea or vomiting.

On physical examination, the affected testicle is mildly enlarged and tender with mild hemiscrotal redness and swelling. The testicle should have a normal vertical lie. The classic Prehn's sign (alleviation of pain by elevating the scrotum) may be seen, although not consistently in the pediatric population.

Atypical Clinical Presentation

In the unvaccinated male, consider mumps as a cause for epididymo-orchitis. Mumps presents with fever, myalgias, and fatigue, often followed by parotitis. Approximately 5–10 days later, the patient may develop fever again and severe scrotal pain, which is more commonly unilateral but may be bilateral.

Although brucellosis infection is rare, up to 20% of patients infected with the *Brucella* bacteria present with epididymo-orchitis. Brucellosis is most commonly contracted via ingestion of unpasteurized dairy products or by handling infected animals on a farm. In addition, patients with underlying genitourinary anomalies or recurrent urinary tract infection (UTI; e.g., patients with spina bifida) may develop epididymo-orchitis due to unusual bacterial causes, such as *Pseudomonas aeruginosa* or *Enterobacter* species.

Differential Diagnosis

See Table 42.1 for causes of painful and painless scrotal swelling.

Diagnostic Confirmation

All patients with suspected epididymo-orchitis should undergo an emergent ultrasound with Doppler to exclude testicular torsion. On ultrasound, epididymo-orchitis may show an enlarged epididymis with increased blood flow, along with normal blood flow to the testis. In sexually active patients, urine should be sent for culture and sensitivity as well as for *C. trachomatis* and *N. gonorrhoeae*. In non-sexually active patients, urine testing is controversial because the utility is limited, given that the etiology is most often viral. However, in patients with increased risk for UTI, such as patients with underlying genitourinary anomalies or a history of UTI, urine should be obtained for culture and sensitivity. Blood tests are generally not indicated, although they may be helpful in high-risk populations.

Treatment

Treatment for epididymo-orchitis depends on the suspected etiology. In prepubertal patients with a suspected viral etiology, treatment is supportive with scrotal support, limited activity, and analgesics. Patients with a likely bacterial etiology, such as those with possible sexually transmitted infection (STI) or with underlying genitourinary anomalies or recurrent UTIs, should be treated with oral antibiotics directed toward the suspected organisms and preventative measures counseling.

Disposition

Nearly all cases of epididymo-orchitis are managed as an outpatient with pain control, scrotal support, oral antibiotics if needed, and outpatient pediatric urology follow-up within a few weeks. For rare cases, such as those caused by suspected brucellosis or in a high-risk patient with a history of resistant or multiple UTIs, consider inpatient treatment for intravenous antibiotics and further workup.

Complications

Complications to epididymo-orchitis are very rare but include scrotal abscess and chronic pain. The vast majority of patients with first-time epididymo-orchitis have no long-term complications.

Key Points

- Epididymo-orchitis typically presents in preteen males with mild to moderate unilateral testicular pain as well as hemiscrotal erythema and swelling.
- Testicular ultrasound with Doppler flow should be obtained, which may show increased blood flow to the epididymis and, more important, should exclude testicular torsion.
- In non-sexually active patients who are otherwise healthy, the cause is usually viral, and the treatment is supportive.
- In sexually active males, test for and treat sexually transmitted infections.

- In patients with a history of recurrent UTIs or genitourinary anomalies, urine culture should be sent with empiric antibiotic treatment pending organism susceptibilities.

Pitfall

- Failure to consider an unusual or early presentation of testicular torsion

Hydrocele

Background

Hydrocele is the accumulation of fluid around the testicle and is the most common cause of painless scrotal swelling in children. Approximately 10% of newborn males have a hydrocele, although it may not be detected until a few weeks or months of life. Hydroceles can be unilateral or bilateral, and they are categorized as communicating (with a congenitally patent processus vaginalis) or noncommunicating. Most noncommunicating hydroceles resolve spontaneously by 24 months of age; those hydroceles that persist or are large will likely require surgical correction. The communicating hydrocele is often associated with inguinal hernia, where a loop of bowel can also protrude into the scrotal sac. A hydrocele with a reducible inguinal hernia remains painless. However, if the bowel becomes entrapped and edematous, this may lead to pain and vomiting, swelling and discoloration of the scrotum, and then the inguinal hernia is considered incarcerated, which is a true genitourinary emergency.

Classic Clinical Presentation

Most hydroceles present within the first year of life. The caregiver may note unilateral or bilateral intermittent swelling, which is worse when the patient is awake, crying, standing, or walking. The swelling often resolves when the patient stops crying, is supine, or is sleeping. Although the classic physical examination finding for hydrocele is transillumination (using the light of an otoscope to light up the hemiscrotum through the hydrocele fluid), transillumination is a nonspecific finding because an incarcerated hernia may also transilluminate.

Atypical Clinical Presentation

An acute hydrocele that does not first present in infancy may be a result of a more acute process such as a viral infection, testicular torsion, torsion of testicular appendage, or malignancy.

Differential Diagnosis

See Table 42.1 for causes of painful and painless scrotal swelling.

Diagnostic Confirmation

Classic presentations of hydrocele do not require any diagnostic testing in the ED. However, if there is concern for other causes of painless scrotal swelling, testing should be directed toward the other possible causes. Ultrasound can help differentiate between an inguinal hernia and a hydrocele, and it can also be helpful to visualize an intrascrotal tumor.

Treatment

Management of most hydroceles includes education of the family and outpatient referral to a pediatric urologist for follow-up and possible surgical repair. Most spontaneously resolve by 2 years of age and do not require surgical intervention.

Disposition

Hydroceles are primarily managed in the outpatient setting by a pediatric urologist, with elective surgery if the hydrocele does not reabsorb spontaneously. A hydrocele with complications such as an incarcerated hernia requires emergent bedside reduction of the hernia and, if non-reducible, may necessitate emergent surgical repair.

Complications

Hydroceles rarely lead to complications. However, a hydrocele may mask serious conditions such as torsion or an incarcerated hernia. Intervention is required to prevent serious sequelae such as bowel or testicular ischemia/necrosis.

Key Points

- A hydrocele typically presents during infancy as intermittent, painless scrotal swelling that can be unilateral or bilateral, often worse with crying.
- Most hydroceles resolve spontaneously by 2 years of age, although those that do not reabsorb may require surgical correction.
- A communicating hydrocele may be associated with an inguinal hernia,

which can become incarcerated and must be treated expeditiously.

Pitfall

- Failure to consider serious alternative diagnoses of testicular swelling, including testicular torsion, tumors, or the presentation of nephrotic syndrome

DISORDERS OF THE PENIS

Similar to scrotal complaints, penile complaints are also common in the pediatric population. The emergency provider must know which diagnoses are true emergencies versus those whereby the family can be reassured and the patient treated as an outpatient. Problems such as paraphimosis, tourniquet syndrome of the penis, and zipper injury of the penis require immediate intervention in the ED. Other diagnoses, such as phimosis and balanoposthitis, can be safely managed by the primary care provider or pediatric urologist.

Balanoposthitis

Background

Balanitis refers to cellulitis of the glans, whereas posthitis refers to cellulitis of the foreskin. When a patient has both, it is termed balanoposthitis. This is one of the most common penile problems in the pediatric population, with an estimated incidence between 3% and 15% of all boys, with more uncircumcised males affected. Although balanoposthitis can occur at any age, the majority of cases are seen between ages 2 and 5 years. Risk factors include being uncircumcised, having poor hygiene, and being in a diaper.

Classic Clinical Presentation

Typically, balanoposthitis presents in a boy less than 5 years old whose chief complaint is swelling and redness of the penis for a couple days. There is usually associated pain, dysuria, or grabbing/itching at the penis and slight penile discharge. Swelling and erythema of the glans (balanitis), swelling and erythema of the foreskin (posthitis), or both (balanoposthitis) may be present. In uncircumcised males, there is often an associated phimosis, making it very difficult to visualize the glans. Figure 42.2 shows a 2-year-old with pain, erythema, and swelling of the foreskin. Upon slight retraction of the foreskin, erythema was noted of the glans, consistent with balanoposthitis.

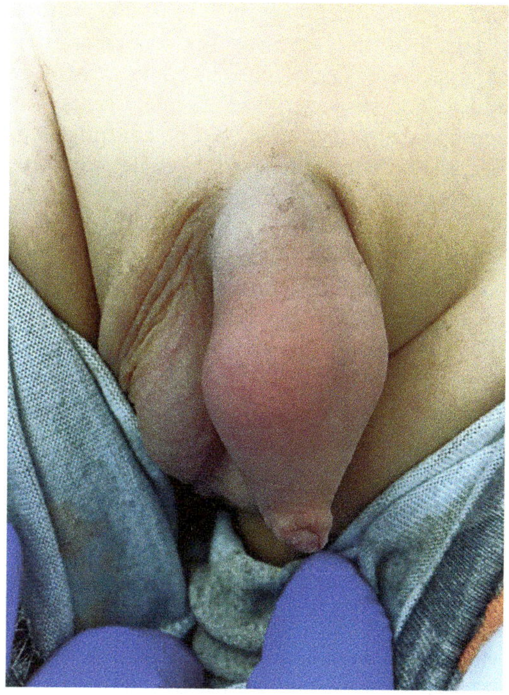

FIGURE 42.2 Two-year-old patient with pain, erythema, and swelling of the foreskin and tip of the glans (glans not shown) consistent with balanoposthitis.

Atypical Clinical Presentation

In some cases of balanoposthitis, in addition to redness and swelling of the glans/foreskin, the examination may show an erythematous papular rash with satellite lesions. In this scenario, the balanoposthitis may be caused by a fungal instead of bacterial infection.

Differential Diagnosis

The clinician should perform a careful history and physical examination to differentiate other causes of erythema and swelling of the penis from balanoposthitis, such as eczema, psoriasis, lichen planus, and herpes virus infection.

Diagnostic Confirmation

The diagnosis is clinical, but urine studies or evaluation for STIs may be indicated based on symptoms and risk factors.

Treatment

For the majority of patients with balanoposthitis, treatment consists of an oral first-generation cephalosporin such as cephalexin, which will cover the most common bacterial pathogens (*Streptococcus*, *Escherichia coli*, and *Staphylococcus aureus*). For cases with a red papular rash and satellite lesions, a topical antifungal cream such as nystatin may be added. For suspected STI in adolescents, the appropriate antibiotics should be administered. For all patients, improved hygiene measures and sitz baths are recommended.

Disposition

Nearly all cases of balanoposthitis are treated as an outpatient with primary care provider follow-up. Recurrent cases should be referred to a pediatric urologist for further management, which usually includes an elective circumcision if the patient is uncircumcised and has a phimosis. Complicated cases, such as those with significant urinary retention due to an associated tight phimosis and swelling from posthitis, may require an emergent urology consult.

Complications

Most cases of balanoposthitis are uncomplicated. For those rare cases with urinary retention due to a tight phimosis and swelling from the balanoposthitis, an emergent urology consult may be indicated. In addition, severe and refractory cases of balanitis may lead to balanitis xerotica obliterans, which is a chronic condition and should be followed by a urologist.

Key Points

- Balanoposthitis is common and presents with erythema and swelling of the glans and/or foreskin.
- This form of cellulitis is typically easily treated with improved hygiene, warm soaks, and an oral first-generation cephalosporin.
- Recurrent cases should be referred to a pediatric urologist for possible circumcision.

Pitfalls

- Do not forcibly retract the foreskin in tight phimosis, which is painful and could induce paraphimosis.
- Failure to consider the possibility of child abuse, particularly if an STI is present in a young child.

Phimosis

Background

Phimosis refers to the inability to fully retract the foreskin past the glans in an uncircumcised male. Phimosis may be physiologic or pathologic. Nearly all young male infants have a physiologic phimosis, but with cleansing and gentle retraction of the foreskin during bathing, the phimosis usually resolves by approximately age 5 years. A pathologic phimosis is one that persists beyond school age or one that is acquired due to scar tissue from recurrent balanoposthitis or forcible foreskin retraction.

Classic Clinical Presentation

Most cases of phimosis present in younger school-age boys whose caregiver has noticed intermittent penile swelling. Upon further questioning, there may be a history of ballooning of the foreskin or dribbling of urine from the penis following urination. The patient or parent may notice that the urine stream may be irregular and spray or be deflected. To help discern whether the phimosis is physiologic or pathologic, determine whether the phimosis has always been present since early infancy or if the parent has noticed that the foreskin has become tighter and difficult to retract with time. On examination, the foreskin may show ballooning with retained urine. As shown in Figure 42.3, the foreskin is difficult to retract, and the clinician may only be able to visualize the tip of the glans and meatus or may not be able to visualize the meatus at all.

Atypical Clinical Presentation

A patient may present with acute urinary retention due to a severe phimosis where the foreskin is nearly completely sealed off. Such

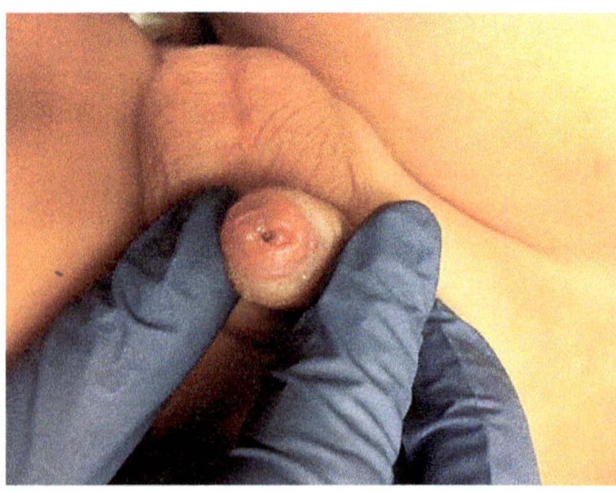

FIGURE 42.3 Five-year-old patient with phimosis whose foreskin could only be retracted slightly to visualize the meatus.

severe cases are caused by a pathologic phimosis, usually due to scar tissue forming after forcible retraction of the foreskin or from recurrent or persistent balanoposthitis.

Differential Diagnosis

Other diagnoses to consider in addition to phimosis include paraphimosis, balanoposthitis, UTI, and lichen sclerosis.

Diagnostic Confirmation

Phimosis is a clinical diagnosis. However, in unusual or complicated cases, urine testing for UTI may be indicated.

Treatment

No treatment is necessary for physiologic phimosis in young asymptomatic children except for gentle retraction of the foreskin and cleansing during the bath. For phimosis that persists into school age, the clinician can offer a medium-potency topical steroid, such as betamethasone, to be used twice a day for at least 4 weeks in addition to gentle retraction of the foreskin while bathing. Topical steroids are only somewhat effective, however, and the family should be counseled that the patient may likely still require outpatient follow-up with a pediatric urologist for possible circumcision depending on the degree of phimosis.

Disposition

Almost all patients with phimosis are managed as an outpatient and should be referred to a pediatric urologist non-urgently. Cases with acute urinary retention due to a severe phimosis may require Foley placement and either admission or close outpatient follow-up with urology.

Complications

Persistent phimosis can lead to recurrent balanoposthitis, recurrent UTI, chronic pain, and an abnormal urine stream.

Key Points

- Phimosis is physiologic in young boys and typically spontaneously resolved by 5 years of age.
- Phimosis often presents in young school-age children as ballooning of the foreskin and penile swelling.
- Topical steroids may loosen phimosis, but circumcision is often required.
- Persistent or pathologic phimosis can lead to recurrent balanoposthitis, UTI, and acute urinary retention.

Pitfall

- Do not forcibly retract a tight phimosis because this can cause trauma to the area, with bleeding, scar tissue, and potential paraphimosis.

Paraphimosis

Background

Paraphimosis occurs in uncircumcised males when the foreskin is retracted proximal to the glans and becomes fixed in that position. This is a true genitourinary emergency that requires emergent intervention. Due to impaired venous and lymphatic drainage, the foreskin and glans become progressively edematous, which may ultimately lead to decreased arterial blood flow and ischemia of the glans.

Classic Clinical Presentation

Paraphimosis classically presents in two age groups with different presentations. In the infant and toddler age groups, the caregiver may retract the foreskin during bathing and forget to return the foreskin back over the glans afterwards. This may go unnoticed for hours until the diaper is changed and penile swelling is seen by the parent. It may also go undetected until the patient is crying and irritable due to pain of unknown etiology. In preteen and teenage males, paraphimosis is most often due to masturbation or vigorous sexual activity, which is typically not easily elicited during the history taking. Regardless of the mechanism, the paraphimosis causes pain, swelling, and may lead to urinary retention. On examination, there is very painful swelling of the shaft and glans distal to the tight constricting ring of foreskin. The swelling appears as a symmetrical ring just proximal to the glans, as shown in Figure 42.4. If the glans or foreskin is dark or purple, necrosis may be imminent.

Atypical Clinical Presentation

Although more rare, there are cases in which a patient, parent, or health care provider who performs intermittent bladder catheterization for neurogenic bladder inadvertently forgets to return the foreskin to the normal position after in and out catheterization, causing paraphimosis.

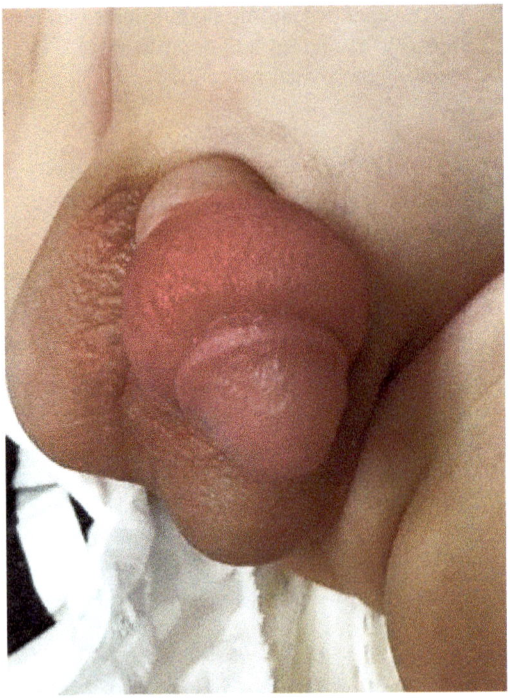

FIGURE 42.4 Two-year-old with a ring of swelling just proximal to the glans and distal to the constricting ring, consistent with paraphimosis.

Differential Diagnosis

In addition to paraphimosis, other causes of penile swelling include phimosis, balanoposthitis, trauma, hair tourniquet syndrome of the penis, and angioedema.

Diagnostic Confirmation

Paraphimosis is a clinical diagnosis. No laboratory or radiographic testing is typically indicated.

Treatment

Once paraphimosis is diagnosed, plan to attempt manual reduction as quickly as possible. A very mild or early case of paraphimosis may not require sedation or analgesia, but this is not the norm. Most cases of paraphimosis are extremely painful and require procedural sedation or a dorsal penile block (in older adolescents) to be successfully reduced.

Once analgesia or sedation is achieved, the emergency physician must first reduce the swelling. A bag of ice can be first placed over the area in 3-minute intervals to avoid cold injury of the tissues. However, the most effective method to reduce the swelling is by manually compressing or squeezing the edema of the edematous glans and foreskin until the skin appears somewhat shriveled. This can be very painful and often takes 3–5 minutes of steady pressure. Other methods have been used to decrease the edema, including spreading granulated sugar over the skin, which acts as an osmotic agent to draw out the edema. However, this method has variable success and takes a significant amount of time. For severe cases of edema, one may use a small 23-gauge needle to create multiple small puncture holes and then attempt compression to alleviate the edema.

Once the swelling has decreased, the paraphimosis is manually reduced by placing both thumbs over the glans and placing the second and third fingers of both hands on the trapped foreskin. Then the thumbs push the glans forward into the foreskin while the second and third fingers bring the trapped foreskin back over the glans into the normal position. This maneuver has been described as "turning a sock inside out." Depending on the severity of the paraphimosis, this pushing may take a few minutes of steady firm pressure until the foreskin is entirely pulled over the glans. In some severe or prolonged cases of paraphimosis, manual reduction may not be successful. In such cases, a more invasive approach such as a dorsal slit procedure may be performed.

Disposition

A patient with paraphimosis that has been manually reduced in the ED can be safely discharged home after the patient is able to spontaneously void. The patient and family should be instructed not to retract the foreskin for approximately 10 days to allow for complete resolution of swelling. Urgent urology referral for possible circumcision should occur. Penile necrosis may require inpatient observation.

Complications

The major complication of an unreduced paraphimosis is necrosis of the penis. Possible complications of manual reduction or surgical reduction include pain, bleeding, and infection.

Key Points

- Paraphimosis is a true emergency; expedited intervention is critical to prevent glans ischemia.

- Reduction should occur with procedural sedation or with a dorsal penile block.
- Complicated cases may require a dorsal slit procedure.
- Urology referral for circumcision should occur in all cases.

Pitfalls

- Failure to recognize penile edema as paraphimosis
- Failure to inquire if a patient is circumcised; a misdiagnosis of cellulitis or focal inflammation may occur

Zipper Injury of the Penis

Background

Penile zipper injury occurs when a portion of the skin of the penis becomes entrapped within the zipper of a patient's pants. It is most common in school-age and teenage boys who are not wearing underwear and hastily zip up their pants. This can also occur in patients with neurocognitive disorders or intellectual disabilities. The penile shaft, foreskin, or glans becomes entrapped between the teeth of the zipper, leading to progressive pain, swelling, and bleeding.

Classic Clinical Presentation

Entrapment is clear on history and physical examination. Often, the patient or caregiver has already attempted to remove the zipper at home by using some type of lubricant, such as petroleum jelly or cooking oil. For any significant amount of trapped skin, this is usually not successful, and the patient usually presents to the ED with the skin stuck within the intact zipper surrounded by a cutout of the pants, which is now very greasy.

Treatment

If the skin is caught between only the teeth of the zipper, it is relatively easy to cut the cloth between the zipper teeth, which will then allow the zipper to come apart. However, in most cases that present to the ED, the penile skin is caught within the zipper fastener, not just the zipper teeth. In this scenario, consider some type of sedation or analgesia (intravenous, intramuscular, or intranasal medications, or via a dorsal penile block in a teenager) prior to attempted zipper release because the procedure is painful and often challenging.

There are several methods described in the literature to release the zipper fastener. The most commonly used technique is to cut the median bar of the zipper by using heavy wire cutters or a bone cutter. However, the angle of the fastener to the trapped skin may not allow enough access to the median bar to be able to use a somewhat bulky tool. Another possible method involves using a small flathead screwdriver. Wedge the tip of the screwdriver in between the faceplates of the zipper and then twist in order to create a gap between the faceplates, which will allow the zipper teeth and penile skin to be released. Needle-nose pliers may also be used to squeeze open the zipper fastener. Operative intervention may rarely be required.

Disposition

After successful bedside zipper release, the patient can be discharged home. The patient and caregivers should be instructed to use topical antibiotic ointment for any open wound, keep the area clean and dry, use oral analgesics, and follow up with the primary care provider to monitor wound healing. Typically, only the skin of the penis is entrapped in the zipper, and no long-term sequelae occur.

Complications

Following penile zipper injury and release of the zipper, patients with any abrasion or crush injury to the skin are at risk for skin infection and should be counseled to keep the area clean and dry.

Key Points

- Procedural sedation and/or dorsal penile block should be used with entrapped penile skin.
- Bedside zipper release can typically occur utilizing a variety of equipment and tools.

Pitfall

- Failure to utilize appropriate analgesia

Tourniquet Syndrome of the Penis

Background

Tourniquet syndrome most commonly affects the fingers or toes of young infants, but it has also been reported involving the penis, clitoris, labia, and even uvula. Sometimes the caregiver will notice the swollen and discolored body part, but often the caregiver has not been able to identify the location of the pain. As the strangulated tissue becomes swollen and ischemic due to impaired blood flow and drainage, the young infant becomes inconsolable. Therefore, when a young infant presents to the ED for excessive crying, it is imperative to perform a thorough physical examination and check for possible hair/thread tourniquets.

Classic Clinical Presentation

Most cases of tourniquet syndrome occur in young infants and toddlers who are unable to verbalize the location of their pain. A thorough examination will reveal a swollen, tender, and either red or dusky digit or penis distal to the tourniquet. Due to the swelling, it is often difficult to see the actual hair or thread unless one spreads open the surrounding skin. If the tourniquet is caused by hair, it is often the long hair of a caregiver such as the mother that has become wrapped around the body part. Tourniquet syndrome can be caused by long thread from clothing as well, often inside a sock or in the covered feet portion of an infant's footed pajamas.

Atypical Clinical Presentation

Tourniquet syndrome can present in older children as well, still most often as a result of a long hair or thread becoming twisted around the penis or digit. Figure 42.5 shows a 9-year-old boy who had mild penile pain 24 hours prior to presentation but then with increasing pain noticed a hair wrapped around a small portion of his foreskin.

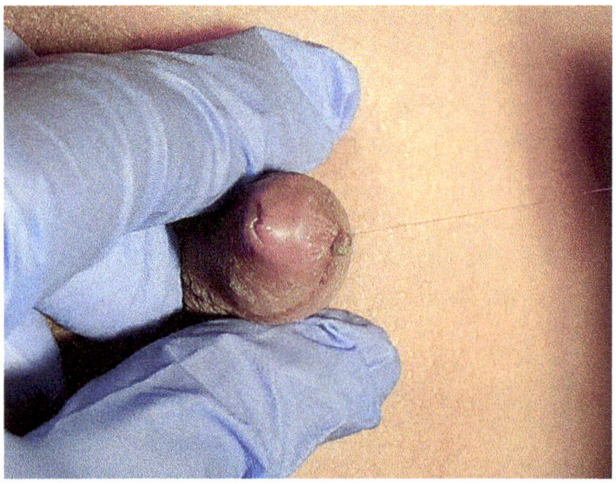

FIGURE 42.5 Nine-year-old with tourniquet syndrome of the penis where only a very small portion of his foreskin was entrapped by a long hair. The hair was successfully removed by applying a hair depilatory agent.

Diagnostic Confirmation

The diagnosis of tourniquet syndrome is made by a careful physical examination. Laboratory or radiographic tests are not indicated.

Treatment

Management of tourniquet syndrome involves the immediate removal of the tourniquet. Sedation and/or analgesia should be administered first. Upon careful inspection, if one can pass a fine forceps or other instrument under the tourniquet, then it can be easily cut with a pair of fine scissors. However, many tourniquets present after there is significant swelling with the hair or thread cutting into the edematous skin. In such instances, it may be extremely difficult to pass an instrument under the tourniquet. If the tourniquet is caused by actual hair, then a depilatory cream (e.g., Nair®) can be applied to the area and rubbed carefully into the hair to dissolve the tourniquet. Note that rubbing the depilatory cream for several minutes into the skin of an infant will likely lead to skin breakdown and some bleeding. It is also important to note that depilatory creams will not work on synthetic fibers from clothing. Rarely, surgical intervention is required if the tourniquet is unable to be removed.

Disposition

In most cases, tourniquets can be successfully removed at the bedside by the emergency physician. If the penis or other body part appears to have good perfusion following removal of the tourniquet, the patient should be discharged home with topical antibiotics and instructions to keep the area clean and dry. The family should be counseled to return to the ED if the penis or body part appears dusky or darkened, becomes more painful, or appears infected.

Complications

If the tourniquet constricts blood flow for a prolonged period of time or if there is failure to remove the tourniquet in a timely manner, the penis can become disfigured, resulting in permanent tissue damage, urethral transaction, or even penile amputation in severe cases.

Key Points

- Tourniquet syndrome is a possible etiology for excessive crying in an infant or young toddler; a detailed physical examination is required.
- Physical examination reveals swelling, tenderness, and skin discoloration distal to the tourniquet.
- Emergent removal is required.

Pitfall

- Failure to recognize the rare case of tourniquet syndrome due to child abuse

Priapism

Background

Priapism is a prolonged erection not occurring with sexual stimulation. The two types of priapism are low-flow (venous) and high-flow (arterial) priapism, which have different etiologies, presentations, and management.

Low-flow priapism is due to the sludging of red blood cells, which leads to venous congestion and ischemia. In children, the most common cause of low-flow priapism is sickle cell disease (all forms including sickle hemoglobin C and sickle thalassemias); additional etiologies include leukemia (with extreme hyperleukocytosis), illicit drug use such as cocaine and cannabis, and medications such as antidepressants and antipsychotics. Low-flow priapism is painful and a true emergency.

High-flow (arterial) priapism is usually due to pelvic or perineal trauma resulting in the overshunting of blood into the cavernous bodies. This can result in priapism for days or even weeks without any ischemia. High-flow priapism is painless and not a true emergency.

Classic Clinical Presentation

Unless there is a history of pelvic or perineal trauma, almost all priapism in children is low-flow (ischemic) and associated with sickle cell disease. Low-flow priapism presents with an obviously painful erection. Often, the corpora cavernosa are painfully erect, but the glans and corpora spongiosum are not completely rigid. Sickle cell patients often present with "stuttering priapism," with recurrent episodes of low-flow priapism of variable duration.

Atypical Clinical Presentation

Determine the type of priapism (low-flow vs. high-flow) by history and physical examination. If the etiology remains questionable, send aspirated blood from the corpus cavernosum for blood gas analysis. Blood aspirated in low-flow priapism will be dark in color with a PO_2 < 30 mmHg, a PCO_2 > 60 mmHg, and a pH < 7.25. Aspirated blood in high-flow priapism will be bright red in color with a blood gas similar to an arterial blood sample. Alternatively, Doppler ultrasound may show decreased blood flow in the cavernous arteries.

Treatment

Most cases of high-flow (arterial) priapism are treated conservatively because these are non-ischemic. In contrast, low-flow priapism should be treated emergently to avoid permanent damage. With suspected low-flow priapism, ascertain the duration of symptoms because low-flow priapism that lasts for >4 hours has a significant risk of impotence. Administer oxygen, intravenous fluids at 1.5 times maintenance, and opioid analgesics. If the patient has sickle cell disease, exchange transfusion should be considered in conjunction with a hematologist. Urologic consultation should be obtained for cases of priapism approaching 4 hours in duration for corporeal aspiration and irrigation with normal saline, intracavernous injection of phenylephrine, or surgical shunting if all other measures fail.

Disposition

High-flow priapism can be managed as an outpatient by urology. In cases of low-flow priapism, detumescence should be achieved prior to discharge. In cases of refractory priapism, a surgical shunting procedure and admission are indicated.

Complications

The main complication from low-flow priapism is permanent tissue damage leading to impotence.

Key Points

- High-flow (arterial) priapism is usually caused by trauma and is not an emergency.
- Low-flow (venous) priapism is a true emergency and is usually due to sickle cell disease, extreme

hyperleukocytosis (leukemia), or drug-induced (antidepressants, antipsychotics, cocaine, and cannabis).

- Low-flow priapism that persists beyond 4 hours is associated with impotence.

Pitfalls

- Failure to recognize that the glans and corpora spongiosum can remain somewhat flaccid in priapism (with erect corpora cavernosa)
- Failure to consult urology when low-flow priapism is approaching 4 hours in duration

Further Reading

Hoffman RJ, Wang VJ, Scarfone RJ, eds. *Fleisher and Ludwig's 5-Minute Pediatric Emergency Medicine Consult.* Philadelphia, PA: Lippincott Williams & Wilkins; 2012.

Liu DR. Pediatric urologic and gynecologic disorders. In: Tintinalli JE, Stapczynski JS, Ma OJ, Yealy DM, Meckler GD, Cline DM, eds. *Tintinalli's Emergency Medicine.* 8th ed. New York, NY: McGraw-Hill; 2016:875–881.

Liu DR. Medical emergencies: Genitourinary. In: Wang VJ, Flood RG, Godambe SA, Hoffman RJ, Liu DR, Vella AE, eds. *Pediatric Emergency Medicine Question Review Book 2017.* 3rd ed. Lulu.com; 2017:81–88.

43

Gynecologic Emergencies

CHISOM AGBIM AND EMILY L. WILLNER

NORMAL AND ABNORMAL NEWBORN GYNECOLOGIC FINDINGS

Background

The newborn genitourinary (GU) examination has several anatomic differences compared to that of an older child or adult female. The term newborn has prominent labia majora, whereas in the preterm female the labia minora and clitoris are more prominent. Hyperpigmentation is common from exposure to in utero maternal estrogen. Newborns may also have vaginal skin tags, which are considered a normal anatomic variant. Gentle separation of the labia minora allows for further characterization of the hymen, which is thick and redundant in newborns due to maternal estrogenization.

Classic Clinical Presentation

Physiologic hyperpigmentation and discharge are normal variants that may be present in the first weeks of life due to in utero maternal estrogen exposure. Vaginal discharge is whitish to yellowish and mucoid, and it resolves after the first few weeks of life.

"Blood in the diaper" is a common complaint in the newborn period. Red color in the diaper may be due to blood from urine, vagina, or stool, or it may be from urate crystals. Urate crystals look orange, reddish, or pinkish on the diaper and are not seen on the GU area on examination. They are classically seen in the urine of breastfed infants in the first few days of life when breast milk volume is low and urine is highly concentrated. Another common benign cause of blood in the diaper is vaginal bleeding from withdrawal from high prenatal estrogen levels. This "mini-menses" presents within the first 2 or 3 weeks of life and is considered normal, although it requires reassurance of parents, who are often alarmed by it. Blood in urine or stool in the neonatal period is uncommon and requires further evaluation.

Diagnostic Confirmation

Well-appearing infants presenting with a complaint of blood in the diaper should have an external genital examination. If there is a small amount of vaginal bleeding on examination and the infant is younger than age 3 or 4 weeks with an otherwise normal examination, then reassurance and no further evaluation is needed. If the diaper appears to have an orange-red color in a breastfeeding neonate, suspect urate and consider no further testing, but evaluate for signs of dehydration. If the diaper appears to have red blood, and no vaginal bleeding is noted with a gentle wipe of the introitus with gauze, a urine sample should be obtained for urinalysis to evaluate for hematuria and pyuria. If those are negative, consider workup for gastrointestinal sources with stool Hemoccult testing.

Ill-appearing, febrile infants, or those with significant bleeding, require an extensive evaluation for infection/sepsis and coagulopathy, including complete blood count (CBC), blood and urine cultures, coagulation studies, and broad-spectrum empiric antibiotics. Neonates with confirmed hematochezia in the first 2 weeks of life should have abdominal radiographs to evaluate for necrotizing enterocolitis. If there are any signs of trauma, the infant should have a thorough evaluation for inflicted injuries.

Treatment

Infants with urate crystals should be evaluated for clinical signs of dehydration. Concerning symptoms include fewer than four or five wet diapers per 24 hours and weight loss of >10% from birth weight. If there is mild dehydration, supplemental feeds with expressed breast milk or formula may be recommended until breastfeeding is well-established, and close pediatrician follow-up is needed. Physiologic vaginal withdrawal bleeding requires no further testing or care, and reassurance should be provided to families. In the case of confirmed gastrointestinal bleeding in a neonate younger than age 2 weeks or heavy vaginal bleeding, a thorough evaluation for coagulopathy should be performed, along with consideration of empiric broad-spectrum antibiotics and consultation with a neonatologist.

Disposition

Well-appearing, hydrated infants with a normal or benign GU condition may be discharged home with primary care follow-up. Emergency providers should have a low threshold for admission if there is any clinical concern for infection or a serious condition.

Key Points

- In utero maternal estrogen exposure and subsequent postnatal withdrawal influence the normal appearance and physiology of the newborn genitalia, causing hyperpigmentation, vaginal discharge, and bleeding.
- A parental complaint of "blood in the diaper" of a well-appearing female neonate should be approached by first identifying the anatomic source to guide workup.
- Vaginal discharge and small-volume bleeding are normal findings in the first few weeks of life due to in utero estrogen exposure.

Pitfall

- Excessive invasive testing in infants with benign conditions (i.e., catheterized urine testing or laboratory testing in an infant with classic vaginal withdrawal bleeding)

OBSTRUCTIVE MÜLLERIAN ANOMALIES (IMPERFORATE OR MICROPERFORATE HYMEN)

Background

Anatomic anomalies of the hymen can occur to varying degrees. An imperforate hymen refers to a thin membrane that completely covers the vaginal opening. Transverse vaginal septae are less common and obstruct the genital tract higher within the vaginal canal, and they can present with similar symptoms as those of imperforate hymen.

Classic Clinical Presentation

Hymen anomalies can be detected as early as the neonatal period and may be noted on routine GU inspection during health surveillance in infancy or childhood. Newborns with an imperforate hymen can be noted to have a thin bulging membrane covering the vaginal opening, as maternal estrogen stimulates vaginal mucus production that is retained behind the imperforate hymen. After the neonatal period, vaginal discharge is minimal, and it may be difficult to see the hymenal membrane on visual inspection. If not detected earlier, at the onset of menarche patients will begin normal menstrual cycles but without vaginal bleeding. Blood from each menstrual cycle will accumulate in the uterus and vaginal canal, causing cyclic lower abdominal pain and, eventually, a lower abdominal mass. This accumulated blood is called hematocolpos; it can cause urinary retention or constipation due to mass effect within the pelvis, which may also be the presenting complaint. Patients who have a partially obstructing hymen or vaginal septum may complain of prolonged menstrual bleeding, difficulty inserting or removing tampons, or pain or difficulty with attempted intercourse.

Diagnostic Confirmation

Diagnosis is made by visualizing the hymenal anomaly on examination, which is classically described as a purplish bulge at the vaginal introitus. Pubertal girls presenting with recurrent lower abdominal pain or unexplained urinary retention should have, with assent and a chaperone, a visual external examination of the genitalia. Hematocolopos can be identified and characterized using ultrasound. Either ultrasound or magnetic resonance imaging can be used to determine the degree of retained blood and identify other associated anomalies.

Treatment

Treatment involves surgical correction by a pediatric gynecologist or general surgeon under general anesthesia. Simple drainage of the material by making a "nick" in the hymen is contraindicated because it does not allow for adequate drainage of the thick fluid, is not definitive, and increases the risk of infection (pyometras). In addition, distinguishing an imperforate hymen from a transverse vaginal septum is important because the latter requires a relatively extensive procedure to reconstruct a functional vaginal tract and also because it has implications in terms of reduced fertility. The procedure is well tolerated and does not require further surgeries once the menstrual cycle has resumed. Because the retained fluid is sterile, antibiotics are unnecessary.

Disposition

Patients presenting with an imperforate hymen require surgical correction by a pediatric gynecologist or surgeon. Repair is urgent but not emergent, unless the hematocolpos is causing a complication requiring more urgent treatment such as urinary retention. Depending on local resources, this may be arranged as an outpatient procedure, or the patient may be admitted to expedite definitive treatment. Bedside drainage should not be attempted.

Complications

Imperforate hymen or vaginal septum may lead to mass effect in the pelvis and lead to urinary retention, urinary tract infections (UTIs), or obstipation. In rare cases of microperforate hymen, the retained menstrual fluid may become infected because bacteria can enter through the perforations. Obstructive Müllerian anomalies increase the risk of developing endometriosis.

Key Points

- The diagnosis of imperforate hymen can be made as early as the newborn period. If left undiagnosed, it will lead to primary amenorrhea with retained menstrual fluid.
- The absence of menarche in a patient with signs of late pubertal development is concerning for a Müllerian tract obstruction.
- Treatment for obstructive Müllerian anomalies is surgical and requires subspecialty consultation.

Pitfalls

- Do not omit a visual examination of the external genitalia in pubertal girls with recurrent abdominal pain or acute urinary retention.
- Bedside drainage or lancing of a suspected imperforate hymen should not be attempted.
- Hematocolpos contains sterile fluid; therefore, antibiotics are not indicated in the absence of infectious symptoms.

URETHRAL PROLAPSE

Urethral prolapse occurs when the inner layer of the distal portion of the urethra protrudes through the external urethral meatus. It is a rare condition that occurs predominantly in prepubertal Black girls and postmenopausal women. The mechanism is thought to be due to low estrogen production and increased intra-abdominal pressure.

Classic Clinical Presentation

Urethral prolapse appears on examination as an edematous doughnut-shaped mass that obscures the urethral opening. Most premenarchal girls with urethral prolapse are asymptomatic, and it is noted during diaper changes or bathing. Associated symptoms can include scant vaginal bleeding, often noted as streaks of blood in diaper or underwear by a caregiver; dysuria; or urinary retention in severe cases.

Differential Diagnosis

In addition to urethral prolapse, the differential for a GU mass in the premenarchal population includes, but is not limited to, sarcoma botryoides, prolapsed ureterocele, polyp, periureteral abscess, cervical prolapse, vaginal prolapse, and rhabdomyosarcoma.

Diagnostic Confirmation

Urethral prolapse is a clinical diagnosis confirmed with the "doughnut" sign, which refers to the round-shaped protrusion of distal urethral tissue and surrounding edema with a clearly visible central urethral opening (the "doughnut hole"). Although swelling is present, urethral prolapse causes minimal or no pain in uncomplicated cases. The diagnosis does not require any additional imaging or laboratory tests. A pediatric urology or gynecology consultation may be needed for diagnostic confirmation in cases in which malignancy or an alternate diagnosis is highly suspected.

Treatment

Prepubertal girls with symptomatic urethral prolapse can be managed medically with topical estrogen therapy (i.e., conjugated estrogens cream, or estradiol 0.01% cream), which is applied sparingly to the prolapsed tissue twice daily following sitz baths. This regimen is continued for 2 weeks but may require a longer duration of treatment if not resolved. Because straining and Valsalva maneuvers contribute to prolapse by increasing intra-abdominal pressure, assess for and treat any concurrent constipation with an appropriate oral regimen to ensure stool is soft and easy to pass. Persistent prolapse lasting more than a few weeks requires a urology consultation to assess for a prolapsed ureterocele.

Medical management is not appropriate for patients with significant bleeding, necrosis, or thrombosis of the urethra. These patients require immediate surgical correction.

Disposition

Girls with urethral prolapse may be discharged from the emergency department. Follow-up within 1 week should be established with the patient's primary care provider. Patients should return to care for urinary retention; pain with micturition; worsening swelling; or if the prolapse does not improve with estrogen creams, sitz baths, and constipation treatment, if indicated. Patients with recurrent urethral prolapse will need a referral for surgical correction.

Complications

Complications of urethral prolapse include recurrence. In rare cases, prolonged urethral prolapse may lead to thrombosis, bleeding, or necrosis. Patients who use topical estrogen cream in treatment of urethral prolapse may develop mild side effects, including temporary breast bud development, scant pubic hair formation, and darkening of the labia. These side effects resolve when the topical therapies are discontinued.

Key Points

- Urethral prolapse is a benign condition that occurs when the distal portion of the urethra protrudes from the urethral meatus.
- Diagnosis is clinical, and treatment includes a combination of estrogen creams and sitz baths.
- Patients presenting with significant bleeding, urinary retention, or thrombosis require immediate surgical management and should not be treated conservatively.

Pitfall

- Manual reduction of urethral prolapse should not be attempted.

LABIAL ADHESION

Background

Labial adhesion (also called labial fusion, labial agglutination, and synechia vulvae) refers to the fusion of the labia minora in the presence of vulvar inflammation and a low-estrogen environment. It is most commonly seen in infants and premenarchal females between ages 3 months and 3 years, with a peak incidence between ages 13 and 23 months. As many as 1–3% of prepubertal females have labial adhesions. Inciting events may include local trauma; poor perineal hygiene; infection; or, less commonly, inflammatory processes such as lichen sclerosis, Beçhet's disease, or following Stevens–Johnson syndrome.

Classic Clinical Presentation

Labial adhesions are rarely symptomatic. Most come to attention when noticed by a caregiver during a diaper change or by a health provider during a physical examination or during an attempt at urethral catheterization. The degree of adhesion is variable and can range from only a small portion of fusion of the labia minora to complete fusion. The key to distinguishing labial adhesion from other diagnoses is a grayish membrane of fibrotic tissue joining the labia minora that is referred to as "raphe" at the point of fusion. The adhesions can be visualized with gentle forward and upward traction of the surrounding perineal tissues. If symptomatic, patients most commonly present with abnormal voiding, urinary frequency, post void dribbling, abnormal discharge, dysuria, or UTI.

Treatment

Treatment for labial adhesion is dependent on the degree of adhesion and accompanying symptoms. No treatment is required for asymptomatic patients or small adhesions that do not affect the urinary stream. These lesions may resolve with the onset of puberty when estrogen production increases.

Topical estrogen (i.e., conjugated estrogens cream, or estradiol 0.01% cream) is the preferred treatment in symptomatic patients. Side effects of topical estrogen cream are mild and transient. The most common side effects include redness, irritation, hyperpigmentation of the vulva, and breast bud development. These effects are minimized with appropriate application over a short duration of time. The cream is applied twice daily at the point of midline fusion. The resolution of labial adhesions has been reported to be 50–59% with topical estrogen. The total duration of therapy has varied in published studies from 2 to 6 weeks; however, a direct relationship between the duration of therapy and resolution of adhesions has not been shown.

Topical betamethasone 0.05% can be offered as a second-line therapy for patients who do not respond to topical estrogens. Betamethasone is applied directly to the raphe twice daily for 4–6 weeks.

Significant adhesions resulting in severe symptoms such as urinary retention are extremely rare, and they are the only indication for manual separation. This procedure should be done with local anesthetic or general anesthesia by an experienced provider who is comfortable with manual separation; therefore, emergency providers should strongly consider a gynecologic specialist consult. No specific surgical technique defines how to surgically separate the labia, although all efforts must be made to minimize tissue trauma during the procedure. Following manual separation, topical estrogen treatment is recommended for 2–4 weeks to promote re-epithelization.

Disposition

Almost all children diagnosed with labial adhesions can be discharged home. Follow-up care should be established with the patient's primary care provider within 1 week of discharge to monitor for improvement. Return precautions should be given for urinary retention, signs of a UTI, or failure to improve with outpatient therapy. Patients presenting with severe symptoms such as urinary retention should be referred to a pediatric subspecialist for prompt surgical correction.

Complications

The most common complication of labial adhesions is abnormal voiding, which resolves when the condition is treated. Side effects from topical estrogen cream include breast bud formation, darkening of the vulvar skin, and vaginal discharge, which all resolve when discontinued.

Key Points

- Labial adhesion is a benign condition caused by vulvar inflammation and a low-estrogen environment.
- Labial adhesion is a clinical diagnosis that does not involve imaging or laboratory testing.
- The majority of labial adhesions can be treated conservatively with topical estrogen treatment.
- Patients with severe symptoms such as urinary retention require subspecialist referral for surgical correction.

Pitfalls

- Failure to inquire about micturition habits while taking initial history.
- Emergency providers should not attempt manual separation of the adhered labia.

PREPUBERTAL VULVOVAGINITIS

Background

Vulvovaginitis is the most common gynecologic complaint in young girls. Nonspecific vaginitis is the ultimate diagnosis in 25–75% of vulvovaginitis complaints in prepubertal females. Factors that contribute to the development of pediatric vulvovaginitis include the proximity of the vulva and the anus; a low-estrogen environment leading to a thin, sensitive epithelium; poor toileting hygiene; and the lack of labial fat pads and hair, causing greater susceptibility to local trauma.

Classic Clinical Presentation

Pediatric vulvovaginitis presents with vaginal irritation, discomfort, itching, and dysuria. Occasionally, vaginal discharge or scant bleeding is present. The parent or child may present for evaluation of persistent discomfort or dysuria after having been treated for UTI or yeast infection. The condition is exacerbated by irritants including soaps, underwear or clothing made of tight or nonbreathable synthetic material, bubble baths, perspiration, wet clothing, and dirt that cause local irritation to the lower one-third of the vagina and vulvar tissue. Another contributing factor is that young girls' small body size on large toilets can cause them to void with their legs pressed together, which can lead to reflux of acidic urine into the vagina, irritation, and post-void "dribbling." Unlike in postpubertal females, candida infections are not common in otherwise healthy prepubertal girls with vaginal itching.

Diagnostic Confirmation

Vulvovaginitis is diagnosed clinically on external examination. The vulvar tissue may be tender and may appear erythematous, and there may be scant discharge from the introitus or superficial excoriations from scratching. Copious, purulent, or foul-smelling vaginal discharge should prompt an evaluation for bacterial infection or foreign body. Well-circumscribed bright erythema is suggestive of Group A *Streptococcus* infection. Providers should take special note of any abnormalities suggestive of sexual abuse, including hymenal tears or posterior notching, bruising, and other evidence of trauma to the introitus. If sexual abuse is suspected, urine and vaginal specimens should be collected for testing, and local child protection and child abuse specialists should be consulted.

Treatment

Treatment for nonspecific vulvovaginitis is focused on removing irritants and improving perineal hygiene. It is important to reinforce a front-to-back wiping technique. Young girls can be advised to sit backward on the toilet seat to urinate, thus opening the legs and minimizing urine reflux into the vagina. Bubble baths, "bath bombs," and bath colorants should be stopped, and after any tub baths the vaginal area should be rinsed with clear water to remove soap residue. Symptomatic relief is provided with sitz baths twice daily; adequate drying of area; the use of a barrier cream such as a zinc oxide diaper ointment; and cotton, nonconstricting underwear. If there is no relief of symptoms within several days with this regimen, or if significant discharge is present, a vaginal culture should be obtained to rule out a specific cause. Vulvovaginitis with vaginal discharge and that is refractory to hygiene measures can be treated with a 10-day course of oral antibiotic therapy (typically amoxicillin or amoxicillin–clavulanate) or with topical antibiotics such as metronidazole or clindamycin to shorten the duration of symptoms. Less commonly, a short course of topical estrogen cream may be prescribed to thicken the vaginal mucosa and to make it more resistant to recurrent nonspecific infections.

If dysuria is present, a urine dipstick or urinalysis may be performed to exclude UTI. Inflammation from vulvovaginitis can cause small numbers of white and red blood cells in the urine, and young girls have difficulty performing a midstream clean catch specimen, so use caution in diagnosing UTI without significant pyuria or nitrites. In the absence of red flags such as fever, abdominal pain, history of UTI, or known urinary tract abnormalities, consider sending a urine culture and not treating with antibiotics unless culture results suggest UTI.

Vaginal foreign bodies can cause vulvovaginitis symptoms. Toilet paper accounts for 79% of cases of vaginal foreign bodies in girls, and it is typically associated with foul-smelling discharge. If suspected, it can be removed with gentle irrigation with warmed normal saline using a syringe connected to an infant or small-gauge Foley catheter or feeding tube. With the patient lying on her back, insert the lubricated Foley tip 1 or 2 cm into the vagina, and slowly instill approximately 200 cc of saline. If irrigation is unsuccessful, if the patient is unable to tolerate vaginal irrigation in the emergency department, or if a foreign body other than toilet paper is suspected, an examination under anesthesia will need to be coordinated with a pediatric gynecologist.

Disposition

Pediatric patients presenting for vulvovaginitis may be discharged from the emergency department. Return precautions should be given for development of bloody or purulent discharge or unexplained fevers. Patients should establish follow-up with their primary pediatrician. Referral or consultation with a specialist is not necessary for simple vulvovaginitis.

Complications

If left untreated, pediatric vulvovaginitis can lead to labial adhesions.

Key Points

- Pediatric vulvovaginitis is a benign condition that is caused by vulvar inflammation and irritation in a low-estrogen environment.
- The diagnosis of pediatric vulvovaginitis is clinical and does not require laboratory testing or imaging.

Pitfalls

- Failure to consider a vaginal foreign body in the differential diagnosis of vulvovaginitis
- Prescribing antibiotics or antifungals for simple pediatric vulvovaginitis without other evidence for infection
- Treatment of a patient with dysuria with antibiotics for presumed UTI in the absence of pyuria or systemic signs of infection

OVARIAN TORSION

Ovarian torsion is the twisting of an ovary on ligaments that hold it in place, leading to the obstruction of blood flow and subsequent edema and tissue damage. Ovarian torsion usually presents in females of childbearing age. In infants and prepubertal girls, it is often associated with an abnormality of the ovary, such as a teratoma or prepubertal cyst, but it is also relatively more likely to occur with a normal ovary in infants and prepubertal girls compared to older females due to hypermobility of an abnormally long fallopian tube, mesosalpinx, or meso-ovarium.

Classic Clinical Presentation

Ovarian torsion presents with acute onset, unilateral abdominal pain, and sometimes vomiting. The lower abdomen is tender, and presentation may mimic appendicitis or pelvic inflammatory disease. Signs and symptoms of ovarian torsion are nonspecific, and the diagnosis can be challenging, especially in younger girls. Laboratory testing is frequently normal, and even sonographic imaging with Doppler may be nonspecific.

Differential Diagnosis

The differential diagnosis for ovarian torsion includes appendicitis, nephrolithiasis, gastroenteritis, hemorrhagic ovarian cyst rupture, pelvic inflammatory disease, and ectopic pregnancy.

Diagnostic Confirmation

The gold standard for diagnosis of ovarian torsion is high-frequency ultrasound with Doppler. However, this test has pitfalls because findings can be nonspecific and often lead to an equivocal study with the inability to radiologically rule out torsion. The diagnostic criteria are wide, and findings can include a unilaterally enlarged ovary or asymmetric ovarian enlargement; heterogeneous appearance of one ovary due to edema; the presence of a simple or complex adnexal mass; present or diminished/absent flow on color Doppler; peripherally displaced follicles due to stromal edema from ischemia; medialization of the ovary; displacement of the uterus from the midline; free pelvic fluid; and the "whirlpool sign," defined as twisting of the ovarian pedicle causing twisting of vessels. Although the absence of vascular flow on Doppler highly suspicious for torsion, the sensitivity of absent arterial flow ranges from 40% to 73%. Venous compression is evident in up to 93% of torsion cases, but it is more difficult to interrogate with Doppler. This venous and lymphatic obstruction causes edema and asymmetric ovarian size.

Treatment

Laparoscopic surgery is the best diagnostic and therapeutic treatment. Surgical correction should be focused on isolated detorsing of the affected ovary without further intervention, instead of oophorectomy, which historically had been favored by pediatric surgeons.

Disposition

Patients with ovarian torsion require prompt evaluation by a pediatric surgeon or a gynecologist. Patients should be kept fasting until a surgical plan is developed. In some cases, patients will require hospital admission for observation and frequent reassessment.

Complications

Untreated ovarian torsion carries the risk of ovarian necrosis and decreased fertility. Unlike testicular torsion, there is no clear target time frame for surgical correction. Ovaries that have been torsed for >10 hours are associated with adenexal necrosis; however, the actual duration of ischemia beyond which the damage is irreversible remains unknown.

Key Points

- Ovarian torsion presents most commonly in females of childbearing age but can affect any age group.
- Ovarian torsion often presents with nonspecific symptoms of lower abdominal pain and vomiting; therefore, providers should maintain an index of suspicion and proceed with ultrasound imaging if there is clinical concern.
- The gold standard of treatment is surgical correction with attempts to conserve the affected ovaries.

Pitfall

- Due to the nonspecific symptoms, there is often a delay in diagnosis of ovarian torsion. Consider the diagnosis in any female with abdominal pain.

INGUINAL HERNIAS AND OTHER GROIN MASSES

Background

Groin masses are relatively rare in females. The most common inguinal mass in females is an inguinal hernia. Inguinal hernias in females are caused by the persistence of a congenital outpouching of peritoneum that extends from the round ligament on the uterus to the labia majora. It is considered the equivalent of the processes vaginalis in males. Persistence of this outpouching predisposes the patient to sliding hernias involving the reproductive tract. Approximately 15–20% of sliding hernias in premenarchal females contain the ovary and/or fallopian tube. If an ovary is within the hernia contents, reduction may be more difficult than with bowel contents, and it can predispose to torsion of the affected ovary. For this reason, it is prudent to obtain an ultrasound in girls presenting with hernia to evaluate for the presence of, and Doppler flow to, the ovary.

Classic Clinical Presentation

Inguinal hernias are recognized as a bulge in the groin that enlarges with increasing intra-abdominal pressure. Although the mass may be large, most hernias are not painful and reduce with palpation. A painful mass in the groin or a mass that cannot be reduced should prompt concern for an incarcerated hernia. Girls are more likely to develop incarceration of an inguinal hernia; the incidence in girls is 17.2%, whereas the incidence in boys is 12%.

Atypical Presentation

In rare instances, bilateral inguinal hernias can be seen in complete androgen insensitivity syndrome. The prevalence of complete androgen insensitivity in females with inguinal hernias has been estimated to be between 0.8% and 2.4%. In these cases, the hernia contains a descending testis, although the external genitalia are female due to androgen insensitivity.

Differential Diagnosis

The differential for groin masses in young females includes Bartholin's cyst, abscess, lymphadenopathy, lymphadenitis, and oncologic causes. Bartholin's cysts emerge from the Bartholin's glands (also called the vestibular glands), which are located in the vulva and secrete mucus for lubrication of the vulva and vagina. Bartholin's gland disorders are rare before puberty. When these glands become obstructed, they can cause fluid backup, resulting in cyst or abscess formation. Diagnosis is made by visualizing a tender swelling arising from the labia minora adjacent to the vaginal opening. Bartholin's abscesses require surgical drainage and/or correction. Antibiotics are not required for drained Bartholin's abscesses in the absence of cellulitis, UTI, pregnancy, immune compromise, signs of systemic illness (fever), or sexually transmitted infection (STI). Uncommonly, abscesses of the labial or perineal region may occur in prepubertal girls.

As noted previously, these rarely involve the Bartholin's gland, and initial treatment is supportive, including antibiotics, sitz baths, good hygiene, and over-the-counter analgesics. If not resolving with conservative measures, drainage may be needed and often requires sedation in young children.

Lymphadenopathy presents as a semimobile, round or ovoid mass located outside the inguinal canal. The movement will be more limited than an inguinal hernia. Lymphadenitis will appear as a tender lymph node located outside of the inguinal canal, often with tenderness and overlying erythema or warmth. An abscess will present similarly, but fluctuance or drainage may be noted. Ultrasound can further characterize the swelling if there is diagnostic uncertainty. Treatment includes supportive therapy and antibiotics when indicated. Procedural drainage of a suppurative inguinal lymph node should not be attempted without a subspecialist consult.

Diagnostic Confirmation

The image modality of choice for inguinal masses is an ultrasound with high-frequency transducer. Unlike in boys, most girls with inguinal hernias should have ultrasound imaging, especially if the hernia cannot be easily or fully reduced, to exclude a herniated or torsed ovary.

Treatment and Disposition

Pediatric hernias involving the ovaries should be referred to a pediatric surgeon or gynecologist for prompt surgical correction.

Complications

Complications of inguinal hernias in girls include incarcerated or strangulated hernia, ovarian torsion or necrosis, and damage to the fallopian tubes.

Key Points

- Inguinal hernias are the most common cause of groin masses in females.
- Sliding inguinal hernias may contain ovarian and fallopian tube contents.
- The differential for groin masses in young females includes Bartholin's gland disorders, abscess, lymphadenopathy, lymphadenitis, and oncologic causes.

Pitfall

- Not obtaining ultrasound to confirm the diagnosis in an undifferentiated inguinal mass

STRADDLE INJURIES

Background

Straddle injuries refer to direct trauma to the groin, genitalia, or perineum after falling on an object that is being straddled. In females, straddle injuries mostly result in injury to the vulva. Accidental falls and sports are the major causes of straddle injuries, with a peak incidence at age 6 years.

Classical Clinical Presentation

Straddle injuries usually present with superficial lacerations, abrasions, skin tears, or hematomas. Copious bleeding is common upon initial injury due to friable vulvar tissue and injury to the subcutaneous internal and external pudendal artery and vein. Bleeding often resolves by the time the patient is examined in the emergency department. Continued bleeding from the introitus or a penetrating injury of the vagina is suggestive of a vaginal laceration, and these patients should be examined and their lacerations repaired under anesthesia by a gynecologist. Patients may have significant anxiety and pain, limiting examination; providers should have a low threshold for examination with mild to moderate sedation in the emergency department, or under general anesthesia with a specialist, to adequately assess and treat the injury. Speculum and digital vaginal examinations in prepubertal girls should *not* be done in the emergency department.

Differential Diagnosis

It is important to perform a thorough external GU examination, including inspection of the vulva, labia majora and minor, urethra, clitoris, vagina, hymen, and anus to rule out further injury to these areas.

Although accidental injury is common, sexual abuse remains in the differential diagnosis for pediatric patients presenting with genital trauma. Injury patterns that do not match the reported mechanism of injury should raise suspicion for abuse. Examination findings that are suspicious for, but not diagnostic of, abuse include bruising, abrasions, or lacerations of the hymen, posterior fourchette, and lateral vaginal walls. Most penetrating vaginal injuries are consistent with sexual abuse.

Diagnostic Confirmation

Providers should have a low threshold for performing an examination under anesthesia, especially for patients unable to cooperate with the examination, those with extensive injuries, and those with injuries that are highly concerning for abuse. An examination under anesthesia with a specialist is superior in detecting occult injury.

Treatment

Hematomas usually involve the labia, mons, and clitoris and can be managed with cold compresses, warm sitz baths, and oral analgesics. Indications for operative treatment include vary large hematomas, involvement of adjacent structures (vagina, mons pubis, and abdominal wall), evidence of necrosis, and rapid expansion.

Small or superficial lacerations of the vulva requiring repair for hemostasis may be closed by an emergency physician, typically using absorbable suture such as chromic gut, under procedural sedation. More complex repairs should be completed by an experienced subspecialist. Indications for repair in the operating room include penetrating injuries, lacerations >3 cm long, vaginal bleeding of an unclear source, lacerations through or above the hymen, and deep lacerations.

Disposition

Patients with straddle injuries that do not require repair can be discharged from the emergency department with advice for sitz baths and gentle hygiene. Providers should ensure that patients can void prior to discharge to rule out occult urethral injury. Young girls are often fearful of the pain of urination, and parents can be advised to have the child urinate while seated in water to minimize discomfort. Patients with extensive injuries should be repaired by a pediatric gynecologist or surgeon under sedation or in the operating room.

If sexual abuse is suspected, providers are mandated reporters. Child Protective Services must be contacted to ensure that the patient will be discharged to a safe environment. Patients for whom a safe discharge plan cannot be ensured require hospital admission. Referral to a local child abuse center is recommended.

Complications

Complications of straddle injuries include urethral strictures and possible bowel or bladder incontinence if injuries are severe and are not recognized and promptly corrected.

Key Points

- Straddle injuries are common accidental injuries, and usually present with superficial lacerations or hematomas.
- Providers should always consider sexual abuse in the differential for straddle injuries.
- Providers should have a low threshold for coordinating an examination under anesthesia with a pediatric gynecologist for patients who cannot tolerate a bedside examination or those with extensive injuries.

Pitfalls

- Failure to provide adequate analgesia and/or sedation when examining females with straddle injury
- Failure to consider timely subspecialty consult and examination under anesthesia

MENSTRUAL DISORDERS

Background

Menstrual disorders and abnormal uterine bleeding are common complaints in teens. In the first few years after menarche, cycles may be anovulatory or irregular. Teens may also present to the emergency department for abnormally heavy or prolonged bleeding, or menstrual cramping.

Classic Clinical Presentation

Normal menstrual patterns in adolescents differ from those in adults. In the first post-menarchal year, average cycle length is 32 days; however, the range considered normal in teens is 21–45 days. Most cycles are ovulatory by the third post-menarchal year. Bleeding lasts 7 days or less, and most teens use three to six pads or tampons per day. It is important to elicit exactly what a patient means when she complains of abnormal menstrual bleeding: Ask about normal and current cycle length, duration of bleeding, and quantification of how heavy bleeding is typically and on presentation. With dysmenorrhea, determine what treatments have been tried at home and any associated symptoms.

Differential Diagnosis

Consider and test for pregnancy in all females of reproductive age. Ovarian dysfunction, structural abnormalities, and coagulopathies should also be considered. STIs may cause or contribute to abnormal uterine bleeding in sexually active teens.

Diagnostic Confirmation

If the bleeding pattern is determined to be abnormal, workup and treatment are indicated. Depending on the clinical status and seriousness of the menstrual abnormality, evaluation and treatment may be initiated in the emergency department or referred for outpatient evaluation. All patients should be evaluated for hemodynamic instability and, if present, have appropriate treatment initiated, including volume resuscitation and preparation for blood transfusion. A physical examination should be done with attention to signs of anemia, bruising, abdominal tenderness or distention, and hepatomegaly or signs of liver failure. An external GU examination should be performed to assess for extent of bleeding. If there is concern for pelvic inflammatory disease and the teen reports past penetrative sexual activity, perform a bimanual pelvic examination and send urine or cervical samples for STI testing. If there is concern for trauma, a speculum examination should be done. Note that pelvic examinations (speculum or bimanual) on virginal girls and teens should *not* be attempted in the emergency department except in very rare cases.

Pediatric patients presenting to the emergency department with abnormally heavy or prolonged bleeding should have a pregnancy test, CBC, and type and screen. Up to 20% of women with heavy bleeding may have a coagulation disorder, so initial testing should include prothrombin time (PT), partial thromboplastin time (PTT), and fibrinogen. In teens with a history of heavy bleeding since menarche, Von Willebrand's testing should be performed. Further testing for thyroid and liver dysfunction can be considered if there is clinical concern. Sexually active teens should have STI (chlamydia and gonorrhea) testing performed.

Treatment

Treatment depends on the severity of the presentation. In patients with severe hemorrhage or hemodynamic instability with anemia, blood transfusion should be given. Hormonal therapies are given to stop bleeding. Intravenous conjugated estrogen may be required for unstable patients or those not tolerating oral intake. Stable patients may be started on combined oral contraceptives containing 35 μg of ethinyl estradiol or an oral progestin (medroxyprogesterone acetate, 20 mg). One pill is typically given three times per day for 7 days. After this, adolescents without contraindications should be instructed to begin once-daily oral contraceptive pills and to continue until follow-up with their primary care physician.

Dysmenorrhea is a common complaint and is best managed with nonsteroidal anti-inflammatory drugs. These are most effective if given at adequate anti-inflammatory dosing (i.e., ibuprofen 10 mg/kg, maximum 600 mg), started 12–24 hours prior to the onset of menstrual bleeding, and continued on a scheduled basis through the first 2 or 3 days of menses.

Disposition

Patients with abnormal uterine bleeding should be admitted if hemodynamically unstable, requiring transfusion for severe anemia, or with significant, ongoing, bleeding. Otherwise, discharge with outpatient follow-up with a primary care physician, gynecologist, or adolescent medicine specialist is appropriate.

Complications

Abnormal uterine bleeding can cause iron deficiency anemia. Even in the absence of severe medical complications, abnormal bleeding and dysmenorrhea can significantly interfere with adolescents' school attendance and participation in sports and activities.

Key Points

- Normal menstrual bleeding patterns are different in adolescents compared to adults.
- If the history is consistent with abnormally heavy or prolonged bleeding, laboratory evaluation with pregnancy test, CBC, PT/PTT, and fibrinogen is indicated. STI testing should be done in sexually active teens.

- Treatment with combined oral contraceptives, progesterone, or intravenous estrogen, if unstable, should be used to stop bleeding.

Pitfall

- Failure to recommend continuation of oral contraceptives at the end of the initial treatment course, which may result in recurrence of bleeding

SEXUALLY TRANSMITTED INFECTIONS AND PELVIC INFLAMMATORY DISEASE

Background

Sexually transmitted infections are commonly diagnosed among adolescent females. Young people aged 15–24 years acquire half of all new STIs, and one in four sexually active adolescent females has an STI, such as chlamydia or human papillomavirus. Considering that there is such a high prevalence in this population, providers should be especially aware of the specific nuances of STI diagnosis and management for adolescent females.

Pelvic inflammatory disease (PID) is a polymicrobial inflammatory condition of the female upper genital tract that is caused by an ascending STI. It involves the endometrium, fallopian tubes, and/or pelvic peritoneum. An estimated one in eight sexually active adolescent girls develops PID before reaching age 20 years. Acute PID can lead to issues with infertility, tubo-ovarian abscesses, chronic pelvic pain, and infertility.

It is of utmost importance that providers take a careful, confidential history with all adolescent patients. This includes escorting caregivers and visitors outside the examination room while inquiring about past sexual history, condom use, high-risk behaviors, and previous history of pregnancy and STIs. Currently, all states allow teens older than age 14 years to consent to testing and treatment for STIs without parental consent or notification. Consent for other reproductive services (contraception, prenatal care, and abortion) varies by state, and clinicians should familiarize themselves with local legislation.

Classical Clinical Presentation

Adolescents frequently present to the emergency department for medical care. It is important to consider STIs and PID for all adolescent females presenting with abdominal pain. Other symptoms can be nonspecific and include vaginal discharge, dysfunctional uterine bleeding, and pelvic pain. Asymptomatic infections are also common.

Diagnostic Confirmation

Confirmatory testing for STIs can be achieved with urine or vaginal swab samples. No single historical, physical, or laboratory finding is both sensitive and specific for the diagnosis of acute PID. If a patient is sexually active with lower abdominal pain, providers should perform a bimanual examination to evaluate for cervical motion tenderness. Speculum examinations are not necessary for diagnosis of STI or PID in this population. If an adolescent has no past history of penetrative intercourse, both the bimanual and speculum examination should be avoided.

The Centers for Disease Control and Prevention has established diagnostic criteria for PID. A low threshold to begin empiric treatment should be maintained for patients presenting with uterine, adenexal, or cervical motion tenderness on bimanual examination with no other apparent cause. Other findings that support the diagnosis include cervical or vaginal mucopurulent (green or yellow) discharge, fever, elevated inflammatory markers on lab, and confirmatory testing. One of the most specific findings for diagnosis is thickened, fluid-filled Fallopian tubes apparent on transvaginal ultrasound or magnetic resonance imaging, although imaging is not necessary to make the diagnosis.

Treatment

Treatment for STIs and PID in adolescent females is outlined by the Centers of Disease Control and Prevention and is identical to that of adults (Table 43.1). Providers should strongly consider empiric treatment for STIs (e.g., directly observed treatment in the emergency department) in this population given the high risk of poor compliance and difficulties coordinating follow-up care among adolescent females.

Disposition

The majority of patients with STIs and PID of mild to moderate severity can be safely discharged from the emergency department with

TABLE 43.1 RECOMMENDED FIRST-LINE TREATMENT FOR SEXUALLY TRANSMITTED INFECTIONS

Disease	Treatment
Chlamydia cervicitis	Azithromycin PO[a]: 1 g orally in a single dose *or* Doxycycline PO: 100 mg orally 2×/day for 7 days
	Infants and children (<45 kg) with urogenital or rectal disease Erythromycin base *or* erythromycin ethylsuccinate PO: 50 mg/kg/day orally (4 divided doses) daily for 14 days
Gonococcal infections	Ceftriaxone PO: 250 mg IM in a single dose *plus* Azithromycin PO: 1 g orally in a single dose
	Children (≤45 kg) with urogenital or rectal disease Ceftriaxone IV or IM: 25–50 mg/kg IV or IM, not to exceed 125 mg IM in a single dose
Pelvic inflammatory disease, mild to moderate outpatient regimen	Ceftriaxone PO: 250 mg IM in a single dose *plus* Doxycycline PO: 100 mg orally 2×/day for 14 days
Pelvic inflammatory disease, severe inpatient regimen	Cefotetan IV: 2 g IV every 12 hours *plus* Doxycycline IV: 100 mg orally or IV every 12 hours *Or* Cefoxitin IV: 2 g IV every 6 hours *plus* Doxycycline IV: 100 mg orally or IV every 12 hours *Or* Clindamycin IV: 900 mg IV every 8 hours Gentamicin IV: loading dose IV or IM (2 mg/kg), followed by a maintenance dose (1.5 mg/kg) every 8 hours; single daily dosing (3–5 mg/kg) can be substituted
Genital herpes simplex (first clinical episode)	Acyclovir PO: 400 mg orally 3×/day for 7–10 days *or* Acyclovir PO: 200 mg orally 5×/day for 7–10 days *or* Valacyclovir PO: 1 g orally 2×/day for 7–10 days *or* Famciclovir PO: 250 mg orally 3×/day for 7–10 days
Bacterial vaginosis	Metronidazole PO: 500 mg orally 2×/day for 7 days *or* Metronidazole gel 0.75%: One 5-g applicator intravaginally 1×/day for 5 days *or* Clindamycin 2% topical cream: One 5-g applicator intravaginally at bedtime for 7 days

[a]Azithromycin is the recommended treatment in pregnancy.
IM, intramuscularly; IV, intravenously.
Source: Adapted from the Centers for Disease Control and Prevention. 2015 Sexually Transmitted Diseases Treatment Guidelines. https://www.cdc.gov/std/tg2015/default.htm.

outpatient follow-up. The decision to hospitalize adolescents with acute PID should be based on the same criteria as those for adults. Criteria for hospitalization for PID include severe illness (nausea, vomiting, or high fever), surgical emergencies, tubo-ovarian abscess, pregnancy, unable to follow an outpatient oral regimen, or failure of outpatient management.

Complications

Complications for a missed diagnosis of STI include the progression to PID, tubo-ovarian abscesses, chronic pelvic pain, and infertility. Pregnant women who have PID are at high risk for premature delivery and preterm morbidity.

Key Points

- One in four sexually active adolescent females has an STI.
- It is of utmost importance that providers take a detailed confidential history privately without other individuals in the room.

- Teens between ages 14 and 18 years (and in many states without a lower age limit) may consent to STI testing and treatment without parental consent or notification.
- Management of STIs and PID follows the same algorithms as used for adults, but it is strongly recommended to consider empiric, directly observed treatment if there is clinical concern for STI/PID, given compliance and confidentiality concerns.

Pitfalls

- Not considering STI or PID in the differential for a postmenarchal female patient presenting with abdominal pain
- Failure to empirically treat adolescents with high suspicion of STI and PID, given challenges with engaging patients to return for treatment.

Further Reading

Bacon JL, Romano ME, Quint EH. Clinical recommendation: Labial adhesions. *J Pediatr Adolesc Gynecol.* 2015;28(5):405–409. doi:10.1016/j.jpag.2015.04.010

Centers for Disease Control and Prevention. Pelvic Inflammatory Disease (PID)—2015 STD treatment guidelines. https://www.cdc.gov/std/tg2015/pid.htm. Published January 11, 2019. Accessed November 18, 2019.

Centers for Disease Control and Prevention. 2015 Sexually Transmitted Diseases Treatment Guidelines. https://www.cdc.gov/std/tg2015/default.htm. Published October 30, 2019. Accessed November 18, 2019.

Dasgupta R, Renaud E, Goldin AB, et al. Ovarian torsion in pediatric and adolescent patients: A systematic review. *J Pediatr Surg.* 2018;53(7):1387–1391. doi:10.1016/j.jpedsurg.2017.10.053

Omole F, Kelsey RC, Phillips K, Cunningham K. Bartholin duct cyst and gland abscess: Office management. *Am Fam Physician.* 2019;99(12):760–766.

44

Obstetrical Emergencies

ANNA MCFARLIN

INTRODUCTION

Pregnancy should be considered in all adolescent females presenting to the emergency department (ED). Roughly half of all teenagers report that they are sexually active. Adolescents participate in risky behavior, including unprotected sex and inconsistent birth control use with high risk for pregnancy.

Due to concerns about confidentiality, transportation, cost, embarrassment, and perception of judgment, teens are less likely to seek care for possible pregnancy. When they do seek care, they are more likely to present to the ED than to a primary care provider. They often present at a much more advanced gestational age compared to their adult counterparts. They may also be more likely to conceal their true concerns during their visit. Emergency providers perceive barriers to providing effective care to these patients, including parental presence, difficulty building rapport in the ED setting, lack of comfort or knowledge about confidentiality laws, and overall discomfort in managing adolescent reproductive health. Often, the possibility of pregnancy is not even considered in this population. Multiple retrospective reviews have shown that neither a sexual history nor pregnancy test are done in the majority of adolescent females in the ED, even in those with abdominal or genitourinary complaints. Last, the menstrual history is particularly unreliable in this population due to anovulatory cycles. These factors often result in a missed diagnosis and/or delayed prenatal care.

Teen pregnancy is associated with an increased risk of both maternal and fetal complications, such as ectopic pregnancy, preeclampsia, preterm birth, preterm premature rupture of membranes, anemia, intrauterine growth retardation and low birth weight, neonatal infections, complications from sexually transmitted infections, miscarriage/stillbirth, and neonatal death. These risks are increased in girls aged 15 years or younger. Teens often experience insufficient prenatal care, nutritional deficiencies, and delays in the diagnosis and treatment of infections. Smoking, drug and alcohol misuse, mood disorders, violence, and an unstable and/or unsafe home environment are more commonly associated with teenage mothers compared with adults. This higher risk of adverse outcomes highlights the importance of early diagnosis of pregnancy and initiation of prenatal care.

Pregnancy should be considered in the differential diagnosis for nearly every chief complaint in the postpubertal adolescent girl. Teenagers may present with a variety of symptoms, including amenorrhea, abdominal pain, nausea, vomiting, dizziness, fatigue, weight changes, urinary problems, irregular periods, and recurrent or vague unexplained presentations. A pregnancy test should be performed regardless of a given history of sexual activity. The possibility of pregnancy should not be excluded in teens with chronic illness or disability. Even in patients with seemingly unrelated complaints, early diagnosis of pregnancy will allow appropriate referrals for prenatal care or abortion services, allow early management of risk factors such as substance use and poor nutrition that can contribute to bad outcomes, and advise avoidance of potentially teratogenic medical interventions during management in the ED.

CONFIDENTIALITY AND CONSENT

Clinicians providing care to adolescents must be aware of issues of confidentiality and consent in this population. Usually, patients younger than age 18 years cannot receive health care services without the consent of a parent or guardian. The exceptions include services for sexually transmitted infection and pregnancy in all states and for contraception, sexual assault, mental health, and substance use depending on specific state law. Regarding pregnancy, confidentiality must be maintained throughout the visit unless there is concern that the patient may harm herself or others. The results of a positive pregnancy test are best shared with the patient alone. At this time, the provider should encourage the teen to share the information with a parent or trusted adult who can offer support and assistance. Some adolescents do not have parental support and are at risk for abuse or being asked to leave their home. If the adolescent is afraid to disclose to the parents, the provider should further explore these concerns and ensure that the adolescent feels safe at home.

There are certain situations in which disclosure is required, regardless of the teen's wishes. Every state has enacted mandatory reporter statutes that include suspected sexual abuse. Many states include any sexual activity (evidenced by pregnancy, sexually transmitted infection, or disclosure) in patients younger than age 13 years or with more than 2 years difference in age between partners in the definition of sexual abuse.

PREGNANT VAGINAL BLEEDING AND/OR ABDOMINAL PAIN PER TRIMESTER

Significant overlap in the differential diagnosis exists between vaginal bleeding and abdominal pain in pregnancy. Both obstetric and and non-obstetric etiologies should be considered.

First Trimester

Approximately 25% of women experience vaginal bleeding in their first trimester; roughly half of those will go on to have a miscarriage (abortion). The differential of bleeding includes abortion, ectopic pregnancy, infection, implantation, and benign bleeding. Bleeding equal to or heavier than a menstrual period, bright red blood, or concurrent abdominal pain increase the risk of pregnancy loss. Light bleeding or spotting does not seem to be associated with miscarriage. Many women with vaginal bleeding progress with normal pregnancies. Typically, all first-trimester vaginal bleeding should be labeled threatened abortion unless an alternative etiology is identified in the ED. Associated abdominal pain, signs of hemodynamic instability, or peritoneal signs require emergent evaluation for ruptured ectopic pregnancy.

A pelvic examination including speculum and bimanual components can help identify causes of bleeding. Non-obstetric causes that may be seen on speculum exam include vaginitis, cervicitis, human papillomavirus lesions, a traumatic laceration, or a cervical polyp. The provider should note whether the cervical os is open or closed and the presence of any visible products of conception. The rate and content of vaginal bleeding should also be noted. All clots should be removed from the vaginal vault, and all specimens should be sent to pathology for confirmation of gestational products.

Trends in quantitative β-human chorionic gonadotropin (β-hCG) levels provide useful information when distinguishing a normal from an abnormal early pregnancy. β-hCG levels should predictably double every 48–72 hours in a normal pregnancy. Decreasing levels in the first trimester indicate a nonviable pregnancy. The discriminatory level (1,500–3,000 mIU/mL) is the level above which an intrauterine pregnancy (IUP) should be visible on transvaginal ultrasonography. An IUP should be visible on transabdominal ultrasonography with β-hCG levels ≥6,500 mIU/mL. Failure to detect an IUP on transvaginal ultrasound in the setting of β-hCG levels >1,500 mIU/mL should raise concern for early pregnancy loss or ectopic pregnancy.

ED ultrasound should evaluate for an IUP. If a bedside study is performed and no IUP visualized, a formal ultrasound by the radiology department should be obtained. A normal fetal heart rate of 120–160 beats per minute (bpm) is reassuring. However, a fetal heart rate of <80 bpm is almost always associated with a future miscarriage. Subchorionic hemorrhage is a common cause of first-trimester vaginal bleeding that can be detected on ultrasound. Although it is associated with miscarriage, the prognosis is good if the hematoma is <25% the size of the gestational sac.

First-trimester bleeding may be the first sign of spontaneous abortion. Approximately one in three women will experience a miscarriage in their life. Common risk factors include advanced maternal age, infections, illicit drug use (particularly cocaine), and medical comorbidities such as uncontrolled diabetes or hypertension. The rate of early pregnancy loss is approximately 10% after an IUP has been detected on ultrasound. This risk increases in the setting of vaginal bleeding. Table 44.1 presents pregnancy complications and diagnostic criteria.

Treatment of stable patients with threatened abortion (vaginal bleeding with normal IUP on ultrasound and closed cervical os) is expectant management and pelvic rest with close obstetrician follow-up. They should be counseled that a spontaneous abortion may still occur; risk of abortion is approximately 35–50% depending on patient demographics, associated symptoms, and severity of bleeding. Best rest does not improve outcomes, but avoidance of activity such as heavy lifting or strenuous exercise is commonly recommended.

Complete spontaneous abortion can be confirmed by an ultrasound showing absence of any products of conception (in a previously confirmed IUP). Contraception may be started immediately after completed abortion. Provision of emotional support with appropriate referrals are essential components of care.

Pregnancy of uncertain location is diagnosed when neither an IUP nor an ectopic

TABLE 44.1 PREGNANCY COMPLICATIONS AND DIAGNOSTIC CRITERIA

Complication	Criteria
Early pregnancy loss	Nonviable IUP within the first trimester
Threatened abortion	Vaginal bleeding in first 20 weeks of gestation with a viable IUP detected on ultrasound; cervical os closed
Spontaneous abortion or miscarriage	Spontaneous loss of pregnancy prior to 20 weeks of gestation
Complete abortion	Complete passage of all products of conception; cervical os closed
Incomplete abortion	Vaginal bleeding with or without pain; open cervical os; products of conception may be seen in the canal
Inevitable abortion	Vaginal bleeding with an open cervical os; no products have passed
Missed abortion	Fetal or embryonic demise without passage of any tissue; closed cervical os; no bleeding
Nonviable pregnancy	Pregnancy that cannot result in live birth (i.e., ectopic or early pregnancy loss)
Viable pregnancy	Pregnancy that can potentially result in a live birth
Pregnancy of uncertain location	Positive pregnancy test; no IUP or ectopic noted on ultrasound (usually diagnosed in setting of β-hCG below the discriminatory zone)
Intrauterine pregnancy of uncertain viability	Ultrasound shows intrauterine gestational sac with no embryonic cardiac activity
Anembryonic gestation (blighted ovum)	Ultrasound shows gestation sac ≥25 mm and no yolk sac or fetal pole
Embryonic demise	Ultrasound shows embryo with crown–rump length ≥7 mm and no cardiac activity

β-hCG, β-human chorionic gonadotropin; IUP, intrauterine pregnancy.

pregnancy is seen on ultrasound. Inability to visualize an ectopic pregnancy or IUP does not rule out ectopic pregnancy. A pitfall lies in not ordering an ultrasound in patients with β-hCG levels below the discriminatory zone. Ectopic pregnancy may still be noted with a β-hCG level ≤1,500, or other soft signs may be suggestive, such as free fluid in the pelvis. Management of patients with pregnancy of uncertain location is expectant management with strict return precautions for increasing bleeding, pain, or dizziness and serial quantitative β-hCG levels. Repeat testing should occur within 48–72 hours.

If products of conception are visible on examination or ultrasound and the cervical os is open, the diagnosis of incomplete abortion may be made. If clot or tissue is noted within the os, it should be gently removed with forceps. These patients may have significant bleeding and pain.

Patients with incomplete, missed, or inevitable abortions can be managed with expectant, medical, or surgical management (uterine aspiration) in consultation with the obstetrician. Patient satisfaction, mental health outcomes, infection rates, and future fertility are similar among these treatments. Patients should be included in the medical decision-making. Expectant management is more than 80–90% effective. However, patients who choose expectant management may experience more days of bleeding and longer time to completion. The majority of women complete expulsion within 1 or 2 weeks. Medical management is most effective in anembryonic gestation or embryonic demise, less so in incomplete abortion. Medical management involves the administration of oral mifepristone (Mifeprex) 200 mg followed by vaginally administered misoprostol (Cytotec) 800 μg 24 hours later. Adverse effects include cramping and heavy vaginal bleeding, as well as nausea and diarrhea. Women who elect for expectant or medical management should be prescribed pain medications and given anticipatory guidance. They should be counseled that close follow-up is needed and surgical intervention may be necessary if complete expulsion does not occur. Retained products of conception can cause significant bleeding, fever, sepsis, and disseminated intravascular coagulation (DIC).

Rh factor should be assessed if Rh status is not known. Rh_0(D) immune globulin (Rhogam) is indicated within 72 hours for all Rh-negative patients with abdominal trauma, ectopic pregnancy, early pregnancy loss, and in those who undergo surgical treatment for miscarriage. There is insufficient evidence for use of Rh_0(D) immune globulin in patients with threatened abortion. The recommended dose is 50–120 μg before 12 weeks of gestation and 300 μg after 12 weeks of gestation or if lower doses are not available.

Second and Third Trimesters

Bleeding can also occur in second and third trimesters arising from a variety of etiologies. Acute hemorrhage places both mother and fetus at risk; the fetus may be compromised by uteroplacental insufficiency and premature birth. Bleeding during this time is usually attributed to placenta previa, placental abruption, or vasa previa. Lower genital tract lesions or early labor are common etiologies of late pregnancy bleeding as well. Minor trauma, such as sexual intercourse or a vaginal examination, can result in spotting or minor vaginal bleeding. Other possible non-obstetric causes of bleeding include hemorrhoids, urinary tract infections, nephrolithiasis, and lower gastrointestinal bleeding. Women with active, ongoing hemorrhage regardless of etiology require stabilization and possible preparation for delivery with prompt obstetrics consult or transfer.

Placenta previa is placental implantation overlying or abutting the internal cervical os. These patients classically present with painless bleeding. Diagnosis is made by ultrasound (transvaginal preferred), commonly in the second trimester. Most resolve by term. Persistent previa in the third trimester requires pelvic rest and, occasionally, hospitalization. Vasa previa occurs when fetal vessels traverse between the internal cervical os and the presenting fetal parts. It is rare but can result in fetal exsanguination. Bleeding is typically painless and often associated with rupture of membranes. Neonatal mortality is high.

Placental abruption occurs with placental separation prior to delivery resulting in loss of fetal perfusion. Risk factors for abruption include trauma (including minor trauma), hypertension, smoking, cocaine abuse, preterm premature rupture of membranes, advanced maternal age, and uterine myomas. Patients typically present with significant abdominal pain, vaginal bleeding, and/or fetal distress.

The amount of vaginal bleeding correlates poorly with the degree of placental separation; a large abruption can be concealed behind the placenta with only minimal or no vaginal bleeding. Ultrasound is only moderately sensitive for abruption; diagnosis is best made clinically with history and physical examination, fetal monitoring, and tocometry. Bleeding can be significant. Emergent delivery is indicated with significant bleeding, severe anemia or coagulopathy, abnormal fetal heart tracing, or maternal instability. Neonatal morbidity and mortality are high.

Significant bleeding from any cause is managed with rapid assessment of maternal and fetal status, fluid resuscitation, replacement of blood products when necessary, and urgent obstetrics consult. In patients with vaginal bleeding later in pregnancy, ultrasound evaluation should be performed prior to attempting a digital examination. Bimanual examination in the presence of placenta previa or vasa previa can provoke exsanguinating hemorrhage by further tearing the placenta or cord. The laboratory evaluation should include a baseline complete blood count, coagulation studies evaluating for possible DIC, and a type and crossmatch. Consider notifying the blood bank to the possibility of massive hemorrhage and need for massive transfusion protocols. Rh immunoglobulin should be administered to patients with bleeding who are Rh negative. Fetal heart rate monitoring and tocometry are indicated if available in the department.

Maternal DIC may result from systemic processes such as sepsis or obstetric processes such as placental abruption. Management focuses on identification of the underlying cause and maternal resuscitation with administration of platelets, blood, and fresh frozen plasma. Alternatively, prothrombin complex concentrate can be given.

Emergent or urgent delivery should be anticipated in the setting of significant vaginal bleeding or abdominal pain once the fetus has reached viability. No specific management scheme exists for patients in the early second trimester because the fetus is nonviable. Some patients with only a small amount of resolved bleeding, maternal hemodynamic stability, reassuring fetal status, and absence of active bleeding or contractions may be managed expectantly after obstetric evaluation. Expectant management in this case may include either discharge home or short-term observation in an antenatal unit. Because most neonatal morbidity and mortality result from complications of prematurity, the main therapeutic strategy is to prolong pregnancy until fetal lung maturity is achieved. Tocolytic agents such as magnesium may treat preterm contractions. Corticosteroids should be administered to women who have bleeding from placenta previa at 24–34 weeks of gestation. Limited data exist regarding outcomes in second-trimester bleeding; perinatal morbidity may approach 25%.

ECTOPIC PREGNANCY

Ectopic pregnancy occurs in approximately 1% or 2% of pregnancies; the fertilized ovum implants outside the uterus, usually in the fallopian tube (rarely in the cervix or abdominal cavity). The most common cause is scarring from salpingitis due to previous pelvic inflammatory disease (PID). Other risk factors pertinent to adolescents include smoking, previous ectopic pregnancy, endometriosis, and use of an intrauterine device for contraception. An ectopic pregnancy, if not recognized and treated, can cause tubal rupture and intra-abdominal exsanguination. It is the leading cause of pregnancy-related maternal death in the first trimester. Teenagers and minorities have the highest mortality from ectopic rupture, due largely to delay in seeking care.

Patients can present with delayed menstrual period, abdominal pain, and/or vaginal bleeding. Because these are not always present, it is imperative that providers have a high index of suspicion for ectopic pregnancy in girls with hypotension with no obvious cause. Patients may also present with nonspecific signs such as syncope. Tachycardia, hypotension, and peritoneal signs are indications of possible rupture. The consequences of missing an ectopic pregnancy can be catastrophic. Misdiagnosis is common; nearly half of women receive a different diagnosis during their initial ED evaluation. With ectopic pregnancy, adolescent girls tend to complain of more pain compared to their adult counterparts.

Diagnosis involves ultrasound and quantitative β-hCG levels. Physical examination is unreliable. If the β-hCG is beyond the discriminatory zone (1,500–3,000 mIU/L), an IUP should be visualized. If no IUP is noted, the pregnancy is presumed to be ectopic. Alternate diagnoses include early pregnancy and spontaneous abortion. In the case of ectopic pregnancy, an extrauterine pregnancy may be visualized on ultrasound. An adnexal mass with echogenicity and associated free fluid in the cul-de-sac is diagnostic. Definitive diagnosis with a β-hCG level below the discriminatory zone and a normal ultrasound without IUP is more difficult and will likely require serial visits (preferably in the outpatient clinic or ED if the clinic is not available). Ultrasound may show free fluid in the pelvis well below the discriminatory zone suggestive of ectopic and so may still be of use. If the patient was previously evaluated, look for prior ultrasound and β-hCG levels with which to compare. With an ectopic pregnancy, the expected doubling of the quantitative β-hCG in 48 hours should not occur.

Patients with an ectopic pregnancy can be managed medically or surgically in close cooperation with obstetrics. In patients deemed hemodynamically stable, conservative medical management with a single intramuscular methotrexate injection (50 mg/m^2 or 1 mg/kg) may be indicated. Alternative multidose regimens also exist. Contraindications for medical management include evidence for rupture, mass ≥3.5 cm, an initial β-hCG level of ≥5,000 mIU/mL, or a medical condition in which methotrexate is contraindicated. Patients must follow closely with obstetrics for serial examinations and β-hCG levels. When treating an adolescent, the clinician must ensure that the teen is willing and able to attend close follow-up (as often as daily clinic visits). Like medical management for incomplete/missed abortion, this process may be prolonged, typically taking 3–7 weeks. Medical management of ectopic pregnancy is more cost-effective than surgical management, with similar outcomes with respect to treatment success and future reproductive outcome. Treatment success is greater the lower the initial β-hCG level.

Methotrexate side effects include nausea, vomiting, diarrhea, stomatitis, and abdominal pain, making future clinical judgments about the possibility of subsequent rupture potentially difficult. If such patients return to the ED, repeat pelvic ultrasound should be obtained to assess for free fluid. Hemoperitoneum could indicate failure of therapy and rupture of ectopic pregnancy.

Patients with a contraindication to methotrexate use, fetal cardiac activity, signs of rupture, or hemodynamic instability should be managed surgically. These patients should be promptly resuscitated with crystalloids and packed red blood cells as needed. Surgical consultation in the unstable patient with a suspected ectopic pregnancy should not be delayed for formal ultrasound. Point-of-care pelvic ultrasound and FAST (focused assessment with sonography for trauma) can be very helpful in this situation to look for free fluid, suggestive of a ruptured ectopic pregnancy.

PREMATURE LABOR AND PREMATURE RUPTURE OF MEMBRANES

Adolescents are at increased risk of preterm labor. Typical presentations include contractions, cramping abdominal pain, pelvic pressure, back pain, an increase or change in vaginal discharge, and/or vaginal bleeding between 20 and 37 weeks of gestation. Diagnosis is made by demonstrating painful contractions lasting longer than 30 seconds and occurring at least four times every 20 minutes with associated change in length or dilation of the cervix. Alternatively, Braxton–Hicks contractions (false labor) are irregular, uncoordinated contractions that are not associated with demonstrable cervical changes.

Premature rupture of membranes (PROM) is the rupture of the amniotic membrane before the onset of labor. This is classified as preterm premature rupture of membranes (PPROM) if it occurs before 37 weeks of gestation. Adolescents demonstrate a higher risk of both PROM and PPROM compared with their adult counterparts. PPROM nearly always leads to premature delivery. Rupture of membranes presents as either a large release of clear vaginal fluid or a regular trickle. Urinary incontinence or excess vaginal secretions can be confused with PROM. Because it is difficult to rule out PROM based on history alone, it is necessary to perform a sterile speculum examination. Digital cervical examination should be avoided because it raises the risk of infection. Diagnosis is made by applying fluid to a microscope slide, allowing it to dry, and observing ferning. Alternatively, testing of the pH of the fluid can be performed; amniotic fluid has a basic pH of 6.5–7.5 compared with the more acidic vaginal secretions (3.5–6.0).

Patients with preterm labor, PROM, and PPROM should be transferred or admitted to an obstetrics unit. Patients with PROM are at increased risk of infection (chorioamnionitis, endometritis, and neonatal sepsis), with the incidence increasing with decreasing gestational age. Group B streptococci screening should be performed if available. If not, consider empirically treating with penicillin G (5 million units intravenously followed by 2.5 million units every 4 hours until delivery) to prevent vertical transmission of this infection to the newborn. In cases of PROM, start a 48-hour course of intravenous ampicillin and erythromycin to reduce the risk of neonatal morbidity.

HYPERTENSIVE DISEASE OF PREGNANCY: CHRONIC HYPERTENSION, GESTATIONAL HYPERTENSION, PRE-ECLAMPSIA/ECLAMPSIA, AND HELLP SYNDROME

Hypertensive disease is one of the most common complications affecting pregnancy. The underlying mechanism may involve abnormal placental development. Hypertensive disorders of pregnancy are associated with increased maternal morbidity and mortality, predominantly because of maternal stroke but also including pulmonary edema, myocardial infarction, acute respiratory distress syndrome, coagulopathy, renal failure, and retinal injury. Hypertensive disorders are responsible for nearly 10% of all maternal deaths. The increased vasospastic state compromises placental perfusion, which leads to an increase in fetal morbidity and mortality as well. Infants born to mothers with hypertensive disease are often born small for their gestational age. Preterm deliveries are common. Placental abruption can occur. The risk of pre-eclampsia is increased in adolescence, especially in girls aged 13–15 years.

During pregnancy, blood pressure readings >140/90 mmHg are considered to be hypertensive. Women with gestational hypertension will have an elevated blood pressure but no proteinuria, edema, or significant laboratory abnormalities (and hypertension resolves after delivery). Pre-eclampsia is defined as hypertension with proteinuria (≥1 or 2+ on urinalysis), pathologic edema, and/or end organ dysfunction. The edema is usually generalized, involving the hands and face, and persists throughout the day. As pre-eclampsia worsens, the degree of hypertension and proteinuria also worsens, eventually accompanied by renal insufficiency. Severe pre-eclampsia (Table 44.2) may be associated with mental status changes, headaches, visual disturbances, elevated liver function tests, abdominal pain, thrombocytopenia, and pulmonary edema. Particularly difficult to detect, women with chronic hypertension may develop superimposed pre-eclampsia with especially high morbidity. HELLP syndrome (hemolysis, elevated liver function tests, low platelets), thought to be a variant of pre-eclampsia, may develop. Diagnostic criteria for HELLP syndrome include microangiopathic hemolysis with increased lactate dehydrogenase (>600 U/L), increased aspartate aminotransferase (>70 U/L), and thrombocytopenia (<100 × 10^9/L). One of the most striking complications of pre-eclampsia is eclampsia, which is a generalized tonic–clonic seizure

TABLE 44.2 PRE-ECLAMPSIA DIAGNOSTIC CRITERIA

Pre-eclampsia	Severe Features of Pre-eclampsia
Blood pressure ≥140/90 mmHg on two separate occasions	Blood pressure >160/110 mmHg
Plus	Creatinine >1.1 mg/dL or 2× baseline
Proteinuria defined as one of the following: ≥300 mg/24-hour collection Protein:creatinine ratio of ≥0.3 mg/dL Random protein dipstick >1 or 2+	Hepatic dysfunction (transaminases ≥2× baseline) or epigastric/right upper quadrant pain
Or	New-onset headache; neurologic or visual disturbances
Any severe feature	Platelet count <100 × 10^9/L Pulmonary edema

due to encephalopathy from underperfusion of the brain.

Pregnant patients with hypertension require a urinalysis and evaluation of hepatic, renal, and hematologic function. When blood pressure increases to >160/110 mmHg, the goal is prevention of seizures and permanent end organ damage. Antihypertensives such as intravenous hydralazine or labetalol should be given to lower blood pressure with a goal 140–150/90–100 mmHg. Dropping blood pressure too low may cause hypoperfusion of the maternal organs and fetus. Hydralazine can be administered in 5- to 10-mg aliquots at 15- to 20-minute intervals. Initial dose of labetalol is 20 mg; if this is not effective in 10 minutes, it can be followed by a second dose of 40 mg, then with 80 mg every 10 minutes, total dosage not exceeding 220 mg. Oral nifedipine is also considered a first-line therapy for reduction in severe elevations of blood pressure in pregnancy. Seizures are treated with magnesium sulfate. The initial loading dose is 4–6 g intravenously over 15–20 minutes, followed by an infusion rate of 1 or 2 g/hour.

Patients with pre-eclampsia with severe features or eclampsia should be admitted for intravenous therapy; definitive treatment is delivery of the fetus. Delivery timing involves balancing the risk of prematurity against worsening pre-eclampsia. To improve maternal outcomes, delivery is generally indicated at 37 weeks of gestation for women who have pre-eclampsia without severe features. Delivery at 34 weeks of gestation is indicated for women with severe features once maternal stabilization has been achieved.

INFECTIONS IN PREGNANCY

Pregnant patients may be more severely affected by a wide range of common bacterial and viral infections that can be dangerous to their health as well as the health of the fetus. These infections can be classified into two major categories: gynecologic infections and systemic infections. Gynecologic infections can cause complications including PROM, preterm delivery, and fetal malformations. Systemic infections such as urinary tract infections and those caused by influenza viruses, HIV, parvovirus, and *Listeria* can have serious, life-threatening implications for the mother and fetus when they occur during pregnancy. Treatment decisions must weigh the benefits of treatment against the risks of antimicrobials during pregnancy.

Gynecologic Infections

See Chapter 43 for presentation of common gynecologic infections. Specific pregnancy-related concerns are mentioned here. Bacterial vaginosis (BV) during pregnancy is associated with an increased risk of spontaneous abortion, preterm labor, PROM, endometritis, and chorioamnionitis. Treatment of asymptomatic patients with BV has not been shown to improve outcomes. Symptomatic pregnant patients should be treated with oral metronidazole 500 mg twice daily for 7 days.

Symptomatic trichomoniasis should be treated. Vulvovaginal candidiasis is uncomfortable but not associated with significant obstetric complications. Intravaginal antifungal treatment may be used to treat symptomatic infections for 7 days.

Gonorrhea and chlamydia can cause significant obstetric complications, including preterm delivery, PROM, spontaneous septic abortion, chorioamnionitis, postpartum infections, perinatal mortality, and neonatal infections. Patients can be asymptomatic or present with vaginal discharge. Concurrent infection with both *Neisseria gonorrhoeae* and *Chlamydia trachomatis* is common. Pregnant women should be treated empirically if infection suspected prior to confirmatory tests with both a single dose of azithromycin 1 g orally and a single dose of ceftriaxone 250 mg intramuscularly.

Chorioamnionitis is an infection of the amniotic fluid, membranes, and placenta. Once a patient is pregnant, any infection in the uterus is termed chorioamnionitis rather than PID. Similar to PID in the nonpregnant patient, it is typically an ascending infection caused by normal vaginal flora. Common organisms include *Escherichia coli*, group B *Streptococcus*, *Bacteroides*, or *Clostridium*. Young age, nulliparity, low socioeconomic status, prolonged labor, and ruptured membranes are risk factors. Diagnosis is clinical. Signs and symptoms include fever, uterine tenderness, tachycardia, purulent vaginal discharge, and leukocytosis. The fetus may demonstrate decreased activity, tachycardia, and decreased beat-to-beat variability on monitoring. Consequences may include neonatal sepsis, placental abruption, premature birth, cerebral palsy, and neonatal death. Maternal complications include sepsis, prolonged labor, need for cesarean delivery, postpartum endometritis, and postpartum hemorrhage. If suspected, empiric antibiotics should be started. Ampicillin plus gentamicin is the most commonly recommended empirical treatment.

HSV -1 and -2 can cause recurrent outbreaks in either the oral or the genital region. Primary infections result in more severe maternal disease manifestations as well as higher fetal morbidity and mortality. Subsequent outbreaks are more common but less severe. Maternal symptoms may include gingivostomatitis, vulvovaginitis, and disseminated herpes (hepatitis, encephalitis, thrombocytopenia, leukopenia, and coagulopathy). Vertical transmission to the fetus is most likely, with genital tract viral shedding at the time of vaginal delivery. In the neonate, HSV can result in several clinical syndromes, including skin, eye, and mouth disease; disseminated disease with a mortality rate of almost 30%; and central nervous system disease with a mortality rate of 4% but a high morbidity. Acyclovir is the recommended treatment (400 mg three times daily). Treatment for primary infections should last 7–10 days; treatment for recurrent outbreaks should last 5 days.

Caused by *Treponema pallidum*, syphilis can present with a wide variety of symptoms depending on the stage (i.e., primary, secondary, and tertiary). Primary syphilis is characterized by a painless genital chancre. If syphilis goes untreated during pregnancy, it can result in spontaneous abortion, stillbirth, fetal hydrops, intrauterine growth restriction, premature delivery, and perinatal mortality. Infants with congenital syphilis can have hepatosplenomegaly, bone abnormalities, petechiae, anemia, jaundice, frontal bossing, palatal deformations, and nasal deformities. The treatment of syphilis is penicillin G. No other antibiotics are effective for the treatment of maternal syphilis and the prevention of congenital syphilis. Desensitization should occur in patients with a reported penicillin allergy. Although parenteral penicillin G is the treatment of choice, the formulation, dose, and duration differ. Providers should be aware of the indications for each formulation of penicillin (benzathine, aqueous procaine, or aqueous crystalline) in order to ensure adequate treatment.

Systemic Infections

Infections of the urinary tract are common in pregnancy and can cause significant maternal and neonatal manifestations. The presence of any urinary tract bacteriuria, including asymptomatic bacteriuria, cystitis, and pyelonephritis, has been associated with adverse outcomes, including preterm birth, PROM, postpartum fever, and neonatal infection. Given the high incidence of progression to pyelonephritis, even patients with asymptomatic bacteriuria should be treated. The most common pathogens are *E. coli*, *Klebsiella*, *Enterobacter*, *Citrobacter*, *Proteus*, *Pseudomonas*, *Enterococcus*, and group B *Streptococcus*. A 3- to 7-day course of nitrofurantoin or cephalosporins is safe and effective in pregnant patients with asymptomatic bacteriuria or cystitis. In general, pregnant patients with pyelonephritis should be hospitalized after a full workup including blood cultures and assessment of renal function. They are at risk of developing bacteremia, acute respiratory distress syndrome (ARDS), septic shock, DIC, preterm labor, PROM, chorioamnionitis, and neonatal sepsis. Treatment is with intravenous fluids and antibiotics (penicillins or cephalosporins) until the patient is afebrile for 48 hours. A very select population of pregnant patients with pyelonephritis, including those with a fetus <24 weeks gestation age, previously healthy, and without fever, vomiting, tachycardia, tachypnea, or hypotension, may be treated as outpatients with very close follow-up.

The management of HIV during pregnancy is complicated and should best be accomplished with assistance from obstetrics and infectious disease. All HIV-positive pregnant women should be treated with antiretrovirals, regardless of viral load. These patients should not start therapy until after 14 weeks to decrease risk of teratogenicity. When a patient with HIV is diagnosed with pregnancy prior to 14 weeks of gestation, they can be discharged with close follow-up. If pregnancy is identified after 14 weeks of gestation, specialist consultation in the ED is indicated. All patients with HIV who present to the ED in active labor should receive intravenous zidovudine as soon as possible, before delivery, to decrease vertical transmission risk.

Waning immunity in pregnancy makes pregnant women more susceptible to common viral illnesses, including upper respiratory tract infections and influenza. These patients commonly present to the ED seeking evaluation and guidance. Pregnant women are at increased risk of complications from the influenza virus, especially respiratory complications such as pneumonia and ARDS. In addition, there is an increased risk of preterm delivery and fetal morbidity. All pregnant patients, regardless of the duration of their symptoms, should be treated with antiviral therapy. Treatment of common upper respiratory infections is supportive, and guidance for appropriate over-the-counter medication use in pregnancy is paramount. Other viral infections can also have devastating consequences. Parvovirus B19 can cause fever, rash, headache, and arthralgias. Vertical transmission can cause fetal demise or hydrops. Patients with cytomegalovirus (CMV) are most commonly diagnosed with a simple viral illness or upper respiratory infection due to nonspecific symptoms of fever, sore throat, fatigue, myalgias, and swollen glands. Infants with congenital CMV may be born with microcephaly, seizures, and/or hepatosplenomegaly.

Listeriosis is a food-borne illness that is much more common in pregnant women than the general population. Caused by *Listeria monocytogenes*, listeriosis can cause gastrointestinal and influenza-like symptoms. Consequences to the fetus can be devastating. Diagnosis is made with blood cultures. All pregnant patients with high suspicion for listeriosis should be admitted for intravenous antibiotics until culture results return. Treatment is high-dose intravenous ampicillin.

COMPLICATIONS OF ABORTION

Compared to adults, adolescents are more likely to delay seeking elective abortion, resort to unskilled providers, use dangerous methods, and delay seeking care for postabortive complications. Most complications are minor and expected, including abdominal cramping and vaginal bleeding. Medical abortions are more likely to result in complications compared with surgical abortions. The most common complication is an incomplete or failed abortion requiring subsequent uterine aspiration or repeated doses of abortifactant. Other complications include hemorrhage, infection, trauma to the cervix or vagina, uterine perforation, or anesthesia-related complications. The rate of cervical trauma after abortion in teens is nearly twice that of their adult counterparts. Girls who present with significant postabortion bleeding or pain should have a hemodynamic assessment, evaluation for significant anemia or infection, and an ultrasound searching for any retained products of conception.

Any type of abortion (including spontaneous, medical, or surgical) can be complicated by an intrauterine infection (septic abortion). Septic abortion can occur when retained products of conception have not been adequately expelled and endometritis develops. Common signs and symptoms include fever, chills, abdominal pain, vaginal bleeding, uterine tenderness, and purulent vaginal discharge. In severe cases, patients can develop signs of severe sepsis and septic shock. The infection frequently spreads from the placenta and endometrium through the myometrium to the peritoneum. Complications can include hemorrhage, lacerations, perforation of the uterus or bowel, tetanus, and severe pelvic infections. Long-term complications may include chronic pelvic pain, infertility, spontaneous abortion in future pregnancies, and an increased risk of future ectopic pregnancies. Evaluation includes cell count, signs of DIC and hemolysis, assessment of renal function, and need for possible anti-D immunoglobulin (Rhogam). Pelvic ultrasound can demonstrate retained products of conception, uterine perforation, or abscess formation. Treatment of septic abortion includes fluid resuscitation for hemodynamic stabilization, culture collection, broad-spectrum parenteral antibiotics, and rapid surgical removal of any retained products of conception.

VOMITING IN PREGNANCY AND HYPEREMESIS GRAVIDARUM

Nausea and vomiting in pregnancy are extremely common; they occur so often that they are considered a "normal" part of pregnancy. Despite the term "morning sickness," nausea and vomiting can affect women at any time of the day or night. Women are generally most affected in their first trimester, but some women experience symptoms throughout their pregnancy. Symptoms can range from mild discomfort, managed by dietary and lifestyle modifications, to severe recurrent vomiting characterized by significant dehydration requiring intravenous fluids and medications. Vomiting is a common presenting complaint to the ED for pregnant women.

Hyperemesis gravidarum (HG), the most severe manifestation of nausea and vomiting in pregnancy, occurs in up to 3% of pregnant patients. It is characterized by intractable vomiting with evidence of starvation or weight loss ≥5% of prepregnancy weight. Evidence for starvation includes ketonuria, renal insufficiency, electrolyte imbalance (hyponatremia, hypokalemia, and hypochloremia), or signs of dehydration (tachycardia, dry mucous membranes, and increased hematocrit or urine concentration). HG has significant morbidity, can lead to adverse birth outcomes, and is the most common reason for hospital admission in early pregnancy. Risks include preterm labor, small for gestational weight infants, vitamin deficiencies, and possible neurodevelopmental effects from fetal malnutrition. Beyond the maternal and fetal consequences of malnutrition, the severity of HG can cause a major psychosocial burden particularly in adolescents, leading to depression, anxiety, loss of identity, social isolation, and even pregnancy termination. Rare but serious complications include Wernicke encephalopathy, acute renal failure, liver function abnormalities, central pontine myelinolysis, esophageal rupture, and pneumothorax.

Alternative diagnoses should always be considered. The aim of treatment is to control symptoms enough to promote quality of life and to enable sufficient oral intake to avoid dehydration and malnutrition. Dietary modifications are first line and moderately effective. These include avoidance of sensory stimuli such as strong odors and heat, eating frequent small meals to avoid an empty or particularly full stomach, avoidance of spicy or high-fat foods, elimination of iron-containing prenatal vitamins, maintenance of adequate hydration, and the addition of a small carbohydrate-rich snack such as crackers before rising in the morning. Alternative therapies including ginger supplementation and acupuncture/acupressure may be used.

Acute treatment is rehydration with crystalloid boluses. Dextrose containing saline may improve symptoms and decrease ketonuria. Thiamine (vitamin B_1) should also be given to reduce the risk of Wernicke's encephalopathy in severe cases. Vitamin B_6, or pyridoxine (10–75 mg/day), is considered first-line pharmacologic treatment when nonpharmacologic options have failed and is available over the counter. Combination vitamin B_6 with doxylamine (10–20 mg) is available by prescription and is currently the only U.S. Food and Drug Administration-approved antiemetic in pregnancy. If pyridoxine/doxylamine is not effective, the next tier of treatment would include either antihistamines (dimenhydrinate or diphenhydramine) or a dopamine antagonist (prochlorperazine, promethazine, metoclopramide, or droperidol). Side effects of these medications may be limiting and include significant drowsiness, dystonic reaction, and dry mouth.

Ondansetron, a serotonin receptor antagonist and the most commonly used antiemetic, has been shown to be as effective as, and perhaps more effective than, previously listed options. Concern has been raised recently about the possibility of congenital anomalies with ondansetron, particularly cleft palate and cardiac malformations. Data from different studies have been contradictory, however, and overall there is insufficient evidence to suggest that it be avoided in pregnancy. There is little evidence to support the use of any one of these medications over any others, and risks/benefits should be considered. When using multiple antiemetics combined, the risks of side effects including prolonged QT, extrapyramidal side effects, and the possibility of neuroleptic malignant syndrome are increased.

AMNIOTIC FLUID EMBOLISM

Amniotic fluid embolism (AFE) is a rare, unpredictable, often fatal complication of late pregnancy. It is one of the main causes of maternal mortality in the United States. The prognosis is poor; most women do not survive. Maternal and fetal survivors tend to have persistent neurologic sequelae. Despite the lack of a definitive understanding, AFE is thought to be caused by an abnormal maternal response to the introduction of amniotic fluid and fetal tissue into the systemic maternal circulation. Vasoactive and procoagulant factors in amniotic fluid trigger endothelial activation, leading to a massive inflammatory insult. This immune response has led AFE to be referred to as anaphylactoid syndrome of pregnancy. It occurs in the intrapartum or immediate postpartum period (generally within 48 hours of birth), more rarely during abortion or abdominal trauma. The classic triad is sudden hypoxia, hypotension, and coagulopathy. Symptoms may also include fetal distress, altered mental status, seizures, multiorgan failure, and cardiovascular collapse. Diagnosis is clinical, based on the presence of these elements and the exclusion of other likely causes.

AFE is primarily a clinical diagnosis. Management includes immediate supportive and resuscitative measures including airway control; correction of hemodynamic instability with fluid resuscitation, blood transfusion, and vasopressors when needed; and correction of coagulopathy with aggressive component replacement. Massive transfusion protocol should be implemented in the setting of ongoing hemorrhage. Given the proposed anaphylactoid pathophysiology of AFE, consideration may be given to the administration of steroids. Prompt delivery (perimortem cesarean section) in the mother who has sustained cardiopulmonary arrest is critical for improved newborn outcome. This not only may be life-saving for the fetus but also in theory may assist in maternal resuscitation by removing venacaval compression.

MOLAR PREGNANCY

Molar pregnancy is an abnormal pregnancy (more common in adolescents) in which a nonviable fertilized egg implants in the uterus. A complete mole is diploid, resulting from the duplication of a single sperm after fertilization of an ovum without chromosomes. Patients with a complete molar pregnancy have very high hCG levels, usually >100,000 mIU/mL, and a higher rate of malignancy (20%). Partial moles have triploid karyotypes, caused by an egg fertilized by two sperm. Patients with complete moles have no fetal tissue; ultrasound demonstrates a central heterogeneous mass described as a "snowstorm" appearance or a "cluster of grapes." Patients with partial moles usually have fetal tissue. Patients with a molar pregnancy may present with vaginal bleeding, anemia, hyperemesis gravidarum, pre-eclampsia before 20 weeks of gestation, or gestational hyperthyroidism due to hyperstimulation of the thyroid by hCG. On examination, the patient may have a uterus larger than expected for estimated gestational age. Molar pregnancies require surgical evacuation and close follow-up with serial β-hCG levels. Given risk of malignancy (gestational trophoblastic neoplasia), an evaluation for metastasis including chest radiograph should be obtained. Patients should be referred to a gynecologic oncologist.

CHEST PAIN IN PREGNANCY

Chest pain may be due to gastroesophageal reflux and benign dyspnea of pregnancy as well as more ominous pathology, including pulmonary embolus (PE), acute myocardial infarction, coronary dissection, aortic disease, and cardiomyopathy. Venous thromboembolus, coronary thrombosus, and vasculitis may occur with hypercoagulable state and hormonal changes induced by pregnancy.

Pulmonary Embolism

Venous thromboembolism (VTE) including PE and deep vein thrombosis, is a significant cause of pregnancy-related morbidity and mortality despite the overall low incidence in pregnancy. The incidence of VTE ranges from 3 to 50 times higher in pregnant women compared with their nonpregnant counterparts. Risk peaks in the immediate postpartum period. The clinical presentation of PE in pregnancy is highly variable. Many of the symptoms of VTE overlap with the normal physiological changes in pregnancy, including dyspnea, tachycardia, and leg swelling. Patients may also present with chest pain, fever, tachypnea, hypoxia, hemoptysis, syncope, cough, or hypotension.

The diagnosis of VTE in pregnancy is controversial and without clear evidence-based recommendations. A lower extremity duplex ultrasound is a noninvasive test that does not expose the patient or fetus to ionizing radiation. Computed tomography pulmonary angiogram (CTPA) is often the recommended diagnosis of choice in PE but exposes the patient and fetus to radiation. A ventilation–perfusion scan may be performed if the patient's chest X-ray is normal, but this test exposes the fetus to higher radiation than CTPA. Magnetic resonance pulmonary angiography is less sensitive and not frequently available.

Inpatient management for anticoagulation therapy should occur with hemodynamic instability, large clots, medical comorbidities, and in women in whom delivery is expected. Low-molecular-weight heparin (LMWH) does not cross the placenta and is the drug of choice for the treatment of VTE in pregnancy. The most commonly used LMWH is enoxaparin at a dose of 1 mg/kg twice daily. In pregnant patients with significant PE, an unfractionated heparin bolus should be given in the ED followed by continuous infusion titrated to goal PTT values until the patient is stabilized, at which time the medication can be transitioned to LMWH. Patients with massive PE and hemodynamic compromise may be treated with thrombolysis and/or embolectomy, but these treatments are relatively contraindicated in pregnancy and their use is controversial.

TRAUMA IN PREGNANCY

The most common causes of trauma during pregnancy include motor vehicle collisions, assaults, and falls. Traumatic injury is the leading cause of non-obstetric maternal death. Fetal death can result from maternal hemodynamic instability, placental abruption, uterine rupture, direct fetal injury, and as a result of preterm birth associated with maternal trauma. Significant uterine injury is rare in the first trimester because the bony pelvis protects the small gravid uterus.

Even minor trauma can be the precipitating factor for preterm labor. With few exceptions, the evaluation of the pregnant trauma patient should proceed in a similar manner as the evaluation of a nonpregnant patient. At all times, priority should be given to maternal assessment and stabilization because fetal outcomes are directly linked to early and aggressive maternal resuscitation. Secondary assessment should include sterile vaginal speculum examination to evaluate for vaginal lacerations or bony fragments that may indicate pelvic fractures. Examine for cervical dilation and for the presence of blood and/or amniotic fluid leakage. If fluid is present, it can be tested for ferning and for its pH (normal vaginal secretions have a pH of 5.0, whereas amniotic fluid has a pH of 7.0). Perform bedside ultrasound to determine fetal position and movement; assess for problems such as placenta previa. After primary and secondary survey, place the patient in the left lateral decubitus position. In a supine pregnant patient, the combined weight of the uterus, fetus, placenta, and amniotic fluid can compress the inferior vena cava enough to obstruct venous blood return to the heart.

Radiologic studies should not be avoided over concerns for the fetus if they are necessary for complete assessment of the mother. No single diagnostic procedure administers a dose of radiation sufficient to threaten the developing fetus, especially during mid- to late pregnancy. Obtain a maternal blood type and Kleihauer–Betke test to assess for fetomaternal hemorrhage—the transfer of fetal blood cells into the maternal circulation. If the maternal blood type is rhesus negative and the fetus is rhesus positive, even a small amount of blood can cause the mother to develop antibodies against the fetal Rh_0(D) antigen. In subsequent pregnancies, this can cause hemolytic disease of the newborn, which, if severe, is associated with total body edema, hepatosplenomegaly, heart failure, and intrauterine death. All rhesus-negative mothers should receive Rhogam after trauma.

Cardiotocographic monitoring is the most sensitive indicator of fetal distress and thus is required for a minimum of 4–6 hours following maternal trauma if the fetus is viable. Until continuous electronic fetal heart rate monitoring is available, perform serial measurements using a Doppler ultrasonography. Normal values range from 120 to 160 bpm; slower rates are far more ominous than faster ones.

Premature labor can affect up to 25% of trauma cases beyond 22 weeks. Signs of preterm labor should be sought in every patient with a viable fetus; signs include vaginal bleeding, contractions, rupture of membranes, and bulging perineum. If risk of delivery is high because of preterm labor or premature rupture of membranes, consider administering steroids (betamethasone 12 mg or dexamethasone 6 mg), antibiotics, and tocolytics (magnesium sulfate). In the setting of a relatively stable mother and nonreassuring fetal heart tracing in a viable fetus (fetal heart rate <100 bpm, prolonged decelerations, or recurrent late decelerations), emergent cesarean delivery should be considered. Maternal trauma is not an absolute contraindication for vaginal delivery. Pelvic fractures have been suggested as a contraindication to vaginal delivery only when the fracture obstructs the birth canal or is unstable; >80% of women who sustain pelvic fracture can deliver vaginally.

POSTPARTUM PROBLEMS

The period just after delivery is a high-risk period. Common presenting complaints include vaginal bleeding or discharge, obstetric wound concerns, breast problems, fever, and abdominal pain.

Postpartum depression usually begins within 4 weeks following delivery, affecting 10–15% of pregnancies. The most feared consequences of postpartum depression include suicide and infanticide. Emergency providers should screen all postpartum women in the ED regardless of chief complaint. Patients may present with unrelated complaints or complaints related to their infant. It is important to keep a high suspicion of postpartum depression in both adolescent mothers presenting themselves as the patient and also when evaluating their neonates in the ED. Depressive symptoms may also manifest as anxiety about the infant's health, concern about their ability to care for the infant, or a lack of interest in the infant.

Peripartum cardiomyopathy is new-onset heart failure near the end of pregnancy or within the first 5 months postpartum. Signs and symptoms include shortness of breath, orthopnea, cough, pedal edema, pulmonary crackles, cardiac murmurs, jugular venous distension, hemodynamic instability, and respiratory distress. ED evaluation and treatment are similar to those of all patients with heart failure. Differential should also include other peripartum pathology, such as PE, AFE, pre-eclampsia/eclampsia, and myocardial infarction. Treatment should focus on respiratory support with supplemental oxygen and/or positive-pressure ventilation as needed, diuresis, afterload reduction, and pressor/inotropic support if required.

Headaches in late pregnancy and postpartum may represent a common benign headache, migraine, or a more pathologic process. Benign postpartum headaches are common due to recent neuraxial anesthesia, sleep deprivation, and hormonal fluctuations. Postdural puncture headaches are typically described as severe and postural in nature, worsening with sitting or standing. ED treatment includes intravenous fluids, caffeine, analgesics, and blood patch in severe/refractory cases. Serious pathology including intracranial hemorrhage, ischemic stroke, and central venous thrombosis is more common in the postpartum period. A low threshold for further evaluation with labs and imaging should be maintained, and any new neurologic symptoms should be taken seriously, even if subtle or subjective. See Chapters 19 and 20 on neurovascular and neurological emergencies, respectively. In the setting of hypertension, pre-eclampsia/eclampsia should be considered.

Postpartum infections such as urinary tract infection, pyelonephritis, mastitis, and endometritis are also common. Workup for most postpartum infections includes blood count, electrolytes and liver enzymes, coagulation studies, and catheterized urinalysis. Patients with endometritis present with abdominal pain, uterine tenderness, fever, and purulent lochia in the first 2 weeks after delivery. Cesarean section is the most significant risk factor. No imaging can definitely diagnose endometritis, but imaging modalities including both ultrasound and CT can be useful to rule out other postpartum complications, such as abscess, hematoma, and fistula. Patients with suspected postpartum endometritis should be admitted for broad-spectrum parenteral antibiotics.

Mastitis is an infection of the breast seen in breastfeeding women, usually in the first 3 months postpartum. Nipple breakdown and poor milk drainage lead to an entry pathway and nidus for bacterial infection from the infant's nasopharynx or the mother's skin. The most common pathogen is *Staphylococcus aureus* (methicillin-sensitive and methicillin-resistant), although *Streptococcus pyogenes* and *E. coli* have also been implicated. Patients present with a painful, swollen, erythematous breast and associated fever, chills, and myalgias. Mild to moderate symptoms lasting <24 hours without fever may be attributed alternatively to simple breast engorgement. Ultrasound may demonstrate a breast abscess. Treatment involves frequent breast emptying with continued breastfeeding, pumping, or manual expression; anti-inflammatory medications; and antibiotics. Incision and drainage are not indicated for associated abscesses.

Excessive vaginal bleeding or hemorrhage can occur up to 12 weeks postpartum. Possible etiologies include lower genital tract lacerations, uterine inversion, and subinvolution of the placental bed. Less common etiologies in the ED include uterine atony, placenta accreta, coagulopathy, and uterine rupture. Uterine inversion occurs when the uterine fundus collapses into the endometrial cavity, essentially turning the organ inside-out. Most cases occur within the first 24 hours after birth; however, up to 10% of cases may not occur until 1 month or more postpartum. Diagnosis may be made on physical examination or by ultrasound. Subinvolution of the placental bed, the most common cause of delayed postpartum hemorrhage, is the failure of blood vessels underlying the placental implantation site to resolve, leading to delayed postpartum bleeding. This is most commonly caused by retained placental tissue or endometritis. Diagnosis is made on transvaginal ultrasound. For all patients with significant postpartum hemorrhage, workup should include a blood count, coagulation studies, and type and screen. The management should focus on simultaneous volume resuscitation with fluids and/or blood as well as hemorrhagic source control. Consideration should be given to uterine tonic agents or an intrauterine balloon tamponade device in the event of massive hemorrhage.

Key Points

- Pregnancy should be considered in all adolescent females, regardless of chief complaint.
- Pregnancy complications are more common in the pediatric patient.
- Diagnostic delay of life-threatening conditions is common in the pregnant child.

Further Reading

Hendriks E, MacNaughton H, Castillo MacKenzie M. First trimester bleeding: Evaluation and management. *Am Fam Physician*. 2019;99(3):166–174.

Pontius E, Vieth JT. Complications in early pregnancy. *Emerg Med Clin North Am*. 2019;37(2):219–237.

Sutton AL, Harper LM, Tita AT. Hypertensive disorders in pregnancy. *Obstet Gynecol Clin*. 2018;45(2):333–347.

Wheaton N, Al-Abdullah A, Haertlein T. Late pregnancy and postpartum emergencies. *Emerg Med Clin North Am*. 2019;37(2):277–286.

Young JS, White LM. Vaginal bleeding in late pregnancy. *Emerg Med Clin North Am*. 2019;37(2): 251–264.

45

Emergency Pediatric Vascular Access

GARRETT S. PACHECO

INTRODUCTION

Obtaining vascular access in pediatric patients is associated with a myriad of challenges. For the child who is conscious, lack of cooperation can foil any efforts at performing this procedure successfully. Furthermore, multiple painful attempts can compromise the present procedural encounter. Failures have potential to negatively impact every attempt at vascular access for that child in the future.

The challenges of vascular access in pediatric patients are exacerbated by a variety of factors. Differences in anatomy complicate the ability to achieve successful vascular cannulation: Vessels are smaller in caliber and therefore often difficult to visualize and palpate. Increased mobility of the vessels leads to high failure rates of cannulation. Dehydration can further complicate the ability to visualize, palpate, and isolate the vessels for a cannula attempt. The presence of critical illness in emergency conditions is also an issue; other predictors of difficult intravenous (IV) access include obesity, prematurity, age younger than 3 years, and weight <5 kg.

In emergency care, vascular access is often needed to obtain blood for laboratory analysis, to provide fluid resuscitation and medication, and for potential blood product administration. The method, site, and size of device used to obtain vascular access are primarily dependent on the conditional needs of the patient. Parent preference as well as agent to be administered also contribute to the decision.

Catheter size is the primary difference for pediatric vascular equipment. Specialized locations used for venous access can also differ based on age. Terminology used to describe the diameter of the device for vascular access includes single-lumen catheters described by gauge (G). Multi-lumen catheters are described by French size (Fr). Being familiar with this equipment and the indication for vascular access will aid the operator in making an informed decision for the patient's vascular access needs.

PERIPHERAL VENOUS ACCESS

Common sites for peripheral venous cannulation are hands, wrists, feet, and the antecubital fossa. The scalp in young neonates and infants is a site less often used. External jugular, saphenous, and axillary veins can also be utilized when needed. Cannulation of the small vessels of the extremities may be nearly impossible due to venous collapse during shock or cardiopulmonary arrest, prompting the provider to try one of these other locations.

Emergency physicians are often called to obtain vascular access if nursing or ancillary staff is unable to successfully cannulate a peripheral vessel. When common peripheral sites have failed, the external jugular vein is an option that provides increased size and visibility. Access can be hindered due to increased mobility and/or ease of compression of the vessel. An infant can receive a 22- or 24-G catheter, whereas an older child may require a 20- or 22-G catheter. The right side provides convenience and is preferred for access. In the young child, a small roll under the shoulder and back that leads to hyperextension of the neck is helpful. The awake child may require gentle restraint in a 30° Trendelenburg position with the head turned away from the side to be punctured. Distal occlusion above the clavicle and the Valsalva maneuver may increase the vessel size. Ultrasound offers an improved view of the vessel that is lateral to the internal jugular vein, and when used it may increase the operator's success.

The greater saphenous vein is often an easy target in emergency vascular access. The vessel lies anterior to the medial malleolus and is best visualized with the foot held in plantar flexion. In the past, when no other peripheral access could be obtained in emergent conditions, the distal saphenous vein was a primary target used for a peripheral venous cut-down. This procedure is completed by making a small transverse incision medial and superior to the medial malleolus. After careful dissection of the vessel, a suture ligature is placed distally while the vessel is cannulated proximally. In the era of intraosseous (IO) devices, this measure is rarely needed.

With technologic advances, devices are available to aid with successful vascular cannulation. Vein finders use infrared technology to identify veins. This technique improves visibility of vessels, thus improving accuracy with cannulation and decreasing pain associated with multiple access attempts. Ultrasound can also be used to guide peripheral and central vascular access. With delineation of the anatomy provided by ultrasound, there is increased accuracy and decreased number of attempts at cannulation required. This modality can also distinguish arterial from venous structures based on pulsatility, appearance with compression, and use of color flow Doppler.

Because venipuncture produces anxiety for the pain associated with the procedure, efforts to decrease pain are paramount for successful venous cannulation. Anesthetic creams, such as 4% lidocaine (e.g., LMX4), applied 30 minutes prior to venipuncture help reduce the pain associated with the procedure. Vapo-coolant sprays can also be utilized (e.g., PainEase). These sprays act by cooling the skin to temporarily reduce pain sensation. Needle-free delivery systems, such as the J-Tip, use compressed gas to inject lidocaine. If needed, anxiolysis via the intranasal route with an agent such as midazolam may help facilitate this procedure. Child life specialists may also ease the patient prior to any procedure attempt. Any technique used to limit pain and anxiety is likely to improve vascular cannulation success.

HYPODERMOCLYSIS

Hypodermoclysis, also known as subcutaneous rehydration, is re-emerging as a technique used in the pediatric patient requiring fluid resuscitation. Subcutaneous rehydration is geared toward the stable child who is unable to tolerate oral rehydration. The child is typically mildly to moderately dehydrated. Ideal candidates for subcutaneous rehydration are children who only require slow fluid resuscitation and are predicted to have difficult IV access.

Subcutaneous rehydration is performed by applying a topical anesthetic (e.g., LMX4) between the scapula. After time has elapsed to achieve adequate anesthesia, a 25-G butterfly needle is inserted at this location and secured, followed by administration of 150 U hyaluronidase subcutaneously (the same dose is used regardless of patient age/weight). At this time, fluid resuscitation with crystalloid can be administered over 1 hour. If needed, fluid administration can be repeated or venipuncture can be attempted.

INTRAOSSEOUS ACCESS

Intraosseous access (i.e., cannulation of the medullary cavity) provides direct, noncollapsible access to the central venous circulation. Fluids and medications infused drain via venous sinusoids into emissary veins and from there to the systemic circulation. In critically ill children, IO placement can be done rapidly and with a high rate of success. Pediatric Advanced Life Support guidelines state that after two unsuccessful IV attempts,

TABLE 45.1 EZ-IO DEVICE SPECIFICATIONS[a]

Specification	Pink Hub	Blue Hub	Yellow Hub
Gauge (G)	15	15	15
Length (mm)	15	25	45
Patient weight (kg)	3–39	≥3	≥40[b]
Patient population	Neonate to school-age child	Preteen, teen, adult	Obese

[a]EZ-IO devices are inserted with a power drill.
[b]Used for patients with excessive tissue over any insertion site. Manufacture recommends considering for proximal humerus in patients at this weight.

the resuscitation team should convert to IO. There may be cases of critical illness or cardiovascular collapse in which IO is a primary access modality while further peripheral venipuncture attempts are made.

Preferred sites for pediatric IO placement are the proximal tibia, distal tibia, distal femur, and proximal humerus. IO needles can be manually inserted with 14–18 G sizes that are 3 or 4 cm in length. A power-driven IO needle such as the EZIO can be used for children as well. The drill-powered device uses a 15-G needle available in three different lengths (Table 45.1). Clinically, the patient may need a different depth for placement than what is recommended by the manufacturer, depending on the amount of subcutaneous tissue.

The subcutaneous tissue overlying the bone at the insertion site needs to be evaluated by the IO operator to determine if the needle selected has the appropriate amount of depth to penetrate the bone. To avoid displacement after IO insertion, the operator should ensure the black 5-mm-depth mark is visible on the needle after the IO enters the periosteum and the soft tissue is pierced. Each hub has the visible black line that needs to be above the skin after the periosteum is accessed. The pink hub has a single black line, whereas the black and yellow hubs have multiple black lines. Once the needle hub enters the medullary space, the operator senses a loss of resistance. At this point, a single black line on the hub chosen should be above the skin. If the black line is not visible after insertion, the needle is not long enough. It is not uncommon for infants with excessive subcutaneous tissue to require the blue (25-mm) needle hub.

Any medication or fluid can be given by IO infusion. Administration under pressure is required to overcome the intrinsic resistance of the marrow cavity. Although any medication can be administered, medications that are particularly injurious to surrounding tissues (e.g., sodium bicarbonate) should only be inserted with IOs ensured to be in appropriate position. Preservative-free (2%) lidocaine can be used for local anesthesia in the child responsive to pain. Systemic analgesia in the form of intranasal fentanyl (2 or 3 μg/kg) may be necessary prior to initiation of the procedure. Lidocaine can be used to make a wheal on the skin. The lidocaine can then be administered at 0.5 mg/kg and allowed to sit in the IO space for 1 minute prior to infusion. It is imperative to monitor the limb for signs of extravasation. Unfortunately, there is no perfect way of stabilizing the needle following insertion. Chest compressions and movement of the patient are common reasons for IO displacement leading to potential extravasation of infusion medications. The IO needle should be removed as soon as alternative IV access is gained.

Contraindications for IO placement include infection at the insertion site, insertion on a bone with a recent IO attempt in the past 24 hours, or bones that have a fracture. Fluid may leak from the previous cortex violation, and there is subsequent risk for developing compartment syndrome.

CENTRAL VENOUS CATHETERS

The umbilical vein can be accessed in the first 7–10 days of life. A size 3.5- or 5-Fr single lumen umbilical catheter is used for the procedure. To prepare the catheter, it should be flushed with normal saline and attached to a stopcock. The umbilical cord is cleaned with antiseptic solution. A loose tie is placed at the base of the umbilical cord around Wharton's jelly or the skin margin. If necessary, this tie can be tightened to prevent excessive bleeding following transection of the cord. However, a strangulating tie may compromise skin perfusion. An incision is made below the umbilical clamp 1 or 2 cm above the skin line. This is a horizontal incision across the cord; one should avoid making an angled incision. The umbilical smiling face composed of vessels will be visible—that is, two eyes (the two muscular umbilical arteries) and mouth (the thin-walled umbilical vein). During emergency resuscitation, the catheter is only advanced in the vein until there is free flow of venous blood on aspiration. This is typically at 2–4 cm. Contraindications to this procedure include neonates with signs of abdominal wall infection/omphalitis, necrotizing enterocolitis, and peritonitis.

With the use of IO devices, central venous catheters (CVCs) are rarely needed in the acute phase of resuscitation encountered in the emergency department. CVCs are necessary when vasoactive IO access has questionable reliability, administration of vasoactive medications/hyperosmolar fluids is needed, or medications are not compatible, and it can also be considered when venous access is required and peripheral access attempts have been unsuccessful. The most common locations for central venous access are the femoral, internal jugular (IJ), and subclavian veins. A child who is not intubated will likely require procedural sedation and analgesia prior to procedure attempt. If the CVC is being inserted to replace an IO, ketamine can be given at 1 or 2 mg/kg through the IO. If no access exists, then 4–6 mg/kg ketamine can be given intramuscularly to help facilitate this procedure.

Ultrasound-guided insertion contributes to increased success and safety when performing central access cannulation. A high-frequency linear array transducer with a small footprint is optimal for pediatric vascular access (Figure 45.1). This probe will allow for best resolution without the need for significant tissue penetration. Transverse (cross-section) or in-line (longitudinal) transducer orientations can be used depending on what vessel is being accessed. Ultrasound can also confirm guidewire placement in the vessel (Figures 45.2), whereas a chest radiograph will aid with determination of adequate and desired tip position of the line. If a high line (IJ or subclavian line) was selected as the vessel to be accessed, a chest radiograph also is obtained to ensure no pneumothorax occurred following insertion of the catheter. If the femoral site was used, a post-insertion cross-table lateral pelvic radiograph is often obtained to ensure the catheter tip lies anterior to the vertebral column.

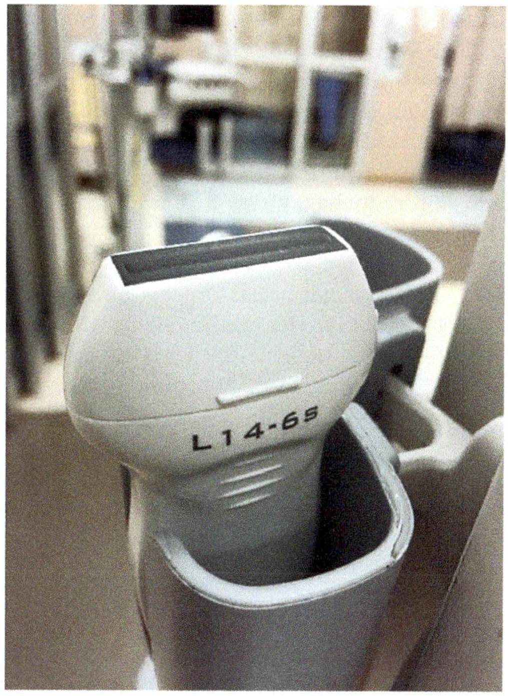

FIGURE 45.1 Lightweight linear array probe with a small footprint provides an advantage for ultrasound guidance of small-caliber pediatric vessels.

The IJ vein has the straightest and shortest route to the right atrium. Ultrasound can be used to assist successful placement. A drawback to this site is the potential discomfort associated with neck access. The subclavian vein has a short distance to the right atrium. The line is in a relatively fixed position, providing comfort and stability. Ultrasound can only be employed if accessing above the clavicle (supraclavicular line); otherwise, traditional landmarks are used. There is risk for iatrogenic injury to the pleura, leading to pneumothorax when high lines are selected.

The femoral vein can be accessed quickly, and ultrasound can be used to accurately identify the vessel to be cannulated medial to the femoral artery. Traditionally, the femoral vein has been a preferred access point in emergency resuscitation due to anatomy familiarity and avoidance of the intrathoracic complications mentioned previously. Infants often have skin that is slack and redundant in the inguinal region. When accessing the femoral vein, the operator should have a method to maintain traction on the skin while inserting the needle into the vessel. Unfortunately, the position in the groin crease limits comfort and mobility, and skin redundancy may decrease stability of the catheter.

The Seldinger technique is used for nearly all central vascular access procedures. The use of a 21- or 22-G finder needle (Figure 45.3) and thin (0.018-in.) flexible-tip wire to establish access is recommended. A common issue that arises with pediatric lines relates to the small size of the flexible-tip wire. The guidewire frequently kinks following dilation. Ensuring the wire moves in and out of the dilator while it is being advanced will prevent kinking at the skin surface. Straightening the J point and the entire flexible-tip wire prior to insertion also prevents kinking when it is inserted through the needle.

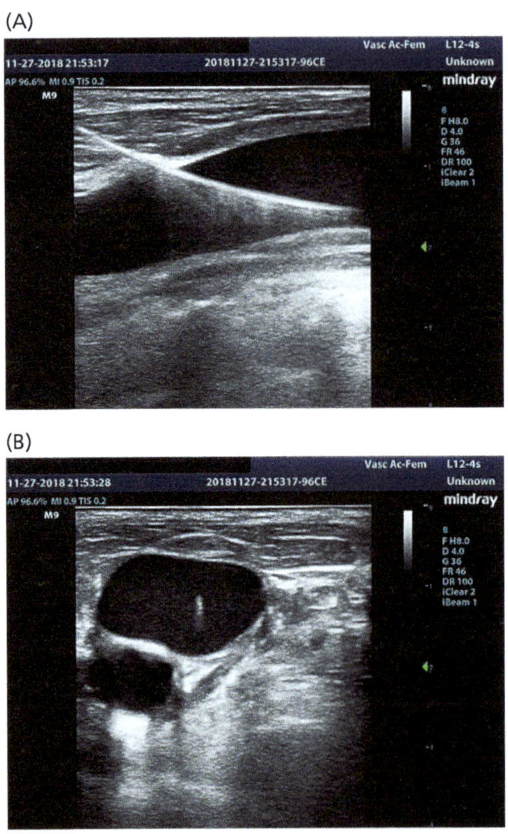

FIGURE 45.2 Longitudinal (A) and cross-section (B) views of guidewire within the vessel.

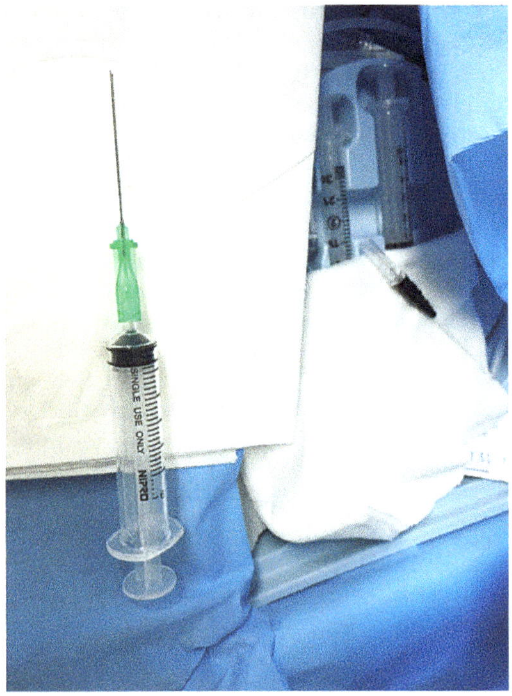

FIGURE 45.3 The typical finder/introducer needles in most pediatric CVC kits are 21 G. A 0.018-in. diameter spring guidewire is included and used for insertion of the catheter by the Seldinger technique.

The size of the CVC selected for use is determined by the size of the vein selected and the therapy required (Table 45.2). A number of height-, weight-, and surface landmark-based formulas exist to attempt to determine length of catheter insertion, but these can be difficult to determine during resuscitation of a critically ill child. Typically, for the cannulation of the IJ vein, 5-cm lines may be used for children <15 kg, 8-cm lines for patients 16–40 kg, and 13-cm lines for those >40 kg. Longer lines may be preferred if the left subclavian or femoral route is used.

As with peripheral lines, ultrasound-assisted CVC placement improves success. The ultrasound machine is optimally positioned across the patient gurney. The patient is placed supine. For high lines, the patient is placed in Trendelenburg position to distend target veins and prevent air embolism. A shoulder roll can be used to extend the neck and improve ease of access to the IJ vein. Turning the head to the contralateral side is helpful with high-line access. There are mixed opinions on the effectiveness of a shoulder roll during subclavian

TABLE 45.2 SIZE AND DEPTH OF CENTRAL VENOUS CATHETERS[a]

Age	CVC Size (Fr)	CVC Depth (cm)[b]
<6 months	3–4	5–8
6 months to 3 years	4–5	8–13
4–5 years	5.5–6.0	8–13
6–9 years	5.5–6.0+	8–13
>10 years	6.0+	13–20

[a]This table serves only as a guide to appropriate-sized CVC. Each child will need to be assessed individually for appropriate catheter diameter to be used and depth to be inserted depending on the particular vessel used for cannulation.
[b]The larger depth is typically reserved for femoral access and, in some instances, left-sided subclavian access.
CVC, central venous catheter.

access: It can increase exposure but also possibly decrease the cross-sectional area of the subclavian vein, making cannulation difficult. Infants and toddlers often have lower extremity vessels that are disproportionately smaller compared to the vessels above the diaphragm. In young children, the femoral vein can be partially or completely overlapped by the femoral artery. Separation and exposure of the femoral vein can be increased by abduction and external rotation of the leg. Often, a small towel roll/bump at the coccyx will help with access to the femoral vessels. With ultrasound evaluation of the vessels prior to the procedure, if too much overlap with the femoral artery exists or the vessel is considered very small, making access difficult, an alternate site should be considered to avoid complication.

COMPLICATIONS

Due to their close proximity, arterial injury may result from central venous access. Ultrasound guidance and using a smaller needle will help decrease these complications. A micropuncture needle can be withdrawn and subsequent pressure applied. This is easiest with the femoral artery compared to the carotid or subclavian artery due to lack of access to provide adequate pressure following accidental arterial piercing. As mentioned previously, with the high-line vessels, the pleura may be injured. The risk is increased for patients receiving positive pressure ventilation because the apex of the lung reaches the lower neck. Another complication to consider is development of vessel thrombosis.

Pediatric vascular access in the emergency department can be challenging. Utilizing technology may aid with peripheral venipuncture. However, it may be necessary to access vessels that increase chances of success or potentially obtain IO or even central venous access for patients who are critically ill.

Further Reading

Church JT, Jarboe MD. Vascular access in the pediatric population. *Surg Clin North Am.* 2017;(97):113–128.

Leung S. A review of pediatric ultrasound-guided peripheral intravenous access. *Clin Pediatr Emerg Med.* 2015;16(4):240–243.

Murphy PC, Arnold P. Ultrasound-assisted vascular access in children. *BJA*. 2011;1(2):44–49.

Scott-Warren VL, Morley RB. Paediatric vascular access. *BJA Education*. 2015;15(4):199–206.

Spandorfer PR. Subcutaneous rehydration: Updating a traditional technique. *Pediatr Emerg Care.* 2011;27(3):230–236.

46

Pediatric Foreign Bodies

You Stuck What? Where?

ANN M. DIETRICH

INTRODUCTION

Foreign bodies are common in children. Children commonly place objects into a variety of orifices, including the nose, ears, gastrointestinal (GI) tract, and vaginal or rectal areas. Children with attention-deficit/hyperactivity disorder (ADHD), autism, or mental health issues are more likely to insert a foreign body into an orifice. Both organic and non-organic objects may be inserted. Most objects do not cause problems, but objects such as magnets, batteries, and long, sharp objects may result in significant adverse events. Also, if one object is present, there may also be other objects in other locations, so a comprehensive evaluation must be conducted.

EAR FOREIGN BODIES

Foreign bodies in the ear can occur in children or adults. Children tend to be more creative, and the most commonly removed objects include beads, paper/tissue, cotton tips, erasers, and popcorn kernels. Adults more commonly have insects in the external auditory canal, although children may also have insects. Anatomically, the external auditory canal is nearly straight in children and becomes adult size at approximately age 9 years with a final sigmoid shape. The external auditory canal has two natural points of narrowing: the bone and cartilage junction and just lateral to the tympanic membrane.

Foreign bodies are uncommon in children younger than age 9 months because they lack a pincer grasp. Children usually present with a witnessed event, a visible foreign body, decreased hearing, otalgia, or otorrhea. Button batteries are of particular concern, with reports of auditory damages to the tympanic membrane and ossicles.

Diagnostic Confirmation

Clinical confirmation is usually accomplished with an otoscopic evaluation to identify the foreign body.

Treatment

The removal may be quite challenging, depending on the age of the child and level of cooperativity. Procedural sedation should be considered to facilitate removal.

Options for removal include the following:

1. Water irrigation—good for small non-organic objects. It is contraindicated for children with a suspected tympanic membrane perforation, removal of organic material, removal

of a battery, or removal of any suspected foreign body that is made of a spongy material that may swell and enlarge with water.
2. Suction—good for objects that are in the distal ear canal. This should be performed with a soft suction-tipped catheter that has a thumb-controlled release valve. Insert the suction against the foreign body under direct visualization and then activate the suction and remove the foreign body, maintaining suction until the foreign body is completely out of the external auditory canal.
3. Forceps removal or cerumen loops—can be used if the child is cooperative and the object is visible.
4. Cyanoacrylate—requires a cooperative patient. Apply a small amount of cyanoacrylate or skin glue to the blunt end of a cotton-tipped applicator. Wait until the glue is tacky and then insert the glue-covered tip against the foreign body under direct visualization and hold in place until the glue dries. Then remove the applicator with the foreign body attached.
5. Ear, nose, and throat (ENT) surgeons have developed a magnet probe for removal of button batteries and ferrous material.

Special Considerations

If a live insect is present and the tympanic membrane is not perforated, prior to attempting removal, kill the insect rapidly by instilling alcohol, 2% lidocaine (Xylocaine), or mineral oil (mineral oil has been shown to be the most effective) into the ear canal.

If the foreign body is Styrofoam and the tympanic membrane is intact, acetone may be used to dissolve the Styrofoam.

Avoid irrigation if a button battery is in the ear (electrical current or battery contents may result in liquefaction tissue necrosis).

Procedure

Prepare well: The first attempt at removal is critical because success rates markedly decrease after the first failed attempt. In addition, as the number of failed removal attempts increases, the complication rate increases and the child's cooperativity rapidly diminishes.

Multiple foreign bodies are not uncommon, especially in small children. Thus, all other orifices of the head should be inspected after removal of a foreign body from the external auditory canal.

Disposition

Emergent ENT consultation should be obtained for button batteries and magnets.

ENT referral as an outpatient may be considered for patients with trauma to the canal or tympanic membrane, a nongraspable foreign body that is tightly wedged in the medial two-thirds of the canal or is suspected of touching the tympanic membrane, foreign bodies with sharp edges (e.g., pieces of glass), or unsuccessful removal attempts.

After a successful removal, otic antibiotic drops on discharge should be given to patients with concurrent otitis externa and should be considered when canal lacerations or trauma are present.

Complications

Complications include damage to the auricular canal, perforation of the tympanic membrane, local inflammation, bleeding, and pain.

Key Points

- Consider a foreign body in any child with ear pain or otorrhea.
- The first attempt is the most critical; a good plan is necessary.
- Whenever one foreign body is identified, conduct a comprehensive examination searching for others.

Pitfalls

- Failure to identify a foreign body in the ear, especially a battery, and emergently obtaining an ENT consult
- Failure to adequately prepare and plan prior to the attempts at foreign body removal

NASAL FOREIGN BODIES

Nasal foreign bodies are common and may present in a variety of ways. Because children younger than age 9 months do not have a pincer grasp, nasal foreign bodies tend to occur in children aged 2–5 years, with boys having a higher incidence. Again, children with autism, ADHD, or cognitive deficits have a higher incidence. Based on the anatomy, nasal foreign bodies tend to be located on the floor of the nasal passage, just below the inferior turbinate, or in the upper nasal fossa anterior to the middle turbinate.

Objects may be organic or inorganic. Common inorganic objects include batteries, magnets, and pieces of toys. Batteries and multiple magnets are dangerous, with preoperative and postoperative septal perforations reported.

Children may present with a witnessed event or the child telling the parents they put something in their nose, but subtle presentations such as unilateral nasal drainage, unilateral foul-smelling drainage, or nasal obstruction are common. Whenever possible, obtain information on the type of foreign body; the approximate time frame it was placed; and the presence of epistaxis, nasal discharge, and systemic symptoms. A comprehensive physical examination should be conducted, including a visual inspection of the nasal cavity using a speculum. The location, shape, and type of foreign bodies should be noted, as well as the presence of any mucosal changes or epistaxis surrounding the object. Superior foreign bodies in the anterior nasal cavity can be obscured by swelling or mucous. Adequate visualization is needed if the history is suggestive or the patient was known to have a foreign object in the nose, such as the back of a nose ring. In addition, the external ear canals should be evaluated for the presence of other foreign bodies because younger children will often insert foreign objects into one or more cavities.

Diagnostic Confirmation

Sometimes, confirmation is easy—the event is witnessed and upon examination a foreign body is seen. Other times, it is not so easy. When a history is obtained for an inorganic object and one is not visualized on examination, a radiograph may be obtained. Although radiographs focused on the nasal bones will capture most objects, depending on an elicited history of other upper airway or aspiration symptoms, one may consider radiographic examination of the neck and chest (including the entire gastric antrum) for complete evaluation. Plain films may help rapidly identify button batteries or magnets (Figure 46.1). If a foreign body is suspected, computed tomography CT is a more sensitive technique than ultrasound.

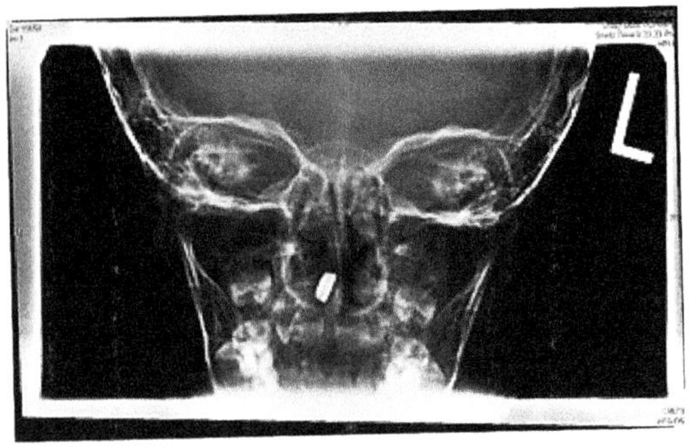

FIGURE 46.1 Nasal foreign body button battery.

Source: Image courtesy of Czer Anthoney Lim.

Treatment

If history of an inserted disc battery or multiple magnets is elicited, it is imperative for the provider to prepare for emergent removal by contacting specialists in otolaryngology and preparing the child and family for a possible sedated/operative procedure (see Figure 46.1). Thermal damage and pressure necrosis caused by these items can quickly result in uncontrolled epistaxis and nasal septal perforation.

Fortunately, most nasal foreign bodies can be removed in the office, urgent care, or emergency department. Consider that attempts at removal may push the nasal foreign body into the pharynx, potentially creating an airway hazard. So carefully analyze the cooperativity of the child, foreign body, and risks prior to attempts. Sedation may increase complications by reducing the gag and cough reflexes.

Before attempting removal, 0.5% phenylephrine may be administered to the affected nostril to decrease mucosal edema.

The most popular, easy to utilize technique is the positive pressure technique. This can be accomplished in several ways. Older children who can cooperate (especially for solid objects such as beads) can be asked to close their mouth, occlude the non-obstructed nostril, and blow. For younger children, the "kiss" technique works very well. In this technique, the parent covers the child's mouth with his or her mouth, plugs the unobstructed nostril with a finger, and gives a rapid, soft puff of air. If the child and parent have difficulty accomplishing the kiss technique, positive pressure may be delivered with an Ambu bag (the mask must be turned upside down to not occlude the nares).

If the initial less invasive methods are unsuccessful, removal through mechanical methods may be attempted. Minimal patient movement and maximal nasal cavity exposure using a nasal speculum and proper lighting are integral for successful removal. It is important that mechanical removal attempts only be made after the foreign body is visualized; blind mechanical attempts may displace the object more posteriorly or cause damage to tissues.

For graspable objects, bayonet or alligator forceps may be utilized for removal. Round, smooth, and other nongraspable objects may be manipulated using a curette, loops, or small suction tips. Some magnetic nose rings are strong enough to attract across the septum, causing septal necrosis if left in place. These can be dislodged by introducing another magnet or ferrous material into the naris, encouraging one magnet to flip. The Foley removal method may be useful for nongraspable or easily friable objects. The distal portion of a small-diameter (5 or 6 Fr) Foley is positioned passed posteriorly adjacent to the foreign body, the balloon is inflated, and the Foley is retracted. Commercially available products utilize a rigid stylet to facilitate positioning and removal. Pretreatment with pledgets soaked in lidocaine and epinephrine has the dual advantage of anesthetizing the mucosa and decreasing mucosal bleeding.

Other alternatives include the use of cyanoacrylate applied to the end of a swab, held to the foreign body and then removed (good for solid objects). In addition, advances continue to evolve: ENT surgeons have developed a magnet probe to assist with removal of button batteries and other ferrous materials.

Disposition

Consultation should be emergently obtained for button batteries or magnets. If resources are unavailable at the facility, patients may require transfer to a facility with pediatric operative capability. Consultation with the otolaryngology service will guide management.

Urgent consultation with an ENT subspecialist should be obtained when the foreign body cannot be removed, adequately visualized, or when a tumor or mass is suspected. The foreign body should be removed or ENT consulted for any foreign body that cannot be removed in the emergency department. Otolaryngology (ENT) follow-up may be arranged for patients with significant delay to presentation or if there are signs of erosion or infection in the area of the lodged object following removal.

Following removal of the foreign body, a repeat examination should occur to note the presence of any additional foreign objects and any damage or bleeding in the area from the object or removal. Routine antibiotics are not indicated. Antibiotics with skin and sinus flora coverage may be considered for foreign bodies presenting after significant delay or for patients requiring multiple attempts at removal, resulting in mucosal injury. Parents should be instructed to schedule a visit with the child's primary care physician within 48 hours for a recheck. Parents should be instructed to return to the emergency department if the child has persistent epistaxis or pain or if unilateral purulent discharge or other signs of infection develop.

Complications

Most complications are minor (epistaxis, sinusitis, and otitis media) and occur in approximately 10% of cases. Button batteries may result in septal perforations.

Barotrauma to the ear is a theoretical risk of positive pressure ventilation, but it has not been reported. Appropriate infection-control precautions should be taken because when the nasal foreign body is expelled, it will be covered with mucus and possibly blood.

Button batteries must be removed from the nose immediately because of the danger of liquefaction necrosis of the surrounding tissue.

Key Points

- Consider a nasal foreign body in a child with nasal obstruction or unilateral drainage/bleeding.
- Button batteries and magnets in the nose require emergent removal.
- The "kiss" technique is an effective initial strategy for removal.

Pitfalls

- Failure to carefully plan, resulting in the foreign body being pushed back into the oropharynx
- Failure to consult ENT for button battery in the nose

GASTROINTESTINAL FOREIGN BODIES

Gastrointestinal foreign body ingestions are common, especially in children, and have the potential to result in a life-threatening situation. Almost half of the foreign bodies ingested, reported by the American Association of Poison Control Centers, occur in children younger than age 5 years, with the vast majority unintentional and occurring in the home setting. The most common foreign body ingested is a coin, but a wide variety of other possible objects, such as batteries, magnets, and small toys, may be ingested. Although the majority of ingested foreign bodies pass through the gastrointestinal (GI) tract uneventfully, 10–20% will require an intervention, most commonly endoscopy, to prevent adverse events such as impaction, ulceration, perforation, and potentially death.

High-risk foreign bodies include long objects, sharp objects, batteries, and magnets (Table 46.1). The most dangerous foreign bodies are button/disc batteries and small powerful magnets. Button/disc batteries may result in devastating injuries if lodged in the esophagus for even a short period of time. The highest risk is with larger lithium-based batteries, but all may cause serious damage. Children with a suspected button/disc battery ingestion will require emergent management; a battery lodged in the esophagus requires removal without delay.

Unfortunately, not all magnets are benign when ingested. Neodymium magnets (composed of iron, boron, and neodymium and 5–10 times more powerful than traditional magnets) are a potentially devastating health hazard for children, with a high risk of intestinal obstruction and perforation because loops of bowel may be trapped between multiple magnets. A single swallowed magnet in combination with another metallic object, most notably a button/disc battery, may also cause severe injury.

TABLE 46.1 CLASSIFICATION OF INGESTED FOREIGN BODIES

Low Risk	High Risk
Length <5 cm	Length >5 cm
	Sharp/pointed
Width <2 cm	Width >2 cm
	Button battery
	Magnet

Classic Clinical Presentation

Sometimes the presentation is easy—a parent or caregiver witnesses the ingestion—but most often, in younger children, the diagnosis is more challenging. Older children may be able to convey the site of discomfort, but this is not reliably predictive of the location of the object.

The presentation depends on the age of the child, what was ingested, and the time that has elapsed since the ingestion. Presenting symptoms may include coughing and choking, chest pain, refusing to eat, drooling, vomiting, abdominal pain, respiratory distress (especially foreign bodies located in the proximal esophagus), or blood-tinged saliva. Thus, a careful history regarding the potential material ingested (especially button batteries, magnets, or objects with sharp points), quantity ingested (if known), prior history of dysphagia/similar episodes, GI surgeries, and symptoms the child has been experiencing should be obtained from the child (if able to communicate) or guardian. Fever and peritonitis may be a presentation of foreign body perforation.

Vital signs are an important initial assessment item; check for fever, tachycardia, and any evidence of hypoxia. Note the position of the child: tripoding or preferential positioning. Also identify any signs of perforation (crepitus and rigid abdomen). In the majority of situations, the physical examination will be normal, but that does not exclude a foreign body.

Imaging

A high degree of suspicion and early imaging for identification can improve outcomes. Plain radiographs can be very valuable as an initial imaging choice. Radiopaque material, such as coins or batteries, may be easily detected and localized. However, objects such as thin bones, plastic, glass, thin fragments of aluminum (pull tabs), and wood are not radiopaque and may not be seen. Secondary complications that may indicate an underlying foreign body include aspiration, prevertebral soft-tissue emphysema (cervical esophageal perforation), hydrothorax, pneumothorax, or hydropneumothorax (perforation of thoracic esophagus); free mediastinal or peritoneal air may also be seen on plain radiographs. Handheld metal detectors can be useful in locating metallic foreign bodies. In a systematic review (11 studies), the sensitivity for detecting a coin using metal detectors was 99.4% and the accuracy of identifying location was 99.8%.

Button disc batteries are critical to identify and may be distinguished from a coin when seen on a radiograph by their characteristic two-layer appearance when seen on-end or a circle-within-a-circle appearance when seen front-to-back.

CT scanning may be useful in situations in which complications are suspected or when a foreign body is suspected but not identified on plain radiography. Sensitivity and accuracy of CT are higher than those of radiography (97% and 98% vs. 47% and 52%, respectively). Fluoroscopic contrast esophagram and CT with oral contrast may be beneficial for localization of radiolucent foreign bodies, but their ideal use is not clearly defined.

Treatment

Fortunately, the vast majority of foreign bodies pass through the GI tract without complication. The decisions regarding the need for and timing of an intervention are dependent on several factors: patient age and clinical condition, the location and characteristics of the ingested material, time since ingestion, and the technical capabilities of the endoscopist and facility. Children who have swallowed a low-risk foreign body and who are asymptomatic and previously healthy typically will do well. If the object is still in the esophagus but low risk, a repeat film in 6 hours may allow for safe passage into the stomach and obviate the need for intervention. Esophageal foreign bodies that remain lodged require consult for endoscopic removal.

All esophageal button batteries require emergent removal (ideally in <2 hours). In addition, any symptomatic child with an esophageal or stomach button battery requires emergent consultation for endoscopy. Honey (dosed at 10 mL every 10 minutes) or sucralfate (dosed at 10 mL every 10 minutes) has been advocated to coat the battery and delay hydroxide generation and exposure. Honey should not be given to children younger than age 1 year secondary to the potential risk of infantile botulism. Once in the stomach, most batteries will pass through the GI tract without incident. An exception is a large-diameter (>20 mm) battery remaining in the stomach longer than 24–48 hours, documented by repeat imaging, which should be removed (even if asymptomatic). Magnet and button battery co-ingestions also require emergent removal. Table 46.2 provides recommendations.

As mentioned previously, not all magnets are benign when ingested. Any single magnet ingestion, in an asymptomatic patient, may be managed in one of two ways: consultation with a GI specialist for removal or use of serial radiographs to monitor its passage. If serial radiographs are to be used, the family needs to be warned that the child should not wear any clothing with metallic snaps or put metal objects on their body or near their body. In addition, parents should carefully monitor the child's environment to avoid a metal co-ingestion. Children who have ingested multiple

TABLE 46.2 FOREIGN BODY INGESTIONS

Emergent Removal	Urgent Removal	Other Considerations
Esophageal disk batteries, sharp objects	Stomach foreign bodies that are long (>5 cm) or wide (>2 cm)	Elective removal of stomach foreign bodies that do not pass within 3 or 4 weeks
Esophageal obstruction		
Symptomatic stomach disk batteries	Single magnet in esophagus; consult gastrointestinal for removal	Single magnet, asymptomatic patient; monitor with serial radiographs
Esophageal/stomach multiple magnets	Single magnet in stomach; removal or serial radiographs	
Esophageal/stomach magnet and metallic object		
Multiple magnets in intestines		

magnets or a magnet and a metallic foreign body that are in the esophagus or stomach require emergent GI consult for removal. If a child ingests multiple magnets or a magnet and a metallic object and they are past the stomach and the child is symptomatic, surgery should be consulted. Children who are asymptomatic require surgery/GI consult to determine the best procedure for removal.

Objects that are longer than 5 cm or wider than 2 cm also require urgent consultation for potential endoscopy.

Some centers will remove small esophageal foreign bodies, especially coins, with a bougie or a balloon catheter, but these require substantial experience and expertise.

Endoscopy is also typically used to remove large, sharp/pointed, or other high-risk objects from the stomach or in patients for whom continued passage of the object through the GI tract poses a risk. Objects in the lower GI tract should be managed in conjunction with a specialist, who may recommend surgical removal.

Medical management of foreign body ingestion is not recommended. Emetics and meat tenderizers are usually ineffective.

Disposition

Patients/caregivers should be instructed on the signs and symptoms of subsequent potential complications and instructed to return for evaluation for abdominal pain, vomiting, or fever. Radiographs every 3 or 4 days to monitor progress through the GI tract may be beneficial for button batteries that have made it into the stomach and beyond. Asymptomatic children who have ingested a single magnet that is in the stomach or beyond may be carefully followed as an outpatient. The family should be advised to not allow the child to wear any clothes with metal on them (no snaps on pants, belt buckles, or metal clips of any kind) and to return emergently for any symptoms.

Complications

Fortunately, complications are uncommon. The pyriform sinus and cervical esophagus are the most common sites of esophageal perforation (mortality rate >20%) and usually secondary to a sharp object.

Esophageal button batteries may have devastating consequences secondary to direct corrosive action through the leaking of alkaline solution which leads to liquefaction necrosis, with esophageal damage in as early as 1 hour. Perforation may occur as early as 6 hours after ingestion. Long-term complications include fistulas and scarring. Once button batteries are in the stomach, most pass without issue, but they still require careful monitoring because there may still be potential for injury.

Multiple magnets may be attracted to each other and trap bowel between them, leading to perforation, necrosis, obstruction, peritonitis, or sepsis. Magnets may also be attracted to ferromagnetic objects, again with the potential to lead to perforation, necrosis, or obstruction.

Key Points

- Most esophageal ingestions are benign, and the object passes through the GI tract without problems.
- Esophageal button batteries may have devastating consequences and should be removed as quickly as possible.
- More than one magnet or a magnet with a metallic object may result in bowel ischemia, necrosis, or obstruction.

Pitfalls

- Failure to remove an esophageal button battery in a timely manner
- Failure to identify a button battery or magnet as the ingested object

VAGINAL/RECTAL FOREIGN BODIES

Background

Both vaginal and rectal foreign bodies are uncommon. Symptoms secondary to a vaginal foreign body are responsible for approximately 4% of pediatric gynecologic outpatient visits. Small pieces of toilet paper are the most common foreign body (up to 80%), but other objects include safety pins, hair grips, pencils, small jam jars, especially in the intellectually challenged or young child. The majority of the incidents are accidental, but they may also be intentional in older children to induce abortion or as a contraceptive device. Girls with developmental delays and behavioral disorders are, as for other foreign bodies, at a higher risk of having retained vaginal foreign objects. Sexual abuse should also be considered for both vaginal and rectal foreign bodies.

Fortunately, most foreign bodies inserted into the rectum do not cause significant injury even if they are large, sharp, or pointed. Common rectal foreign bodies include thermometers, rectal tubes, anal packs, light covers, enema tips and covers, suppository wrappers, and oral or topical medication used inappropriately in the rectum. Sexual abuse must also be considered when a rectal foreign body is suspected.

Classic Clinical Presentation

Frequently, the history of insertion may not be available (~50% of the time), especially for vaginal foreign bodies. Vaginal foreign bodies typically present with bleeding or foul-smelling vaginal discharge. The most frequent symptoms reported are vaginal discharge, often bloody, purulent, or foul smelling; pain in the lower abdomen and suprapubic region; urinary frequency; burning sensation; and dysuria. Clues to the presence of a foreign body may also include vaginal discharge recurrence or resistance to antibiotic therapy. Systemic infection and perforation rarely occur with vaginal foreign body. Physical examination may be nonspecific and reveal irritation or discharge. Knee–chest positioning may reveal a small object, but frequently an examination under anesthesia is required to locate and remove the foreign body.

Rectal foreign bodies in children may present with rectal pain, abdominal pain, rectal bleeding, inability to have a bowel movement, or rectal discharge. Physical examination may reveal a mass in the lower quadrants of the abdomen, or on rectal examination the foreign body may be visualized. External examination may reveal evidence of trauma, purulent discharge, or evidence of a foreign body.

Differential

For prepubertal girls who present with vaginal discharge, other diagnoses that should be considered include trauma, sexual abuse, vaginitis, precocious puberty, rectovaginal fistula, local vaginal neoplasm, sarcoma botryoides, ovarian neoplasms such as granulosa cell tumor and germ cell tumor, or exposure to exogenous estrogen.

For rectal foreign bodies, maintain a high degree of suspicion for sexual abuse.

Imaging

Plain radiography may be helpful if the foreign body is radio-opaque, but it's use is otherwise limited. Ultrasound, which is safe and well tolerated by children, may be helpful and reveal nonspecific echogenic changes and indentation of the posterior bladder wall, but it is challenging and associated with interobserver variation. A pelvic CT may potentially be helpful, but it has a high risk of radiation exposure. The best and most accurate imaging modality is pelvic magnetic resonance imaging (MRI). However, MRI is limited by a lack of availability in emergency departments, time, cost, and need for sedation in toddlers and younger children. Unfortunately, even with the use of imaging modalities, a foreign body may not be identified.

Treatment

Consultation with pediatric surgery or gynecology for timely removal is warranted if a foreign body is identified or suspected. Vaginal irrigation is often well tolerated in cooperative children and is effective if the object is located in the distal vagina. If a specific diagnosis is unclear, an examination under anesthesia remains the gold standard, offering the dual advantages of diagnosis and extraction at the same time.

Rectal foreign bodies should be managed in consultation with GI or surgery.

Disposition

All patients require consultation with the appropriate specialist for removal.

Key Points

- Suspect a vaginal foreign body with vaginal discharge, especially if the discharge does not resolve with appropriate treatment.
- Consider sexual abuse in any child with vaginal or rectal foreign body.
- Consultation with gynecology (vaginal) or surgery (rectal) may be required if a foreign body is suspected.

Pitfalls

- Failure to consider a foreign body in a child with vaginal discharge or a child with rectal pain and discharge
- Failure to consider sexual abuse with a rectal or a vaginal foreign body

Further Reading

Fung BM, Sweetser S, Wong Kee Song WM, Tabibian JH. Foreign object ingestion and esophageal food impaction: An update and review on endoscopic management. *World J Gastrointest Endosc.* 2019;11(3):174–192. doi:10.4253/wjge.v11.i3.174

Kramer RE, Lerner DG, Lin T, et al.; North American Society for Pediatric Gastroenterology, Hepatology, and Nutrition Endoscopy Committee. Management of ingested foreign bodies in children: A clinical report of the NASPGHAN Endoscopy Committee. *J Pediatr Gastroenterol Nutr.* 2015;60(4):562–574.

47

Pediatric Procedures

MEGHAN R. CAIN AND MARK S. MANNENBACH

THORACOSTOMY

Indications

Bedside thoracostomy procedures include needle thoracostomy, catheter thoracostomy, and tube thoracostomy (Table 47.1). The ability to perform these procedures is critical in emergency care. As with most procedures, they are less likely required in children. The most common indication is blunt thoracic trauma, but these procedures may be utilized to manage complications related to airway intervention as well as vascular access procedures.

TABLE 47.1 INDICATIONS FOR THORACOSTOMY

Hemothorax	Traumatically induced
Pneumothorax	Traumatically induced and seen on initial chest radiograph
	Large and symptomatic with underlying lung disease
	Large and/or symptomatic without underlying lung disease
Empyema	Large
	Persistent after treatment with IV antibiotics

IV, intravenous.

Procedural Landmarks

In regard to landmarks for catheter placement, it is particularly important to avoid breast bud tissue in prepubertal females not only for cosmetic reasons but also to avoid any risk of abnormal breast development during puberty. Special attention should be given to choosing a site that is at least several centimeters away from the outer edge of the areola. Also, deliberate attention should be given to avoiding subcutaneous dissection near the breast bud and areolar areas.

Either the second intercostal space in the midclavicular line or an over-the-needle catheter at the fifth intercostal space slightly anterior to the midaxillary line can be used for emergent needle decompression.

The choice of device for thoracostomy should be considered not only in regard to the ease of insertion but also in terms of effectiveness. The use of a pigtail catheter has been compared to traditional thoracostomy tubes for the management of primary spontaneous pneumothorax, traumatic pneumothorax, and parapneumonic effusions.

Pigtail catheters have similar outcomes compared to large-bore chest tubes in patients with primary spontaneous pneumothorax. The smaller pigtail catheters are easier to place and also have a lower complication rate. Patients report less pain with smaller catheters, and lower narcotic administration in children has been demonstrated.

For the treatment of children with parapneumonic effusions, pigtail catheters and chest tubes have been shown to be equally efficacious, with similar rates of drainage failure and with a lower incidence of pneumothorax as a complication. Viscous empyema drainage may be less successful with pigtail catheters. Similarly, a traumatic hemothorax may not be adequately drained with a smaller pigtail catheter.

Several guidelines for selection of an appropriately sized chest tube can be referenced. The display of tables on equipment carts regarding approximate chest tube size based on age or weight may help providers remember which tube to select (Table 47.2).

Other adjuncts, such as the Broselow–Luten (length-based) resuscitation tape, may also be useful. Mnemonics for appropriate equipment choices have been helpful for many providers. Variations of the "1-2-3-4 rule" have been adopted in many ready references, with "1" representing the uncuffed endotracheal tube (ET) size, "2" times the ET tube size representing the nasogastric tube or urinary catheter in French size, "3" times the ET tube size representing the depth of insertion of the endotracheal tube at the lip in centimeters, and "4" times the ET tube size representing the chest tube in French size.

The finger thoracostomy technique often advocated for use in the care of adult patients is simply not an option when placing a chest tube in many children. The size of the provider's finger is larger than the intercostal space will allow. Consider inserting a fine curved hemostat in the end of the thoracostomy tube to allow for penetration through the chest wall similar to the over-the-needle technique utilized for peripheral intravenous (IV) placement. The curve of the hemostat can be used to direct the tube toward the desired location while preventing direct contact between the sharp edges of the open hemostat and the lung tissue. This technique allows for accommodation of the more highly compliant chest wall of children and does not lead to the creation of an entry site that is too large to keep the tube in place.

TABLE 47.2 CHEST TUBE SIZE SELECTION BY AGE

Age (Weight)	Size (Fr)
Newborn (<5 kg)	8–10
0–1 year (5–10 kg)	10–14
1–2 years (10–15 kg)	14–20
2–5 years (15–20 kg)	20–24
5–10 years (20–30 kg)	24–28
>10 years (30–50 kg)	28–40

Anticipating Complications

- When placing a thoracostomy catheter, avoid the neurovascular bundle found along the inferior border of each rib.
- Anticipate the presence or creation of a pneumothorax for all intubated pediatric patients and have equipment immediately available to treat a tension pneumothorax.
- Pay close attention to acute changes in end-tidal CO_2 concentration or capnography waveform as evidence of tension pneumothorax even before the development of cardiovascular compromise.

Key Points

- Develop readily accessible references to ensure accurate choice of appropriate-sized equipment for pediatric thoracostomy.
- Consider using a pigtail catheter rather than a large-bore catheter in the setting of a spontaneous pneumothorax or traumatic pneumothorax.

Pitfalls

- Be certain to understand the landmarks involved in appropriate placement of a thoracostomy device to avoid complications.
- Pay close attention to the anatomy of the prepubertal female patient to avoid any potential damage to the developing breast tissue.

NEEDLE CRICOTHYROTOMY

Indications

Needle cricothyrotomy is a last-ditch rescue airway for pediatric patients with an obstruction above the cricothyroid membrane that is unable to be ventilated or oxygenated with traditional airway techniques. In infants, this membrane is only 3 mm in length, which may not be sufficient in size for traditional surgical cricothyrotomy. The age range for which needle technique is recommended over surgical is controversial, with sources citing anywhere from infancy up to 12 years of age. There are no true contraindications because this is the last option available. Relative contraindications include significant trauma to the airway, especially in the case of tracheal transection.

Procedure setup begins with appropriate identification of anatomic landmarks. This can be particularly difficult in small children, in whom the laryngeal prominence is not fully developed. Running a finger along the anterior neck in the caudal direction can help identify the cricoid cartilage as a small bump or bulge. The cricothyroid membrane lies just above this prominence. The area should be cleaned prior to needle insertion.

The basic procedure involves using a large-bore angiocatheter (14 or 16 G) to enter the trachea via the cricothyroid membrane. A saline-filled syringe should be attached to the catheter during insertion, which allows for visualization of bubbles when the needle has entered into the correct space. After the trachea is entered, the needle should be held in place while the catheter is advanced to the hub. The catheter should be held at all times, or a suture can be used to secure the location.

Once placed, the catheter can be attached to a bag-valve device for oxygenation. There are several setups to allow for connection between the angiocatheter and the ventilation device. The most common connections include using the adapter from a 3.0 endotracheal tube or a 3-mL syringe and the adapter from a 7.0 endotracheal tube. The ventilation device should be attached to a 100% oxygen source. Oxygen can be delivered with a bag-valve device, but this rigid setup is prone to becoming dislodged. Ventilation with the bag should occur at 10–12 breaths per minute.

Alternatively, the catheter can be connected directly or via IV tubing to a Y-connector or stopcock, which is then connected to a standard wall oxygen supply. The oxygen source should be 10–12 L/min for children and 15 L/min for adolescents or adults. This setup allows for ventilation by opening and closing the in-line valve. While ventilating the patient, be sure to allow for adequate expiration because a rapid respiratory rate may lead to barotrauma of the chest, especially in patients with upper airway obstruction. Recommended inspiratory:expiratory (I:E) ratios are dependent on whether or not the patient has upper airway obstruction. In children, the standard I:E ratio is 1:4 or 1:5 without upper airway obstruction and 1:9 if upper airway obstruction is present.

Anticipating Complications

There are several potential complications from this procedure largely arising from the inexperience of the provider. Common procedural complications such as hemorrhage and infection apply to this as well. Ideally, a midline approach and sterile or clean technique should prevent these complications. If hemorrhage were to happen, the likely only treatment is a definitive airway obtained by an otorhinolaryngology surgeon. Other complications, such as subcutaneous emphysema and tracheal perforation, are secondary to improper angiocatheter placement. If these occur, replacement of the catheter into the proper location should be prioritized. If the catheter is improperly placed, a second attempt should be performed while awaiting definitive surgical intervention.

Key Points

- Needle cricothyrotomy is a rescue airway for infants and children aged younger than 12 years.
- Needle cricothyrotomy is temporizing until a more definitive airway can be achieved.
- The simplest method involves a large-bore angiocatheter attached to the bag valve with the adapter from a 3.0 ET tube.
- If the cricothyroid membrane cannot definitively be located, a lower intercartilaginous tracheal space can be safely used.
- A bag-valve or a high-flow oxygen setup can be used.

Pitfalls

- Landmark identification: Be comfortable finding the cricothyroid membrane to ensure subglottic placement.
- Equipment discomfort: Know what is available in your institution and be ready to use it.

- Depth of catheter insertion: Ensure you are drawing back on a syringe while inserting the catheter. This is a very small airway; even a few millimeters can affect appropriate placement.
- Catheter integrity: Once inserted, the catheter will easily kink; ensure the hub is secure at all times.
- Ventilation limitations: Due to the small size of the catheter, more oxygenation will be achieved than ventilation. To allow for exhalation, you may need to disconnect and use manual pressure to decompress the chest.

LUMBAR PUNCTURE

Indications

Lumbar punctures (LPs) are routinely performed by those who practice emergency medicine. In the pediatric patient, the typical reason for completion of an LP is due to concern for meningitis. Fever in a young infant with or without a bulging anterior fontanelle typically prompts this procedure to be performed. Older children may also have fever, headache, neck pain, mental status changes, or meningismus demonstrated by the presence of pain with neck flexion (Brudzinski's sign) or pain on the extension of the knee with hips flexed to 90° (Kernig's sign) as indications for completion of a LP.

Contraindications

Contraindications to the performance of LP include concern for infection in the tissues near the proposed puncture site, hemodynamic or respiratory instability, severe coagulopathy, evidence of spinal cord trauma or compression, and signs of pending cerebral herniation. If increased intracranial pressure due to a space-occupying lesion is suspected, caution in the performance of the LP should be exercised. Focal neurologic findings should be interpreted as a sign of suspected herniation and the LP should be deferred. With an emphasis on reducing radiation exposure to children, practitioners may be hesitant to perform imaging studies prior to an LP, but this must be considered when there is concern for increased intracranial pressure.

However, if infection is suspected, appropriate antibiotic therapy should be given and not delayed until imaging is completed or until cerebrospinal fluid (CSF) is obtained.

With the decreased incidence of bacterial meningitis in children over time, there are simply fewer opportunities to perform a lumbar puncture.

The use of ultrasound-assisted guidance for the performance of an LP can improve success. In adults, ultrasound decreases traumatic procedures and the number of attempts for LP.

Anesthetic use has been shown to improve success and decrease pain scores.

As for most procedures, success is determined by understanding the anatomy involved before attempting the procedure. The upper aspect of the posterior and superior iliac crests is to be palpated with an imaginary line between them visualized. This line intersects the midline just above the fourth lumbar spine. The interspaces between L3–L4 and L4–L5 tendons can be easily identified, with one site chosen for the puncture.

The appropriate depth of insertion of the spinal needle is often challenging to determine when performing an LP in younger children and infants. The classic "pop" often found in adults is not necessarily appreciated in younger patients. Deliberate slow advancement of the needle until a change in resistance is appreciated may optimize success.

The distance from the level of the skin to the spinal fluid sac is estimated to be between 1 and 2 cm in infants younger than age 6 months.

The "stylet out" technique improves success in young children and decreases traumatic and unsuccessful LPs. This technique begins with the stylet in during the initial push through the skin, and then the stylet is removed during needle advancement. This technique allows the provider to visualize CSF flow out of the needle while relying less on the "pop" that is less frequently felt in young children.

Anticipating Complications

Complications during and following the LP are generally infrequent but must be anticipated. Special attention should be given to the monitoring of the patient's airway during the procedure, especially for infants. Although studies have not demonstrated a significant difference in success rates between various positioning of children undergoing LP, the potential for airway compromise in infants certainly would be reduced without the forced neck flexion often used with an infant in the lateral recumbent position. Consider using the sitting position for all patients, including infants, because measurement of opening pressure is often not needed for this patient population.

The complication of post spinal or post LP headache has been proposed to occur in up to 25% of pediatric patients. Previous recommendations regarding the use of bed rest or supine positioning have not been shown to reduce the incidence of this complication. Factors associated with reducing this complication include reinsertion of the stylet prior to needle withdrawal, insertion of the needle perpendicular to the dura, and use of a smaller needle size for the procedure. The use of an "atraumatic needle" compared to a "cutting needle" has also demonstrated lower rates of headache after the completion of an LP.

Treatment of post spinal headache can include the following:

- Bed rest and treatment of both pain and nausea. This is adequate for most patients experiencing headache after a LP.
- Intravenous caffeine
- Epidural blood patching, which involves injection of 5–15 mL of autologous fresh blood into the epidural space at the same level where the procedure was completed

Key Points

- Prompt administration of antibiotics should be prioritized for children with suspected meningitis.
- Clear attention to identifying children with suspected increased intracranial pressure should be given prior to performance of an LP.
- Deliberate attention to safe positioning and monitoring of children and especially infants must be given to avoid complications and specifically airway compromise. Holding patients at the level of the shoulders to avoid neck flexion is strongly recommended. Consideration of the sitting position for infants may be helpful in achieving safety during the procedure.
- The utilization of some form of anesthetic has been shown to optimize success for LP.
- The use of an "atraumatic needle" may reduce the incidence of post LP headache.

Pitfalls

- Inadequate positioning of the child prior to the procedure may lead to multiple attempts or complications in regard to airway compromise.
- Inadequate analgesia prior to the procedure may be a contributing factor to unsuccessful attempts.
- Inappropriate needle size may lead to post LP headache.

Further Reading

Abo A, Chen L, Johnston P, Santucci K. Positioning for lumbar puncture in children evaluated by bedside ultrasound. *Pediatrics.* 2010;125:e1149–e1153.

Baxter AL, Fisher RG, Burke BL, et al. Local anesthetic and stylet styles: Factors associated with resident lumbar puncture success. *Pediatrics.* 2006;117:876–881.

Hanson AL, Ros S, Soprano J. Analysis of infant lumbar puncture success rates. *Pediatr Emerg Care.* 2014;30:311–314.

48

Procedural Sedation and Pain Management

ROSALIA HOLZMAN AND JENNIFER MITZMAN

There are many conditions in the emergency department that require pain management or procedural sedation due to significant pain or complexity. There are also a number of procedures and conditions that will require pain control or anxiolysis in children due to development and behavioral factors. This chapter discusses pharmacologic intervention, including narcotic and non-narcotic medications; non-pharmacologic interventions; procedural sedation; and nerve blocks.

PHARMACOLOGIC PAIN CONTROL

Background

Recognition and anticipation of pain can be challenging in children. Physiologic signs of pain include elevated heart rate, elevated respiratory rate, elevated blood pressure (if measured), or subtle pupillary dilation. Behavioral signs include facial expressions such as grimacing, furrowed brow, or nose wrinkling. Parents may also help identify discomfort.

Clinical Application

Commonly performed painful procedures in the emergency department are indicated in Box 48.1. Consideration of pain control should reflexively be part of procedure planning.

There are many different pharmacologic pain control options, including topical, oral, intravenous (IV), and intranasal (IN) administrations. Box 48.2 lists commonly used medications. Each agent has both advantages and disadvantages related to time of onset and duration. Tables 48.1–48.4 present the timing, selection, and dosing of various agents.

Topical agents include EMLA, lidocaine–epinephrine–tetracaine (LET), lidocaine (LMX), and ethyl chloride. Dosing and timing are described in Table 48.1. Each of these agents carries the benefit of painless application. This can help build rapport with pediatric patients and their families as they see the medical team taking simple steps to mitigate pain. The main drawback to EMLA and LMX is dosing based on body surface area, which increases the calculation needed to ensure a safe dosing window. This is particularly relevant when using them for a larger area. EMLA also carries a risk of methemoglobinemia, whereas LMX is not indicated in children younger than age 2 years. EMLA is designed for intact skin, making it suitable for anesthetizing skin prior to attempting venipuncture or lumbar puncture. LET gel is indicated for disrupted skin and is commonly used for laceration repairs. The epinephrine in LET causes skin blanching due to local vasoconstriction. Ethyl chloride's onset of action is

BOX 48.1

COMMONLY PERFORMED PAINFUL PROCEDURES IN THE EMERGENCY DEPARTMENT

- Fracture reduction
- Burn care (debridement, dressing changes)
- Tube thoracostomy (large caliber or pigtail)
- Laceration repair
- Abscess care (including incision and drainage, repacking)
- Lumbar puncture
- Foreign body removal
- Placement of an intravenous catheter (central or peripheral)
- Placement of an intraosseous line
- Dislocation reduction
- Venipuncture
- Joint injection

immediate but short-lived. It also carries a risk of permanent hypopigmentation of the skin.

Oral analgesics commonly used in pediatrics include non-opioid medications such as sucrose solution, acetaminophen, and ibuprofen, as well as a number of opioid analgesics alone or in combination with acetaminophen (Table 48.2). Acetaminophen is well tolerated, sold over-the-counter, and widely available. Combined narcotic/acetaminophen medication should not be used with other acetaminophen-containing products. Ibuprofen is widely available but carries gastrointestinal side effects including nausea, vomiting, ulcers, and bleeding, making it less well tolerated than acetaminophen. Sugar solutions are also non-opioid and widely available to decrease pain in infants.

BOX 48.2

COMMONLY USED MEDICATIONS

- Lidocaine/prilocaine cream (EMLA)
- Lidocaine–epinephrine–tetracaine gel (LET)
- Lidocaine (LMX)
- Ethyl chloride (Pain Ease)
- Acetaminophen
- Ibuprofen
- Sucrose solution
- Ketorolac
- Morphine
- Fentanyl
- Oxycodone
- Hydromophone
- Ketamine

Hydrocodone/acetaminophen has an opioid component and an onset of action of approximately 30 minutes when taken orally. Side effects include gastrointestinal discomfort, nausea, and vomiting, but neurologic changes such as drowsiness may also occur. Dosing is driven by the acetaminophen component, and in some patients that threshold is reached before adequate opioid effects are reached. This dosing mismatch can limit efficacy. Oxycodone is available as a stand-alone opioid or in combination with acetaminophen. It also takes effect in less than 30 minutes. Oxycodone is more sedating than hydrocodone. Dosing mismatch with acetaminophen can occur with this medication as well when used in combination.

Codeine is no longer recommended by the World Health Organization for pain control in children due to inconsistencies with metabolism and desired pain control. Deaths have been reported in ultra-rapid metabolizers.

Ketorolac, as a nonsteroidal anti-inflammatory drug, is an excellent non-opioid IV analgesia. Similar to ibuprofen, it can cause bleeding, gastrointestinal side effects, and decreases renal perfusion. Morphine is well tolerated and mid-range in duration of analgesia of the opioid narcotics listed in Table 48.3. Fentanyl is the quickest in onset as well as the shortest acting. This can be uniquely beneficial for shorter procedures, including those that would not necessarily require pain control in an adult. Narcotic medications can cause cardiovascular and respiratory depression as well as drowsiness and sedation. Patients should be monitored for these side effects, and ventilatory support and/or medication reversal with naloxone may rarely be necessary.

TABLE 48.1 TOPICAL AGENTS

Medication	Usage	Dose/Route	Maximum Dosing	Timing of Onset	Duration
EMLA[a]	Intact skin	Topical covered by occlusive dressing	By BSA	1 hour	3–4 hours
LET	Disrupted skin, wound repair	Topical, does not need an occlusive dressing	3–5 mg/kg of lidocaine	20 minutes	30–60 minutes
LMX	Abraded skin	Topical ± occlusive dressing	By BSA	30 minutes	60 minutes
Ethyl chloride	Cools intact skin and minor wounds	Spray for 4–10 seconds from 4–8 in. away	Stop when skin pales	Immediate onset	1 minute

[a]EMLA maximum dosing: 0–3 months or <5 kg: maximum dose 1 g; 3–12 months and >5 kg: maximum dose 2 g; 1–6 years and >10 kg: maximum dose 10 g; 7–12 years and >20 kg: maximum dose 20 g.
BSA, body surface area; LET, lidocaine–epinephrine–tetracaine.

Intranasal medication is well tolerated in children because it can be administered quickly and does not require IV access (Table 48.4). IN ketamine dosing is for sub-dissociative analgesia. These medications work well for painful assessments, including radiographic imaging to evaluate for fracture or acute appendicitis. Escalation to IV access and dosing may occur when indicated.

Ibuprofen should frequently be a first-line therapy because many studies have demonstrated analgesic equivalence and fewer side effects compared to opiates (even in postoperative or fracture pain). However, for some patients, this will not provide adequate pain relief. Inadequate pain control and formation of pain memory, conversely, can lead to future pain dysregulation. Short-term pain control in the form of a single or a few doses while in the emergency department does not seem to be associated with addiction. Utilizing medication longer than necessary or at larger than required doses can increase risk of dependence and addiction. The risk of narcotics at discharge should be weighed carefully because most pediatric patients do not require outpatient narcotics. If prescribed, narcotics should quickly be replaced by acetaminophen and/

TABLE 48.2 ORAL AGENTS

Medication	Class/Indication	Dose/Route	Maximum Dosing
Acetaminophen	Non-opioid	10–15 mg/kg q4–6 hours PO or up to 20 mg/kg PR	Infants 60 mg/kg/day Children 75 mg/kg/day
Ibuprofen	NSAID	10 mg/kg q6-8 hours PO	40 mg/kg/day
Sucrose	Non-opioid	20–50% sugar in 0.2- to 2-mL doses q6 hours PO	Unknown
Hydrocodone/ acetaminophen	Opioid	0.1–0.2 mg/kg of hydrocodone q4–6 hours PO	Driven by acetaminophen component
Oxycodone	Opioid	0.05–0.015 mg/kg of oxycodone q4–6 hours	Maximum dosing driven by acetaminophen component if given in combined form

NSAID, nonsteroidal anti-inflammatory drug.

TABLE 48.3 INTRAVENOUS AGENTS

Medication	Class/Indication	Dose/Route	Maximum Dosing	Timing
Ketorolac	Non-opioid NSAID	0.5–1 mg/kg q6 hours Also can be given IM	<50 kg maximum: 15 mg IV q6 hours	Variable onset, peaks in 2 or 3 hours
Morphine	Opioid	0.05–0.1 mg/kg IV	10 mg IV per dose	Onset in 15–20 minutes
Fentanyl	Opioid	1–2 μg/kg IV	100 μg per dose	Onset in 5–15 minutes
Hydromophone	Opioid	0.015 mg/kg IV	0.2 mg/kg per dose	Onset in 10–20 minutes

IM, intramuscularly; IV, intravenously; NSAID, nonsteroidal anti-inflammatory drug.

or ibuprofen, and the extra pills should be discarded.

Key Points

- Do not withhold pain medication for surgical consultation.
- Give pain medications in triage for pediatric patients reporting moderate pain (>6/10). This can be done utilizing triage order sets, physician in triage models, or by requesting prompt evaluation for these patients while they are simultaneously triaged.
- Utilize topical anesthetics when feasible.

Pitfalls

- Failure to utilize pain control whenever it is appropriate and urgency allows
- Giving insufficient time for the medication to work
- Withholding narcotics when indicated, or utilizing a narcotic when an equivalent non-narcotic option would suffice

NON-PHARMACOLOGIC PAIN CONTROL

Background

Non-pharmacologic interventions are very useful and effective in the pediatric patient. They are commonly used in conjunction with medication but may be the only intervention required. Parental involvement is helpful. Simple distractions and child-friendly techniques can help the child feel more in control of the environment and mitigate anxiety.

Professional child life specialists who help children understand and cope with illnesses, procedures, and hospitalizations should be used if available. Child-friendly techniques include comfortable positioning for examination and procedures and honest explanations in age-appropriate language of what they child may see, hear, or feel when in the emergency department. Medical play can be helpful. For example, a stuffed animal or toy with an IV or a cast can be used to show patients what is meant by terms that may be unfamiliar to them. Distraction techniques are quite effective.

Clinical Application

Offering choices when possible will aid in cooperation. For example, the patient can be asked if they would like to sit with a family member or on the examination table. Allowing a family member to be with the patient for procedures when possible is also comforting.

Child-friendly language is also important, and examples are illustrated in Table 48.5.

TABLE 48.4 INTRANASAL AGENTS

Medication	Class/Indication	Dose/Route	Maximum Dosing	Timing
Fentanyl	Opioid	1.5–2 μg/kg IN	100 μg per dose; divide equally between each nostril	Onset in 5–15 minutes
Ketamine	Non-opioid	0.5–1.0 mg/kg IN	Not well-established	Onset in 10–20 minutes

IN, intranasally.

TABLE 48.5 CHILD-FRIENDLY LANGUAGE

Traditional Language	Child-Friendly Language
"I am going to give you a shot."	"I need to give you medicine with a small needle."
"IV"	"Small plastic straw"
"This feels like _____."	"Tell me how this feels to you."
"Be a big girl/boy."	"When I count to three, blow the bad feelings away from your body."
"Don't cry."	"That was really hard."

Table 48.6 includes a number of strategies useful with different age groups. Simple relaxation techniques, such as counting to 10 or taking deep breaths, can be taught at a young age. Of note, screen time is particularly effective in decreasing pain and improving success of procedures. In addition, giving children some control in the form of simple/feasible choices can also be quite powerful and mitigate anxiety. For example, asking a child if they want to be told right before the needlestick or not can give the child a sense of control over overwhelming circumstances.

Key Points

- Do not lie about what is going to happen. Early in the visit, use caution when predicting clinical course because changing course may be interpreted by some children as lying. This is damaging to trust and the therapeutic relationship.
- Utilize screen time as a powerful distraction for many age groups.
- Offer the patient as much control and decision-making power as is age appropriate and possible.

Pitfalls

- Failure to combine non-pharmacologic techniques with appropriate pharmacologic techniques
- Using language that is too scary or incomprehensible to the patient or their family

TABLE 48.6 AGE-BASED DISTRACTION TECHNIQUES

Age Group	Interventions
Infants	Dim lighting when possible Toys such as keys, rattles, or badges Swaddling Side lying positioning Sucking on a pacifier or feeding when possible
Toddlers	Music, books, stories Coloring, stickers, bubbles Ice or heat packs Fun Band-Aids
School-age children	Music, books, or television Teach a simple relaxation technique Squeeze balls Talk to them about friends or favorite things Have them tell you a joke
Adolescents	Engage in ongoing conversation Allow texting, television, playing a game, or talking to a friend Teach a simple relaxation technique Allow as much control as possible

PROCEDURAL SEDATION

Background

Procedural sedation is used in children to control behavior and allow safe completion of a procedure. It may be required in children even if the procedure is not painful. The procedural sedation continuum has discrete stages that can be unpredictable and challenging to separate clinically. It is vitally important that anyone performing procedural sedation in children be capable of rescuing the child from deeper than intended sedation and be adequately trained in pediatric resuscitation, including airway management. (See Chapter 5 on pediatric airway management.)

Clinical Application

The first step in procedural sedation is carefully considering the situational dynamics. Is the procedure primarily painful or scary for the child? The agent should be chosen based on the need for pain control, anxiolysis, as well as consideration of the developmental age of the patient and any other complicating circumstances or history. Family presence during sedation must not endanger the family member or provide a distraction to the procedure. The emergency department should also have the appropriate equipment and personnel to perform the procedure safely. Patient assessment should include a detailed risk assessment of sedation based on the patient's history, physical examination, and the indication for sedation. A prior history of sedation (and complications) should also be obtained.

The following subgroups of patients may be at risk for complications:

- Patients younger than age 1 year
- Patients being sedated for a procedure that will manipulate the airway or gastrointestinal tract
- Patients with signs or symptoms of obstructive sleep apnea
- Patients with American Society of Anesthesia class 3 or higher physical status
- Patients with active upper respiratory infections

Patients in these subgroups may not be appropriate for bedside sedation in the emergency department. The risk versus benefit should be carefully weighed and operative sedation considered.

Table 48.7 lists commonly used procedural sedation agents.

Ketamine is the most commonly used agent in pediatric patients because it has both sedating and dissociative properties coupled with analgesia. Using a single agent for pain and

TABLE 48.7 PROCEDURAL SEDATION AGENTS

Medication	Properties	Dosing	Side Effects
Ketamine[a]	Analgesia, dissociation, sedation	1–2 mg/kg IV initial dose 0.5–1 mg/kg IV additional doses 4–5 mg/kg IM	Nausea and vomiting Agitation Nystagmus Very rarely laryngospasm
Propofol	Sedation	0.5–1 mg/kg IV initial dose 0.25-0.5 mg/kg IV additional dose	Apnea Respiratory depression Lack of analgesia
Etomidate	Sedation	0.1–0.2mg/kg IV initial dose 0.05 mg/kg IV additional dose	Myoclonus Localized pain Nausea and vomiting
Midazolam	Sedation	0.05–0.1 mg/kg IV initial dose 0.2–0.3 mg/kg IN initial dose	Headache Nausea and vomiting
Nitrous oxide	Anxiolysis	30–50% NO blended with O_2 inhaled	Nausea and vomiting Seizures

[a]Commercially available in different concentrations. 10 mg/1 mL should be used with IV administration. 100 mg/1 mL should be reserved for IM administration and clearly labeled to avoid dosing errors.
IM, intramuscularly; IN, intranasally; IV, intravenously.

anxiety avoids the potential for cumulative effects or drug interactions of multiple agents.

The most common side effects of ketamine include nausea/vomiting, nystagmus, and hallucinations. Respiratory depression occurs less commonly with ketamine than with other sedation agents. Approximately 1% or 2% of patients may require nasal airway, oral airway, or, rarely, unanticipated endotracheal intubation. Laryngospasm is a rare but dreaded complication of ketamine. It is more common with intramuscular than with IV administration, and it occurs most frequently with initial medication administration and just prior to waking. If possible, an IV should be placed once the patient is safely sedated to treat potential complications.

Propofol is the shortest acting of the agents but does not have analgesic properties. An additional agent should be utilized in painful procedures. Propofol provides ideal sedation for anxiety in a procedure that is not expected to be painful. Clinical and subclinical respiratory depression may occur in approximately one-third of patients sedated with propofol. Burning and pain with injection commonly occur. In addition, myoclonus is a common side effect. Families should be warned prior of these side effects prior to administration.

Etomidate is readily available and has a rapid onset, but it carries slightly higher rates of subclinical respiratory depression compared with propofol.

Midazolam can be administered IV or via mucosal atomizer device for IN administration. IN midazolam is safe and effective at achieving sedation and can be performed without IV access. IN administration may burn, and some children may find it noxious, which may initially increase agitation.

Nitrous oxide is very short-acting and wears off nearly immediately on removal of the face mask. It can be used safely without IV access. It manages both pain and anxiety with a very low adverse event rate and minimal side effect profile. It preserves cardiopulmonary status well. However, it requires a scavenger and is not available in all practice environments.

Following sedation, all patients should have a documented discharge check-in. This should include a post-procedural assessment of the patient. Children should be awake and tolerating oral intake prior to discharge.

Key Points

- Consider carefully the goals and timeline of procedural sedation in order to choose the correct medication(s).
- Procedural sedation should be performed only by those qualified in pediatric resuscitation.

Pitfalls

- Failure to plan for deeper than intended sedation and rare complications

NERVE BLOCKS

Background

Regional anesthesia has been shown to be effective and safe, and it decreases the need for both systemic analgesia and sedation. Procedural sedation carries its own risk and can also be time-consuming. In the adult population, a fair amount of regional anesthesia can be performed based on anatomy and landmarks. This is more difficult to accomplish in infants and children because some of these landmarks can vary or be absent based on their age and stage of development. Children may have limited capacity to communicate when the anesthesia becomes effective. These limitations can be overcome with the use of ultrasound guidance. A higher body water content leads to improved success in visualizing nerves and other structures with ultrasound.

When planning to use regional anesthesia in pediatric patients, in addition to risks and benefits, there are a few other points to consider. Pain control may not be the limiting factor in proceeding with a laceration repair or fracture/dislocation reduction. A successful block requires not only the proper equipment and technique but also the support and cooperation of the patient. Anticipated pain, needles, or manipulation of the affected area can create a fair amount of anxiety for the patient. This is where adjuncts should be involved, such as distraction or utilization of child life specialists, along with consideration for further anxiolysis such as with oral or IN midazolam.

Another key consideration is the utility of regional anesthesia, or even local infiltration

TABLE 48.8 COMMONLY USED LOCAL ANESTHETIC AGENTS

Medication	Onset (Minutes)	Duration (Minutes)	Concentration (%)	Maximum Dosing (with Epinephrine)
Bupivacaine (amide)	10–15	200+	0.25–0.5	3 mg/kg (5 mg/kg)
Chloroprocaine (ester)	5	45	1–2	8 mg/kg
Lidocaine (amide)	5	30–60	0.5–2	4 mg/kg (7 mg/kg)
Mepivacaine (amide)	3	45–90	0.5–1	4 mg/kg
Prilocaine (amide)	5	30–90	4	5 mg/kg
Ropivacaine (amide)	5–15	200+	0.5	3 mg/kg

with an injection, when topical anesthetics can be as effective. Topical agents such as LET work well on disrupted skin and can negate the need for further anesthetics prior to the procedure (see Table 48.1). This is most often useful for smaller wounds or facial lacerations.

As in systemic analgesia and procedural sedation, there are also potential adverse events of which to be aware. Hypersensitivity reactions to the anesthetics are rare. Systemic toxicity is a serious side effect to be wary of in both adults and children; however, in infants and small children, the early signs and symptoms can be subtle. Anesthetic toxicity is dose dependent, placing infants and children at increased risk for toxicity. Recommendations are to dose based on body weight (Table 48.8). Of note, amide local anesthetics (e.g., lidocaine and bupivacaine) are cleared by the liver; however, hepatic enzymes are not at full adult activity until the end of the first year of life and, as such, use of an ester local anesthetic in such infants may be considered. Early symptoms of systemic toxicity include perioral paresthesias, tinnitus, and visual changes, all of which can be difficult for a child to report. Symptoms can progress to seizures, myocardial collapse, dysrhythmias, and cardiac arrest if not identified early. To further minimize risks of toxicity, ensure proper weight-based dosing and perform negative aspiration prior to every injection.

Clinical Application

Facial/Dental Blocks

There are multiple types of facial and dental nerve blocks that can be used in both adult and pediatric patients. For each of these procedures, have the patient seated with the head of the bed at approximately 45° and consider restraint versus distraction with younger patients. These procedures are not typically performed with ultrasound guidance. Most are similar in technique for pediatric patients as for adults, but a description of each block is included. Universal precautions should be utilized for all blocks but are not necessarily demonstrated in the figures presented in the following sections.

Infraorbital Nerve Block

This block anesthetizes the ipsilateral upper lip, nasal alae, and lower eyelid. It is most useful for laceration repairs (especially those involving the vermillion border).

Procedure Intraoral approach: Identify the infraorbital notch, and the infraorbital foramen should lie approximately 0.5 cm inferiorly. Use another finger to retract the upper lip. Insert the needle into the mucolabial fold anterior to the apex of the first premolar and advance toward the infraorbital foramen.

Extraoral approach: Identify the infraorbital ridge along the midline 0.5 cm inferior to the orbit (as shown in Figure 48.1). For each, inject between 1 and 2 mL of anesthetic.

Inferior Alveolar Nerve Block

This block can be used to anesthetize the ipsilateral mandibular teeth, skin of the chin, and lower lip. It can also involve the lingual nerve, which will affect the side of the tongue and can pose a risk for lingual injury with young pediatric patients because the anesthesia persists after the procedure.

Procedure Identify the coronoid notch by grasping the extraoral posterior ramus with

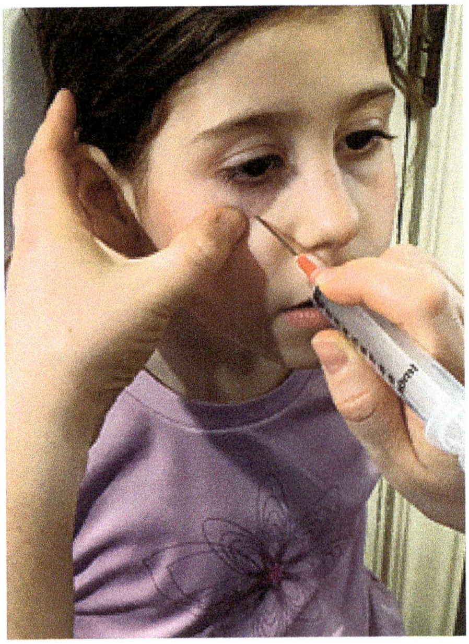

FIGURE 48.1 Infraorbital nerve block: extraoral approach.

one finger and the intraoral anterior ramus with another finger (Figure 48.2). The deepest area palpated is the coronoid notch. Insert the needle here and advance until contacting bone, then slightly withdraw the needle, aspirate, and slowly inject 1–2 mL of anesthetic.

Mental Nerve Block

This block involves the buccal gingiva anterior to the mental foramen and the ipsilateral mucosa and skin of the lower lip.

Procedure Locate the mental foramen by palpation. It should be between the two lower premolar teeth in adolescents or between the first and second primary molars in children (Figure 48.3). Insert the needle in the buccal fold near the foramen while aspirating, and then slowly inject 1–3 mL of anesthetic.

Ophthalmic Nerve Block

This involves the supraorbital, supratrochlear, and infratrochlear nerves leading to anesthesia of the forehead and anterior scalp. Providers can consider using this with large or multiple lacerations to this area; however, for small and simpler wounds, topical agents should be the anesthesia of choice.

Procedure Identify the supraorbital notch, which can be palpated midline on the superior orbit. Inject anesthetic at the level of the eyebrow (Figure 48.4). Apply pressure inferior to the injection site to avoid anesthetic drainage into the eyelid.

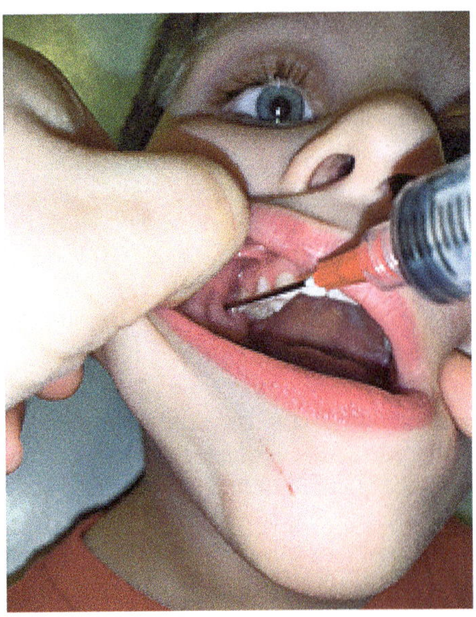

FIGURE 48.2 Inferior alveolar ridge block: inserting a needle into the coronoid notch.

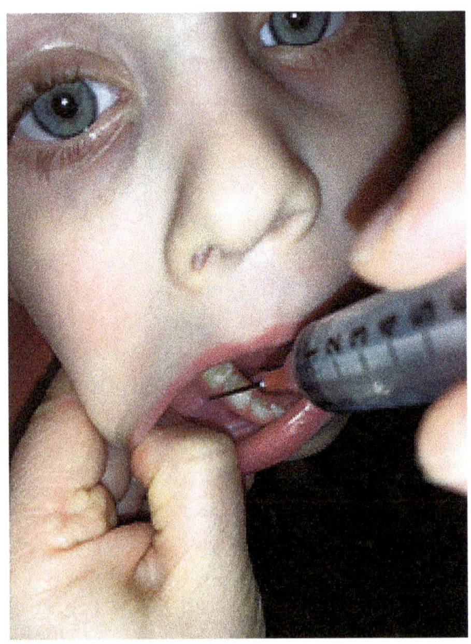

FIGURE 48.3 Mental nerve block.

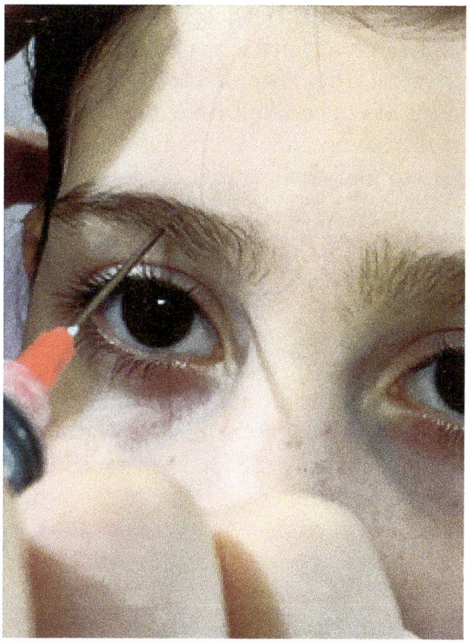

FIGURE 48.4 Ophthalmic nerve block.

Auricular Nerve Block

This is used to provide anesthesia to the entire ear. It can be particularly useful with extensive lacerations requiring repair, hematoma drainage, or when local filtration would create too much distortion or obstruction of existing landmarks. Lidocaine *without* epinephrine should be used.

Procedure Using a 25- to 27-gauge needle, insert the needle above the ear in the midline and advance along the superior–posterior border of the ear and, after aspiration, inject approximately 3–5 mL along that track (Figure 48.5). Next, without removing the needle, create a second track along the superior–anterior border of the ear and repeat. For the lower aspect of the ear, repeat these initial two steps but with the needle inserted in the midline inferior to the ear and creating tracks along the inferior–posterior and inferior–anterior borders with subsequent anesthetic administration.

Supraperiosteal Infiltration (Dental Block)

This block is for anesthesia of individual teeth. It can be used for the maxillary teeth in adolescents and adults. However, in children it can be used for the maxillary as well as mandibular teeth due to porous characteristics of the mandibular bone in children compared to adults.

Procedure Retract the lip. With the needle bevel toward the bone, insert the needle into the mucobuccal fold and advance toward the apex. This should be approximately 1 cm in a preschool-aged child and 1.5 cm in a school-aged child. Withdraw the needle when it contacts the periosteum, and after aspiration, slowly inject 1–2 mL of the anesthetic. For children with permanent teeth, if there is

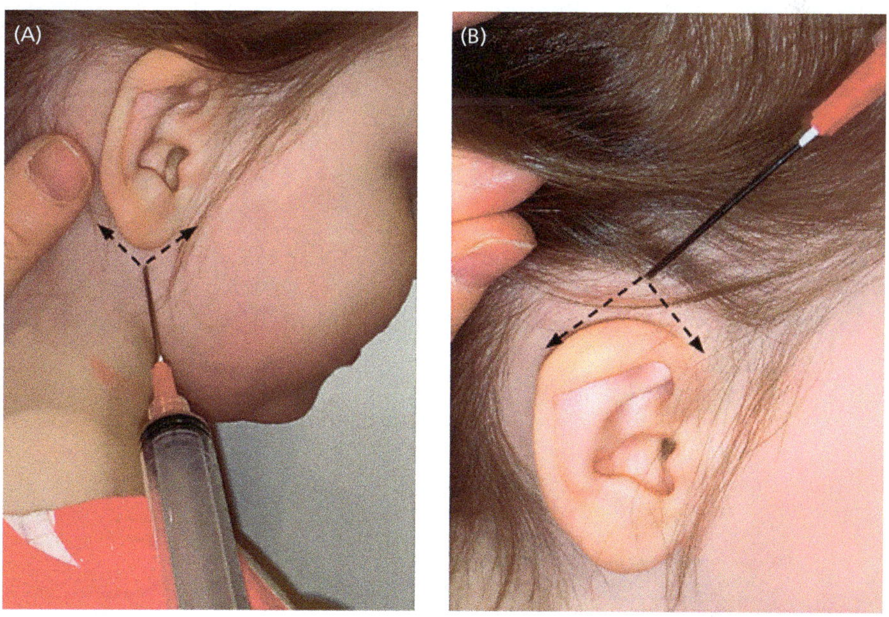

FIGURE 48.5 A AND B Auricular nerve block.

inadequate anesthesia to the central incisors, consider injecting medially and laterally to the apex of the tooth because there can be innervation from adjacent teeth.

Upper Extremity

The median, ulnar, and radial nerve blocks are the most commonly used in the emergency department, and iatrogenic risk can be minimized with ultrasound guidance. These blocks provide anesthesia to their respective distribution territories (Figure 48.6) and can be used with fractures, reductions, and large lacerations. Anatomic landmarks can be difficult to locate given their small size and developmental immaturity, so ultrasound guidance is recommended. When using ultrasound, blocks are done more commonly in-plane versus out-of-plane for visualization of the entire needle while performing the block (Figure 48.7). Importantly, make sure to perform as complete of a neurologic examination of the upper extremity as possible prior to performing the regional anesthesia.

Intra-Articular Shoulder Block

This block can negate the need for a procedural sedation in shoulder dislocation reductions. It also provides pain relief prior to procedure, as well and adequate anesthesia during and afterwards. This type of block requires a fair amount of cooperation from the patient, however, so recommendations are to limit this procedure to more cooperative adolescents.

Procedure Insert a 20- or 22-gauge needle perpendicularly to the acromion process in the sulcus created by the dislocation. Ultrasound can also be used to help identify the correct location. Using a transverse posterior approach with a linear transducer, the glenoid labrum and displacement of the humeral head can be identified. It can often take up to 15 minutes for full anesthetic effect to be in place to proceed with reduction.

Median Nerve Block

The median nerve provides sensation to the radial aspect of the palm, the palmar surface of the thumb, along with the second, third, and the radial half of the fourth finger. It travels just medial to the brachial artery; courses deep to the flexor digitorum superficialis at the mid-forearm; and then becomes superficial at the wrist, lying between the palmaris longus and flexor carpi radialis tendons.

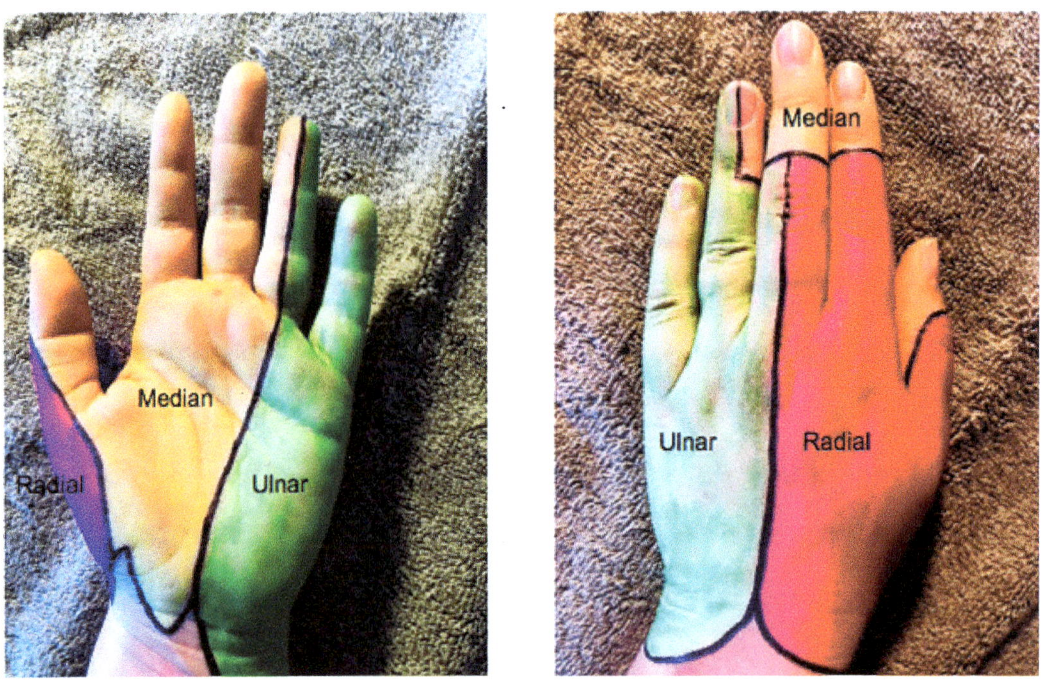

FIGURE 48.6 Hand distribution of the sensory branches of the radial, median, and ulnar nerves.

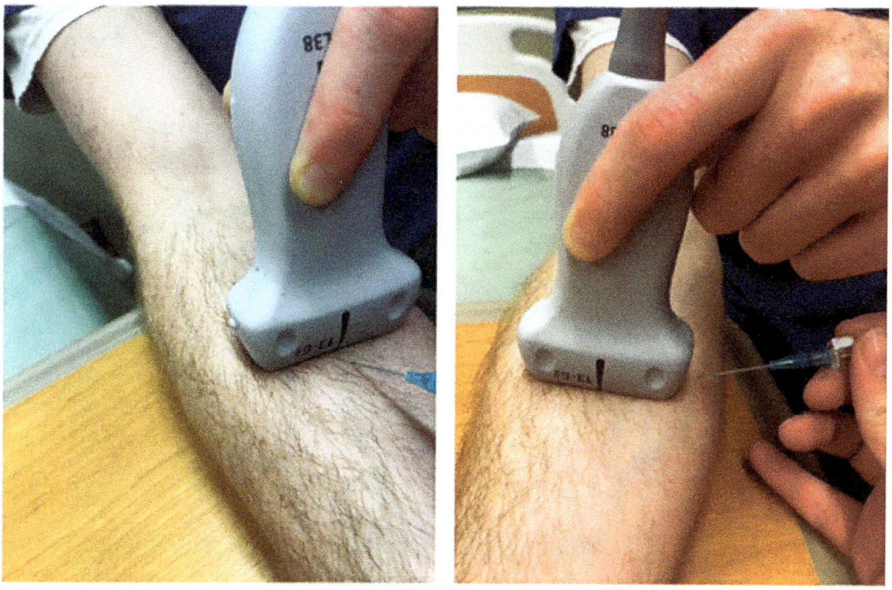

FIGURE 48.7 Needle approaches for ultrasound-guided nerve blocks.

Procedure Using the ultrasound, place the transducer transversely to the volar aspect of the forearm. In the midline of the forearm, the nerve should be identified as a round or oval hyperechoic structure and will be 1 or 2 cm deep and medial to the pulsating radial artery. Either insert the needle medially to the transducer and advance the needle until near the nerve or insert it mid-transducer (out-of-plane but a shorter distance to the nerve) and similarly advance. After negative aspiration, inject anesthetic to infiltrate around the nerve.

Radial Nerve Block

The radial nerve provides sensation to the dorsum of the thumb, second finger, third finger, and the radial half of the ring finger (proximal to the distal interphalangeal joint). On entering the forearm, the nerve divides into a superficial and a deep branch, with the superficial being the sensory branch. It follows the radial artery to the wrist.

Procedure Place the ultrasound transducer transversely over the volar aspect of the wrist. Move the probe proximally to the upper third of the forearm, keeping the radial artery in view. The superficial branch should be visible as a round hyperechoic structure lateral to the radial artery. Insert the needle under ultrasound visualization, and after negative aspiration, infiltrate the area surrounding the nerve with anesthetic.

Ulnar Nerve Block

Sensation from the ulnar nerve is provided to the ulnar aspect of the dorsal and palmar surface of the hand along with the fifth finger and the ulnar side of the fourth finger. At the level of the elbow, the nerve runs between the medial epicondyle and olecranon process and then courses along the medial forearm. Along the distal forearm and toward the wrist, it travels next to the ulnar artery, and at the wrist it lies lateral to the flexor carpi ulnaris tendon and medial to the ulnar artery. This block can be performed using anatomic landmarks at either the elbow or the wrist, or it can be done in the mid-forearm with ultrasound guidance.

Procedure Using ultrasound guidance, place the transducer transversely on the volar aspect of the wrist and identify the ulnar nerve, which should be a round and hyperechoic object adjacent to the pulsating ulnar artery. Trace the nerve proximally to the mid-forearm, and inject while using the in-plane or out-of-plane approach with visualization of the needle.

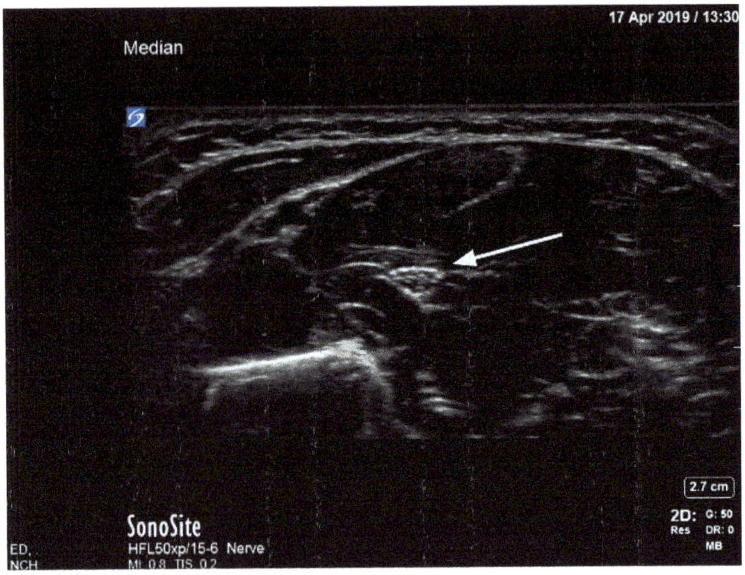

FIGURE 48.8 Ultrasound visualization of median nerve in the mid-forearm.

Hematoma Block

This is most commonly performed for analgesia prior to wrist fracture reductions; however, it can also be used for injuries involving the humerus, ankle, and sternum.

Procedure Landmarks can be palpated, allowing for needle insertion into the hematoma surrounding the fracture, aspiration of blood, and subsequent injection of 5–10 mL 1% lidocaine based on the patient's weight. This can be more difficult in the setting of significant soft tissue swelling or the patient's body habitus; however, ultrasound guidance can be utilized. Place the transducer over the fracture in parallel to the involved bone and follow the needle under guidance into the fracture space. Aspirate a small amount of blood and inject the anesthetic. This ultrasound-guided technique also minimizes risk of inadvertent vascular injection.

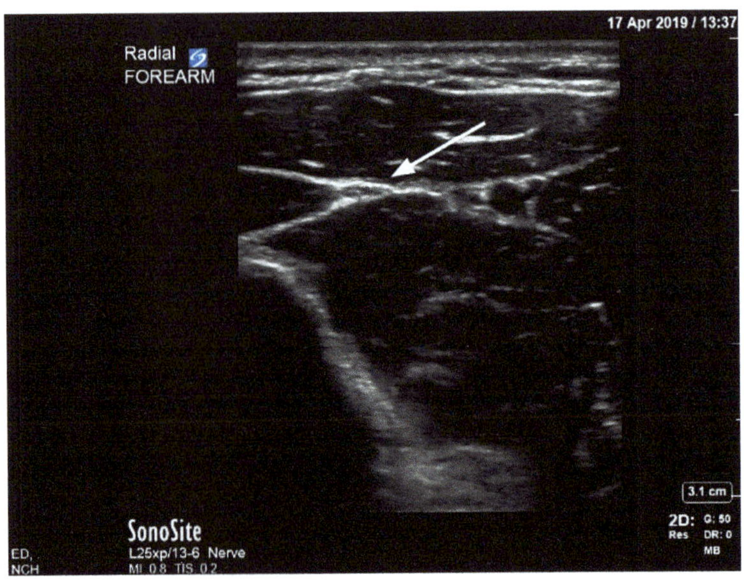

FIGURE 48.9 Ultrasound visualization of the radial nerve in the mid-forearm.

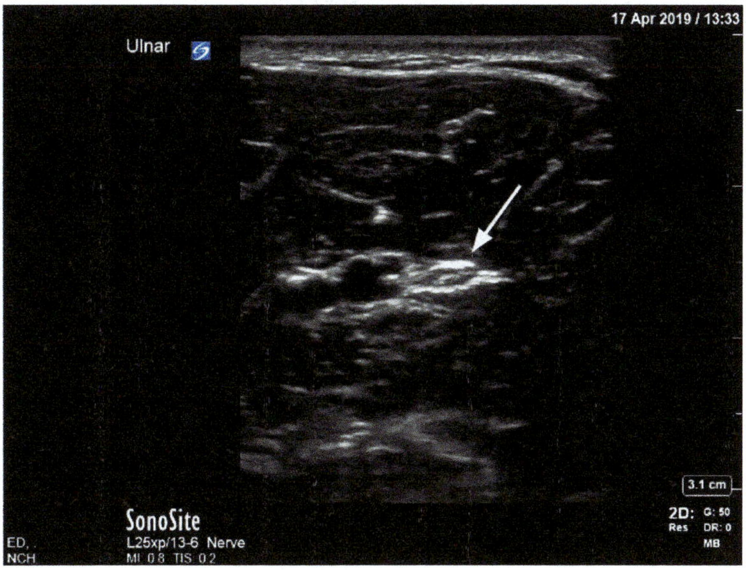

FIGURE 48.10 Ultrasound visualization of the ulnar nerve in the mid-forearm.

Finger Digital Blocks

Digital nerve blocks allow for effective analgesia for finger lacerations, reductions, incision and drainage, along with nail bed injury repairs, partial amputations, and drainage of paronychia. Analgesia can be accomplished via a single injection along the palmar aspect or two separate injections into the adjacent web spaces.

Single Injection Insert the needle at the midline palmar surface overlying the metacarpal phalangeal crease and advance the needle into the flexor tendon. After aspiration, inject anesthetic *without* epinephrine; this should provide anesthesia to the entire digit. Inject 0.75–3 mL of anesthetic, a volume sufficient to moderately distend the skin at the injection site.

Double Injection (Web Space) In the fourth and fifth digits, often palmar and dorsal blocks are needed for complete analgesia. Approximately 1 cm distal to the web space, insert the needle perpendicular to the finger on the lateral side of the finger, inject one-third of the anesthetic, and then redirect toward the dorsal surface of the finger and inject another third; redirect again toward the palmar surface and inject the final third. Repeat this on the medial side of the finger.

Toe Digital Blocks

Nerve blocks to the toes are also very useful and can be using for laceration repair, nail bed injuries, ingrown nails, partial amputations, incision and drainage, and reductions.

Procedure The methods are similar to those for the fingers. For toes 2–5, a single dorsal midline injection at the base of the phalanx can be used. For anesthesia of the great toe (hallux), use a circumferential ring block. This involves four anesthetic injections, with each creating a track using approximately 1–2 mL. One track runs from the plantar to dorsal aspect along with the medial aspect of the base of the hallux, and another is performed similarly to the lateral aspect. In addition, 1–2 mL is injected perpendicularly across the base of the hallux on the dorsal aspect from lateral to medial and again along the plantar aspect, creating a circumferential ring of anesthetic. In total, only 4–8 mL of anesthetic should be used.

Key Points

- Regional anesthesia can decrease the use of systemic analgesics and procedural sedation in pediatric patients in the emergency department.
- There are procedures for regional anesthesia for most areas of the body;

however, some are more easily utilized in an emergency department setting.

- To ensure a successful procedure, ultrasound guidance assists in proper location and technique, and the use of child life specialists along with other methods of distraction aid in the cooperation of the patient.
- Prior to performing nerve blocks, consider placing topical anesthetic such as LMX cream.
- When applicable, consider using LET as an alternative to injection with an additional needle.

Pitfalls

- A nerve block requires a needlestick and may not obviate procedural anxiety.
- Pediatric patients may be unable to describe onset and effectiveness of the block.
- Although ultrasound guidance can improve accuracy, the procedure will still require appropriate cooperation from the patient.

Further Reading

Delvi MB. Ultrasound-guided peripheral and truncal blocks in pediatric patients. *Saudi J Anaesth.* 2011;5(2):208–216.

Goodwin SA, Burton JH, Gerardo CJ, et al. Clinical policy: Procedural sedation and analgesia in the emergency department. *Ann Emerg Med.* 2014;63;247–258.

Illinois Emergency Medical Services for Children. *Pediatric Pain Management in the Emergency Setting.* Chicago, IL: Illinois Emergency Medical Services for Children; 2013.

University of Florida College of Medicine–Jacksonville Department of Emergency Medicine, Pain Assessment and Management Initiative (PAMI): A Patient Safety Project. Pediatric Pain Management in the Acute Care Setting. https://pami.emergency.med.jax.ufl.edu. Accessed June 2016.

Zempsky WT, Cravero JP; American Academy of Pediatrics Committee on Pediatric Emergency Medicine and Section on Anesthesiology and Pain Medicine. Relief of pain and anxiety in pediatric patients in emergency medical systems. *Pediatrics.*2004;114(5):1348–1356.

49

Emergency Care of Children with Medical Complexity

CHRISTIAN D. PULCINI, ANNIQUE HOGAN, AND ERON FRIEDLAENDER

INTRODUCTION

Advancements in pediatric care have led to a significant increase in the number of children living longer (or living into adulthood) with medical complexity. Children with medical complexity are generally defined as those with multiple significant chronic health problems involving multiple organ systems, which result in functional limitations, high health care needs or utilization, and often require need for, or use of, medical technology. Although children with medical complexity represent less than 1% of the pediatric population, they account for a large proportion of health care utilization among children, including acute care and emergency department settings. Many of these children receive a majority of their specialty and outpatient care at tertiary care children's hospitals, but evidence indicates that 80–90% of encounters for emergency care are at community emergency departments. Furthermore, many of the complex, chronic conditions that characterize children with medical complexity are becoming more clinically relevant to all providers as this subgroup of children mature into adulthood. Therefore, it has and will become increasingly relevant for all emergency providers to be prepared to evaluate and manage what have been traditionally pediatric conditions, technologies, and complications among children in this population. In this chapter, a case-based approach is used to illustrate more common and challenging patient scenarios when evaluating and treating children with medical complexity in the emergency department. We hope that this information is practical and assists emergency care providers in providing high-quality care for children with medical complexity.

CASE 1: TEMPERATURE INSTABILITY

Isaiah is a 4-year-old male patient with a history of agenesis of the corpus callosum, septo-optic dysplasia (with resulting pituitary axis dysfunction), gastric tube (G-tube) dependence for feeding, and adrenal insufficiency who presents with an elevated temperature of 37.2°C (his baseline is 34.8°C). He also is reportedly less interactive than normal.

TEMPERATURE INSTABILITY (FEVER AND HYPOTHERMIA)

A fever is 37.2°C? In patients with conditions affecting their autonomic axis, the traditional definition of fever as >38°C may not accurately reflect an infectious illness. Core temperature fluctuations may be a stable homeostatic state for some, and for others, a significant temperature drop or elevation from baseline may be of concern. Confirming normal vital signs for each patient, through either record review or caregiver report, provides essential reference points. Importantly, patients with medical complexity may have serious bacterial illnesses in the absence of temperature change; caregiver suspicion, feeding intolerance, skin mottling, increased seizures, tachycardia, or change in level of alertness or activity are common presenting findings concerning for infection in this medically fragile group of patients.

Differential Diagnosis

Isaiah's history is concerning for acute infection. Sepsis is challenging to recognize given the absence of customary vital signs and mental status changes, but it is critically important to consider. Poor airway clearance abilities and frequent micro-aspiration in patients with low airway tone raise suspicion for aspiration pneumonia given the increased supplemental oxygen requirements. Similarly, progression of a viral upper respiratory infection to pneumonitis is highly likely in this context. Patients without bladder control are at risk for urinary tract infections (UTIs) that may evolve into urosepsis. A careful physical examination will help identify additional potential focal sources of infection: dental abscesses, otitis media, or cellulitis.

Diagnostic Confirmation

Given a risk of serious bacterial illness, inflammatory markers including procalcitonin and lactate, along with blood cultures, assist in risk stratification. A two-view chest radiograph, urinalysis, and urine culture are similarly of diagnostic value. For patients with a tracheostomy, respiratory cultures can be obtained if there is consideration of tracheitis.

Treatment

Broad-spectrum parenteral antibiotics should be administered as soon after collecting cultures as possible when concern for serious bacterial illness exists. If a clearly identified source allows for a more tailored approach, antibiotic choice may be determined with greater discrimination. Consider past infections and known colonization with specific organisms, such as pseudomonas, when choosing an empiric treatment plan. Warming and cooling measures may provide comfort, and antipyretics and fluid resuscitation are indicated by clinical picture.

Clinical Algorithms

Refer to the Children's Hospital of Philadelphia (CHOP) pathway library at https://www.chop.edu/pathways-library for pathways that may be helpful, including sepsis, fever without central venous catheter, and stress dose steroid administration.

Disposition

Depending on hemodynamic and respiratory status, home-based family resources and comfort help dictate appropriate disposition. Notably, many medically fragile patients have home care providers who are comfortable escalating supportive services. Importantly, however, many of these patients have potential for rapid decline and require positive airway pressure with continuous positive airway pressure (CPAP) or bilevel positive airway pressure (BiPAP) along with aggressive airway clearance procedures (albuterol, inhaled saline, chest physical therapy, chest vest, etc.) until their illness reaches a symptomatic plateau. Close follow-up with a provider who knows the child is universally important for any child being discharged home. For any serious bacterial infection that causes clinical concern and need for admission, transfer to a pediatric specialty center is advisable.

Complications

Isaiah's adrenal insufficiency is highly relevant to his treatment plan. Stress dose steroids are recommended. Often, patients with medical complexity have a standing protocol known to their caregivers for dose and timing. If the patient is ill-appearing with or without fever, steroids should not be delayed for consultation or because of difficulty accessing medical records.

Key Points

- Temperature instability in children with medical complexity, especially in those with underlying autonomic dysfunction, is not a reliable indicator of serious bacterial infection.
- A thorough history and examination may be more challenging in this population; an understanding of specific

risks in a given patient will help direct a plan of care.
- Treatment and disposition need to be tailored to home-based resources and the potential for rapid clinical change requiring increasing level of care.

Pitfalls

- Overwhelming infection may not present with fever.
- Delaying treatment of potential serious bacterial infection due to difficulty in assessment, intravenous access, or obtaining outside consultation.

CASE 2: GASTROJEJUNOSTOMY TUBE MALFUNCTION

Maria is a 4-year-old former 26-week premature female with a history of necrotizing enterocolitis requiring operative intervention, gastrojejunostomy (GJ) tube dependence, significant global developmental delay, episodic hypoglycemia, and failure to thrive; she presents with feeding intolerance. Her feeds have stopped flowing easily during infusion, and she has become restless and irritable. She has no fevers and maintains normal voiding and output. There have been no recent formula or medication changes, and feeding rate and volume have been unchanged.

GASTROJEJUNOSTOMY TUBE MALFUNCTION/DISCOMFORT WITH FEEDS

Differential Diagnosis

The differential diagnosis includes bowel obstruction especially with a history of abdominal surgery, intussusception around the jejunostomy tube (J-tube) tip, infectious illness (whether gastroenteritis, UTI, or other), tube displacement, obstruction within the tube ("clogging"), malabsorption in the context of intake changes, constipation, gastroparesis, and gastritis/gastroesophageal reflux.

Diagnostic Confirmation

Initial assessment of a patient with concern for feeding intolerance begins with consideration of a possible surgical abdomen. Early recognition of volvulus, peritonitis, or intestinal perforation is essential to limit morbidity and mortality. Ill-appearance, poor perfusion, hemodynamic or respiratory compromise, altered mental status, abdominal distention, tenderness, and guarding suggest a need for expeditious imaging. Supine and upright plain radiographs of the abdomen can be done quickly and at the bedside to screen for pneumoperitoneum or obstruction. Ultrasound or computed tomography (CT) with contrast will further detail an intestinal lesion and grade of obstruction. Plain radiographs with gastrograffin may be used to highlight tube placement. Ultrasonography is the preferred imaging study to identify intussusception. Urinalysis and culture, as well as stool cultures, are recommended in the appropriate clinical context. Constipation, reflux, and dismotility are recognized through careful discussion of symptoms. Consider a glucose check and basic metabolic panel in patients with excessive gastrointestinal (GI) losses, evidence of moderate to severe dehydration, or in patients at risk for adrenal insufficiency. Notably, some children present very well-appearing to the emergency department with "clogging" of the tube due to the formula passing through the tube being high in lipids. This is often obvious when flushes are attempted, and the family usually is aware of the protocol on how to unclog the tube (often with an enzymatic solution such as Clog Zapper).

Treatment

Volvulus and pneumoperitoneum require immediate operative intervention; urgent surgical consultation is recommended for findings of intussusception and bowel obstruction. Intractable vomiting may be relieved with a sump drain along with venting of the G-tube. Correction of dehydration with isotonic solutions followed by maintenance fluids follows clinical indication. Toxic-appearing patients and those with suspicion or evidence of peritonitis require broad-spectrum parenteral antibiotics targeted at gram-negative and anaerobic enteric pathogens. Stress dose hydrocortisone is essential in the context of adrenal crisis. Dislodged J-tubes without additional complication require skilled interventional radiology for reinsertion; for individuals dependent on J-tube feeds for a majority or the entirety of their hydration and nutrition needs, admission on maintenance fluids is necessary until procedure completion. Note that if the GJ-tube is completely dislodged, immediate placement of a Foley catheter into the stoma is crucial to preserve the catheter tract. UTI, constipation, gastritis, and reflux may require admission for care initiation if dehydration, weight loss, or pain prohibit safe discharge. It is imperative that patients with medical complexity demonstrate tolerance of feeds/oral intake prior to being discharged. In the case of internal obstruction of the tube ("clogging"), a variety of techniques, including strong flush pressure, carbonated solutions, and enzymatic formulations such as Clog Zapper, can be utilized safely. Confirmation that feeds can run through the tube after unclogging is often necessary.

Clinical Algorithms

For figures and guidance for common G/GJ-tube problems, see https://www.chop.edu/clinical-pathway/gastrostomy-g-gj-j-complications-clinical-pathway and https://www.chop.edu/clinical-pathway/g-j-or-g-tube-displacement-clinical-pathway.

Complications

Most children with medical complexity require pediatric subspecialist care to manage GJ-tube and related feeding complications. Hypoglycemia, dehydration, and sequelae from missed home medications occur when enteral intake needs are not transitioned to parenteral infusion. In addition, GJ-tube tracts, even those that are long-standing, may close precipitously unless stented open with a Foley catheter as a temporizing measure.

Key Points

- Feeding intolerance can be due to a wide spectrum of disease, from an emergent bowel obstruction to the uncomfortable but less urgent constipation.
- In the setting of hypoglycemia, feeding intolerance is an emergency.
- It should be ensured that patients are able to tolerate feeds before leaving the medical setting under almost all circumstances.
- Maintain stoma patency with a Foley catheter if a GJ-tube is completely dislodged.
- Begin intravenous fluids to maintain hydration and for medication administration if there will be delay in replacing the J-tube.

Pitfall

- Feeding intolerance may reflect abdominal catastrophe or systemic infection without the classic symptoms, signs, and vital sign changes familiar in other patient populations.

CASE 3: TRACHEOSTOMY COMPLICATIONS

George is a 2-year-old male with a tracheostomy and ventilator dependence due to a cerebrovascular accident at birth (neonatal stroke, unknown etiology), with resulting right-sided hemiparesis and mild developmental delay. He presents with increased secretions from the tracheostomy site and intermittent increased supplemental oxygen requirement. He has remained playful and interactive and without fever.

TRACHEOSTOMY COMPLICATIONS

Differential Diagnosis

Mechanical complications of the tracheostomy may present with acute medical decline or subacute changes related to changes in respiratory secretions, ability to adequately clear sections with suctioning, leaking from the stoma site, or escalating respiratory support requirements. Considerations include mucus plugging, dislodgment, granuloma formation, outgrowing tracheostomy size, and trauma from a tracheostomy change. Alternatively, infection of the tracheostomy site, the trachea itself, or lower in the respiratory tract may present with difficulty maintaining airway clearance and need for greater than baseline respiratory support; consider cellulitis and abscess around the stoma, tracheitis, viral pneumonitis, and pneumonia. Significant bleeding from the tracheostomy may indicate invasion of the innominate artery requiring immediate surgical intervention; only a surgical specialist should manipulate the tracheostomy in such cases, and medical resuscitation should occur in parallel.

Diagnostic Confirmation

The time course of symptom development (acute or subacute) along with characterizing the changes in quality/character of sections and changes in needed respiratory support are elemental to beginning an evaluation. Deep suctioning with re-evaluation allows for airway clearance as well as collection of respiratory cultures for Gram stain, bacterial culture, and viral panels. Examination of the tracheal stoma will direct further investigation of poor sizing or cellulitis and abscess formation, which may be a clinical diagnosis confirmed with ultrasonography. Suspected pathology from within the trachea (granuloma formation or airway injury) requires a bedside scope by otorhinolaryngology (ENT).

Treatment

Patients with acute respiratory failure unresponsive to suctioning and ventilation through the tracheostomy require an emergent tracheostomy change. In a patient with evidence of overwhelming invasive infection, immediate broad-spectrum parenteral antibiotics should be initiated with consideration of organisms with which the patient is known to have had prior infection. Children with an increase in baseline suctioning needs along with evidence of a local tracheal infection or lower airway viral process may have the support at home with nursing and skilled caregivers to maintain aggressive pulmonary toilet as an outpatient. Subspecialty recommendation is critical for plan of care decision-making regarding intratracheal lesions or upsizing of the tracheostomy tube.

Disposition

Degree of illness, associated respiratory or hemodynamic compromise, home care service support, and family preference guide disposition planning.

Complications

Skilled individuals should replace a tracheostomy and perform all suctioning. Inability to replace the tracheostomy correctly may result in false tracts with poor ventilation and oxygenation. Respiratory therapists and surgical specialists may provide needed support.

Key Points

- Immediate change of the tracheostomy tube should occur with dislodgement or obstruction.
- Common tracheostomy complications include displacement, granuloma formation, and infection.

Pitfall

- Delay in expeditious tracheostomy change to correct a mechanical obstruction may prevent optimal ventilation or oxygenation.

CASE 4: VENTRICULOPERITONEAL SHUNT COMPLICATIONS

Emily, a 9-year-old female with a ventriculoperitoneal (VP) shunt for treatment of congenital hydrocephalus and a baclofen pump to ease the discomfort of spastic quadriplegia, presents with vomiting. The emesis is nonbilious and has increased in frequency over the course of the day. She has had normal stool output and no fevers. She is more tired and less active, but she remains alert and appropriate.

VENTRICULOPERITONEAL SHUNT COMPLICATIONS

Differential Diagnosis

The differential diagnosis includes proximal malfunction due to shunt obstruction or tubing discontinuity, distal malfunction secondary to pseudocele, constipation or discontinuity, or infection.

Diagnostic Confirmation

Symptoms and signs of shunt malfunction guide evaluation for shunt integrity and functioning using imaging and/or tapping of the shunt. Typical symptoms of shunt malfunction include headache, irritability, and vomiting. Signs predictive of shunt malfunction include hypertension with bradycardia, irregular respirations, depressed mental status, and focal neurologic deficits such as sundowning. Head CT with a shunt protocol is optimal for assessing malfunction concerns. A shunt series may be helpful if tubing discontinuity is suspected. A neurosurgeon may choose to "tap the shunt" as a more nuanced procedure to identify a proximal obstruction that may not show on head CT. Regarding the choice of imaging, low-dose CT is becoming the standard of care. If it is not available, comparable imaging is preferred for immediate comparison because changes can be more readily recognized on the same imaging modality. Concern for infection necessitates sampling of cerebrospinal fluid (CSF) either directly from a shunt reservoir or through a traditional lumbar puncture; a neurosurgeon should guide decision-making.

Treatment

There is a spectrum of clinical compromise with a shunt malfunction. Altered mental status, focal neurologic changes, and hemodynamic instability reflect potential for imminent life-threatening herniation and a need for emergent surgical intervention. Temporizing supportive care with neuroprotective measures including Decadron, Diamox, 3% saline, intubation with mild hyperventilation, and raised head of bed to 30° should be instituted. CSF may also be withdrawn from a shunt reservoir to immediately decompress mass effect until definitive operative care. Individuals with less emergent presentations may be medically stabilized in a pediatric intensive care unit while awaiting neurosurgical mediation. Concern for shunt infection dictates broad-spectrum parenteral antibiotics once cultures are pending. Of note, some shunts are programmable. If a child has a programmable shunt, consultation with a neurosurgeon is necessary to confirm or change settings. Furthermore, if the child requires magnetic resonance imaging (MRI), the MRI technologist will need to know this information.

Clinical Algorithms

See the CHOP VP shunt pathway at https://www.chop.edu/clinical-pathway/ventricular-shunt-obstruction-infection-clinical-pathway.

Disposition

A VP shunt malfunction in a pediatric patient requires immediate pediatric neurosurgical consultation.

Complications

Sedation to support a patient lying still for head imaging will contribute to a change in mental status, making close observation for deterioration more challenging. Consultation with an anesthesiologist may be necessary.

Key Points

- VP shunt malfunction is a surgical emergency.
- Head CT is the diagnostic study of choice to evaluate for shunt malfunction, and it should be obtained as quickly as possible regardless of radiation exposure.
- Temporizing neuroprotective medical interventions are indicted in emergent situations while definitive correction is pending.

Pitfalls

- Failure to recognize a shunt malfunction in a timely way may delay care and increase morbidity and mortality risks.

BACLOFEN PUMP COMPLICATIONS

Background

Intrathecal baclofen (ITB) is delivered through a surgically implanted, computer-programmed infusion pump to help reduce spasticity and severe dystonia resulting from spinal cord injury, cerebral palsy, or multiple sclerosis. Approximately 25% of patients experience a complication related to this device.

Differential Diagnosis

Complications include catheter dislodgment, pump failure, CSF leaks, hemorrhage, and infection. Mechanical/programming errors are also common; importantly, catheter migration, battery failure, and improper dose delivery have consequential effects. Withdrawal from baclofen is a medical emergency and presents with exaggerated rebound spasticity and rigidity, fever/hyperthermia, tachycardia, hypertension, hyperthermia, and altered mental status, with potential progression to rhabdomyolysis, multiple organ system failure, and death. Alternatively, an adverse reaction to baclofen may present with hypotension, hypoventilation, increased or decreased muscle tone, seizures or tremors, altered mental status, peripheral edema, constipation or diarrhea, urinary retention or frequency, or pruritus. CSF leaks may occur within the abdominal cavity or at the site of a catheter tear. These require surgical intervention. Infections of the implant, most commonly with *Staphylococcus aureus*, require targeted antibiotics, vigilant monitoring, and potential catheter removal and replacement. Given the broad range of symptoms caused by both withdrawal and overdose (in combination with already medically fragile children), all etiologies need to be considered, including serious bacterial infections, trauma, or other causes consistent with the individual child.

Diagnostic Confirmation

Plain radiographs may be sufficient to confirm catheter placement; pump injection studies with contrast may be required to evaluate for CSF leak. Neurosurgeons may need to interrogate the pump to confirm its integrity. Clinical suspicion is essential to identifying any complication and must be addressed with urgency.

Treatment

Concern for symptomatic baclofen withdrawal due to pump failure is managed with confirmation of ITB programming, medication concentration, dosing, and amount of available drug. The pump may simply require refill. If medication is unable to be drawn through the side post, a presumed catheter disconnection or obstruction is confirmed and requires surgical revision. If the pump is incapable of delivering the needed dose, a single bolus of the drug is delivered while definitive pump interrogation is pending. Baclofen overdose requires discontinuation of ongoing baclofen dosing and supportive intensive care, largely for respiratory support.

Disposition

Most issues involving the baclofen pump will require transfer to a tertiary care facility for evaluation and treatment.

Complications

Depending on the particular complication, patients are at risk for significant illness and compromise, requiring urgent neurosurgical and pediatric intensive care support.

Key Points

- Most issues involving the baclofen pump are mechanical or infectious and require neurosurgical or other specialty consultation.

Pitfall

- Failure to recognize worsening withdrawal of overdose. The complications of such can quickly become life-threatening.

CASE 5: INCREASED FUSSINESS

Chi is a 16-year-old male with trisomy 18, chronic kidney disease, mild aortic valve dysfunction, seizure disorder, and failure to thrive who presents with increased fussiness over 2 days. He has had no fever, vomiting, coughing, or injury. His intake has been at baseline. He has no new medications or changes in routine.

"FUSSINESS"

Background

"Fussiness" is a common pediatric complaint often used to describe changes in mood, or in some instances mental status, especially in nonverbal individuals with limited communication skills. Importantly, it may serve as an indication to caregivers that a patient with medical complexity is in pain, ill, or depressed.

Differential Diagnosis

A thorough and exhaustive history and physical examination may bring attention to an occult infection (dental abscess, decubitus ulcer, or UTI), discomfort [corneal abrasion, occult fracture from routine care in the context of severe osteopenia or abuse, tetany from hypocalcemia, poorly fitting orthotics, a decubitus ulcer, constipation (even with a normal stooling pattern), gastroesophageal reflux, or bowel obstruction], or a mood disorder some patients are unable to articulate in words but rather do so through behavior changes. At times, screening laboratory investigation, including inflammatory markers, lipase, urinalysis, and imaging, may help determine a need for ongoing evaluation or support decision-making in support of conservative serial outpatient examinations.

Diagnostic Confirmation

This is largely dependent on findings from the history and physical examination. Some patient with clear irritability of unknown cause may require admission for close observation.

Treatment

The treatment is dependent on etiology. Treatment should follow standard medical practice.

Disposition

Depending on the level of concern and degree of symptomatology, inpatient or outpatient management is case dependent.

Complications

Complications may occur with lack of vigilance to history, physical examination, and maintaining a broad differential of consideration.

Key Points

- Fussiness is a common pediatric complaint, notably among those who are nonverbal and use behaviors as their primary means of communication.
- A thorough history and physical examination should be performed to elicit etiology and reduce unnecessary testing.
- The differential diagnoses should include common pediatric and child-specific conditions.

Pitfall

- Non-accidental trauma occurs at much higher rates among children with special health care needs in general, and vigilance is required to identify such victims.

Further Reading

Temperature Instability

Children's Hospital of Philadelphia. ED Pathway for Evaluation/Treatment of Infants >28 Days of Age and Children with Suspected Severe Sepsis. https://www.chop.edu/clinical-pathway/sepsis-emergent-care-clinical-pathway.

Gastrojejunostomy Tube Malfunction

Children's Hospital of Philadelphia. Clinical Pathway for Management of Gastrostomy Tube Complications. https://www.chop.edu/clinical-pathway/gastrostomy-g-gj-j-complications-clinical-pathway.

Children's Hospital of Philadelphia. ED Pathway for Care of the Child with G-J or G-Tube Displacement. https://www.chop.edu/clinical-pathway/g-j-or-g-tube-displacement-clinical-pathway.

50

Pediatric Ingestions and Toxicologic Exposures

VINCENT CALLEO AND RICHARD CANTOR

INTRODUCTION

Pediatric ingestions and toxicologic exposures are extremely common. Nationally in 2017, there were approximately 1.3 million calls to poison control centers for pediatric exposures. Although many of the children for whom calls were made to poison control centers were able to remain home with parental observation, a substantial number required evaluation by health care professionals. Only a small cohort of toxicologic exposures resulted in death, but severe toxicity was frequently seen and required substantial medical interventions.

The vast majority of exposures in children aged 0–5 years are unintentional. For children aged 6–12 years, the ratio of accidental to intentional ingestions starts to shift more toward intentional ingestions. During the ages of 13–19 years, the vast majority of exposures are intentional and rarely accidental.

The basics of medical stabilization should be applied to the acutely poisoned patient. The airway should be secured in an altered patient unable to protect from aspiration or those with respiratory difficulty; however, the decision to intubate must be carefully considered with certain ingestions, such as salicylates. In general, respiratory and circulatory support may be indicated depending on substance and severity of the ingestion.

After stabilization, early identification and treatment of hypoglycemia are paramount (see Chapter 21 on fluid and electrolyte emergencies). Hypoglycemia is very common in children after ingesting a number of medications.

After completing an evaluation for hypoglycemia, an electrocardiogram (ECG) should be performed. When evaluating a poisoned patient, the ECG is so important that it should be regarded as a vital sign. Countless substances may lead to ECG changes. Some ECG changes are benign, whereas others are markers of toxicity and may pose imminent life threats to the patient. The most frequent changes that affect a patient clinically are QRS prolongation and QTc prolongation. Careful attention should be paid to these intervals when looking at the ECG of a poisoned patient.

After initial primary survey and stabilization, a secondary survey and evaluation for toxidromes should be performed.

Pupil size should be evaluated and documented. Many substances cause miosis, whereas others cause mydriasis. However, polypharmacy can lead to mixed pupillary findings.

Bowel sounds should be evaluated in multiple quadrants because they assist in toxidrome diagnosis and also screen for contraindication to whole bowel irrigation.

Assessing reflexes and muscle tone are two integral parts of the physical examination for poisoned patients. Exposure to various agents may lead to hypo/hyperreflexia. If a patient is extremely rigid or flaccid, it provides insight into the primary process affecting the patient.

Body temperature and skin findings should be evaluated. Hyperthermia without diaphoresis or diaphoresis without temperature changes should be noted. Whenever possible, core body temperatures should be obtained.

GASTROINTESTINAL DECONTAMINATION

The most common form of gastrointestinal (GI) decontamination is administration of activated charcoal (AC); the other main GI decontamination techniques are orogastric lavage and whole bowel irrigation (WBI). There are several forms of extracorporeal removal of xenobiotics, including hemodialysis and exchange transfusion. Although AC administration is far more common than the other methods of GI decontamination and more frequently used than extracorporeal removal methods, each method has a role in the proper clinical setting.

Activated charcoal binds to many medications and helps decrease absorption, thereby limiting toxicity. For a single dose in a pediatric patient, most clinicians use 1 g/kg (maximum 50 g). Many medications have delayed absorption (many extended-release drug formulations), whereas others slow gut motility and impede absorption time. In both of these cases, giving AC, even after the traditional 2-hour mark, may significantly diminish the amount of available drug and improve patient outcomes. There are even some cases in which multiple doses of AC are beneficial. However, this only applies to certain situations, and consulting a toxicologist may be helpful when trying to determine when this is indicated.

Perhaps the major limitation with AC in the pediatric population is compliance; many patients will not drink AC due to its texture and flavor. AC can be mixed with other substances that children find more palatable, such as chocolate milk. Once mixed, it can also be administered through a bottle or sippy cup, if needed. Another limitation of AC is that will not bind well to metals or liquids and is ineffective with these ingestions.

Administration of AC should only be done once a careful analysis of the risk:benefit ratio has been performed. The major risk of AC is aspiration, and it should not be given to altered patients with poor airway protection. Aspiration pneumonitis is a severe potential complication. Patients who are intubated with a protected airway may be good candidates for AC through a nasogastric tube; however, patients should not be routinely intubated solely for AC administration.

Orogastric (OG) lavage and WBI are rarely used and are typically only initiated in the setting of large, potentially fatal ingestions. Neither is without risk, and there is little literature describing significant benefits of either procedure. OG lavage is particularly difficult to successfully perform in pediatrics because the OG tube is smaller than that used in adults. This makes it more difficult to recover pills. If remaining medication is present from the ingestion, comparing the size of the pill to the fenestrations in the OG tube can help determine if there is any chance of success with lavage.

WBI can potentially be beneficial in the setting of large life-threatening overdoses of certain medications, such as calcium channels blockers, iron, and extended-release buproprion. Bowel sounds must be confirmed prior to administration. WBI is normally performed with polyethylene glycol solution, and the volumes vary depending on the size of the patient. Once initiated, WBI is normally continued until the patient has clear rectal effluent. Before initiating OG lavage or WBI, either toxicology or the poison control center should be consulted.

COMMON TOXIDROME RECOGNITION AND TREATMENT

Patients should be evaluated for signs of a toxidrome to facilitate diagnosis, particularly in an undifferentiated ingestion.

Cholinergic Toxidrome

The cholinergic toxidrome is seen when patients are exposed to substances that increase levels of acetylcholine; many substances accomplish this by inhibiting acetylcholinesterase. Some substances that cause this toxidrome are organophosphates and carbamates. Miosis, increased lacrimation, hypersalivation, nausea, vomiting, increased bowel sounds, urinary incontinence, diarrhea, and diaphoresis are common findings. Bronchorrhea, bradycardia, and bronchospasm are sometimes seen in severe cholinergic toxidromes and are worrisome findings because they can cause life-threatening complications.

Initial treatment of cholinergic symptoms starts with titrating atropine until excessive secretions cease and patients no longer have symptomatic bradycardia (not pupil size). Pediatric atropine dosing is 0.02 mg/kg intravenously (IV) and can be repeated every 5 minutes until clinical improvement occurs (with a maximum dose of 0.5 mg per dose). Dosing can be increased to 0.05 mg/kg IV every 5 minutes. In organophosphate toxicity, pralidoxime should be given to abort pathological toxic effects (in consultation with a toxicologist).

Anticholinergic Toxidrome

Many medications can cause anticholinergic toxicity. Some of the most common agents seen are diphenhydramine and benztropine. With this toxidrome, clinicians will see essentially the opposite of the cholinergic toxidrome. Symptoms include agitation, mydriasis, dry mucous membranes, tachycardia, decreased bowel sounds, bladder distention, anhidrosis, and hyperthermia. Hyperthermia is normally secondary to increased muscle movement from motor agitation coupled with the inability to perspire.

Supportive care is the mainstay of management. Fluid resuscitation and body temperature stabilization, with cooling measures as needed, are pivotal. Benzodiazepines are normally effective for agitation; IV benzodiazepines, such as midazolam or diazepam, are typically the agents of choice due to their rapid onset of action of approximately 5 minutes.

Physostigmine may be used when benzodiazepines are insufficient to treat agitation. Physostigmine inhibits acetylcholinesterase and results in increased acetylcholine. Dosing is typically 0.02 mg/kg, with a maximum dose of 2 mg. Physostigmine should be given slowly (over 10 minutes) to avoid precipitating seizures. One way to do this is to mix physostigmine in a 50-mL bag of normal saline and run in through a pump over 10 minutes.

Prior to giving physostigmine, an ECG should be performed. If the QRS is prolonged, physostigmine should not be given. Cardiac monitoring should occur during physostigmine administration because bradycardia may occur. Atropine may be required if cholinergic symptoms develop, and dosing should be titrated to secretions and bradycardia. A toxicologist or the poison control center should be contacted for guidance prior to giving physostigmine.

Sympathomimetic Toxidrome

The sympathomimetic toxidrome typically results from enhanced adrenergic activity. Numerous substances can precipitate a sympathomimetic toxidrome. Cocaine and methamphetamine both increase catecholamines and are common causes of this toxidrome. Symptoms include agitation, mydriasis, tachycardia, tachypnea, increased bowel sounds, diaphoresis, and hyperthermia. A key distinguishing feature between the sympathomimetic toxidrome and the anticholinergic toxidrome is the skin; sympathomimetic patients are normally extremely diaphoretic whereas patients who are anticholinergic typically have extremely dry skin.

A sympathomimetic toxidrome requires excellent supportive care, including IV fluids. Rhabdomyolysis commonly occurs from increased muscle use and agitation. Benzodiazepines are often required for agitation. Escalation of care up to intubation may be required in severe cases. As with the anticholinergic toxidrome, patients can become very hyperthermic and may require aggressive cooling measures.

Opioid Toxidrome

One of the most commonly seen toxidromes is the opioid toxidrome. Patients of any age can be exposed to opioids. Pediatric patients can be exposed to a plethora of xenobiotics, both legal and illegal. Common pain medications to which patients are exposed are hydrocodone and oxycodone. In addition, medications such as methadone and buprenorphine are frequently prescribed, especially during the current opioid epidemic. The major receptor to which opioids bind and cause clinical effects is the μ-receptor. Once a substance binds to the μ-receptor, this can lead to miosis, bradycardia, bradypnea, and altered mental status. The degree of physiologic effect is largely dependent on dose and formulation.

Early supportive care must be optimized. Mild bradypnea and somnolence may simply require monitoring, but obtundation and respiratory cessation require immediate intervention. Emergent airway support is indicated with bag mask ventilation. However, intubation may be required if patients do not respond to antagonist medication.

Naloxone is an opioid receptor antagonist that competitively inhibits binding at the opioid receptor and can reverse the opioid toxidrome and restore spontaneous respiration. IV administration is most commonly used in the emergency department (ED) and it has a rapid onset. In apneic patients, high-quality bag mask ventilations should be performed prior to naloxone administration to help decrease the incidence of flash pulmonary edema. Naloxone may precipitate opiate withdrawal in a chronic user, so ideally the dose should be slowly titrated to reversal of respiratory depression. Repeat doses may be required, and a naloxone drip can be used with persistent/recurrent apnea. Toxicology consultation is recommended.

Sedative–Hypnotic Toxidrome

Physicians should be able to rapidly identify and treat the sedative–hypnotic toxidrome. This toxidrome typically occurs with substances that cause sedation and/or drowsiness; although there are various mechanisms through which this can occur, one of the most common ways is through interaction with γ-aminobutyric acid (GABA) receptors. Benzodiazepines, barbiturates, and ethanol can all precipitate this toxidrome. When seen clinically, sedative–hypnotic patients frequently have decreased coordination and ataxia. Slurred speech is routinely seen as well. Respiratory depression can occur in large overdoses, although this is more commonly seen with polypharmacy ingestions.

Sedative–hypnotic toxidromes are normally managed well with supportive care. Respiratory depression may occur with significant toxicity and require intubation. For patients with no history of chronic benzodiazepine use who ingest benzodiazepines acutely, flumazenil, a reversal agent, may be used (with caution) as an antidote. If patients use benzodiazepines routinely, they are at risk for developing benzodiazepine-resistant seizures if they receive flumazenil. Dosing for flumazenil is typically 0.01 mg/kg up to 0.2 mg for an initial dose. Consulting with a toxicologist or the poison control center is recommended when considering flumazenil.

MEDICATION OVERDOSES

Acetaminophen

Acetaminophen ingestion is one of the most common overdoses. With timely identification and treatment, outcomes are excellent. However, unlike most medications, acetaminophen does not normally exhibit telltale signs in the early stages of ingestion. Therefore, if the clinician does not have acetaminophen ingestion on the differential, it is difficult to find and properly treat an acetaminophen overdose. Fortunately, significant accidental ingestions are extremely rare; exceptions to this occur when caregivers miscalculate dosing and frequency. An acetaminophen level is critical to make the diagnosis. Early detection and treatment initiation are associated with the best outcomes. When acetaminophen is ingested in therapeutic doses, it is broken down into nontoxic metabolites primarily through sulfation and glucuronidation. Even with appropriate doses, a small amount of its toxic metabolite, NAPQI, is generated, but it is rapidly converted to a nontoxic metabolite by combining with glutathione. In the overdose setting, glucuronidation and sulfation are overwhelmed, and large amounts of acetaminophen are converted to NAPQI.

NAPQI usually starts causing damage in zone 3 of the liver (centrilobular necrosis). Hepatocyte death can produce synthetic dysfunction of the liver and lead to transaminitis, elevated prothrombin time/international normalized ratio (INR), and hypoproteinemia. In severe poisonings, acetaminophen toxicity can result in multisystem organ failure and subsequently death.

Acetaminophen toxicity normally occurs in four stages. In stage 1, there may be GI symptoms (nausea, vomiting, and abdominal pain) for the first several hours after ingestion, although sometimes patients have no complaints. Stage 2 is a quiescent phase in which patients may seem to improve clinically; this typically occurs 6–24 hours after ingestion, although it is not always present. Stage 3 involves multisystem organ failure and occurs 12–72 hours after ingestion in most circumstances. After stage 3 is complete, stage 4 commences and has one of two outcomes: death or recovery. Patients who do not die normally have a full recovery.

When assessing for acetaminophen toxicity, several laboratory tests should be ordered and trended. An acetaminophen level should be obtained. However, clinicians should be aware of the time when the acetaminophen level is drawn in relation to when the ingestion occurred. If the level is drawn before 4 hours post ingestion, it should be repeated at the 4-hour mark. However, the time of ingestion is often loosely approximated or simply unknown. In this case, an elevated level should be repeated and trended to be sure it is not increasing. Liver function tests, including aspartate aminotransferase and alanine aminotransferase, should be ordered and trended if the patient has an elevated acetaminophen concentration. Coagulation studies, including an INR, should be checked and trended in patients with supratherapeutic acetaminophen levels, transaminitis, or patients being treated for toxicity. Checking a venous blood gas may also be useful as part of the initial workup and repeated as needed.

Supportive care should be optimized when treating acetaminophen overdoses. Although acetaminophen is normally rapidly absorbed, activated charcoal should be considered if patients present within the first 2 hours of ingestion and can safely receive this intervention. Activated charcoal may be considered later than 2 hours in patients with polypharmacy ingestions because GI motility may be reduced and subsequently cause delayed acetaminophen absorption. Patients should receive adequate IV fluid resuscitation.

The mainstay of treatment for acetaminophen toxicity is *N*-acetylcysteine (NAC). NAC works by replenishing the body's glutathione stores. It detoxifies NAPQI and also partially reactivates the sulfation pathway for acetaminophen metabolism. If started within the first 8 hours of acetaminophen ingestion, NAC makes the likelihood of injury infinitesimally low. Treatment of acetaminophen toxicity is based on the Rumack–Matthew nomogram; this tool looks at acetaminophen concentrations in relation to time after ingestion. If patients are above the treatment line, they are at risk for adverse outcomes and should receive NAC. Although this tool is indispensable for acute overdoses, it has no use for chronic ingestions or ingestions for which the time is unknown. With chronic cases or unknown ingestion times, treatment should be based on other parameters, such as acetaminophen levels, liver function tests, and INR measurements. Increases in the aforementioned markers should prompt consideration of NAC therapy (although NAC can raise the INR up to a value of approximately 1.9).

NAC is available in both oral and IV formulations. The oral version is normally used in acute ingestions without marked liver function test (LFT) or INR elevations. It does have a rotten egg smell, and this is normally one of the barriers faced when giving it to children. Antiemetics administration prior to initiating therapy should be considered because it may decrease vomiting. IV NAC is used more commonly than oral, and it should be the formulation of choice if patients already have transaminitis. Administration can cause anaphylactoid reactions in rare cases; this normally occurs with the first dose. Dosing regiments can vary, but normally IV NAC is given over 21 hours. The first dose is 150 mg/kg given over 1 hour, the second dose is 50 mg/kg given over 4 hours, and the third dose is 100 mg/kg given over 16 hours. In young pediatric patients, this can lead to the administration of large fluid volumes, and clinicians should consider having the solutions concentrated by the pharmacist. Normally, NAC is administered until the acetaminophen level is negative and the LFTs have a negative downward trend. However, if there are any questions regarding dosing or treatment duration, clinicians should contact the local toxicology team or the poison control center.

Salicylates

Although salicylates have been used for more than a century, large overdoses deeply concern even the most seasoned toxicologists. Perhaps the most easily accessible form of salicylate is aspirin. Fortunately, given its concentration and formulation, very few young children accidentally consume enough aspirin to result in significant toxicity. The same cannot be said for older children and adolescents, for whom the exposures are routinely intentional. However, there are products on the market, such as oil of wintergreen, that have extremely high concentrations of salicylate and can cause severe toxicity with as much as a single sip. Knowing the amount of product consumed and the concentration of salicylate in the product are quintessential pieces of information to gather when risk-stratifying patients after an ingestion has occurred.

From a mechanistic standpoint, salicylates cause damage in the overdose setting by uncoupling oxidative phosphorylation; in essence, the patient loses the ability to undergo aerobic metabolism. This can rapidly lead to clinical deterioration, particularly in young patients. Salicylate toxicity has three main stages: Patients normally start with a respiratory alkalosis, followed by a mixed respiratory alkalosis and metabolic acidosis, and ending with a mixed metabolic and respiratory acidosis. Initially, patients normally have a respiratory alkalosis due to direct stimulation of the respiratory center by the salicylates; this may lead to hyperpnea and/or tachypnea. As toxicity progresses, uncoupling of oxidative phosphorylation occurs, which leads to a mixed acid–base status with a metabolic acidosis and respiratory alkalosis. Finally, once the toxicity worsens to its final stage, patients become fatigued and can no longer sustain an appropriate respiratory alkalosis to balance the metabolic acidosis; at this point, patients become acidotic with a respiratory and metabolic acidosis. When the blood pH starts to decrease, more salicylate molecules are able to enter the brain which leads to deleterious outcomes.

Nausea and vomiting are often seen early after a large salicylate ingestion. Some patients may complain of tinnitus, whereas others state their hearing is muffled. Patients may complain of shortness of breath; this may be from hyperpnea or tachypnea or possible due to pulmonary edema secondary to direct salicylate toxicity. On physical examination, clinicians should pay close attention to vital signs. Increased respiratory rates are common, as is deep breathing. Clinicians should also pay very close attention to temperature; hyperthermia is a very poor prognostic indicator for patients with salicylate toxicity, and patients with elevated temperatures may have an unfortunate outcome, despite aggressive management. Patients can also have altered mental status, commonly secondary to neuroglycopenia.

When evaluating a patient for salicylate toxicity, laboratory studies are very important. Routine blood work should include a basic metabolic panel (BMP), blood gas, and salicylate level. One should also order an acetaminophen level because it is a common co-ingestant with salicylates and is otherwise difficult to detect. When looking at a patient's BMP, one may see a decrease in bicarbonate levels if the patient is becoming acidotic. In addition, some laboratory assays show false elevations in chloride levels if there is a large amount of salicylate in the serum. Blood gases are extremely important when assessing a patient with a salicylate ingestion. In early stages of salicylate toxicity, patients often will have a low pCO_2 and a pH that is slightly alkalotic. This will likely change as toxicity progresses, with the pH decreasing and pCO_2 eventually increasing as the patient begins to fatigue.

Salicylate levels are extremely useful in assessing patients with suspected salicylate overdoses. Peak serum concentration times vary depending on the formulation of the ingested substance. Liquid formulations, such as oil of wintergreen, tend to have rapid absorption and subsequent early peaks in serum levels. When pills are ingested, time to peak levels can vary. Typically, levels will start to rise within the first 4 hours of ingestion. However, clinicians should be careful in cases of polysubstance ingestions because gastric emptying may be delayed. Salicylates can cause pylorospasm and thus delay gastric emptying. Once levels start to rise, they should be trended until the patient has tolerated a PO trial and has two salicylate levels trending downwards, both of which are <20.

Treating patients with salicylate toxicity requires excellent supportive care. If the patient is hypoxic, supplemental oxygen should be administered. Because intubation impairs the ability of salicylate toxic patients to help buffer their serum pH, these patients should not be intubated until it becomes absolutely necessary. If a patient must be intubated, it should be performed by the most senior provider after providing adequate pre-oxygenation; ketamine may be a good medication to consider utilizing because it preserves respiratory drive. Prior to intubation, the provider should note what the patient's respiratory drive was prior to fatiguing and attempt to match it. An astute clinician will pay attention to both the ventilator rate and the tidal volume if a salicylate toxic patient requires intubation. Frequent blood gases should be obtained after intubation to ensure the patient's pH is not worsening.

In patients who are intravascularly depleted, a 20 mL/kg bolus of normal saline should be considered. Patients who are altered and have a blood sugar <300 mg/dL should receive a bolus of dextrose in an attempt to improve mentation; this is especially important with younger patients because they are more prone to neuroglycopenia. An ECG should also be obtained to ensure there are no abnormalities with the QRS and QTc intervals.

In patients with a patent airway or patients who are intubated, AC should be administered. Multiple doses may be beneficial because salicylates can form pharmacobezoars that delay absorption; multidose AC may decrease the amount of drug a patient will absorb systemically. Note, however, that salicylate overdose patients should not be intubated solely for the purpose of administering AC. WBI may be beneficial in patients with ingestions of pills containing salicylates; it should not be used if liquid forms of salicylates are ingested. The risks of performing WBI should be carefully considered before initiating this therapy.

One treatment for salicylate overdose is sodium bicarbonate. This is typically accomplished by giving a 1 mEq/kg bolus of sodium bicarbonate. After this, 3 ampules of sodium bicarbonate should be added to 850 mL of D5W and run at 1.5 times maintenance rate. This helps trap the salicylate ions in the urine, which aids in excretion; more important, it helps change serum pH and prevents the uncharged salicylate molecules from entering the brain and worsening toxicity.

In severe cases of salicylate overdoses, extracorporeal removal of salicylate should be considered. Guidelines typically recommend intermittent dialysis for salicylate levels >100 or levels >90 with impaired renal function. It is also recommended for patients with altered mentation, new-onset hypoxia, or a pH <7.2. However, if the initial salicylate level is elevated at 70 or higher and the patient does not look well clinically, involving nephrology early is recommended. Salicylate levels should be repeated hourly to monitor the rate of rise; a rapidly rising salicylate level in an ill-appearing patient should lead clinicians to consider prompt dialysis. If there are any questions regarding the proper treatment of patients with salicylate ingestions, the local toxicology team or poison control center should be contacted for further guidance.

Sulfonylureas

Sulfonylurea medications are available in several forms, including long-acting formulations. For several reasons, pediatric patients are at an increased risk for hypoglycemia when consuming these medications. First, pediatric patients have lower stores of glycogen compared with adults. In addition, children do not undergo gluconeogenesis as efficiently as adults. These two factors, combined with relatively higher mg/kg dosing with the ingestion of a single pill, amplify the probability that a sulfonylurea can cause problems in pediatric patients.

Sulfonylureas are commonly prescribed for patients with type II diabetes to increase the release of insulin. Sulfonylureas ultimately lead to a change in the membrane potential of the β islet cells of the pancreas and, through a cascade of events, lead to increased insulin release. If the body has too much insulin intravascularly, this can precipitate severe, and sometimes life-threatening, hypoglycemia.

Hypoglycemia manifests in several ways and can often imitate a myriad of medical conditions. Patients with hypoglycemia can have fatigue, somnolence, headache, anxiety, lethargy, focal neurologic deficits, and seizures. Whenever a patient presents with altered mentation, checking a glucose level is extremely important, especially if the patient may have been exposed to a sulfonylurea. If hypoglycemia is rapidly identified, it can usually be quickly corrected, leading to substantial clinical improvement.

Treating patients with sulfonylurea overdoses requires aggressive supportive care and diligent glucose checks. If a patient presents soon after ingesting a sulfonylurea, giving a dose of AC is suggested if the patient can safely tolerate it. Otherwise, GI decontamination is not generally recommended. If a patient presents with hypoglycemia but has a normal Glasgow Coma Scale score and can protect their airway, allowing the patient to eat or drink something with glucose is a very reasonable approach to help correct hypoglycemia. However, many patients with hypoglycemia are not able to protect their airway or tolerate a PO trial; these patients should receive dextrose-containing fluid. Younger patients should receive lower concentrations of dextrose, such as D5 or D10, to help minimize the risk of IV infiltration. Frequent fingerstick glucose checks should be done on patients with hypoglycemia, and if the glucose levels are still low, additional dextrose boluses should be administered. If a patient requires more than two boluses, dextrose-containing maintenance fluids should be initiated for sustained control of hypoglycemia.

If a patient has persistent hypoglycemia despite adequate dextrose administration, octreotide should be administered. Octreotide works by blocking calcium entrance into the β islet cells; this results in decreased endogenous insulin release. Dosing for pediatric patients is normally 1 μg/kg subcutaneously every 6 hours as needed, with a dose maximum of 50 μg/kg.

All children with a potential sulfonylurea ingestion should be admitted to the hospital for monitoring, even without hypoglycemia. Sulfonylureas can cause delayed hypoglycemia, and admission for 24 hours with frequent monitoring and glucose checks is recommended.

Tricyclic Antidepressants

Although the use of tricyclic antidepressants (TCAs) has decreased in recent years, overdoses on these medications can be catastrophic, especially in small children.

There are several mechanisms of toxicologic effects with TCA overdoses. Sodium channel blockade can lead to cardiac conduction disturbances. Interaction with GABA receptors can contribute to seizures. Blockade of α_1 receptors can cause hypotension and reflex tachycardia. Anticholinergic properties may also cause patients to become altered and have an anticholinergic toxidrome.

Patients with TCA overdoses will commonly be altered unless the ingestion was just prior to presentation. Significant TCA overdoses decompensate rapidly. Patients can develop altered mentation, tachycardia, hypotension, cardiac dysrhythmias, ECG changes, hemodynamic instability, and seizures. Any of these abnormalities should be rapidly identified and treated to prevent deleterious outcomes.

Rapid assessment and stabilization should occur after a TCA ingestion. Intubation is frequently required. Emergent ECG should be performed to evaluate for QRS prolongation.

Sodium bicarbonate is a mainstay of treatment for patients with TCA overdoses. Patients with a QRS >100 msec are at increased risk of seizure. Should the patient have a seizure, the blood pH will drop, which leads to increased toxicity. In an acidic environment, more uncharged drug is able to cross the blood–brain barrier, which worsens toxicity. By administering sodium bicarbonate, the QRS should improve due to the sodium in the solution, and the blood pH is improved by the bicarbonate. Typical bolus dosing for patients with a widened QRS interval is 1 or 2 mEq/kg. Bolus dosing can be repeated every few minutes until the QRS narrows. Once this is achieved, a sodium bicarbonate drip can be started with the goal to titrate to a blood pH between 7.50 and 7.55.

If a patient becomes hypotensive, norepinephrine is generally the preferred choice because it possesses more α agonism than epinephrine. This can increase vasoconstriction and improve blood pressure in hypotensive patients. If a patient has persistent cardiac dysrhythmias despite sodium bicarbonate, lidocaine can be considered; it may bind to the sodium channels more readily than TCAs and displace them. Patients with a widened QRS and/or a history of TCA ingestion should never receive physostigmine because fatalities have been reported in this patient cohort. Persistently hemodynamically unstable/peri-arrest patients should receive intralipid.

β-Blockers and Calcium Channel Blockers

Many older patients are on a number of medications that are extremely toxic to young children in very low doses. A grandparent's medication is also frequently more accessible to children through lack of childproofing in packaging and location.

Cardiac medications, particularly β-blockers and calcium channel blockers, can cause significant morbidity and potential mortality in a child. β-Blockers work by blocking the action of endogenous catecholamines at the β receptors in the heart. Calcium channel blockers, on the other hand, work by blocking the calcium channels in the heart. Non-dihydropyridine calcium channel blockers, such as verapamil and diltiazem, do this more effectively than dihydropyridine calcium channel blockers. Calcium channel blockers are able to directly decrease heart rate and blood pressure, whereas β-blockers primarily decrease heart rate, and hypotension is very rarely seen in the absence of bradycardia with β-blockers.

Patients with toxicity secondary to a β-blocker or calcium channel blocker overdose may present with lethargy, shortness of breath, chest discomfort, vomiting, and confusion. With certain medications, such as propranolol, seizures can occur. Patients will also likely present with hypotension and bradycardia with calcium channel blockers, although initial reflex tachycardia may be seen with dihydropyridine calcium channel blockers. For patients with β-blocker overdoses, bradycardia is common, and this may lead to subsequent hypotension. Hyperglycemia may be present in calcium channel blocker ingestion due to inhibition of insulin release from the pancreas.

Mild cases of calcium channel or β-blocker toxicity can be treated with supportive care. Crystalloid IV fluid boluses can improve blood pressure and heart rate. Atropine may transiently treat bradycardia but is short-acting and not always effective. Glucagon may improve hemodynamics after a β-blocker overdose but causes significant vomiting and can worsen the clinical picture; if glucagon is used, antiemetics should be given concomitantly.

Calcium increases cardiac inotropy and is commonly used to treat both calcium channel and β-blocker overdoses. Calcium gluconate is preferred in children due to the potential complication of vascular sclerosis with calcium chloride if extravasation occurs.

If patients have refractory hypotension despite the previously discussed therapies, high-dose insulin treatment is indicated. Although the exact mechanism is unclear, it is theorized to work by increasing delivery of glucose to the heart and by increasing contractility, which may cause improved hemodynamics. This therapy normally takes approximately 30–45 minutes to start working once it is initiated. Dosing for high-dose insulin therapy involves a 1 U/kg bolus of regular insulin, followed by 1 U/kg/hr dosing; depending on the patient's hemodynamic status, this can be titrated up to 10 U/kg/hr. Patients on this therapy should receive frequent glucose checks with a dextrose infusion. The insulin may have to be concentrated to avoid fluid overload.

Vasopressors may be required to manage hypotension and bradycardia. Vasopressors typically are started simultaneously with high-dose insulin, given their rapid onset, and are titrated down once the high-dose insulin starts to take effect. Epinephrine is commonly used in pediatrics for both β-blocker and calcium channel blocker overdoses; however, norepinephrine can also be used. Dosing for epinephrine is typically 0.05 μg/kg/min and can be titrated up to 1 μg/kg/min, depending on the patient's size.

In severe cases of β-blocker and calcium channel blocker overdose, some patients will unfortunately be refractory to all of the previously discussed therapies. In such cases, intralipid may be considered in a hemodynamically unstable or coding patient. However, extracorporeal membrane oxygenation is likely a more effective treatment, and it should be explored soon after a toxic patient arrives in the ED to maximize the likelihood of arranging treatment prior to the patient's decompensation.

GI decontamination is often helpful in patients with calcium channel blocker and β-blocker overdoses, especially if the medication is a long-acting drug. AC can be considered if the patient has an appropriate mental status. In cases of large verapamil or diltiazem overdoses, along with extended-release β-blockers, WBI may be beneficial. Delayed gut absorption may worsen a patient's clinical picture, and using WBI to decrease the gut burden of a drug may be life-saving. This should be considered on a case-by-case basis, and the local toxicology service or poison control center can assist in decision-making in these situations.

OPIOID OVERDOSES

The United States is currently facing an opioid epidemic, with countless individuals using both prescription and illicit opioids. Many older people have chronic pain, and a large number of them take opioid pain medication to help mitigate their symptoms. Ingestion of opioid medications in opioid-naive pediatric patients can be catastrophic. There are numerous formulations and concentrations of opioids on the market, including immediate- and extended-release preparations. Knowing the concentration of medication ingested and its formulation is critical for properly risk-stratifying patients, and asking these questions can help save a child's life.

Opioids work through a number of mechanisms, but the main therapeutic effect derives from agonism of the μ-receptors. In the overdose setting, patients frequently have respiratory depression, miosis, hypotension, bradycardia, and altered mental status. Fortunately, most patients with opioid overdoses do well if they are treated early and effectively. Supportive care, including airway support, is paramount. Naloxone is normally an effective antidote for opioids in an accidental ingestion setting, and dosing is 0.1 mg/kg/dose. In opioid-naive patients, providers should not be afraid of precipitated withdrawal so the disadvantages of naloxone are few in this setting. Patients who are apneic should be provided adequate bag mask ventilation prior to naloxone administration to help decrease the incidence of flash pulmonary edema.

When dispositioning a pediatric patient who ingested an opioid, risk-stratifying the patient based on the dose and formulation of medication is key. Any pediatric patient who may have ingested a long-acting opioid should be observed for 24 hours in the hospital with continuous oximetry and cardiac monitoring. Patients exposed to a single tablet of an immediate-release opioid, such as hydrocodone or oxycodone, should be monitored for a minimum of 6 hours. If a patient develops any symptoms during that time, the observation period is extended past 6 hours until they are back at baseline; providers should be sure patients are asymptomatic for a minimum of 6 hours since the last dose of naloxone. This is further complicated depending on the time of presentation to the ED. Providers who encounter patients with opioid ingestions who present to the ED at nighttime should strongly consider observing them until the morning, even if it past the 6-hour mark, because it is very difficult for families to assess a sleeping child for altered mental status and respiratory depression. Opioids can be extremely dangerous in the overdose setting, and providers should exercise caution when treating patients who have been exposed to these medications.

COMMON HOUSEHOLD ITEMS

There are countless items in the average household that, although they seem fairly innocuous because they are readily available, possess significant toxicity with exposures. When obtaining a history from a patient or family member, a skilled provider will remember to ask about any household substances with which the patient may have had contact. This will help increase the accuracy of the history and thereby allow the clinician to more rapidly and effectively treat the patient.

Eye drops are common in many households. Many eye drops contain chemicals that are members of the tetrahydrolozine family. These medications trigger peripheral α-receptors when used topically and cause vasoconstriction that helps remedy red eyes. However, when ingested, they can cause central α_2 agonism. This can lead to bradycardia, hypotension, bradypnea, and depressed mental status. This particular ingestion can mimic an opioid overdose, and providers should keep it on their differential diagnosis when working up a pediatric patient with altered mental status. Treatment is mainly supportive, although high-dose naloxone can be tried. This sometimes results in reversal of toxicity until the naloxone wears off; in some cases, high-dose naloxone may obviate the need for intubation in a small child.

Bleach is also common in most households. Household bleach usually contains sodium hypochlorite. If a small child drinks household bleach, the child will normally do very well provided only a small volume was consumed; larger volumes increase the likelihood of potential toxicity. If the bleach is industrial strength, its toxicity is significantly increased. When ingested, bleach can be very caustic and cause structural damage to the esophagus. If a child has ingested bleach, providers should be on the lookout for a triad of symptoms: vomiting, drooling, and stridor. If two of the three symptoms are present, a gastroenterologist should be consulted for an upper endoscopy to evaluate for any injury. If the patient has one or none of these symptoms, is well-appearing, and can tolerate PO without difficulty, it is unlikely they will go on to develop further toxicity. Treatment for bleach consumption is typically supportive.

Although the majority of people do not realize it, toxic alcohols are common in many homes. Ethylene glycol is one of the main ingredients in antifreeze, and methanol is commonly added to dry gas and certain windshield washer fluids. Just one sip of any of these substances is enough to cause severe toxicity in a pediatric patient. These substances can lead to a high anion gap metabolic acidosis. Ethylene glycol can cause renal injury, whereas methanol can lead to ocular toxicity. Any patient who has a suspected ingestion should receive an immediate workup that includes a BMP, venous blood gas, and measured serum osmolality; ethylene glycol and methanol levels are helpful, but many institutions cannot obtain these in a clinically significant timely manner. If the patient has any signs of acidosis or an elevated osmolality gap, the patient should be treated with fomepizole. Patients with methanol ingestions can be given folic acid, and patients with ethylene glycol ingestions can be given thiamine and pyridoxine to help augment metabolism of toxic metabolites. Ultimately, most patients with elevated ethylene glycol or methanol levels, or those with a large osmolality gap and metabolic acidosis, will need dialysis, so contacting a nephrologist early is advantageous to help prevent delays in care.

Hydrofluoric acid is also available in many homes. It is contained in many rust removers and wheel cleaners. Highly concentrated hydrofluoric acid is extremely toxic, and significant toxicity can result even from small dermal exposures. As little as 2% body surface area exposure of concentrated hydrofluoric acid can make patients extremely ill. Hydrofluoric acid is a weak acid and exerts its toxicity when the fluoride anion binds to positive cations, such as calcium and magnesium, in the body. This can produce localized pain and, more important, can lead to severe hypocalcemia and hypomagnesemia; the latter two can cause lethal cardiac dysrhythmias. An ECG should be obtained and trended to ensure no cardiac toxicity is arising. Any exposure to hydrofluoric acid should be taken very seriously with local decontamination. Large-bore IVs should be established because large doses of calcium and magnesium may need to be administered to help prevent a deleterious outcome. Any hydrofluoric acid exposure should prompt a call to the local toxicology group or poison center for further advice on management.

ONE PILL KILLS

A number of medications can be lethal in very small amounts. The weight of the patient plays a major role in determining lethality of a substance with a single dose; lighter patients are more likely to become toxic because the mg/kg dose is higher. Most "one pill kill" substances have a low minimum lethal dose, which means the mg/kg dose expected to cause toxicity can be rapidly achieved by ingesting a small amount of substance. Prescription medications, over-the-counter medications, supplements, and household chemicals can all lead to severe toxicity and possibly death with relatively small ingestions. A number of these medications were mentioned previously, including β-blockers, calcium channel blockers, sulfonylureas, opioids, oil of wintergreen, toxic alcohols, and hydrofluoric acid. There are many others, and a few are mentioned in this section.

A number of prescription drugs can cause death with an ingestion of as little as one pill, including antidepressant medications. As previously mentioned, TCAs can easily lead to mortality at low doses. Another medication class that can lead to severe toxicity at low doses is the monoamine oxidase inhibitors (MAOIs). These medications have a narrow therapeutic window; thus, toxicity can occur at relatively low doses. Certain MAOIs can be life-threatening at doses as little as 2 or 3 mg/kg. MAOIs such as phenelzine are available in 15-mg tablets. Therefore, if a 15-kg child takes two tablets of this medication, there is the potential for severe toxicity.

MAOIs work by preventing the breakdown of catecholamines; this in turn leads to an increase in epinephrine, norepinephrine, serotonin, and dopamine. When this occurs, a hyperadrenergic state ensues. This can manifest with fever, tachycardia, dysrhythmias, hypertension, diaphoresis, and seizures. In the most severe cases, patients can develop hemodynamic instability. Unfortunately, no antidote exists for MAOI ingestions. Rather, good supportive care is paramount. Some of these patients will require multiple doses of benzodiazepines for adequate control of symptoms. Unless the patient is actively seizing, using agents such as midazolam or diazepam is recommended; both of these have rapid times to onset, and using them may prevent dose stacking of medications. Patients may need active cooling if they become hyperthermic.

Antimalarials are another type of medication that can be lethal at low doses. Medications such as chloroquine can be extremely lethal in low doses. Chloroquine works by subduing sodium currents. These medications can lead to central nervous system (CNS) depression, seizures, hypotension, and dysrhythmias. QRS widening may be seen, and sodium bicarbonate may be a beneficial therapy to try if this occurs. Seizures should be treated with benzodiazepines, and this may also be advantageous if the patient has any agitation or tachycardia. Vasopressor may be required as well. Although not a first-line therapy, if a patient has cardiovascular collapse, intralipid should be considered.

Clove oil is a substance that is lethal in minuscule amounts. Many people use clove oil as a local anesthetic to treat ailments such as tooth pain. For a small child, consuming as little as 5 mL of concentrated clove oil can result in significant morbidity and mortality. The compound in clove oil that is responsible for toxicity is eugenol. After metabolism, eugenol's metabolites are hepatotoxic. However, studies suggest that damage can be mitigated if NAC is administered soon after the ingestion. High anion gap metabolic acidosis can sometimes arise with ingestion of this substance, although the exact mechanism for its origin is unknown. Clove oil ingestion may also lead to CNS depression; in some cases, mentation becomes so altered that intubation is required.

Isoniazid is extremely dangerous at low doses, and it can cause severe toxicity with minute doses. Isoniazid is commonly used by individuals being treated for tuberculosis. Although an exact pediatric dose of toxicity has not been established, extrapolating from adult data of toxicity starting at 35–40 mg/kg, a 10-kg patient could become critically ill if four or five tablets are ingested. The amount of GABA in the brain is decreased in the overdose setting, and this can lead to life-threatening seizures that may be resistant to benzodiazepines; pyridoxine administration should be strongly considered for any suspected isoniazid ingestions because it helps restore GABA and terminate seizure activity.

A number of other substances can also have catastrophic consequences in low doses. If questions or concerns arise regarding the lethality of a substance, providers should immediately call a poison control center for guidance.

RECREATIONAL DRUG USE AND DRUG SCREENING

Recreational drug use is highly prevalent in the United States. Chemists and drug dealers are extremely adept at creating new drugs or adding substances to existing drugs; this means a shrewd provider must be on the lookout for different toxidromes and patterns to help with drug recognition. This section presents a brief discussion of some of the more commonly used drugs of abuse and different management options.

Two of the most commonly used stimulant drugs are cocaine and amphetamines. These drugs lead to increased levels of catecholamines. If either of these drugs is used in isolation, a sympathomimetic toxidrome normally occurs. However, if either of these "upper" drugs is mixed with a "downer" (e.g., heroin), a mixed clinical picture can result. Patients who present with a sympathomimetic toxidrome are normally managed with good supportive care, including IV benzodiazepines (preferably midazolam or diazepam due to their rapid onset).

As many US states move to legalize marijuana, either medicinally or recreationally or both, it stands to reason that accidental ingestions of marijuana may arise. The active component of marijuana, tetrahydrocannabinol (THC), is commonly used in many edible products. Concentrations of THC vary with each product, and it is difficult to predict the clinical effects if a young pediatric patient consumes even small amounts of an edible product. Pediatric patients who accidentally ingest THC-containing products can have a number of findings, including altered mental status, slurred speech, nystagmus, ataxia, and decreased respiratory drive. Treatment is largely supportive.

Vaping is a relatively new phenomenon that bears mentioning given the recent increase in e-cigarette or vaping product use associated lung injury (EVALI). Although most EVALI injuries occur in patients who vape THC, they have occurred in patients who exclusively vape nicotine products. The exact pathophysiology of illness is unknown, but many believe it is due in part to the excipients in the vaping solution. Patients with EVALI can have a myriad of symptoms and signs on examination, including shortness of breath, decreased exercise tolerance, decreased oxygen saturations, and bilateral ground glass opacities. Treatment is largely supportive, and this disease process is a diagnosis of exclusion. However, in confirmed cases of EVALI, steroids may improve the clinical course. Consultation with the local toxicology group or poison control center may help with diagnosis and disposition.

One final item that bears mentioning is the utility of urine drug screens (UDS). UDS are often routinely ordered by providers for any child with altered mental status. As with any test, the provider should have a clinical question they are trying to answer with the UDS. UDS frequently have false positives and false negatives, and they are rarely useful in clinical decision-making for an acutely ill patient. It is essential to remember that a positive test does not necessarily mean the patient is actively intoxicated and a negative test does not mean a patient is not intoxicated; rather, the decision regarding drug intoxication should be based on a clinical examination. Cocaine normally does not have false positives; however, a positive result may simply mean the patient used cocaine within the past 3 days, so clinical correlation is required. UDS may be helpful if there are concerns for potential child abuse/neglect, and providers may want to send positive results for confirmatory testing. If a provider is concerned for recreational drug ingestion but the UDS is negative, a comprehensive drug screen (with greater sensitivity and specificity) can be ordered, although this normally takes several days to obtain results and is often followed by the admitting team or outpatient pediatrician.

Further Reading

Nelson LS, Howland MA, Lewin NA, Smith SW, Goldfrank LR, Hoffman RS. eds. *Goldfrank's Toxicologic Emergencies*. 11th ed. New York: McGraw-Hill; 2019.

51

Drowning

MARK ZHANG AND EMILY ROSE

INTRODUCTION

Drowning is the second leading cause of accidental death in children worldwide (after motor vehicle accidents). In addition, many children survive drowning events—some without significant sequelae, whereas others survive neurologically devastated. The challenge for emergency providers is to successfully and adequately resuscitate potential survivors while ensuring an optimal neurological outcome.

Drowning is most common in children younger than age 5 years (associated with inadequate supervision or inappropriate barriers) and adolescents and young adults between the ages of 15 and 25 (associated with risk-taking behaviors). Epilepsy is associated with a 10-fold increase in risk of drowning. Cold water immersion may precipitate arrhythmia in congenital long QT syndrome type 1 and lead to a drowning event in an otherwise good swimmer.

Approximately half of all drowning events occur in swimming pools. Approximately half of all infant drownings occur in bathtubs and have a significant association with child neglect or even inflicted injury (see Chapter 53 on child abuse).

MANAGEMENT

Early continuous cardiopulmonary resuscitation (CPR) is extremely important for the prehospital care of the acutely drowned patient. Routine cervical spine immobilization is not required unless significant trauma is suspected.

In the emergency department, resuscitation of the acutely drowned patient is primarily respiratory and supportive care. Aspiration of liquid washes out surfactant, and patients may develop bronchospasm, pulmonary edema, shunting, and persistent hypoxia. Hypoxic insult may result in multiorgan system failure. All symptomatic patients should be admitted to the hospital after a drowning event because significant pulmonary irritation and edema may occur.

Oxygen should be administered if hypoxia is present. Patients may develop acute bronchospasm from pulmonary irritation which may require bronchodilators. Positive pressure ventilation may be required to assist in ventilator effort and oxygenation. Intubation may be required in the unresponsive, apneic, or those in severe distress. Ventilator settings should be lung protective with tidal volumes of 5 or 6 mL/kg.

Circulatory support should be given. Active warming, intravenous fluid resuscitation, and vasopressors should be administered as indicated. Mild hypothermia (32–35°C) may be passively rewarmed with warm fluids, warm/humidified oxygen, active movement, and passive external warming (removing wet clothing, blankets). Moderate hypothermia (28–32°C) will require (in addition to the previous suggestions) cardiac monitoring, minimization of movements to prevent arrhythmias, and both active external (heating blankets, forced air) and minimally invasive rewarming techniques (bladder lavage). For the severely hypothermic patient (<28°C), consider yet more invasive warming techniques (peritoneal or thoracic lavage) and extracorporeal membrane oxygenation (ECMO). In general, patients with circulatory compromise (systolic blood pressure <90 mmHg or ventricular arrhythmias), core temperatures of <28°C, and no obvious coexisting conditions (e.g., trauma) can be candidates for ECMO. There is no benefit to prophylactic antibiotics or steroids after a drowning event.

The underlying etiology of the drowning event should be considered and if a possible underlying medical trauma condition exists that should be concomitantly treated. Underlying cardiac arrhythmias (particularly prolonged QT syndrome), seizure disorder, or other medical emergency may have triggered the drowning event. Both the medical history and the physical examination should investigate for the potential of underlying conditions and the possibility of traumatic injury, particularly non-accidental injury in a younger child and spinal cord injury in an older child.

Labs and imaging are not routinely indicated after a drowning incident. However, a child requiring resuscitation should have both obtained to assist with critical care. The chest X-ray findings do not directly correlate with clinical severity. It requires approximately 11 mL/kg of aspirated material to impact volume status and double that amount to impact electrolytes; most drowning victims aspirate approximately 3 or 4 mL/kg of liquid (or may have laryngospasm and not aspirate any liquid). Hypoxic injury can cause insult to any organ, and sequelae include multiorgan system failure and elevated intracranial pressure. These complications require supportive management.

LENGTH OF RESUSCITATION

Each individual drowning event is unique, and there is no one risk factor that reliably predicts outcome. The age and underlying health of the patient, circumstances of the drowning event, length of time in the water, temperature of the water, and time to initiation of CPR all contribute to the ultimate outcome. There are multiple case reports of excellent outcomes despite prolonged submersion times. These cases all had significant hypothermia and utilized ECMO for continued resuscitation and support. Excepting the hypothermic patient, prolonged resuscitation after drowning events typically results in a neurologically devastated survivor. The literature supports the conclusion that resuscitation for >30 minutes in warm water submersions or >60 minutes in ice-water submersions or requiring three doses of epinephrine is unlikely to result in a neurologically good outcome. But be wary of the hypothermic patient. This patient is potentially salvageable with a good outcome if resuscitated well with the assistance of ECMO, particularly if early CPR was administered and hypoxia occurred prior to the onset of ischemic injury.

HYPOTHERMIA

Hypothermia on presentation warrants a focused discussion. Hypothermia is neuroprotective *only* when it occurs prior to the onset of ischemia. In most drowning incidents, a hypothermic patient simply correlates with a prolonged immersion time. Notably, there are many case reports of patients with severe hypothermia (core temperature as low at 13.7°C) who have survived with excellent neurologic outcome. The most impressive survival cases utilized ECMO early and had good outcomes despite prolonged resuscitation efforts (up to 9 hours). Early mobilization of resources and initiation of ECMO in a hypothermic drowning patient are critical to optimal outcomes in the appropriate patient. Resuscitation of a hypothermic patient should continue until the patient is rewarmed to approximately 32°C and absence of cardiac motion confirmed by bedside ultrasound (if available).

KEY POINTS

- Witnessed submersions with short time to resuscitation have the best prognosis.

- Prolonged CPR and epinephrine requirements are poor prognosticators.
- Pediatric drowning victims do not need routine cervical immobilization.
- The child who is able to follow commands has a nearly 100% survival rate.
- Patients may be discharged with a normal pulmonary examination and oxygenation 4 hours after the drowning event.
- Symptomatic patients should be admitted after a drowning event.

PITFALLS

- Failure to consider foul play, particularly in bathtub drownings
- Failure to consider a traumatic or medical etiology of drowning
- Failure to rewarm the patient to 32°C prior to terminating the resuscitation
- Failure to admit patients with hypoxemia or pulmonary symptoms

52

Mental Health Emergencies

GENEVIEVE SANTILLANES AND SHILPA AGRAHARKAR

INTRODUCTION

A substantial and increasing proportion of emergency department (ED) visits by children and adolescents are related to mental health disorders. Although diagnosing specific psychiatric disorders is not realistic during brief ED visits, emergency medicine clinicians are responsible for the initial evaluation and stabilizing treatment for patients with mental health emergencies. Emergency medicine clinicians must distinguish whether behavioral signs and symptoms result from a psychiatric disorder or another process such as intoxication or an underlying non-psychiatric illness. In many EDs without readily available mental health consultants, emergency medicine clinicians provide initial treatment of severe symptoms and must determine which patients can be safely discharged without emergent evaluation by a mental health professional and which patients require emergent mental health consultation or transfer to a specialized center for further evaluation. For patients with milder symptoms, emergency medicine clinicians should also be able to discuss options for outpatient mental health treatment. Because training in pediatric mental health is typically limited, many emergency medicine clinicians feel unprepared to treat pediatric mental health disorders. In this chapter, we provide a framework for clinicians in the approach to children and adolescents with mental health emergencies.

Comparison with Adults

Assessment of the child or adolescent with mental health complaints varies from the assessment of adults in multiple dimensions. Many mental health disorders present very differently in children and adults. Youth with mental health disorders often present with somatic symptoms and may be unable to verbalize their feelings. Clinicians accustomed to caring for adults may not recognize depression or trauma-related symptoms, for example, in a young child because the manifestations are quite distinct from a typical adult presentation. The differential diagnosis varies by age; certain disorders, such as schizophrenia, are uncommon prior to later adolescence and would be very unusual in a prepubertal child.

Children's words and actions must be interpreted in light of their developmental status. Their understanding of events is critical. Children may demonstrate risky behavior without understanding that the behavior is dangerous. Or they may report negative thoughts as "hearing voices."

Although an assessment for exposure to events with the potential to cause psychological trauma is important in patients of all ages, it is critical in youth with behavioral and mental health complaints. Last, the home environment must be assessed. Parents or other caretakers must be capable of monitoring the child and obtaining any needed follow-up care.

ANXIETY

Background

Anxiety disorders are the most common mental health disorders with a lifetime prevalence of approximately 30%. Initial presentation of anxiety disorders often occurs in childhood. Key features of specific anxiety disorders are presented in Box 52.1.

Anxiety disorders can be challenging to recognize because fear and worry are normal. Particularly in children, transient fears are a common and normal phase of development. Anxiety disorders occur when worries and fears are persistent, excessive, and lead to distress or impairment of normal functioning. Consideration of developmental stage is critical in determining if symptoms are consistent with an anxiety disorder or a normal developmental stage. Significant distress with every brief separation from a parent is normal in 9- to 12-month-old infants but would not be typical in a 4-year-old child.

Classic Clinical Presentation

Children and adolescents with anxiety commonly present to EDs with somatic complaints. Typical complaints are abdominal pain, nausea, headache, chest discomfort, and shortness of breath. Symptoms are frequently chronic and recurrent. Typically, pediatric patients with somatic symptoms of anxiety are school-age through adolescent patients. Frequently, patients have been previously seen in the ED or other medical settings for similar symptoms. Patients may present both for management of pain or other uncomfortable symptoms and for evaluation to determine the cause of the symptoms.

Atypical Clinical Presentations

Another potential presentation in the patient with an anxiety disorder is a behavioral outburst when faced with an anxiety-provoking situation (e.g., a patient with out-of-control behavior when about to be left at a new school for the first time). Upon review of the events leading up to the incident once the patient is calmer, it may be evident that the patient has chronic symptoms of anxiety and that severe anxiety precipitated the behavioral outburst.

Patients may also present with panic attacks. Panic attacks present with some combination of the following symptoms: chest pain or discomfort, rapid heart rate, nausea or vomiting, a choking sensation, shortness of breath,

BOX 52.1

ANXIETY DISORDERS

Generalized anxiety disorder: Persistent, excessive worry about multiple domains that causes distress or interferes with normal functioning

Separation anxiety disorder: Persistent fears around separation from parents that often leads to clinginess and school refusal; can lead to somatic symptoms due to separation or anticipated separation

Panic disorder: Recurrent panic attacks

Social anxiety disorder: Persistent anxiety about social situations or being embarrassed or judged by others

Phobias: Excessive and persistent fear of a specific object or situation that can lead to avoidance behaviors

Agoraphobia: Persistent fear of multiple situations in which escape from the situation would be difficult; often leads to avoidance or a need to be accompanied by another person

hyperventilation, carpopedal spasms, lightheadedness, facial or hand numbness, shaking, sweating, and a fear that one is dying.

Differential Diagnosis

Somatic symptoms of anxiety are often nonspecific and may overlap with symptoms also seen in other medical disorders, particularly disorders with chronic, recurrent symptoms. Disorders to consider include the following:

- Primary and secondary causes of headache
- Abdominal migraine
- Gastrointestinal disorders
- Arrhythmias
- Asthma and other respiratory disorders
- Hyperthyroidism
- Pheochromocytoma (rare)

Medical disorders to consider in patients with symptoms of a panic attack include the following:

- Hyperthyroidism
- Electrolyte abnormalities causing carpopedal spasm: hypocalcemia, hypokalemia, hypophosphatemia, and hypomagnesemia
- Diabetic ketoacidosis, aspirin overdose, or other causes of acidosis leading to rapid breathing
- Asthma and other respiratory disorders
- Arrhythmias
- Intoxication or drug withdrawal
- Other cardiovascular disorders
- Pheochromocytoma (rare)
- Pulmonary embolism (rare in children and adolescents)

Treatment

When treating panic attacks or acute behavioral outbursts due to severe anxiety, coaching patients in slow deep breathing or other behavioral techniques often suffices to help patients calm themselves. A small dose of a benzodiazepine in the ED may sometimes be appropriate for the patient with an acute panic attack to help them relax and focus on behavioral calming techniques. However, benzodiazepines should not be prescribed for home use. Discuss behavioral techniques for use at home with the patient and caregiver.

If anxiety is recognized as the etiology of symptoms, unnecessary and potentially harmful testing and treatment can be avoided. Patients and families can be reassured that symptoms are not due to a dangerous underlying physical disorder. Emphasize that somatic symptoms are not imagined or faked. Convey that you understand that the symptoms are distressing and do not minimize their discomfort. One approach is to discuss how stress and anxiety affect the nervous system, resulting in uncomfortable physical sensations such as headache or abdominal pain. Many families believe that mental health disorders are stigmatizing. It is important to normalize mental health disorders and emphasize that mental health disorders are common and treatable but that without appropriate treatment can lead to significant morbidity.

Ongoing treatment of anxiety disorders is best managed by the patient's primary physician or a mental health clinician. If possible, provide outpatient mental health resources to discharged patients. Cognitive–behavioral therapy is effective in the treatment of anxiety disorders. Selective serotonin reuptake inhibitors are also effective, but they should be prescribed by a clinician who is able to follow up with the patient and monitor response. It is appropriate for the emergency clinician to discuss outpatient treatment so that patients and families are aware that effective treatment options are available and are motivated to seek outpatient treatment.

Disposition

Usual disposition is home. Admission is indicated if an emergent medical etiology warranting admission cannot be excluded. Admission may also be indicated for coexisting suicidality.

Complications

Untreated anxiety tends to be a chronic, remitting disorder. Children and adolescents with untreated anxiety are more likely to develop depression and substance use disorders. Lost productivity due to anxiety often manifests in children as poor school performance, school refusal, or absenteeism. Anxiety disorders may also result in difficulties with social interactions.

Patients with anxiety are, of course, still at risk of other medical illnesses. Attributing new or changing symptoms to the patient's underlying anxiety could result in a missed or delayed diagnosis. On the other hand, unrecognized anxiety manifesting as somatic complaints can lead to unnecessary medical workups and treatments that can be costly, painful, and associated with risks of side effects and complications.

Key Points

- Anxiety is common in children and adolescents.
- Anxiety often presents with somatic complaints such as abdominal pain, chest discomfort, or headache.
- Evaluate patients with new or changing symptoms to ensure that a coexisting medical disorder is not present.
- Emphasize to patients and families that symptoms are not imagined or faked.
- Normalize anxiety and other mental health disorders and emphasize that effective treatment is available.

Pitfalls

- Attributing symptoms of a medical disorder to anxiety
  - Somatic symptoms of anxiety are nonspecific and overlap with symptoms of other medical disorders.
  - A thorough history and physical examination often reveal clues to medical illness.
- Excessive workup when history and examination are most consistent with anxiety
- ED prescription of ongoing benzodiazepines or other sedatives

DEPRESSION AND SUICIDALITY

Background

Childhood depression and suicidal ideation are on the rise, with visits to pediatric EDs for suicidal ideation or suicide attempts doubling from 2007 to 2015. Depression is increasingly common among adolescents, with almost one in eight adolescents experiencing at least one depressive episode in the past calendar year. Furthermore, suicide is the second leading cause of death among adolescents. The majority of adolescents with depression are not in treatment, and the prevalence of depression and suicidal ideation continues to rise. Suicidal ideation among preteens and children is also on the rise. One recent study found that 7% of children presenting to pediatric EDs for medical complaints screen positive on a suicide screening tool. Emergency clinicians increasingly see children with depression and suicidal ideation either as presenting complaints or as part of their clinical picture. With many hospitals lacking readily accessible child, or even adult, psychiatrists, care falls to ED clinicians.

Classic Clinical Presentation

The classic clinical presentation of depression in children and adolescents is very different than that seen in adults. Adolescents are much more likely than children to present with depression. Among adolescents, more than children, the presentation of depression can be similar to a typical adult presentation, with vocalized depressed mood, crying, and sadness. Adolescents with depression are more likely to present with a variety of rebellious behaviors. Like adults, substance use and abuse can also be comorbid; depression and suicidal ideation are much more dangerous when substance use is involved, likely due to an increase in impulsive behaviors.

Often, and more frequently than in adults, children and adolescents with depression complain of somatic symptoms, such as abdominal pain, frequent headaches, or other minor pain. Somatic symptoms may, in fact, be the reason for ED presentation. Particularly with children, this is likely because they are unable to articulate their feelings as adults or adolescents could.

Atypical Clinical Presentation

Less than 2% of children younger than age 12 years have a diagnosis of depression. Most often, there is a stressor that can be pinpointed, in addition to symptoms of depressed mood, irritability, tearfulness, difficulty concentrating, feeling worthless, fatigue, appetite changes, and difficulty sleeping. Often, the child does not disclose a change in mood but, rather, comes to clinical attention after an episode of self-harm, suicide attempt, or a significant change in behavior. Irritability is seen much more frequently in children and adolescents with depression than in adults.

Children also frequently present with psychotic features, often stating that they are "hearing voices" saying negative things about them. These auditory hallucinations, when probed further, are frequently simply negative self-thoughts. The irritability and psychotic complaints often lead to a misdiagnosis of bipolar disorder or schizophrenia. In adults, these symptoms may be evidence of a bipolar or psychotic disorder, whereas in children they are a classic presentation of depression.

Differential Diagnosis

Differential diagnosis is broad and depends on the specific presentation. Medical conditions that can mask as depression include hypothyroidism, severe anemia, viral illnesses including mononucleosis, and vitamin D or folate deficiency. Psychiatrically, many disorders share symptoms with depression. A careful screening for trauma is always important, but it is particularly important with children who may be depressed. Depressed and irritable youth with a history of trauma may be suffering from posttraumatic stress disorder (PTSD), and treatment should then be tailored to PTSD. More important, children need to be assessed for ongoing abuse and to ensure current safety. Substance abuse can mimic or coexist with depression, necessitating an assessment for substance use. Anxiety is very frequently comorbid with depression, and treating one without treating the other would be inadequate. As mentioned previously, psychotic features are frequently present, and although rare, it is important to rule out bipolar disorder or psychosis.

Treatment

First and foremost is risk assessment. The primary goal for the emergency clinician is to ensure that if the child is discharged, they are not at imminent risk of harm to self or others. If the emergency clinician believes that discharge is not safe, the child requires emergent evaluation by a mental health clinician or arrangement for inpatient care. If a child is determined to be safe for discharge, the next goal is to ensure that the child is connected to ongoing treatment with a mental health clinician for treatment, including therapy. Options for therapy include cognitive–behavioral therapy, interpersonal therapy, supportive therapy, and others. Selective serotonin reuptake inhibitors are the first-line medications. A discussion of options for outpatient treatment is appropriate, but medication should be prescribed by a psychiatrist or pediatrician who has an ongoing outpatient relationship with the child.

Clinical Algorithm

When a child presents to the ED with depression, the ED clinician must assess if the child is suicidal. A quick and helpful suicide risk screening tool is the ASQ (Box 52.2). The ASQ toolkit is available at no cost on the National Institute of Mental Health's website (see Further Reading). The toolkit includes the screen, suggested scripts for clinicians, and a guide for further evaluation of patients who screen positive.

Suicidal ideation can be active or passive. Patients with active suicidal ideation want to kill themselves. Patients with passive suicidal

BOX 52.2

ASQ SUICIDE RISK SCREENING TOOL

1. In the past few weeks, have you wished you were dead?
2. In the past few weeks, have you felt that you or your family would be better off if you were dead?
3. In the past week, have you been having thoughts about killing yourself?
4. Have you ever tried to kill yourself? If yes, how? When?

If the patient answers YES to any of the above, ask the following acuity question:

5. Are you having thoughts of killing yourself right now? If yes, please describe.

Source: Questions reproduced from the ASQ Suicide Risk Screening Tool. The screening tool and other materials are freely available on the National Institutes of Mental Health website at https://www.nimh.nih.gov/research/research-conducted-at-nimh/asq-toolkit-materials/index.shtml.

ideation have thoughts that they do not care if they live or die, but not that they want to kill themselves. For example, an individual with passive suicidal ideation might say "I just don't want to be alive anymore," whereas an individual with active suicidal ideation would say "I want to kill myself." If there is concern for suicidal ideation, a psychiatrist, if available, should be consulted. If a psychiatrist is not accessible, the ED clinician will need to begin a risk assessment.

Components of the risk assessment include the following:

- Collateral information from the family or caregiver
  - Necessary whether or not they accompanied patient
  - Find out the caregiver's understanding of how the child is doing and elicit the caregiver's concerns
- Access to lethal means of suicide
  - Ask the child and caregiver
  - Ensure lethal methods are secured regardless of disposition
- Assess if suicidal ideation is passive or active
- If active suicidal ideation
  - Consult a psychiatrist
  - Assess if they have a method (means of hurting themselves) such as an overdose or jump from a height
  - Assess if they have a plan (e.g., "I would jump off the roof in my apartment building, which I know is unlocked.")
- Assess for intent (they had the intention of carrying out their plan until for whatever reason they stopped)

In addition to details about the suicidal ideation, consider other risk factors when making a decision about safety.

Chronic risk factors include the following:

- Prior suicide attempt
  - Greatest risk factor
  - Carefully evaluate patients with a history of suicide attempt for current suicidal ideation
- Lower socioeconomic status
- Fewer social supports or social obligations
- Parental conflict
- Family history of suicide death

The following are other risk factors:

- Recent suicides in the news or at their school
- Recent loss of relationship
- Pain
- Severe anxiety
- Recent medical diagnosis
- Feeling of being a burden
- Escalating self-harm

Disposition

Disposition depends on the evaluating clinician's evaluation of the child's risk. Determining low, medium, or high risk of suicide requires a careful consideration of all acute and chronic risk factors, along with supportive factors that mitigate risk. Actively suicidal patients with plan and intent are likely to be high risk for suicide and are unlikely to be safe for discharge. Children with depression who deny suicidal ideation are more likely to be at low or moderate risk for suicide; discharge is likely to be appropriate if the caregiver agrees and wants to take the child home.

Without outpatient care, it is unlikely that depression will self-resolve, and the patient may present again with worsening depression or even suicidal ideation. Discharged low-risk patients should be given a referral or a list of clinics to contact for an appointment. At the very least, the pediatrician should be informed that the child was evaluated for depression so that the pediatrician can make a referral. For discharged patients deemed to be at moderate risk, a follow-up appointment should be given. If that is not possible, give a list of clinics that provide children's mental health services and arrange a telephone check-in by an ED clinician because even telephone follow-up soon after a crisis has been shown to lower suicide risk.

In addition, for patients with depression or suicidal ideation who are discharged, a staff member should assist the patient and caregiver to make a safety plan. Ideally, the staff person would be a social worker or another clinician comfortable making safety plans with children. A safety plan is not a "contract for safety" but, rather, helps the child and family plan ahead so that symptoms do not worsen in the future.

Safety plans include the following:

- Thinking about and listing triggers
- Thinking about and listing coping skills
- Naming people and places that help the child feel better or can be resources
  - If already connected to therapy, this should include the therapist
- A crisis number the child can call
- Thinking of ways to make the environment safer
  - Removing lethal means of harm such as guns, knives, and pills

If a child is deemed to be at high risk of suicide, a psychiatric admission should be strongly considered. Legal requirements for involuntary psychiatric admission vary by state but generally are based on safety concerns for the child or for others.

Complications

Suicide and suicide attempt are the most significant and most dangerous complications of depression. Suicide is the second leading cause of death for adolescents in the United States, and approximately 4% of adolescents have made a suicide attempt. Furthermore, almost one in five adolescents has engaged in nonsuicidal self-injury, such as cutting or scratching without any intent of killing themselves, often as a result of depression.

Other complications of depression include an increase in substance use and other risky behaviors. Comorbid substance abuse is particularly dangerous because substance use increases impulsivity, which increases the likelihood of suicide. Lower school attendance, a decline in grades, obesity, and increased social isolation and withdrawal can also complicate depression.

Universal Suicide Screening

Universal screening for suicidal ideation in EDs is extremely important in prevention of suicide, particularly because many adolescents may not see primary care doctors regularly. Although suicide is often associated with depression, it can also occur in many other psychiatric disorders. The ASQ (see Box 52.2) frequently identifies suicidality in children without a history or current diagnosis of depression.

Key Points

- Depression in children rarely presents with an expressed complaint of low mood.
  - Typical symptoms include irritability, auditory hallucinations, and somatic complaints.
  - Adolescents may present similarly to children or adults.
- Risk assessment is the most important task for EDs.
- Medications should be initiated by a clinician with an ongoing relationship and ability to follow up with the child.
- Give discharged patients a list of clinics providing outpatient mental health treatment.

Pitfalls

- Failing to do a suicide screen on all adolescents
  - Suicide screening identifies at-risk youth presenting for other reasons.
- Assuming symptoms are not due to depression if a child does not endorse a low mood
- Failing to provide appropriate follow-up

PSYCHOSIS

Background

Psychosis is a symptom, not a diagnosis. Psychosis is a break with reality in which a patient has difficulty determining what is real and what is not. They may hear auditory hallucinations or see visual hallucinations, or they may believe that things happening in the world around them have greater salience or meaning than is actually true. For example, if two people in a row are wearing a red backpack, they may place importance on the color red and believe there is a meaning to it. Or if several people on the street happen to look up at the patient, the patient may become paranoid, believing that people are after them or want to hurt them. These can be very terrifying experiences for the individual having them.

Classical Clinical Presentation

Many other psychiatric disorders that are much more common in children and adolescents than schizophrenia and bipolar disorder can present with symptoms of psychosis or symptoms mimicking psychosis. Consider these other diagnoses first when evaluating a child with psychotic symptoms.

Major depressive disorder and generalized anxiety disorder can present with psychotic features, and patients frequently complain of auditory hallucinations. When probed, the "hallucinations" are frequently negative thoughts about self or anxious worries that present to the child as auditory hallucinations. For example, a child with significant anxiety around peers may report hearing voices that say "No one in school likes you." This may initially sound psychotic, but if probed further, frequently the patient is able to state that these are their own anxious, often overwhelming, negative thoughts about themselves.

Obsessive–compulsive disorder (OCD) frequently appears similar to a primary psychotic process. Patients may experience anxious negative self thoughts but also frequently have rigid obsessions and compulsions that appear to be psychotic in nature. For example, a patient with OCD may hoard bizarre objects, such as urine or trash, resulting in the person appearing disorganized or bizarre.

Children with PTSD may appear to break from reality when they dissociate or when triggered by fear or a reminder of their trauma. They may become rageful with no apparent clear cause. Without a careful history and evaluation, children responding to perceived fear secondary to their trauma may appear to be paranoid or delusional.

Immaturity can also lead to symptoms concerning for psychosis. For example, a child with a fear of the dark and an overactive imagination might present with visual hallucinations that when probed further are simply "seeing shadows in the dark." Imaginary friends to whom children talk are developmentally appropriate at certain ages. These shadows and imaginary friends may continue to older ages in children with intellectual disability or autism spectrum disorder (ASD) than in non-developmentally delayed children, but they should not be considered psychotic in nature. It is also developmentally appropriate to have hypnagogic or hypnopompic hallucinations when going to sleep or waking up from sleep, respectively. These can be quite scary to the child and, subsequently, the parent, but they should not be considered psychotic.

Numerous substances may result in psychosis, some only while the individual is intoxicated and others for a period after acute intoxication.

Atypical Clinical Presentation

Frequently, non-psychiatrists evaluating patients with psychosis first consider schizophrenia, other disorders in the primary psychotic family, or a manic episode of bipolar disorder. Although these may be typical disorders in adults presenting with psychosis, they are unusual in children with psychotic symptoms. Particularly in children, psychosis does not always equal a primary psychotic diagnosis.

Whereas the prevalence of schizophrenia in the adult population is approximately 1 in 200, the prevalence of childhood-onset schizophrenia (onset before age 13 years) is approximately 1 in 10,000. When a child presents with psychosis, schizophrenia should be close to the bottom of the differential. In addition, whereas bipolar disorder frequently presents in adolescence, it is very rare in childhood. Manic episodes of bipolar disorder are often accompanied by psychotic symptoms, but diagnosis requires an extended period of mood change (irritability or euphoria), with several other symptoms that can include grandiosity, racing thoughts, and pressured speech.

Differential Diagnosis

Psychosis does not automatically indicate that a patient has schizophrenia or bipolar disorder. Hallucinations reported by children are much more likely to be secondary to anxiety or depression rather than due to a primary psychotic process. Similarly, mood changes that appear to occur very acutely and without apparent cause do not necessarily indicate that the child is psychotic. Remembering this can avoid initiation of medications that have side effects and will not be helpful in treating the underlying disorder.

Multiple psychiatric disorders can present with psychotic symptoms or symptoms mimicking psychosis, including the following:

- Major depressive disorder
- Generalized anxiety disorder

OCD

PTSD

Immaturity/developmental stage

Bipolar disorder (rare in young children)

Schizophrenia (very rare before adolescence)

Medical etiologies must be considered as well. If patients are disoriented, consider whether they have delirium, not psychosis. The following is a non-exhaustive list of medical diagnoses to consider:

Substance use or withdrawal

Infectious encephalitis or meningitis

Autoimmune disorders including lupus, anti-NMDA encephalitis, and acute demyelinating encephalomyelitis

Head injury

Thyrotoxicosis

Atypical seizures or post-ictal state

Acute intermittent porphyria or other metabolic diseases

Thyroid disorders

Steroid-producing tumors

Brain tumors or other space-occupying lesions

Treatment and Disposition

Treatment of psychotic processes depends on the etiology. Treat the underlying etiology, such as anxiety or depression, rather than the symptom of psychosis. Regardless of etiology, if there is concern that psychosis is impeding the patient's ability to function and care for themselves, a psychiatric evaluation is necessary to determine if the patient requires admission.

Medical workup is often warranted in children presenting with an apparent first episode of true psychosis. Evaluate for ingestion of any substances. Based on the presentation, consider brain imaging, lumbar puncture, and laboratory studies.

Key Points

- Psychotic symptoms in children are rarely due to schizophrenia or bipolar disorder.
- Bipolar disorder and schizophrenia are more common in adolescents than in children, but even in adolescents, psychotic symptoms are much more likely due to another cause.
- Common etiologies of psychosis or symptoms mistaken for psychosis include normal developmental behavior, intellectual disability, ASD, depression, anxiety, OCD, and PTSD.
- Treat the etiology of the psychosis rather than the symptom of psychosis itself.

Pitfalls

- Attributing all auditory or visual hallucinations to psychosis secondary to bipolar disorder or schizophrenia
- Placing more importance on the "psychotic" symptoms rather than the etiology of these symptoms

TRAUMA-RELATED DISORDERS AND SYMPTOMS

Background

A history of exposure to potentially traumatic events is very common, particularly among youth with mental health-related emergencies. Examples of potentially traumatic events include child maltreatment, exposure to domestic or community violence, and natural disasters. It is estimated that two-thirds of individuals in the United States experienced at least one potentially traumatic event in their childhood. A history of exposure to trauma does not inevitably lead to distress. However, traumatic events, particularly repeated traumatic events at an early age, have the potential to lead to emotional dysregulation and elevate the risk of both internalizing symptoms (e.g., anxiety and depression) and externalizing symptoms (e.g., aggression and oppositional behaviors).

Classic Clinical Presentation

A patient's history of trauma may be obvious. Examples include children brought by Child Protective Services for evaluation after removal from the home for physical abuse or patients brought for evaluation after sexual assault. Patients with a disclosed history of trauma may present for somatic symptoms relating to anxiety or depression. Or a patient with a known history of PTSD may present for psychiatric evaluation after an exacerbation of symptoms.

The classic patient with a post-traumatic disorder or trauma-related symptoms has experienced a traumatic event in the past, but the traumatic event is not ongoing. Examples are veterans after their return from combat or patients who have suffered a traumatic event such as a sexual assault. In classic PTSD, patients with exposure to a traumatic event have functional impairment due to intrusion symptoms (e.g., nightmares or flashbacks), avoidance of triggers, alterations in arousal and activity (e.g., hypervigilance or difficulty sleeping), and negative alterations in thoughts or mood.

Atypical Clinical Presentation

Children with histories of trauma often do not manifest findings classic for PTSD. Another example of a pediatric trauma-related disorder is a case in which a child with a history of physical abuse and neglect and exposure to domestic violence is brought to the ED by foster parents for increasing oppositional behavior.

In other cases, trauma is not disclosed or recognized but impacts the ED visit and contributes to patient or family distress. For example, a history of sexual abuse may lead to a variety of unexpected reactions when a patient is asked to undress for an examination. Or a patient may become unexpectedly angry, anxious, or withdrawn when questioned about a particular topic.

Psychiatrists and other mental health clinicians are increasingly recognizing "complex trauma," which occurs in individuals who remain in or frequently return to traumatic environments. Examples include children who have been abused repeatedly or had numerous serious disruptions in home environment resulting in frequent changes in primary caregivers. Patients with complex trauma may not present with classic symptoms of PTSD, such as flashbacks and nightmares, and may not meet diagnostic criteria for PTSD. More likely, they present with a wide range of symptoms, including aggression, behavioral dysregulation, mood lability, and impulsivity. Youth with complex trauma are frequently mischaracterized as having bipolar disorder or schizophrenia because their moods and behaviors seem to shift inexplicably. Profound changes in mood and behavior may be due to triggers that reactivate trauma-related symptoms. Children and adolescents may not be able to explain what triggered them and may not even fully understand or acknowledge what led to their shift in mood and behavior.

Treatment

Knowing that a history of exposure to traumatic events is common, approach all patients as if they may have a history of trauma. Be sensitive to patient and family distress, and offer support if they exhibit signs of distress. An assessment for trauma is an important component of the history in pediatric patients with mental health emergencies and is imperative in any child or adolescent with a significant history of aggression or behavioral outbursts. Because exposure to trauma in childhood is very common and has the potential to impact health, consider screening all patients for trauma.

Be aware that patients with agitation may have a history of trauma. Childhood trauma can result in emotional dysregulation that can contribute to agitation and aggression. Being mindful of the possibility can aid clinicians in avoiding interactions that could retraumatize patients. Physical restraints can be quite triggering, especially in youth with a history of sexual trauma, and should be avoided if possible. If restraints are absolutely necessary, a debriefing after the event is particularly important in children with a history of trauma.

If patients disclose a history of trauma, ensure that they are now in a safe environment. Some new disclosures (e.g., child maltreatment or endangerment) may require reporting to authorities. If the traumatic history is causing ongoing distress or impairment, refer patients to a mental health professional for ongoing care.

Key Points

- Traumatic events in childhood are common.
- Youth with complex trauma often do not present with classic PTSD symptoms, but they often present with emotional dysregulation, behavioral outbursts, and aggression.
- Avoid restraint in youth with a history of trauma, particularly sexual trauma, if possible.

Pitfalls

- Failing to screen for a history of trauma in youth with behavioral or mental health symptoms, particularly those with behavioral outbursts and aggression

- Assuming rapid shifts in behavior or mood are due to bipolar disorder or schizophrenia
  - Youth with complex trauma may have seemingly inexplicable shifts in mood or behavior. These shifts may be due to triggers that the youth cannot articulate.

AUTISM SPECTRUM DISORDER

Background

Youth with ASD frequently present to EDs for care. In 2014, 1 in 59 children in the United States had ASD, according to the Centers for Disease Control and Prevention. Emergency clinicians are not expected to diagnose ASD or provide chronic management. However, emergency clinicians must be comfortable with the assessment and treatment of acute complaints in patients with ASD.

Characteristics of ASD include deficits in communication and social interaction and restricted and repetitive patterns of behavior, activities, or interests. These characteristics are present from an early developmental period. Milder communication deficits such as difficulty adjusting behavior to the appropriate social context may not be immediately obvious during a brief ED interaction. Conversely, severely affected patients may be nonverbal. Behavioral symptoms that may result in challenges with ED assessment include difficulty with transitions, need to adhere to routine, and hyperreactivity to sensory input.

For several reasons, patients with ASD are at risk of delayed diagnosis of medical conditions and injuries. An inability to effectively communicate symptoms may result in delayed presentation for care or missed or incorrect diagnoses. In addition, parents may be reluctant to bring youth with ASD to the ED, knowing that the visit will be stressful.

Classic Clinical Presentation

Children and adolescents with ASD are frequently brought to the ED for acute medical complaints and injuries unrelated to their diagnosis of ASD. Although the chief complaint may be unrelated, their ASD may require that the assessment be tailored to their specific needs. Medical assessment may be complicated by the patient's challenges with communication and because a change in routine, the unpredictability of an ED visit, and the sensory overload of the ED are stressful to patients with ASD.

Atypical Clinical Presentation

Patients with ASD may also present to the ED for behavioral symptoms such as agitation or aggression that cannot be managed at home or school. It is critical to recognize that behavioral symptoms may have a medical etiology. Patients may present with behaviors such as head banging or aggression when they have pain or other discomfort that they are unable to verbally communicate. Do not automatically attribute changes in behavior to the patient's ASD without considering other etiologies.

Differential Diagnosis

A wide variety of medical conditions may present nonspecifically in the nonverbal or minimally verbal child. Nonspecific symptoms may include restlessness, headbanging, decreased appetite, change in sleeping patterns, changes in vocalizations, or change in activity level.

Workup should be based on the history provided by the caretakers and a physical examination. The following etiologies merit specific mention:

Dental issues: Patients with ASD frequently are not able to tolerate regular dental examinations and oral care, and they may present with previously unrecognized painful caries or dental abscesses.

Constipation: Constipation is common, particularly in children with developmental issues, and may lead to significant discomfort.

Appendicitis: Appendicitis is common, particularly in the second decade of life, and symptoms may be nonspecific in nonverbal children.

Injury: Patients may have accidental injuries that go unnoticed because the patients are unable to communicate. However, the possibility of inflicted (abusive) injury must be considered because children with developmental delay and behavioral challenges are at increased risk of nonaccidental trauma.

Side effects of medications

Treatment

General Principles

Enlisting the help of parents is key. Ask parents how best to communicate with their child.

Visual communication is more effective for some patients, and some families will have their own visual communication systems.

Ask parents what is unsettling and what is soothing for their child. Some patients with ASD are very distressed by changes in routine. Knowing what to expect in the ED can be helpful. EDs are highly stimulating environments that may be unsettling to patients with hypersensitivity. Minimize unnecessary stimuli when possible. Quiet, dim rooms may be helpful. Limit the number of providers interacting with the child. Encourage use of any soothing items brought from home (e.g., a fidget spinner or weighted blanket). Utilize distractions that have been helpful for the patient in the past. Watching favorite videos or listening to music on a phone or tablet may be distracting. If available, enlist child life specialists or occupational therapists experienced in treating patients with ASD.

Prolonged sitting in a busy waiting room may be distressing to the patient with ASD and may result in agitation or a behavioral outburst. Consider alternatives such as prioritizing rooms for patients with special needs, including those with ASD. Alternatively, parents may prefer to wait outside with their child and receive a phone call when the patient's examination room is ready. Although these alternatives may seem to be disruptive to ED flow or unreasonable uses of staff time, if the evaluation occurs more smoothly, the change in procedures may benefit ED staff as well as the patient and family.

Approach to the Patient with ASD Presenting with Change in Behavior or Agitation

Strongly consider if agitation or other changes in behavior are due to physical discomfort. A detailed history and review of symptoms from parents or other caretakers may be helpful. Ask parents how the child usually reacts to pain or illness and what triggers have led to changes in behavior in the past.

If pain is thought to be likely, consider treatment with acetaminophen, ibuprofen, or other pain medication. Consider medication if agitation is not alleviated with calming measures. Ask parents about prior experiences with medication. If the patient is on home medications that are calming, consider an extra dose of the patient's home medication. Clonidine, risperidone, olanzapine, and chlorpromazine are reasonable choices. Avoid use of benzodiazepines in patients with ASD due to risk of disinhibition. Diphenhydramine may be considered, although this is also occasionally disinhibiting. Physical restraint and intramuscular medication administration are overwhelming and upsetting and should be the last resort, utilized only when necessary for safety.

Approach to the Patient with ASD Presenting with Another Medical Complaint

Patients with ASD often present to EDs for medical complaints unrelated to their ASD. The inability to communicate symptoms or tolerate procedures typically performed in the ED can complicate the medical evaluation.

Many patients with ASD are sensitive about their personal space. Approach the patient gradually, desensitizing them to your presence. Save examinations that may be unsettling for last. Breaking down procedures into small steps, describing in detail what will occur, and allowing breaks may facilitate the examination. When possible, allow patients to examine equipment such as otoscopes before use. When time allows, have parents prepare their child for unfamiliar procedures such as diagnostic imaging.

Patients with ASD are at risk of delayed diagnoses of medical conditions, so do not skip necessary evaluations because the examination is challenging. However, consider which specific procedures will aid in diagnosis or otherwise benefit the patient and which procedures are performed based on routine or protocol. For example, although obtaining a temperature or a pulse oximetry reading may be very distressing to a patient with ASD, those tests are necessary in the patient presenting with a week of worsening cough and shortness of breath. However, temperature and pulse oximetry may not be relevant in the patient with an acute witnessed arm injury who needs an X-ray. In that case, skipping the temperature and pulse oximetry and focusing on obtaining an X-ray may be more productive.

Allowing extra time for explanation and breaks may ultimately result in time savings for the clinician and a less distressing visit for the child. Procedural sedation may sometimes be necessary for procedures that would be tolerated by neurotypical children of the same age.

Disposition

Disposition will depend on the specific presentation.

Psychiatric Admission

Many psychiatric facilities do not accept patients with ASD, making disposition challenging when patients present with increased aggression or other behavioral changes unable to be managed at home. Knowing resources in your area is helpful.

Medical Admission

When patients with ASD present with medical or surgical disease, their specific needs may factor into disposition decisions. For example, if a patient with autism requires a procedure that generally occurs in an outpatient setting (e.g., dressing changes), admission to perform the procedure under sedation may be required if the patient cannot tolerate outpatient procedures. On the other hand, inpatient admission may be very stressful to children with inflexible routines. If inpatient admission can be safely avoided, patients may be better managed at home with a plan to return to the ED for worsening symptoms.

Complications

Patients with ASD are at risk of delayed or missed diagnoses due to delayed presentation for care and challenges with evaluation.

Patients with ASD are at risk of agitation due to lack of routine, overstimulation, and challenges with communication. If agitation progresses, patients are at risk for being physically and chemically restrained.

Key Points

- ASD is common.
- Patients have challenges with communication and social interaction.
- Change in routine may result in anxiety and agitation.
- Communicate in detail what to expect during the ED visit.
- Patients with limitations in communication may present with nonspecific symptoms when ill or in discomfort.

Pitfalls

- Attributing all behavioral symptoms to autism
  - Patients may demonstrate behaviors such as head banging, aggression, or poor sleep when in discomfort.
- Failing to enlist the help of parents
  - Parents know their child the best and can often anticipate what will be upsetting to their child and suggest strategies to calm the child.
- Failing to allow extra time for evaluation or to allow breaks if the child is overwhelmed
- Not performing an adequate evaluation
  - Patients with autism are at risk of delayed or missed diagnoses.
  - Consider how to modify ED procedures to accommodate a patient's needs without compromising care.

ACUTE AGITATION

Background

Agitation, an unpleasant state of excessive arousal, is a symptom rather than a specific disease process. Similar to pain, the symptom of agitation should be treated while the etiology is investigated.

Classic Clinical Presentation

The presentation of agitation varies dramatically based on the patient's age, ability to communicate, and the severity of agitation. Agitation is a state of hyperarousal, often manifested by behaviors such as pacing, fidgeting, hand wringing, and other excessive motor behaviors. Patients may appear tense with clenched fists or other aggressive body language. Speech may be loud, sarcastic, aggressive, or threatening.

Agitation exists on a continuum. Patients may initially appear anxious or restless but able to engage with clinicians. As patients become increasingly agitated, they may become aggressive, violent, and unable to engage in conversation.

Typically, the pediatric patients who require intervention for agitation are teenagers. Classically, the teenage patient with agitation is under the influence of a disinhibiting (e.g., alcohol) or stimulating (e.g., amphetamine) substance or has an underlying psychiatric disorder such as psychosis or a developmental disorder such as ASD. It is important to remember that teenagers presenting with agitation often have a history of trauma such as abuse, neglect, or family disruption.

Atypical Clinical Presentation

Although the classic pediatric ED patient with agitation is a teenager, younger children may require intervention for agitation. Young children with agitation frequently have communication challenges such as intellectual disability or ASD or have a history of severe trauma.

Differential Diagnosis

Agitation is a symptom with multiple potential causes. Critically, the symptoms of agitation may overlap with symptoms of delirium, a state of cerebral dysfunction that may manifest with an altered level of consciousness, confusion, or disorientation. Delirium is a medical emergency and should not be attributed to a psychiatric disorder. Patients with agitation are alert, oriented, and, although they might misperceive events, not generally confused.

Patients presenting with symptoms of agitation may require emergent treatment due to an underlying medical disorder, such as the following:

- Hypoxia or hypercarbia
- Metabolic derangements (e.g., hypoglycemia)
- Encephalopathy
- Head injury
- Thyrotoxicosis
- Atypical seizures or post-ictal state
- Encephalitis, meningitis, or other central nervous system infection
- Autoimmune encephalitis (e.g., anti-NMDA receptor encephalitis)
- Intoxication or toxic exposure
- Withdrawal from alcohol or other substances
- Akathisia from antipsychotics or other medications

Psychiatric, developmental, and cognitive disorders that may present with agitation include the following:

- Psychosis
- Mania
- Developmental or cognitive impairments
- ASD
- Other communication disorders
- Disruptive behavior disorders
- Attention-deficit/hyperactivity disorder
- Anxiety
- Depression
- PTSD
- Emotional dysregulation due to history of psychological trauma (complex trauma)

Treatment

Prompt treatment is critical because agitation is uncomfortable for patients and can progress to aggression and violence. Efforts to prevent agitation should occur in patients at high risk of agitation, such as patients with ASD, acute psychosis, or a history of agitation or aggression. Quiet, less stimulating rooms may be helpful. Communicating expectations and providing updates can decrease patient and family anxiety. Attending to the patient's comfort with food, blankets, or distractions demonstrates to the patient that you are trying to help and may prevent agitation or help patients with early agitation to calm themselves.

Early recognition of agitation allows for intervention when patients may be more able to regain control of their emotions and behaviors. Seek and treat the underlying cause of agitation.

The least coercive and least restrictive management of agitation possible should be employed, with physical restraint and involuntary medication administration used only as last resorts, when necessary for patient or staff safety. Coercive measures generally increase, rather than decrease, agitation. Be aware that many youth with agitation have histories of trauma; physical restraint and other coercive measures can retraumatize patients.

Attempt verbal de-escalation whenever a patient demonstrates signs of agitation or verbalizes that they are feeling tense, anxious, or restless. Box 52.3 lists important principles of verbal de-escalation. Even if more restrictive measures must be used, verbal de-escalation should be attempted simultaneously.

One clinician should establish communication with the patient. Multiple people speaking simultaneously can be overwhelming. Tailor attempts at verbal de-escalation to the patient's developmental level. Remain calm and respectful, and speak in a quiet, even voice, using simple language and allowing the patient time

> **BOX 52.3**
> **TEN DOMAINS OF VERBAL DE-ESCALATION**
>
> 1. Respect personal space.
> 2. Do not be provocative.
> 3. Establish verbal contact.
> 4. Be concise.
> 5. Identify wants and feelings.
> 6. Listen closely to what the patient is saying.
> 7. Agree or agree to disagree.
> 8. Lay down the law and set clear limits.
> 9. Offer choices and optimism.
> 10. Debrief the patient and staff.
>
> *Source:* Reprinted from Richmond JS, Berlin JS, Fishkind AB, Holloman GH Jr, Zeller SL, Wilson MP, Rifai MA, Ng AT. Verbal de-escalation of the agitated patient: Consensus statement of the American Association for Emergency Psychiatry Project BETA De-escalation Workgroup. West J Emerg Med. 2012;13(1):17–25. Adapted from a box originally published in Fishkind A. Calming agitation with words, not drugs: 10 commandments for safety. Current Psych. 2002;1(4)32–39.

to process what is being said. Body language should be neutral and nonthreatening. Maintain a safe distance from the patient. Both the clinician and the patient should have access to the exit—feeling trapped worsens agitation. Listen to patients and identify their needs. Communicate limits in a clear but respectful manner.

Family members may serve as a calming presence or may further agitate the patient. Separate family members who seem to escalate the agitation, but whenever possible, allow the presence of soothing family members. Especially for youth with ASD and developmental disabilities, guidance from parents or other caretakers can be invaluable. Parents generally can identify their child's triggers and know what is calming.

Physical restraint should be utilized only as a last resort, when needed for immediate safety concerns, and restraints should be released as soon as the patient is able to control their behaviors. Administer medication to achieve a calmer state if physical restraint is necessary.

Clinical Algorithm

Concurrent with attempts at verbal de-escalation, offer oral medication early, choosing medications based on the underlying etiology, if known. Involuntary intramuscular administration of medications should be avoided when possible, but if intramuscular medications must be given, they should be directed at suspected etiology. If the child takes medications for a mental health disorder, an extra half or full dose of their usual medication can be helpful.

There is not strong evidence or even expert consensus to support any particular medication. Benzodiazepines and diphenhydramine are options, but both can be disinhibiting; avoid these medications in patients at risk of paradoxical reactions. For this reason, benzodiazepines are not generally recommended for patients with ASD and developmental disabilities. Clonidine is an α_2 agonist that is used in some centers, particularly for patients with attention-deficit/hyperactivity disorder. Antipsychotics such as haloperidol, olanzapine, chlorpromazine, and risperdone are also commonly used. First-generation antipsychotics such as haloperidol are less preferred by many experts due to their side effect profile.

In 2019, a workgroup of child and adolescent psychiatrists published recommendations to guide the use of medication in agitated pediatric patients. Table 52.1 details the workgroup's recommended medications. Figure 52.1 is a flowchart to aid clinicians in choosing an appropriate medication based on etiology of agitation.

Disposition

Disposition is based on underlying etiology and the patient's ability to control their behaviors.

Complications

Physical restraint is a complication that may often be avoided by early recognition and intervention to help patients manage their own behaviors. Physical restraint is potentially traumatizing to the patient and family members. Physical restraint may also result in patient or staff injury; patient deaths after restraint have also been reported. Furthermore, physical

TABLE 52.1 MEDICATIONS FOR TREATMENT OF AGITATION

Medication (Class)	Dose (Standard Adolescent Dose and Weight-Based Child Dose)	Maximum Daily Dose	Time to Peak Effect	Notes/Monitoring
Diphenhydramine (antihistamine)	PO/IM 12.5–50 mg 1 mg/kg/dose	Child: 50–100 mg Adolescent: 100–200 mg	PO: 2 hours	Avoid in delirium. Can be combined with haloperidol or chlorpromazine if concern for EPS. Can cause disinhibition or delirium in younger or DD youth.
Lorazepam (benzodiazepine)	PO/IM/IV 0.5–2 mg 0.05–0.1 mg/kg/dose	Child: 4 mg Adolescent: 6–8 mg depending on weight/ prior exposure	IV: 10 minutes PO/IM: 1–2 hours	Can cause disinhibition or delirium in younger or DD youth. Can be given with haloperidol, chlorpromazine, or risperdone. Avoid giving within 1 hour of olanzapine (especially IM due to risk of respiratory suppression).
Clonidine (α_2 agonist)	PO: 0.05–0.1 mg	27–40.5 kg: 0.2 mg/day 40.5–45 mg: 0.3 mg/day >45 kg: 0.4 mg/day	PO: 30–60 minutes	Monitor for hypotension and bradycardia. Avoid giving with benzodiazepine or atypical antipsychotic due to hypotension risk.
Chlorpromazine (antipsychotic)	PO/IM 12.5–50 mg (IM should be one-half of PO dose) 0.55 mg/kg/dose	Child <5 years: 40 mg/day Child >5 years: 75 mg/day	PO: 30–60 minutes IM: 15 minutes	Monitor for hypotension and QT prolongation.
Haloperidol (antipsychotic)	PO/IM 0.5–5 mg (IM should be one-half of PO dose) 0.55 mg/kg/dose	15–40 kg: 6 mg >40 kg: 15 mg[a]	PO: 2 hours IM: 20 minutes	Monitor for hypotension. Consider ECG or cardiac monitoring for QT prolongation, especially for IV administration. Note EPS risk with doses >3 mg/day, with IV dosing having very high EPS risk.
Olanzapine (antipsychotic)	PO/IM: 2.5–10 mg (IM should be one-fourth to one-half of PO dose)	10–20 mg[a]	PO: 5 hours (range, 1–8 hours) IM: 15–45 minutes	Avoid giving within 1 hour of benzodiazepine given risk of respiratory suppression.
Risperidone (antipsychotic)	PO/ODT 0.25–1 mg 0.005–0.01 mg/kg/dose	Child: 1–2 mg Adolescent: 2–3 mg[a]	PO: 1 hour	Can cause akathisia (restlessness/agitation) at higher doses.
Quetiapine (antipsychotic)	PO 25–50 mg 1–1.5 mg/kg/dose (or divided)	>10 years: 600 mg[a]	PO: 30 minutes to 2 hours	More sedating at lower doses. Monitor for hypotension.

[a]Depending on prior antipsychotic exposure.
DD, developmental disability; ECG, electrocardiogram; EPS, extrapyramidal symptoms; PO, oral; IM, intramuscular; IV, intravenous; ODT, orally dissolving tablet.
Source: Adapted from Gerson R, Malas N, Feuer V, Silver GH, Prasad R, Mroczkowski MM. Best practices for evaluation and management of agitated children and adolescents (BETA) in the emergency depart-

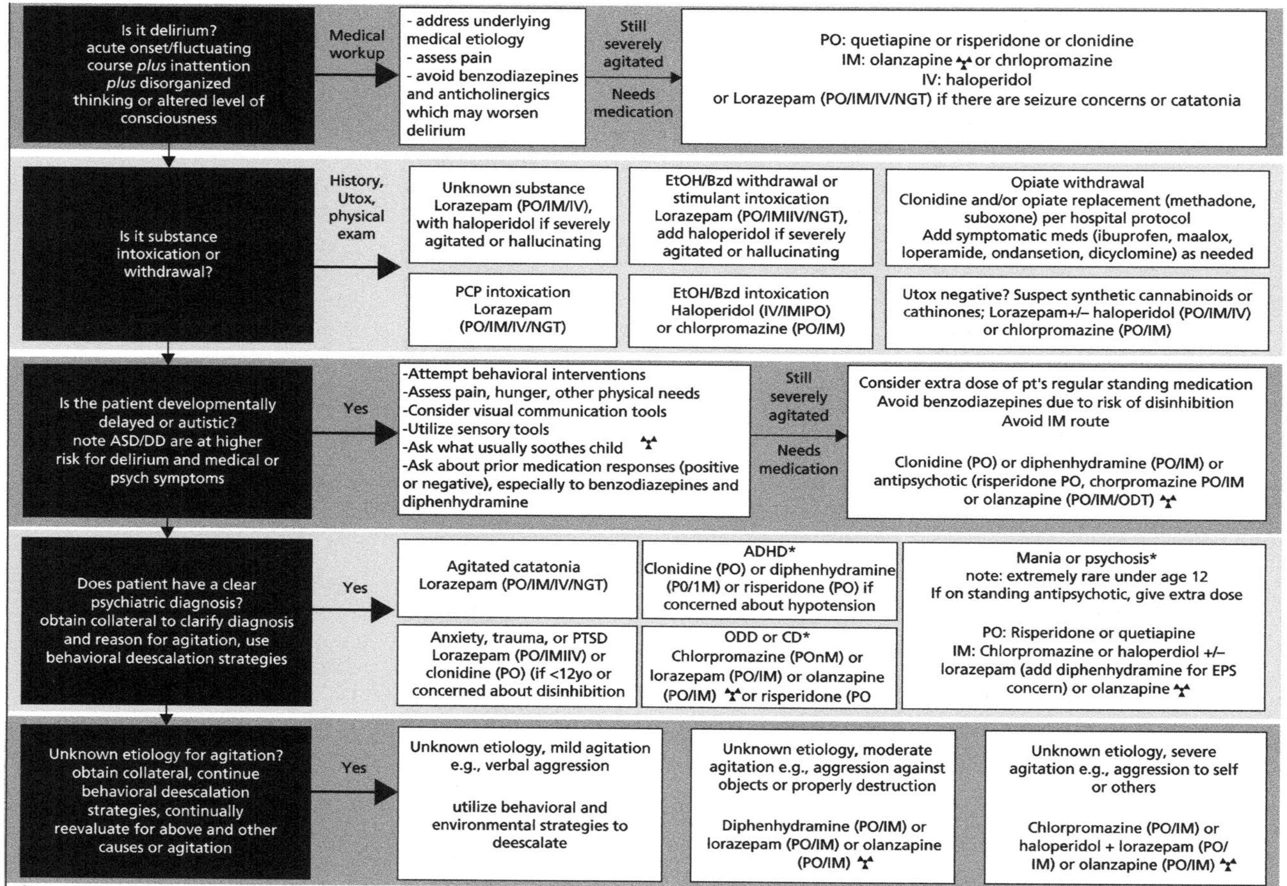

Figure. Clinical decision flow chart.
PO, by mouth; *IM*, intramuscular; *IV*, intravenous; *NGT*, nasogastric tube; *EtOH*, ethanol; *Utox*, urine toxicology; *PCP*, phencydidine; *EPS*, extrapyramidal symptoms; *ASD*, autism spectrum disorder; *DD*, developmental disability; *BZD*, benzodiazepines; *ODT*, orally dissolving tablet; *PTSD*, post-traumatic stress disorder; *ADHD*, attention deficit hyperactivity disorder; ODD, oppositional defiant disorder; CD, conduct disorder; pt, patient.
*For these etiologies, in absence of consensus, medication options are listed alphabetically; ☢ Do not give olanzapine and benzodiazepines within one hour of each other.

FIGURE 52.1 Flowchart to guide choice of medication for treatment of agitation. ADHD, attention-deficit/hyperactivity disorder; ASD, autism spectrum disorder; BZD, benzodiazepine; CD, conduct disorder; DD, developmental disability; EPS, extrapyramidal symptoms; EtOH, ethanol; IM, intramuscular; IV, intravenous; NGT, nasogastric tube; ODD, oppositional defiant disorder; ODT, orally dissolving tablet; PCP, phencydidine; PO, by mouth; pt, patient; PTSD, post-traumatic stress disorder; Utox, urine toxicology.

Source: Reprinted from Gerson R, Malas N, Feuer V, Silver GH, Prasad R, Mroczkowski MM. Best practices for evaluation and management of agitated children and adolescents (BETA) in the emergency department: Consensus statement of the American Association for Emergency Psychiatry. *West J Emerg Med.* 2019;20(2):409–418.

restraint, involuntary medication administration, and other coercive measures undermine trust in clinicians, resulting in difficulty engaging the patient in further evaluation. Patients who require physical restraint and sedating medications often have longer ED lengths of stay.

Key Points

- The goal of intervention is to decrease patient distress and help the patient regain control of their own behaviors.
- Be attuned to early signs of agitation.
- Utilize the least restrictive and least coercive intervention possible.
- Consider whether the patient is physically uncomfortable.
  - Attend to basic needs such as food, a beverage, or a blanket.
- Utilize verbal de-escalation techniques.
- Offer oral medication early, based on likely etiology.
  - Consider an extra dose of the patient's home medication or ask what has worked in the past.
- Parents and other caretakers frequently know the patient's triggers and the best calming measures.

Pitfalls

- Failing to recognize patients at high risk of agitation
  - Take measures to prevent agitation in high-risk patients.
- Failing to intervene early when patients demonstrate early signs of agitation
  - Agitation exists on a spectrum. Patients will be most able to regain control of their symptoms and behaviors if treated at an early stage.
- Worsening symptoms by administering a disinhibiting medication
  - Benzodiazepines and diphenhydramine can cause a paradoxical reaction, particularly in patients with ASD and developmental disabilities. Ask about past reactions. Consider other medications in high-risk patients.

Further Reading

Chun TH, Mace SE, Katz ER. Evaluation and management of children and adolescents with acute mental health or behavioral problems. Part I: Common clinical challenges of patients with mental health and/or behavioral emergencies. *Pediatrics.* 2016;138(3):e20161570; Part II: Recognition of clinically challenging mental health related conditions presenting with medical or uncertain symptoms. *Pediatrics.* 2016;138(3):e20161573.

Gerson R, Malas N, Feuer V, Silver GH, Prasad R, Mroczkowski MM. Best practices for evaluation and management of agitated children and adolescents (BETA) in the emergency department: Consensus statement of the American Association for Emergency Psychiatry. *West J Emerg Med.* 2019;20(2):409–418.

Marsac JL, Kassam-Adams N, Hildenbrand AK, et al. Implementing a trauma-informed approach in pediatric health care networks. *JAMA Pediatr.* 2016;170(1):70–77.

National Institute of Mental Health. Ask Suicide-Screening Questions (ASQ) Toolkit. https://www.nimh.nih.gov/research/research-conducted-at-nimh/asq-toolkit-materials/index.shtml

Richmond JS, Berlin JS, Fishkind AB, et al. Verbal de-escalation of the agitated patient: Consensus statement of the American Association for Emergency Psychiatry Project BETA De-escalation Workgroup. *West J Emerg Med.* 2012;13(1):17–25.

53

Child Abuse

RHIANNON MAIN, LAURA JACOBSON, AMY YOUNG, AND TIM YOUNG

BACKGROUND

Child maltreatment evokes strong emotions and is one of the most challenging pediatric conditions. The emergency department (ED) is frequently the site of initial evaluation when a child is the victim of an acute inflicted injury. Abused children may present to the ED for vague complaints that could be attributed to a more benign illness such as a viral infection, but have evidence of abusive injuries. This evidence is sometimes overt but often subtle. Recognition of these injuries may save the child's life, spare them from years of psychological and physical suffering, and prevent long-term morbidity such as intellectual disability and need for chronic medical care. In this way, emergency providers are at the front line of child abuse detection. Although not as readily apparent, the recognition of child abuse is as life-saving as securing an airway or aggressively treating sepsis.

Emergency providers face barriers to child abuse recognition, including (1) time pressure, (2) fear of disrupting family dynamics, (3) fear of having to explain actions to parents, (4) uncertainty regarding the likelihood of abuse, and (5) fear of the obligation of going to court. As emergency providers, we are trained to do a focused assessment and manage an acute problem or potential life threat. We employ advanced pattern recognition to determine whether a child is critically ill or has a life-threatening condition. We form this impression from the history we are given and the appearance of the patient in front of us ("sick" or "not sick"). However, in the setting of child abuse, this approach fails for several reasons. We are typically given a history that is false. We must be willing to doubt the history based on our objective findings. The trauma that has occurred to the patient may be subacute or ongoing, lessening the apparent acuity or severity of the patient we see in front of us. The workup and steps that need to be taken to manage these subtle indicators of child abuse may seem to be "going overboard." However, an ED encounter may be the best or only opportunity to recognize child abuse and intervene. This means protecting the child from a dangerous social situation or potential injurer, not necessarily an injury that has already occurred. We are trained to evaluate injuries based on the extent of the current injury itself, but with child abuse we must also consider potential future injuries. Assessing a child's safety means searching for evidence of previous and current injury and involving people and institutions that can help us evaluate social factors. Approaching potential child abuse with the same urgency as midgut volvulus, open fracture, or any other life-threatening emergency means being able to "switch gears" to this approach in the middle of a busy shift. In the same way that fever in a newborn triggers specific tests and treatment, an unexplained, suspicious, or potential sentinel injury should trigger certain actions, including taking a more detailed history; doing a more thorough skin, scalp, mouth, and genitourinary examination; and ordering more tests and asking for more help than we are used to for a child who appears well in the moment. An unexplained subconjunctival hemorrhage should alarm us just as the symptoms of a transient ischemic attack do in an adult. A bruise on the ear should trigger us just as deep anterior T-wave inversions do on an adult electrocardiogram. We must also remember that we are mandatory reporters and that we are liable if we do *not* report. It may be helpful to know that most child abuse reporting does not result in the removal of a child from the home. It is not our responsibility to try to explain findings that do not make sense, but it is our responsibility to report a suspicion and protect a child from escalating dangers in the home.

CLASSIC CLINICAL PRESENTATION

The hallmark of child abuse is the presentation of an injury that does not match the given mechanism or is unexplained. An implausible or changing explanation for an injury is also a red flag. When taking a history, it is important to allow the adult to state what happened in their own words. Avoid the temptation to "fill in the blanks" with what you think may have logically happened. Injuries may be unwitnessed, or blame may be attributed to siblings or even family pets. The presentation may be delayed. However, this is often not the case, especially in more severe injuries. Such injuries are likely to present to the ED. A common misconception is that an abuse perpetrator would be calloused to a child's needs and try to hide the injured child and thus hide their actions. In the setting of a significant injury, a perpetrator often realizes that the child needs help and assumes medical personnel will trust their false history. The perpetrator often seeks medical attention for the child immediately after the injury occurs. A delayed presentation signals additional neglect of the child's needs, but an immediate presentation does not make abuse less likely.

Although a large variety of injuries in children can be abusive, several injury patterns merit special alarm. These include patterned bruises, certain fracture patterns such as metaphyseal or posterior rib fractures, and fractures in non-ambulatory children. Bruises may appear as patterned petechial rupture outside of the area where the child was struck with an object. Petechiae may also outline hand marks. Strangulation may cause petechiae on the neck. It is helpful to remember the mantra "those who don't cruise rarely bruise," meaning that any bruise should be considered suspicious in a child who is not yet cruising (taking steps while holding onto objects for support). A thorough skin examination under good lighting is key to bruise detection. Time must be deliberately taken for this examination despite typical ED time pressures. When this can occur outside of the caregiver's presence, it will cause less stress for the clinician and provide the chance to take forensic pictures.

Bruising is the most common "sentinel" injury, presenting before subsequent life-threatening inflicted injuries. The TEN-4 clinical decision rule states that bruising on the *t*orso, *e*ars or *n*eck in children younger than age 4 years is especially concerning for abuse, as is any bruising in a child younger than age *4* months. Children of this age would not be expected to be able to pull to a stand or take steps, which makes accidental bruising unlikely. The mnemonic FACES can be added to TEN-4 to remember additional high-yield areas to examine for abusive injuries (Figure 53.1). Examine the entirety of the skin, paying special attention to the locations listed in the mnemonic, as well as the genitourinary area. Remember that there are three frenula in the mouth, including inside the upper lip, lower lip, and under the tongue. These can be torn by blunt facial trauma or from force-feeding. In order to recognize implausible explanations, an emergency physician must be familiar with basic developmental milestones. For example, a 1-month-old rolling off of a bed would usually be an implausible scenario based on typical development (Figure 53.2).

T	Torso
E	Ears
N	Neck
4	Any bruise under 4 months of age
F	Frenula
A	Angle of the mandible
C	Cheeks
E	Eyelids
S	Subconjunctiva

FIGURE 53.1 TEN-4 FACES rule for high-suspicion bruising in children younger than age 4 years.

ATYPICAL CLINICAL PRESENTATION

Severe child abuse can present in a variety of forms. An adult may bring a child to the ED because the child "stopped breathing," had a seizure, or has a change in mental status. A child who has been severely injured may present in cardiac arrest. For an infant who has been shaken, there may be no signs of external trauma. Surprisingly, many abusive injuries, including femur fractures and abdominal injuries, may not show obvious visual signs of injury. Do not expect to see bruising in the shape and pattern of fingertips ("fingertip" bruising) at the site of injury. To better detect injuries, include more than just visual inspection. Incorporate palpation and test full passive range of motion of extremities to elicit any tenderness. The chief complaint may be vague, such as "fussiness," "lethargy," or "poor feeding." Because the history is false or lacking, these cases may seem to have a medical cause but in fact are traumatic presentations and should be treated similarly to any other trauma. Once there is suspicion for child abuse, the emergency clinician must shift the approach from medical to trauma, which will mean not only a complete trauma-style primary and secondary evaluation but also potentially involving a surgeon, activating a trauma team, or transferring to a trauma center depending on the institution.

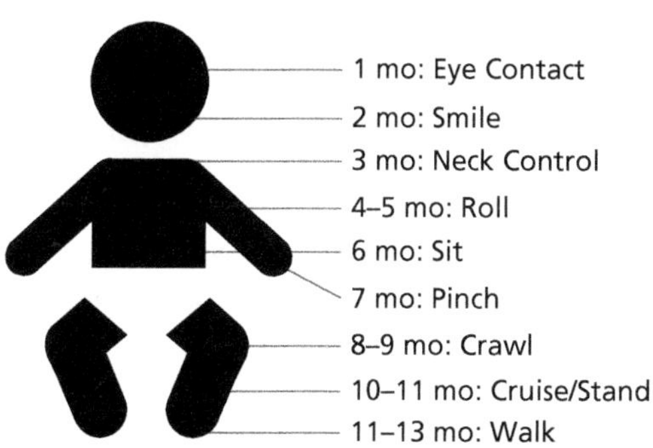

FIGURE 53.2 Simplification of development milestones for easy recall.

Source: Courtesy of Tom Sherwin, Loma Linda University Medical Center, Loma Linda, CA.

Well-groomed, appropriate-appearing parents abuse their children. Many abusers are first-time offenders and have no criminal record. A "gut impression" based on interactions with parents can be misleading. Regardless of parental appearance, emergency physicians must consider the child's safety. This means objectively taking a step back and considering whether the injury is consistent with the proposed mechanism, despite any general impression of concern obtained from parents. It is not the physician's responsibility to determine intent.

In addition to acute trauma, children who are abused have often suffered chronic or subacute trauma. In this way, the emergency medicine heuristic of "sick/not sick" fails. Although the child in front of you may not appear "sick," there may be a life-threatening social situation at home. Previous injuries may have already healed or be in the process of healing. This shifts the focus from searching for only acute injuries that will affect medical management to also evaluating for subacute trauma such as healed fractures or chronic subdural hematomas. Discovering these injuries may affect the child's disposition and help move them out of a dangerous situation to a safe environment. The presence of prior injuries is very helpful when trying to determine the plausibility of a single, acute injury. For example, single fractures can present a diagnostic dilemma in young, newly ambulatory patients, but when a skeletal survey reveals additional healing fractures, the concern for child abuse becomes much clearer.

DIFFERENTIAL DIAGNOSIS

It is helpful to be aware of common child abuse mimics. This knowledge may save a clinician and family time and trouble. For instance, a toddler's fracture is a non-displaced spiral fracture, most commonly of the tibia, that has a seemingly insignificant mechanism but a characteristic presentation and radiographic appearance. It usually results from a torsional force on the bone from a minor fall, one in which the child twists on a planted foot. A trampoline fracture is another pattern that may be mistaken for abusive trauma. Typically, the child suffers a transverse, non-displaced proximal tibia fracture as a result of a "double bounce" from a larger child or adult on a trampoline or in a bounce house. Impetigo or ecthyma may look like burns; phytophotodermatitis, Mongolian spots, or cultural practices such as cupping or coining may be mistaken for abusive bruising. Dirt may be mistaken for a bruise but is easily removed with an alcohol swab.

Although knowledge of child abuse mimics may prevent unnecessary workup or reporting when a known mimic is present, it is important to not be too hasty to ascribe a presentation to a mimic when the presentation does not fit the classic scenario. An injury with an appearance or pattern often attributed to a non-abusive cause should not be assumed to be accidental when it occurs in an unusual setting. For example, a supracondylar fracture in a child who does not run is unusual. Toddler's fractures generally do not occur in non-ambulatory children. A young infant may be unwilling to use an arm due to an abusive fracture rather than a nursemaid's elbow. Many child abuse reports will ultimately be designated as unsubstantiated or undetermined; this is to be expected, and the clinician should remember that suspicion, not definitive evidence, is the bar for reporting. When a situation is unclear, reporting is the best option.

DIAGNOSTIC CONFIRMATION

An essential part of the workup in all cases of suspected child abuse is a report with the state child protection agency. This may come from a social worker or directly from the clinician. This should be considered part of the workup, not the result of a definitive diagnosis of abuse. If your hospital's practice is to file a report through a consultant social worker, be clear about your concerns, plainly communicate that you are asking for a report to be filed, and state the concerns you want the report to convey. Although a consultant social worker can be helpful in the reporting process, reporting is ultimately the responsibility of the treating physician.

The realization that reporting to a state child protection agency is a mandatory part of the workup may relieve clinician anxiety related to reporting. Child protection agencies do not reflexively remove children from the home. Other services may be offered to a family based on a home visit and evaluation. Reports may collectively uncover a pattern that helps provide appropriate services to the family.

The workup of suspected child abuse is to an extent age-dependent. Testing mirrors typical trauma workups with the caveat that the goal is to identify not just clinically important findings but also forensically relevant ones that might affect the child's disposition or future placement. This may be life-saving. For example, child abuse literature has identified a threshold level of 80 IU/L for liver enzymes for abdominal imaging. This is a lower threshold than that for children who are victims of blunt force non-abusive trauma. A clinically inconsequential liver injury found in a child following a motor vehicle collision would have no forensic importance because the mechanism is not in question. This is not true for child abuse. A liver injury found in addition to a brain injury might support the diagnosis of child abuse and provide valuable evidence to protect a child. It is also important to recognize that decision rules such as the Pediatric Emergency Care Applied Research Network (PECARN) pediatric head injury prediction rule should not be applied in child abuse because their goal is to find clinically, not forensically, important injuries. In addition, such decision rules often include mechanism, which is falsely minimized in child abuse.

Labs to order include a complete blood count, complete electrolytes with liver enzymes, lipase, amylase, coagulation studies, urinalysis, and urine drug screen. A skeletal survey should also be ordered for nonverbal children and includes at least 19 images in order to be

TABLE 53.1 DIAGNOSTIC TESTING

Factor	Testing
Younger than age 3 years	CT head, CBC, CMP, UA with reflex to culture, UDS, PTT/INR, lipase/amylase, skeletal survey
Older than age 3 years + verbal	CBC, CMP, UA, UDS, lipase/amylase
Older than age 3 years + nonverbal	Add skeletal survey and head CT
Liver enzymes >80 IU/L	CT abdomen/pelvis
Chest trauma	CT chest
Many bruises	CK
Significant external head trauma at any age	CT head

CBC, complete blood count; CK, creatine kinase; CMP, complete metabolic panel; CT, computed tomography; INR, international normalized ratio; PTT, partial thromboplastin time; UA, urine analysis; UDS, urine drug screen.

consistent with standard practice: 3 images of the skull, 2 oblique rib images, 2 views of the spine, 8 images of the distinct regions of the extremities, as well as at least 1 view each of the hand and foot. An example guide to diagnostic ordering is provided in Table 53.1.

Fractures found on a skeletal survey that strongly suggest inflicted injury include bucket handle or corner fractures, posterior rib fractures, any fracture in a non-ambulatory child, and multiple fractures including those in mixed stages of healing. Healed rib fractures characteristically appear as round calluses at the site of a previous fracture (Figure 53.3).

It is important to differentiate several imaging tests that are easily confused. A skeletal survey is a defined series of images that provides a thorough evaluation of the skull, trunk, and each limb. A "babygram" is a colloquial term for a single radiograph of an infant's body that may demonstrate fractures. However, this radiograph is a grossly incomplete evaluation for abusive fractures. Its main utility lies in uncovering obvious, potentially abusive fractures in an infant who is currently too sick to undergo a skeletal survey. A bone scan generally refers to a nuclear medicine study that is more often used in the setting of osteomyelitis or cancer than in child abuse. Although it may help show subtle bone injuries, it is not the first imaging test of choice for an abuse evaluation.

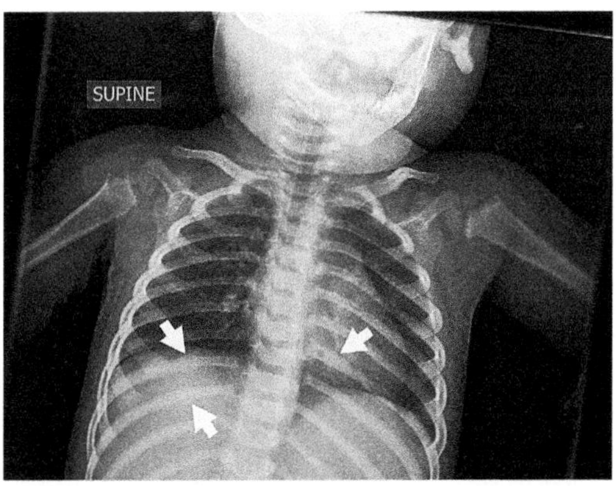

FIGURE 53.3 Healed posterior rib fractures.

To help determine when a particular fracture does not match the stated mechanism, it is necessary to understand how mechanism usually relates to fracture type (Figure 53.4).

Photos of external injuries such as burns, bruises, hematomas, and subconjunctival hemorrhages are a helpful addition to the medical record. They can be considered analogous to a computed tomography (CT) head scan, labs, and skeletal survey for internal injuries. They may prove helpful for a child abuse pediatrician, especially when evaluating the patient after external injuries have healed or faded, in order to form a more definitive impression of the likelihood of abuse. Many electronic health record software systems facilitate importing photos into the chart. Labeling the patient's name, body part, and time and date is important. Using a ruler or forensic scale card will help orient to size and standardize color.

TREATMENT

Once life-threatening conditions are stabilized in accordance to trauma principles and a workup is initiated, the next challenge a clinician faces is explaining the plan to caregivers. Allying oneself with the parent is a useful strategy. It is also helpful to employ preconsidered scripts (Table 53.2).

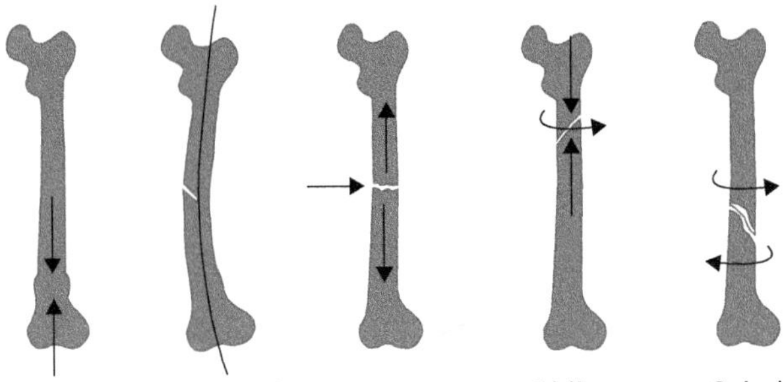

FIGURE 53.4 Fracture mechanism. A torus or buckle fracture typically results from compression. A greenstick fracture results from bending. A transverse fracture occurs from traction or a perpendicular shearing force. An oblique fracture results from twisting and compression. A spiral fracture results from twisting.

Source: Courtesy of Tim Young, Loma Linda University Medical Center, Loma Linda, CA.

TABLE 53.2 COMMON QUESTIONS AND ANSWERS REGARDING POSSIBLE CHILD MALTREATMENT

Question	Answer
"Why is a child protection agency involved?"	"I am required to report unusual or unexplained injuries. Right now, I cannot explain this injury. I hope you can understand that this is part of my job."
"Why does he need blood work and X-rays?"	"We have found an injury that is unexpected based on what happened to (him). We need to look for other possible injuries."
"Why are you ordering all this?"	"Your child has an injury that I do not understand based on what you have told me. I need to obtain more information with labs, radiographs, and consultations in order to understand it."
"Why do I need to wait in the ER so long? Can you just call me for results?"	"Right now I know that both of us are wanting to keep your child safe; waiting for more information and consultations is an important step in doing so."
"What do you think happened doctor?"	"Your child has an injury that I cannot explain. Has he been under the care of anyone else that you think may have hurt him?"
"Does CPS have to be involved?"	"We have found an unexplained injury. I know that you must be concerned about how this happened to your child. So we are contacting some people who can help us figure that out."
"Why can't you just give us a splint and send us home?"	"I am concerned that there are injuries we could miss. We are going to obtain more labs and images, and the social worker will be by to speak with you. We want your child to be safe and make sure we are not missing anything."
"Why are you trying to get my child taken from me?"	"When we see these kinds of injuries, I am required to report them to social services. That alone does not mean that your child is going to be taken from you, but a social worker will need to interview you and your family for safety reasons."

CPS, Child Protective Services; ER, emergency room.

At-risk siblings will need evaluation for abusive injuries as well. Obtaining an adequate social history and communicating sibling status with your state's child protection agency ensures that at-risk siblings can be referred for an urgent evaluation. It is also important to remember that child abuse is a crime and that law enforcement for the region in which the crime occurred should be notified. This is in contrast to the report made to the child protection agency, which should be the agency that covers the child's place of residence.

CLINICAL ALGORITHM

Any algorithm applied will depend on resources available and should be vetted through local agencies and child abuse specialists. Existing hospital protocols should be followed.

DISPOSITION

An abused child may require admission to a pediatric center for additional testing, which can include specialized imaging such as magnetic resonance imaging or a dilated fundus examination by a qualified ophthalmologist. If a safe environment is available or secured by child protection agency workers and the child's workup is complete, discharge with outpatient follow-up at a child abuse assessment center with a child abuse pediatrician and a forensic interview may be an appropriate option. When available, it is helpful to discuss workup, disposition, and follow-up with a child abuse pediatrician, who may recommend testing that can be more easily obtained in the ED than in an outpatient setting.

COMPLICATIONS

The complications of child abuse may include lifelong neurologic devastation leading to long-term care at chronic health facilities, depression and mental illness including behavioral problems, as well as socioeconomic problems such as early incarceration and unemployment. Researchers are discovering important information about adverse childhood experiences (ACEs), some of which include physical abuse, emotional abuse, sexual abuse, emotional neglect, and physical neglect. It appears that ACEs have a strong influence on health and can disrupt early brain and physical development, leading to increased risk of health problems in adulthood, including heart disease, lung disease, liver disease, autoimmune disease, suicide, and even early death. Recognition of "sentinel" injuries such as suspicious fractures or bruising before devastating injuries occur may have an enormous impact on a child's ultimate health.

KEY POINTS

- Emergency physicians provide frontline care for abused children. Recognition of sentinel injuries may save a child's life.
- Often, the ED is the most appropriate or only option to obtain timely lab testing and imaging. Inability to complete this workup should prompt transfer to a capable facility.
- Involvement of child protection agencies occurs in the workup/evaluation phase of child abuse management and is triggered by suspicion, not a definitive diagnosis.

PITFALLS

- Failure to perform a child abuse-specific examination, including examination of skin and other high-risk areas
- Ordering an incomplete workup
- Not considering a report to a state's child protection agency an essential part of the workup
- Failure to recognize red flags and consider child abuse in a differential diagnosis
- Failing to document important injuries
- Failing to approach an abused child as a trauma victim
- Not seeking help from child abuse pediatricians who are available

CHILD SEXUAL ABUSE

Background

Child sexual abuse is a pervasive form of child abuse. Unlike adult sexual assault, which often presents after an acute incident, child sexual abuse is more often chronic in nature and delayed in its presentation. Child sexual abuse often begins at an early age when the child is unable to emotionally process the abuse as a violation. Most perpetrators are someone with whom the child is familiar.

Classic Clinical Presentation

Classically, a child's disclosure is the factor that prompts presentation to the ED.

Alternatively, the disclosure may come indirectly from another source. The sexual assault, whether acute or chronic, may involve the perpetrator forcing or coercing the child to engage in sexual acts that may or may not include penetration.

Another common presentation occurs when a parent asks for a child to be evaluated due to concern for sexual abuse by another family member or close acquaintance of the family without the child's disclosure. This may happen for a variety of reasons. The parent or caregiver may have noticed a physical symptom, such as bruising, bleeding, or a rash to the genital area. This may also occur when parents have split custody, and one parent reports that the child has genital irritation or a new behavior after returning from the other parent's care. Often, the patient will have a normal external physical examination in the ED, and parents should be made aware that this does not exclude sexual abuse. A report should be made to the child protection agency to document the parent's concern.

Atypical Clinical Presentation

Sexual abuse is more difficult to detect when it presents with vague somatic complaints such as abdominal pain; malaise; myalgias; enuresis; sleep disorders; or behavioral problems such as poor school performance, truancy, depression, or promiscuity. A more easily recognized presentation is a child acting out their victimization on other children. Often, children displaying sexualized behaviors are victims of child sexual abuse. A report made to a child protective agency will allow for evaluation of the child's safety and provide services.

Another form of sexual abuse, sex trafficking, is perhaps even more difficult to recognize in the ED. Human trafficking is the use of force, fraud, or coercion to obtain some form of labor or benefit from another person. Sex trafficking is human trafficking that obtains benefit from sexual exploitation. It is a crime in the United States and according to international law. It may take many forms, including prostitution, pornography, and labor in a massage parlor or strip club. A number of sex trafficking victims are children; victimization begins at an average age of 13 years. Regardless of the use of coercion or force, any child younger than age 18 years who is involved in prostitution is a victim of sex trafficking. Victims of sex trafficking are unlikely to identify themselves to emergency care providers out of fear for potential consequences. Some clues may aid in recognizing child sex trafficking. Usually, an older person will accompany the patient. This person may claim to be a family member or close friend. The person may have a controlling demeanor and refuse to leave the patient's side, allow the patient to answer questions, or allow the patient to have any control of their possessions. The patient may not speak English and may appear dazed, distant, or afraid. The patient may make poor eye contact and may be unable to identify a place of residence. These findings are not universal; it is important to recognize that not all children will view themselves as victims. Some may seem streetwise and perceive that they are in control of the situation.

If trafficking is suspected, the clinician must separate the patient from the accompanying person. It can be helpful to state that this is standard procedure for patients of this age. When speaking privately with the patient, it will benefit the clinician to keep questions nonjudgmental and respectful. If the patient speaks a language with which the clinician is not fluent, an interpreter is essential. The term "sex trafficking" is generally unhelpful and should be avoided. A better approach is to start simply, with a general question such as "Have you ever been forced to do something you didn't want to do?" Physical examination should target the skin because bruising and other signs of physical abuse may be present. Tattoos or other forms of "branding" may also be evident. A genitourinary examination may reveal signs of sexual abuse. When sex trafficking is suspected, contact a child protection agency and law enforcement. The National Human Trafficking Resource Center hotline (1-888-373-7888) may provide assistance, but it is important to note that this is not a reporting agency and does not satisfy the clinician's obligation to report to a child protection agency or law enforcement. Law enforcement will often provide a more immediate response for children in immediate danger. Law enforcement may request sample collection, and sexually transmitted infection testing and treatment may be needed. The patient may benefit from psychiatric evaluation and in some cases may require inpatient medical or psychiatric management.

Differential Diagnosis

Some findings that raise concern for child sexual abuse have a differential diagnosis that includes medical conditions. Blood found in the diaper may have multiple alternative causes. This may occur in newborns during maternal hormone withdrawal or in older children when labial adhesions open from minor trauma. Urate crystallization in the diaper may also mimic blood, but typically has a more salmon-colored, chalky appearance. This occurs normally in newborns due to a high level of excreted uric acid, but can also occur in older infants with dehydration. In toddlers and school-age children, straddle injuries, urethral prolapse, vaginal foreign bodies, and precocious puberty may cause bleeding. Pelvis radiographs or an ultrasound may reveal a vaginal foreign body. Vulvovaginitis may present with labial erythema, and commonly occurs in young girls who are learning self-wiping. Genital ulcers may be aphthous ulcers or a component of Behçet's disease and are not definitive for abuse. Rectal dilation is common with procedural sedation, especially with deep sedative–hypnotics such as propofol. This knowledge can prevent surprise and sexual abuse concerns when a child is sedated for another reason and this examination finding is incidentally noted. Molluscum contagiosum may have a similar appearance to genital warts. Genital warts themselves can be transmitted from nongenital skin contact and may not always be abusive, but they should be reported so that a detailed investigation can be done.

As with child physical abuse, it is advisable that clinicians not ascribe concerns for sexual abuse to a mimic haphazardly. Unclear cases need expert consultation. In many locations, involvement of a child protection agency or law enforcement is a necessary step in the referral process to a child abuse pediatrician, who can perform a more thorough evaluation and colposcopic examination.

Diagnostic Confirmation

Unlike adult sexual assault, a time-sensitive sample collection usually is not required in cases of pediatric sexual assault. Often, the sexual assault occurred remotely and there has not been acute genital contact. In the more rare presentation when the abuse has included body fluid exposure, a forensic DNA sample collection may be requested by law enforcement. Because the sample is legal evidence, it will require appropriate chain of custody and should only be collected when law enforcement has a mechanism in place to handle it. It is generally requested when the incident occurred within 72 hours. Law enforcement bears the burden of cost and sample processing.

Even when sample collection is not required, an external genitourinary examination should be done. Prior to performing the examination, it is important to clarify parent expectations. Often, a parent may have the unreasonable expectation that an external examination will definitively exclude sexual assault. The examination may be normal in cases of sexual abuse for several reasons: Genital injuries heal quickly, children may be inappropriately touched without penetration, and penetration can occur without injury. A preemptive statement that a normal external examination does not exclude sexual abuse is helpful. It is also worth stating that the child may receive a more detailed colposcopic examination by a child abuse practitioner in the future. The external ED examination will cause apprehension in the pediatric patient. Informing the patient why it is being performed and what is happening may ease anxiety. Helpful statements include, "We are looking at your private area because Mom is here and she brought you to the doctor to make sure you are healthy." Asking the parents the words that they use in their home to reference the genitalia may assist in communication with the child. A neutral third-party chaperone, such as a nurse, should be present for the comfort of the child, to assist in positioning, and for witness documentation. The patient should be examined in a supine position with the hip flexed in a frog-leg position. A more advanced examination can be done by placing the female child in a prone knee-to-chest position. This allows structures to adjust with gravity and may provide a better view. In the majority of examinations of victims of child sexual abuse, the external examination is unrevealing. When a finding is discovered, it is best to document it in the medical record in a descriptive way rather than a diagnostic one.

In cases in which sexual abuse is unclear and the external examination is unrevealing, testing may be better left to the assessment center visit with the child abuse pediatrics team. Most children should have urine nucleic acid testing such as polymerase chain reaction for chlamydia and gonorrhea. If body fluid exposure is known to have occurred, the child will need testing to include syphilis serum testing, hepatitis B and C testing, HIV testing, and a pregnancy test. Chlamydia and gonorrhea swabs can be done if extragenital contact has occurred. If herpetic lesions are present, they should be unroofed for sampling and the fluid sent for culture. If available, an infectious disease specialist may also be consulted in these cases. The child will need follow-up at 6 weeks, 3 months, and 1 year. When appropriate evaluation and testing are not possible, the child should be transferred to an appropriately equipped facility.

Treatment

When an emergency physician has suspicion for child sexual abuse, a report to the relevant child protection agency should be filed. When the abuse is clear, law enforcement will often provide a more immediate response to concerns and should be notified. If the abuse is occurring at home, the state's child protection agency should be involved. As with child physical abuse, the child protection agency where the child lives is the appropriate one to contact, whereas law enforcement where the crime occurred is appropriate to contact. Law enforcement will be required to handle a specimen when collection is needed. Law enforcement is also the appropriate agency to contact when a crime has occurred outside of the home and the home environment is not in question.

In the case of penetration or body fluid contact, the child will need appropriate sexually transmitted infection treatment. A common regimen is ceftriaxone and azithromycin. HIV prophylaxis is also required. In addition, the child will need follow-up at a child abuse assessment center for forensic interviews and evaluation by a child abuse pediatrics team.

Clinical Algorithm

As with child physical abuse, a child sexual abuse algorithm may be a beneficial care resource but will reflect local practice and resources and should be vetted through specialists.

Disposition

Once the child is found to be medically stable for discharge, placement will be done in conjunction with the child protection agency. This may result in removal from parents' custody or placement in foster care. The child protection agency may require an urgent response to the ED in order to determine placement. In some instances, the patient will be cleared for discharge with a home evaluation arranged by the child protection agency at a timeline dictated by the urgency of the presentation.

Complications

Complications of child sexual abuse are mostly psychological, including depression, other mental illness, and behavioral problems. The child may act out abuse on other children. Pregnancy or sexually transmitted infections may occur.

Key Points

- Child sexual abuse is usually a chronic phenomenon, occurring over a longer duration of time, and is less commonly a single isolated event.
- Perform an appropriate examination with a chaperone present.
- Sexual abuse concerns are best reported to the appropriate child protection and law enforcement agencies so that correct referral processes can occur.

Pitfalls

- Allowing personal discomfort to prevent one from performing an appropriate examination
- Not involving law enforcement and ensuring that a report is filed
- Allowing the child to leave the ED without a clear safety plan in place
- Not remembering that child perpetrators are often abused themselves and also require an evaluation

Further Reading

Child Physical Abuse

Kellogg ND; American Academy of Pediatrics Committee on Child Abuse and Neglect.

Evaluation of suspected child physical abuse. *Pediatrics.* 2007;119(6):1232–1241.

Pierce MC, Kaczor K, Aldridge S, O'Flynn J, Lorenz DJ. Bruising characteristics discriminating physical child abuse from accidental trauma. *Pediatrics.* 2010;125(1):67–74.

Section on Radiology, American Academy of Pediatrics. Diagnostic imaging of child abuse. *Pediatrics.* 2009;123(5):1430–1435.

Child Sexual Abuse

Becker HJ, Bechtel K. Recognizing victims of human trafficking in the pediatric emergency department. *Pediatr Emerg Care.* 2015;31(2): 144–147.

Kellogg N; American Academy of Pediatrics Committee on Child Abuse and Neglect. The evaluation of sexual abuse in children. *Pediatrics.* 2005;116(2):506–512.

54

Medical Legal Aspects

Assessment and Treatment of Minors in the Emergency Department

MADELINE JOSEPH

BACKGROUND

Children and adolescents may present to the emergency department (ED) without a guardian for several reasons, such as emergencies occurring during school or lack of guardian availability so that relatives, family friends, or day care or school personnel accompany children to the ED. Also, runaway youths, immigrant children living in the United States, and children for whom a guardian or other resources for medical care are not available during disasters may seek care in the ED. In addition, adolescents may seek medical care in the ED for health concerns that develop related to behaviors that their parents or guardians disapprove of, including sexual activity, substance abuse, interpersonal violence, and mental illness.

The Emergency Medical Treatment and Labor Act (EMTALA) mandates that any individual, including minors, presenting to an ED in a hospital receiving federal funding be offered a medical screening examination to determine whether an emergency medical condition exists. Such screening should be performed for minors in conjunction with making every effort to obtain consent without delaying treatment of an emergency medical condition to obtain such consent.

CLINICAL APPLICATION

A 14-year-old male with a history of diabetes was brought to the ED via rescue and was escorted by the police because he had been arrested and was acting combative; rescue checked his blood glucose, which was >700 mg/dL. Upon arrival to the ED, the patient was sleepy, easily aroused, but refused to talk to the medical team in the ED or give any guardian contact information. Upon further evaluation, the patient was diagnosed with hyperosmolar hyperglycemia without acidosis, with his glucose being 1,100 mg/dL. It was determined that he needed to be admitted to a pediatric intensive care unit with endocrinology consult; both of these services were not available at the treating hospital.

This case raises the following questions:

1. Can the ED team treat this minor patient without consent from a guardian?
2. Who would sign the transfer documents on behalf of the minor to be able to transfer him to the medical facility that can provide the needed care?
3. Can the police consent for treatment and transfer because this minor patient is arrested and no caregivers accompanied him?

Although the minor patient was involved in the juvenile justice system, the ED team determined that the patient's condition was considered an emergency. State laws generally define an emergency as "any threat to the minor's life or health." In this case, an emergency medical condition was declared; thus, the hospital must provide treatment, stabilization, and even transfer for definitive care. The ED team continued to attempt to obtain contact information for the guardian by asking the patient and checking previous ED visits in the electronic medical records. This plan followed the "emergency exception rule" or "doctrine of implied consent," which assumes that were a guardian present, he or she would consent to treatment in the best interest of the child. On the other hand, if, after a medical screening examination is performed, no emergency medical condition is identified and the minor is not legally authorized to consent, non-emergency care should be delayed until a parent or guardian can be contacted to provide legal consent. Otherwise, the practitioner may be vulnerable to legal action. Of note, the wide use of cellphones has facilitated obtaining phone consent rapidly with a witness listening to the conversation, thus preventing care from being delayed.

When a minor patient is involved with the juvenile justice system, state laws vary with regard to who can provide consent for medical care. For example, in Florida and Pennsylvania, the detention center must obtain consent from the minor's parent or legal guardian to obtain routine care, whereas in California, the courts may remove this right from the parent or guardian.

CONDITIONS THAT CAN BE TREATED WITHOUT CONSENT IN THE EMERGENCY DEPARTMENT

Considering the unique nuances of each state's laws, and constant change of these laws, providers should be aware of their state's specific current statutes regarding minors' authority to consent for specific medical conditions. These conditions include

- reproductive health concerns such as pregnancy or sexually transmitted infections;
- mental health concerns; and
- substance abuse.

Of note, federal law supports adolescents' freedom to confidentially seek family planning services through Title X of the Public Health Service Act. As a result, in all states, minors of any age may consent for and receive confidential family planning services at Title X-funded sites.

EMANCIPATION AND MINOR DOCTRINES

Laws vary from state to state regarding legal emancipation and mature minor doctrines, which can grant minors the right to seek health care independent of parental consent. ED physicians should be aware of their state laws regarding these issues. The following factors may allow a minor to be considered legally emancipated:

- Being married or married and divorced
- Being enrolled in the armed services
- Being financially independent
- Parent failing to fulfill parental support obligations
- Pregnant or who has borne a child: In a few states, laws support consent for care for their children but not for themselves.

The mature minor doctrine, which has been adopted in various forms in some states, allows a minor of a certain age, commonly aged 12 years or older, who demonstrates understanding of medical evaluation and treatment, to provide consent without seeking previous emancipation. In states without these laws, the standard remains that parents or other custodial guardians acting in the best interest of the child consent for treatment of non-emergency medical conditions. In the latter, assent from the minor patient for permission for medical evaluation and treatment should also be sought when parents are not available.

KEY POINTS

- EMTALA mandates that any individual, including minors, presenting to an ED be offered a medical screening examination to determine whether an emergency medical condition exists.
- Such screening should be performed for minors in conjunction with making every effort to obtain consent without delaying emergency care.

- Minors of any age may consent in all states for and receive confidential family planning services at Title X-funded sites.
- Laws vary from state to state regarding legal emancipation and mature minor doctrines.

PITFALLS

- Delaying care for minors until consent is obtained by the parents or legal guardian in emergency medical conditions
- Assuming that a pregnant minor can consent for her child regardless of the specific state laws

LEGAL RESOURCES

English A, Ford CA. The HIPAA privacy rule and adolescents: Legal questions and clinical challenges. *Perspect Sexual Reprod Health*. 2004;36(2):80–86. https://www.guttmacher.org/journals/psrh/2004/hipaa-privacy-rule-and-adolescents-legal-questions-and-clinical-challenges. Accessed February 1, 2020.

Guttmacher Institute: Provides an overview of minors' consent law and state policies. http://www.guttmacher.org/statecenter/spibs/spib_OMCL.pdf. Accessed February 1, 2020.

Further Reading

Benjamin L, Ishimine P, Joseph M, Mehta S. Evaluation and treatment of minors. *Ann Emerg Med*. 2018;71:225–232.

Sullivan DJ. Minors and emergency medicine. *Emerg Med Clin North Am*. 1993;11:841–851.

APPENDIX 1

Resuscitation Medications

Pediatric Code Drugs and Adjuncts			GRAY (premie/ neonate) [3–5 kg]	PINK (small infant) [6–7 kg]	RED (infant) [8–9 kg]	PURPLE (toddler) [10–11 kg]	YELLOW (small child) [12–14 kg]	WHITE (child) [15–18 kg]	BLUE (child) [19–23 kg]	ORANGE (Large Child) [24–29 kg]	GREEN (Adult) [30–100 kg]	Special Notes
Drug	Indication	Example Dose										
Rapid Sequence Induction (RSI)			5 kg			10 kg					50 kg	
Atropine	RSI/Bradycardia	0.0 2mg/kg	0.1 mg			0.2 mg					0.5 mg	Max 0.5 mg/dose, may be needed in younger and with succinylcholine
Etomidate	RSI/Induction	0.3 mg/kg	1.5 mg			3 mg					15 mg	
Ketamine	RSI/Induction	1–2 mg/kg (IV)	NA			10–20 mg					50–100 mg	IM route: 3-4mg/kg, not in <3 mo of age
Rocuronium	RSI/Paralytic	1 mg/kg	5 mg			10 mg					50 mg	
Succinycholine	RSI/Paralytic	2 mg/kg IV	10 mg			20 mg					100 mg	Do not use in hyperkalemia or myopathies
Vecuronium	RSI/Paralytic	0.1 mg/kg	0.5 mg			1 mg					5 mg	
Arrhythmias/Code/Resuscitation												
Epinephrine	Vfib/Vtach/PEA/ Brady Arrest	0.01 mg/kg IV	0.05 mg			0.1 mg					0.5 mg	Max 1 mg/dose
Synchronized cardioversion	Supraventricular tachycardia (SVT) or ventricular tachycardia (V-tach) with a pulse	0.5–1 J/kg, then 2 J/kg	5 J			10 J					50 J	

(continued)

Defibrillation	Pulseless Vfib/ Vtach	2 J/kg, then 4 J/kg, max 10 J/kg	10 J, 20 J, max 50 J	20 J, 40 J, max 100 J	100 J, 200 J	Max 200 J or 360 J (depending on machine)
Adenosine	SVT	0.1 mg/kg	0.5 mg	1 mg	5 mg	Max initial dose 6 mg then subsequent doses 12 mg
Amiodarone	V-tach	5 mg/kg (max 300 mg)	25 mg	50 mg	250 mg	Max 300 mg, may repeat bolus to max of 15 mg/kg (absolute max of 2.2 g/24 h)
Lidocaine	V-tach	1 mg/kg	5 mg	10 mg	50 mg	May repeat dose
Procainamide	V-tach	15 mg/kg (over 15–30 min)	75 mg	150 mg	750 mg	
Magnesium	Torsades de Pointes	20–50 mg/kg (max 2 gm)	250 mg	500 mg	2 gm	Max 2 gram/dose
Calcium Chloride 10%	Hyperkalemia/ Arrest	20 mg/kg	100 mg	200 mg	1 gm	Hypocalcemia may impact cardiac contractility, particularly in <1 year
Bicarbonate	Acidosis/Arrest/ TCA OD	1 mEq/kg of 8.4% sodium bicarbonate; <2 yrs: use 4.2% sodium bicarbonate	5 mEq	10 mEq	50 mEq	<2 years: use 4.2% (0.5 mEq/mL) sodium bicarbonate at 1 mEq/kg
Esmolol	SVT/rate control	0.5 mg/kg IV bolus, 25–500 mcg/kg/min infusion				
PGE1	Maintain PDA open	0.1 mcg/kg/min	0.5 mcg/min	N/A	N/A	
Phenylephrine	Tet Spell	5–20 mcg/kg/dose	30 mcg/dose	100 mcg/dose	500 mcg/dose	
Hypertonic saline 3%	Elevated ICP/ traumatic brain injury	3–5 mL/kg	25 mL	50 mL	250 mL	

Mannitol	Elevated ICP	0.5–1 gm/kg	5 gm	10 gm	50 gm	
Naloxone	Opiate Overdose	0.1 mg/kg	0.5 mg	1 mg	4 mg	
Glucose (D5)	Hypoglycemia	10 mL/kg	50 mL	100 mL	500 mL	
Glucose (D10)	Hypoglycemia	5 mL/kg	25 mL	50 mL	250 mL	
Glucose (D25)	Hypoglycemia	2 mL/kg	N/A, do not use	20 mL, (controversial use, D10 is preferred)	100 mL	
Glucose (D50)	Hypoglycemia	1 mL/kg	N/A, do not use	N/A, do not use	50 mL	
Normal Saline/ Lactated Ringers	Hypotension	10–20 mL/kg	50–100 mL	200 mL	1,000 mL	neonates may be volume-sensitive
Packed Red Blood Cells (pRBC)	Trauma/Anemia	5–10 mL/kg	25–50 mL	100 mL	500 mL	
Platelets	Bleeding with thrombocytopenia or abnormal platelet function	10–15 mL/kg	50 mL	1 unit	5 units	May also dose 1 unit per 10 kg over 15 kg
Tranexemic acid	Hemorrhage in Trauma	15 mg/kg bolus (max 1 g), 2 mg/kg/hr infusion (doses not well established)	75 mg bolus, 10 mg/hour infusion	150 mg bolus, 20 mg/hour infusion	750 mg bolus, 100 mg/hour infusion	Off-label use
Vasopressors and Inotropic Support						
Norepinephrine	Warm Shock	0.05–2 mcg/kg/min , titrate by 0.02 mcg/kg/min q5 min	5 mcg/min	10 mcg/min	50 mcg/min	
Epinephrine	Cold Shock	0.1–1 mcg/kg/min IV, titrate by 0.02–0.05 mcg/kg/min q10–15 min	2.5 mcg/min	5 mcg/min	25 mcg/min	Child are more commonly in cold shock and epinephrine is the preferred vasopressor in cold shock (over norepinephrine)

(continued)

Dopamine	Poor perfusion/ shock	2–20 mcg/kg/min IV, titrate by 5 mcg/kg/min q5–10 min	50 mcg/min	100 mcg/ min	500 mcg/ min	
Phenylephrine	Shock	0.1–1 mcg/kg/min	2.5 mcg/min	5 mcg/min	25 mcg/ min	
Dobutamine	Inotropic support	2–20 mcg/kg/min IV, titrate by 2.5 mcg/kg/min q10 min	50 mcg/min	100 mcg/ min	500 mcg/ min	
Vasopressin	Shock	0.17–8 milliunits/ kg/min	10 milli-units/min	20 milli-units/min	100 milli-units/min	
Milrinone	Inotropic support	0.25–0.75 mcg/kg/ min IV +/- con-troversial loading dose of 50 mcg/ kg; titrate by 0.005 mcg/kg/min q10–15 min	2.5 mcg/min	5 mcg/min	25 mcg/ min	Slow bolus over 10–60 min
Hydrocortisone	Shock	1–2 mg/kg (or 25 infants, 50 mg children or 100 mg adolescents) IV	25 mg	25 mg	100 mg	vasopressor resistent, adrenal insufficiency

Status Epilepticus First-line Anti-epileptics

Lorazepam (Ativan)	Seizure	0.1 mg/kg IV q 5 min × 3 (max 4mg/ dose)	0.5 mg IV	1 mg IV	4 mg IV	
Diazepam (Valium)	Seizure	0.2 mg/kg IV (max 10 mg IV); rectal (diastat): 2–5 yrs: 0.5 m/kg 6–11 yrs: 0.3 mg/kg >12 yrs: 0.2 mg/kg max: 20 mg/dose (PR)	1 mg IV	2 mg IV	10 mg IV	

Midazolam (Versed)	Seizure	0.15 mg/kg IV; 0.2 mg/kg IM/IN; buccal (0.4–0.5 mg/kg)	0.75 mg IV	1.5 mg IV	7.5 mg IV	
Second-line Anti-epileptics						
Fosphenytoin	Seizure	20 PE/kg IV at 3 mg/kg/min	100 PE	200 PE	1000 PE	Max 1500 mgPE/dose; max rate 3 mgPE/kg/min (max 150 mgPE/min)
Phenytoin (Dilantin)	Seizure	20 mg/kg gtt at 1 mg/kg (max 50 mg)/min	100 mg	200 mg	1 gram	
Levatiracetam	Seizure	20 mg/kg; may repeat up to 60 mg/kg	100 mg	200 mg	1 gram	Max 4500 mg/dose
Valproic Acid (Depakote)	Seizure	15–20 mg/kg IV	100 mg	200 mg	1 gram	Do not use in <2 years; Max 3000 mg/dose
Phenobarbital	Seizure	20 mg/kg (max 1 g)	100 mg	200 mg	1 gram	Predominantly used in neonates/young infants
Refractory Status Epilepticus						
Pyridoxine (INH tox)	Seizure (INH Toxicity)	1 gm/gm INH (5 gm if unk INH dose); pyridoxine dependent seizures <1y: 100 mg	pyridoxine dependent seizures <1y: 100 mg			
Midazolam drip	Refractory status epilepticus	0.2 mg/kg bolus, then 0.05–2 mg/kg/hour	1 mg bolus, then 0.5 mg/hour	2 mg bolus, then 1 mg/hour	10 mg bolus, then 5 mg/hour	Initiate after two benzodiazepines and two second-line anti-epileptic medications

(continued)

Propofol drip	Refractory status epilepticus	2 mg/kg bolus, then 1–15 mg/kg/hour	10 mg bolus, then 25 mg/hour			20 mg bolus, then 50 mg/hour					100 mg bolus, then 250 mg/hour	Initiate after two benzodiazepines and two second-line anti-epileptic medications
Ketamine drip	Refractory status epilepticus	0.5–2 mg/kg bolus, then 0.5–2 mg/kg/hour	5 mg bolus, then 5 mg/hour			10 mg bolus, then 10 mg/hour					50 mg bolus, then 50 mg/hour	Initiate after two benzodiazepines and two second-line anti-epileptic medications

*Adapted from Broselow Pediatric Emergency Medicine Tape, Los Angeles County + University of Southern California Department of Emergency Medicine, PediStat

RSI = rapid sequence induction, ICP = intracranial pressure, TCA = tricyclic antidepressant, PDA = patent ductus arteriosus, Vfib = ventricular fibrillation, Vtach = ventricular tachycardia, TET = tetralogy of Fallot defect, INH = isoniazid, OD = overdose, PE = phenytoin equivalents

Compiled and reviewed by Samuel Beckerman, Mimi Lu and Liza Kearl

A special thank you to LAC + USC pharmacist Jacklyn Chong for her review of the medication dosing and administration

APPENDIX 2

Common Pediatric medications and doses

Drug	Dose	Comments
	Pain	
Acetaminophen	15 mg/kg q4–6 hr	
Ibuprofen	10 mg/kg q6 hr	
Morphine	0.1 mg/kg IV/SQ	
Hydromorphone (Dilaudid)	0.05 mg/kg IV	
Fentanyl	1 mcg/kg IV/IN	
Ketamine	0.1–0.3 mg/kg IV	
	Anti-emetics	
Ondansetron (Zofran)	2 mg (<15 kg) 4 mg (>15 kg) PO/ IV or 0.15 mg/kg PO/IV	
Metoclopramide (Reglan)	0.1–0.2 mg/kg IV/PO (max 10 mg)	
Prochlorperazine (Compazine)	0.1 mg/kg PO q6h 0.3 mg/kg PO q8–12h or 0.1–0.15mg/kg IV q3–4h (max 10 mg/dose)	Effective headache medication
	Croup	
Dexamethasone	0.2–0.6 mg/kg (max 16 mg)	
Nebulized epinephrine (1 mg/mL concentration))	0.5 mL/kg (max 5 mL)	For stridor with rest or respiratory distress
Racemic Epi	0.25–0.5ml (2.25% neb in 3ml NS)	For stridor with rest or respiratory distress
	Asthma	
Albuterol	2.5 mg (<15 kg), 5 mg (>15 kg) q 20 min, can escalate to continuous (max 20–30 mg/hour though higher doses may be beneficial in severe cases	
Ipratropium (Atrovent)	250 mcg < 15 kg, 500 mcg (>15 kg) q 20 min, max 3 doses in 24 hours	
Magnesium	50 mg/kg (max 2 g over 20 mins)	
Terbutaline	2–10 mcg/kg IVP or 0.01 mg/kg SQ (max 250 mcg)	
Epinephrine (1 mg/1 mL)	0.01 mg/kg IM q15 min (max 0.5 mg)	
Prednisone	1 mg/kg/day bid PO (max 60 mg)	
Methylprednisolone	2 mg/kg IV/IM (max 80 mg) then 0.5 mg/kg IV/IO q6hr (max 120 mg/day)	
Dexamethasone	0.6 mg/kg (max 16 mg)	

(continued)

Procedural Sedation		
Ketamine	1–2 mg/kg IV, 4 mg/kg IM	
Propofol	0.5–2 mg/kg IV	
Midazolam (Versed)	0.15 mg/kg IV	
Etomidate	0.15 mg/kg	
Methohexital (Brevital)	1 mg/kg IV	
Anaphylaxis/Allergy		
Epi 1 mg/1 mL	0.01 mg/kg IM q15 min prn (max 0.5 mg)	* Epinephrine is the only effective management of anaphylaxis, see chapter 23 on dermatologic emergencies
Epi 0.1 mg/mL	0.1 mcg/kg/min gtt (max of 10 mcg/min)	
Benadryl	1 mg/kg (max 50 mg)	
Famotidine (Pepcid)	0.5 mg/kg (max 20 mg)	
Dexamethasone	0.6 mg/kg (max 16mg)	
Acute Agitation	See chapter 52 for algorithm on the management of the acutely agitated child	
Diphenhydramine	1 mg/kg; 12.5–50 mg PO/IM	Avoid in delirium, peak effect in 2 hours
Haloperidol (Haldol)	0.5–5 mg (IM should be <1/2 of po dose), 0.05–0.15 mg/kg	
Olanzapine (Zyprexa)	2.5–10 mg (IM should be <1/2 of po dose)	
Chlorpromazine (Thorazine)	12.5–50 mg (0.55 mg/kg/dose)	
Risperidone (Risperdal)	0.25–1 mg (0.5–0.01 mg/kg/dose)	
Antibiotics		
Amoxicillin	45 mg/kg/dose BID, max: 1.5–2g/dose	high dose: otitis media, sinusitis, pneumonia
Amoxicillin	25 mg/kg BID, max 1 gram/day	standard dose: pharyngitis
Amoxicillin clavulanate (Augmentin ES) 600mg/5mL	45 mg/kg/dose BID (max: 1.5–2g/dose)	high dose: otitis media, sinusitis, pneumonia
Ampicillin/sulbactam (Unasyn)	50 mg/kg q6h IV	dosed on ampicillin component
Azithromycin (100 mg/5mL)	10 mg/kg day 1, then 5 mg/kg day 2–5	
Trimethoprim sulfate (Bactrim) 40 mg/5 ml	TMP 3–6 mg/kg BID	In children > 2 mo. Old. Dosed on TMP component, (maximum single dose 160 mg TMP)
Cefazolin (Ancef)	25mg/kg IV q 8 hours	maximum single dose 1–2 grams
Cefdinir (Omnicef); (125 or 250/5mL)	7 mg/kg BID or 14 mg/kg once daily	max: 600 mg/day. Can cause bright red stools
Cefotaxime	50 mg/kg IV	Maximum 2 grams/dose
Ceftriaxone	50 mg/kg IV (100 mg/kg for meningitis)	Maximum 1–2 gram/dose

Cephalexin (Keflex), (125 or 250 mg/5ml)	25–100 mg/kg/day divided tid-qid	
Clindamycin (75 mg/5mL)	10 mg/kg q8h PO or IV	
Gentamicin	2.5 mg/kg IV q 8 hours	Or 4–9 mg/kg q 24 hour (extended interval dosing)
Piperacillin/tazobactam (Zosyn)	100 mg/kg IV q8h	Dosed on piperacillin component
Rifampin	20 mg/kg/day divided bid	Maximum 600 mg/dose
Vancomycin	15 mg/kg IV q6h	

Po: per os, IM: intramuscular, IV: intravenous, IN: intranasal, SQ: subcutaneous, NS: normal saline,
Compiled and reviewed by Samuel Beckerman, Mimi Lu and Liza Kearl
A special thank you to LAC + USC pharmacist Jacklyn Chong for her review of the medication dosing and administration

APPENDIX 3

Age and weight based pediatric resuscitation equipment

Pediatric Resuscitation Equipment

	GRAY (premie/ neonate)	PINK (small infant)	RED (infant)	PURPLE (toddler)	YELLOW (small child)	WHITE (child)	BLUE (child)	ORANGE (Large Child)	GREEN (Adult)	Special Notes
Weight (kg)	3–5 kg	6–7 kg	8–9 kg	10–11 kg	12–14 kg	15–18 kg	19–23 kg	24–29 kg	30–100 g	
Approximate Age	0–1 mo	1–6 mo	6–12 mo	12–18 mo	18–36 mo	36–48 mo	5–7 yo	8–9 yo	>10 y/o	
Blood Pressure Cuff	Neonatal #5/Infant	Infant/ Child	Infant/ Child	Child	Child	Child	Child	Child	Small Adult	
Bag-Valve Mask (BVM)	Infant/ Child	Infant/ Child	Infant/ Child	Child	Child	Child	Child	Child	Adult	
Non-Rebreather	Pediatric	Pediatric	Pediatric	Pediatric	Pediatric	Pediatric	Pediatric	Pediatric	Pediatric/ Adult	
Oral Airway (mm)	50	50	50	60	60	60	70	80	80	
Laryngoscope Blade (mac/ miller)	00/0	1	1	1 or 1.5	2	2	2	2 or 3	3–4	mnemonic: "use a 2 at 2, and 3 in 3rd grade"
Endotracheal Tube (cuffed, >1mo)	N/A	3–3.5	3–3.5	3.5–4	4	4.5	5	6	6.5–7.5	(Age/4)+3.5, mnemonic: "use a 5 at 5"

(continued)

Endotracheal Tube (uncuffed)	GA (wks)/10	3.5+	3.5+	4+	4.5+	5+	5.5+	N/A	N/A	(Age/4)+4, +use cuffed tubes outside of neonatal period
Stylet (endotracheal tube) (F)	6	6	6	6	6 or 10	10	10 or 14	14	14	
Endotracheal Tube Depth (cm)	9–10.5 or 6 +wt (kg)	10.5–11	10.5–11	11–12	13.5	14–15	16.5	17–18	18–23	Tip to Lip (cm) 3xETT size
Glidescope blade/baton	#0 (2 kg), #1 (3 kg), #2 (4 kg), small	#2, small	#2, small	#.2.5, small	#2.5, small	#2.5, small	#2.5, small	#3, small	#3, large	
Laryngeal Mask Airway (LMA)	1	1.5	1.5	2	2	2	2.5	2.5	3	
Chest Tube (F)	10–12	10–12	10–12	16–20	20–24	20–24	24–32	28–32	28–38*	3–4x ETT size; *smaller tubes are better tolerated. Pigtail catheter may be used for pneumothorax
Intravenous (IV) Catheter (ga)	22–24	22–24	22–24	20–24	18–22	18–22	18–20	18–20	16–20	
Intraosseus (IO) Catheter (ga)/color	18/15	18/15	18/15	15	15	15	15	15	15	Most commonly proximal tibia, distal femur, humerus
Central Line	3 F, 8 cm	4 F, 12 cm	4 F, 12 cm	4 F, 12 cm	5 F, 12 cm	5 F, 12 cm		7 F		Length should be measured prior to placement of internal jugular and subclavian lines. Femoral lines use longer catheters and placement depth is less precise
Suction Cather (F)	5	8	8	10	10	10	10	10	10–12	
Nasogastric Tube (F)	5	8	8	8–10	10	10–12	10–12	12	12	2x ETT size
Urinary Catheter (F)	5	8	8	8–10	10	10–12	10–12	12	12	2x ETT size

*Adapted from Broselow Pediatric Emergency Tape, The American Heart Association (AHA), Pediatric Advanced Life Support (PALS), Los Angeles County + University of Southern Calironia Department of Emergency Medicine Compiled and reviewed by Samuel Beckerman, Mimi Lu, and Liza Kearl

APPENDIX 4

Normal Pediatric Vital Signs

PEM Appendix: Normal Pediatric Vital Signs

	Normal Vital Signs								
	GRAY (premie/ neonate) [3–5 kg]	PINK (small infant) [6–7 kg]	RED (infant) [8–9 kg]	PURPLE (toddler) [10–11 kg]	YELLOW (small child) [12–14 kg]	WHITE (child) [15–18 kg]	BLUE (child) [19–23 kg]	ORANGE (Large Child) [24–29 kg]	GREEN (Adult) [30–100 kg]
Approximate Age	0–1 mo	1–6 mo	6–12 mo	12–18 mo	18–36 mo	36–48 mo	5–7 yo	8–9 yo	>10 y/o
Respiratory Rate (breaths/min)	30–60	30–60	24–50	24–40	24–40	22–34	18–34	18–30	16–24
Heart Rate (beats/min)	100–180	100–160	100–160	100–140	80–130	80–130	70–120	70–110	60–100
Systolic Blood Pressure (mmHg)*	60	70	70	75	75	80	80	90	90
Diastolic Blood Pressure (mmHg)	40	45	45	50	50	55	55	60	60
Urine Output (cc/kg/hr)	3–10	6–14	8–18	10–22	12–28	15–36	19–46	24–58	30–200

*Estimated lowest normal systolic blood pressure for ages 1–10 y.o. = 2 × (age in years) + 70

APPENDIX 5

Pediatric Vaccination Schedule

Birth	1 month	2 month	4 month	6 month	12 month	15 month	18 month	19–23 month	2–3 years	4–6 years
HepB	HepB			HepB						
		RV	RV	RV						
		DTaP	DTaP	DTaP		DTaP				DTaP
		Hib	Hib	Hib	Hib					
		PCV13	PCV13	PCV13	PCV13					
		IPV	IPV	IPV						
				Influenza (Yearly)*						
					MMR					MMR
					Varicella					Varicella
					HepA§					

https://www.cdc.gov/vaccines/schedules

INDEX

Page numbers followed by *b*, *f*, and *t* indicate boxes, figures, and tables, respectively.